Textbook of
NURSING FOUNDATION

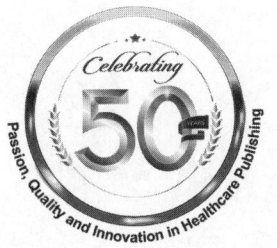

Textbook of NURSING FOUNDATION

I and II Including First Aid

As per INC New Syllabus

THIRD EDITION

I Clement
Doctor of Philosophy in Nursing (PhD) MSc (Nursing) Medical Surgical Nursing
MA (Sociology) MSc (Physiology) MA (Child Care and Education)
Postgraduate Diploma in Hospital Administration

Professor and Principal
Department of Medical Surgical Nursing
Columbia College of Nursing
Bengaluru, Karnataka, India

Formerly, Professor and Principal
VSS College of Nursing
Bengaluru, Karnataka, India

Professional Life Member
PhD Society of India, Chennai, Tamil Nadu
Nursing Research Society of India, New Delhi
Trained Nurses Association of India, New Delhi
Christian Medical Association of India, New Delhi
Indian Society of Psychiatric Nursing, Bengaluru
Medical Surgical Nursing Society of India, Chennai
Indian Society of Neuroscience Nursing, New Delhi
Asian Association of Cardiac Nurses, Kolkata, West Bengal

Health Organization Member
Indian Red Cross Society, Bengaluru
St. Johns Ambulance Association, Bengaluru
General Secretary, Indian Society of Medical Surgical Nurses

Assignments and Examiner
Faculty of Nursing, RGUHS, Bengaluru, Karnataka, India
LIC Inspector, Chief Squad, Observer
Research Guide, RGUHS, Bengaluru
Examiner, Paper-setter, valuator other Universities in India
Professional Activity and Editorial
Indian Journal of Practical Nursing
National Editorial Advisory Board, New Delhi
Nurses of India (former) Bengaluru
Chairman-Souvenir Committee, Florence Nightingale Awards-2012

Winner
Florence Nightingale Awards—2013
Rajiv Gandhi Education Excellence Award
National Mahila Rattan Gold Medal Award, New Delhi

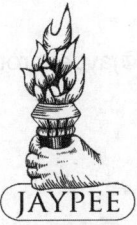

JAYPEE BROTHERS MEDICAL PUBLISHERS
The Health Sciences Publisher
New Delhi | London

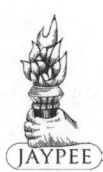 **Jaypee Brothers Medical Publishers (P) Ltd**

Headquarters

Jaypee Brothers Medical Publishers (P) Ltd
EMCA House, 23/23-B
Ansari Road, Daryaganj
New Delhi 110 002, India
Landline: +91-11-23272143, +91-11-23272703
+91-11-23282021, +91-11-23245672
Head Office: 011-43574357
Email: jaypee@jaypeebrothers.com: www.jaypeebrothers.com

Corporate Office

Jaypee Brothers Medical Publishers (P) Ltd
4838/24, Ansari Road, Daryaganj
New Delhi 110 002, India
Phone: +91-11-43574357
Fax: +91-11-43574314
Email: jaypee@jaypeebrothers.com

Overseas Office

J.P. Medical Ltd
83 Victoria Street, London
SW1H 0HW (UK)
Phone: +44 20 3170 8910
Fax: +44 (0)20 3008 6180
Email: info@jpmedpub.com

Website: www.jaypeebrothers.com
Website: www.jaypeedigital.com

© 2021, Jaypee Brothers Medical Publishers

The views and opinions expressed in this book are solely those of the original contributor(s)/author(s) and do not necessarily represent those of editor(s) of the book.

All rights reserved. No part of this publication may be reproduced, stored or transmitted in any form or by any means, electronic, mechanical, photocopying, recording or otherwise, without the prior permission in writing of the publishers.

All brand names and product names used in this book are trade names, service marks, trademarks or registered trademarks of their respective owners. The publisher is not associated with any product or vendor mentioned in this book.

Medical knowledge and practice change constantly. This book is designed to provide accurate, authoritative information about the subject matter in question. However, readers are advised to check the most current information available on procedures included and check information from the manufacturer of each product to be administered, to verify the recommended dose, formula, method and duration of administration, adverse effects and contraindications. It is the responsibility of the practitioner to take all appropriate safety precautions. Neither the publisher nor the author(s)/editor(s) assume any liability for any injury and/or damage to persons or property arising from or related to use of material in this book.

This book is sold on the understanding that the publisher is not engaged in providing professional medical services. If such advice or services are required, the services of a competent medical professional should be sought.

Every effort has been made where necessary to contact holders of copyright to obtain permission to reproduce copyright material. If any have been inadvertently overlooked, the publisher will be pleased to make the necessary arrangements at the first opportunity. The **CD/DVD-ROM** (if any) provided in the sealed envelope with this book is complimentary and free of cost. **Not meant for sale.**

Inquiries for bulk sales may be solicited at: jaypee@jaypeebrothers.com

Textbook of Nursing Foundation

First Edition:
Second Edition: 2017
Third Edition: **2021**

ISBN: 978-81-948028-4-6

Printed at Rajkamal Electric Press

Dedicated to

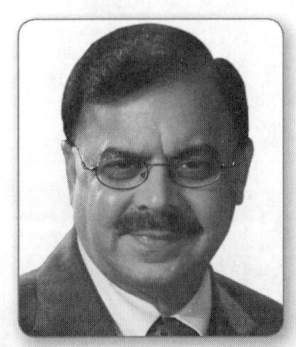

Shri Jitendar P Vij
(Group Chairman)

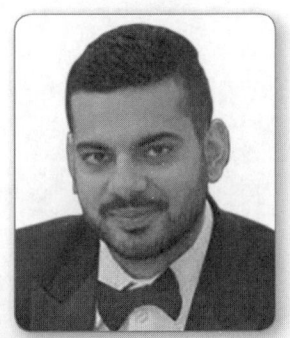

Mr Ankit Vij
(Managing Director)

Jaypee Brothers Medical Publishers (P) Ltd.
New Delhi, India

Preface to the Third Edition

It gives me immense pleasure to draft this third edition of *Textbook of Nursing Foundation*. First of all I would like to thank my Lord Almighty for his wonderful blessing to complete this project in time. This book has been devised as per revised Indian Nursing Council (INC) syllabus; it is divided into nursing foundation I and II including first aid. This book has 32 chapters, each framed with review questions and multiple choice questions (MCQs), designed to create interest in chapter for the student to review after reading each chapter. Each chapter is prepared with adequate tables and diagrams for better understanding of the content. All the descriptions are framed basis latest information, findings and evidence-based research, and contents are drafted in the simple form of english, and facilitate reading from the examination point of view. Even the present year student can also utilize this book, since entire book will be a boon for those about to take this following academic year. I wish all the readers best of luck for their examination.

I Clement

Preface to the First Edition

Nurses are noble living beings; with their rich services, they serve the people; right from the birth till death, nurses provide care. It gives me immense pleasure to introduce this *Textbook of Nursing Foundation* which will be a great help for budding nurses, all nursing students, and faculties to prepare them as a complete nurse. I am proud and privileged to be a nurse. Through my journey in nursing profession, I have portrayed in this book, depicted in a simple and easy manner and in step-by-step fashion which I have experienced in my nursing profession.

All the contents explained in the textbook are included as per the Indian Nursing Council syllabus which will be a complete pack of knowledge boost for the upcoming nursing students; contents are thoroughly updated as per scientific principles of nursing. This book will definitely lay a strong basic knowledge foundation for all budding nurses, pictures are presented in such a manner so that theory is integrated with practice and students who go through will definitely have a strong idea about the nursing procedures.

Textbook of Nursing Foundation deals with patient care, bridges the gap between the information contained at large. It presents with basic concepts of nursing foundation, basic nursing procedures, special needs of the individual and health and hospital-related topics.

This book consists of five sections: Section-I: Basic Concepts of Nursing Foundations (Chapters 1 to 6); Section-II: Nursing Foundation Procedures (Chapters 7 to 31); Section-III: Medical Surgical Procedures (General) (Chapter 32); Section-IV: Special Needs (Chapters 33 to 45) and Section-V: Special Units (Chapters 46 to 51).

I Clement

Acknowledgments

I am thankful to the Lord Almighty who strengthens me with his abundant blessing through innumerable means, helping me in all my accomplishment. My heartfelt thanks to Shri Sommana, Former Minister of Karnataka and Chairman of VSS Group of Institutions for his constant support and encouragement.

My sincere thanks to my guru Dr BT Basvanthappa, Principal, Rajarajeshweri College of Nursing, Bengaluru, Karnataka, India and Professor PV Ramachandran, Chairman, College of Nursing, Sri Ramachandra University, Chennai, Tamil Nadu, India, a great philosopher and internationally renowned teacher of nursing, who helped me in discovering the world of knowledge. I am thankful to Ms Shylaja Sommana, Managing Directors: Dr BS Naveen, Dr BS Arun and Ms Divya from VSS Group of Institutions, Bengaluru, Karnataka, India, for their support and encouragement.

I am also grateful to Dr BC Bhagavan, Syndicate Member of RGUHS, Bengaluru, Professor, Department of Surgery, Kempagowda Institute of Medical Sciences, Bengaluru, Karnataka, India and Dr Aswathnarayanan MLA, Deputy Chief Minister of Karnataka, Chairman, Padmashree Group of Institutions, Bengaluru, Karnataka, India.

Special thanks to Dr TV Ramakrishnan, Professor of Anesthesiology and Head of Clinical Services, Department of Accident and Emergency Medicine, Sri Ramachandra University, Chennai, India; Dr Jeyaseelan Manickam Devadassan, Syndicate Member, The Tamil Nadu Dr. MRG Medical University, Chennai, Dean, Annai JKK Sampoorani Ammal College of Nursing, Erode, Tamil Nadu, India; Dr Tamilmani, Principal, Annai JKK Sampoorani Ammal College of Nursing, Erode, Tamil Nadu, India, Professor Mrs Jessie Sudarsanum, Head, Department of Medical Surgical Nursing, Annai JKK Sampoorani Ammal College of Nursing, Erode, Tamil Nadu, India and all my teachers and students.

I convey my sincere thanks to my beloved parents, brothers and sisters and my wife Nisha Clement for her continuous support and constant encouragement in each step of my life. I take this opportunity to thank my little ones, Cibin, Cynthia and Cavin. I extend thanks to my beloved friend and brother, Mr Regi T Kurien, USA.

Special thanks to Shri Jitendar P Vij (Group Chairman), Mr Ankit Vij (Managing Director), Mr MS Mani (Group President), Dr Madhu Choudhary (Publishing Head–Education), Ms Pooja Bhandari (Production Head), Ms Sunita Katla (Executive Assistant to Group Chairman and Publishing Manager), Ms Seema Dogra (Cover Visualizer), Mr Rajesh Sharma (Production Coordinator), Mr Omprakash Mishra (Typesetter), Ms Geeta Barik (Proofreader), Mr Radhey Shyam Singh (Graphic Designer) of M/s Jaypee Brothers Medical Publishers (P) Ltd, New Delhi. I would also like to thank Mr Venugopal V (Associate Director-South), Mr Santhosh Kumar (Author Coordinator, Bengaluru), and other staff members of M/s Jaypee Brothers Medical Publisher (P) Ltd, Bengaluru branch.

Contents

1. **Introduction** — 1
   - Terminology *1*
   - Concept of Health *2*
   - Definition of Health *2*
   - Dimensions of Health *3*
   - Multiple Facts of Health—WHO *3*
   - Maslow's Hierarchy of Needs *4*
   - Health–Illness Continuum *4*
   - Models of Health and Illness *5*
   - Biopsychosocial Aspects of Health and Illness *7*
   - Determinants of Health *7*
   - Factors Influencing Health *8*
   - Concept of Disease *9*
   - Cultural Factors in Health and Disease *10*
   - Causes and Risk Factors for Developing Illness *10*
   - Concepts of Health, Illness and Sick Behaviors *11*
   - Illness-Illness Behavior *12*
   - Stages of Illness Behavior *12*
   - Impact of Illness on Patient *13*
   - Impact of Illness of Family *13*

2. **Health Care Delivery System** — 16
   - Terminology *16*
   - Definition *17*
   - Concept of Health for All *17*
   - Levels of Illness Prevention *17*
   - Levels of Health Care *18*
   - Health Care Delivery System in India *19*
   - Health Care Services *20*
   - Health Care Team *20*
   - Health Care Agencies *21*
   - Hospital: Types, Organization and Functions *22*
   - Classification of Hospitals *24*

3. **History of Nursing and Nursing as a Profession** — 27
   - Terminology *27*
   - History of Nursing *28*
   - History of Nursing in India *28*
   - History of Florence Nightingale *30*
   - The Nightingale's Pledge *30*
   - Contributions of Florence Nightingale *31*
   - Definitions of Nursing *31*
   - Objectives, Concepts and Philosophy of Nursing *32*
   - Values of Professional Nursing *33*
   - Basic Nursing Principles *33*
   - Nursing Science *33*
   - Nursing as a Profession *34*
   - Characteristics of a Professional Nurse *34*
   - Qualities of Professional Nurse *34*
   - Role and Functions of a Nurse *35*
   - Scope of Nursing *36*
   - Categories of Nursing Personnel *37*

Patient-centered Nursing Care (Nursing Procedures) *38*
Nurse as a Member of Health Care Team *39*
Values of Professional Nurse *39*
Concept of Professionalism in Nursing *41*
Issues Related to Nursing Profession *41*
Caring and Advocacy *41*
Extended Role of Nurse *42*
Ethical Issues in Nursing *42*
Code of Ethics *42*
Ethical Principles *43*
Ethical Dilemmas *45*
Ethical Decision Making *45*
Statements of Ethical Responsibility *46*
Professional Etiquettes for Nurses *46*
Legal Issues in Nursing *47*
Integrating Nursing Service and Nursing Education *48*

4. **Communication and Nurse–Patient Relationship**   **50**
Communication: Levels, Elements, Types, Models, Process and Factors Affecting Communication *50*
Levels of Communication *52*
Principles of Communication *52*
Communication Process *53*
Basic Communication Skills *54*
Factors Affecting Communication Process *54*
Nonverbal Communication *56*
The Best Model *57*
Barriers in Communication *57*
Interpersonal Relationship *59*
Therapeutic Nurse–Patient Relationship *61*
Communication in Nursing *65*
Communication in the Hospital *66*
Nurse–Client Helping Relationship *67*
Communicating Effectively with Patient, Family and Team Members *68*
Communication within Nursing Process *68*
Maintaining Effective Human Relation with Vulnerable Group *69*
Ten Commandments of Communicating *71*
Patient Teaching: Importance, Purpose, Process and Role of Nurse *71*

5. **Documentation and Reporting**   **74**
Terminology *74*
Meaning of Records and Reports *75*
Definitions of Records and Reports *75*
Purpose Recording and Reporting *76*
Principles of Recording and Reporting *76*
Types of Records, Reports and Registers in Nursing *78*
Common Record Keeping Forms *79*
Computerized Documentation *79*
Legal Implications of Records and Reports *80*
Role of a Nurse in Recording and Reporting *80*
Minimizing the Legal Liability through Effective Record Keeping *81*
Change-of-Shift Report *82*
Incident Report *83*
Transfer Report *84*

6. **Health Assessment**   **86**
Terminology *86*
Definition *87*
Purpose and Factors Affecting Health Assessment *87*
Principles of Health Assessment *87*
Responsibilities of Nurse in Health Assessment *87*
Methods of Physical Examination *88*

Health History *90*
Mental Health Assessment *92*
Preparation of the Patient *92*
Preparation of the Environment *93*
Admission Assessment *93*
Shift Assessment *94*
Focused Assessment *94*
Physical Examination Procedure *100*
Head to Toe Examination *102*
Role of Nurse in Health Assessment *105*
Recording of Health Assessment *105*

7. Vital Signs 108
Terminology *108*
Guidelines for Assessing Vital Signs *109*
Vital Signs Measurement *109*
Principles of Vital Signs *110*
Body Temperature: Physiology, Regulation and Factors Affecting Body Temperature *110*
Assessment of Body Temperature: Sites, Equipment, Techniques and Special Considerations *112*
Types of Thermometer *114*
Care of Thermometer *114*
Oral Temperature *114*
Axillary Temperature *115*
Rectal Temperature *117*
Fever (Pyrexia) *118*
Care of Fever *119*
Temperature Alterations: Hyperthermia, Heat Cramps, Heat Exhaustion, Heat Stroke, Hypothermia *120*
Rigor *123*
Hot and Cold Applications *124*
Pulse *135*
Respiration *137*
Alterations in Respiration *139*
Blood Pressure *140*
Alteration in Blood Pressure *141*

8. Equipment and Linen 144
Terminology *144*
Definition *145*
Concept of Equipment Maintenance *145*
General Principles of Instrument Care *145*
Cleaning and Disinfection of Equipment Maintenance *145*
Inspecting Equipment for Safety Hazards *146*
Teaching the Client About Safe Use of Equipment *146*
Types of Materials Used in Hospital *146*
Patient Care Equipment *146*
Monitoring Equipment Used *147*
Tubes and Catheters Used in Hospital *148*
Life Support and Emergency Equipment *149*
Care of Linen *150*
Care of Rubber Goods *151*
Care of Enamel Ware *152*
Care of Stainless Steel Instruments *153*
Care of Surgical Sharp Instruments *154*
Care of Fiberoptics with Camera Item *154*
Care of Suction Machine *155*
Care of Refrigerator *155*
Care of Glass Instruments *156*
Care of Kitchen *156*
Disinfecting Ward Equipment *156*
Care of the Sanitary Annexes *156*
Hospital Furnitures *157*

Sterilization Techniques *157*
Physical Methods of Sterilization *158*
Hot Air Oven *159*
Radiation Method of Sterilization *160*
Chemical Disinfectants *160*

9. Infection Control in Clinical Setting — 163
Acronyms and Abbreviations *164*
Infection Control: Nature of Infection, Chain of Infection and Transmission *164*
Defenses Against Infection: Natural and Acquired *168*
Hospital-acquired Infection/Nosocomial Infection *170*
Barrier Nursing *174*
Universal Precautions: Standards and Safety Pecautions *176*
Asepsis *177*
Surgical Asepsis *178*
Transmission-based Precautions *180*
Role of the Nurse in Infection Control *181*
Transportation of Infectious Patients *183*
Decontamination of Equipment and Unit *183*
Personal Protecting Equipment *184*
Biomedical Waste Management *184*
Ill Effects of Biomedical Waste *188*
Elements of Biomedical Waste Management *189*
Safety and Health Issues in a Nutshell *191*
Nurses' Role and Responsibility in BMW *192*

10. Comfort, Rest and Sleep, and Pain — 194
Terminology *194*
Comfort Measures *194*
Bed Making *195*
Unoccupied Bed or Closed Bed *198*
Open Bed *199*
Occupied Bed *200*
Operation Bed *201*
Cardiac Bed *201*
Fracture Bed *202*
Amputation Bed *202*
Comfort Devices *203*
Pillow *203*
Back Rest *203*
Rolls *204*
Footrests *204*
Sand Bags *205*
Air and Water Mattresses *205*
Rings *205*
Bed Cradles *205*
Bed Blocks *206*
Air Cushion *206*
Positions *206*
Supine/Dorsal Position *207*
Dorsal Recumbent Position *208*
Lithotomy Position *208*
Prone Position *208*
Lateral Position *209*
Sims' Position *209*
Knee-Chest/Genupectoral Position *209*
Trendelenburg's Position *210*
Fowler's Position *210*
Complementary/Alternative Therapies of Health *214*
Uses of Complementary Therapy *214*
Nurses' Role in Complementary Therapies *214*

Integrative Approach in Health Care *215*
Biofeedback *215*
Non-pharmacological Therapies *215*
Nurses' Role in Pain Management *216*

11. Promoting Safety in Health Care Environment — 218
Terminology *218*
Definition *219*
Objective/Goals of Patient Safety *219*
Safety in Health Care Environment *219*
Patient Safety in the Hospital *220*
Optimum Environment for the Patient *220*
Influence of External Environment *220*
Therapeutic Environment *221*
Hospital Cleaning *222*
Reduction of Physical Hazards: Fire and Accidents *223*
Five Steps to Improve Safety *224*
Care of Patients Unit *224*
Furnishing Patient's Unit *225*
Disinfection of the Unit *226*
Safety Devices: Restraints *227*
Side Rails *229*
Trapeze *230*
Falls Risk Assessment *230*
Patient Fall Prevention and Assessment *232*
Common Errors in Patient Safety *233*
Role of Nurse in Safe and Clean Environment *234*

12. Hospital Admission and Discharge — 236
Admission to Hospital Unit *236*
Unit and Its Preparation *238*
Admission Procedure *238*
Special Considerations *239*
Medicolegal Issues *239*
Patient's Bill of Rights *240*
Role and Responsibilities of Nurse in Admission *241*
Transfer Procedure *242*
Discharge Planning *243*
Discharge from Hospital *243*
Types: Planned Discharge, Lama, Abscond, Referrals and Transfer *243*
Discharge Procedure *244*
Care of Unit After Discharge *245*

13. Mobility and Immobility — 247
Terminology *247*
Definition *248*
Basic Elements of Normal Movement *248*
Benefits of Exercise *248*
Mobility *249*
Factors Affecting Mobility *249*
Effects of Mobility *250*
Complications of Immobility *252*
Providing Care to Clients with Immobility *253*
Nursing Management *253*
Body Mechanics *254*
Nursing Process in Body Mechanics *256*
Range of Motion Exercise *257*
Lifting and Transferring *258*
Log Rolling *261*
Transferring Patient from Bed to Wheelchair *262*
Transfer from Wheelchair to Bed *263*

Transfer from Bed to Stretcher and Stretcher to Bed 263
Plaster Casts 263
Cast Application 264

14. Patient Education   267
Concept of Patient Education 267
Definition 267
Therapeutic Patient Education 267
Value of Patient Education 268
Competencies of Health Educator 268
Objectives of Patient Education 268
Need of Patient Education 269
Benefits of Patient Education 269
Importance of Patient Education 269
Principles of Patient Education 270
Elements of an Educational Program 271
Effective Patient Teaching Strategies 271
Patient Education Methods 272
Evaluating Patient Learning 272
Barriers in Patient Education 272
Tips to Improve Patient Education 273
Nurses' Role in Patient Education 273

15. Hygiene   275
Terminology 275
Definition 275
Types of Hygiene 275
Factors Influencing Hygiene Practices 276
Personal Hygiene 276
Head to Toe Care 278
Oral Hygiene 279
Bed Bath 282
Care of Eyes, Nose and Ears 284
Care of Hands, Feet and Nails 285
Back Care/Back Massage/Back Rub 286
Assessment of Pressure Ulcers Using Braden Scale and Norton Scale 287
Care of Pressure Points/Bedsore 289
Care of Hair 291
Hair Combing 292
Hair Wash/Bed Shampoo 293
Pediculosis Treatment 294
Care of the Perineum 295
Clothing 296
Care of Dentures 296
Care of Hearing Aid in Nursing 298
Care of Contact Lens in Nursing 298

16. Nursing Process   301
Terminology 301
Critical Thinking and Nursing Judgement 301
Components of Critical Thinking 302
Importance of Critical Thinking 302
Critical Thinking in Nursing 303
Special Skills Required for Critical Thinking 303
Characteristics of Good Critical Thinker 303
Critical Thinking Through Nursing Practice 304
Levels of Critical Thinking in Nursing 305
Nursing Process Overview: Application in Practice 306
Steps in the Nursing Process 307
Benefits of Nursing Process 308
Nursing Assessment 309
Data Collection 309

Nursing Diagnosis *310*
Nursing Planning *313*
Nursing Implementation *314*
Nursing Evaluation *315*
Nursing Care Plan *317*

17. Nutritional Needs — 321
Terminology *321*
Nutrition and Health *322*
Nutritional Assessment *324*
Care of Patient with Dysphagia *325*
Care of Patient with Anorexia *326*
Care of Patient with Nausea *326*
Care of Patient with Vomiting *327*
Diet in Sickness *328*
Therapeutic Diet *329*
Hospital Diet *329*
Full Fluid Diet *331*
Soft Diet *331*
Normal Diet *331*
Feeding the Helpless Patient *332*
Nasogastric Tube Insertion *332*
Gastric Gavage *334*
Gastrojejunostomy Feeding *335*
Breastfeeding *337*
Artificial Feeding *337*
Total Parenteral Nutrition *338*
Gastric Analysis *340*

18. Elimination Needs — 343
Terminology *343*
Urinary Elimination *343*
Definition *343*
Physiology of Urine Elimination *344*
Characteristics of Urine *344*
Diagnostic Examination *344*
Factors Affecting Urinary Elimination *345*
Common Alterations in Urinary Elimination *346*
Urinary Retention *346*
Urinary Incontinence *347*
Monitoring Urinary Output *348*
Use of Urinal *349*
Catheterization of the Urinary Bladder *349*
Bladder Irrigation *351*
Catheter Care *353*
Collecting Urine Specimen *354*
Collecting a Single Voided Specimen *355*
24 Hours Urine Collection *356*
Urine Culture *357*
Urine Testing *358*
Role of Nurse in Urinary Elimination *361*
Bowel Elimination *361*
Factors Affecting Bowel Elimination *361*
Common Problems in Bowel Elimination *362*
Constipation *362*
Diarrhea *363*
Flatulence *364*
Insertion of a Flatus Tube *364*
Use of Bedpan *365*
Enema *366*
Bowel Wash *369*

Stool: Routine and Culture 371
Colostomy Irrigation 372
Barium Enema 373
Role of Nurse in Bowel Elimination 375

19. Diagnostic Testing 377
Terminology 377
Salient Features of Diagnostic Testing 379
Complete Blood Count 379
Serum Electrolytes 381
Liver Function Test 382
Lipid/Lipoprotein Profile 383
Serum Glucose: AC (Fasting Plasma Glucose), PC (Postprandial Plasma Glucose), HbA1C (Glycated Hemoglobin A1C) 384
Monitoring Capillary Blood Glucose (Glucometer Random Blood Sugar) 384
Specimen Collection 385
Urine Collections from Catheter 386
Urine Culture 387
Stool: Routine and Culture 388
Sputum Culture 389
Blood Smear 390
Blood Culture 390
Throat Swab 391
Vaginal Swab/Smear 392
Urine Testing 392
Endoscopies 394
Radiological Studies 409

20. Oxygenation Needs 425
Terminology 425
Review of Cardiovascular Physiology 426
Review of Respiratory Physiology 427
Factors Affecting Respiratory Functioning 427
Respiration: Types, Assessment, Management 429
Care of Patient with Dyspnea 429
Need of Oxygen Therapy 431
Acute Diseases Affect Blood Oxygen Level 431
Factors Affecting Oxygenation 431
Alterations in Oxygenation: Hypoxia 432
Care of Oxygen Cylinders 433
Oxygen Administration 434
Nasal Cannula 434
Nasal Catheter 435
Oxygen Mask 435
Oxygen Tent 436
Home Oxygen Therapy 438
Airway Management 438
Oropharyngeal Airway 438
Nasopharyngeal Airway 440
Endotracheal Tubes 441
Tracheostomy Tubes 441
Artificial Airway Management 442
Nursing Process in Airway Management 444
Coughing Techniques 445
Suctioning Procedure 445
Tracheostomy Suctioning 447
Steam Inhalation 448
Postural Drainage 449
Pulse Oximetry 453
Water Seal Chest Drainage 454
Cardiopulmonary Resuscitation 459

21. Fluid, Electrolyte and Acid-Base Balances — 464
Terminology *464*
Review of Physiological Regulation of Fluid, Electrolyte, and Acid-Base Balances *464*
Fluid Intake *465*
Sources of Water Intake *465*
Physiology of Body Fluids *466*
Factors Affecting Fluid Movement *467*
Mechanisms Controlling Fluid and Electrolyte Movement *467*
Regulation of Fluids and Electrolytes or Homeostatic Mechanism *468*
Fluid Imbalances *469*
Electrolytes *471*
Importance of Electrolytes *472*
Electrolyte Imbalances *474*
Acid-Base Balances *482*
Acid-Base Imbalances *482*
Intravenous Catheter Insertion *483*
Maintenance of IV System *486*
Administering Medications by Heparin Lock *487*
Intravenous Cutdown *488*
Blood Transfusion *490*
Fluid Restriction *492*

22. Administration of Medications — 495
Terminology *495*
Introduction to Medication Administration *496*
Sources of Drugs *496*
Drug Information Sources *497*
Drug Administration *497*
Factors Influencing Medication Action *498*
Route of Administration *499*
Medication Orders and Prescriptions *499*
Systems of Measurement *500*
Medication Dose Calculation *501*
Ten Rights of Medication Administration *502*
Errors in Medication Administration *503*
Care of Medicine and Medicine Cupboard *505*
Oral Medication *507*
Syringes and Needles *508*
Injections *509*
Intramuscular Injection *513*
Subcutaneous Injection *515*
Intradermal Injections *516*
Intravenous Injection *517*
Intravenous Infusions *518*
Transdermal Route *522*
Transmucosal *523*
Rectal Rectum *523*
Topical *523*
Special Drug Delivery Systems *523*
Instillation of Ear Drops *524*
Instilling Nasal Drops *525*

23. Sensory Needs — 528
Terminology *528*
Concept of Sensory Integration *529*
Definition *529*
Functioning of Sensory Organs *529*
Components of Sensory Experience *530*
Factors Influencing Sensory Function *530*
Sensory Assessment *531*
Nurses, Responsibility in Sensory and Thought Disturbances *532*

Sensory Alterations *532*
Sensory Deprivation *533*
Sensory Overload *533*
Nursing Process Application in Sensory Problems *533*
Communicating Patients with Aphasia *534*
Communicating Patient's Artificial Airway *535*
Communicating Visual Impairment *535*
Communicating with Hearing Impairment *537*
Care of Unconscious Patient *538*
Nursing Care Plan for Unconscious Patient *540*

24. Care of Terminally Ill, Death and Dying — 546
Terminology *546*
Loss *547*
Grief *548*
Types of Grief *548*
Manifestations of Grief *549*
Stages of Grief *550*
Grief Process *550*
Theories of Grief and Loss *551*
Kubler-Ross Five Stages of Dying *551*
Six 'R's of Mourning *552*
Factors Influencing Loss and Grief Responses *552*
Grief, Bereavement and Mourning *552*
Counseling and Supporting Grieving Relatives *553*
Care of Dying *554*
Death *556*
Hygienic Care of Dead Body *558*
Care of the Body After Death *558*
Documentation of Death *559*
Medicolegal Issues *559*
Advance Directives: Euthanasia, Will, Dying, Declaration, Organ Donation, etc. *560*
Autopsy *561*
Postmortem Care *561*
Embalming *562*

25. Self-concept — 564
Terminology *564*
Definition *564*
Concept of Self-concept *564*
Domains of Self-concept *565*
Positive Health Concept *565*
Development of Self-concept *566*
Factors Affecting Self-concept *566*
Self-concept Theory *567*
Carl Rogers and the Self-concept Theory of Personality *568*
Erikson's Theory *568*
Components of Self-concept *568*
Body Image *569*
Role Performance *569*
Self-esteem *570*
Identity *570*
Assessment of Self-concept *570*
Nursing Process *570*
Self-concept Disturbance: Low Self-esteem *571*
Situational Low Self-esteem *571*
Disturbed Body Image *573*

26. Sexuality — 576
Terminology *576*
Sexual Health Concerns *578*

Definitions *578*
Sexual Development Throughout Life *579*
Circles of Sexuality Model *581*
Components of Sexuality *581*
Characteristics of Sexual Health *581*
Characteristics of a Sexually Healthy Person *582*
Importance of Sexual Health *583*
Sexual Orientation *584*
Consequences of Poor Sexual Health *584*
Improve their Sexual Health *585*
Sexual Response Cycle *585*
Physiological and Sexual Response in Women *586*
Physiological Changes and Sexual Response in Men *586*
Nurse's Responsibility in Collecting the Sexual History *587*
Nurse's Responsibility *588*
Prevention of Sexually Transmitted Diseases *589*
Prevention of Unwanted Pregnancy *590*
Prevention of Sexual Harassment *590*
Prevention Sexual Abuse *590*
Sexual Health Education *591*
Advantages of Nurses in Sexual Health Services *592*
Nurses Responsibility in Sexual Health *592*

27. **Stress and Adaptation**   **594**
Terminology *594*
Meaning of Stress *595*
Sources of Stress *595*
Symptoms of Stress *595*
Types of Stress *596*
Types of Stressors *596*
General Adaptation Syndrome (Hans Selye, 1945) *597*
Local Adaptation Syndrome *597*
Strategies of Stress Management *598*
Role of Nurse in Stress Management *599*
Adaptation *599*
Concept of Crisis and Resolution *600*
Crisis Intervention *601*
Nursing Process Application in Crisis Intervention *603*
Grief and Resolution of Grief *605*
Maladaptive Grief Responses *605*
Recreation and Diversional Therapies *606*

28. **Cultural Diversity and Spirituality**   **608**
Terminology *608*
Concepts: Culture, Subculture and Multicultural *609*
Cultural Competence *610*
Providing Culturally Responsive Care *611*
Psychosocial Care and Assessment *612*
Cultural Diversity *612*
Transcultural Nursing *614*
Models of Transcultural Nursing *616*
Nurses' Competences to Provide Transcultural Care *617*
Spirituality and Nursing *618*
Meaning and Definition *619*
Lifespan Consideration in Spiritual Health *619*
Characteristics of Spirituality *621*
Factors Affecting Spiritual Health *621*
Spiritual Dimensions of Nursing *623*
Age-specific Spiritual Interventions *623*
Dealing with Spiritual Distress/Problems *624*

29. Nursing Theories 627
Terminology 627
History of Nursing Theories 628
Definition 629
Nursing Metaparadigm 630
Components of Nursing Theories 630
Purposes of Theories and Conceptual Model 630
Goals of Theoretical Nursing Models 631
Basic Characteristics of a Theory 631
Nursing Theories Important 631
Theoretical Models of Nursing Practice 631
Kinds of Theories 631
Types of Theory (by Abstraction) 632
Development of Nursing Theories 633
Paplau's Theory (1952) 633
Henderson's Theory (1955) 634
Orem's Theory 636
Neuman's Theory (1972) 637
Rogers Theory (1970) 638
Roy's Theory (1979) 639
Linking Theories with Nursing Process 639
Use of Theories in Nursing Practice 640

30. First Aid and Emergencies 642
Terminology 642
Introduction to First Aid 644
The Management of the Case 647
Golden Rules of First Aid 647
First Aid Kit 648
Wounds 649
Hemorrhage 654
Shock 655
Musculoskeletal Injuries: Fractures, Dislocation, Muscle Injuries 657
Rice Treatment for Acute Musculoskeletal Injury 661
Dislocation 661
Injuries to the Joint and Muscles 663
Transporting Casualities 663
Lifting Casualties 666
Unconsciousness 668
Respiratory Emergencies and Basic CPR 671
First Aid for Foreign Bodies in the Eye, Ear, Nose, and Throat 675
Basic Cardiac Life Support 678
Burns and Scalds 681
Bites and Stings 684
Poisoning 685
First Aid in Convulsions 688
Fainting 688
Epistaxis 688
Electric Shock 689
Hanging, Strangling and Throttling 689
Bandaging First Aid 690
Types of Bandages 691
Special Bandages 692
Slings 692
Binder 693
Community Emergencies 693

31. Meeting Needs of Perioperative Patients 697
Terminology 697
Definition and Concept of Perioperative Nursing 698
Preoperative Nursing 700

Intraoperative Phase: Threater—Set-Up, Equipment and Role of Nurse *703*
Postoperative Nursing *705*
Postoperative Complications *709*
Perioperative Nursing Process *710*
Wounds *711*
Dressing: Suture Care *714*
Suturing the Wound *715*
Surgical Dressing *715*
Suture Removal *717*
Care of Drains *718*

32. Surgical Procedures   **722**
Abdominal Paracentesis *722*
Thoracentesis *724*
Lumbar Puncture *726*
Bone Marrow Biopsy and Aspiration *728*
Surgical Dressing *730*
Liver Biopsy *732*
Wound Care *733*

Appendices
Appendix 1: Abbreviations and Symbols   737
Appendix 2: Temperature Conversion Table   739
Appendix 3: Laboratory Values   740

Glossary   741

Index   749

CHAPTER 1

Introduction

LEARNING OBJECTIVES

- Concept of health—definitions (WHO), dimensions
- Maslow's hierarchy of needs
- Health-illness continuum
- Factors influencing health
- Causes and risk factors for developing illness
- Illness—types, illness behavior
- Impact of illness on patient and family

TERMINOLOGY

- **Acute illness:** Illness characterized by symptoms that are of relatively short duration, are usually severe and affect the functioning of the clients in all dimensions.
- **Adaptation:** Process by which changes occur in any of a person's dimensions in response to stress.
- **Etiology:** Identification of the cause of a problem. The cause may be direct or a contributing factor in the development of client problem or need.
- **Health:** Dynamic state in which an individual adapts to internal and external environments so that there is a state of physical, emotional, intellectual, social and spiritual well-being.
- **Health behavior:** Activities through which a person maintain, attains or regains behavior as an expression of personal health beliefs.
- **Health-belief model:** Conceptual framework that predicts a person's health behavior as an expression of personal beliefs.
- **Health-illness continuum:** Scale by means of which a personnel's level of health can be described, ranging from high level wellness to severe illness. The scales take in to account the presence of risk factors.
- **Health promotion:** Activities directed toward maintain or enhancing the health and wellbeing of clients.
- **Health promoting behavior:** Considered a third subcategory of health behavior and through assessment, reveal needs for vehicular safety, home safety, domestic violence recognition, recreational safety, occupational safety and health.
- **Holistic health:** A system of compressive or total care that considers the physical, emotional, social, economical and spiritual needs of the person, the response to the illness, and the effect of the illness on the person's ability to meet self-care needs.
- **Models:** Models are graphic or symbolic representations of phenomena that objectify and present certain perspectives or points of view about nature or function or both.
- **Concept:** Concepts are the elements or components of a phenomenon necessary to understand the phenomenon and derived from impressions the human mind receives about phenomena through sensing the human environment.
- **Philosophy:** A philosophy is statement of belief and values about human being and their world.
- **Theory:** Theory refers to a set of logically interrelated concepts, statement, proposition and definitions which have been derived from philosophical beliefs of scientific data and from which questions or hypothesis can be deduced, tested and verified.
- **Health:** A state of physical, mental and social well-being, and the absence of disease or other disorders. It involves constant change and adaptation to stress.
- **Community:** Community as a group of inhabitants living together in a somewhat localized area under the same general regulations and having common interests, functions, needs and organizations.
- **Nursing:** Nursing is an art, science and profession by which we render, serve to human being to help him to regain or to keep a normal state of body and mind and when it cannot accomplish this, it help him for the relief from physical pain, mental anxiety or spiritual discomfort.
- **Community health:** Community (public) health is a science and art of preventing disease, prolonging life and promoting health and efficiency through organized effort.
- **Community health nursing:** Community health nursing is a synthesis of nursing and public health practice applied of promoting and preserving the health of people. The practice is general and compressive. It is not limited to a particular age group or diagnosis, and continuing, not episodic.

- **Profession:** A profession is an occupation with moral principles that are devoted to the human and social welfare. The service is based on specialized knowledge and skill developed in a scientific and learned manner.
- **Quality care:** The degree of which health services for individuals and populations increase the likelihood of desired health outcomes and are consistent with current professional knowledge.
- **Health care team:** Health care team refers to health personal in all of the departments of a health care facility, who provides health care services. They are doctors, nurses, technicians and paramedical staff.
- **Primary nursing:** In primary nursing, a professional nurse has total responsibility for a particular patient or group of patients. The model's purpose is to provide continuity and coordination of care.
- **Primary health care:** It is an essential health care based on practical, scientifically sound and socially accepted methods and technology, made universally acceptable to individuals and families in the community involving their full participation and at a cost that the community and country can afford to maintain at every stage of their development.
- **Health center:** It is defined as an institution for the promotion of health and welfare of the people in a given area, which seeks to achieve health work through coordination with welfare and relief organizations.
- **Comprehensive health care:** Comprehensive health care is the combined (integrated) curative, preventive, promotive and restorative care made available to the people without distinctions of caste, creed or economic status from birth to death (from womb to tomb).
- **Primary health center:** Primary health center is an institution for providing comprehensives health care, e.g. preventive, promotive and curative services, to the people living in a defined geographical area. It seeks to achieve its purpose by grouping under one roof or coordinate all the health work of that area.
- **Health for all:** Health for all has been defined as attainment of a level of health that will enable every individual to lead a socially and economically productive life.
- **Community development block:** Community development is a process which is designed to promote better living of the whole community, with the active participation by the community itself along with governmental efforts.
- **Community health nurse:** Community health nurse is person plays important role in helping people learn to care themselves and to work with other community residents to develop the capacity or infrastructure needed to ensure essential health care for everyone.
- **Disease:** Any deviation from or interruption of the normal structure or function of any part, organ or system of the body, manifesting with a characteristic set of signs and symptoms.

INTRODUCTION

- Health in its broadest sense is a dynamic state in which the individual adapts to changes in internal and external environments to maintain a state of well-being. The internal environment includes many factors that influence health, including genetic and psychological variables, intellectual and spiritual dimensions and disease processes.
- The external environment includes factors outside the person that may influence health, including factors outside the person that may influence health, including the physical environment, social relationships, and economic variables because both environments continuously change, the person must to maintain a state of well-being.
- Health and illness therefore must be defined in terms of individual. Health can include conditions that the client or nurse may have previously considered to be illness. Health is also closely related to an individual's work place and home life and stressors can be the result of those environments.

CONCEPT OF HEALTH

Health is considered by many as the opposite of illness or disease. For some, it means a well developed or adequately nourished body, capable of various activities and able to withstand physical stress. All communities have their concepts of health integrated as a part of their culture. Widely differing culture groups share the concept of health as a state of balance and harmony.

The WHO has defined health as a "State of complete physical, mental, social, spiritual well-being, and not merely absence of disease or infirmity. The concept of positive wholeness or completeness is emphasized and health is seen as more than a physical state. An individual's health is never static and is always in a dynamic equilibrium with his environment.

Physical well-being is measurable although it is varying ranges and validity. As regards mental well-being, measurable standards vary from culture to culture and hence the criteria for mental wellbeing may differ from one country to another or from place to place within the same country. There is also difference of opinion as to what is precisely meant by social well-being. Social well-being may be regarded as a state of predisposing condition of health.

DEFINITION OF HEALTH

- WHO definition of health: Health is a state of complete physical, mental and social well-being and not merely the absence of disease or infirmity.

- **Wellness:** It is a state of high-level health. One can achieve this by balancing their focus amongst the various dimensions of health.
- **Holistic health:** It is an understanding that all the aspects of wellness are interrelated. Lifestyle choices can impact your health physically, mentally, emotionally, socially and spiritually. Examples are what to eat, and when to exercise.

DIMENSIONS OF HEALTH

Traditionally health has been defined in terms of the presence or absence of disease. Nightingale defined health as a state of being well and using every power the individual possess to the fullest extent. It reflects concern for the individual as a total person functioning physically, psychologically and socially.

Environmental determinants: Environment has the direct impact on the health of individual, family or community. Internal or external and physical, biological and psychosocial components of environment influence the mental, social, spiritual and physical well-being of individuals, Environmental pollution has become a global threat. We must find the ways to reduce and manage the pollution as well as waste. It is worth mentioning that Florence Nightingale had also given importance to environmental factors in the maintenance of the health and care of the sick. Air, water, noise, radiation, housing, waste management, etc. all affect the health status and quality of life.

Political system: Political system has a great effect on the social climate in which we live. Political influences have the power and authority to regulate much of our surroundings—in that health care is also included. Implementation of any health programme cannot be conducted properly without the strong political will. In our country health is a subject of concurrent list, so there is a need of coordination between the union and state governments in the health-related matters.

Behavioral determinants: Health is the mirror of a person's lifestyle because faulty and ill habits have the adverse effect on the health of the individual. It is an established fact that culture and ethnic heritage shape much of our lifestyle including the health care.

Socioeconomic determinants: Socioeconomic conditions have the major impact on the health status of any country. Education, economy, occupational opportunities, housing, nutritional level, per capita income, etc. determine the health care system and health resources.

Health care delivery system determinants: The health care delivery system plays a great role in the field of health, this is considered as a disease-oriented system, but in our country which has the second largest population in the world, providing health care services at the grass-roots level is a difficult task. Besides the above-mentioned determinants women's issue, ageing population, agriculture, social welfare, rural development, urban improvement, etc. also have a major impact on the health of the nation, its families and individuals.

MULTIPLE FACTS OF HEALTH—WHO

- **Health a tridimensional state:** "Health is a state of complete physical, mental and social wellbeing and not merely the absence of disease or infirmity".
- **Health a fundamental right:** "The enjoyment of the highest attainable standards of health is one of the fundamental rights of every human being, without distinction of race, religion, and political belief, and economic and social condition".
- **Health for peace and security:** "The health for all people is fundamental to the attainment of peace and security and is dependent upon the fullest cooperation of individuals".
- **Health a government responsibility:** "Government have a responsibility for the health of their people, which can be fulfilled only by the provision of adequate health and social measures".
- **Health and health information:** "The extension to all people of the benefits of medical, psychological, and related knowledge is essential to the fullest attainment of health".
- **Health and people cooperation:** "Informed opinion and active cooperation on the part of the public are of the utmost importance in the improvement of health of the people".
- **Health and health care:** "Unequal development in different countries in the promotion of health and control of disease, especially communicable disease is a common danger".
- **Health and child development:** "Healthy development of the child is of basic importance. The ability to live harmonically in changing total environment is essential to such development".
- **Health gain for all:** "The achievement of any state in the promotion and protection of health is of value to all".

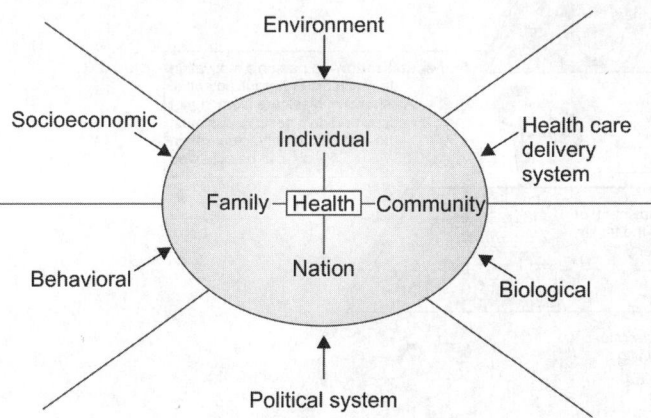

Fig. 1.1: Dimensions of health.

MASLOW'S HIERARCHY OF NEEDS

Maslow's hierarchy of needs is a motivational theory in psychology comprising a five-tier model of human needs, often depicted as hierarchical levels within a pyramid. From the bottom of the hierarchy upwards, the needs are: physiological, safety, love and belonging, esteem, and self-actualization.

Maslow stated that people are motivated to achieve certain needs and that some needs take precedence over others. Our most basic need is for physical survival, and this will be the first thing that motivates our behavior. Once that level is fulfilled the next level up is what motivates us, and so on.

- **Physiological needs**—these are biological requirements for human survival, e.g. air, food, drink, shelter, clothing, warmth, sex, sleep. If these needs are not satisfied the human body cannot function optimally. Maslow considered physiological needs the most important as all the other needs become secondary until these needs are met.
- **Safety needs**—protection from elements, security, order, law, stability, freedom from fear.
- **Love and belongingness needs**—after physiological and safety needs have been fulfilled; the third level of human needs is social and involves feelings of belongingness. The need for interpersonal relationships motivates behavior. Examples include friendship, intimacy, trust, and acceptance, receiving and giving affection and love. Affiliating, being part of a group (family, friends, work).
- **Esteem needs**—which Maslow classified into two categories: (i) esteem for oneself (dignity, achievement, mastery, and independence) and (ii) the desire for reputation or respect from others (e.g. status, prestige). Maslow indicated that the need for respect or reputation is most important for children and adolescents and precedes real self-esteem or dignity.
- **Self-actualization needs**—realizing personal potential, self-fulfillment, seeking personal growth and peak experiences. A desire "to become everything one is capable of becoming".

HEALTH–ILLNESS CONTINUUM

- According to Neuman (1990), health on a continuum is the degree of client wellness that exist at any point in time ranging from an optimal wellness condition, with available energy at its maximum, to death, which represents total energy depletion.
- According to health-illness continuum model, health is a dynamic state that continuously alters as a person adapts to changes in the internal and external environments to maintain a state of physical, emotional, intellectual, social, developmental and spiritual well-being.

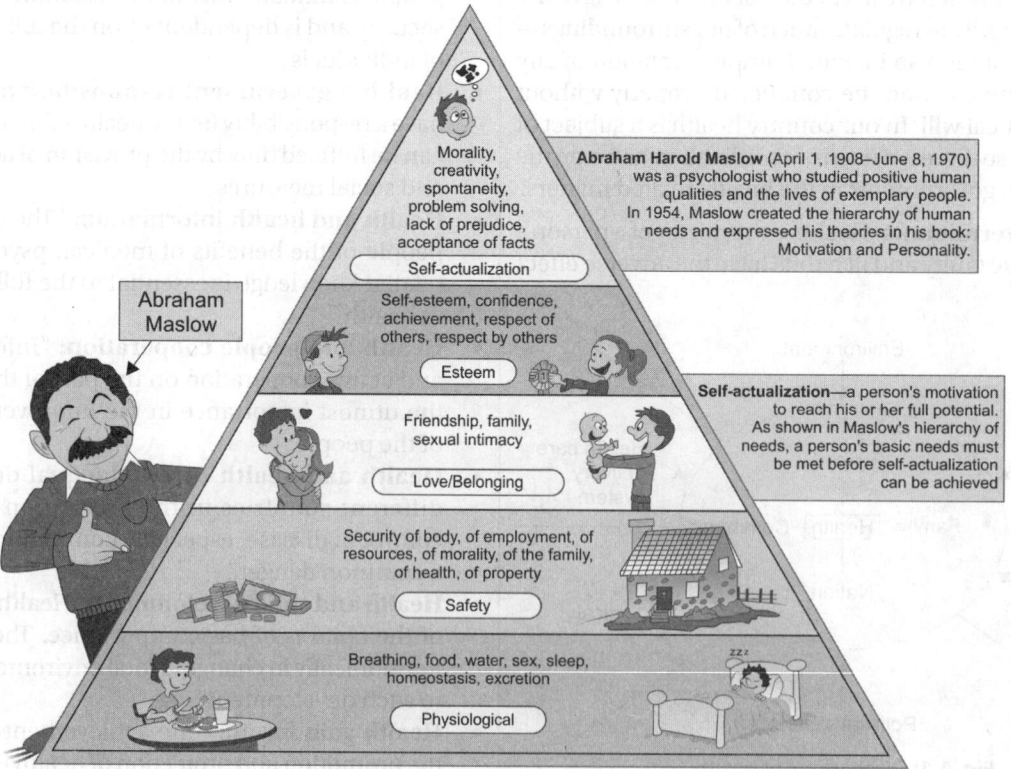

Fig. 1.2: Maslow's hierarchy of needs.

- The continuum is thought of a complex, dynamic process that includes physical, psychological and social components. There are adaptive or maladaptive behavioral responses to internal and external stimuli.
- Health and illness tend to merge but may represent pattern of adaptive change along the continuum. The direction of change may be reversible, depending on the quality of the individual's adaptive efforts.
- The individual at the illness end of the continuum is characterized by feeling of uncertainty, helplessness, loss of control, loss of identity and incapacity for problem solving.
- As the patient is in the sick role, there is incapacity to meet other social roles, the person has sought diagnosis and get treatment.
- Less far along the illness end of the continuum, as illness behavior are brought in to play, the person may be tired, rundown and irritable with complains of loss of sleep, appetite, dependence, self-absorption, minor illnesses such as colds, infections, headaches andbackaches.
- Between illness and wellness there is the ambiguous area where no symptoms are present and the person is neither especially well nor especially ill.
- At the health end of the continuum, as health behaviors are utilized, the persons are not only unaware of disease and without pain, fatigue or somatic complications but also tend to be resistant to infections, industrious, vigorous and physically agile, with a strong sense of identity and autonomy, caring out usual social roles and needing no health care.
- The goal in preventive health care is to maintain equilibrium between health and illness, with balance in favor of maximum wellness for the individual.

MODELS OF HEALTH AND ILLNESS

Health–Wellness Model

- It was developed by Dunn (1997), the high level wellness model is oriented toward maximizing the health potential of an individual.
- This model requires the individual to maintain a continuum of balance and purposeful direction within the environment.
- It involves progress toward a higher level of functioning open-ended and expanding challenges to live at the fullest potential

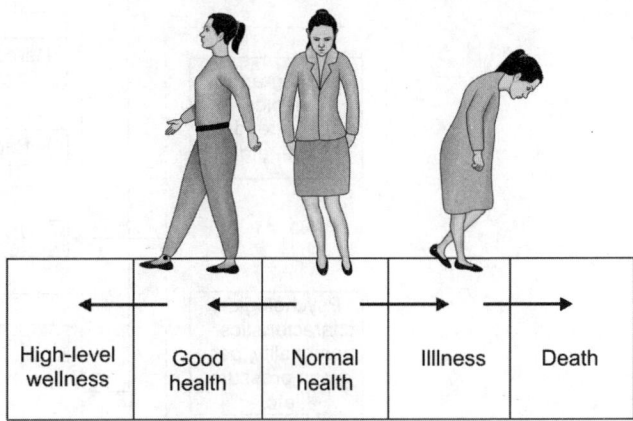

Fig. 1.3: Health–Wellness model.

Agent-Host-Environmental Model

- The agent-host-environmental model of health and illness originated in the community health work of level, etc.
- According to this approach the health or illness of an individual or group depends on the dynamic relationship of the agent, host and environment.
- The agent is any internal or external factors that its presence or absence can lead to disease or illness or disease.
- The host is the person or persons who may be susceptible to a particular illness or diseases.
- The environment consists of all factors outside of the host. It includes physical environment, social environment and biological environment.

Health Belief Model

- Rosenstoch's (1794) and Bakerand Maiman's (1975) health belief model addresses the relationship between a person's belief and behavior.

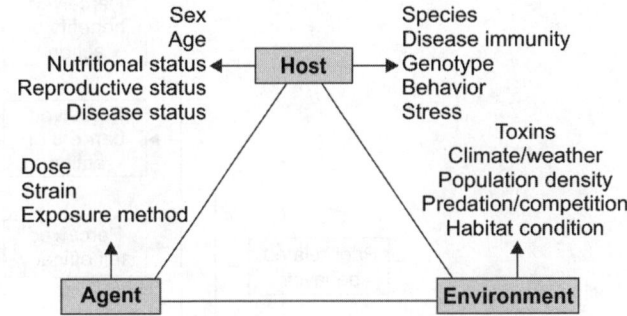

Fig. 1.5: Agent-Host-Environmental model.

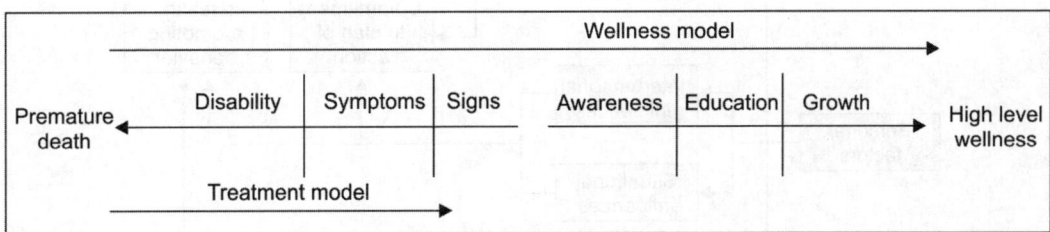

Fig. 1.4: Health-Illness continuum.

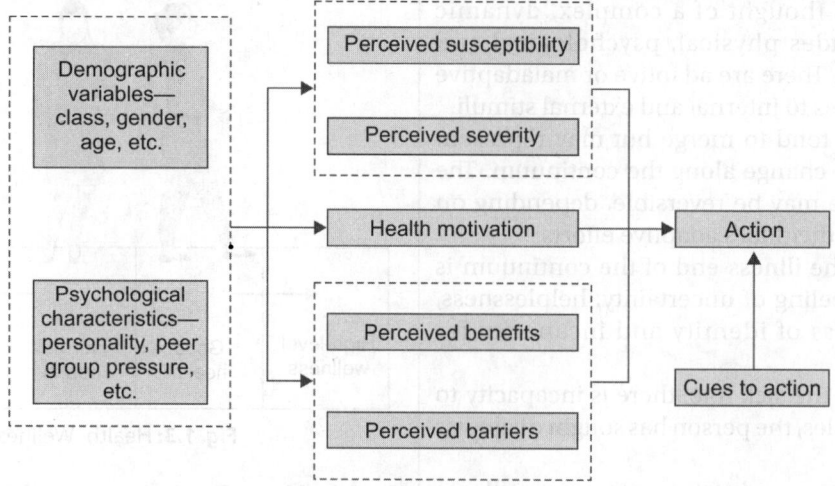

Fig. 1.6: Health belief model.

- It provides a way of understanding and predicating how clients will behave in relation to their health and how they will comply with health care therapies.
- The first component in this model involves the individual's perception of susceptibility to an illness.
- The second component is the individual's perception of the seriousness of the illness. This perception is influenced and modified by demographic and sociopsychological variables, perceived threats of the illnesses, and cues to action.
- The third component: The likelihood that a person will take preventive action- is the person's perception of the benefits of taking action.

Health Promotion Model

- The health promotion model proposed by Pender (1996). It was designed to be a complementary counterpart to models of health protection.
- Health promotion is directed at increasing a client's level of well-being.

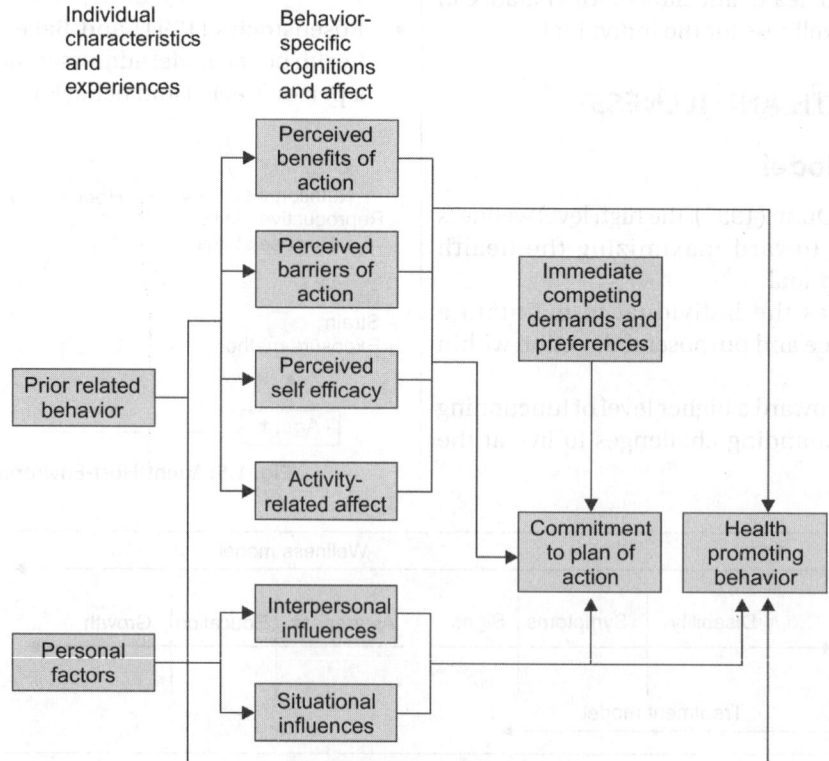

Fig. 1.7: Health promotion model.

- The model also organizes cues into a pattern to explain the likelihood of a client's participation in health-promotion behavior.
- The focus of this model is to explain the reasons that individuals engage in health activities. It is not designed for use with families or communities.

BIOPSYCHOSOCIAL ASPECTS OF HEALTH AND ILLNESS

Physical, social, cultural and psychological factors interact dynamically and have an important influence on patient care needs. There are needs common to everyone, no matter their sociocultural background, so-called human needs. These needs when they are not met create tensions and these tensions may give rise to anxiety that can hamper recovery if not relived.

Developmental Needs

- **Prenatal:** This stage determines many characteristics of the person and to some extend the requirements for use of adaptive resources throughout life.
- **Neonatal:** Developmental tasks are mostly physical, foundations are begun at this time for later personality responses.
- **Infancy:** This is a time of much physical, but foundations are begun at this time for later personality reponses.
- **Childhood:** Marked physical growth continues during this time. There is the beginning of role identification and moving out from the family to the peer group and community.
- **Adolescence:** Many physical and emotional changes occur as growth and maturation continues, changing hormonal activity and search for identity are major stresses for the adolescent.

- **Young adulthood:** Physical maturation is completed. There are many psychosocial stresses related to family and community roles during this stage.
- **Middle adulthood:** Developmental tasks are mostly psychosocial, reacting to reassessment of goals, physical stamina and hormone output beginning to decline.
- **Older years:** Physical conditioning is generally declining, and decreased sensory acuity may be noticeable. Developmental takes are related to sharing accumulated experiences and evaluating achievements.

Cultural Influences

- Culture may be thought of as the total way of life of a people, the social legacy the individuals acquire from his or her groups.
- The culture concept is cardial to an understanding of ourselves and our world.
- Custom and group habits are referred to as folkways and mores. Folkways are the accustomed and time-honored ways of doing things, the social habits that become routine and that are often performed without thinking.
- The patient's cultural background helps to determine the way the relationship with the physician or nurse in perceived and facilitates or impedes interaction or communication.

Religious Aspects

- Religion traditionally has focused on a God beyond the individual and has concentrated itself with relating the individual and has concerned itself with relating the individual to that God.
- Religious beliefs are seldom held to oneself but are part of group processes, so that there is immediate family or group support for the patient.
- It helps the patient's own attitude or belief that recovery is possible and that there are forces available to facilitate the healing process.
- It is important if the nurse is to be of help, to understand not only the spiritual needs of the patient but also the means and methods that organized religion has for meeting those needs.

DETERMINANTS OF HEALTH

Environmental determinants: Environment has the direct impact on the health of individual, family or community. Internal or external and physical, biological and psychosocial components of environment influence the mental, social, spiritual and physical well-being of individuals, Environmental pollution has become a global threat. We must find the ways to reduce and manage the pollution as well as waste. It is worth mentioning that Florence Nightingale had also given importance to environmental factors in the maintenance of the health and care of the sick. Air, water, noise, radiation, housing, waste-management, etc. all affect the health status and quality of life.

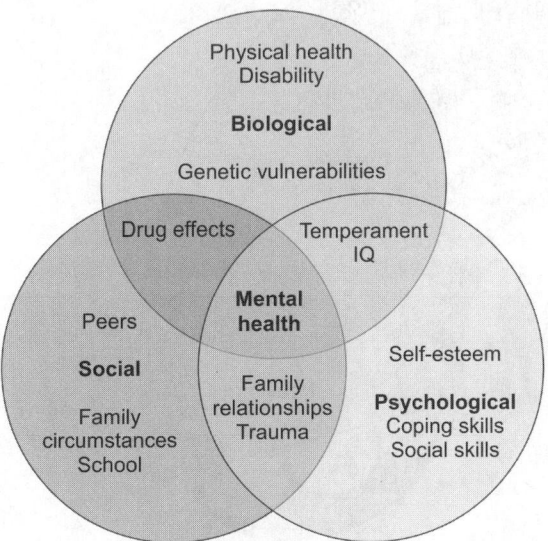

Fig. 1.8: Biopsychosocial model.

Political system: Political system has a great effect on the social climate in which we live. Political influences have the power and authority to regulate much of our surroundings in that, health care is also included. Implementation of any health programme cannot be conducted properly without the strong political will.

Behavioral determinants: Health is the mirror of a person's lifestyle because faulty and ill habits have the adverse effect on the health of the individual. It is an established fact that culture and ethnic heritage shape much of our lifestyle including the health care.

Socioeconomic determinants: Socioeconomic conditions have the major impact on the health status of any country. Education, economy, occupational opportunities, housing, nutritional level, per capita income, etc. determine the health care system and health resources.

Health care delivery system determinants: The health care delivery system plays a great role in the field of health, this is considered as a disease-oriented system, but in our country which has the second largest population in the world, providing health care services at the grass-roots level is a difficult task. Besides the above-mentioned determinants women's issue, ageing population, agriculture, social welfare, rural development, urban improvement, etc. also have a major impact on the health of the nation, its families and individuals.

FACTORS INFLUENCING HEALTH

Health influenced by various factors which interact with each other and determine the health status of many individual, family and community at large at any given point of time. These factors known as determinants of health. According to WHO expert committee on community health nursing. Technical report series 558 (1974) and Blum, these factors are categorized as human biology, Environment, lifestyle, health and health allied resources.

Human Biology

- **Genetic inheritance:** Hereditary or genetic predisposition to specific illness is a major physical risk factor. For example, a person with a family history of diabetes mellitus is at risk for developing the disease later in life. Other documented genetic risk factors include family history of cancer, coronary disease and renal disease.
- **Age:** Age increases susceptibility to certain illness. For example, the risk of cardiovascular disease increases with age for both sexes. The risk of birth defects and complications of pregnancy increase in women bearing children after age 35. Age risk factors are often closely associated with other risk factors such as family history and personal habits.
- **Race:** Race increases susceptibility to certain illness. For example, the risk of sickle cell anemia is more common in Africans and Mediterranean people.
- **Self-concept:** Self-concept implies individual's perception of his or physical, intellectual and social abilities.

Environment

The physical environment: The physical environment includes atmospheric pressures, gravity, light and sound

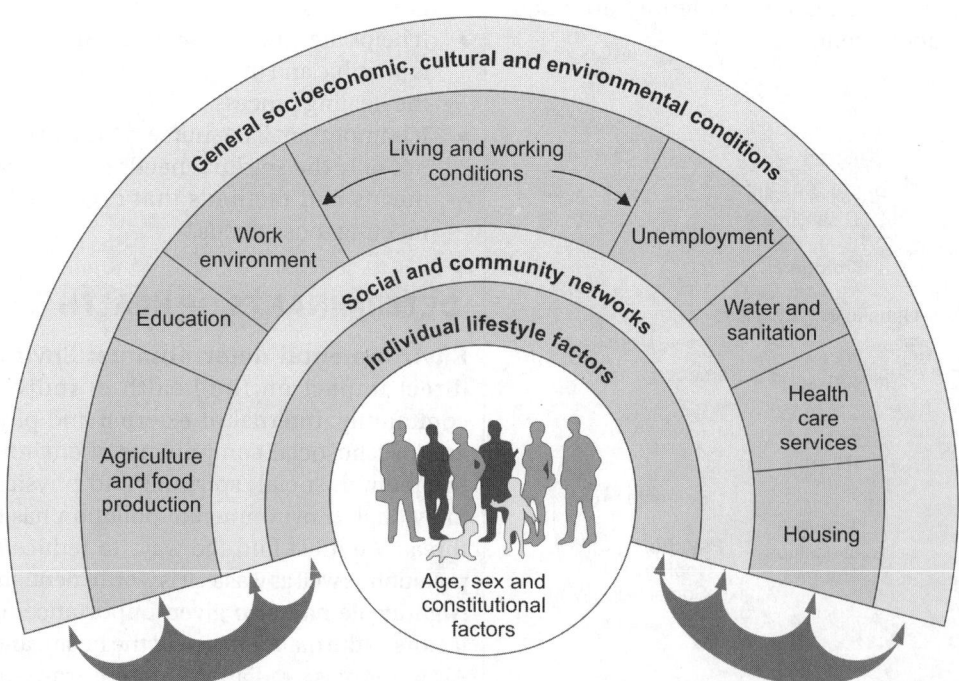

Fig. 1.9: Socio-economic, cultural and environmental factors affecting on health.

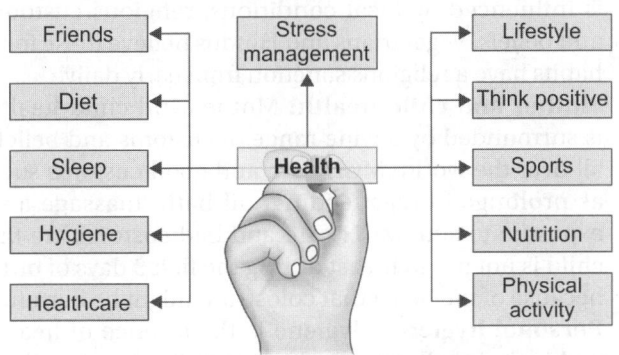

Fig. 1.10: Intrinsic and extrinsic factors affect on health.

waves, temperature, humidity, wind velocity, solar radiation, electromagnetic fields and seasonal variations, etc. The variety of pollutants are found to pollute air, water, food and soil, and are the cause of various acute and chronic diseases, e.g. gastrointestinal, respiratory, skin cancer, cardiovascular diseases, etc.

The biological environment: Most of the plants and animals are useful to human being to promote health but are the same time, they produce diseases like malaria, insect bites and allergic reactions.

The social environment: The social environment include other people and social institutions, sociocultural events, religious beliefs, moral and ethical values and social rules and regulations, pertaining to living society, socioeconomic support system.

Life-style: Many activities, habits and practices involve risk factors, the stresses of life crises and frequent life changes also risk factors. Health practices and behaviors can have positive or negative effects in health. Practices with potential negative effects are risk factors these include overeating or poor nutrition, insufficient rest and sleep and poor personal hygiene. Other habits that put a person at risk for illness include smoking, alcohol or drug abuse, and activities involving a threat of injury such as skydiving or mountain climbing. Some habits are risk factors for specific diseases. For example, excessive sunbathing increases the risk of skin cancer, and being overweight increases the risk of cardiovascular disease.

Prolonged emotional stress may increase the chance of illness. Emotional stress may occur with events such as divorce, pregnancy and arguments. Job related stresses, e.g. many overtax a person's cognitive skills and decision making ability leading to mental overload or burnout.

Health and Health Allied Resources

- **Health services:** Health services are directly concerned with improvement of health status of people. Health services can also contribute on socioeconomic development of people because sound health can improve and increase the physical, intellectual and emotional capacity of people to get educated, work and earn for their livelihood improve their lifestyle which will further reinforce their health.
- **Socioeconomic conditions:** Socioeconomic conditions have significant influence on community health. In developed countries like America, UK and Canada, there has been significant reduction in the morbidity and mortality rates and increases in longevity at birth because of socioeconomic developments. Socioeconomic conditions include economic status, education, occupation and living standards.
- **Political system:** The political system has a very strong role in health promotion of people in the country. The health care delivery system is determined by the political system though there is constitutional control. Decisions pertaining to health policy, allocation of funds, programs, manpower development, infrastructure, health technology and delivery of health services are made by the ruling party within the parliament system.
- **Health related services:** The health related services include education governmental policies; social welfare developmental programmes, food and agriculture, industry, communication and broadcasting rural and urban development and transportation facilities. The health related services needs to have balanced approach between National health policy and voluntary health promotes active participation.

CONCEPT OF DISEASE

Disease can be considered as something more than mere deviation from health, each disease being a distinct entity, with distinguishing qualities in its pathologic process, its

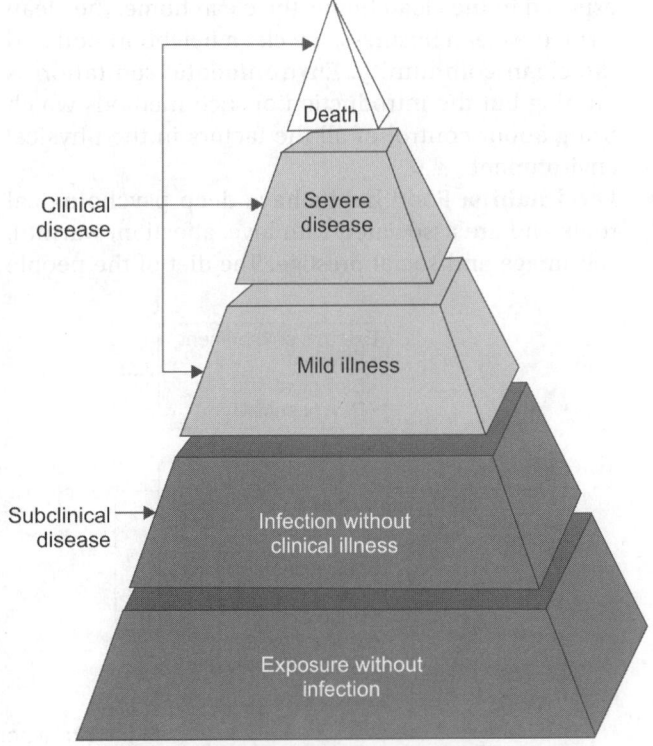

Fig. 1.11: Concept of disease.

typical clinical appearance and often its characteristic epidemiologic pattern of distribution in terms of time, place and person. The concept of disease also may vary from one society to another society. There will be no difficulty in distinguishing an illness which is severe enough to necessitate bed rest and treatment, but milder condition of disease and in apparent or subclinical conditions which do not make these individual take to bed are likely to be missed or ignored. Just like the border-line health conditions, diseases of mild nature and in apparent or subclinical conditions are supposed to lie in the middle of a spectrum. At one end of this spectrum is "optimal health" and at the other end "serious disease" and in between those two ends, various grades of health and disease are located. The milder the disease or the more border - line the health, the more difficult it is to differentiate between health and disease.

CULTURAL FACTORS IN HEALTH AND DISEASE

The member of a particular society quite unconsciously agrees upon a common pattern of living. It includes basic rules for living together. These rules could be understood as the culture of the society. The behavior pattern of a particular culture are not biologically inherited but socially acquired through learning.

Concept of etiology and cure: Supernatural causes like wrath of God and Goddess, breach of taboo, past sins, evil eye and spirit or ghost intrusion. Physical causes include the effects of weather, water and impure blood.

- **Environmental sanitation:** Sanitation is the science of safe-guarding health. It is the quality of living that is exposed in the clean home, the clean home, the clean farm, the clean business, the clean neighborhood and the clean community. Environmental sanitation is nothing but the introduction of such methods which bring about control of all the factors in the physical environment.
- **Food habits:** Food habits have deep psychological roots and are associated with love, affection, warmth, self-image and social prestige. The diet of the people is influenced by local conditions, religious customs and beliefs. Vegetarians and Hindus believe these food habits have a religious sanction from early daily.
- **Mother and child health:** Mother and child health is surrounded by a wide range of customs and beliefs all over the world. MCH care and good customs such as prolonged breastfeeding, oil bath, massage and exposure to sun. MCH care and bad customs are the child is not put to breast during the first 3 days of birth because of the belief that colostrum might be harmful.
- **Personal hygiene:** Hygiene is the science of health and includes all factors which contribute to healthful living. Personal hygiene includes all those personal factors which influence the health and well-being of an individual. The practice of an oil bath is a good Indian custom. Circumcision is a prevalent custom among Muslims which has a religious sanction.
- **Sex and marriage:** Sexual customs vary among different social, religious and ethnic groups. Orthodox Jews are forbidden to have intercourse for seven days after the menstruation ceases, these custom have an important bearing in family planning. Marriage is sacred. It is the usual social custom in India to perform marriages early at about the age of puberty. Child marriages are fortunately disappearing. The high rate of venereal diseases in Himachal Pradesh is attributed to the local marriage customs.

CAUSES AND RISK FACTORS FOR DEVELOPING ILLNESS

An illness is the response, the person has to disease. It is an abnormal process in which the person's level of functioning is changed compared with a previous level.

Internal Variables

- **Developmental stage:** A person's thought and behavior patterns change throughout life.
- **Intellectual background:** Knowledge about body functions and illnesses, educational background and

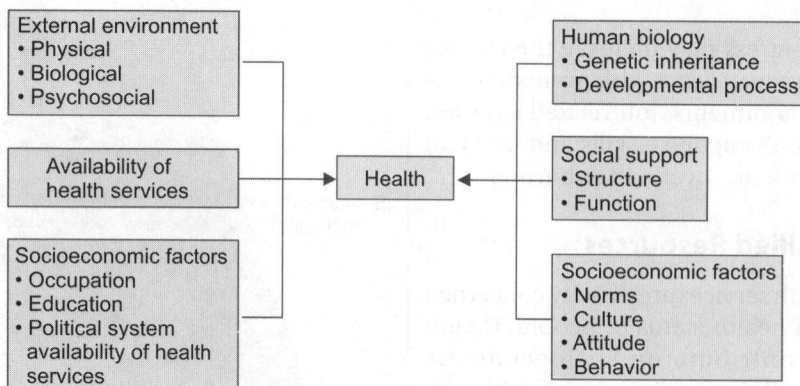

Fig. 1.12: Factors affecting health.

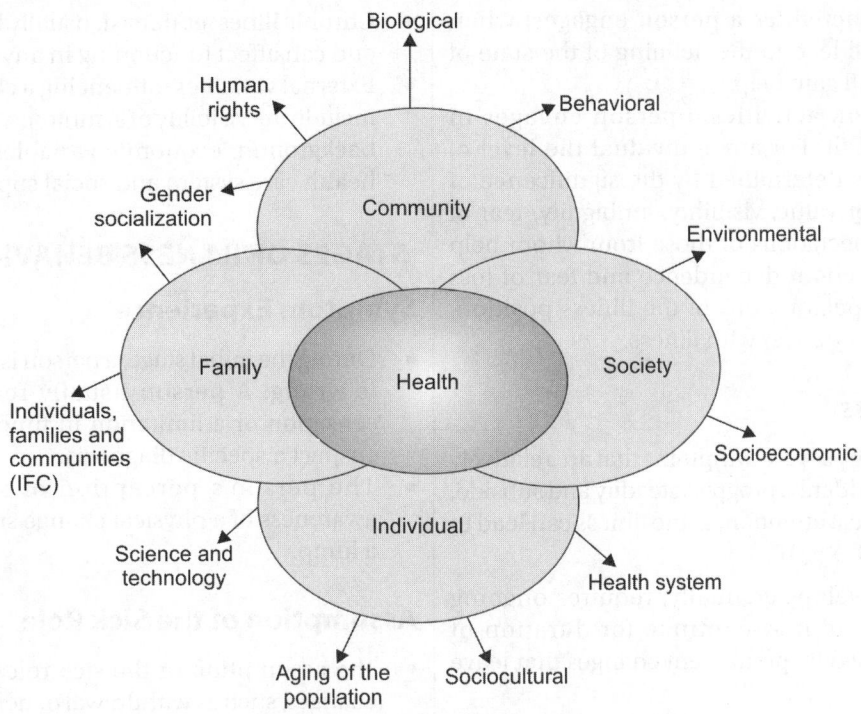

Fig. 1.13: Determinants of health.

past experiences, all influence the health beliefs and practice of patients.
- **Emotional and spiritual factors:** The patient's degree of calm or stress can influence health beliefs and practices. Spiritual beliefs also influence whether and how a patient seeks or avoids healthy behavior.

External Variables

- **Family practices:** The way that patient's families use health care services, their perceptions of the seriousness of diseases and their preventative care behaviors can influence the health beliefs and practice.
- **Socioeconomic factors:** Social relationships, economic level and psychosocial factors influence health beliefs and practice.
- **Cultural background:** It influences beliefs, values and customs. It influences the approach to the health care system, personal health practices and nurse-patient relationship.

Factors affecting a patient's health status:
- Smoking
- Nutrition
- Alcohol use
- Habituating drug use
- Driving
- Exercise
- Sexuality and contraceptive use
- Family relationships
- Risk factor modification
- Coping and adaptation.

CONCEPTS OF HEALTH, ILLNESS AND SICK BEHAVIORS

- It is useful for the nurse to be aware of the behavioral components of health, illness and sick role behavior.
- Every person develops a system of health beliefs and attitudes, and these tend to fall within the framework provided by society or cultural heritage.
- Health behavior activities a person engages in, when feeling well, to take measures to prevent disease and illness or to detect them before symptoms occur.

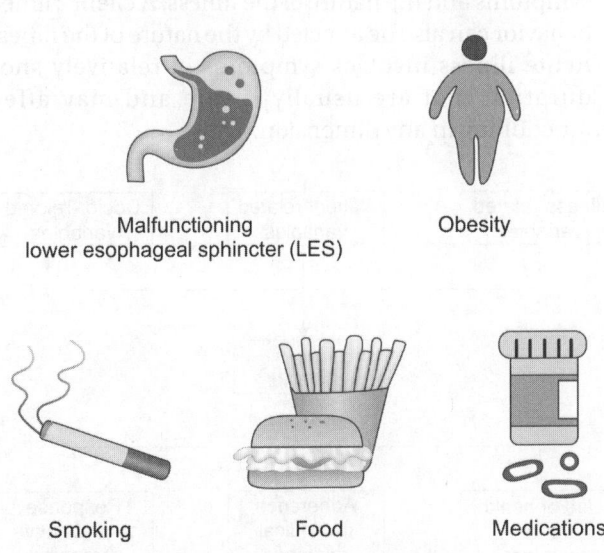

Fig. 1.14: Major causes of illness.

- Illness behavior activities a person engages, when feeling ill, that will lead to the defining of the state of health and that will gain help.
- Sick-role behavior, activities a person engages in believing himself ill. For any individual the level of health behavior is determined by the significance of symptoms- danger value, visibility, ambiguity, fear of unknown, the expectations of those from whom help is sought, feeling about dependence and fear of loss of control, the expectorations of the illness position, including past experiences with illness.

Concepts of Illness

Acute: Characterized by severe symptoms that are relatively short-lived, appear suddenly, progress steadily and subside; may not require medical attention; acute illness can lead to chronic illness, i.e. MI → CHF.

Chronic: Usually develops gradually, requires ongoing medical attention, and may continue for duration of person's life. Are caused by permanent changes that leave residual disability.

Remission: When symptoms subside.

Exacerbation: When symptoms reappear or worsen.

ILLNESS-ILLNESS BEHAVIOR

- Illness is not merely the presence of disease process. Illness is a state in which a person's physical, emotional, intellectual, social, developmental or spiritual functioning is diminished or impaired compared with that person's previous experiences.
- Illness behavior involves the ways persons monitor their bodies, definite and interpret their symptoms, take remedial actions, and use their health care system.
- The important internal values influencing the way clients behave when they are ill are their perceptions of symptoms and the nature of the illness. A client's illness behavior can also be affected by the nature of the illness.
- Acute illness involves symptoms of relatively short duration that are usually severe and may affect functioning in any dimension.
- Chronic illnesses persist, usually longer than 6 months, and can affect functioning in any dimension.
- External variables influencing a client's illness behavior include the visibility of symptoms, social groups, cultural background, economic variables, accessibility of the health care system and social support.

STAGES OF ILLNESS BEHAVIOR

Symptom Experience

- During the initial stage, a person is aware that something is wrong. A person usually recognizes a physical sensation or a limitation in functioning but does not suspect a specific diagnosis.
- The person's perception of symptoms includes awareness of a physical change such as pain, a rash, or a lump.

Assumption of the Sick Role

- The assumption of the sick role results in emotional changes, such as withdrawal or depression, and physical changes.
- Emotional changes may be simple or complex, depending on the severity of the illness, the degree of disability and anticipated length of the illness.

Medical Care Contact

- If symptoms persist despite home remedies, become severe or require emergency care, the person is motivated to seek professional health services.
- In this stage the client seeks expect acknowledgement of the illness, as well as treatment in addition, the client seeks an explanation of the symptoms, the cause of the symptoms, the course of the illness for future health.
- Client's illness can be validated at any point on the health illness continuum. A health professional may

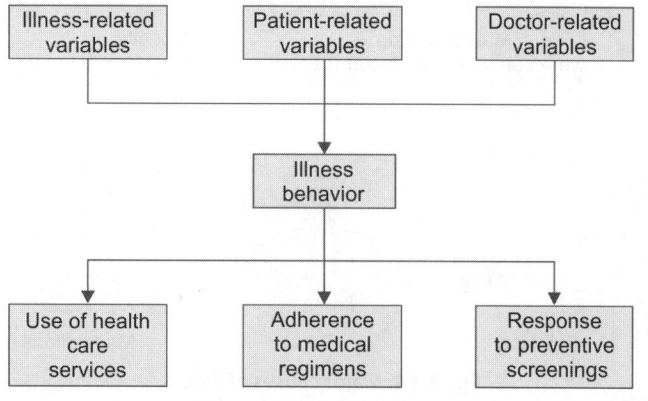

Fig. 1.15: Illness behavior.

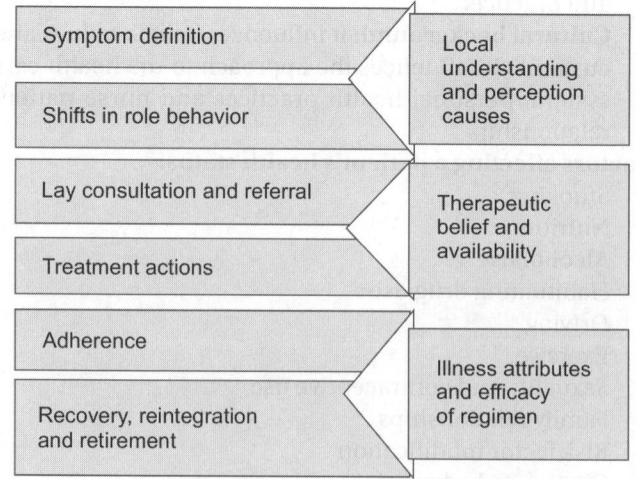

Fig. 1.16: Stages of illness behavior.

determine that they do not have an illness or that illnesses are present and may belief threatening.

Dependent Client Role

- After accepting the illness and seeking treatment, the client enters the fourth stage of illness behavior.
- In this stage, the client depends on health care professionals for relief of symptoms. The client accepts care, sympathy and protection from the demands and stresses of life.
- It is socially permissible for clients in the dependent role to be relieved of normal obligations and tasks.

Recovery Stage

- The final stage of illness behavior-recovery and rehabilitation-can arrive suddenly, such as when a fever subsides.
- The recovery is not prompt, long-term care may be required before the client is able to resume an optimal level of functioning.
- In the case of chronic illness, the final stage may involve an adjustment to a prolonged reduction in health and functioning.

Impact of illness on patient
- Behavioral and emotional changes
- Changes in patient role within family
- Disturbance of family dynamics
- Severe illness may affect physical appearance and functioning
- Emotions of guilt, anger, anxiety

Impact of illness on family
- Acute and chronic illness changes family functioning
- Feelings experienced go up and down
- Sometimes family members withdraw from each other—fear feelings may not be okay
- Family members uncertain how to treat and relate to sick member
- Shift of responsibilities within family

IMPACT OF ILLNESS ON PATIENT

Physical changes from a disease may affect the appearance. These changes can turn a positive self-image into a poor one. Mood disorders such as depression and anxiety are common complaints of people with chronic conditions, but they are extremely treatable.

Chronic illness can also influence the ability to work. Morning stiffness, decreased range of motion, and other physical limitations may force to change the work activities and environment. A decreased ability to work may also lead to financial problems.

Stress can build and can shape the feelings about life. Prolonged stress can lead to frustration, anger, hopelessness, and, at times, depression. The person with the illness is not the only one affected; family members are also influenced by the chronic health problems of a loved one.

IMPACT OF ILLNESS OF FAMILY

Behavioral and Emotional Changes

- People react differently to illness. Individual behavioral and emotional reactions depend on the nature of the illness, the client's attitude toward's it, the reaction of others to it, and the variables of illness behavior.
- Severe illness, particularly one that is life threatening, can lead to more extensive emotional and behavioral change, such as anxiety, shock, dental, anger and withdrawal.

Main categories	Subcategories
Disease onset crisis	Confusion
	Disease related tension
	Distress
Disease burden	Finance problems
	Treatment problems
	Patient's physical and mental state
	Caregiver exhaustion
	Knowledge deficit
	Family issues
	Lack of support
Living in the shadow of death	Disease progress and disabilities
	Fear of patient's death
	Waiting for patient's death

Impact of Family Roles

- When an illness occurs, the roles of client and family may change. Such a change may be subtle and short-term or drastic and long-term.
- An individual and family generally adjust more easily to subtle, short-term changes in most cases they know that the role change is only temporary.
- Long-term changes, however, require an adjustment process similar to the grief process. The client and family often require specific counseling and guidance to assist them in coping with role changes.

Impact on Body Changes

- Some illnesses result in changes in physical appearance, and client's and families react differently to these changes.
- When changes in body image occur, such as results from a leg amputation, the client generally adjusts in the following phases: Shock, withdrawal, acknowledgment, acceptance and rehabilitation.

- Withdrawal is an adaptive coping mechanism that can assist the client in making the adjustments.

Impact of Self-concepts

- Self-concept is individual's mental image of themselves, including how they view their strengths and weaknesses in all aspects of their personalities.
- Self-concepts depend on parts of body image and roles but also include other aspects of the psychological and spiritual self.
- Self-concept changes because of illness may no longer meet the expectations of the family, leading to tension or conflict.

Impact of Family Dynamics

- Family dynamics is the process by which the family functions, makes decisions, give support to individual members, and copes with everyday changes and challenges.
- If a parent in a family becomes ill, family activities and decision making often come to a habit as the other family members wait for the illness to pass, or they delay action because they are reluctant to assume the ill person's roles or responsibilities.

CONCLUSION

Health is a fundamental human right. The World Health Organization defines it as a "state of complete physical, psychological and social well-being and not merely the absence of disease or infirmity". The health of individuals, however, is also linked to the environment in which they live and especially to their ability to adapt and integrate into their life context. The relationship with the environment is extremely important because it is that interaction that outlines the concept of normality compared to pathology. Such normality needs to be contextualized by gender, geographical origin and by the individuals' living conditions: as a matter of fact, what is normal for a young person may differ from what is normal for a senior one. A disease is a physical or mental disturbance involving symptoms, dysfunction or tissue damage, while illness (or sickness) is a more subjective concept related to personal experience of a disease. There are many diseases that can afflict the human body, ranging from common colds to cancers.

■ BIBLIOGRAPHY

1. Craven R, Himle C. Fundamentals of Nursing, 2nd edition. Philadelphia: Lippincott, 1996.
2. Harkness-Hood G, Dincher JR. Total Patient Care: Foundations and Practice of Adult Health Nursing, 8th edition. St. Louis: Mosby-Year Book, Inc, 1992.
3. Lindberg J B, et al. Introduction to Nursing: Concepts, Issues and Opportunities. Philadelphia: JB. Lippincott Co, 1990.
4. Potter PA, Perry AG. Fundamentals of Nursing: Concepts, Process and Practice, 3rd edition. St. Louis: Mosby-Year Book, Inc, 1993.
5. Purtilo R. Health Professional and Patient Interaction, 4th edition. Philadelphia: W.B. Saunders, 1990.
6. Timby BK, Lewis LW. Fundamental Skills and Concepts in Patient Care, 5th edition. Philadelphia: JB Lippincott, Co, 1992.

■ REVIEW QUESTIONS

Long Essays

1. Define health promotion; discuss in detail about the levels of prevention of diseases.
2. Define health; explain the determinants of health.
3. Define illness; describe the factors affecting illness behavior.
4. Define hospital; explain the functions and classifications of hospital.
5. Define immunity; discuss in detail about the types of immunity.
6. What are the stages of impact of illness behavior? Explain in detail.

Short Essays

1. Define health team. Discuss the functions of each member.
2. Define profession and characteristics of nursing profession.
3. Discuss the scope of nursing.
4. Explain the qualities and functions of a nurse.
5. Define ethics; explain the code of ethics in detail.
6. Enumerate the legal responsibilities of the nurse.

Short Answers

1. Describe informed consent.
2. Discuss the ethical responsibilities of a nurse.
3. What is professional etiquette?
4. List out the ethical principles.
5. What are the criteria of profession?
6. Discuss the values of professional nursing.

■ MULTIPLE CHOICE QUESTIONS

1. **The word hospital is derived from:**
    a. Latin word hospice
    b. French word hospital
    c. Both (a) and (b)
    d. None of the above
2. **Inflammatory response, phagocytosis is:**
    a. Second line defense
    b. Fourth line defense
    c. First line defense
    d. Third line defense
3. **Illness is great impact on:**
    a. Behavior and emotions
    b. Self control
    c. Family dynamics
    d. All of the above
4. **Public hospital, voluntary hospital is classified on the basis of:**
    a. Clinical basis
    b. Objective basis
    c. Management basis
    d. Ownership/control basis

5. **National Health Policy developed in the year:**
   a. 1983
   b. 2000
   c. 1986
   d. 1981
6. **PHC and subcenter are responsible for providing which level of health care:**
   a. Tertiary health care
   b. Primary health care
   c. Specialized health care
   d. Critical care
7. **Which is the following is tertiary protection?**
   a. Health promotion
   b. Specific protection
   c. Early diagnosis and treatment
   d. Disability limitation

ANSWERS

1. a   2. a   3. d   4. c   5. a   6. b   7. d

CHAPTER 2

Health Care Delivery System

LEARNING OBJECTIVES

- Levels of illness prevention—primary (health promotion), secondary and tertiary
- Levels of care—primary, secondary and tertiary
- Types of health care agencies/services—hospitals, clinics, hospices, rehabilitation centers, extended care facilities
- Hospital types, organizations and functions
- Health care teams in hospitals—members and their roles

TERMINOLOGY

- **Health services** consist of medical professionals, organizations, and ancillary health care workers who provide medical care to those in need. Health services serve patients, families, communities, and populations. They cover emergency, preventative, rehabilitative, long-term, hospital, diagnostic, primary, palliative, and home care.
- **Hospitals:** Hospitals are the ultimate "catch-all" healthcare facility. Their services can vary greatly depending on their size and location, but a hospital's goal is to save lives. Hospitals typically have a wide range of units that can be loosely broken into intensive care and non-intensive care units.
- **Primary prevention** includes those measures that prevent the onset of illness before the disease process begins. Immunization against infectious disease is a good example.
- **Secondary prevention** includes those measures that lead to early diagnosis and prompt treatment of a disease. Breast self-examination is a good example of secondary prevention.
- **Tertiary prevention** involves the rehabilitation of people who have already been affected by a disease, or activities to prevent an established disease from becoming worse.
- **Hospice care** involves a core team of skilled experts and volunteers who provide medical, psychological, and spiritual care when cure is no longer possible. Hospice care is usually based at home so that families take part in the patient's care**.**
- **Independent providers:** These are nurses, therapists, aides, homemakers, and companions who are privately employed by the people who need their services. The patient or family must recruit, hire, and supervise these providers.
- **Ambulatory surgical centers:** Ambulatory surgical centers, also called outpatient surgical facilities, allow patients to receive certain surgical procedures outside a hospital environment. These environments often offer surgeries at a lower cost than hospitals while also reducing the risk of exposure to infection—since patients are there for surgery, not to recover from sickness and disease.
- **Nursing homes:** Nursing homes offer a living situation for patients whose medical needs aren't severe enough for hospitalization, but are too serious to manage at home. Some nursing homes offer services for heavier medical needs, such as speech and occupational therapy.
- **Tele-health** refers to the use of electronic communication technology to facilitate long-distance health care and health education.

INTRODUCTION

Health Care Delivery System (HCDS) is a societal response to the determinants of health. The concept of health care system includes the involvement of the people, organizations, agencies, and resources that provide services to meet the health needs of the individual, community, and population. The fundamental premise of the HCDS is to value human life, promote, restore, and maintain the health of the population and that is focused and organized around the health needs and expectations of people. The effectiveness of health care system depends upon human, materials, finance, availability and accessibility of resources. The optimal HCDS integrates the different health services encompasses the management and delivery of quality and safe health services. Moreover, in the balanced health care system people receive a continuum of health promotion, disease prevention, diagnosis, treatment, disease management, rehabilitation and palliative care services, through the different levels and sites of care within the health system, and according to their needs throughout the life course.

DEFINITION

Health care delivery system is defined as the aggregate of institutions, organizations and persons who enter, the health care system, who has responsibility that include the promotion of health, prevention of illness, detection and treatment of disease and rehabilitation.

CONCEPT OF HEALTH FOR ALL

- The World Health Assembly in its 30th meeting in 1977 decided the goal of Health for All (HFA) and defined that "Main social targets of Governments and WHO in the coming decades should be the attainment of all citizens of the world by the year 2000 of a level of health that will permit them to lead socially and economically productive life."
- Attainment of a level of health that will enable every individual to lead a socially and economically productive life.

Health for All Goals

- Realization of highest possible of health which includes physical, mental and social well-being.
- Attainment of minimum level of health that would enable to the economically productive and participate actively in social life of community in which they live.
- Removal of obstacles to health such as unemployment, ignorance, poor living conditions, standards and malnutrition, etc.
- Health care services are within the reach of all in the country.

Strategies for Health for All

The Alma Ata declaration called for global strategy to provide guidelines for member countries to refer. In 1981, the WHO after consultations with member countries developed a global strategy for Health for All. The global strategy provides common broad framework which can be modified and adopted by countries according to their needs. The global strategy for HFA is based on the following principles.
- Health is a fundamental human right and a worldwide social goal and an integral part of social and economic development of the communities.
- People have right and the duty of participate individually and collectively in the planning and implementation of their health care.
- The existing gross inequality in the health strategies is of common concern of all countries and must be drastically reduced.
- Government has responsibility for the health of their people.
- Countries and people must become self-reliant in health matters.
- Governments and health professionals have the responsibility of providing health information to people.
- There should be equitable distribution of resources within and among the countries but should be allocated most to those who need most.
- Primary health care would be the key to the success of HPA and it has to be the integral part of the country's health system.
- Development and application of appropriate technology according to health care system of the nation.
- Research in the field of biomedical and health services must be conducted and findings should be applied soon.

The National Health Policy echoes the WHO a call for HFA and the Alma Ata declaration. It had laid down specific goals in respect of various health indicators by different dates such as 1990 and 2000 AD.
- Reduction of infant mortality from the level of 125 (1978) to below 60.
- To raise the expectation of life at birth from the level of 52 years to 64.
- To reduce the crude death rate from the level of 14 per 1000 population to 21.
- To reduce the crude birthrate from the level of 33 per 1000 population to 21.
- To achieve a net reproduction rate of one rural population.

LEVELS OF ILLNESS PREVENTION

The disease process, in many instances, is susceptible to interruption in order to limit its further progress or the speed of its progression. As disease involves interaction of host, agent and environment prevention can be achieved by altering one or more of these three elements so that interaction does not take place or is interrupted in favor of the host.

Effective preventive measure requires that the disease process be interrupted as early in its course as possible. The interaction between the agent and the host can be avoided either by the elimination of the agent in the environment or by converting the human host susceptible or immune to the attack of the agent. Those attempts to bring about changes in the three elements before the disease stimulus is produced are grouped under one type of prevention namely primary prevention. When the disease stimulus has already been practiced and the disease process has crossed over to the period of pathogenesis two types of prevention, namely secondary and tertiary prevention.

1. **Primary prevention**: Primary prevention can be defined as "action taken prior to the onset of disease which removes the possibility that a disease will ever occur". It signifies intervention in the prepathogenesis

The Levels of Prevention

	Primary prevention	Secondary prevention	Tertiary prevention
Definition	An intervention implemented before there is evidence of a disease or injury	An intervention implemented after a disease has begun, but before it is symptomatic	An intervention implemented after a disease or injury is established
Intent	Reduce or eliminate causative risk factors (risk reduction)	Early identification (through screening) and treatment	Prevent sequelae (stop bad things from getting worse)
Example	Encourage exercise and healthy eating to prevent individuals from becoming overweight	Check body mass index (BMI) at every well checkup to identify individuals who are overweight or obese	Help obese individuals lose weight to prevent progression to more severe consequences

phase of a disease or health problem or other departure from health.

Primary prevention is applied at the prepathogenic period; it includes health promotion and specific protection

- **Health promotion:** The first level of prevention is by promoting and maintaining the health of the host by nutrition, health education, good heredity and other health promotion activities.
- **Specific protection:** It may be directed towards the agent like disinfection of contaminated particles, materials, water, food, and other particles on the assumption that the agent has escaped into these vehicles or environment. Specific protection can also be achieved by immunizations to increase the resistance of the host so that the host will be able to withstand the onslaught of the agent. This is done by the active and passive immunizations.

2. **Secondary prevention:** Secondary prevention can be defined as "action" which halts the progress of a disease at its incipient stage and prevents complications. The specific interventions are early diagnosis, e.g. screening tests, case finding programs) and adequate treatment. The secondary prevention done by early diagnosis and treatment. Early diagnosis and prompt treatment comes under secondary prevention. If primary prevention fails or when suitable measures are not available (as in cancer) the disease stimulus is bound to be produced. Early detection of the disease is possible by periodic examinations of population groups who are at special risks like antenatal mothers, growing children, industrial workers, etc.

Monitoring of persons middle age and above is one of the modern methods of early detection of cancer. In many instances, this detection of the diseases condition is possible only after the onset of the signs and symptoms. Early detection of the disease ensures prompt treatment so that the disease will not progress further.

3. **Tertiary prevention:** When the disease process has advance beyond its early stages, it is still possible to accomplish prevention by what might be called "Tertiary prevention". It signifies intervention in the late pathogenesis phase. Tertiary prevention can be defined as "all measures available to reduce or limit impairment and disabilities, minimize suffering caused by existing departures and disabilities, minimize suffering caused by existing departures from good health and to promote the patient's adjustments to irremediable conditions". Tertiary prevention includes disability limitation and rehabilitation.
   - **Disability limitation:** It is necessary that the disability that is caused by limited by active medical or surgical treatment so that there is no further deterioration of the disease process.
   - **Rehabilitation:** Those with permanent disability as in the case of leprosy, tuberculosis, polio, mental retardation, etc. will not be able to lead an independent life unless they are rehabilitated. This level will be needed only when have failed in the application of previous levels of prevention.

LEVELS OF HEALTH CARE (FIG. 2.1)

Primary healthcare: Primary healthcare denotes the first level of contact between individuals and families with the health system. According to Alma Ata Declaration of 1978, Primary Healthcare was to serve the community it served; it included care for mother and child which included family planning, immunization, prevention of locally endemic diseases, treatment of common diseases or injuries, provision of essential facilities, health education, provision of food and nutrition and adequate supply of safe drinking water.

In India, Primary Healthcare is provided through a network of subcenters and Primary Health Centres in rural areas, whereas in urban areas, it is provided through Health posts and Family Welfare Centres. The subcenter consists of one Auxiliary Nurse Midwife and Multipurpose Health Worker and serves a population of 5,000 in plains and 3,000

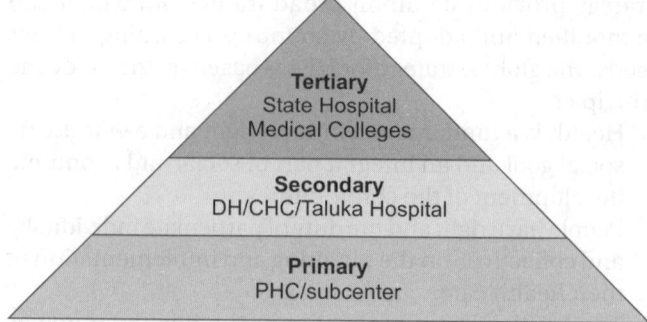

Fig. 2.1: Tier of health care in India. The health care services in India are organized at three levels, each level is supported by the higher level, to which the patient is referred.

persons in hilly and tribal areas. The Primary Health Center (PHC), staffed by Medical Officer and other paramedical staff serves every 30,000 population in the plains and 20,000 persons in hilly, tribal and backward areas. Each PHC is to supervise six subcenters.

Secondary health care: Secondary Healthcare refers to a second tier of health system, in which patients from primary health care are referred to specialists in higher hospitals for treatment. In India, the health centres for secondary health care include District hospitals and Community Health Centre at block level.

Tertiary health care: Tertiary Health care refers to a third level of health system, in which specialized consultative care is provided usually on referral from primary and secondary medical care. Specialized Intensive Care Units, advanced diagnostic support services and specialized medical personnel on the key features of tertiary health care. In India, under public health system, tertiary care service is provided by medical colleges and advanced medical research institutes.

HEALTH CARE DELIVERY SYSTEM IN INDIA

Service delivery systems should also consider the whole spectrum of care from promotion and prevention to diagnostic, rehabilitation and palliative care, as well all levels of care including self-care, home care, community care, primary care, long-term care, hospital care, in order to provide integrated health services throughout the life course. WHO is supporting countries in moving towards universal health coverage through improving the efficiency and effectiveness of their health service delivery systems.

The health care system is intended to deliver the health care services. It constitutes the management sector and involves organizational matters. It operates in the context of the socioeconomic and political framework of the country. The health care delivery system in India has different components to it and **Figure 2.2** below explains the existing pattern.

I. **Health problems**
   - Communicable disease problem.
   - Nutritional problems.
   - Environmental and sanitation problem.
   - Medical care problems.
   - Population problems.

II. **Resources**
   - Health manpower.
   - Money and material.

III. **Health care services**
   - Comprehensive care.
   - Accessible care.
   - Acceptable care.
   - Provide scope for community participation.
   - Available at a cost community and country can afford.

IV. **Health care system**
   - Public sector.
   - Private sector.
   - Indigenous system of medicine.
   - Voluntary health agencies.
   - National health programs.

Public Sector

- Primary Health Center (PHC)
- Hospitals.
  - Community health center
  - Rural hospital
  - Strict hospital
  - Specialist hospital
  - Teaching hospitals.
- Health insurance schemes—ESI (1948), Central government schemes (1954).
- Other agencies—defensive and railways.

Private Sector

- Private hospitals—polyclinics, nursing homes and dispensaries.
- General practitioners and clinics.

Indigenous Systems of Medicine

- Ayurveda and Siddha.
- Unani and Tibbi.
- Homeopathy.
- Unregistered practitioner.

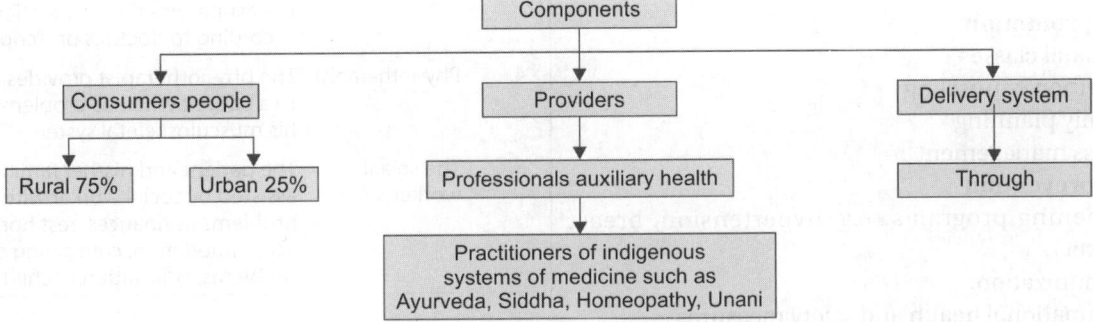

Fig. 2.2: Health care delivery system in India (existing).

Voluntary Health Agencies

- Indian Red Cross Society (1920).
- Hindu Kusht Nivaran Sangh (1950).
- Indian Council for Child Welfare (1952).
- Tuberculosis Association of India (1939).
- Bharat Sevak Samaj (1952).
- Central Social Welfare Board (Aug 1953).
- Kasturba Memorial Fund (1944).
- Family Planning Association of India (1949).
- All India Women Conference (1929).
- All India Blind Relief Society (1946).
- Professional Bodies (CMAI, TNAI).
- International Agencies.

Health Programmes in India

- National Malaria Eradication.
- National Filaria Eradication.
- National Tuberculosis Programme.
- National Leprosy Eradication.
- Genuea Worm Eradication.
- National Blind Control.
- National Diabetes Control.
- National Mental Illness Control.
- Iodine Deficiency Control.
- Diarrheal Disease Control.
- STD Control.
- Minimal Needs Program.
- MCH and Family Planning.
- Universal Immunization.
- Cancer Control Programme.

HEALTH CARE SERVICES

Health service delivery systems that are safe, accessible, high quality, people-centered, and integrated are critical for moving towards universal health coverage. Service delivery systems are responsible for providing health services for patients, persons, families, communities and populations in general, and not only care for patients. While patient-centered care is commonly understood as focusing on the individual seeking care (the patient), people-centred care encompasses these clinical encounters and also includes attention to the health of people in their communities and their crucial role in shaping health policy and health services.

- **Health promotion**
  - Prenatal classes
  - Nutrition counseling
  - Family planning
  - Stress management
- **Illness prevention**
  - Screening programs (e.g. hypertension, breast cancer)
  - Immunization
  - Occupational health and safety measures
  - Mental health counseling
  - AIDS control program.
- **Primary care**
  - School health units
  - Routine physical examination
  - Follow up for chronic illnesses (e.g., diabetes, epilepsy)
- **Diagnosis**
  - Radiological procedure (e.g., CT scans, X-ray studies)
  - Physical examination
  - Laboratory investigations
- **Treatments**
  - Surgical intervention
  - Laser therapies
  - Pharmacological therapy
- **Rehabilitation**
  - Cardiovascular programs
  - Sports medicine
  - Mental illness program.

HEALTH CARE TEAM

Healthcare is a team effort. Each healthcare provider is like a member of the team with a special role. Some team members are doctors or technicians who help diagnose disease. Others are experts who treat disease or care for patients' physical and emotional needs. Health team consists of a group of people who coordinate particular skills in order to assist a patient or his family. The personnel who comprise a particular team will depend upon the needs of the patient. **Figure 2.3** shows health care team members.

Sl. No.	Team	Description
1.	The physician	In hospital setting, the physician is responsible for the medical diagnosis and for determining the therapy required by the person who is ill or injured. A physician is a person who is legally authorizes to practice medicine in particular jurisdiction.
2.	The nurse	A nursing team composed of personnel who provide nursing services to the patient and family. The team leader head nurse is responsible for delegation of duties to members of her team and care given to the patients.
3.	Dietitian	Dietitian designs special duties and they supervise the preparation of meals according to doctor's prescription.
4.	Physiotherapist	The physiotherapist provides assistance to a patient who has problem related to his musculoskeletal system.
5.	The social worker	The patient and his/her family are assisted by social worker with such problems as finances, rest home accommodation, counseling or marital problems, adaptation of children.

Contd...

Contd...

Sl. No.	Team	Description
6.	The occupational therapist	The occupational therapist assists patients with some impairment of function to gain skills as they relate to activities of daily living (ADL) and helping with a skill that is therapeutic.
7.	Paramedical technologist	It includes laboratory technologist and radiologic technologists. **Laboratory technologist** examines and study specimen such as urine, faces, blood and discharges from wound. **Radiologic technologist** assists in wide variety of X-ray procedures, from simple chest radiography to more complex fluoroscopy. Through use of radio active materials, nuclear medicine technologists can provide diagnostic information about functioning of the patients liver, etc.
8.	The pharmacist	The pharmacist prepares and dispenses pharmaceuticals in hospital and community settings. The role of pharmacist in monitoring and evaluating the actions and side effects of medications on patients are becoming increasingly prominent.
9.	Respiratory therapist	Respiratory technologist is skilled in therapeutic measures used in care of patients with respiratory problems. These therapists are knowledgeable about oxygen therapy devices, intermittent positive pressure breathing respirators, artificial mechanical ventilators and accessory devices used for inhalation therapy.

HEALTH CARE AGENCIES

Types of health care agencies: Health care is provided in various settings.

- **Outpatient services:** Patients who don't require hospitalization can receive health care in a clinic. An outpatient setting is designed to be convenient and easily accessible to the patient. Outpatient services are generally directed at primary and secondary health centers.
- **Clinics:** Clinics involve a department in a hospital where patients not requiring hospitalization, receive medical care.
- **Hospitals:** Hospitals have been the major agency of health care system. Hospitals are classified as i. Public, ii. Private, iii. Military

  A Public Hospitals are financed and operated by the government agency at the local, state or national level. Hospitals provide services at free of cost.

  Private Hospitals are owned and operated by churches, corporations, individuals and charitable organizations. Private hospitals are operated on a for-profit-basis.

  Military Hospitals provide medical care for the armed forces and their families.
- **Hospice care:** Care designed to give supportive care to people in the final phase of a terminal illness and focus on comfort and quality of life, rather than cure. The goal is to enable patients to be comfortable and free of pain, so that they live each day as fully as possible. Aggressive methods of pain control may be used. Hospice programs generally are home-based, but they sometimes provide services away from home—in freestanding facilities, in nursing homes, or within hospitals. The philosophy of hospice is to provide support for the patient's emotional, social, and spiritual needs as well as medical symptoms as part of treating the whole person.
- **Rehabilitation care:** Rehabilitation is care that can help to get back, keep, or improve abilities that you need for daily life. These abilities may be physical, mental, and/or cognitive (thinking and learning).
  - Assistive, which are tools, equipment, and products that help people with disabilities move and function.
  - Cognitive rehabilitation therapy to help you relearn or improve skills such as thinking, learning, memory, planning, and decision making.
  - Mental health counseling
  - Music or art therapy to help you express your feelings, improve your thinking, and develop social connections.
  - Nutritional counseling.
  - Occupational therapy to help you with your daily activities.
  - Physical therapy to help your strength, mobility, and fitness.
  - Recreational therapy to improve your emotional well-being through arts and crafts, games, relaxation training, and animal-assisted therapy.
  - Speech-language therapy to help with speaking, understanding, reading, writing and swallowing.
  - Treatment for pain.
  - Vocational rehabilitation to help you build skills for going to school or working at a job.

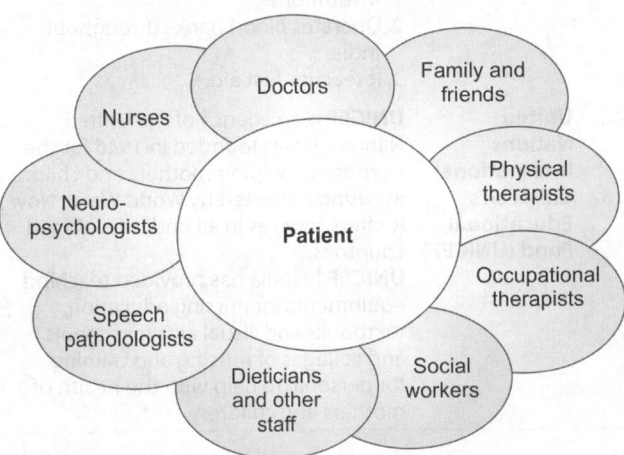

Fig. 2.3: Health care team members.

Health Care Organizations

Sl. No.	Team	Description
1.	World Health Organization (WHO)	The World Health Organization is a specialized agency of the United Nations. It was organized in 1948 to achieve the highest possible level of health for all people. More than 150 countries are members of WHO and help to finance the financial requirement the health care activities around the world. The WHO is also active in nursing education and practice in a number of ways in India: • It has offered guidance in setting up programme of nursing education • It has promoted training for auxiliary nursing personnel. • The WHO promotes public health in many ways around the world.
2.	The International Red Cross Society	The International League of Red Cross was formed in 1919 after World War I. It works closely with national societies during times of national disasters, providing expertise and conducting seminars to help these societies to improve their administrations and services. A super global body made up of the above League and national societies is the **International Conference of Red Cross**'s activities. The body meets once in four years. It supports unity in the work of all of these organizations and promotes governmental support of the Red Cross Activities.
3.	The Indian Red Cross Society	The Indian Red Cross Society was established in 1920, with major aims of helping others from a neutral point. It gives relief to needy and suffering people at times of major disasters and in times of wars. **Aims:** Prevention of disease, promotion of health and care of the sick in any kind of situation. **Functions** 1. Gives financial aid to social welfare institutions. 2. Operates blood banks throughout India. 3. It teaches first aid.
4.	United Nations International Children's Educational Fund (UNICEF)	UNICEF is an agency of the United Nations. It was founded in 1946 for the purpose of helping mothers and children in country affected by World War II. Now it offers services in all underdeveloped countries. UNICEF in India has provided teaching equipments for nursing education, textbooks and visual aids for schools and colleges of nursing and training for personal to help with the health of mothers and children.

Contd...

Sl. No.	Team	Description
5.	USAID (United States Agency for International Development)	**USAID was started in 1961**. It provides grants and loans for a number of projects designed to improve the health of the people. The US government presently extends aid to India through three agencies. **Agencies of United States:** 1. United States agency for International Development (USAID), 2. The public law -food for peace programme, 3. The US export – import Bank. **USAID on Health in India:** 1. Malaria eradication programme, 2. Medical education, 3. Nursing education 4. Health education, 5. Water supply and sanitation, 6. Control of communicable diseases, 7. Nutrition, 8. Family planning.
6.	UNDP (United Nations Development Programme)	The United Nations Development programme was established in 1966 contributes towards increasing the pace of development in the third world countries. It supports all phases of socioeconomic development including agriculture, industry, education, health and social welfare. It is the main source of funds for technical assistance. The basics objective of the UNDP is to help poorer nations develop their human and natural resources more fully.

HOSPITAL: TYPES, ORGANIZATION AND FUNCTIONS

The English word 'Hospital' originates from the Latin word "HOSPILE" and also some viewed that it comes from the French word 'Hospitale' as do the words 'Hostel' and 'Hotel'. The three words hospital, hostel, hotel, all are derived from same source, are used in different sense but basically the meaning of the word will be the same. For example, in hotel, hotel authorities take care of the clients, who wish to stay there and client will receive the hospitality according to their ability. In hostel also, the hostel authorities are expected to treat their clients by providing basic amenities and other facilities as needed by their clients. In the same, hospital authorities also receive their clients as their guests and are expected to show hospitality than those of hotel or hostel. Likewise, all these three institutions are meant treating their clients but style of treatment will be different. Now, the term 'Hospital' means an establishment temporary space occupied by the sick or injured. In other words, the hospital is an institution in which sick or injured persons are treated.

Definition

- **According to WHO,** "The hospital is an integral part of a social and medical organizations, the function of which

is to provide for the population complete health care, both 'curative' and 'preventive' and whose outpatient services reach out to the family and it's environment; the hospital is also a center for the training of health workers and biosocial research".
- **According to Steadman's Medical Dictionary,** "Hospital is an institution for the care, cure and treatment of the sick and wounded, for the study of diseases and for the training of doctors and nurses".
- **According to Blakiston's New Gould Medical Dictionary,** "Hospital is an institution for medical facility primarily intended, appropriately staffed, and equipped to provide diagnostic and therapeutic service in general medicine and surgery or in circumscribed field or fields of restorative medical care, together with bed care, nursing care and dietic service to the patients requiring such care and treatment".

Objectives of the Hospital

As stated in the definition and philosophy of the hospital, its main objective is to:
- Provide optimum health services to all people irrespective of race, color, caste and creed, and regardless of socioeconomical status.
- Provide care, cure, and preventive services to all people irrespective of race, color, caste, creed and economic and social status.
- Protect the human rights of clients while taking care in its jurisdiction in all areas of its services.
- Provide training for professional's, i.e. doctors, nurses, pharmacists, dentists and others technical personnel who are involving in health care services.
- Provide in-service/continuing education in all discipline professional/technical personnel involving health care. For updating their knowledge, skills, etc.
- Participate/conduct research and investigations in basic and applied biomedical, social and technological sciences that will benefit patient care, improve the community health status, the management of hospital services and the education of individual who perform the required service.
- Define its leadership role in the community and possibly the region depending upon its size, type and facilities in relation to regional area planning of hospital.

Scope of Hospital

As stated in the objectives of the hospital, an optimum health care services have the basis of scientific method and should be applied in a personalized manner with full recognition and attention to personal dimensions in client, needs and are carried out within a framework of social responsibility. It should be available and accessible to everyone who needs it through his own community. **The optimum health services consist of following elements.**
- **Team approach:** The care of the needy person will be taken by the team of professional members (Doctors, Nurses, etc.) arid paraprofessionals, technicians under the leadership of medically qualified persons with integration and coordination.
- **Contents of service:** A spectrum of services that includes diagnosis, specific treatment, rehabilitation, education and prevention.
- **Coordination:** Clients' care will cover the coordinated efforts of all agencies which have the required facilities at all levels.

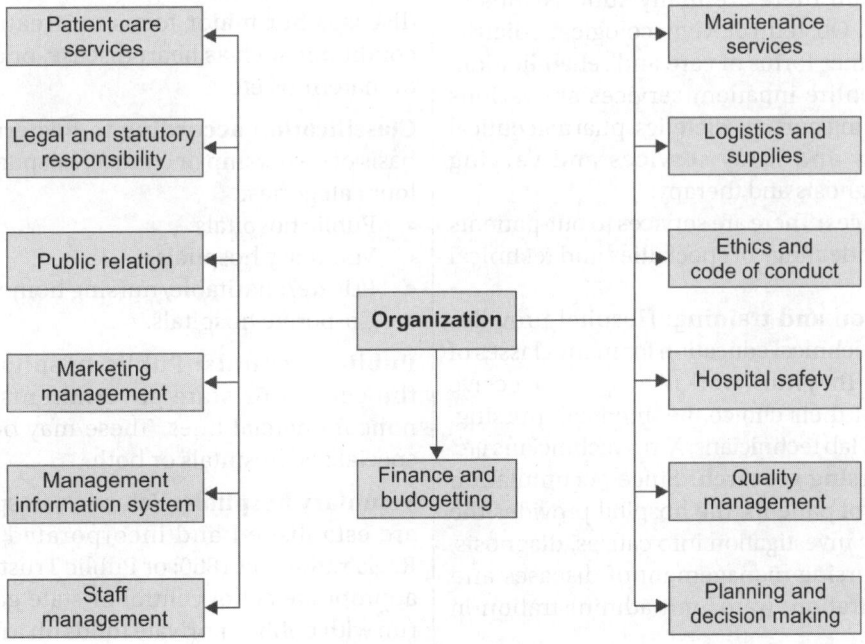

Fig. 2.4: The organization function.

- **Continuity of care:** Continuity of client care will be available and rendered by the particular agency with specific services whenever needed.
- **Integration:** Organization of the hospital care of both ambulatory and non-ambulatory patients into a continuum with common integrated services.
- **Evaluation and research:** Periodic evaluation programs and provision of conducting research included in the optimum health services for adequacy in meeting needs of the patients and the community.

Functions of the Hospital

- **Patient care:** Care of the sick and injured, and restoration of the health of a diseased person without any discrimination.

Functions of Hospitals

1. The main function of a hospital is treatment of patients
2. At the same time, a hospital provides preventive measures for health protection of people, prophylaxis of diseases, prevention of relapses and complication of diseases
3. It carries out large work on medical and social rehabilitation of patients
4. Large work is done by a hospital on examination of capacity for work
5. Training of medium-level medical personnel and students
6. Improvement of qualification of medical workers and research work is conducted in hospital

- **Diagnosis and treatment of disease:** There are diagnosis and treatment services to in-patients. Within this broad function there are many subdivisions of Medical, Surgical, Obstetrical, Gynecologic, Pediatric, Psychiatric and other forms of care and rehabilitation. Involved in the entire inpatient services are various modalities, including nursing, dietetics, pharmaceutical skills, laboratory and X-ray services and varying refinement of diagnosis and therapy.
- **Out-patient services:** There are services to out-patients with an equally wide range of specialties and technical modalities.
- **Medical education and training:** Hospital provides professional and technical education for many classes of health personnel. They must work in hospital to receive proper training of their choice, i.e. medical, nursing, pharmacy, dental, lab technicians, X-ray technicians etc.
- **Medical and nursing research:** Since accumulation of different types of patients, the hospital provides the basis for scientific investigation into causes, diagnosis, treatment and nursing management of diseases and hospital administration, ward/unit administration in hospitals.
- **Prevention of disease and promotion of health:** Hospital provides services to surrounding populations that may be preventive care and promoting their health. There are many ways that hospitals as centers for technical skills can offer services to people before they are sick or can protect patients from the hazards of disease beyond that for which they have come to the hospital.

CLASSIFICATION OF HOSPITALS

Hospitals have been classified in many ways. Each hospital is distinct in its characteristic as it differs in structure, functions, performance and the community it serves. However, we can classify the hospitals into different types, depending upon different criteria **(Fig. 2.5)**. The most commonly accepted criteria for classification of the modern hospital are according to:

- Length of stay of patient (long-term and short-term)
- Clinical basis
- Ownership/control basis
- Objectives
- Size
- Management
- System of medicine.

Classification according to length of stay of patient: A patient stays for a short-term in a hospital for treatment of disease that is acute in nature, such as pneumonia, peptic ulcer, gastroenteritis, etc. A patient may stay for a long-term in a hospital for treatment of diseases that are chronic in nature, such as tuberculosis, leprosy, cancer, psychosis. The hospital according to long-term and short-term also known as chronic-care hospital and acute care hospitals respectively.

Classification according to clinical bases: These are hospitals licensed as general hospital; treat all kinds of diseases but major focus on treating speed disease or conditions such as heart disease, or cancer, or ophthalmic or maternity, etc.

Classification according to ownership control: On the basis of ownership or control, hospitals can be divided into four categories:
- Public hospitals.
- Voluntary hospitals.
- Private/charitable/nursing homes.
- Corporate hospitals.

Public hospitals: Public hospitals are those run by the central or state governments or local bodies on noncommercial lines. These may be general hospital or specialized hospitals or both.

Voluntary hospitals: Voluntary hospitals are those which are established and incorporated under the Societies Registration Act 1860; or Public Trust Act 1882 or any other appropriate act of central or state governments. They are run with public or private funds on a noncommercial basis.

Private nursing hospitals/Nursing homes: Private nursing hospitals/nursing homes are generally owned by

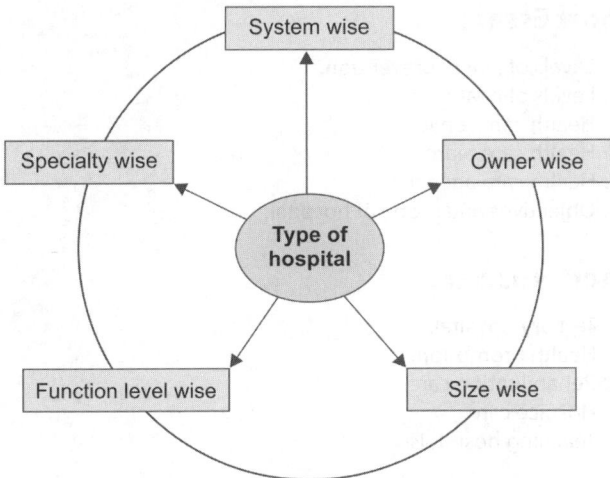

Fig. 2.5: Classification of hospital.

an individual doctor or a group of doctors. They run the hospital or nursing home on a commercial basis. They accept patient suffering from infirmity, advanced age, illness, injury, chronic, disability, etc. But do not admit patient suffering from communicable disease, alcoholism, drug addiction or mental illness. Usually they prefer patient from wealthy families.

Corporate hospitals: Corporate hospitals are hospitals which are public limited companies formed under the companies act. They are normally run on commercial lines. They can be either general or specialized or both (e.g. Hinduja Hospital, Mallya Hospital, Apollo Group of Hospitals).

Classification According to the Objectives: According to the objectives, hospitals can be classified into three categories:
1. Teaching-cum-research hospitals.
2. General hospitals.
3. Specialized hospitals.

Teaching-cum-Research Hospital

Teaching cum research hospital is a hospital to which a college is attached for medical Nursing/dental/pharmacy education. The main objective of these hospitals is teaching based on research and the provision of health care is secondary, e.g. AIIMS, New Delhi, PGMERI, Chandigarh, JIPMER, Pondicherry, KR Hospital, Mysore, Victoria hospital, Bangalore belong to this type.

General Hospitals

General hospitals are those which provide treatment for common diseases and conditions. All establishments permanently staffed by at least two or more doctors which can offer inpatient accommodation and provide active medical and nursing care for more than one category of medical discipline such as general medicine, general surgery, obstetrics and gynecology, pediatrics etc. The main objective of these hospitals is to provide medical care to the people. While teaching and research is secondary and incidental, e.g. all district and taluks or PHC or rural hospitals belong to this type.

Specialized Hospitals

Specialized hospitals are hospitals providing medical and nursing care primarily for only one discipline or a specific disease or condition of one system. In other words, these hospitals concentrate on a particular aspect or organ of the body and provide medical and nursing care in that field, e.g. tuberculosis, ENT, ophthalmology, leprosy, orthopedics, pediatrics, cardiology, mental health psychiatric, oncology, STDs, maternal, etc. The specialized department, administration attached to a general hospital will not be considered as specialized hospital.

Isolation Hospitals: Isolation hospital is a hospital in which the persons are suffering from infections/communicable diseases requiring isolation of the patients, e.g. Epidemic Diseases Hospital, Bengaluru.

Classification According to Size: On the basis of health committee report, it is recommended that the following pattern of development of hospitals to be adopted according to size, i.e. bed strength.
- Teaching hospital 500 (bed to be increased according to the number of students).
- District hospital 200 (may be raised up to 300 beds depending upon population).
- Taluks hospital 50 (may be raised depending upon population to be served).
- Primary health centers 6 (may be increased up to 10 depending upon needs).

Classification According to Management

- Union government/government of India: All hospitals administered by the government of India, e.g. hospital run by the railways, military/defense, or public sector undertakings of the central Government.
- State governments: All hospitals administered by the state/union territory. Government authorities and public sector undertaking operated by the state/union territories including the police, prison, irrigation department and etc.
- Local bodies: All hospitals administered by local bodies, i.e. municipal corporation, municipality, zila parishad, panchayat, e.g. corporation maternity homes.
- Autonomous bodies: All hospitals established under special act of parliament or state legislation and founded by the central/state government/union territory, e.g. AIIMS, New Delhi, PGI, Chandigarh, NIMHANS, Bengaluru.
- Private: All private hospitals owned by an individual or by a private organization, e.g. MAHE, Manipal, Manipal Hospital, Bengaluru, Hinduja hospital, Mumbai.

- **Voluntary agencies:** All hospitals operated by a voluntary body/a trust/charitable society registered or recognized by the appropriate authority under central/state government laws. This includes hospitals run by missionary bodies and cooperatives.

Classification According to System: According to the system of medicine, we can classify the hospital as follows:
- Allopathic hospitals.
- Ayurvedic hospitals.
- Homeopathic hospitals.
- Unani hospitals.
- Hospitals of other systems of medicine.

CONCLUSION

Health of an individual or group affects its work output and efficiency, good health is not only essential for a normal life and activities, but it is the basic factor for a happy life. Nurses care for individuals who are healthy and ill, of all ages and cultural backgrounds, and who have physical, emotional, psychological, intellectual, social and spiritual needs. The profession combines physical science, social science, nursing theory, and technology in caring for those individuals. Health promotion concerns are those activities directed towards maintaining or enhancing the health and well-being of individuals and their families. The student learns the role of patient advocate as he/ she provides information needed to make health care decisions and then supports the patient in that decision. The student learns and teaches health practices that promote and enhance optimum functional levels of wellness. Such practices include, but are not limited to, nutrition, diet, exercise, drug therapy and complementary therapies.

BIBLIOGRAPHY

1. Craven R, Himle C. Fundamentals of Nursing, 2nd edition. Philadelphia: Lippincott; 1996.
2. Harkness -Hood G, Dincher JR. Total patient care: Foundations and Practice of Adult Health Nursing, 8th edition. St. Louis: Mosby-Year Book, Inc, 1992.
3. Lindberg J B, et al. Introduction to nursing concepts, issues and opportunities, Philadelphia: JB Lippincott Co, 1990.
4. Potter PA, Perry AG. Fundamentals of Nursing Concepts, Process and Practice, 3rd edition. St. Louis: Mosby- Year Book, Inc, 1993.
5. Purtilo R. Health Professional and Patient Interaction, 4th edition. Philadelphia: W.B. Saunders; 1990.
6. Timby BK, Lewis LW. Fundamental Skills and Concepts in Patient Care, 5th edition. Philadelphia: JB Lippincott, Co, 1992.

REVIEW QUESTIONS

Long Essays

1. Define health care delivery system, discuss in detail about health care delivery system in India.
2. Define hospital; explain the types and functions of hospital.

Short Essays

1. Levels of illness prevention.
2. Levels of health care.
3. Health care services.
4. Health care team.
5. Health care agencies.
6. Objectives and scope of hospital.

Short Answers

1. Tertiary hospital.
2. Health promotion.
3. Rehabilitation care.
4. Hospice care.
5. Teaching hospitals.

MULTIPLE CHOICE QUESTIONS

1. **The concept of health care system includes the involvement of:**
   a. People
   b. Organizations and agencies
   c. Resources that provide services
   d. All of the above

2. **The World Health Assembly in its 30th meeting held in the year ———— decided the goal of Health for All (HFA).**
   a. 1976
   b. 1977
   c. 1978
   d. 1979

3. **Health promotion is a first level of prevention is by promoting and maintaining the health of the host by:**
   a. Nutrition
   b. Health education
   c. Good heredity and other health promotion activities
   d. All of the above

4. **Service delivery systems should also consider the whole spectrum of care from promotion and prevention to:**
   a. Diagnostic
   b. Rehabilitation
   c. Palliative care
   d. All of the above

5. **Hospice care is designed to give supportive care to people in the final phase of:**
   a. Terminal illness
   b. Acute illness
   c. Chronic illness
   d. Systemic illness

6. **Classification hospital according to the system of medicine, we can classify the hospital as follows:**
   a. Allopathic hospitals
   b. Ayurvedic hospitals
   c. Homeopathic hospitals and unani hospitals
   d. All of the above

7. **Classification of hospitals according to the objectives is the following, except:**
   a. Teaching-cum-research hospitals
   b. General hospitals
   c. Private hospitals
   d. Specialized hospitals

ANSWERS

| 1. d | 2. b | 3. d | 4. d | 5. a | 6. d | 7. c |

CHAPTER 3
History of Nursing and Nursing as a Profession

LEARNING OBJECTIVES
- History of nursing, history of nursing in India
- Contributions of Florence Nightingale
- Nursing: Definition—Nurse, nursing, concepts, philosophy, objectives, characteristics, nature and scope of nursing/nursing practice, functions of nurse, qualities of a nurse, categories of nursing personnel
- Nursing as a profession: Definition and characteristics/criteria of profession
- Values: Introduction—Meaning and importance
- Code of ethics and professional conduct for nurses

TERMINOLOGY
- **Nursing:** Nursing is an art, science and profession by which we render, serve to human being to help him to regain or to keep a normal state of body and mind and when it cannot accomplish this, it help him for the relief from physical pain, mental anxiety or spiritual discomfort.
- **Profession:** A profession is an occupation with moral principles that are devoted to the human and social welfare. The service is based on specialized knowledge and skill developed in a scientific and learned manner.
- **Professional conduct:** A professional conduct is behaving with a real sense of dignity and respect for the service given for the patient.
- **Beneficence:** The state or act of intentionally doing or producing good. The principle of beneficence involves duties to prevent harm, remove harm, and promote the good of another person. The obligation of health care professionals to seek the well-being or benefit of other patients. Duties of beneficence concern the welfare of others.
- **Competent:** A legal concept that describes people who are able to make decisions for themselves. Minors are presumed to be incompetent, except under certain specified conditions. The corollary medical-ethical term is decisional capacity.
- **Confidentiality:** The professional-client promise not to reveal information without consent.
- **Durable power of attorney for health care:** An advance directive that goes into effect in the event that a patient who has completed such a document loses decisional capacity. Allows an individual to name a person(s) who is empowered to make health care decisions when the individual becomes incapacitated.
- **Emancipated minor:** A teenaged minor, who is legally, independent of parental control and who can thus give informed consent to medical treatments.
- **Ethics committees:** An interdisciplinary group that deals with conflicts of values in patient care in acute and long-term settings. Such committees discuss policy issues (e.g., regarding withholding and withdrawing of life-sustaining treatments) respect for patient dignity.
- **Expanded role:** Expanded role of nursing means enlargement of nurse with the bonders of nurse.
- **Empathy:** Intellectual and emotional awareness and understanding of another person thoughts, behaviors and feelings
- **Nurse anesthetics:** A nurse who completed the course of study in an anesthesia school and carries out pre-operative status of clients.
- **Nurse practitioner:** Is a nurse who has completed either as certificate program or a master's degree in a specialty and is also certified by the appropriate specialty organization. She is skilled at making nursing assessments, performing PE, counseling, teaching and treating minor and self-limiting illness.
- **Sympathy is** balancing someone's feeling especially in his sorrow or trouble
- **Informed consent:** The legal and ethical requirement that no significant medical procedure can be performed until the competent patient has been informed of the nature of the procedure, risks and alternatives, as well as the prognosis if the procedure is not done. The patient must freely and voluntarily agree to have the procedure done.
- **Nonmaleficence:** The state of not doing harm or evil; see also beneficence.

- **Privileged communication:** Information communicated to an attorney, physician, spouse, or counselor that may not be revealed, even in court, without the consent of the person who made the statement.
- **Proxy consent:** Voluntary informed consent given on behalf of another who is for some reason incapable of giving it for himself or herself.
- **Abortion:** Expulsion or removal of a usually nonviable fetus. (a fetus that cannot live outside the uterus at that time).
- **Active euthanasia:** The ending of another person's life by an aggressive method to end suffering.
- **Assault:** A deliberate act wherein one person threatens to harm another without consent and the victim feels the attacker has the ability to carry out the threat.

INTRODUCTION

Nursing has been called the oldest of the arts and the youngest of the profession. The word nurse evolved from the Latin word nutritious, which means nourishing. The roots of medicine and nursing are intertwining and found in mythology, ancient eastern and western cultures and religion. Nursing, besides being a honorable profession, is one of the oldest arts and an essential modern occupation. Nursing is one of the greatest of humanitarian services and all people whether ill or well, rich or poor, literate or illiterate, young or old, at work or at play, in or out of hospital, are in some way or other, directly or indirectly closely associated with it. Nursing has its own body of knowledge scientifically based and humanitarianism that promises expanded benefits to people and society. It assists the individual or family to achieve their potential for self-direction for health.

HISTORY OF NURSING

The word "nurse" originally came from the Latin word "nutrire", meaning to suckle, referring to a wet-nurse; only in the late 16th century did it attain its modern meaning of a person who cares for the infirm. From the earliest times most cultures produced a stream of nurses dedicated to service on religious principles. Both Christendom and the Muslim World generated a stream of dedicated nurses from their earliest days. In Europe before the foundation of modern nursing, Catholic nuns and the military often provided nursing-like services. It took until the 19th century for nursing to become a secular profession.

Nursing has been called the oldest of the arts and the youngest of the profession. The word nurse evolved from the Latin word nutritious, which means nourishing. The roots of medicine and nursing are intertwining and found in mythology, ancient eastern and western cultures and religion. Nursing is defined by various authors at various times. Hansderson says "nursing is primarily assisting the individuals (sick or well) in the performances of those activities, contributing or its recovery (or to a peaceful death) that he would perform unaided, if he had the necessary strength, will or knowledge. The unique contribution of nursing is to help the individual to be independent or such assistance as soon as possible.

Nursing, besides being a honorable profession, is one of the oldest arts and an essential modern occupation. Nursing is one of the greatest of humanitarian services and all people whether ill or well, rich or poor, literate or illiterate, young or old, at work or at play, in or out of hospital, are in some way or other, directly or indirectly closely associated with it. Nursing has its own body of knowledge scientifically based and humanitarianism that promises expanded benefits to people and society. It assists the individual or family to achieve their potential for self-direction for health.

HISTORY OF NURSING IN INDIA

Nursing in India is the practice of providing care for patients, families, and communities in that nation to improve health and quality of life. History indicates that the principles and practices of nursing in India are ancient. Prior to the 20th century, Indian nurses were usually young men, with women acting as midwives for assisting with child birth. The acceptance of nursing as a profession in India is improved a lot with good quality of education and clinical exposure to students.

1905: Association of Nursing Superintendents was constituted/formed.

1908: Trained Nurses Association of India was established/formed.

1909: Bombay Presidency Nursing Association was formed. Missionary Nurses North India Board set up under Medical Missionary Association of India.

1911: The South Indian Board was established INAI affiliated to International Council of Nurses.

1912: The First Nurses Registration Act was enacted in Madras Presidency.

1930: The Christian Nurses Auxiliary formed by the missionary nurses.

1934: The Bengal Nurses Act was enacted for the nurses, midwives and H.V. of undivided Bengal.

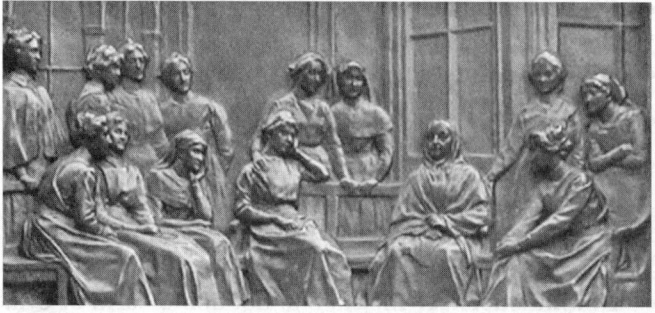

Fig. 3.1: Florence Nightingale's organized teaching of nursing.

1936: The Mid India Board of Education affiliated to Christian Nurses league, Christian Nurses Auxiliary Association was affiliated to TNAI.

1941: Standardized pay scales and terms of services were established in Madras. State nursing superintendent, appointed at state level (Madras).

1942: The Auxiliary Nursing Service (ANS) was established. One nursing superintendent was appointed as nursing advisor at DGHS, Government of India, to organize nursing services.

1943: Establishment of School of Nursing Administration for Military Nursing Services Health Survey and Development Committees (Bhore) constituted by Government of India. Study groups worked on proposal for university education in nursing in India. CMC Vellore and Madras General Hospital started courses to train nursing tutors. Commissioned rank was given to the Indian Military Nursing sisters.

1946: Bhore Committee submitted report, recommendations made on improvement of various aspects of nursing profession: Nursing education, working conditions, nursing services in hospital and community and deputing nurses for higher education to abroad, etc. Establishment of the College of Nursing at Delhi (now Rajkumari Amrit Kaur College of Nursing) under the Union Ministry of Health to start university nursing education programme for the first time in India leading to Bachelor's degree in nursing, i.e. BSc (Hons.) Nursing.

1947: Indian Nursing Council Act was passed (31.12.1947) on the basis of recommendations of Bhore Committee. Degree programme for nursing started in Vellore.

1948: The first meeting of Indian Nursing Council (INC) was held.

1950: The INC took decision to establish ANM programme to meet the requirement of workers in nursing.

1951: Establishment of urban field teaching center was started at College of Nursing, Delhi in collaboration with existing MCH centers of Municipal Corporation, Delhi for teaching of urban community health nursing.

1952: Establishment of residential field teaching center for teaching community health nursing in the rural area under College of Nursing, Delhi in collaboration with primary health center, Najafgarh.

1953: Ms Edith Buchanan, vice principal, College of Nursing (RAK), Delhi was sent to Columbia University to earn her Doctorate in Education (D. Ed.) through WHO fellowship.

1954: Government of India constituted committee to review conditions of services, emoluments, etc., of nursing profession (Shetty committee). Shetty Committee Report was published, recommended nursing staff norms of hospital community and other improvements in nursing.

1955: Establishment of child guidance clinic at College of Nursing (RAKCON) for providing services and strengthening community health nursing and pediatric nursing. Ms Margaretta Craig, principal, College of Nursing, Delhi attended ICN meeting in France, to present a paper on the need for nursing research in India.

1959: Dr Edith M. Buchanan, succeeded in establishing the long cherished "Master of Nursing" degree programme at (RAK) College of Nursing, New Delhi under University of Delhi (October 1959). Healthy Survey and Planning Committee (Dr LN Mudaliar) was constituted by Government of India to review the progress made in health since, Bhore committee recommendation.

1961: Mudaliar Committee report published made some recommendations to improve nursing profession.

1963: A WHO assisted technical project was undertaken at the INC to Revise the GNM course. Dr Buchanan, succeeded in sending Mrs Sulochana Krishnan, one of the first graduates of this newly established, M.N. degree programme, to earn the D. Ed. degree from Columbia University.

1964: Dr. Marie Furguson, a public health nurse came to the College of Nursing, Delhi was able to create greater appreciation and understanding of the need and value of research in planning nursing administration and education with senior leaders of the country conducted "Activity studies to define the nursing and non-nursing functions of nursing personnel."

1965: A WHO publication on 'Guide for School of Nursing' in India was published.

1966: TNAI established research section under the Chairmanship of Ms Margarata Craig. TNAI conducted 'Time study' with the co-operation of Ms Anna Gupta, principal, RAKCON, under the supervision of Dr Sulochana Krishnan.

1969-71: INAI and VHAI, CHAP conducted study on survey on the socioeconomic status of nurses in India.

1973: Kartar Singh Committee report on multipurpose workers and Health and family planning department published and recommended ANM and LHVs were redesignated and health workers (F) and health assistant (F) to cover the required population at rural area for providing proper health services.

1975: Shrivastav Committee report on 3 tier-plan of health care delivery system to rural area was recommended.

1976: Dr Marie Farell and Dr Aparna Bhaduri of Rajkumari Amrit Kaur College of Nursing, New Delhi, conducted seminars on nursing research for educationists at Delhi, Mussoorie (Uttarakhand) and Yarcaid to strength the nursing research in India.

1978: Government Nurses Association of Karnataka established.

1981: Dr Farrel and Dr Bhaduri's book 'Health Research'-A Community based Approach' published by World Health Organization.

1986: The Nursing Research Society of India (NRSI) was established to promote research within and around nursing environment. Dr (Mrs) Inderjit Walia was founder president. Mrs Uma Hunda was its secretary. M Phil in nursing programme started at RAKCON, under Delhi University.

1987: Reports of the expert committee on health and manpower planning, production and management (Bajaj Committee) published. This committee also dealt with nursing service conditions norms and nurse's emoluments, etc.

1988: RAKCON, New Delhi was designated as World Health Collaboration Center for nursing Developments reports of the high power committee on nursing and nursing profession published. Dr Ruth Hurner book "Nursing Education in India" published on the basis of survey.

1991: Author registered PhD in nursing at Bangalore University.

1992: PhD in nursing programme started at RAKCON, under Delhi University. Mrs Asha Sharma got registered for the Doctoral course.

HISTORY OF FLORENCE NIGHTINGALE

- Florence Nightingale was born May 12, 1820 in Florence, Italy. She was an English social reformer and statistician and is credited with being the founder of modern nursing.
- She was born into a rich upper-class family and was known to have a very serious demeanor but was very charming to those who met her.
  Nightingale's most famous contribution occurred during the Crimean War. On October 21 of 1854, Nightingale and a staff she trained, were sent to care for wounded soldiers at the Ottoman Empire.

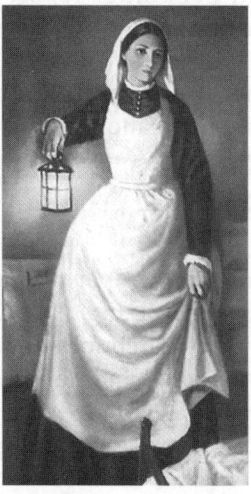

Fig. 3.2: Florence Nightingale.

- During her first winter serving as a nurse the death toll for soldiers was at an all time high. After the arrival of Nightingale and her staff of 34 volunteer nurses, there was a significant decline in the death rate of soldiers.
- Nightingale believed that the majority of deaths came from poor nutrition, lack of supplies, stale air, and overworked soldiers. When she returned home she collected data and evidence which she then presented before the Royal Commission in hopes to resolve these issues.
- Her experience while serving as a nurse during the war later influenced her career, as she became a strong advocate for sanitary living conditions for soldiers.
- Nightingale gained the nickname "The Lady with the Lamp" from her hard work and dedication. The times wrote, "She is a "ministering angel" without any exaggeration in these hospitals, and as her slender form glides quietly along each corridor, every poor fellow's face softens with gratitude at the sight of her.
- When all the medical officers have retired for the night and silence and darkness have settled down upon those miles of prostrate sick, she may be observed alone, with a little lamp in her hand, making her solitary rounds.
- In 1857, the Nightingale fund was established to train nurses as a form of recognition for Nightingale's work during the war.
- Nightingale used the £45,000 from the fund to open Nightingale Training School at St Thomas Hospital.
- The school is now known as Florence Nightingale school of nursing and midwifery Nightingale died on August 13, 1910 at the age of 90.

THE NIGHTINGALE'S PLEDGE

- I solemnly pledge myself before God and in the presence of this assembly, to conscientiously practice my profession.
- I will respect all life, dignity, rights of man in the practice of my calling.
- I will zealously seek, to nurse those who need care irrespective of nationality, race, creed, color, age, sex, politics or social status.
- I will collaborate and coordinate with health team, and devote myself to the welfare of my patients, my family and my country.
- I will endeavor to fulfill my rights and privileges as a good citizen, and take my share of responsibility to promote health, to prevent illness, to restore health, and to alleviate suffering.
- I will constantly endeavor to increase my knowledge and skills in nursing, and to use them wisely.
- I will be active in assisting others, in safeguarding and promoting the health, and happiness of mankind.

CONTRIBUTIONS OF FLORENCE NIGHTINGALE

Miss Florence Nightingale knows of her devotion to the services to the poor and the sick and is also aware of what she did for humanity and to raise the status of nursing profession. Florence Nightingale was born in a wealthy English family, on 12th May 1820. As she grew off, she became interested in people and in politics. She had great desire to become a nurse though her parents were not keen on her becoming one.

- She was dissatisfied with the dealt routine lifestyle of the upper class women of their days. She had an active mind and an interest in her surroundings beyond household and socials events.
- She had received a classical education equal to that of men of her day. This education provided her with an understanding of the circumstances of the world in which she lived.
- She became aware of the inadequate care being provided in hospitals, when she accompanied her mother on visits to the ill. What Nightingale saw in the hospitals intrigued her and made her want to become more involved.

In 1846, in spite of the concerns of parents and friends Nightingale became to visit and care for the sick in her community. In addition, she visited hospitals in England and throughout Europe. Out of her experiences she recognized that nurses required knowledge, training and discipline, if they were to be effective. Nightingale learned about the school at Kaisersworth and in 1850, she was admitted to the training program. The three years of training she received were rigorous but helped her clarify what was lacking in the current training of English nurses. After her training, in 1853 she was appointed as Superintendent of the Institution for the Care of the Sick Gentlewomen in London.

She had an opportunity to give her best service to the wounded soldiers in the Crimean War in 1854. Florence Nightingale and her nurses attended thousands of wounded and dying soldiers. Every night Florence Nightingale walked about with a lamp in her hand to help the suffering soldiers. At this time she helped them to write letters to their families and last messages for those who were dying. She was rightly known as "The Lady with the Lamp". Nightingale and a small band of untrained nurses went to the British hospitals at Scutari in Turkey. She found the patients were laid on the floor in bloody uniforms. Equipments and facilities were not present adequately. With great compassion, she set about the task of organizing and cleaning the hospital and provided care to the wounded soldiers.

Through her efforts and the help of others, Nightingale introduced numerous improvements in the military hospital. Her efforts were largely responsible for traumatic reductions (42% to 2%) in the wartime death rate of British Soldiers.

She also founded the first training school for nurses (St. Thomas Hospital, London, 1860). Throughout the publication of countless articles and papers, she shared her ideas about nursing and nursing education. Miss Nightingale was the first to mention **Holism** (treating the whole patient) in nursing and the first who stated that a unique body of knowledge is required to practice professional nursing.

After the war, she worked to bring about better health conditions in the British army. Nightingale almost single-handedly tried to change health care in England. Nightingale was the founder of modern nursing education. She established the Army Medical School at the Fort Pitt. Despite her ill health she worked for the development of nursing services without taking sufficient rest.

Florence founded a training school for nurses in 1860 at St. Thomas Hospital London. The funds, which were raised by the British people for her service in the Crimean War, were used for this training school. She was very much interested in improving the conditions of the army in India also. She planned a complete public health program, which was practiced in all hospitals and in the fields of nursing. She died peacefully in her sleep at the age of 90 (13th May 1910). In recognition of her meritorious help to mankind she was offered the Order of Merit in 1907. She was the first lady recipient for such an honor.

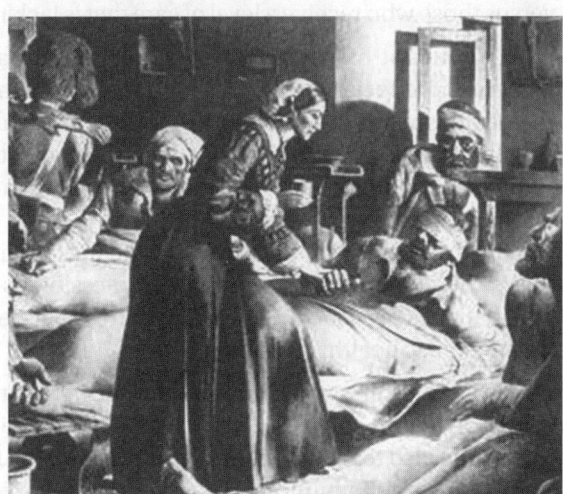

Fig. 3.3: Direct patient care by Florence Nightingale during Crimean War.

DEFINITIONS OF NURSING

- **International Council of Nursing (ICN) 1973:** Nursing is to assist the individual (sick or well) in the performance of those activities contributing to health, its recovery (or to a peaceful death) that he would perform unaided, if he had the necessary strength, will or the if he had the necessary strength, will or the knowledge and to do this in such a way as to help him gain independence as rapidly as possible.
- **Florence Nightingale:** Nursing defined as the act of utilizing the environment of the patient to assist him in his recovery.

- **Canadian Nurses Association-1987:** Nursing practice as a dynamic, caring and helping relationship in which the nurse assists the client to achieve and obtain optimal health.
- **American Nurses Association:** Nursing practice as direct goal oriented and adaptable to service the needs of the individual, the family and community during health and illness.

OBJECTIVES, CONCEPTS AND PHILOSOPHY OF NURSING

Objectives of Nursing

- To prepare nurses who will give expert bedside nursing care in the hospital and community.
- To provide integration of health and social aspect of theory and practice in generalized public health nursing.
- To provide an adequate, sound scientific foundation to understand the functioning of body and mind in health and disease.
- To prepare nurses who will be able to work cooperatively with team members.
- To provide opportunities through curricular and extracurricular activities for full development of personality of each individual student.
- To ensure opportunities for initiative and resourcefulness and sense of responsibility for oneself.

Concept of Nursing

- **The art of nursing:** Professional nursing practice is grounded in the art of nursing, described as taking a holistic, client-centered focus; being caring and ethical in interactions with patients, families and colleagues; having above-average interpersonal skills; and making sound judgments based on experience and knowledge, thus averting potential problems.
- **Competence:** Professional practice demands competence in relation to knowledge and technical skills. This requires not only a broad base of knowledge, but also depth of knowledge in a chosen area of practice, a desire and ability to continue developing that knowledge base and to share it with others and critical thinking in decision-making.
- **Attributes of practice:** Professional practice reflects a particular approach to one's work, with collaboration by far most salient characteristic. Professional nursing practice means working in partnership with other nurses and health professionals in providing client care, being highly organized in managing activities and time, having the ability to manage many complex tasks simultaneously, working autonomously as appropriate and having an open mind and nonjudgmental manner.
- **Personal commitment:** In describing this element of professional practice, respondents referred to the importance of having confidence in one's abilities and taking responsibility for one's actions, including having a sound understanding of the boundaries and limitations of nursing practice. Having a balanced lifestyle and supporting the advancement of the profession were also considered important characteristics of a professional nurse.

Philosophy of Nursing

The philosophy of the nursing profession is defined by four basic concepts. The nursing profession is built upon four key concepts: 1. person, 2. environment, 3. health, and 4. nursing. These four concepts encompass the key elements of nursing philosophy and practice and define the means by which individuals should be viewed and treated within the nursing profession. The four concepts are interrelated and each is built upon the foundation of the concept that precedes it.

Person: In nursing theory, human beings are considered in terms of their physiological, psychological, social, spiritual and cultural selves. People are evaluated in terms of their individual place in society as well as their relationships to their family, community and society as a whole. Additionally, human beings are viewed in terms of their individual needs and how nursing practice is applied to meet these needs. The purpose of nursing and nursing theory is to identify how a particular individuals needs are either met or not met, to predict future needs and to prioritize those needs in order of importance.

Environment: The environment concept of nursing comprises all the internal and external factors that act on human beings and affect their behavior and development. This includes psychological, spiritual, social, physical and cultural forces as well as the environment in which nursing care is provided. The idea behind this concept is that the environment influences individual and collective health and that individuals who experience a positive, comfortable nursing environment are more likely to demonstrate good health versus those who receive a level of care that is lacking.

Health: The concept of health refers to an individual's physical, mental and social well-being and at what point they are on the health spectrum, which ranges from good health to poor health or death. Health is considered to be affected by genetic factors, environmental factors, lifestyle factors and external mechanisms such as bacteria. A person's place on the health spectrum is constantly changing and in a nursing context, it is the responsibility of nursing professionals to identify the patient's place on the spectrum and to take steps to help that person's health improve.

Nursing: Nursing refers to the process of caring for the health of human beings and assisting individuals in meeting their needs while also teaching them the basics of caring for themselves. The responsibilities of the nursing profession are to promote good health, to prevent disease when possible, to promote healing in those who are ill and to ease the suffering of dying patients. The concept of nursing extends beyond the health care facility to the community and society as a whole, and views individual health and the environment as closely related. Nursing is defined as care that is tailored to the needs of individuals and that is provided in an efficient and effective manner.

VALUES OF PROFESSIONAL NURSING

To be successful, nurses must be equipped with certain tools and abilities. These skills are developed over time as a nurse gains experience and confidence.

- **Confidentiality and autonomy:** Nurses have to have an awareness of legislation on patient confidentiality and the policies of their own organization. Nurses should not breach confidentiality, unless the circumstances are exceptional—for instance, if the patient is threatening harm to himself or others. Nurses must not discuss patients' details outside of the care setting, and must take care of notes, paper and computer files. Nurses should make all efforts to promote the patient's rights to make her own decision whenever possible.
- **Protection from harm:** The nurse's conduct must protect the patient from harm. She must not undertake something she thinks might cause harm to the patient even if she has been told or asked to do so by another person. The nurse is accountable for her own actions, and might be asked' to explain these in later proceedings. If the nurse sees anything she fears may endanger the patient, she must immediately report this to management.
- **Professional development:** The nurse has a duty to keep up to date with all developments that may have an impact on her job. She must attend professional development and training activities. Part of her duty may involve training and mentoring new and junior staff. Nurses must meet training requirements and pay any fees needed to maintain licensing.
- **Dedication:** Professional nursing is a difficult profession with many stressful scenarios. Nurses must work long shifts and deal with many vastly different issues on a daily basis. The combination of long work hours, constant care of patients, and the stress of seeing death can cause nurses to unravel. Thus, professional nurses need to be calm, collected and level-headed, able to quickly handle a multitude of problems effectively. Nurses are responsible for patient quality of care and the execution of the health care plan. A dedication to the job is essential for a nurse to fulfill her nursing duties.
- **Systems thinking:** A nurse is faced with a plenty of situations throughout each workday. Each patient has individual problems and requires a different approach. Nurses are expected to develop individualized decisions of care depending on the patient and the specific circumstances
- **Caring:** Nurses are required to take care of the patient throughout the entire health care process. Their goal is to make the healing process and painless and comfortable as possible, without inflicting any unnecessary grief for the patient. In the case of imminent death, nurses must console the patients and the families in order to ease the transition. According to the American Association of Critical Care Nurses, these duties of care giver include "vigilance, engagement, and responsiveness of caregivers, including family and healthcare personnel."
- **Ethnic and religious sensitivity:** Nurses take care of patients from a variety of ethnic and religious backgrounds. Professional nurses must be sensitive to the specific requirements of various cultures and religions in order to facilitate the patient's health care. Nurses must demonstrate a desire to respect various practices while continuing to adhere to professional standards.

BASIC NURSING PRINCIPLES

- **Safety:** It is the protection to hazards to patients and members of the health team from the possible mechanical, chemical, thermal, bacteriological and psychological injuries.
- **Therapeutic effectiveness:** It is the result of the work, that is, whether the purpose of the procedure is fully achieved or out.
- **Comfort:** Every nursing procedure is aimed for the comfort of the patient. It should give the satisfaction to the patient, relatives, and nurse on completion of the work.
- **Use of resources:** The use of time, energy and material should be economic. A procedure should not be cancelled due to the want of one or two items required if they are not extremely essential. In such situations adjustment can be done by improving materials with the available resources.
- **Good workmanship:** It is the skill in doing procedures. There is great difference, in doing things by a fresh hand and an experienced hand. Such skills or the art of doing procedure are developed only by doing the same repeatedly. Nursing is learning by doing and not merely by reading.
- **Individuality:** The likes and dislikes of the individual are unique. So when we are planning nursing care to a person, his needs are to be anticipated and problems are to be identified and feelings are to be considered.

NURSING SCIENCE

Science is a body of knowledge based on a large number of carefully collected facts, which have been arranged and classified in such a way as to establish certain laws and principles. Nursing science is derived from scientific thinking about the discipline or field of nursing and the practice of the profession of nursing. Nursing science is a basic to any professional discipline in the development of a body of knowledge that can be applied of its practice.

Such knowledge is often expressed in terms of concepts and theories.

Steps of Scientific Method

- **Description:** Clarifying ideas, phenomena, experiences or circumstances that are not well understood, for example, describing what pain really means to patients. This clarification is accomplished by presenting new information.
- **Exploration:** Exploring how ideas of interest are related, for example, what is the relationship between pain and patients physical and psychological conditions?
- **Explanation:** Explaining often within the context of an existing theory, the 'whys' of events or occurrences for example, why does pain occur more frequently and severely in persons whose physical and psychological resources are improvised or reduced.
- **Prediction and control:** Knowing and foretelling correctly what will happen and also how to make it happen on command and with some regularity for example in what specific ways can the nurse control the severity of pain for patients?

NURSING AS A PROFESSION

Profession has been defined as that requires extensive education or a calling that requires special knowledge, skill and preparation. Profession is an occupation with moral principles that are devoted to the human and social welfare. Professional nursing is a service devoted to the promotion of human and social welfare.

Professionalism refers to professional character, spirit or methods. It is a set of attributes, a way of life that implies responsibility and commitment. Professionalization is the process of becoming professional that is of acquiring characteristics considered to be professional. Professional nurse is a health worker, a graduate from a recognized school who is identified by law as a registered nurse whether graduated from a baccalaureate (BSc) or a diploma program.

Criteria for profession: Specialized education is an important aspect of professional status. In modern times, the trend in education for the professions that shifted towards programs in colleges and universities.

- **Body of knowledge:** As a profession, nursing is establishing as a well-defined body of knowledge and expertise. A number of nursing conceptual frameworks contribute to the knowledge base of nursing and give direction to nursing practice, education and ongoing research.
- **Service orientation:** Nursing as a tradition of service to others. This service, however, must be guided by certain rules, policies or codes of ethics. Today, nursing is also an important component of the health care delivery system.
- **Ongoing research:** Since the 1970's nursing research has focused on practice related issues. Increasing research in nursing is contributing to nursing practice. Nursing research as a dimension of the nurse's role directed to nursing education and practice.
- **Code of ethics:** Ethical code change as the needs and values of society change. Nursing has developed its own codes of ethics and in most instances has set up means to monitor the professional behaviors of its members.
- **Autonomy:** A profession is autonomous, if it regulates itself and sets standards for its members. Providing autonomy is one of the purposes of a professional association. To be autonomous, a professional group must be granted legal authority to define the scope of its practice, describe its particular functions and roles and determine its goals and responsibilities in delivery of its services.

CHARACTERISTICS OF A PROFESSIONAL NURSE

- Good physical and mental health.
- Truthful and efficient in technical competence.
- Cleanliness, tidy, neat and well groomed.
- Confidence in others and itself.
- Intelligence.
- Open minded, cooperative, responsible, able to develop good interpersonal relations.
- Leadership quality.
- Positive attitudes.
- Self-belief towards human care and cure.
- Convey cooperative attitudes towards co-worker.
- Responsible towards family and society.

QUALITIES OF PROFESSIONAL NURSE

Devotion is the most important quality of any person who wishes to take up nursing as a profession and it should be treated with great care and consideration. Impassiveness is a quality much needed so that the nurse is calm and serene even under pressure of work and during emergency. Some other essential qualities of a nurse are described below:

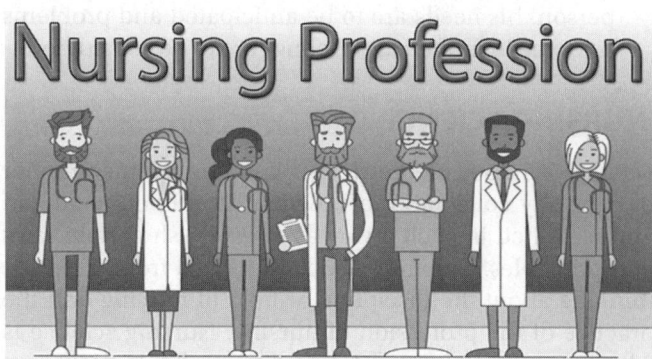

Fig. 3.4: Nurse plays vital role in health care delivery system.

- **Honesty:** A nurse's reliability and integrity must never be questionable. Avoid exaggeration and confess mistakes frankly. So that they may be rectified immediately. Always think of the patient's safety first rather than your possible punishment. Honesty is the most important quality on which others qualities depend.
- **Loyalty:** This quality is practiced towards the school, fellow nurses, senior officers, patients in fact, everybody and everything within the hospital. Hospital matters should not be discussed outside. The patient's affairs should be treated with strict confidence. Disloyalty destroys the entire edifice of the hospital service and the profession itself. Loyalty builds a nursing service of the highest quality.
- **Discipline and obedience:** A nurse must understand the necessity of self-discipline, so that she trains herself to carry out vital orders immediately and accurately without question. At no time she should argue with the staff in authority. A calm, well poised nurse, who has her own emotions under control, inspires confidence and respect. A nurse should never refuse to carry out a legitimate order issued by a senior staff. If there is any point of argument it can be taken up later.
- **Courtesy:** This is a simple form of consideration of others which is practiced towards patients and their relatives, senior officers and fellow nurses. It does not require any extra time, and is much appreciated by all.
- **Dignity:** To be dignified and to maintain a professional attitude towards each other and towards patients is essential. Peals of laughter, loud and immature conversation, anger and argumentation lower a nurse's dignity.
- **Personal appearance:** This is of major importance. A nurse, who appears healthy, neat, well groomed and meticulous about her personal hygiene, immediately creates a favorable impression on patients and colleagues alike. Jewelry, excessive cosmetics, improper shoes, worn out, poorly fitting or soiled uniforms completely ruin the professional appearance.
- **Tact, sympathy, sense of humor and patience:** These are all attributes which a nurse needs to develop, along with tolerance and breadth of outlook. All these help her enormously in dealing with her patients and her fellow nurses.
- **Optimistic outlook:** Without forcing cheerfulness, a nurse may still exude an aura of security and contentment by looking and acting as though she enjoys doing her work, and by maintaining genuine interest in the patient and his welfare. A quick warm smile may be more therapeutic than a dose of medicine.
- **Observation and adaptability:** If these do not come naturally, a nurse may consciously develop these qualities. It is important to be observant of the small things which add to a patient's comfort or those things which may indicate a change of condition. A sharp eye to see out-of order or out-of-place equipment, lack of cleanliness in the ward, is the quality which makes a responsible nurse.
- **Gentleness and quietness:** Develop a gentleness of touch and quietness in handling the patient and equipment, with quick but smooth movements. These increase the patient's comfort and confidence.
- **Economy:** This is the characteristic of an ideal nurse. Equipment and supplies, water and electricity which the nurse controls are valuable material. These must be preserved carefully as if they were personal property not only for the sake of the patients and the hospital, but also for our country.
- **Sense of responsibility:** The most difficult characteristics to acquire is a sense of responsibility. This is the quality which produces reliable and efficient leaders. The nursing profession in India today is in great need of responsible leaders. But still more important are the thousands of nurses each of whom in her own place understand and shoulders her share of responsibility.
- **Adaptability:** To adapt one to existing conditions and living with others counts for much in making of a good nurse.

ROLE AND FUNCTIONS OF A NURSE

Nurses assume a number of roles when they provide care to patients. Nurses often carry out these roles concurrently not exclusively of one another. For example, the nurse may act as a counselor while providing physical care and teaching aspects of the care.

- **Care giver:** The caregiver role traditionally included those activities that assist the patient physically and psychologically while preserving the patient's dignity. Care giving encompasses the physical, psychological, developmental, cultural and spiritual levels.
- **Communicator:** In the role of communicator, nurses identify patient's problems and then communicate these verbally or in writing to other members of the health team. The nurse must be able to communicate clearly and accurately in order for a client's health care needs to be met.
- **Teacher:** As a teacher, the nurse helps the client learn about their health and the health care procedures they need to perform to restore or maintain their health. The nurse assesses the client's learning needs and readiness to learn, sets specific learning goals in conjunction with the client, enacts teaching strategies, and measures learning.
- **Client advocate:** A client advocate acts to protect the client. In this role the nurse may represent the client's needs and wishes to other health professionals, such as relaying the client's wishes for information to the physician.
- **Counselor:** The nurse counsel's primarily healthy individual with normal adjustments difficulties and focuses on helping the person to develop new attitudes, feelings and behaviors by encouraging the client to look

at alternative behaviors, recognize the choices, and develop a sense of control.

- **Change agent:** The nurse acts as a change agent when assisting others that is clients, to make modifications in their own behavior. Nurses also often act to make changes in a system, such as clinical care, if it is not helping a client return to health. Nurses are continually dealing with change in the health care system.
- **Leader:** The leader role can be employed at different levels individual client, family, groups of clients, colleagues or the community.
- **Manager:** The nurse manager also delegates nursing activities to ancillary workers and other nurses, and supervises and evaluates their performance.
- **Case manager:** Nurse case managers work with the multidisciplinary health care team to measure the effectiveness of the case management plan and to monitor outcomes. Each agency or unit specifies the role of the nurse case manager.
- **Research consumer:** Nurses often use research to improve client care. In a clinical area, nurses need to (a) have some awareness of the process and language of research, (b) be sensitive to issues related to protecting the rights of human subjects, (c) participate in the identification of significant researchable problems, and (d) be a discriminating consumer of research findings.
- **Expanded career roles:** Nurses are fulfilling expanded career roles, such as those of nurse practitioner, clinical nurse specialist, nurse midwife, nurse educator, nurse researcher and nurse anesthetist.

SCOPE OF NURSING

There was a time when professional nurses had very little choice of service because nursing was centered in the hospital and bedside nursing. Career opportunities are more varied now for a numbers of reasons. The list of opportunities available is given under:

- **Staff nurse** provides direct patient care to one patient or a group of patients. Assists ward management and supervision. She is directly responsible to the ward supervisor.
- **Ward sister or nursing supervisor:** She is responsible to the nursing superintendent for the nursing care management of a ward or unit. Takes full charge of the ward. Assigns work to nursing and non-nursing personnel working in the ward. Responsible for safety and comfort of patients in the ward. Provides teaching sessions if it is a teaching hospital.
- **Department supervisor/Assistant nursing superintendent:** She is responsible to the nursing superintendent and deputy nursing superintendent for the nursing care and management of more than one ward or unit. Example: Surgical department and out-patient department.
- **Deputy nursing superintendent:** She is responsible to the nursing superintendent and assists in the nursing administration of the hospital.
- **Nursing superintendent:** She is responsible to the medical superintendent for safe and efficient management of hospital nursing services.

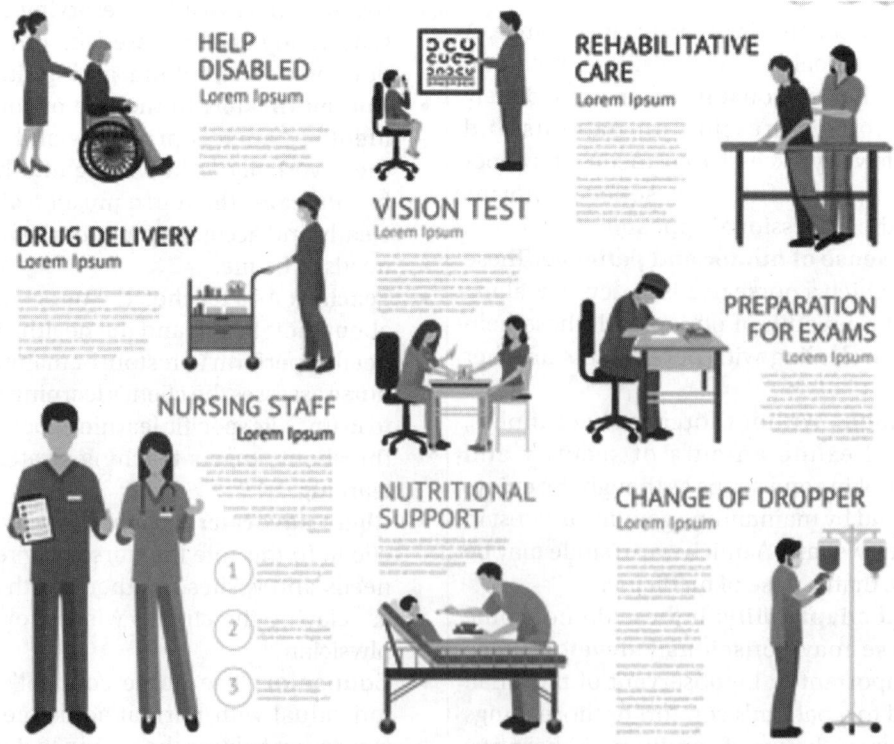

Fig. 3.5: Roles and responsibilities of a nurse.

History of Nursing and Nursing as a Profession

- **Director of nursing** She is responsible for both nursing service and nursing educations within a teaching hospital.
- **Community health nurse (CHN):** Services rendered mainly focusing Reproductive Child Health programme.
- **Teaching in nursing:** The functions and responsibilities of the teacher in nursing are planning, teaching and supervising the learning experiences for the students. Positions in nursing education are clinical instructor, tutor, senior tutor, lecturer, and associate professor, reader in nursing and professor in nursing.
- **Industrial nurse:** Industrial nurses are providing first aid, care during illness, health educations about industrial hazards and prevention of accidents.
- **Military nurse:** Military nursing service became a part of the Indian Army by which means nurses became commissioned officers who are given rank from lieutenant to major general.
- **Nursing service abroad:** Attractive salaries and promising professional opportunities, which cause a major increase for nursing service in abroad.
- **Nursing service administrative positions:** At the state level the Deputy Director of Nursing at the state health directorate. The highest administrative position on a national level is the Nursing Advisor to the Govt. of India.

CATEGORIES OF NURSING PERSONNEL

Nursing personnel are among the largest no of health care professionals working in the various fields of health care they work from the lowest level of care to the highest level. They work in the varied settings namely: 1. Hospital / Clinical areas, 2. Community area, 3. Educational settings, 4. Holistic setting.

Nursing Personnel in Nursing Service

- Nursing director
- Nursing superintendent
- Deputy nursing superintendent
- Departmental in charge
- Head nurse
- Charge nurse
- Senior staff nurse
- Auxiliary nurse midwife
- Nursing aids.

Nursing Director

- Formation of the aims and the objectives policies of the new nursing services
- Staffing based on the nursing requirement according to the accepted standards of the medical standards
- Planning and directing the nursing care
- Coordinating the interdepartmental activities
- Maintaining the supplies and the equipment
- Budgeting
- Keeping records and reports.

Chief Nursing Officer

- Chief Officer for all the staff nurses in hospital. She does planning, coordination, supervision, controlling, reporting to higher medical officer and delegating the work schedules to other nurses.
- Follows and adapts policies, which helps to recruit, assign and allocate the required staff at the right place and time.
- Explains the job description, supervision and delegating responsibilities to each staff nurse.
- Conducts nursing audit, does anecdotal reporting to evaluate nursing care.
- Make all staff observes and follows code of ethics and regulation of the hospitals.
- Has authority to terminate any nurse if she misbehaves or violates hospital regulations.
- Encourages and participates in all round development of nurses, especially in nursing research activities.

Head Nurse

- To plan the duty roster specific to the ward, implement PCS and allocate ward in charge to specific wards.
- To control and coordinate the activities of the specific wards.
- To plan all the activities done by ward in charge in advance, delegate responsibilities and supervise the activities in the wards.
- To supervise the nursing care being rendered for all patients and to take frequent status updates.
- To conduct nursing rounds with ward in charges to assess the problem, plan care, clarify issues, fulfill the requirements and guide the ward in charge.
- To maintain the enrolment register of all the staff and ward in charge, and ensure that all the staff reported duty in time.
- To allocate the alternative staff in case of absenteeism.
- To conduct meeting with the subordinate staff, and provide guidance, and teaching to improve her nursing care.

Ward In-charge

- Report to the head nurse for any issue.
- Plan control and supervise the activity of the subordinates and also ensure that the staff are allocated at required areas and provide good care to the patients.
- Ensure ward cleanliness, safety and security for all the patients in the ward.
- Oversee the patients' conditions regularly and to care for the concerns of doctors who take care of the patients.
- Conduct ward rounds with staff nurse and plan her daily activities accordingly.
- Coordinate the shift schedule, day/night off in the coordination with the head nurse.
- Meet the health care needs of all patients in the ward.

Senior Staff Nurse

- Senior nurses work under the ward in- charge. They have to report to the duty in time and sign in the register.
- They provide individual care to patients who are seriously ill and are assisted by the junior nurses.
- They report the patient care to ward in- charge regularly.
- They write and record the patient details on the nurse's record.
- They maintain the patient care sheet, which has patient identification data, doctor sheet, diagnostic sheet, etc.

Graduate Nurse/Staff Nurse

- The nurse directly provides patient care.
- Learns the policies of the hospital and ward, and works according to the standards of care.
- Provides health education and direct skilled work. She works under the supervision of the senior nurse and holds authority over the Nursing Assistants and the Aids.

Nurses Working in the Community Areas

- The nurses working in the community level are also a large part of the health care delivery system.
- They work at various levels and provide care to various levels. They can be broadly classified as:

Community Health Workers

Community health nurse: There are various community health nurse levels in various states of India generally they can be classified as:
- DPHNO: District public health nursing officer
- BPHN: Block public health nurse
- PHN: Public health nurse/Lady health visitor
- ANM: Auxiliary nurse midwife/Female health workers

ANM (Auxiliary nurse midwife/Female health workers)

Roles and Responsibilities
- Registers and cares for the prenatal and postnatal mothers at home.
- Registers and follows up all the eligible couples.
- Provides nutritional advice and immunization to mother and children.
- Carries out family planning services and including the distribution of the contraceptives.
- Provides treatment to minor ailments.
- Notifies communicable diseases.
- Maintains the records and registers all the services provided and vital events like birth and death.
- Participates in the various disease control programmes.
- Conducts surveys of all subcenter areas and maintains records about every family.
- Coordinates activities with the block level
- Functions in the field of administration and supervision, education training personnel, health services and research.

Nursing Personnel in Nursing Education

- The Dean
- Principal
- Vice Principal
- Reader
- Professor
- Associate Professor
- Lecturer
- Assistant Lecturer
- Clinical instructor

Nursing Personnel in Community Health Service

- Community Health Nurse
- Public Health Nurse
- Village Health Nurse
- Auxiliary Nurse Midwife
- Health Worker-Female
- Health Worker-male
- Dais

PATIENT-CENTERED NURSING CARE (NURSING PROCEDURES)

Procedure means a method of carrying out a treatment. Details of procedure differ in various hospitals, though underlying principles are same. Nursing techniques is the skillful handling of patient with the least discomfort, the skillful handling of sterile apparatus without contamination and elimination of unnecessary movements so as to ensure the maximum speed with the highest efficiency.

Nurse is a primary member of the unit. She should have an interest to work and should radiate joy while doing it. She follows the systematic and orderly way of doing procedures; organizing correct equipments before procedure observe the patient's condition and document the details promptly and properly.

Patient: Patient is considered as an individual holistic approach. While delivering the patient's care. Patient's physical, mental comfort should be considered. Adequate explanation, providing continuous observation is essential in quality nursing care.

The environment: The therapeutic environment should be pleasant to give care and to receive care. The environment should help the patient for faster recovery. The environment should be clean, neat, appropriate temperature, adequate light, well ventilated; noise and draughts should be avoided. The ward or room should be left in order after carrying out procedure.

Equipment: Adequate equipments are important for the effective patient care. All the equipments for a procedure should be clean and in good working condition. After use of all equipments, it should be washed, scrubbed, dried, boiled, aired, etc. All broken equipment should be reported and replacement obtained.

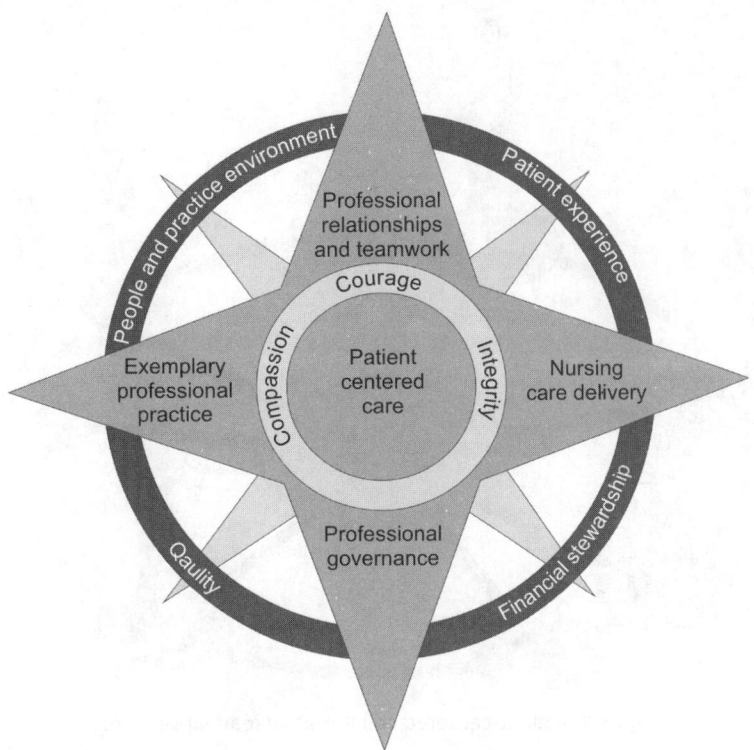

Fig. 3.6: Patient-centered care.

The Five Essential Steps in Every Procedure

Preliminary assessment of the patient and situation includes: Check the doctor's order to note any specific instructions in doing the procedure. General condition of the patient, self-care ability, the mood of acceptance, hygienic status, position to be changed, need of the procedure and assistant. Preparation and organization of articles includes according to the order of use, the nurse must have a thorough knowledge about the details of the procedure. On the basis of judgment a thoughtful nurse will collect and organize all the articles to meet the needs throughout the procedure and concentrate in the performance.

Performance of the procedure the nurse obtained knowledge from the classrooms, books and demonstrations, and by assisting senior sisters in the ward in the beginning. The sincere effort in the part of students and junior staff in learning, observing and practicing is the real method of developing knowledge and skill in doing procedures. Aftercare of patients and articles make the patient comfortable, the effect of the treatment is observed and proper recording is made in the chart. All the articles are well cleaned and sterilized (if needed) replace in the proper place and ready for the next use.

NURSE AS A MEMBER OF HEALTH CARE TEAM

The health team in a health care system may be as simple as consisting only of three members, the doctor, the nurse and the patient or it may be a large team consisting of members of many other specialized fields of care like physical therapists, occupational therapists, dieticians and people who look into the spiritual and social needs of the patient.

Each member of the team possesses unique knowledge and skill which he/she contributes to the total health care system. There are also many areas of shared knowledge and skill, e.g. communication skills, anatomy, physiology, psychology and sociology. The essence of the team concept is that all members work cooperatively for individual family or a community towards their common goal of attaining the highest level of health possible.

VALUES OF PROFESSIONAL NURSE

To be successful, nurses must be equipped with certain tools and abilities. These skills are developed over time as a nurse gains experience and confidence.

- **Confidentiality and autonomy:** Nurses have to have an awareness of legislation on patient confidentiality and the policies of their own organization. Nurses should not breach confidentiality, unless the circumstances are exceptional- -for instance, if the patient is threatening harm to himself or others. Nurses must not discuss patients' details outside of the care setting, and must take care of notes, paper and computer files. Nurses should make all efforts to promote the patient's rights to make her own decision whenever possible.
- **Protection from harm:** The nurse's conduct must protect the patient from harm. She must not undertake

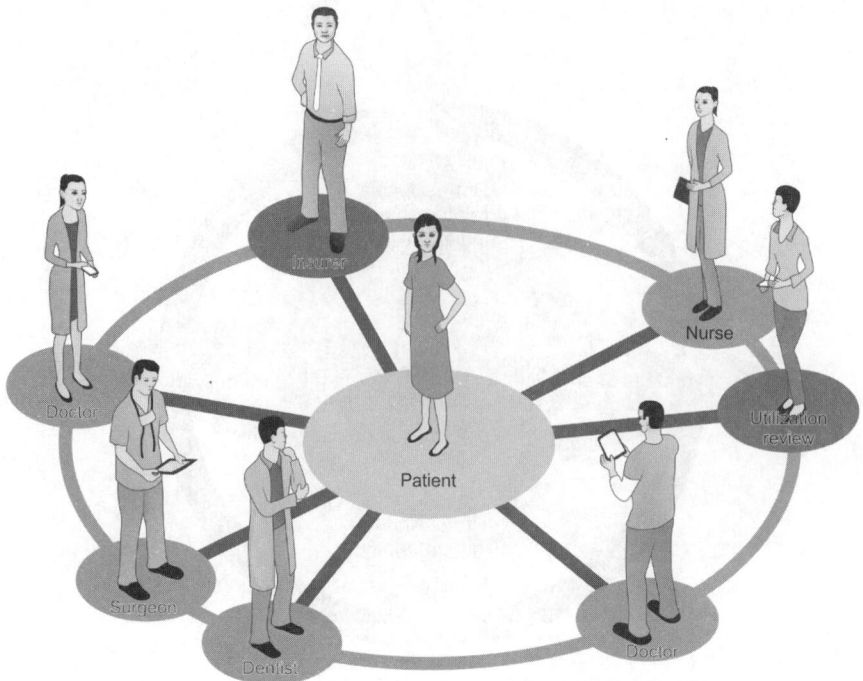

Fig. 3.7: Patient-centered collaborative team approach.

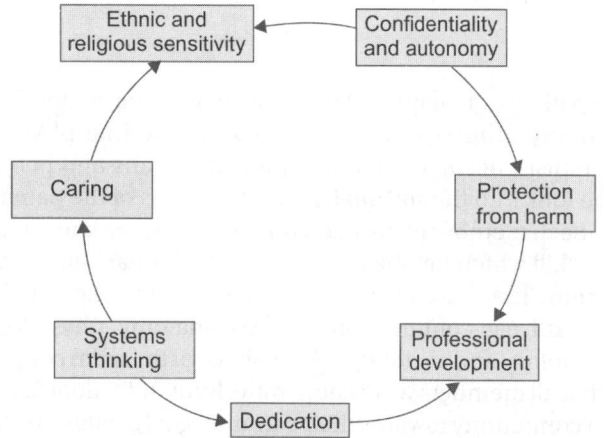

Fig. 3.8: Professional standards of nursing.

something she thinks might cause harm to the patient even if she has been told or asked to do so by another person. The nurse is accountable for her own actions, and might be asked to explain these in later proceedings. If the nurse sees anything she fears may endanger the patient, she must immediately report this to management.

- **Professional development:** The nurse has a duty to keep up to date with all developments that may have an impact on her job. She must attend professional development and training activities. Part of her duty may involve training and mentoring new and junior staff. Nurses must meet training requirements and pay any fees needed to maintain licensing.
- **Dedication:** Professional nursing is a difficult profession with many stressful scenarios. Nurses must work long shifts and deal with many vastly different issues on a daily basis. The combination of long work hours, constant care of patients, and the stress of seeing death can cause nurses to unravel. Thus, professional nurses need to be calm, collected and level-headed, able to quickly handle a multitude of problems effectively. Nurses are responsible for patient quality of care and the execution of the health care plan. A dedication to the job is essential for a nurse to fulfill her nursing duties.
- **Systems thinking:** A nurse is faced with a plenty of situations throughout each workday. Each patient has individual problems and requires a different approach. Nurses are expected to develop individualized decisions of care depending on the patient and the specific circumstances.
- **Caring:** Nurses are required to take care of the patient throughout the entire health care process. Their goal is to make the healing process and painless and comfortable as possible, without inflicting any unnecessary grief for the patient. In the case of imminent deal, nurses must console the patients and the families in order to ease the transition. According to the American Association of Critical Care Nurses, these duties of care include "vigilance, engagement, and responsiveness of caregivers, including family and healthcare personnel."
- **Ethnic and religious sensitivity:** Nurses take care of patients from a variety of ethnic and religious backgrounds. Professional nurses must be sensitive to the specific requirements of various cultures and religions in order to facilitate the patient's health care. Nurses must demonstrate a desire to respect various practices while continuing to adhere to professional standards.

CONCEPT OF PROFESSIONALISM IN NURSING

The art of nursing: Professional nursing practice is grounded in the art of nursing, described as taking a holistic, client-centered focus; being caring and ethical in interactions with patients, families and colleagues; having above-average interpersonal skills; and making sound judgments based on experience and knowledge, thus averting potential problems.

Competence: Professional practice demands competence in relation to knowledge and technical skills. This requires not only a broad base of knowledge, but also depth of knowledge in a chosen area of practice, a desire and ability to continue developing that knowledge base and to share it with others and critical thinking in decision-making.

Attributes of practice: Professional practice reflects a particular approach to one's work, with collaboration by far most salient characteristic. Professional nursing practice means working in partnership with other nurses and health professionals in providing client care, being highly organized in managing activities and time, having the ability to manage many complex tasks simultaneously, working autonomously as appropriate and having an open mind and nonjudgmental manner.

Personal commitment: In describing this element of professional practice, respondents referred to the importance of having confidence in one's abilities and taking responsibility for one's actions, including having a sound understanding of the boundaries and limitations of nursing practice. Having a balanced lifestyle and supporting the advancement of the profession were also considered important characteristics of a professional nurse.

ISSUES RELATED TO NURSING PROFESSION

Issues refer to the items for consideration or questions for discussion. Various issues in nursing profession maybe related to profession, education, practice and nurses themselves.

Various issues related to nursing profession are:
- Status of nursing in society in health care delivery system.
- Values reflected in our nursing performances.
- Attitudes, humane approach and concern shown in the behavior patterns of nurses.
- Quality in nursing hand in hand between education and practice.
- Unique functions of nursing.
- Different levels of nurses required in the country.
- Emphasis from traditional to primary health care approach.
- Evidence-based nursing research.
- Nurses in administration.
- Expanded and extended roles of nurses.
- Globalization in the profession.
- Nursing leadership in bringing changes in health scenario according o community demands.

CARING AND ADVOCACY

In the role of client advocate, the nurse protects the client's human and legal rights and provides assistance in asserting those rights if the need arises. For example, the nurse may provide additional information for a client who is trying to decide whether to accept treatment. The nurse may also defend clients' rights in a general way by speaking out against policies or actions that might endanger client's well-being or conflict with their rights. As protector the nurse helps maintain a safe environment for the client and takes steps to prevent injury and protect the client from possible adverse effects of diagnostic or treatment measures. Confirming that a client does not have an allergy to a medication and providing immunization against disease in a community-based practice are examples of the nurse's protective role

- **Advocacy skills:** The ability to successfully support a cause or interest on one's own behalf or that of another requires a set of skills that include problem solving, communication, influence, and collaboration. Each of these skills will be discussed below.
- **Problem solving:** Advocacy is focused on addressing problems or issues in need of a solution. The steps in the advocacy process are first to identify the issue(s) to be addressed and develop goals and a strategy to address the issue(s). Once the strategy is identified, a plan of action is developed to organize advocacy efforts and establish a time line for completing each activity that supports the strategy. Most advocacy initiatives involve approaching decision makers with requests for action to address the identified issue.
- **Communication:** Most advocacy initiatives involve bringing individuals and groups together to address an issue or concern. Advocates need to communicate clearly and concisely and to structure the message to fit both the situation and the intended audience. Advocates must be comfortable with verbal, written, and electronic formats. Communication regarding the issue should be factual and consistent.
- **Influence:** To facilitate change or solve an issue, the advocate must be able to influence others to action. Influence is the ability to alter or sway an individual's or group's thoughts, beliefs, or actions; it is essential to the advocacy process. Influence is built on competence, credibility, and trustworthiness. Keeping the best interests of those involved in the situation builds trust and credibility.
- **Collaboration:** In addition to demonstrating the skills described above, the advocate must also establish positive, collaborative relationships with others to garner the support necessary to address the issue.

Collaboration is working with other individuals or groups to achieve a common goal. It differs from cooperation which involves groups working together to achieve their own individual goals. In collaboration, the individuals or groups involved develop common goals, along with common strategies and activities that will achieve that goal. Collaboration is built on trust, mutual respect, and credibility.

EXTENDED ROLE OF NURSE

The nurses in India are also prepared and more privileged to face the changes and ready to accept the challenging roles and functions of the nurse as perceived in the globe because of the development in the education and training system. The following roles and positions perceived as in the globe are given below.

- **Nurse educator** works in schools of nursing, staff development departments. They provide the educational program for student's nurses and nurses, teach clients about the self-care and home care.
- **Clinical nurse specialist** specializes in managing specific diseases and they function as clinicians, educators, managers, consultants and researchers.
- **Nurse practitioners** are certified to provide health care to clients in out-patient or community settings.
- **Certified nurse-midwife** is certified by the American College of Nurse-Midwives to provide independent care for women during normal pregnancy, labor and delivery.
- **Nurse anesthetist,** having advance training in anesthesiology, provides surgical anesthesia to the client under the supervision of an anesthesiologist during minor surgery with baccalaureate degrees or master's degree.
- **Nurse administrators** manage client care within the healthcare agencies in a middle level or upper level management position.
- **Nurse researcher** with Doctoral degree investigate nursing problem to improve care and to define and expand the scope of nursing practice.

Advancements in science increase health needs of the society and thereby expect changes in the role of nurses and thus increases the scope for nurses

ETHICAL ISSUES IN NURSING

Ethics are the rules or principles that govern right contact. Ethics are designed to protect the rights of human being. Ethics are characteristics of a healthy profession. The code of ethics will state what kind of conduct is expected from the members of a profession, what are the responsibilities of its members towards those whom they serve, their co-worker, the profession and the society as a whole.

Nursing Ethics

The nursing ethics provide professional standards for nursing activities which protect the nurse and the patient.

In 1973, the International Council for Nurses (INC) adopted code of ethics. The fundamental responsibility of the nurse is fourfold- To promote health, to prevent illness, to restore health and to alleviate suffering.

The need for nursing is universal. Inherent in nursing is respect for life dignity and rights of men. It is unrestricted by considerations of nationality, race, creed, color, age, sex, politics or social status. Nurses render health services to the individual, the family and the community, and coordinate their services with those of related groups.

CODE OF ETHICS

The code of ethics will state what kind of conduct is expected from the members of a profession, what are the responsibilities of its members towards those whom they serve, their co-workers, the profession and the society as a whole. The nurse will adjust better if she understands what a wrong/right behavior in different situations is. The first such code of ethics, called the international code of nursing ethics, was adopted by the grand council of the international council of nurses at Sao Paulo, Brazil in 1953. it was later revised in Frankfurt, Germany in 1965 and then became known as ICN code of ethics.

Nurses and People

The nurse's primary responsibility is to those people who require nursing care. The nurse holds in confidence personal informations and use judgment in sharing this information.

- The nurse's primary responsibility is to those people who require nursing care.
- The nurse, in providing care, promotes an environment in which the values, customs and spiritual beliefs of the individual are respected.
- The nurse holds in confidence personal information and uses judgment in sharing this information.

Nurses and Practice

The nurse maintains the highest standards of nursing care possible within the reality of a specific situation. The nurse when acting in a professional capacity should at all times maintain standards of personal conduct which credit upon the profession.

- The nurse carries personal responsibility for nursing practice and for maintaining competence by continual learning.
- The nurse maintains the highest standards of nursing care possible within the reality of a specific situation.
- The nurse uses judgment in relation to individual competence when accepting and delegating responsibilities.
- The nurse, when acting in a professional capacity, should at all times maintain standards of personal conduct which reflect credit on the profession.

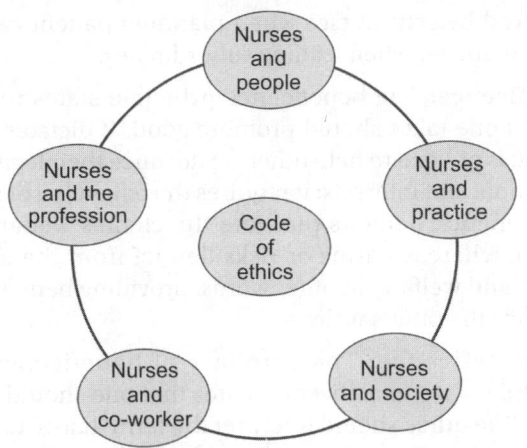

Fig. 3.9: International Council of Nursing (ICN) code of ethics for nurses.

Nurses and Society

The nurse shares with other citizens the responsibility for initiating and supporting action to meet the health and social needs of the public.

Nurses and Co-worker

The nurse maintains a cooperative relationship with co-workers in nursing and other fields. The nurse takes appropriate action to safeguard the individual when his care is endangered by a co-worker or any other person.
- The nurse sustains a cooperative relationship with co-workers in nursing and other fields.
- The nurse takes appropriate action to safeguard the individual when his care is endangered by a co-worker or any other person.

Nurses and the Profession

The nurse acting through the professional organization participates in establishing and maintaining equitable social and economic working conditions in nursing.
- The nurse plays a major role in determining and implementing desirable standards of nursing practices and nursing education.
- The nurse is active in developing a core of professional knowledge.
- The nurse, acting through the professional organization, participates in establishing and maintaining equitable, social and economic working conditions in nursing.

The international code of nursing ethics is given below:
- The fundamental responsibility of a nurse is to conserve life and to promote health. Every nurse is a teacher of health by example.
- A nurse must be adequately prepared to practice nursing and be willing to continue to learn new ideas by reading, and attending meetings.
- The nurse must learn to respect authority.
- The nurse must carry out the doctor's orders accurately and sustain confidence in the doctor, and all members of the health team.
- The nurse should report any unusual conditions or symptoms to the doctor or the in-charge nurse.
- The religious beliefs of a patient should be respected.
- The nurse should hold confidential all information given to her.
- When a patient requires continued nursing care, the nurse must remain with the patient until adequate relief is available.
- The nurse has the obligation to give conscientious service and, in return, is entitled to just remuneration.
- A patient should always be called by his full name.
- Punctuality is very important for every nurse.
- Obedience is very important in observing rules and regulations.
- Every nurse must have respect for authority and for rules and regulations.
- Economy is important for all nurses to practice.

ETHICAL PRINCIPLES

Ethical principles actually control professionalism nursing practice much more than to ethical theories. Principles encompass basic promises from which rules are developed. Principles are the moral norms that nursing, as a profession, both demands and strives to implement to every day clinical practice. Ethical principle that the nurse should consider when making decisions are as follows:
- Respect for persons.
- Respect for autonomy.
- Respect for freedom.
- Respect for beneficence (doing good).
- Respect for nonmaleficence (avoiding harm to others).
- Respect for veracity (truth telling).
- Respect for persons.
- Respect for justice (fair and equal treatment).
- Respect for rights.
- Respect for fidelity (fulfilling promises).
- Confidentiality (protecting privileged information).

Respect for persons: Respect for persons not only applies to clinical situations, but also to all life's situations. It directs individuals to treat themselves and others with a respect inherent to man's humanness. It requires recognition on a sense that all mankind shared a common human destiny.

The respect to persons needs to be simplified as it affects nursing practice.

Autonomy: Autonomy that individuals are able to act for themselves to the level of their capacity. It is the right of individual to govern their actions according to their own purpose and reason. Respect for autonomy requires that persons honor another's right to govern him or her. The legal doctrine of informed consent is the direct reflection of autonomy. So it requires that health personnel obtain a patient's informed consent for treatment and for participation in research. The followings are required for a patient to give informed consent for either:

Disclosure: Adequate presentation of relevant information about the proposed treatment or study.

Understanding: Adequate comprehension of the disclosed information.

Ethical principle	Summary	Example from pediatrics
Autonomy	Self-determination; includes reliability, disclosure, informed consent, confidentiality and promise observance	Obtaining consent from parents for a medical procedure (such as lumbar puncture), with assent from older children about the same procedure
Beneficence	Acting from the essence of sympathy and kindness to benefit others	Providing a broad-spectrum antimicrobial therapy to a child with bacterial meningitis
Nonmaleficence	Non-harming or inflicting the least harm possible to reach a beneficial outcome	Changing the broad-spectrum antimicrobial therapy to penicillin in a child with *Streptococcus* group B bacterial meningitis after obtaining antibiotic susceptibility testing results
Justice	Acting out of fairness for individuals, groups and society, with fair allocation of healthcare resources	Having the optimal treatment available for all children who present with meningitis in any hospital in the community
Autonomy	Self-determination; includes reliability, disclosure, informed consent, confidentiality and promise observance	Obtaining consent from parents for a medical procedure (such as lumbar puncture), with assent from older children about the same procedure
Beneficence	Acting from the essence of sympathy and kindness to benefit others	Providing a broad-spectrum antimicrobial therapy to a child with, bacterial meningitis

Voluntary agreement: Free assent, influenced by external controlling factors.

Competence: Adequate decision making capacity. There are three type of autonomy, i.e. freedom of action, freedom of choice and effective deliberation.

Freedom: The principle of individual freedom decrease that patients be exempt from control by others to select and pursue personal health goals. Nurses as a group believe that patient should have greater freedom of choice within the nation's health care system. This principle should be observed by staff nurses when planning patient care; by nurse manager when leading subordinates.

Beneficence: The beneficence principle states that the actions one takes should promote good. It dictates that a person is obliged to help others to advance their legitimate and important interests; it requires the balancing of harms and benefits. Benefits promote the client's welfare and health, whereas harms or risks detract from the client's health and welfare. In other words, providing benefits that enhance the others welfare

Nonmaleficence: The corollary of beneficence, the principle of nonmaleficence states that one should do no harm. The nurse should interpret the term 'harm' to mean emotional and social as well as physical injury. Harm is thwarting, defeating, or setting back one person's interest through invasive action by another. Many nurses find it difficult to follow the principle when performing treatment and procedures that bring discomfort and pain to patients.

Veracity: Veracity concerns truth telling an incorporates the concept that individuals should always tell the truth. It requires professional caregivers to provide with accurate, reality-based information about their health status and care or treatment prospect. Truth telling is an ethical concern for nurse, because truth is the basis for mutual trust between patient and nurse, and trust is the basis for patient's hope of benefit from nursing services. Nurse Managers use this principle when they give all the facts of a situation, truthfully and assist their employees to make decisions.

Justice: Justice concerns the issue that persons should be treated equally and fairly. This principle of justice requires treating others fairly and giving persons their due. When there are resources to distribute in healthcare, nurses should allocate them in such a way that equal shares go to equal recipients. The following problems complicate the application of justice:

- Not everyone is equal in every way; sometimes there are situations in which it seems that one person should receive a greater or lesser share than another.
- Resources are limited. There is not always enough for each person to receive an equal share.

Questions of justice relate to the fairness with which benefits and burdens are distributed among people. Experience in turn found various principles have to be proposed to guide fair distribution of society's good are as follows:

- Each person should receive an equal share.
- The amount given to each person should be proportional to his or her need.
- The amount given to each person should be proportional to the amount of his or her work effort.
- The amount given to each person should reflect the value of his or her work product.
- The amount given to each person should reflect his to her value to society.
- The amount given to each person should be determined by free market exchange. These principles usually arise

in times of short supplies or when there is competition for resources of benefits.

Rights: Right is an entitlement to behave in certain way under circumstances, such as nurse's entitlement to freely express personal beliefs and preferences by voting in a political election. Another right is the prerogative to define another's behavior in selected situations, such as manager's prerogative to give assignments to subordinates. A right is also a claim to a specific good, service or prerequisite such as tea break time. Right is also used to mean agreement with justice, law and morality. So right may be mental rights or legal rights related to respective profession.

- The patient has the right to every consideration of his privacy concerning his own medical care program.
- The patient has the right to expect that all communications and records pertaining to his care should be treated as confidential.
- The patient has the right to expect that within its capacity a hospital must make reasonable response to the request of a patient for services.
- The patient has the right to obtain information as to any relationship of his hospital to other healthcare and educational institutions in so far as his care is concerned and any professional relationships among individuals, by name, who are treating him.
- The patient has the right to be advised if the hospital proposes to engage in or perform human experimentation affecting his care or treatment and has the right to refuse to participate.
- The patient has the right to expect reasonable continuity of care.
- The patient has the right to examine and receive an explanation of his bill regardless of source of payment.
- The patient has the right to know what hospital rules and regulations apply to his conduct as a patient.

Fidelity: Fidelity is keeping one's promises or commitments. The principle of fidelity holds that a person should faithfully fulfill his duties and obligations. Fidelity is important in a nurse because a patient's hope for relief and recovery rests on evidence of caregiver's conscientiousness. Nurse, Managers abide by this principle when they follow through on any promise they have previously made to employees, such as promised leave, a certain shift to be worked or a promotion to perception within the unit.

Confidentiality: Confidentiality is the duty to respect privileged information. The principle of confidentiality provides that caregivers should respect a patient need for privacy and use personal information about him or her only to improve care. Nurses should practice confidentiality to decrease patient vulnerability and share from widespread knowledge of personal information divulged during care.

ETHICAL DILEMMAS

A dilemma is defined as situations requiring a choice between two equally desirable or undesirable alternatives. In ethical dilemma, each alternative course of action can be justified by two ways in which a person views the course of action based on his or her value system. Issues in healthcare delivery practices present different alternatives based on whether the issue or course of action is viewed by the patient, the health care agency, the legal system or the nurse. Increasingly, staff nurses and nurse managers face difficult decisions caused by tensions between technological capabilities, budgetary structures, and quality of life concerns. Nurses in all clinical and functional specialties face the following ethical dilemmas:

- Need to ration patient care to conserve scarce resources.
- Need to make treatment and care decisions for terminally ill patients.
- Need to obtain patients informed consent for care and treatment orders and measures such as:
  - Do not resuscitate order.
  - Withholding/withdrawing nutrition and fluids.
  - Starting/discontinuing life support system.
- Response to patient request for assisted suicide.
- Need to balance the patients need for confidentiality and privacy against society's needs for protection from unreasonable risk.
- Need to protect autonomy rights of children and incompetent adults concerning consent for research participation.
- Need to protect justice rights of patients who participate in random trials of experimental treatment. Usually the dilemma occurs when opposing views are seen for the solution of an issue and a decision must be made. There is no set of procedures or easy answers for how an ethical dilemma should be resolved. Ethical decision making is needed in all steps of the nursing process and all phases of the nursing management process. Ethical reasoning is similar to the nursing process in that it requires critical thinking skills. A nurse can best resolve ethical dilemma, by systematically considering all options for solving the dilemma. A ethical dilemma occurs as a result of conflict between moral principles that support different courses of action.

ETHICAL DECISION MAKING

Nurse's decisions are increasingly constrained by ethical issues. Ethical decision making involves reflection on the following:

- Who should make the choice?
- Possible options or courses of action,
- Available options,
- Consequences, both good and bad, of all possible options,
- Rules, obligations and values that should direct choices, and
- Desired outcomes.

When making decisions, nurses need to combine all of these elements using an orderly, systematic, and objective method. There are various models for ethical decision making. Perhaps the easiest ethical decision making model to remember and to implement in practice is the "moral model" developed by Thirona and Halloraw as follows:

M—Massage the dilemma. Identify and define the issues in the dilemma. Consider the opinions of all major players in the dilemma as well as their value system. This includes patient's family members, nurses, doctors, priest and any other interdisciplinary healthcare team member.

O—Outline the options. Examine all options including those less realistic and conflicting; this stage is designed only for considering options and not for making final decision.

R—Resolve the dilemma. Review the issues and options, applying the basic principles of ethics to each option. Decide the best option based upon the views of all those concerned in the dilemma.

A—Act by applying chosen action. This step is usually the most difficult as it requires actual implementation. While the previous steps had only allowed for dialogue or discussion.

L—Look back and evaluate the entire process including the implementation. No process is complete without a thorough evaluation. Ensure that those involved are able to follow through on the final option. If not, a second decision may be required and process must start again at the initial step.

Another exchange of traditional model of ethical decision making are as follows:
- Identify the problem.
- Gather data to analyze the causes and consequence of the problem.
- Explore the optional solutions to the problem.
- Evaluate the optional solution.
- Select the appropriate solution from all the options.
- Implement the selected solution.
- Evaluate the result.

STATEMENTS OF ETHICAL RESPONSIBILITY

- Caring demands, the provision of helping services that is appropriate to the needs of the client and significant to others.
- Caring recognizes the client's membership in a family and community, and provides for the participation of significant others in his or her care.
- Caring acknowledges the reality of death in the life of every person, and demands that appropriate support provided to the dying person and family to enable that to prepare for, and to cope with death when it is inevitable.
- Caring acknowledges that the human person has the capacity to face up to health needs and problems in his or her own unique way, and directs nursing action in a manner that will assist the client to develop, maintain or gain personal autonomy, self-respect and self-determination.
- Caring, as a response to a health need, requires the consent and the participation of the person who is experiencing the need.
- Caring dictates that the client and significant others have the knowledge and information adequate for free and informed decisions concerning care requirements, alternative and preferences.
- Caring demands that the needs of the client supersede those of the nurse.
- Caring acknowledges the vulnerability of a client in certain situations and dictates restraint in actions which might compromise the client's rights and privileges.
- Caring involving a relationship which is, in itself therapeutic, demands mutual respect and trust.
- Caring acknowledges that information obtained in the course of the nursing relationship is privileged and that is requires the full protection of confidentiality unless such information provides evidence of serious impending harm to the client or to a third party, or is legally required by the courts.
- Caring requires that the nurse represents the needs of the client and that the nurse takes appropriate measures when fulfillment of these needs is jeopardized by the actions of other persons.
- Caring acknowledges the dignity of all persons in the practice of educational setting.
- Caring acknowledges respects and draws upon the competencies of others.
- Caring establishes the conditions for the harmonization of efforts of different helping professionals in providing required services to clients.
- Caring seeks to establish and maintain a climate of respect for the honest dialogue needed for effective collaboration.
- Caring establishes the legitimacy of respectful challenge and or confrontation when the service required by the client is compromised by incompetency, incapacity or negligence or when the competencies of the nurses are not acknowledged or appropriately utilized.
- Caring demands the provision of working conditions which enable nurses to carry out their legitimate and responsibilities.
- Caring demands resourcefulness and restraint accountability for the use of time, resources, equipment, and funds, and requires accountability to appropriate individuals and/or bodies.
- Caring requires that the nurse bring to the work situation in education, practice, administration or research, the knowledge, affective and technical skills required, and that competency in these areas be maintained and updated.
- Caring commands fidelity, oneself, and guards the right and privilege of the nurse to act in keeping with an informed moral conscience.

PROFESSIONAL ETIQUETTES FOR NURSES

Etiquette is a code of good manners that a nurse should follow. The nurse is an important member of the health team that must work in co-operation and harmony for the care of the sick. For a smooth functioning and a good interpersonal relationship, you as a nurse should follow certain essential good manners.

- The nurse should be courteous to all. Be gentle and polite in your talk.
- The nurse should greet your seniors, co-workers, your patients, etc. with appropriate words and according to the time of the day, e.g. good morning, good evening.
- The nurse should address the seniors with proper title, e.g., sir, madam, sister, mister, miss, etc.
- Stand up when people of higher rank enter your room.
- Stand up when answering questions in the class room.
- Open the door for the senior and stand aside for them to pass.
- Excuse yourself when overtaking a senior person.
- Stand aside and give way to senior when you cross them on the ways, e.g. in the corridors, on the staircases, etc.
- Maintain silence wherever and whenever necessary, e.g. class room, library, study room and dormitories.
- Keep your dress neat and tidy (series arranged and the hair put up).
- While on duty never use any form of jewellery that may interfere with work.
- Obey seniors without arguing.
- Help the seniors to carry a heavy load if you find them on the way.
- Say "thank you" when someone is doing a favor for you, and also when someone corrects you.
- Get prior permission from the sister in charge before you take any article from any department.
- Do not delay the answers to the questions. Give the answer immediately and appropriately.
- Always be punctual.
- Avoid thumb sucking and nail biting.
- In an assembly, let the senior take the seat first.
- Keep eye contact and sit face to face when listing to someone.
- Say "Excuse me" even if you hurt others accidentally.
- Never let others secret go out of you.
- Always close the door after getting into a room or when you get out of the room, if so desired.
- Knock at the door and wait for the answer before you enter into other's room.
- Do not cover the mouth while talking to others. Cover your mouth when you cough or sneeze.
- Excuse yourself before you interfere with others engaged in talking or doing some work.
- The nurse should not give and receive any gifts or present especially from the patients and their relatives.

LEGAL ISSUES IN NURSING

The law constitutes body of principles recognized or enforced by public and regular tribunals have the administration of justice. The law is the body of principles recognized and applied by the state and the administrations of justice. Law is that portion of the established thought and habit which has gained district and formal recognition and the shape of uniform rules backed by the authority and power of the government.

Types of Laws

- **Civil law** includes rules and regulations that specify the required course of action to be followed by an individual in business and social relationships with others. It is concerned with relationships among people and the protection of a person's rights.
- **Criminal law** defines offences that affect public welfare and security and impose penalties. It includes rules forbidding conduct that is injurious to public order and specifying punishments to be administered to individual who exhibits injurious conduct.

Common Legal Issues

- Wrong medications, wrong dosage, wrong route of administration and wrong concentration.
- Mistaken identity-Prepare the wrong patient for an operation, to exchange babies in the labor room.
- To exchange dead bodies in the mortuary.
- Failure to communicate.
- Maintenance of record.
- Giving explanation and getting the concerned.
- Bums and false.
- Counting sponges and instruments during surgery.
- Loss or damage to patient's property and fame.
- Euthanasia or mercy killing—Taking positive step to kill a person in order to end his suffering is a murder.

Law and Nurse

- **Responsibility of appointing and assigning:** The nurse administrators have responsibility for staffing and supervising nursing units to ensure safe, effective patient care. Therefore, they have the authority to temporarily reassign a nursing employee to compensate for emergency staff shortages.
- **Responsibility in quality control:** A nurse manager's legal responsibility for quality control of nursing service imposes a duty to observe report and correct the incompetence of any patient care provider.
- **Responsibility for equipment:** To protect the patients and employees from injury, a nurse manager must ensure that all patient care equipments are fully functional and that defective equipment is promptly repaired or replaced.
- **Responsibility for observation and reporting:** Consequently nurses have a legal duty to observe patients frequently and report findings that have diagnostic or treatment value for the patient's physician and other members of the patient's treatment team.
- **Responsibility to protect public:** The nurse has a legal duty to protect the public from injury by dangerous patients. The manager must ensure that nursing

personnel follow the procedures to alert community members to the presence of a potentially dangerous patient in their midst.
- **Responsibility for record keeping and reporting:** Nurses have legal responsibility for accurately reporting and recording patient's conditions, treatments and response to care. The medical record is an information source document that should be used to plan care, evaluate care, allocate costs, educate personnel, research care measure, and substantiate legal claim.
- **Responsibility for death and dying:** Nurses must be aware of legal definition of death because they must document all events that when the patient is in their care.

INTEGRATING NURSING SERVICE AND NURSING EDUCATION

The field of nursing education basically involves both theoretical and practical knowledge, by theory we mean the most advanced and valid knowledge available that can be generated and applied to many situations. In nursing, the curriculum that is formulated should have a proper framework of theory and practice, the theory which is taught, should help nurses within their field to analyze, synthesis data, organize concepts, principles, suggest new ideas and relations, and even speculate about future nursing. The nursing education to be effective, it needs a good practice, therefore best of good nursing education is whether it can guide for excellent nursing practice. Nursing education and nursing service are both sides of a same coin, so both are equally important, therefore their needs, something called integration which is proper blending of nursing education and practice or service in nursing curriculum.

The nurse educator should choose an appropriate method to teach and practice, whatever the subjects taught about nursing. The nurse educator should make sure the topic meets the objectives of three domains-Cognitive, affective and psychomotor and merging of three appropriately selection of teaching methods in a more realistic situation to the students, supervision of the nursing practice and evaluating this skill is most important. Integrating nursing service is important to give a quality nursing care.

The main goal of education is to equip a person with necessary skill to live effectively and productively in the world of tomorrow. A professional nurse should be productive and humanistic, skillfully blending nursing education (science) with nursing practice (art). Future of nursing as a discrete discipline rests upon strong links between education and every sphere of practice. The difficulties that the new graduates experiencing in making the transition from students to qualified nurses highlights the need for more bridges between education and practice. Preceptor ship is one strategy for assisting new graduates.

The challenge to nursing is to discover strategies to achieve an appropriate balance between artistic and scientific components of nursing. An exploration of the difference between practical and theoretical knowledge, reflection on, in practice and alternative ways of knowing such as maxims, connoisseurship, tacit knowledge which show that all practice is not based on theory. Expertise takes time and cannot be taught. Nurses are urged to move away from perspective rule driven curricula to find ways to provide the impetus for the creative, individualized, context responsive caring, human service oriented, humanistic, critical thinking, human science education that should form the basis of education.

The professional task becomes precondition for ensuring that the training program is really designed to meet the population health needs. The training programs, professional profile and educational program objectives should provide basis for nursing practice in all three levels of health care. Such as primary, secondary and tertiary health care. The advancement to adopted and develop professional skill as specialist is essential. So that the nurses can be prepared as clinical consultants, administrators and as researches in the various fields of nursing practice in order to make both nursing education and practice, identical three principles are fundamental importance.

Another legitimate way of knowing is intuition. The skills required for this are pattern recognition, similarity recognition, common sense understanding, and skilled know-how, sense of salience and deliberations rationality. Intuition is an artistic element, which is unique and cannot be taught but can be enhanced and refined by experience. A number of factors have emerged as significant in enhancing the relationship between nursing educations and nursing practice. In a practice oriented profession such as nursing education and practice are inseparable.

CONCLUSION

Nursing is responsible for encouraging the health of individuals, families, and communities in medical and community settings. Nurses are actively involved in health care research, management, policy deliberations, and patient advocacy. Nurses with post baccalaureate preparation assume independent responsibility for providing primary health care and specialty services to individuals, families, and communities. Nursing encompasses autonomous and collaborative care of individuals of all ages, families, groups and communities, sick or well and in all settings. Nursing includes the promotion of health, prevention of illness, and the care of ill, disabled and dying people. Advocacy, promotion of a safe environment, research, participation in shaping health policy and in patient and health systems management, and education are also key nursing roles.

The profession of nursing has a set of values that act as a standard to guide nursing behavior. The profession expects its members to know, understand, and internalize these values. The interaction of personal, professional and patient values enter into the process of decision making. In an effort to achieve sound ethical and legal decision-making, the faculty directs the student toward the formulation of professional values. Within this framework, the faculty emphasizes that students are directly accountable for their behavior.

BIBLIOGRAPHY

1. Arnold E, Boggs K. Interpersonal relationships: Professional communication skills for nurses, 2nd Ed. Philadelphia: Saunders, 1995.
2. Becker BG, Fendler DJ. Vocational and Personal Adjustments in Practical Nursing, 7th Ed. St. Louis: Mosby-Year Book, Inc, 1994.
3. Craven R, Himle C. Fundamentals of Nursing, 2nd Ed. Philadelphia: Lippincott, 1996.
4. Dietz LD, Hehozky AR. History and Modern Nursing, 2nd Ed. Philadelphia: FA. Davis Co., 1993.
5. Donahue MP. Nursing the Finest Art: An Illustrated History. St. Louis: Mosby Year Book, Inc, 1986.
6. Gordon M. Nursing Diagnosis: Process and Qualification, 3rd ed. New York: McGraw-Hill, 1993.
7. Harkness-Hood G, Dincher JR. Total Patient Care: Foundations and Practice of Adult Health Nursing, 8th Ed. St. Louis: Mosby-Year Book, Inc, 1992.
8. Miller B, Keane C. Encyclopedia Dictionary of Medicine, Nursing, and Allied Health, 6th ed. Philadelphia: Saunders, 1997.
9. Publication Manual of the American Psychological Association. Washington, DC: American Psychological Association, 1994.

REVIEW QUESTIONS

Long Essays

1. Define health promotion, discuss in detail about the levels of prevention of diseases.
2. Define health, explain the determinants of health.
3. Define illness; describe the factors affecting illness behavior.
4. Define hospital; explain the functions and classifications of hospital.
5. Define immunity, discuss in detail about the types of immunity.
6. What are the stages of impact of illness behavior, explain in detail.

Short Essays

1. Define health team; discuss the functions of each member.
2. Define profession and characteristics of profession.
3. Discuss the scope of nursing.
4. Explain the qualities and functions of a nurse.
5. Define ethics; explain the code of ethics in detail.
6. Enumerate the legal responsibilities of the nurse.

Short Answers

1. Describe informed consent.
2. Discuss the ethical responsibilities of a nurse.
3. What is professional etiquette?
4. List out the ethical principles.
5. What are the criteria of profession?
6. Discuss the values of professional nursing.

MULTIPLE CHOICE QUESTIONS

1. The word "nurse" originally came from the Latin word "nutrire" meaning to:
   a. Suckle
   b. Care giver
   c. Comforter
   d. Advisor
2. Trained Nurses Association of India was established/formed in the year:
   a. 1906
   b. 1907
   c. 1908
   d. 1909
3. Mudaliar Committee report published made some recommendations to improve nursing profession in the year:
   a. 1959
   b. 1961
   c. 1969
   d. 1972
4. A WHO publication on "Guide for School of Nursing" in India was published in the year:
   a. 1962
   b. 1963
   c. 1964
   d. 1965
5. The nursing profession is built upon the following key concepts, *except*:
   a. Person
   b. Environment
   c. Health and nursing
   d. Profession

ANSWERS

1. a   2. c   3. b   4. d   5. d

CHAPTER 4

Communication and Nurse–Patient Relationship

LEARNING OBJECTIVES

- Communication: Levels, elements and process, types, modes, factors influencing communication
- Methods of effective communication/therapeutic communication techniques
- Barriers to effective communication/non-therapeutic communication techniques
- Professional communication
- Helping relationships (Nurse–Patient relationship): Purposes and phases
- Communicating effectively with patient, families and team members
- Maintaining effective human relations and communication with vulnerable groups (children, women, physically and mentally challenged and elderly)

INTRODUCTION

Communication is the basic element of human interactions. It is one of the most vital components of all nursing practice. A great deal of nursing practice involves interpersonal communication skills and all the established of relationship essential for successful functioning. For example: communication between the nurse and other members of health team, personnel in other health care agencies or the public. Communication is also a component of therapy, nurses who communicate effectively are able to initiate change that promotes health, establish a trusting relationship with patients and with others, and to prevent legal problems associated with nursing practice **(Fig. 4.1)**.

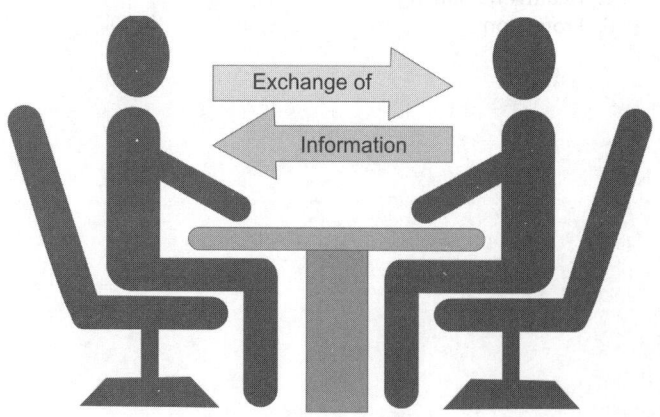

Fig. 4.1: Communication process of exchange of information.

COMMUNICATION: LEVELS, ELEMENTS, TYPES, MODELS, PROCESS AND FACTORS AFFECTING COMMUNICATION

The communication has been derived from Latin word communis, which implies common. Communication is an exchange of facts, ideas, opinions or emotions by two or more persons. Communication is much more than simply transmission of information. It also involves interpretation and understanding of the message. It is an interchange of thoughts and informational intercourse through words, letters, symbols or message.

Definition

- Communication is the process of exchanging information, thought, ideas and feeling from one individual to another.
- Communication is the process by which a message is passed from the sender to the receiver with the objective that the message sent is received and understood as intended.
- Communication is the process of passing information and understanding from one person to another to bring about commonness of interest, efforts, purpose and attitudes.
- Communication is the sum total of the entire things one person does when he wants to create understanding in the mind of another.
- Communication means the interchange of thoughts or informations conveyed to a person in such a way that

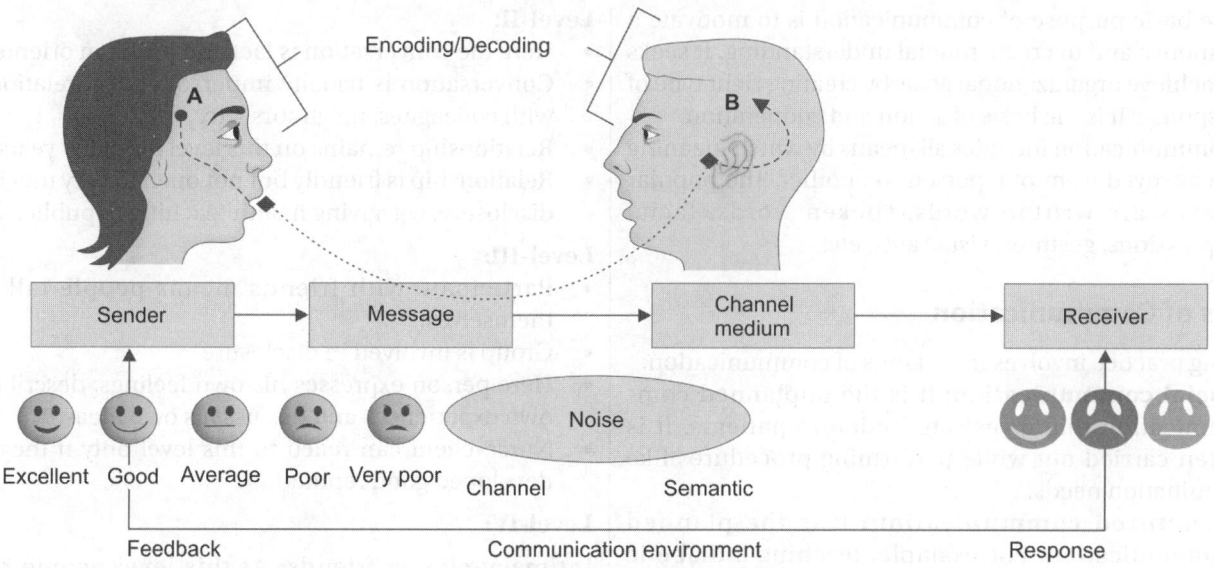

Fig. 4.2: Communication process model.

the meaning received is equivalent to those which the interior of the message intended.

Nature of Communication

- Communication is a two ways or reciprocal process involving exchange of ideas, facts and opinions. The process is not complete unless the receiver has understood the message and his response is known to the sender. Communication involves both informational and understanding. It provides for a feedback mechanism. It is a meeting of minds.
- Communication is a cooperative process involving two or more persons. One person alone cannot communicate. The end-result of communication is mutual understanding.
- The communication is continuous or never-ending process. A manager has to be always in touch with his subordinates and superiors in order to get things done. Communication is also a dynamic activity.
- Communication is pervasive function. It applies to all phases of management and all levels of authority. It travels up and down and also from side to side.

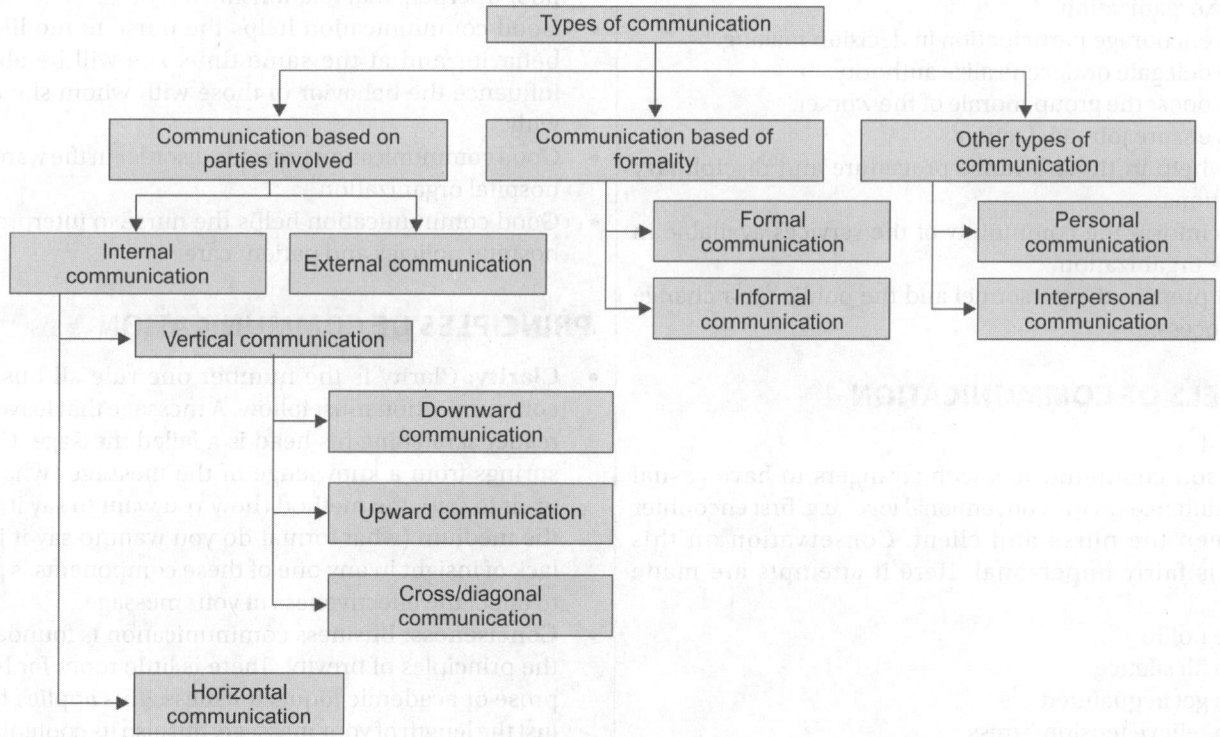

Fig. 4.3: Types of communication.

- The basic purpose of communication is to motivate a response and to create mutual understanding. It seeks to achieve organizational goals by creating right type of response. It is the basis of action and cooperation.
- Communication includes all means by which meaning is conveyed from one person to another. The popular means are written words, spoken words, facial expressions, gestures, visual aids, etc.

Kinds of Communication

Nursing practice involves three kinds of communication:
1. **Social communication:** It is the unplanned communication that gives satisfaction to patients. It is often carried out while performing procedures like elimination needs.
2. **Structured communication:** It is the planned communication. For example, teaching a diabetic patient self administration of insulin injection.
3. **Therapeutic communication:** It is the planned or unplanned communication that is used by nurses in many situations to relieve anxiety and fear in the patients.

Purpose of Communication

- To transfer information between all classes of employees to have a common understanding among them.
- To interpret and adopt policies in the organization.
- To include motivation, cooperation and coordination in the employees.
- To improve employer-employee relationship.
- To recruit, select, train and develop the personnel in the organization.
- To encourage participation in decision making.
- To delegate or decentralize authority.
- To boost the group morale of the worker.
- To ensure job satisfaction.
- To help in the grievance procedure and disciplinary actions.
- To inform the community of the services available in the organization.
- To prepare the personnel and the public for a change process.

LEVELS OF COMMUNICATION

Level-I
A person communicates with strangers to have casual acquaintances in the conventional level, e.g. first encounter between the nurse and client. Conservation on this level is fairly impersonal. Here it attempts are made to:
- Be polite
- To fill silence
- To get acquainted
- To relieve tension/stress
- To convey incidental information.

Level-II:
- Here the conversation is fact and problem oriented.
- Conversation is usually impersonal, e.g. relationship with colleagues, neighbors, etc.
- Relationship remains on this level for many years.
- Relationship is friendly but not open to very much self-disclosure, e.g. giving health teaching to public.

Level-III:
- Participate with friends means people talk with themselves.
- Group is involved in disclosure.
- Here person expresses his own feelings, describes his own experiences and discuss his own ideas.
- Nurse-client can reach to this level only it they have developed good reputation.

Level-IV:
Intimacy-closest friends: At this level people reveal themselves but not they expose themselves intimately in a way that involves risk. Intimate relationships are characterized by communication of feelings and deeply felt mutual understanding, e.g. two close friends.

Importance of Communication

- Communication is important for the nurses to understand and to exchange ideas to the patient and their relatives, the doctors and other members of the health team.
- It reduces the interpersonal tensions and improves the interpersonal relationship.
- Poor communication results in poor patient care and poor interpersonal relationships.
- Good communication helps the nurse to modify her behavior and at the same time, she will be able to influence the behavior of those with whom she deals with.
- Good communication prevents disorder in the ward and hospital organization.
- Good communication helps the nurse to interpret the hospital policies and patient care.

PRINCIPLES OF COMMUNICATION

- **Clarity:** Clarity is the number one rule all business communication must follow. A message that leaves the reader scratching his head is a failed message. Clarity springs from a knowledge of the message (what you want to say), the method (how you want to say it), and the medium (what format do you want to say it in). A lack of insight in any one of these components is going to affect the effectiveness of your message.
- **Conciseness:** Business communication is founded on the principles of brevity. There is little room for lyrical prose or academic loquaciousness. This applies to not just the length of your message, but also its contents. Try to use short sentences and short words. Avoid jargon and

words that send the reader to the dictionary (unless you sell dictionaries!). Adopt this principle for intra-team as well as client focused communication.
- **Objectivity:** Business communication must always have a purpose. This purpose must be apparent to any who glances through your message. Before you put a single word to paper, ask yourself: "what am I trying to achieve with this message?". This will help you stay on course through the message creation process and effect a remarkable improvement in the message efficacy.
- **Consistency:** Imagine that you're reading a book that starts out as a serious medieval romance, turns into a supernatural screwball comedy around the half-way mark, before finally finishing as an avant-garde, high-brow literary exegesis. Without a doubt, such a book will leave you confused and even angry. This is the reason why all business communication must have consistency of tone, voice and content. A humorous satire on one page, a serious explanation on another will alienate your readers. Although you can stray from the set tone from time to time – a few humorous jokes can help lighten the mood – the overall theme must remain consistent.
- **Completeness:** Each message must have a clear and logical conclusion. The reader shouldn't be left wondering if there is more to come. The message must be self-sufficient, that is, it must hold good on its own without support from other messages. This is particularly apt for blog posts which often end abruptly and leave the reader scratching his head.
- **Relevancy:** Every message you send out must be contextually cohesive with previous/future messages. The message must also be relevant to your primary offering. A blog post about Kobe Bryant's free-throw record followed by a webinar on inbound marketing will only leave your readers confused. So make sure that everything you write in a business setting is contextually related and relevant.
- **Audience knowledge:** Lastly, your message must have a thorough understanding of your primary audience. Everything else—clarity, completeness, objectivity—results from your knowledge of your audience. Always know who you are writing for as it will influence the tone, voice and quality of your message.

COMMUNICATION PROCESS

Communication is the two way process involving the sending and receiving of a message. Since the purpose of communication is to elicit a response the process in ongoing. The receiver of the message becomes the sender of the response and the original sender becomes the receiver.

The basic elements of communication are:
- **The sender:** The sender is on the individual or group who wishes to convey the message to another. He is the initiator of the communication process and is sometimes called the source encoder. The individual or group sending the message must have a reason for communicating and must put it in a form that can be transmitted. Encoding means translating the thoughts into specific signs and symbols. Effective encoding depends on a clear message delivered at a right place at right time and phrased in such a way as to attract the receiver's attention.
- **The message:** It is the information that is selected and conveyed by the sender. It requires the sender's decision about what will be side, how, when and where it will be said and the selection of words in a language that can be understood by the receiver.
- **The channel:** It is the means by which the message is transmitted. For example: through the visual, auditory and tactile senses. It is important that the channel be appropriate for the message to make the intent of the message clear. Talking face to face with person may be more effective in some instances than telephoning or writing the message. Recording message on tapes or communicating by radio or television may be appropriate for larger audiences.
- **Receiver:** The receiver is the individual to whom the message is transmitted. This individual is sometimes called the decoder. He interprets and decodes the sender's message into information that has meaning. Understanding is the key to the decoding process. The intended meaning will be communicated when the sender and the receiver have common knowledge and experience.
- **The feedback:** It is the message that the receiver returns to the sender. It is also called feedback. The receiver's verbal and non verbal responses to the sender reveal the receiver understanding of the message. It helps the sender to recognize whether the meaning of his message has been received as intended.

Communication is not successful until the message received has been understood and acted upon appropriately.

Mode or Forms of Communication

- **Verbal communication:** The spoken and/or the written words are the most preferred modes for conveying information of one's ideas, thoughts and feelings to others. The words used vary among individuals according to culture, socioeconomic background, age and education. Examples of written words are:

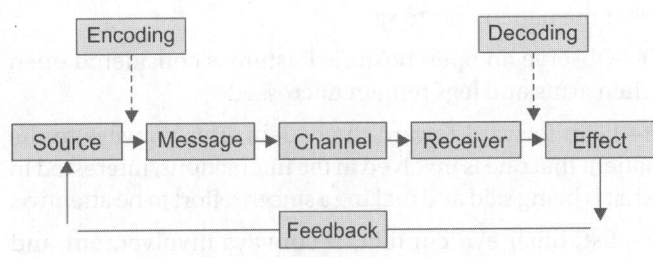

Fig. 4.4: Elements of communication process.

notes, letters, records, forms, news papers, books and magazines.
- **Nonverbal communication:** It is exchange of a message without the use of words. About 80 to 90% communication is nonverbal. It tells others more about what a person is telling than what is actually said because it is controlled less consciously than verbal behavior. Nonverbal communication either reinforces or contradicts what is said verbally.

BASIC COMMUNICATION SKILLS

The word skill means expertness or great proficiency in doing something which comes from training and practice. Apart, from knowledge and technical skill certain other skills are needed for communication.

Human relation skills: Human relation skills include acquisition of such distinct social traits like courtesy, fact, friendliness, speaking skills, etc. These traits are acquired by the individuals and by these traits interpersonal relationship and adjustments, etc. are attained. It is not that, everyone possesses these traits. But there is always room for improvement, if there are efforts on the part of the individuals to recognize these as essential social qualities. Human relation skill is not learned as such but is included during the formative stages of learning.

Listening skills: Listening skills means ability to listen to others. It is an aural skill, and it requires alertness, attentiveness, inquisitiveness, etc. as essential qualities. One must listen well what is being said to him and recognize what tone it connotes, what is the meaning of accompanying gestures, movements of the body etc. Listening is just not simply hearing. A good listener has to be a good observer. A good listener should have the qualities such as:
- Face the person who talks.
- Maintain good eye contact.
- Maintain a natural, well relaxed posture that indicates your interest, e.g. leaning forward towards the other. If the listener repeatedly looks at the watch indicates that she is neither interested in the talk nor relaxed.

Active listening Active listening is good listening and it means to be attentive listening to what the client is expressing verbally and nonverbally. Several nonverbal skills have been identified to facilitate attentive listening and presented the acronym SOLER.

S—Sit squarely while facing the patient. This gives the message that the nurse is there to listen and interested in what the patient has to say.

O—Observe an open posture. Posture is considered open when arms and legs remain uncrossed.

L—Lean forward toward the patient. This conveys to the patient that one is involved in the interactions, interested in what is being said and making a sincere effort to be attentive.

E—Establish eye contact. It conveys involvement and willingness to listen to what the patient has to say.

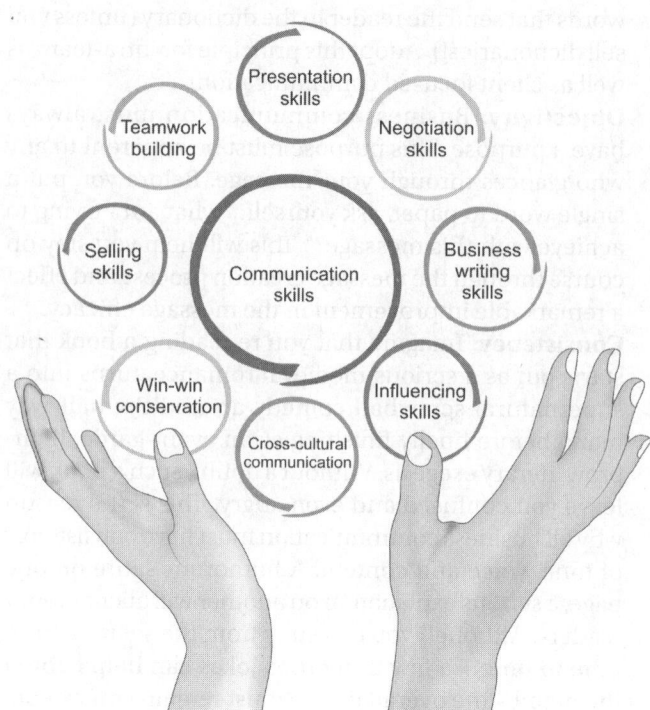

Fig. 4.5: Communication skills.

R—Relax whether sitting or standing during the interaction, the nurse should communicate a sense of being relaxed and comfortable with the patient. Restlessness and forgetting to communicate conveys a lack of interest and a feeling of discomfort.

Writing and reading skills: To develop this one must know the language and should have good vocabulary to clarify his thought which are expressed through writing. The words chosen should be simple but powerful to express the meaning correctly. Writing should be legible and devoid of ambiguity. The writing skill requires reading skill also. The tonal control, the pitch etc. should be kept under control but audible. A touch of emotionality and concern should be there in writing and reading in all the cases.

Drawing skill: Drawing skills requires control of the hand movement and of fingers. Drawing should be simple with minimum of times and maximum of force in the line. There should be meaning and justification in selecting colors.

FACTORS AFFECTING COMMUNICATION PROCESS

In addition to the factors such as a person's socio-cultural background, language, age, education, limitations and attributes of nonverbal communication, the following factors affects the communication process.

Ability of the Communicator

The person's ability to speak, hear, see and comprehend stimuli influences the communication process. The receiver of a message also needs to interpret the message. Even if a patient is free of physical impairments the nurse needs to determine how many stimuli the patient is capable of receiving in a given time frame. The nurse must be careful not to talk too quickly or present too many ideas at once, particularly when offering health instructions.

Perceptions

It is the personal view of events, i.e. each person's sense, interprets and understands the events differently. Perceptions are formed by experience and expectations. It is important in many situations to validate or correct the perceptions of the receiver.

Attitude

It is the tendency or predisposition to act in a particular direction to a thing, a person or an event. Attitudes are communicated convincingly and rapidly to others. The attitude classified in to facilitating attitudes and inhibitive attitudes.

Facilitating Attitudes

- Caring and warming attitudes convey a feeling of emotional closeness, in contrast to impersonal distance. Caring involves giving feelings, thoughts, skills and knowledge.
- Respect is an attitude that emphasizes the other person's worth and individuality. A nurse conveys respect by listening open-mindedly to what the other persons is saying even if the nurse disagrees.
- Acceptance emphasizes neither approval nor disapproval. An accepting attitude allows clients to express personal feelings freely and to be themselves. The nurse may need to restrict acceptance in situations where client's actions are harmful to themselves or to others.

Inhibitive Attitudes

- Condensation: It is an attitude that conveys superiority over other persons.
- Lack of interest: This also inhibits the communication by indicating a lack of concern or a belief that what the person is saying is not important. Lack of interest in the form of not listening to patient or skipping the care to patient may be conveyed by the nurse.
- Coldness: This is the opposite of caring and warmth. Nurses convey this attitude to clients by appearing more interested in the technical and procedural aspects of nursing than in concerns of the persons receiving the therapy.

Knowledge

Knowledge of handling different level persons is essential for communication. An amount of knowledge a source has about the subject matter will affect his message content materials be communicated with maximum effectiveness.

Time

The time factor in communication includes the events that precede and follow the interaction. Nurses' use of time can facilitate or inhibit a client's communication.

Personal Space

Personal space is the distance between the people in interactions with others. Proxemics is the study of distance between people in their interactions. Communication utters in accordance with four distance, each with close and a far phase, described by Hall.
- Intimate: Physical contact to one and half feet.
- Personal: One and half to four feet.
- Social: Four to twelve feet.
- Public: Twelve feet and beyond.

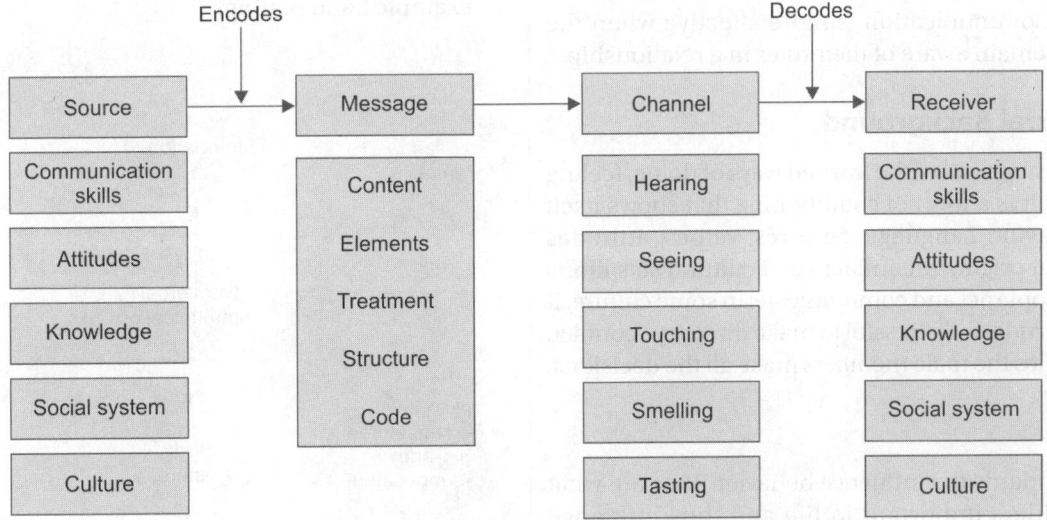

Fig. 4.6: Factors affecting communication process.

Environment

People usually communicate most effectively in a comfortable environment. Warm and comfortable environment facilitates good communication. The setting also influences communication. If the room lacks privacy or is hot, noisy or crowded, the communication process can break down. Environmental distraction can impair and distort communication.

Territory

Territoriality is the drive to gain, maintain and defined as exclusive right to an area of space. It provides people with a sense of identity, security and control. Client often feels the need to defend their territory when others invade it.

Emotions

Emotions are person's subjective feeling about events. The way a person relates or communicates with others is influenced by emotions. Emotions also affect a person's ability to interpret messages. For example a client may feels great fear in remembering, all postoperative instructions offered by the nurse.

Self-esteem

Self-esteem also influences communication patterns, people whose self-esteem is high communicate honestly, with confidence and with congruence (agreement or coinciding) between verbal and nonverbal messages. Those with low self-esteem or under high stress tend to give double messages. The relationship between self-concept and communication is susceptible to change.

Roles and Relationships

The roles and the relationship between sender and the receiver affect the communication process. Choice of words, sentence structure and tone of voice vary considerably from role to role. Communication is more effective when the participants remain aware of their roles in a relationship.

Socio-cultural Background

Culture is the sum total of the learned ways of doing, feeling and thinking. It is a form of conditioning that shows itself through behavior. Language, gestures, values, attitudes reflect cultural origin. The influence of cultural sets limits for the way people act and communicate. In some culture, it is considered rude or distressful to make direct eye contact. In some families the male members make all the decisions.

Values

These are standards the influence behavior. They are what person considers important in life and thus influence expressions of thoughts and ideas.

NONVERBAL COMMUNICATION

- **Physical appearance including adornment:** Personals appearance, body shapes, size, hair styles, clothing and adornments are sometimes rich sources of information about a person. Clothing may convey social and financial status, culture, religion and self concepts. Adornments such as jewellery, perfume, or cosmetics may reveal addition information's. How the person dresses is often an indicator of how the person feels. The nurse needs to be sensitive to sudden changes in a patient's dress; that may be a signal of loss of self-esteem or feeling better.
- **Posture and gait:** The way people walk and carry themselves are often reliable indications of self-concept; mood and health, e.g. erect posture and an active, purposeful walk suggest a feeling of well-being, while tense posture suggests anxiety or anger.
- **Facial expressions:** The face is the most expressive part of the body. Feeling of joy, sadness, fear, surprise, anger and disgust can be conveyed by facial expressions. Many facial expressions convey a universal meaning, e.g. a smile conveys happiness.
- **Eye contact:** The eyes may provide the most revealing and accurate of all communication signals, because they are a point on the body. Mutual eye contact acknowledges recognition of the other person and willingness to maintain communication. Total lack of eye contact may signal low self-esteem, while too much eye contact (staring) is inappropriate, e.g. a patient who feels weak or defenseless often avoids eye contact.
- **Body movements:** Body movements may sometimes take the place of speech, e.g. a shrug of the shoulders to say, I don't know. Some of the basic communication gestures are same throughout the world and convey the same message, e.g. nodding the head is almost universally used to indicate yes, and the hand shake is a victory sign.
- **Touch:** Touch is the most personal form of communication because it brings people into a close relationship, example hand patting.

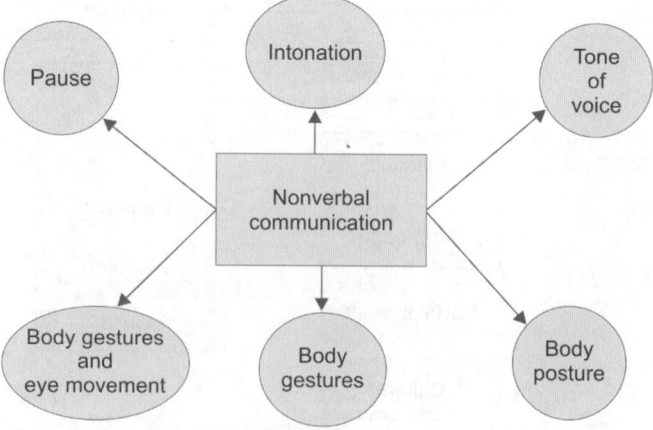

Fig. 4.7: Types of nonverbal communication.

- **Tone of voice:** It can cause people to listen to speech or to be inattentive and unresponsive. An individual's personal warmth, honesty and competence is often displayed by the tone he uses with others.
- **Symbols:** A symbol is a sign that represents ideas.
- **Signals:** A signal is a sign to give instructions or warning, e.g. the patient puts on the signals light when he wishes to call a nurse, traffic signals etc.,

THE BEST MODEL

- Begin with nonverbal cues. Soften (smile, open arms, forward lean, touch with arm, handshake, eye contact, nod).
- Establish information gathering with informal talk.
- Support with emotional channels.
- Terminate with positive notes.

The BEST model fills this void. It includes comprehensive verbal and nonverbal ways of communicating, along with emotional support, showing empathy is important to facilitate any clinical interview; empathy increases efficiency and information gathering, and shows respect. Time spent in listening helps to clarify your patient's agenda and draws attention to their imminent needs. This in turn builds patient's confidence.

Begin with nonverbal cues: Communication starts well before talking, for example; in clinic when you call a patient to your consulting room, there is nonverbal communication when you look at each other's face and gesture. Soften is a mnemonic for a series of nonverbal gestures that makes people more responsive to us. A smile indicates a friendly and open attitude. Smiling puts patients at ease and helps them feel comfortable in an environment that can be stressful. An open body posture can convey a sense of being open minded and allows patient to feel they can reach you. Learning forward slightly while talking shows your interest and encourages patients to talk. Take care not to get too close or invade personal space, though.

Eye contact is the strongest nonverbal gesture and indicates you are listening to what your patient, colleague, or relative has to say. Even when it's your turn to speak, you continue to listen with your eyes. If you realize by your patient's facial expression that you have said something incorrect, correct yourself. Nodding shows you have listened carefully, and encourages the other person to keep talking. More than two third of face conversation is based on body language. This is the aspect that often goes wrong. Leaving patients unsatisfied. It has been estimated that physicians interrupt patients within 23 seconds as they to explain their problems. Be conscious of that.

Establishing Information Gathering with Informal Talk: Informal gathering is an art. Actively control, not by talking more or stopping conversation but by guiding conversations towards relevant topics, at the same time interpreting symptoms. Another good skill is to talk to patients while examining them. If often puts patients at ease, helping them to relax.

Support with emotional channels: There is Chinese proverb "words are just words, and without heart, they have no meaning". Support your conversation with emotional channels, listen to the unsaid, share feelings and transmit a message heart to heart, allowing nonverbal, two way communication. Empathy is important in any trusting relationship with patients. Your eyes, face and gestures should all support you in demonstrating your continued interest in your patients. Keep nodding while the other person is talking, or when you're talking to emphasize important issues. Concentrate on what is being said and put your emotional energy into addressing patient's concerns. In some cases, you may need to get past the tone of voice in order to listen effectively. Do not dismiss that patient if their tone portray them as a complainer, as they may be angry or distressed. Before you do that, listen and make sure there are no legitimate issues you need to address.

Terminate with positive note: Terminate conversation on a positive note. It is good to summarize briefly what you discuss and ask if there are any other concerns. If you have been listening carefully, you will be able to fine at least a few relevant points that you can convert to positives. Try to instill hope. Keeping these BEST steps in mind will help you do a swift consultation and maximize patient satisfaction. It is hard to consciously think of these initially but if practiced for three weeks, a good proportion of these steps ought to infuse your practice. Remember, effective communication has a positive impact on patients. They will feel more involved and empowered in their treatment. This also allows complaints redressals, and increased time efficiency, so follow the BEST model for the best results.

BARRIERS IN COMMUNICATION

Though communication is essential, perfect communication is rarely achieved in practice. There are obstacles which continuously block and distort the flow of ideas and information. Some of these barriers to communication are given below.

- **Badly expressed messages:** Very often the message is expressed in poorly chosen words or empty phrases, lack of coherence, poor organization of ideas, awkward sentence structure. There is use of inappropriate language, poor vocabulary and ambiguous words. The lack of clarity and precision lead to misunderstanding, costly errors and unnecessary clarification. Different people drive different meanings from the same words or symbols due to difference in their education, experience and orientation.
- **Organizational distance:** A complex of faulty organization structure involving several layers of supervision, a long chain of command, and complex line staff relations impedes the interchange of ideas and information. At every layer of the structure the message gets distorted. Long communication lines, presence of specialties and distance between top management

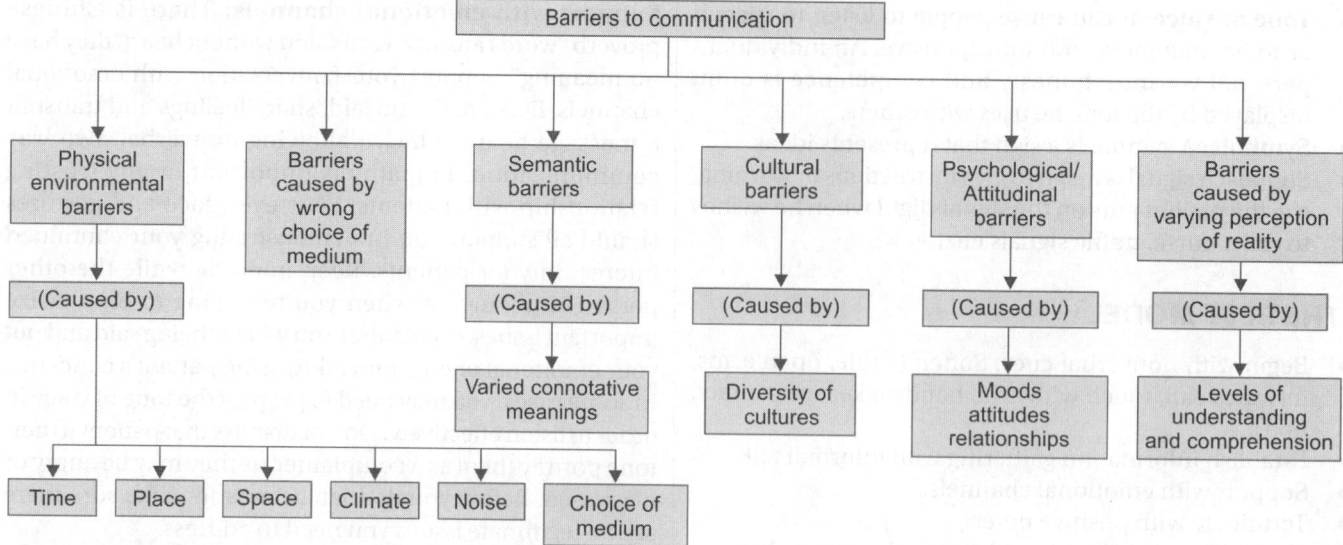

Fig. 4.8: Barriers to communication.

and workers create difficulties in communication. It is necessary to make improvements in the organization structure in order to overcome these difficulties.

- **Status and position:** Vertical communication is hampered by difference in the status and position of the superior and subordinate. Status refers to the regard and attitude of member of the organization towards a position and its occupant. Status arises on account of formal position in the hierarchy, job title, salary and other privileges. Supervisors tend to keep information to themselves and they do not want to listen to subordinates. Subordinates are reluctant to seek clarification for fear of loss of prestige. Effective communication becomes difficult when people become strong conscious of status and position. Subordinates tend to tell the boss what is pleasant and withhold unpleasant information.
- **Inattention:** Many people simply do not pay adequate attention to the message. They do not listen to the spoken words attentively or they fail to read the message carefully. Generally, people pay attention to the information which confirms their beliefs and ignore those conflicts with what they believe. Such selective listening hampers effective communication.

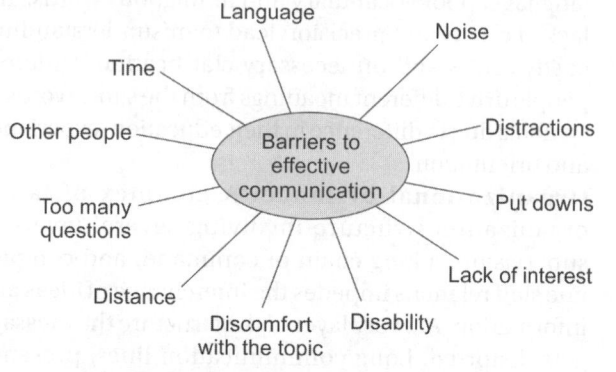

Fig. 4.9: Barriers to effective communication.

Sometimes people pay perfunctory attention because they are victims of communication overload or because the information is solicited. Communication overload arises when people possess more information than they can assimilate or cannot adequately respond to the messages directed to them. Inattention also arises due to lack of interest, over stimulation, tendency to criticize the mode of delivery or noting everything. The source of communication and the way in which it is presented also determine the degree of attention paid to it. Listening is the most neglected skill of communication.

- **Poor retention (screening or filtering):** Successive transmissions of the same message are decreasingly accurate. At each level, the message is screened by receiver and only such information is passed further which gives a favorable impression of the sender. Such filtering arises due to the fact that no one likes to show his mistakes to others. Noise can distort communication at every step in the communication process. In order to overcome the barrier of filtering, it is necessary to develop a well-designed feedback system and rapport with subordinates. The manager should listen to subordinate with an understanding attitude.
- **Perception:** When people with different perceptions communicate, they have trouble in getting the meaning across. Every one perceives the message from his own angle or viewpoint. Perceptions of people differ due to differences in their needs, education, social back ground, interest, etc. in the absence of an open mind and willingness to see things through the eyes of others; people perceive the same information differently. When the communicator does not enjoy trust and credibility, he fails to convey his ideas to others. Differences in value judgments and references frames also inhibit communication.

- **Resistance to change:** Human being by nature prefers to maintain status quo and generally resist new ideas. When the communication contains a new idea, the receiver may not take it seriously or may receive it according to his own convenience. Everyone likes to receive the information which confirms his present belief and tends to ignore anything that is contrary to such belief. A manager should provide sufficient time and assistance to make subordinates receptive to change.

How to overcome the barriers of communication:
Effective communication is essential for successful interpersonal relationship. Breakdown in communication are not only expensive and time consuming, they also are injurious to team-work and morale. It is, therefore, necessary to take steps to ensure effective communication. Though, it may not possible to eliminate these barriers altogether, effort must be made to achieve adequate communication. The following measures can be adopted for this purpose.

- **Clarify the idea:** The communicator must be quiet clear about what he wants to communicate. He should know the objective of his communication. Very often the communicator mistakes the form of communication for its subject matter. Too much attention is paid to media and devices and too little to purpose and content. The mind of the message should be clearly formulated in the mind of the communicator. It should be expressed in as simple and precise language as possible so that the receiver can understand it easily and quickly. The message should be concise, concrete and correct. Technical terms should be avoided and the language of the listener should be used. This obviously requires a familiarity with the language patterns of the receiver.
- **Completeness of the message:** The information is not supplied, people assumptions about the message must be complete, timely and adequate in all respects, and otherwise it is likely to be misunderstood. No important details should be omitted and underlying assumptions must be clarified. If all the information is not supplied, people make assumption about the missing information. This can distort the meaning. Incomplete communication delays action spoils relations and increases costs. The message should be relevant to the nature and purpose of the communication.
- **Understand the receiver:** The communicator must become aware of the total physical and human setting in which the message will be received. Before conveying the message he must find out the needs, feelings, receptivity, perceptions and understanding levels of the communicate. The message should be designed from the viewpoint of the receiver. The sender of the message must work at the problems from the receiver's point of view. This is called empathy in communications.
- **Use appropriate channels:** The media and channels used in communication must be appropriate to the message, the receiver and the purpose of communication. A judicious combination of formal and informal channels and written and oral media will help to improve the effectiveness of communication. Use of multiple channels, certain amount of repetition and participation of subordinates is essential for an orderly flow of information.
- **Consistency in communication:** The message should be consistent with objectives, policies and programmes of the organization. This will avoid chaos and confusion in the organization. Different messages should not mutually conflict. Whenever it is necessary to amend the old message; this fact should be started in the new message to avoid confusion and chaos. Communication should be supported by actions and behavior to ensure credibility in communications. Actions speak louder than words. If actions are contrary to communications, people do not take them seriously.
- **Feed back:** Communication should be a two-way process. The communicator should try to know the reactions of the receiver. The use of feedback mechanism invokes effective participation of subordinates and it help to make future communications more effective. There should be continuous evaluation of the flow of communication in different directions. A feedback system helps to build up mutual understanding and distortions of message can be avoided. Feedback indicates the return flow of communication.
- **Simplified structure:** The communication system can be strengthened by simplifying the procedure, reducing the layer, making constructive use of grapevine and regulating information flow. Lines of communication should be as short and direct as possible and the number of levels should be minimized. Regulating the flow of information eliminates communication overload and ensures an optimum flow of information to members of organization. Filtering of information should be discouraged. The communication system should be tailor made to the needs and characteristics of the enterprise.
- **Improve listening:** The sender of the message as well as receiver must listen with attention, patience and empathy. The communicator can gather useful information for future messages by good listening. Generally, manager suffers from bad listening and they need to avoid value judgments. They must develop awareness of actions and their impact on others. They must develop the habit of empathic listening to secure free and frank responses.
- **Mutual trust and confidence:** Communication is an interpersonal process. Therefore, it can be made effectively by developing mutual trust, respect and confidence among the members of the organization.

INTERPERSONAL RELATIONSHIP

The nurse is an important member of a team that must work in cooperation and harmony for the care of patients. She should be familiar with the plan of organization of the hospital and of the nursing department. The nurse must feel accountable to the organization, should be honest, dependable and willing to carry out the prescribed treatment and care for the patient. She should maintain her position and dignity. She should not accept verbal orders from the physician (medical personnel). There should be a team spirit. The nurse should have respect for the senior and concern and caring attitude towards fellow nurses, juniors and other supporting staff. She should maintain a healthy and good relationship with various departments.

Skills of Interpersonal Relationship

- **Verbal communication:** What we say and how we say it.
- **Nonverbal communication:** What we communicate without words, body language is an example.
- **Listening skills:** How we interpret both the verbal and nonverbal messages sent by others.
- **Negotiation:** Working with others to find a mutually agreeable outcome.
- **Problem solving:** Working with others to identify, define and solve problems.
- **Decision making:** Exploring and analyzing options to make sound decisions.
- **Assertiveness:** Communicating our values, ideas, beliefs, opinions, needs and wants freely.

Principles of Interpersonal Relationship

- Respect every one's individuality. Each member of a team is as important as the other.
- Do not impose anything on anybody.
- Keep emotion under control.
- Do not be afraid to admit ignorance.
- Do not give and take any personal favor.
- The team leader should not make any excuse regarding his or her responsibility.
- Develop habits of listening and focus attention on the problems.
- Do not do or say anything that will disturb other's faith.
- Be impartial to others and practice justice.
- The members of team should be loyal, honest, dependable and willing to carry out the directions of the team leader.
- There should be team spirit or we feeling among the members. The members should work for the interest of the group.
- There should be mutual understanding between the members; they should be willing to give and take corrections.

Elements of professional communication: Professional appearance, demeanor, and behavior are important in establishing the nurse's trustworthiness and competence. A professional is expected to be clean, neat, well groomed, conservatively dressed and scent and odor free. Professional behavior should reflect warmth, friendliness, confidence and competence. Elements which are present in the professional communication are:

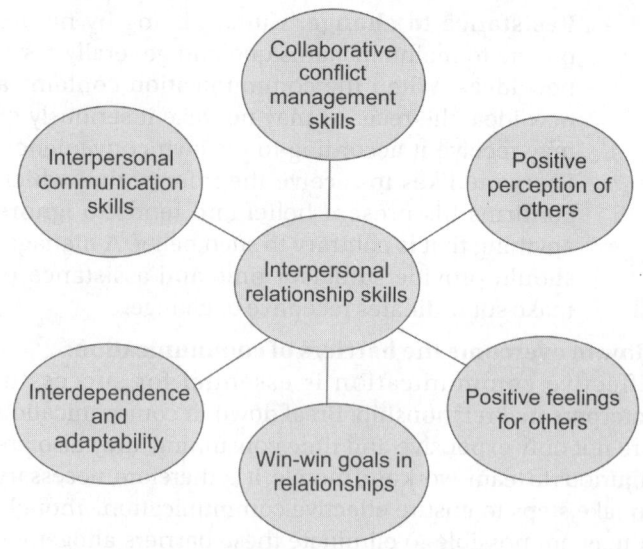

Fig. 4.10: Interpersonal relationship skills.

- Courtesy
- Use of names
- Privacy and confidentiality
- Trustworthiness
- Autonomy and responsibility
- Assertiveness.

Courtesy: Common courtesy is part of professional communication. To practice courtesy the nurse says hello and goodbye, knocks on doors before entering and uses self-introduction. The nurse also states his or her purpose, addresses people by name, says please and thank you to team members and apologizes for inadvertently making an error or causing someone distress.

Use of names: Self introduction is important in communication. The nurse's failure to give a name, indicate status or acknowledge the client can create uncertainty about the interaction and convey an impersonal lack of commitment or caring. Addressing other by name conveys respect for human dignity and uniqueness. Avoid referring to clients by diagnosis, room number or other attribute, which is demeaning and sends the message that the nurse does not care enough to know the person as an individual.

Privacy and confidentiality: Maintaining confidentiality is an important aspect of professional behavior. It is essential that the nurse safeguard the client's right to privacy by carefully protecting information of a sensitive, private nature. Sharing personal information or gossiping about others violates nursing ethical codes and practice standards. It sends the message that the nurse cannot be trusted and damages interpersonal relationships.

Trustworthiness: Trust is relying on someone without doubt or question. Being trustworthy means helping others without hesitation when help is needed. To foster trust, the nurse communicates warmth and demonstrates consistency, reliability, honesty and competence. Sometimes it is not easy for a client to ask for help. Trusting

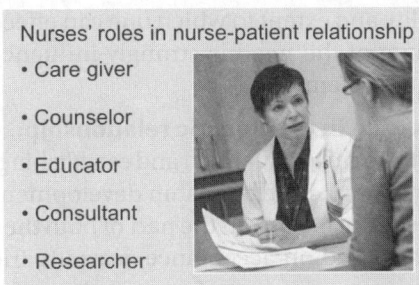

Fig. 4.11: Role of nurse in Nurse–patient relationship.

another person involves risk and vulnerability but it also faster's open, therapeutic communication and enhances the expression of feeling, thoughts and needs.

Autonomy and responsibility: Autonomy is the ability to be self-directed and independent in accomplishing goals and advocating for other. Professional nurses make choices and accept responsibility for the outcomes of their actions. They take initiative in problem solving and communicate in a manner that reflects what they really need and want. Autonomy can be beneficial to the client because people who seek health care are often concerned about losing control of decisions that influence how they live.

Assertiveness: According to Darley, assertiveness comprises respect for others, respect for yourself, self-awareness and effective, clear, and consistent communication. Assertiveness conveys a sense of self assurance while also communicating respect for the other person. Nurses can teach assertiveness skills to others as a means for promoting personal health. Assertive people express feeling and emotions confidently, spontaneously, and honestly. They make decisions and control their lives more effectively than non assertive individuals. Assertive responses are characterized by feelings of security, competence, power, optimism and professionalism. They are good tool for dealing with criticism, change, negative conditions in personal or professional life and conflict or stress in relationship.

Role of Nurse in Interpersonal Relationship

- The patient in the hospital experience new and unfamiliar surroundings. It is uptown the nurse to see that the patient feels at ease and adjusts to the hospital routine and the new environment, to help, to cooperate and accept treatment necessary for regaining health.
- The patient is an important person in the hospital. Treat him as an individual, call him by his name. Help him to overcome fear and anxiety. The nurse should be dignified, cheerful and courteous. Be pleasant with patients but not too familiar. Treat them with sympathy and firmness to gain respect and admiration. Personal appearance is very important in establishing a good nurse patient relationship. The nurse should not talk or discuss personal affairs or about other patients or hospitals. The nurse—patient relationship must be professional and one of absolute trust, irrespective of caste, creed, or social status. She should not accept any personal gift from patients.
- The nurse is an important member of a team that must work in cooperation and harmony for the care of patients. She should be familiar with the plan of organization of the hospital and of the nursing department.
- The nurse must feel accountable to the organization, should be honest, dependable and willing to carry out the prescribed treatment and care for the patient. She should maintain her position and dignity. She should not accept verbal orders from the physician (medical personnel). There should be a team spirit.
- The nurse should have respect for the senior and concern and caring attitude towards fellow nurses, juniors and other supporting staff. She should maintain a healthy and good relationship with various departments.

THERAPEUTIC NURSE-PATIENT RELATIONSHIP

In any nurse-client relationship it is the responsibility of the nurse to establish and maintain appropriate boundaries. Maintaining professional boundaries is an essential component in the provision of safe, competent and ethical nursing care. Nurses must exercise professional judgment when establishing a therapeutic relationship with the client taking into consideration the clients cultural, spiritual, mental and biophysical needs. The nurse-client relationship is the foundation upon which nursing is established. It is the relationship in which both the participation must recognize each other as unique and important human being.

Definition

- Nurse-client relationship is a helping relationship that is therapeutic in nature, is established to meet the needs of clients and is based up on trust and respect.
- A therapeutic nurse-client relationship is established and maintained by the nurse through the use of professional nursing knowledge, skills and caring

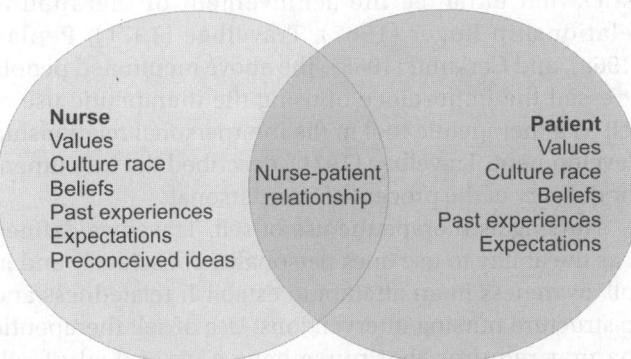

Fig. 4.12: Factors influencing nurse-patient relationship.

attitudes and behaviors in order to provide nursing services that contribute to the client's health and well-being.
- The therapeutic nurse-patient relationship is the process by which nurses provide care for clients in need psychological intervention.
- Interpersonal communication techniques-Both verbal and nonverbal are the tools of psychological intervention.
- Therapeutic relationships are goal oriented and goal directed at learning and growth promotion in an effort to bring about some type of change in clients life.

Goals of a Therapeutic Relationship

- Facilitate communication of distressing thoughts and feelings.
- To assist client with problem solving to help daily living.
- Help client examine self-defeating behaviors and test alternatives.
- Promote self care and independence.

Nurses Role and Therapeutic Communication

Nurse helps the client to cope-up with strategies dealing with specific situation such as:
- Helping the client to identify what is troubling the client.
- Encourage to discuss about the changes needed to make in the client.
- Explore the feeling about the aspects that cannot be charged, alternative modes of coping.
- Discuss alternative strategies for creating changes the client desires to make.
- Discuss the benefits and consequences of each alternative.
- Assist the client to select an alternative.
- Encourage the client to implement the change.
- Provide positive feedback for the client's attempts to create change.
- Assist the client to evaluate outcomes of the change and make modifications as required.

Conditions essential to development of therapeutic relationships: Several theorists have identified characteristics that enhance the achievement of therapeutic relationship Roger (1967), Travelbee (1971), Peplau (1969), and Carkhuff (1968). The above mentioned people stressed the importance of using the therapeutic use of self as a therapeutic tool in the interpersonal relationship development. Travelbee (1971), described the instrument for delivery of the process of interpersonal

Nursing as therapeutic use of self, Travelbee defined it as the ability to use ones personality consciously and in full awareness in an attempt to establish relatedness and to structure nursing interventions. Use of self therapeutic manner requires that nurse have a great deal of self awareness and self understanding, nurses must understand that the ability and extent to which one can effectively help others in time of the need is strongly influenced by this internal value system.

Conditions used in therapeutic relationship:
- **Rapport:** Getting acquainted and establishing rapport is the primary task in relationship development. Rapport implies special feeling on the part of both the client and the nurse based on acceptance, warmth, friendliness, common interest, sense of trust and non-judgmental attitude.
- **Trust:** Trust is the basis of a therapeutic relationship, trust cannot be presumed, it must be earned, and trustworthiness is demonstrated through the nursing interventions that convey a sense of warmth and caring of client. Without establishing trust, helping relationship will not progress beyond; it will be a kind of mechanical relationship only to meet the superficial needs of a client. For example, to establish trust, a nurse can:
    - Provide blanket when the client feels cold.
    - Keeping promises.
    - Provide food when the client is hungry.
    - Being honest.
    - Ensuring confidentiality.
- **Respect:** To show respect is to believe in the dignity and worth of an individual, nurse should be able to respect him and should consider him/her worthwhile and treat as human being. The nurse can convey respect by:
    - Calling by name.
    - Spending time with client.
    - Allowing sufficient time for the client to answer the questions.
    - Promoting an atmosphere of privacy during therapeutic interventions without client.
- **Genuineness:** The concept of genuineness refers to the nurses ability to be open, honest and real in interactions with the client, the nurse who possesses the quality of genuineness responds to the client with truth and honesty, client feel more comfortable revealing personal information to the nurse.
- **Empathy:** Empathy is a process where in an individual is able to see beyond outward behavior and sense accuracy another inner experience at a given time. With empathy, the nurse can accurately perceive and understand the meaning and relevance of the client's thoughts and feelings. A relationship is defined as a state of being related or state of affinity between two individuals.
- **Power:** The power of the nurse comes from the authority of own position in the health care system, specialized knowledge, influence with other health care providers and the client's significant others, and access to privileged information.
- **Intimacy:** Intimacy related to the kind of activities nurses perform for and with the client which create personal and private closeness on many levels. This can involve physical, emotional and spiritual elements.

Types of Relationship

- **Social relationship:** It is a most common kind of relationship; both individuals are equally involved in this relationship and are concerned with meeting their own needs through the relationship.
- **Intimate relationship:** It is a relationship between two individuals committed to one another, caring for and responding each other.
- **Therapeutic relationship:** The nurse and client work together toward the goal of assisting the client to regain the inner resources to meet the life challenges and facilitate the growth.

Therapeutic Communication Techniques

Sl. No.	Technique	Description
1.	Using silence	Accepting pauses or silences that may extend for several seconds or minutes without interjecting any verbal response.
2.	Proving general leads	Using statements or questions that (a) encourage the client to verbalize, (b) choose a topic of conversation and (c) facilitate continued verbalization.
3.	Being specific and tentative	Making statements that are specific rather than general, and tentative rather than absolute.
4.	Using open-ended questions	Asking broad questions that lead or invite the client to explore (elaborative, clarify, describe, compare, or illustrate) thoughts or feeling. Open-ended questions specify only the topic to be discussed and invite answers that are longer than one or two words.
5.	Using touch	Proving appropriate forms of touch to reinforce caring feelings. Because tactile contacts vary considerably among individuals, families and cultures, the nurse must be sensitive to the differences in attitudes and practices of clients and self.
6.	Restarting or paraphrasing	Actively listening for the client's basic message and then repeating those thoughts and / or feelings in similar words. This conveys that the nurse has listened and understands the client's basic message and also offers clients a clear idea of what they have said.
7.	Seeking clarification	A method of making the client's broad overall meaning of the message more understandable. It is used when paraphrasing is difficult or when the communication is rambling or garbled. To clarify the message, the nurse can restate the basic message or conflicts confusion and ask the client to repeat or restate the message.
8.	Perception checking or seeking consensual validation	A method similar to clarifying verifies the meaning of specific words rather than overall meaning of a message.
9.	Offering self	Suggesting one's presence, interest, or wish to understand the client without making any demands or attaching conditions that the client must comply with to receive the nurse's attention.
10.	Giving information	Providing, in a simple and direct manner, specific factual information the client may or may not request. When information is not known, the nurse states this and indicates who has it or when the nurse will obtain it.
11.	Acknowledging	Giving recognition, in a nonjudgmental way, of a change in behavior, an effort the client has made, or a contribution to a communication. Acknowledgment may be with or without understanding, verbal or nonverbal.
12.	Clarifying time or sequence	Helping the client clarify an event, situation, or happening in relationship to time.
13.	Presenting reality	Helping the client to differentiate the real from the unreal.
14.	Focusing	Helping the client expand on and develop a topic of importance. It is important for the nurse to wait until the client finishes stating the main concerns before attempting to focus. The focus may be an idea or a feeling; however, the nurse often emphasizes a feeling to help the client recognize an emotion disguised behind words.
15.	Reflecting	Directing ideas, feelings, questions, or content back to clients to enable them to explore their own ideas and feelings about a situation
16.	Summarizing and planning	Stating the main points of a discussion to clarify the relevant points discussed. This technique is useful at the end of an interview or to review a health teaching session. It often acts as an introduction to future care planning.
17.	Stereotyping	Offering generalized and oversimplified beliefs about groups of people that are based on experiences too limited to be valid. These responses categorize clients and negate their uniqueness as individuals.

Contd...

Contd...

Sl. No.	Technique	Description
18.	Agreeing and disagreeing	Akin to judgment response, agreeing and disagreeing imply that the client is either right or wrong and that the nurse is in a position to judge this. These responses deter clients from thinking through their position and may cause a client to become defensive.
19.	Being defensive	Attempting to protect a person or health care services from negative comments. These responses prevent the client from expressing the true concerns. The nurse is saying you have no right to complain. Defensive responses protect the nurse from admitting weaknesses in the health care services, including personal weaknesses.
20.	Challenging	Giving responses that make clients prove their statement or point of view. These responses indicate the nurse is failing to consider the client's feelings, making the client feel it necessary to defend a position.
21.	Probing	Asking for information chiefly out of curiosity rather than with the intent to assist the client. These responses are considered prying and violate the client's privacy. Asking why is often probing and places the client in a defensive position.
22.	Testing	Asking questions that make the client admit to something. These responses permit the client only limited answers and often meet the nurse's need rather than the clients.
23.	Rejecting	Refusing to discuss certain topics with the client. These responses often make clients feel that the nurse is rejecting not only their communication but also the clients themselves.
24.	Changing topics and subjects	Directing the communication into areas of self-interest rather than considering the client's concerns is often a self-protective response to a topic that causes anxiety. The responses imply that the nurse considers important will be discussed and that clients should not discuss certain topics.
25.	Unwarranted reassurance	Using clichés or comforting statements of advice as a means to reassure the client. These responses block the fear, feelings and other thoughts of the client.
26.	Passing judgments	Giving opinions and approving or disapproving responses, moralizing or implying one's own values. The responses imply that the client must think as the nurse thinks, fostering client dependence.
27.	Giving common advice	Telling the client what to do. These responses deny the client's right to be an equal partner. Note that giving expert rather than common advice is therapeutic.

Therapeutic Communication Phases

Phase	Task	Skills
Pre-interaction phase	The nurse reviews pertinent assessment data and knowledge, considers potential areas of concern and develops plan for interaction.	Organized data gathering: limitations and seeking assistance as required.
Introductory phase		
Opining the relationship	Both client and nurse identify each other by name. When the nurse initiates the relationship, it is important to explain the nurse's role to give the client an idea of what to expect. When the client initiates the relationship, the nurse needs to help the client express concerns and reasons foe seeking help, vague, open-ended questions, such as what's on your mind today? Are helpful at this stage.	A relaxed, attending, attitude to put the client at ease. It is not easy for all clients to receive help.
Clarifying the problem	Because the client initially may not see the problem clearly, the nurse's major task is to help clarify the problems.	Attending listening, paraphrasing, clarifying, and other effective communication techniques discussed in this chapter. A common error at this stage is to ask too many questions of the client instead focus on priorities.
Structuring and formulating the contract (obligation to be met by both the nurse and client)	Nurse and client develop a degree of trust and verbally agree about (a) location, frequency and length of meeting, (b) overall purpose of the relationship, (c) how confidential material will be handled, (d) takes to be accomplished, and (e) duration and indications for termination of the relationship.	Communication skills listed above and ability to overcome resistive behaviors if they occur.

Contd...

Contd...

Phase	Task	Skills
Working phase	Nurse and client accomplish the tasks outlined in the introductory phase, enhance trust and rapport, and develop caring.	Listening and attending skills, empathy, respect, genuineness, concreteness, self-disclosure, and confrontation. Skills acquired by the client are non-defensive listening and self-understanding
Exploring and understanding thoughts and feelings	The nurse assisting the client to explore thoughts and feelings and acquires and understanding of the client. The client explores thoughts and feelings associated with problems, develop the skill of listening and gains insight into personal behavior.	
Facilitating and taking action	The nurse plans programs within the client's capabilities are considers long- and short-term goals. The client needs to learn to take risks (i.e., accept that either failure or success may be the outcome). The nurse needs to reinforce successes and help the client recognize failures realistically.	Decision-making and goal setting skills. Also, for the nurse: reinforcement skills; for the client: risk taking.
Terminal phase	Nurse and client accept feedings of loss. The client accepts the end of the relationship without feelings of anxiety or dependence.	For the nurse: summarizing skills; for the client: ability to handle problems independently.

COMMUNICATION IN NURSING

Communication is the basic element of human interactions that allows people to establish, maintain and improve contacts with others. It constitutes the foundation of interaction among human beings. Nursing is a communicative intervention and the foundation lies in the communicative attitude. This attitude is manifested in the striving for mutual understanding, coordination and co-action. An individual who comes to a health agency has came because he needs help in relation to his health; the nurse and other health professionals are there to provide the help he needs.

Communication is the process by which one person conveys thoughts, feelings and ideas to another. It is a tool that provides a mean for one person to understand another, to accept and be accepted, to convey and receive information, to give and accept directions to teach and to learn. Communication is part of the art of nursing- the intentional creative use of oneself, based on skill and expertise, to transmit emotion and meaning to another. It is a process that requires interpretation, sensitivity, imagination and active participation.

Need of communication in nursing: A critical component of nursing practice is the ability to communicate effectively. Nurses interact with many persons in the course of their profession. Competency in communication helps the nurse maintain effective relationship within the entire sphere of professional practice and helps to meet legal, ethical and clinical requirement.

Communication Skills help the Nurse in Many Ways

- Generate trust between the nurse and clients.
- Provides the nurse with professional satisfaction.
- It is also a means for bringing about change.
- It is a foundation of relationship between the nurse and other members of the health team.
- Induces human being to put forth greater efforts in their work performance.

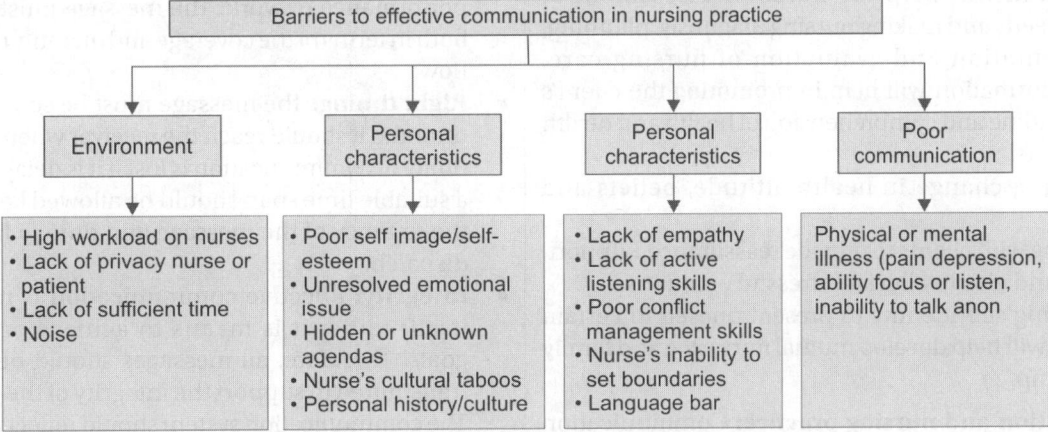

Fig. 4.13: Barriers to effective communication in nursing practice.

- Serves as a lubricant fostering the smooth operation of the management process.
- Provides basis for leadership action.
- Provides means of coordination.

Purpose of Communication in Nursing System

- To transfer information between all classes of employees to have a common understanding among them.
- To interpret and adopt policies in the organization.
- To include motivation, cooperation and coordination in the employees.
- To improve employer-employee relationships.
- To recruit, select, train and develop the personnel in the organization.
- To encourage participation in decision-making.
- To delegate or decentralize authority.
- To boost the group morale of the workers.
- To ensure job satisfaction.
- To help in the grievance procedure and disciplinary actions.
- To inform the community of the services available in the organization.
- To prepare the personnel and the public for a change process.
- To improve public relation with the government and other agencies.
- To get feedback from the personnel and the public for improvement.

Communication Functions in Nursing

Communication is one of the important nursing skills. It allows nurses to understand clients better, attain healthy behaviors. Nurses competence on their ability to send timely and intelligent messages as client's needs dictate and on their ability to understand their communications. Therapeutic communication with the clients involves planned, deliberate interactions that foster a helping relationship. By effective communication the nurse helps the client adapt to change resulting from health alterations.

- **Seeking information and giving information:** seeking information will help the nurse in assessment of nursing needs and making nursing diagnosis, planning, implementation and evaluation of nursing care. Giving information will help in promoting the client's understanding and comprehension of health and health care aspects.
- Influencing change in health attitude, beliefs and actions.
- Interacting with clients to provide reassurance, support, comfort and also to alleviate stressful emotions.
- Establishing self-identity to present oneself in certain ways that will help develop mutual nurturing and family relationship.

Communication and nursing practice: Communication is the basic element of human interactions that allows people to establish, maintain and improve contacts with others. It constitutes the foundation of interaction among human being. Nursing is a communicative intervention and the foundation of nursing lies in the communicative attitude. This attitude is manifested in striving for mutual understanding, coordination and coaction. Communication can be used for influencing as well as obtaining information. A nurse who is able to communicate effectively can bring about positive changes in the health care system, establishing cordial relations with patients, among other things and can also help prevent legal problems. Communication skills help the nurse in many ways:

- Generate trust between the nurse and clients.
- Provides the nurse with professional satisfaction.
- Communication is also a means for bridging about change.
- Communication is the foundation of relationship between the nurse and other members of the health team.
- Communication serves as a lubricant fostering the smooth operation of the management process.
- Communication provides basis for leadership action.
- Communication provides means of coordination.

COMMUNICATION IN THE HOSPITAL

Communication being vital to the success of management, an effective communication system must be developed by every organization. A good system of communication must fulfill the following requirements. Essentials of good communication

- **Clarity:** The basic objective of communication is to create mutual understanding and cooperation. This can be possible only when the message is properly understood by the receiver. Message can be properly understood when it is expressed in as clear and unambiguous language as possible. The sender must use simple and commonly understood words so that the receiver can comprehend the message without difficulty.
- **Adequacy:** Organization members must be provided with all the information that is needed for effective performance of work. The message must be complete both in terms of the coverage and quantity of information flow.
- **Right timing:** The message must be sent at the proper time and it should reach the receiver when required. The utility of communication is lost if it is delayed. Therefore, a suitable time span should be allowed keeping in view the urgency of the message and time to be taken in its dispatch.
- **Integrity:** Effective communication is not an end in itself; rather it is means to achieve organizational goals. Therefore, all messages should be formed and transmitted to support the integrity of the organization. The communication system should reflect the objectives and polices of the organization.

- **Participation:** The receiver must be involved in the planning and transmission of message. Such participation helps to promote mutual trust and confidence. It also improves listening and understanding on the part of organization members.
- **Strategic use of grapevine:** The grapevine can be used to transmit information not considered appropriate for the formal communication. Constructive use of informal channels helps to improve the speed and effectiveness of formal communication.
- **Two-way communication:** A good communication system must contain a feedback mechanism. The sender should try to know the reactions of the receiver. (This will enable the management to ascertain whether or not receiver).
- **Economy:** The communication system should not be unreasonably expensive. The cost of communications should be controlled by avoiding irrelevant messages and communication overload.
- **Appropriate channels:** The media of communication should be appropriate to the message and the receiver. An integration system of communication should be developed. It should be tailor-made to the problems and requirements of the organization.
- **Flexibility:** The system of communication must be flexible enough so that it can be adjusted to the changing requirements of the organization.
- **Attention:** The receiver of communication must be attentive and should have open mind. Adherence to the principle of attention will gradually overcome many barriers to communication.

Communication System used in Hospitals

- Periodical talks between employer and employees.
- Sign posts for patients and general public.
- Staff conferences.
- Social gatherings.
- Employee counseling
- Standing orders, protocols
- Handbook.
- Manuals.
- Bulletin boards.
- Suggestion system, complaint book.
- Hospital magazine, bulletin.
- Annual reports.
- Light signaling system.
- Alarm systems.
- Telecommunication systems.
- Enquiry office or public relation office.
- Patient information booklets.

Ten Commandments of Good Communication

- Seek to clarify your ideas before communicating.
- Examine the true purpose of each communication before communicating.
- Consider the total physical and human setting whenever communication takes place.
- Consult with others, when necessary in planning communication.
- Be mindful, while communicating of the overtones as well as the basic content of the message.
- Take the opportunity, when it arises to convey something of help on value to the receiver.
- Follow-up on communications.
- Communicate for tomorrow as well as today.
- Be sure actions support communications.
- Seek not only be understood but also to understand — be a good listener.

NURSE-CLIENT HELPING RELATIONSHIP

Helping relationship is the foundation of clinical nursing practice, the essential element of care with every client in every situation. In such relationship, the nurse assumes the role of professional helper and comes to be known to the client as an individual who has unique health needs, human responses, and patterns of living. The relationship is therapeutic, promoting a psychological climate that facilitates positive change of growth. The nurse establishes, directs and takes responsibility for the interaction and the clients need to take priority over the nurse's needs. A helping relationship between nurse and client does not just happen; it is created with care and skill and is built on the clients trust in the nurse. Nursing theorist Imogene King (1971) calls the nurse-client relationship, learning experiences whereby two people interact to face immediate health problems, to share, if possible, in resolving it, and to discover ways to adapt to the situation.

Nurse community relationship: Many nurses form relationships with community groups by participating in local organizations, volunteering for community services or becoming politically active. Nurses in a community based practice must be able to establish relationships with their community to be effective change agents. Communication within the community occurs through channels such as neighborhood newsletters, public bulletin boards, newspapers, radio, television and electronic information sites.

Elements of professional communication: Professional appearance, demeanor and behavior are important in establishing the nurse's trustworthiness and competence. They communicate that the nurse has assumed the professional helping role, is clinically skilled and is focused on the client.

- Being on time.
- Organized, well prepared and equipped for the responsibilities of the nursing role also communicate one's professionalism.
- Courtesy.
- Use of names.
- Privacy and confidentiality.

- Trustworthiness.
- Autonomy and responsibility.
- Assertiveness.

COMMUNICATING EFFECTIVELY WITH PATIENT, FAMILY AND TEAM MEMBERS

A good way to encourage autonomy is to collaborate with others. Research has show that successful collaboration requires an active and committed involvement by both client and nurse and a joint effort to ward problem solving. Such a relationship will enhance the clients well being and the nurse's feeling of success.

Nurse-patient relationship: Nurse patient relationship is a basic requirement of nursing practice. A nurse who is efficient and skillful uses the holistic approach in caring for a patient with any type of problem. It is an interaction process in which the nurse fulfils the role by using professional knowledge and skill such a way that the nurse is able to help the patient physically, socially and emotionally.

Nurse-family relationship: Many situations, especially those in community and home health settings, require the nurse to form helping relationships with entire families. The same principles that guide one to one helping relationship also apply when the client is a family unit, although communication within families requires additional understanding of the complexities of family dynamics, needs and relationships. Collaboration among nurse, client and family care givers is especially important.

Nurse-health team relationship: Nurses are members of a larger health care community and often function in roles they require interaction with multiple health team members. Many elements of the nurse-client helping relationship are also applied in these collegial relationships, which are focused on accompany the work and goals of clinical setting communication in such relationships may be geared toward team building, facilitating group process collaboration, delegation, supervision, leadership and management. Both social and therapeutic interactions are needed between the nurse and health team members to build morale and strengthen relationships within the work setting. Everyone has interpersonal needs for acceptance inclusion, identity, privacy, power and control and affection.
Nurse-community relationship : Many nurses form relationships with community groups by participating in local organizations, volunteering for community services or becoming politically active. Nurses in a community based practice must be able to establish relationships with their community to be effective change agents. Communication within the community occurs through channels such as neighborhood newsletters, public bulletin boards, news papers, radio, television and electronic information sites.

COMMUNICATION WITHIN NURSING PROCESS

Nursing assessment: Assessment of client's ability to communicate includes gathering data about the many contextual factors that influence communication. The context refers to all the parts of something that help determine its meaning. Situations have several aspects that influence the nature of communication, interpersonal relationships and client needs. These include that participant's internal factors and characteristics, the nature of their relationship, the situation prompting communication, the environment and sociocultural elements present.

Nursing diagnosis: Most individuals experience difficulty with some aspect of communication, most often, the nurse care is directed toward those individuals who experience more serious impairments in communication. The primary nursing diagnostic label used to describe the client who has limited or no ability to communicate verbally is impaired verbal communication.

The related factor for impaired verbal communication focus on the causes of communication disorder. These can be physiological, mechanical, anatomical, psychological, cultural or developmental in nature. For example deaf older adult with untreated cataracts who has the following nursing diagnosis: impaired verbal communication related to limited vision, absent hearing and inability to articulate works.

Planning: Once the nurse has identified the nature of the clients communication dysfunction, several factors must be considered is the care plan is designed. Motivation is a factor in improving communication, and clients often require encouragement to try different approaches that involve significant change. Expected outcomes for the client with impaired communication are important to identify. In general, effective nursing interventions will result in the client experiencing a sense of trust in the nurse and health team.

At times nurses care for well clients whose difficulty in sending, receiving and interpreting messages interferes with healthy interpersonal relationships. Nurses can plan interventions to help such clients improve their communication skills.

Implementation: It carry out plan of care, nurses need to use communication techniques that are appropriate for the client's individual needs. The most basic nursing interventions used in communication are therapeutic communication techniques. Therapeutic communication techniques are specific responses that encourage the expression of feelings and ideas and convey the nurse's acceptance and respect.

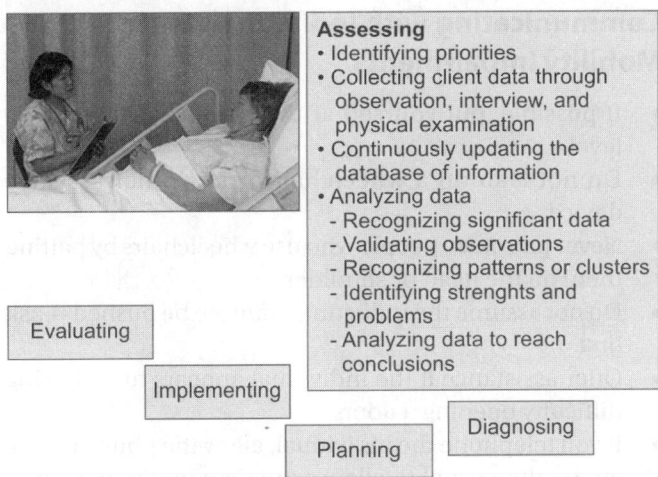

Fig. 4.14: The nursing process assessment—data collection.

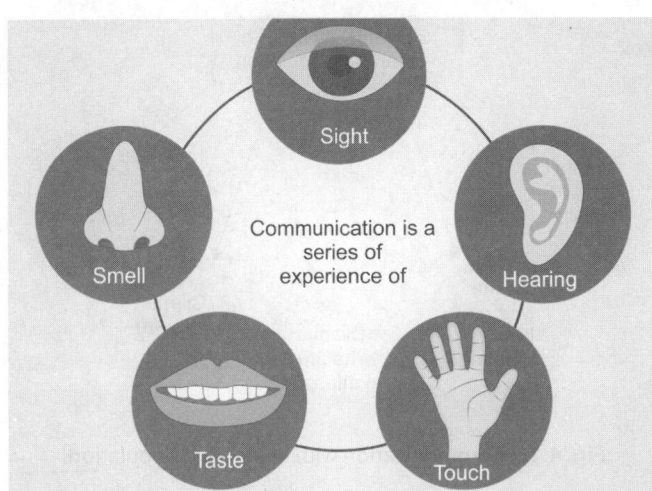

Fig. 4.15: Communication is a series of experience of taste, smell, touch, hearing, taste and sight.

Evaluation: The nurse and client determine whether the plan of care has been successful by evaluating the client communication outcomes established during planning. Nurses can evaluate the effectiveness of their own communication by making process recording, written records of their verbal and nonverbal interactions with clients.

Major Recommendations for Establishing Therapeutic Relationship

- The nurse must acquire the necessary knowledge to participate effectively in therapeutic relationship.
- Establishment of a therapeutic relationship requires reflective practice. The concept includes the required capacities of: self-awareness, self-knowledge, and empathy, awareness of ethics, boundaries and limits of the professional role.
- The nurse needs to understand the process of a therapeutic relationship and be able to recognize the current phase of his/her relationship with the client.
- The entry-level nursing programs must including both theoretical content and supervised practice.
- Organizations will consider the therapeutic relationship as the basis of nursing practice and, over time will integrate a variety of professional development opportunities to support nurses in effectively developing these relationships. Opportunities must include nursing consultation, clinical supervision and coaching.
- Health care agencies will implement a model of care that promotes consistency of the nurse client assignment, such as primary nursing.
- Agencies will ensure that at minimum, 70% of their nurses are working on a permanent fulltime basis.
- Agencies will ensure that nurses worked are maintained at levels conductive to developing therapeutic relationship.
- Staffing decisions must consider client acuity, complexity level, complexity of work environment, and availability of expert resources.
- Organizations will consider the nurse's well-being as vital to the development of therapeutic nurse-client relationship and support the nurse as necessary.
- Organization will assist in advancing knowledge about therapeutic relationship by disseminating nursing research supporting the nurse in using these findings, and supporting his/ her participation in the research process.
- Agencies will have a highly visible nursing leadership and establishes and maintains mechanisms to promote open conversation between nurse and all levels of management, including senior management.
- Resources must be allocated to support clinical supervision and coaching processes to ensure that all nurses have clinical supervision and coaching on a regular basis.
  Organization are encouraged to include the development of nursing best practice guidelines in their annual review of performance indicators/quality improvement, and accreditation bodies are also encouraged to incorporate nursing best practice guidelines into their standards.

MAINTAINING EFFECTIVE HUMAN RELATION WITH VULNERABLE GROUP

Communicating with Individuals Who are Blind or Visually Impaired

- Speak to the individual when you approach him or her.
- State clearly who you are; speak in a normal tone of voice.
- When conversing in a group, remember to identify yourself and the person to whom you are speaking.
- Never touch or distract a service dog without first asking the owner.
- Tell the individual when you are leaving.
- Do not attempt to lead the individual without first asking; allow the person to hold your arm and control her or his own movements.

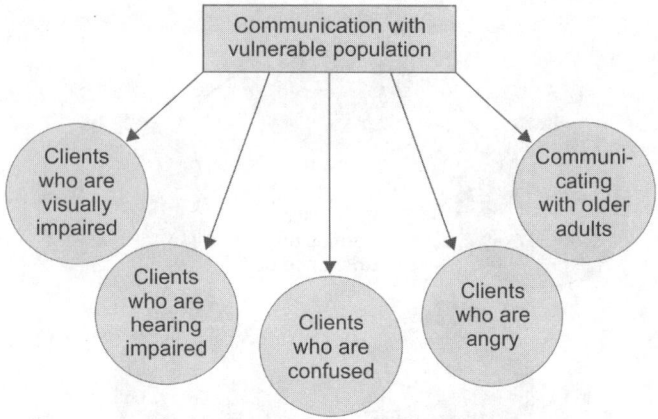

Fig. 4.16: Communication with vulnerable population.

- Be descriptive when giving directions; verbally give the person information that is visually obvious to individuals who can see. For example, if you are approaching steps, mention how many steps.
- If you are offering a seat, gently place the individual's hand on the back or arm of the chair so that the person can locate the seat.

Communicating with Individuals Who are Deaf or Hard of Hearing

- Gain the person's attention before starting a conversation (i.e. tap the person gently on the shoulder or arm).
- Look directly at the individual, face the light, speak clearly, in a normal tone of voice, and keep your hands away from your face. Use short, simple sentences. Avoid smoking or chewing gum.
- If the individual uses a sign language interpreter, speak directly to the person, not the interpreter.
- If you telephone an individual who is hard of hearing, let the phone ring longer than usual. Speak clearly and be prepared to repeat the reason for the call and who you are.

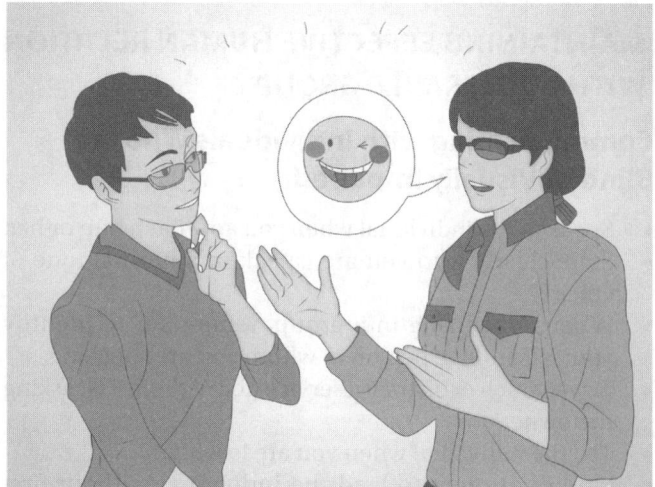

Fig. 4.17: Communication with individual who has impaired hearing.

Communicating with Individuals with Mobility Impairments

- If possible, put yourself at the wheelchair user's eye level.
- Do not lean on a wheelchair or any other assistive device.
- Never patronize people who use wheelchairs by patting them on the head or shoulder.
- Do not assume the individual wants to be pushed — ask first.
- Offer assistance if the individual appears to be having difficulty opening a door.
- If you telephone the individual, allow the phone to ring longer than usual to allow extra time for the person to reach the telephone.

Communicating with Individuals with Speech Impairments

- If you do not understand something the individual says, do not pretend that you do. Ask the individual to repeat what he or she said and then repeat it back.
- Be patient. Take as much time as necessary.
- Try to ask questions which require only short answers or a nod of the head.
- Concentrate on what the individual is saying.
- Do not speak for the individual or attempt to finish her or his sentences.
- If you are having difficulty understanding the individual, consider writing as an alternative means of communicating, but first ask the individual if this is acceptable.

Communicating with Individuals with Cognitive Disabilities

A cognitive impairment is a disability that affects a person's ability to process information. This may be due to an intellectual disability a person was born with or it may be due to an acquired brain injury, such as through a stroke or injury to the head. People with a cognitive impairment or learning disability vary greatly in their abilities, so always respond to the individual's needs rather than making assumptions about their abilities

- If you are in a public area with many distractions, consider moving to a quiet or private location.
- Be prepared to repeat what you say, orally or in writing.
- Offer assistance completing forms or understanding written instructions and provide extra time for decision-making. Wait for the individual to accept the offer of assistance; do not "over-assist" or be patronizing.
- Be patient, flexible and supportive. Take time to understand the individual and make sure the individual understands you.

TEN COMMANDMENTS OF COMMUNICATING

1. Speak directly to the person, rather than through a companion or sign language interpreter who may be present.
2. Offer to shake hands when introduced. People with limited hand use or an artificial limb can usually shake hands and offering the left hand is an acceptable greeting.
3. Always identify yourself, and others who may be with you, when meeting someone with a visual disability. When conversing in a group, remember to identify the person to whom you are speaking. When dining with a friend who has a visual disability, ask if you can describe what is on his or her plate.
4. If you offer assistance, wait until the offer is accepted. Then listen or ask for instructions.
5. Treat adults as adults. Address people with disabilities by their first names only when extending that same familiarity to all others. Never patronize people in wheelchairs by patting them on the head or shoulder.
6. Do not lean against or hang on someone's wheelchair or pet a service animal. Bear in mind that people with disabilities treat their chairs as extensions of their bodies. And so do people with guide dogs and help dogs. Never distract a service animal from its job without the owner's permission.
7. Listen attentively when talking with people who have difficulty speaking and wait for them to finish. If necessary, ask short questions that require short answers, or a nod of the head. Never pretend to understand; instead, repeat what you have understood and allow the person to respond.
8. Place yourself at eye level when speaking with someone in a wheelchair or on crutches.
9. Tap a person who has a hearing disability on the shoulder or wave your hand to get his or her attention. Look directly at the person and speak clearly, slowly, and expressively to establish if the person can read your lips. If so, try to face the light source and keep hands, drinks and food away from your mouth when speaking. If a person is wearing a hearing aid, don't assume that they have the ability to discriminate your speaking voice. Never shout at a person. Just speak in a normal tone of voice.
10. Relax. Don't be embarrassed if you happen to use common expressions, such as "See you later" or "Did you hear about this?" that seem to relate to a person's disability.

PATIENT TEACHING: IMPORTANCE, PURPOSE, PROCESS AND ROLE OF NURSE

Teaching is a system of activities intended to produce learning. Teaching is given to enhance specific learning

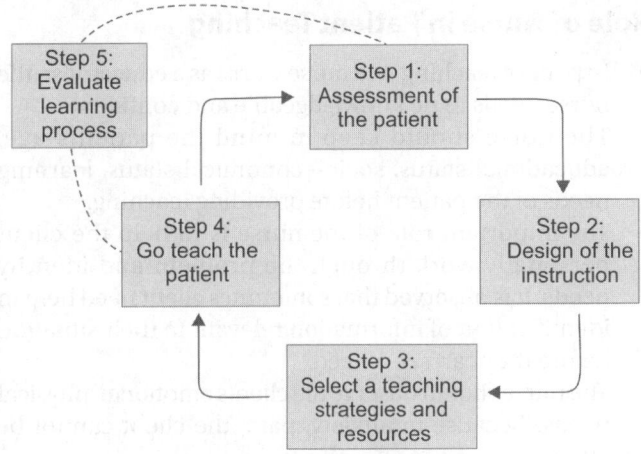

Fig. 4.18: Patient teaching steps.

of patient. Teaching is a system of activities performed to produce learning in client related to health. Teaching can be delivered in the hospital, community, assisted living and long term care facilities.

Definition: Health teaching is defined as a flexible, person-oriented process in which the helping person provides information and support to client with a variety of health related learning needs.

Purposes of Patient Teaching

Patient teaching involves teaching about reducing the health risk factors, increasing client's level of wellness and taking specific protective health measures. The purpose of patient teaching is:
- To promote health.
- To protect health.
- To maintain health.
- To identify relevant health care needs of client.
- To provide emotional and cognitive support during teaching learning process.
- To keep nurse knowledgeable.
- To raise self confidence of a nurse in teaching.

Importance of Health Teaching

- Providing patient teaching is an important function of nurse. As client has a right to know right information, giving information regarding client's health status is mandatory.
- Patient teaching involves dynamic interaction between client and nurse. Patient teaching is important to communicate information, emotion, perceptions and attitude towards health or disease condition.
- Patient teaching ensures the patient safe transition from one level of care to another. It also helps in making appropriate plans for follow-up education in the client's home.
- As client has right to make informed decisions about his health, giving patient teaching is very important.

Role of Nurse in Patient Teaching

- In patient teaching, the nurse works as a educator so the nurse needs to ne knowledgeable and confident.
- The nurse should keep in mind the patients age, educational status, socio-economical status, learning needs of the patient before providing teaching.
- The important role of the nurse is to help the client personally work through the problem and identify needs. It is observed that sometimes client need help in identification of information relevant to their situation before they can see a need.
- The nurse should observe the clients emotional, physical needs. Because in anxiety, pain, the client cannot be attentive.
- The nurse needs to encourage and motivate the nurse to learn at specific time.
- The nurse needs to provide conductive environment while delivering information to client. She should observe lighting system, ventilation, and temperature and noise free atmosphere.
- The nurse should make the patient to actively involved in patients teaching. Active participation, active learning promotes critical thinking and enables the client to solve problems more effectively.
- The nurse should follow the principles of teaching such as simple to complex; the nurse should organize the content of client teaching.

Guidelines for Effective Patient Teaching

- Development and maintenance of rapport between nurse-clients is important.
- Knowledge of client's previous learning enables nurse to encourage client and facilitate learning skill.
- Time for delivering teaching should be opted as per client's convenience.
- Nurse should have all communication skill such as confidence, good voice and tone, eye contact, speak clearly and concisely.
- Language: Local language should be prepared as it will be easily understood by client.
- Active involvement of client fosters learning.
- Reputation reinforces learning, so at the end of learning summarization of content should be done.
- Teaching that involves number of clients senses often enhance learning such as giving demonstration.
- Use of audio-visual aids foster learning and grasps the client's attention.

CONCLUSION

Nursing is an interaction between nurses and patients, nurses and others health professional, and nurses and the community. The process of human interactions occurs through communication: verbal and nonverbal, written and unwritten, planned and unplanned. Communication between people conveys thoughts, ideas, feelings and informations. for nurses to be effective in their interactions, they must have good communication skills. They must aware of their words and body languages are saying to others. As nurse assumes leadership roles they must be effective in both verbal and written communication skills. And as nurses practice in the 21st century, they must have effective computer and other electronic communication skills.

Interpersonal relationship system explains the interactions and subdivision communication. In nurses application the interpersonal relationship system is inseparable and needed. Imogene king say that the interpersonal relationship system in clinical nursing is essential and cannot be viewed as an individual concept. The nurse-client relationship become safer and effective when nurse understand the nature of the nature of the therapeutic nurse-client relationship. The nurse is responsible boundaries of the relationship and is accountable for own behavior, regardless whether harm was intended. The nurse is also responsible for terminating the relationship in an appropriate manner so that the safety and well-being of the client in protector.

BIBLIOGRAPHY

1. Bradley J, Edinberg MA. Communication in the nursing context, 3rd ed. Norwalk: Appleton and Lange, 1990.
2. Gerrard BA, Boniface WJ, Love BH. Interpersonal skills for health professionals. Reston, VA: Reston Publishing Company, Inc, A Prentice-Hall Company, 1980.
3. Lindberg J B, et al. Introduction to nursing concepts, issues and opportunities, Philadelphia: J.B. Lippincott Co, 1990.
4. Macleod CJ, Hopper L, Jesson A. Progression to counseling. Nursing Times 1991; 87(8):41-43.
5. Perry AG, Potter PA. Clinical Nursing Skills and Techniques, 3rd ed. St. Louis: Mosby-Year Book, Inc, 1994.
6. Potter PA, Perry AG. Fundamentals of Nursing Concepts, Process and Practice, 3rd ed. St. Louis: Mosby-Year Book, Inc, 1993.
7. Timby BK, Lewis LW. Fundamental Skills and Concepts in Patient Care, 5th Ed. Philadelphia: J.B. Lippincott, Co, 1992.
8. Vortherms RC. Clinically improving communication through touch. Journal of Gerontological Nursing 1991; 17(5):6.
9. Wilkinson S. Confusions and challenges, communication skills among nurses: A research review. Nursing Times 1992; 88(35):24-28.

REVIEW QUESTIONS

Long Essays

1. Define communication, explain communication process in details.
2. Discuss the barriers of communication and ways to overcome the barriers.
3. Explain therapeutic communication techniques with examples.
4. Enumerate maintaining effective human relation with vulnerable group.

Short Essays

1. Levels of communication.
2. Principles of communication.
3. Forms of communication.
4. Factors affecting communication.
5. Interpersonal relationship in nursing.
6. Therapeutic Nurse-Patient relationship.
7. Nurses role and therapeutic communication.
8. Therapeutic communication phases.
9. Communication in the hospital.

Short Answers

1. Kinds of communication.
2. Elements of communication.
3. Communication skills.
4. Nonverbal communication.
5. Skills of IPR.
6. Principles of interpersonal relationship.
7. Importance of health teaching.

MULTIPLE CHOICE QUESTIONS

1. **Communication includes all means by which meaning is conveyed from one person to another by:**
   a. Written words and spoken words
   b. Facial expressions
   c. Gestures and visual aids
   d. All of the above
2. **Goals of a therapeutic relationship:**
   a. Facilitate communication of distressing thoughts and feelings
   b. To assist client with problem solving to help daily living
   c. Promote self care and independence
   d. All of the above
3. **Communication system used in hospitals, *except*:**
   a. Periodical talks between employer and employees
   b. Sign posts for patients and general public
   c. Health education
   d. Staff conferences
4. **Cognitive impairment is a disability that affects a person's ability to process information:**
   a. Process information
   b. Recall information
   c. Retrieve information
   d. None of the above
5. **The best model explains the:**
   a. Begin with nonverbal cues. Soften (smile, open arms, forward lean, touch with arm, handshake, eye contact, nod).
   b. Establish information gathering with informal talk.
   c. Support with emotional channels and terminate with positive notes.
   d. All of the above

ANSWERS

1. d   2. d   3. c   4. a   5. d

CHAPTER 5

Documentation and Reporting

LEARNING OBJECTIVES
- Documentation: Purposes of reports and records
- Confidentiality
- Types of client records/common record-keeping forms
- Methods/systems of documentation/recording
- Guidelines for documentation
- Do's and Don'ts of documentation/legal guidelines for documentation/recording
- Reporting: Change-of-shift reports, transfer reports, incident reports

TERMINOLOGY

- **Standing order**: Standing orders are the directions and orders of specific nature. On the basis, in the non-availability of doctor, the nurse and health workers provide treatment to patients, at home, hospital or health institution and community.
- **Family folder:** Family folder provides essential and complete information about the family to complete information about the family to the community health nurse to plan, organize and to implement nursing care to the family.
- **Record:** It is a written communication relevant to a client's health care and management. It is a continuing account of the client's health care needs.
- **Informed consent:** It is a person's agreement to allow something to happen based on full disclosure of facts needed to make an intelligent decision. The consent must be given voluntarily by a mentally competent adult.
- **Incident report:** An incident report is field when something arises that can or did cause injury and which was not dealt with good care, so the detail incidental report should give by the particular staff or person.
- **Contract:** A contract is a written or oral agreement between two people in which there is a mention of goods or services exchanged.
- **Documentation**: In the medical record, it provides the only credible proof in court to prove the appropriate care was given and the standards of care was met with.
- **Patient care standards:** These are guides for collaborative practice responding the predicted care requirement for patients. They are based on an analytical and problem solving of assessment, planning, intervention and evaluation.
- **Field review:** It is a method; appraisal of worker is done by the personnel officer by collecting oral rating about them from the supervisor at the place of work. The personnel officer later writes his notes and invites the supervisor to make additions or corrections.
- **Protocol:** A protocol is a written plan specifying the procedures to be followed during care of a client with a selected clinical condition or situation.

INTRODUCTION

Documentation is the process of communicating in written form about essential facts for the maintenance of continuous history of events over a period of time. Recording and reporting are the other ways of documentation. Record is the permanent written communication that documents information relevant to a client's health care management. Record means all documents facilitates evaluation of the program and provides continuity from the time the institution is established.

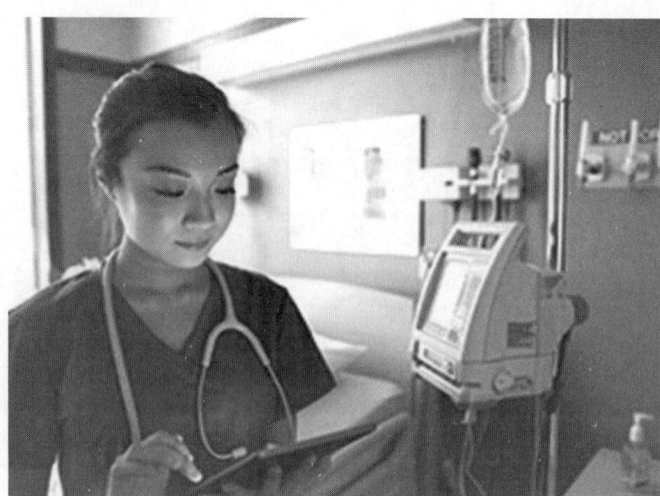

Fig. 5.1: Documentation in patient care.

MEANING OF RECORDS AND REPORTS

- Records and reports are a practical and indispensable aid to the doctor, nurse and paramedical personnel in giving the best possible service to individual, family and to the community.
- Documentation is important in health care today. Documentation is defined as anything written or presented that is relied on as a record of proof for authorized persons.
- A medical records should be comprehensive declaration of the individual family and community health status and needs, as well as the service provided for the client care.
- Recorded facts have a value and scientific accuracy for more than mere impression of memory and these are guidelines for better administration of family health services.
- Records are the means of communication between the health workers and the family, for example, any health or socioeconomic problem observed by the health workers during home visit is recorded, which may require the attention of the doctor or other members of the health team.
- Family records serve as a guide to nursing care as they are major practice tools today in the community health practice.
- Consumerism, accountability and quality assurance plays a vital role on legal written documents. It is necessary to have adequate records to record the care provided and other information which will help to assess and improve the quality of care given.
- Records have been shown not only to help ensure effective service but at the same time to save effort and money. The doctor who knows, what has been done before, can plan his therapy wisely and effectively.
- Records and reports express or presenting the facts, records, means record is the written presentation of information.
- Patient's clinical record is a brief account of the personal and medical history of the patient, results of diagnostic tests, findings of medical examination, treatment, nursing care, daily progress notes are recorded.
- A record is a permanent written communication that documents information relevant to a client's health care management. Health records give information about members, activities carried out, and achievements.

DEFINITIONS OF RECORDS AND REPORTS

Records

- Records are written formal and legal individual family and community. It may provide information about personal socioeconomic, psychological environmental and health.
- Records are facts and figures, arranged in a logical order that a new worker may be able to maintain continuity if service to individuals families and communities.
- A record or documentation is defined as anything written or printed that is relied on as a record of proof for authorized persons.
- A record or documentation is defined as anything written or printed that is relied on as a record of proof for authorized persons.
- It is a written communication that permanently documents information relevant to a client's health care management. It is a continuing account of the client's health care needs.

Reports

- Reports offer a summary of activities or observations seen, performed or heard is exchanged among health care team members, clients and family members.
- A Report summarizes the services of the nurses or the agency. Reports may be in the form of an analysis of some aspect of a service. Reports are usually written daily, weekly, monthly and yearly.
- Report is an oral or written account by one member to another in the health team which includes the end of shift handing over report.

Importance of Report and Records

- It provides facts of health services.
- It provides a basis for analyzing needs and direct towards goal achievement.
- Provides a basis for short- and long-term planning.
- It prevents duplication of services and helps to follow-up services effectively.
- It helps the nurse to evaluate the care and teaching which she has given.
- It enables the nurse to judge the quality and quantity of work done.

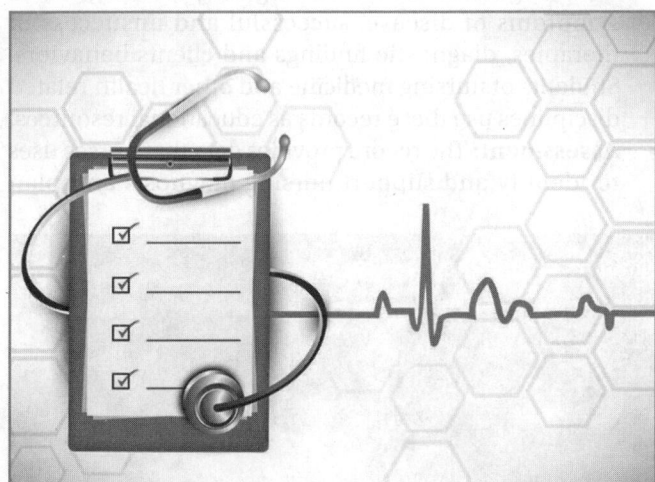

Fig. 5.2: Recording and reporting are the vital role of a nurse.

- It serves as a guide to professional growth.
- Records help to become aware of and recognize their health needs of the individual and the family.
- Records can be used as a teaching tool to the individual and family.
- The record serves as a guide for diagnosis, treatment and evaluation for the doctors.
- The record helps identify families needing service and those prepared to accept help.
- The record helps the supervisor evaluate the services rendered, teaching done and person's actions and reactions.

Reports

- Complete report establishes the nurse's accountability in being sure that client care is uninterrupted.
- It provides a baseline for comparison during the next shift.
- It shares significant information about family members as it relates to client's problems.
- It relay to staff significant changes in the way therapies are given.
- It evaluates results of nursing and medical care measures.
- It describes instructions given in teaching plan and clients' families and community response.

PURPOSE RECORDING AND REPORTING

Recording

- **Communication:** The record is a means by which health care team members communicable and contributes to health of an individual family and community.
- **Financial billing:** The client care record is a document that shows the extent to which health care agencies should be reimbursed for services. It is client's bill.
- **Educational:** The record contains variety of information, including medical and nursing diagnosis, signs and symptoms of disease, successful and unsuccessful therapies, diagnostic findings and clients behaviors. Students of nursing medicine and other health related disciplines use these records as educational resources.
- **Assessment:** The record provides data that nurses uses to identify and support nursing diagnosis and plan

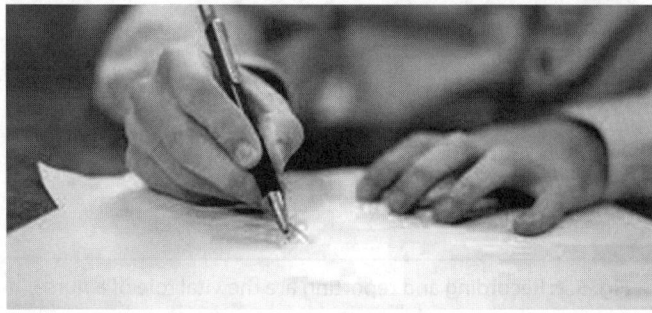

Fig. 5.3: Writing record needs to be prompt and accurate.

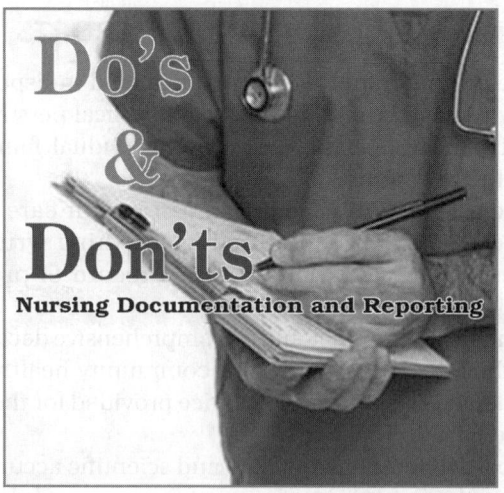

Fig. 5.4: Nurse needs to know do's and don'ts in documentation.

proper investigations of care. Information from the record adds to the nurse's observations and assessment.
- **Research:** Statistical data relating to the frequency of clinical disorders, complications, use of specific medical and nursing therapies, deaths and recovery from illness can be gathered from client's records.
- **Auditing and monitoring:** A regular review of information in client records gives a basis for evaluation of the quality and appropriateness of care provided in an institution.
- **Legal administration:** A medical record must be accurate because it is a legal document. Accurate documentation is one of the best defenses for legal claims associate with nursing care.

Reporting (Written Reports)

- To show the kind and amount of services rendered over a specified period.
- It helps to illustrate progress in reaching goals.
- It acts as an aid in studying health conditions.
- It aids in planning.
- It helps to interpret the services to the public and to the other interested agencies.

PRINCIPLES OF RECORDING AND REPORTING

Recording

- Records should be written clearly, accurately, appropriate and legibly.
- Nurses should develop their own method of expression and form in record writing.
- Records are confidential documents, so it should be handled carefully.
- Care to be taken not to make any errors on the records if anything is crossed out, it should be dated and initialed.
- All records should be written with black ink or typed for better legibility.

- Record should be written in chronological order as to date and time. When recording medications and treatments, note exact time and date on which they are carried out.
- Records should be written immediately after an interview.
- Record system is essential for efficiency and uniformity of services.
- Record should provide for periodic summary to determine progress and to make future plans.
- Select relevant facts and the recording should be brief and accurate.

Care of the Records

- The records are kept under the safe custody of the nurse in each ward.
- No individual sheet is separated from the complete record.
- Records are kept in a place, not accessible to the patients and visitors.
- Records are never sent out of the hospital without the doctor's permission.
- All the records should be handled carefully. Careless handling can destroy the records.
- Records are not handled over to the legal.
- All the hospital personnel are legally and ethically obligated to keep in confidence all the information provided in the records.

Principles of Record Writing

- Since the clinical record is a legal document, it is essential that they should be written clearly, accurately, appropriately and legibly.
- The individual who writes them should sign all entries.
- Care to be taken not to make any error on the records. If anything is crossed out, it should be dated and initialed.
- All records should be written with black ink or typed for better legibility.
- Records should be written in chronological order as to date and time. When recording medications and treatments, note exact time and date on which they are carried out
- Records are written continuously with no blank spaces. If any space is left out, it should be crossed out, dated and signed.
- Lengthy corrections of records are written as amendments.
- Each page of the record should be properly identified with the name, age, I.P. No., OP No. Date, etc.
- Use only standard abbreviations.
- Records should be truthful, brief and complete. It should include all the services given to the patients, the observations made on the patient from day to day and the results of treatments, etc.

General Rules of Recording

- Keep separate records or charts for each individual patient.
- It is a legal document; write it, in English, clearly, accurately, appropriately and legibly.
- Name, age, ward, date and in-patient number should be written on each page.
- All entries should be signed by the individual who makes the entry.
- All entries should be written in blue or black ink.
- Chart nursing-care and medications and other treatments only after giving them.
- It should be reliable and accurate.
- Information about patients and their care must be factual.
- Correct spelling is also important for accurate recording.
- Nurses should not allow others to record for her.
- Use only standard abbreviations.
- Do not use ditto marks or chemical formula in charting.
- Each patient should have a daily note, written by nurses on all shifts.
- The information within a record should be complete.
- Concise data are easy to understand.
- Lengthy notes are difficult to read.
- Record immediately after performing nursing activities. It should have correctness.
- It should be organized in a logical format or order.
- Nurses should maintain confidentiality of patents' record.
- Do not use blank space in the record. Keep it crossed.

Nurses Responsibility in Recording

- Generally, nurses' notes contain the following information.
- Treatment and nursing care given by various members of the health team.
- Doctor's orders carried out by nurses.
- Nursing needs met by nurses as per doctor's order.
- Observations, e.g. vital signs, physical signs and behavioral patterns of patient.
- Response of patient to treatment and nursing care.
- Health advice given by nurses and other staff.
- Independent nursing functions are also recorded.

Principles of Reporting

- Report should be truthful, accurate, appropriate, clear, confidential, brief, complete and legible.
- Good reports will indicate the efficiency of the health team in carrying out their assignments.
- Good reports will avoid duplication of work.
- Good reports will help the relieving personnel to plan the future care of the patient's without wasting time unnecessarily.

- Patient receives better care when the reports are through and give all pertinent data.
- Good report tells us about the problems relating to supplies and equipments.
- Use only standard abbreviations.
- All entries should be signed by the individual who writes them.

Nurse's Responsibility in Record Keeping

Nurses have legal responsibility for accurately reporting and recording patient's conditions, treatments and responses to care. The medical record is a written or computerized account of a patient's illness and treatment that includes information submitted by all members of the patient health care team. The medical record is an information source document that should be used to plan care, evaluate care, allocate costs, educate personnel, research care measure and substantiate legal claims.

TYPES OF RECORDS, REPORTS AND REGISTERS IN NURSING

Types of Records

- **Cumulative or continuing records:** The system utilizing one record for home and clinic services in which home visits are recorded in red and clinic visit in blue ink helps coordinate the service and save the time of all the personnel concerned. Continuing record save time and much filling space by avoiding repetition.
- **Family records:** All the records which relate to members of one family should be placed which relate to members of one family should be placed in the single family folder. In this way, the doctor and health workers can see the total situation and give effective economical service to the family as a whole. The family folder which contains all the individual records of one family.
- **Anecdotal records:** It is a brief description of an observed behavior that appears significant for evaluation purposes, done by the community health nurse during home visit. It provides information about particular one incident.
- **Clinical records:** It is used in the hospital; investigations special treatments and procedures are written and signed.
- **Doctor order sheet:** Doctor Orders regarding medications, investigations, special treatments and procedures are written and signed.
- **Nurses sheet:** Nurses notes are a record of treatments and nursing measures carried out by the nurses, their effects, the observations made on the patient.
- **Other records:** TPR chart, lab report sheet, diet sheets, concern form intake output chart, anesthesia chart, physiotherapy sheet, special treatment sheets, etc.

Types of Reports

- **Oral report:** Oral report is sometimes used as an emergency and followed by a written report later. An oral report is made by the nurse who is assigned to patient care to another nurse who is supposed to relieve her.
- **Written report:** It should concentrate on the past, present and future state of the patient or event. Description and conclusions of action, the influence further planning and decision making are necessary.
- **24 hours report:** Nursing supervisor and nursing administration personnel need to be kept informed of what is happening in all patient care areas.
- **Census report:** The daily census or the number of patients is admitted in the hospital. This report helps in planning of health care services and knows about the morbidity and mortality statistics.
- **Accidental report:** Writing a detailed report on mistakes or accidents that has taken place in the care of patients. It should be promptly informed to the higher authorities by writing accidental report.
- **Change of shift report:** At the end of each shift nurses report information about their assigned clients to the nurses working on the next shift.
- **Transfer report:** It involves communication of information about clients from the nurse on the sending to the nurse on the receiving unit.
- **Other report:** It includes reports among the members of the nursing team, reports between the head nurse and her assistant, reports between the head nurse and the nursing superintendent, reports to the physician, evaluation reports, etc.

Types of Registers

The register usually provides only an indication of the total volume of service and of the types of cases seen. It gives no idea of quality of services or the results achieved. It is necessary to keep each register up-to-date and accurate. A good record system provides all the information available from the usual clinic register. Register maintains the statistics. In all community health centers, hospital system

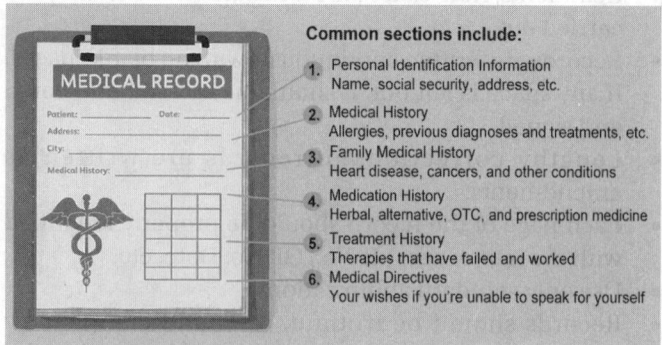

Fig. 5.5: Components of patient details.

and education institutions maintain registers. Every hospital maintains registers such as birth and deaths, register for operations and delivery, census register, register for the admission and discharges, OPD attendants, etc.

In community health care, daily clinic attendance register, immunization register, family planning registers, birth registers and death registers, etc.

COMMON RECORD KEEPING FORMS

Common Forms on the Chart

- Admission nursing history forms
- Graphic sheets and flow sheets
- Client care summary or kardex
- Acuity records
- Standardized care plans
- Discharge summary

Admission nursing history forms: Comprehensive. Gather baseline assessment data when a patient is admitted to a nursing care unit. Compare any changes in patient's condition. For example: Patient's allergies, primary spoken/written language, advance directives, disabilities, and mobility/fall risk and medication reconciliation.

Flow sheets and graphic records: Permit concise documentation of nursing info and patient data over time. Useful for documentation of routine observations or repeated specific measurements for a patient such as vital signs, I and O, hygiene measures, medicine administration, and pain assessment.

Patient education record: Identifies patient's knowledge base about his or her diagnosis, treatment, and medications. Standards for patient education include assessment of needs, functional abilities, learning styles, and readiness to learn.

Client care or kardex: Now many are computerized. Summary prints out for each patient during each shift. Has two parts: an activity and Tx section and nursing care plan section. Includes: Basic demographic area, primary medical diagnosis, allergies, nursing care plan.

Acuity records: Method of determining the intensity of nursing care required for a group of patients. Used as a guide to determine staffing needs. Determines the hours of nursing care and number of staff required for a nursing unit. Allows nursing staff to compare patients with one another. For example: Acuity level 1- means patient returning from surgery and requires frequent monitoring.

Standardized care plans: Computerized. Incorporate several nursing diagnosis or problems in a single care plan. Based on agency standards of nursing practice and are established guidelines used to care for patients with similar health problems. Improve continuity of care. Disadvantage: increased risk that unique, individualized therapies needed by patients will go unrecognized.

Discharge summaries: A comprehensive process with emphasis placed on preparing a pt. for discharge from a health care organization. Important to ensure that a patient's condition results in desirable outcomes. Involve family and caregiver as well.

COMPUTERIZED DOCUMENTATION

Change commonly occurs within the healthcare environment. Technological advancements significantly contribute to these changes and assists nurses in meeting professional and organizational goals. The transition from paper to electronic documentation, in particular, can address some of the issues that nurses are currently experiencing, and help nurses to meet complex health care demands. Although this change is necessary, the implementation of electronic documentation can be challenging for nurses. The application of Kurt Lewin's Change Management Theory provides a structured approach that can help nurses to overcome these challenges, as well as other barriers that impede the transition to electronic documentation. Throughout this paper I have examined Lewin's Force Field Analysis Model and demonstrated how it could be used to plan, implement, and evaluate the transition from paper to electronic documentation. I believe that the implementation of electronic clinical documentation is essential to enhance the quality of nursing care. Lewin's theoretical framework can be used to help nurse informaticists manage this change and successfully implement electronic documentation in practice settings.

Advantages of electronic charting: Electronic health records (EHRs, also known as electronic medical records) have distinct advantages over paper. Mentioned most often is the not insignificant benefit that provider orders are legible and clear. Nurses no longer have to waste time consulting with one another, trying to decipher someone's dreadful handwriting, and fewer errors related to misinterpreted orders should follow. Nurses also like being able to find information about previous episodes of care

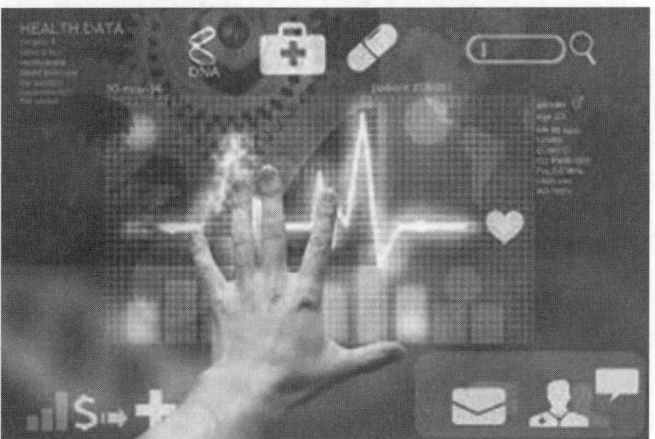

Fig. 5.6: Digital recording of patient's data.

(hospitalizations or visits) easily and having all information about a patient integrated in a single place.

Electronic charting is the wave of the future. There will be a computer at every bedside, and every nurse will type her notes. Electronic charting has some distinct advantages over paper charting, but there are some disadvantages too. A computer makes it very easy to keep a chart readable and accessible, but it is very easy to become accustomed to the ease of a computer. Most computers eventually crash, and in a world that doesn't stop, like health care, nurses have to know how to keep going.

Legibility: Electronic charting is always legible because it is done on a computer screen. There is no question about what an order says or what a note indicates because typeface is not in question. Abbreviations and terms that go against hospital standards can also be automatically edited out of electronic charting to avoid confusion that paper charting can cause. Furthermore, all entries into the record are automatically time- and date-stamped so that an accurate record of the patient's treatments can be followed.

Prompting: Nurses can be prompted by the computer to ask certain questions for their charting or to give certain medications. The computer serves as a guide to help the nurse give proper and safe care. Having a computer function in this way is a definite advantage when a nurse has a high case load and can easily make a mistake or overlook an item to chart. A computer can remind her to check an important assessment and make all the difference to a patient's outcome.

LEGAL IMPLICATIONS OF RECORDS AND REPORTS

Legal Records

- **Incidental reports:** The nurse has a moral and legal responsibility to report to the health agency any accidents, losses or unusual occurrences. The primary purpose is to ensure that there is a record of the details of the incident and subsequent action taken, in the event that legal proceedings are instituted.
- **Informed consent:** One of the most fundamental rights of patients is the right to consent to treatment. It is indeed a well established principle of law that an adult of sound mind has the right to decide what shall or shall not be done to his body. In emergency when treatment is matter of life and death and the patient is unable to give permission/consent may be implied.

Legal Implication in Record Maintenance

- Informed consent is essential before surgery or investigation for the patients.
- Confidential record and report should be shown to authorize persons only.
- Registration of births, deaths and stillbirths are the important vital events.

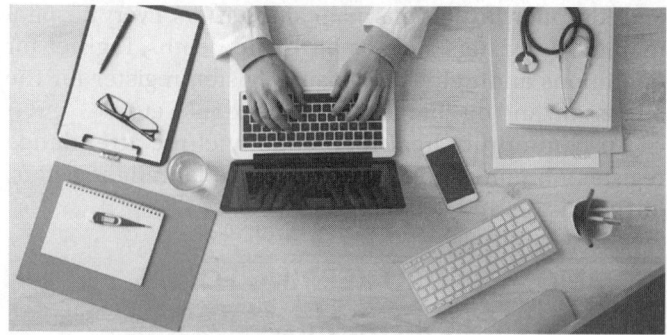

Fig. 5.7: Data entry by using software.

- Medicines should be administered as per the order of physician and also under supervision.
- Checking of labels, appearance of drug and also should be charted accurately before administration.
- Recording and reporting accidents, errors and incompetent behaviors.
- Identification of babies in labor ward by disks.
- Identification of dead bodies in mortuary.

Legal Approaches in the Community

- **Individual approach:** Birth, death report individual health record, immunization chart, maternal description, etc. all records and reports have legal importance.
- **Community approach:** Records and reports present the legal basis through which changes can be levied against medical administration of political system coming in the implementation of health programs, mistakes in the evaluation and medical and administrative inactivity.
- **Nursing approach:** Preserving the individual and family health records of the patients, maintaining the confidentiality and privacy of the records. Records related to medicolegal cases, dying declaration and will, etc. should be handled carefully for giving witness whenever needed.

ROLE OF A NURSE IN RECORDING AND REPORTING

Records and reports are the essential components of implementation and evaluation of community health activities. It is necessary for the community health that nurse to have thorough knowledge of their maintenance.

Securing Record Information

- Records are started in the center or at home at a time when the individual is seeking some service or when the health worker recognizes the need for service. The nurse and the individual should be comfortably seated in a private quiet area so that confidential information can be given and kept at a professional level.
- The record should show chronologically to what extent progress is being made towards the goal of better health

Documentation and Reporting

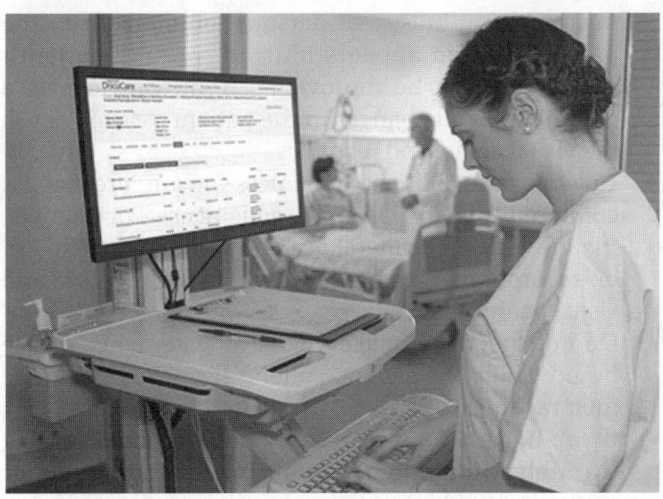

Fig. 5.8: Updating the patient's data in clinical setting.

for the individual and the family. This is particularly important in regard to better nutrition and sanitation.
- The individual and family cooperation in making out the record is important. Explain the reason for making the record, how the record will be used and the confidential nature of the record.

Record Filing: Correct filing of records is essential. Hours of time and effort are served when records are set up and maintained in a systematic planned and organized manner. Some agencies file records alphabetically and others use a numerical system.

Precautions in the Maintenance: The community health nurse should take following precautions in the maintenance of records and reports:
- The records should be kept carefully at a clean place.
- The records should be protected against mice, termites and insects, etc.
- Good filing system should be developed for the records and reports.
- Records should be easily available on time.
- Confidential record and report should be shown to authorize persons only.

School Health Records: It is essential to maintain complete, accurate and continuous health records of school children. It also helps to evaluate the school health services and assist in further development and improvement of health services rendered to school children. It should include information about identification and personal aspect, personal and family health history, findings of physical and medical examination, findings of routine investigations and screening services rendered and the prognosis.

MINIMIZING THE LEGAL LIABILITY THROUGH EFFECTIVE RECORD KEEPING

The nursing record is where we write down what nursing care the patient receives and the patient's response to this, as well as any other events or factors which may affect the patient's wellbeing. These 'events or factors' can range from a visit by the patient's relatives to going to theater for a scheduled operation.

How to Keep Good Nursing Records

The patient's record must provide an accurate, current, objective, comprehensive but concise account of his/her stay in hospital. Traditionally, nursing records are handwritten. Do not assume that electronic record keeping is necessary.
- Use a standardized form. This will help to ensure consistency and improve the quality of the written record. There should be a systematic approach to providing nursing care (the nursing process) and this

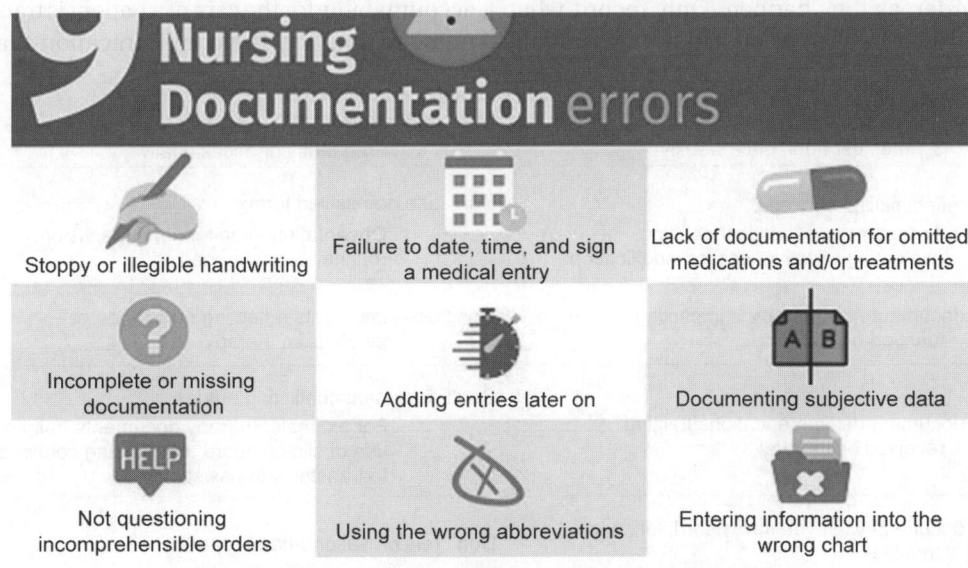

Fig. 5.9: Common documentation errors in nursing practice.

should be documented consistently. The nursing record should include assessment, planning, implementation, and evaluation of care.
- Ensure the record begins with an identification sheet. This contains the patient's personal data: name, age, address, next of kin, career, and so on. All continuation sheets must show the full name of the patient.
- Ensure a supply of continuation sheets is available.
- Date and sign each entry, giving your full name. Give the time, using the 24-hour clock system. For example, write 14:00 instead of 2 pm.
- Write in dark ink (preferably black ink), never in pencil, and keep records out of direct sunlight. This will help to ensure they do not fade and cannot be erased.
- On admission, record the patient's visual acuity, blood pressure, pulse, temperature, and respiration, as well as the results of any tests.
- State the diagnosis clearly, as well as any other problem the patient is currently experiencing.
- Record all medication given to the patient and sign the prescription sheet.
- Record all relevant observations in the patient's nursing record, as well as on any charts, e.g. blood pressure charts or intraocular pressure phasing charts. File the charts in the medical notes when the patient is discharged.
- Ensure that the consent form for surgery, signed clearly by the patient, is included in the patient's records.
- Include a nursing checklist to ensure the patient is prepared for any scheduled surgery.
- Note all plans made for the patient's discharge, e.g. whether the patient or career is competent at instilling the prescribed eye drops and whether they understand details of follow-up appointments.

Writing Tips

- Ensure the statements are factual and recorded in consecutive order, as they happen. Only record what you, as the nurse, see, hear, or do. Do not use jargon, meaningless phrases, or personal opinions (e.g. "the patient's vision appears blurred" or "the patient's vision appears to be improving"). If you want to make a comment about changes in the patient's vision, check the visual acuity and record it.
- Do not use an abbreviation unless you are sure that it is commonly understood and in general use. For example, BP and VA are in general use and would be safe to use on records when commenting on blood pressure and visual acuity, respectively.
- Do not speculate, make offensive statements, or use humor about the patient. Patients have the right to see their records!
- If you make an error, cross it out with one clear line through it, and sign. Do not use sticky labels or correction fluid.
- Write legibly and in clear, short sentences.
- Remember, some information you have been given by the patient may be confidential. Think carefully and decide whether it is necessary to record it in writing where anyone may be able to read it; all members of the eye care team, and also the patient and relatives, have a right to access nursing records.

Keep the nursing records in a place where they can be accessed easily; preferably near to where the nursing team meets at shift change times. This will ensure that records are available for handover sessions and also those they are easily accessible to the rest of the eye care team. The handover may take place with the patient present, if appropriate. Indeed, nursing records can only be accurate if patients have been involved in decision making related to their care. File the nursing records in the medical notes folder on discharge. Ensure that the whole team knows if nursing records are stored elsewhere.

CHANGE-OF-SHIFT REPORT

Change-of-shift report is the time when responsibility and accountability for the care of a patient is transferred from one nurse to another. The communication that ensues during

Do use objective measures: 3 Times per hour, once weekly	Don't use vague terms: Frequently or occasionally
Do reflect skilled services: Assessment, education/teaching, evaluating effectiveness, or modification	Don't use non-skilled terms: Observation, monitoring, supervision, routine, or unchanged
Do document how therapy is impacting function on the unit	Don't use statements reflecting no change or benefit from therapy
Do document recommendations/training received by therapy	Don't document conflicting entries: For example, therapy documents trained on use of sliding board, but nursing continues to transfer with assist of two
Do document what you saw, heard, felt, and smelled	Don't rely on second-hand reports

Fig. 5.10: Guidelines of do's and don'ts in documentation.

this process is linked to both patient safety and continuity of care giving. While many nurses already recognize the value of bringing report to the patient's bedside and have practiced in this manner, this remains relatively uncommon. Typically, nurse change-of-shift report has occurred at a nurses' station, conference room, or hallway and may be face to face, audio-taped, recorded on a telephone service, or in a written format. When report is given away from the bedside, the opportunity to visualize the patient and include the patient and family in an exchange of information and care planning is lost. Yet, patients and families, also stewards of patient safety, are given an opportunity to hear and participate in the exchange of information when report is brought to the bedside. Welcoming patients and families into the report process may be a new and challenging process for nursing staff.

In nursing, a **change-of-shift report** is a meeting between nursing staff members at the change of shift in which patient information is exchanged. Report is generally given by the nurse in charge of one shift to those coming on for the next, and in some facilities, nurse assistants participated in report, though the charge nurse is primarily responsible for making the report. During report, the outgoing nurses discuss with the oncoming nurses the condition of each patient and any changes that have occurred to the patient during the shift. The purpose is not to cover all details recorded in the patient's medical record, but to summarize individual patient progress. Most reports will include new arrivals, discharges, and deaths.

While report is necessary in order to communicate important information between nurses, various problems are posed by the giving of report. Nurses in many places are legally not permitted to leave the facility until they have given report. Walking off the job may be considered abandonment, which may be grounds for revocation of the nurse's license. At the same time, facilities are not legally required in all places to pay nurses for the extra time beyond their shift they are forced to stay over to complete report. It is not uncommon for nurses to attend report in their own time before and after a shift. While privacy laws require report to be given in a location where patients, visitors, and non-nursing staff cannot hear the report, some facilities prohibit family members from visiting patients during report times.

INCIDENT REPORT

An incident report is a form that filled up in order to record the details of accidents, patient injury and other unusual events that occur in a health care facility such as a hospital or nursing home. It is also called an **accident report** which documents the exact details of the accident or unusual event while the information is still fresh in the minds of those who witness the event.

Purpose of an Incident Report

- To document the exact detail of an accident or unusual incident that occurred in a health-care institution.
- To be used in the future when dealing with liability issues stemming from the incident.
- To protect the nursing staff against unjust accusation.
- To protect and safeguard the client in case of negligence on the part of the nurse.
- Helps in the evaluation of nursing care to ensure safe care to all patients.

Function/Purpose

An incident report is not part of the patient's chart, but it may be used later in litigation. A report has two functions:
- It informs the administration of the incident so management can prevent similar incidents in the future.
- It alerts administration and the facility's insurance company to a potential claim and the need for investigation.

When to Report

Incidents that must be reported and documented include:
- Exposure Incidents: Skin, eye, mucous membrane or parental contact with blood or other potentially infectious materials that may result from the performance of an employee's duties.
- Accident/Injury: Patient, visitor, employee slips or falls, or other incident, which results or may result in injury.
- Event, behaviors, or actions: Incidents that are unusual, contrary to agency policy or procedure or which may result in injury.
- Vaccine adverse event reporting system: Reaction to vaccine administered at agency.
- Medication reaction: Reaction to any drug administered at or provided by health department.

Tips for Reporting Incidents

- Include essential information, such as identity of the person involved in the incident, the exact time and place of the incident and the name of the doctor you notified.
- Document any unusual occurrences that you witnessed.
- Record the events and the consequences for the patient in enough detail that administrators can decide whether or not to investigate further.
- Write objectively, avoiding opinions, judgments, conclusions, or assumptions about who or what caused the incident. Tell your opinions to your supervisor later.
- Describe only what you saw and heard and the actions you took to provide care at the scene. Unless you saw a patient fall, write "found patient lying on the floor".
- Do not admit that you are at fault or blame someone else. Steer clear of statements like "better staffing would have prevented this incident".
- Do not offer suggestions about how to prevent the incident from happening again.
- Do not include detailed statements from witnesses and descriptions of remedial action; these are normally part of an investigative follow-up.

Incident Report

EMPLOYEE DETAILS

NAME	
DEPARTMENT	
PHONE NUMBER	

DESCRIPTION OF INCIDENT

Location:	
Date:	**Incident Details**
Time:	(How the incident happened, factors leading to the event, and what took place. Be as specific as possible.)
Police Notified: ☐ Yes ☐ No	

Incident Causes:	Follow Up Recommendations:

Incident reports are necessary for documenting details of the occurrence while they are most present in the minds of the witnesses and incident reporter. The information that is included in the report can be useful for decision-making on future incidents, identify behavioral patterns and identifying larger issues. To maintain a safe and healthy work environment, a thorough investigation should be undertaken following an incident in order to initiate corrective actions.

REPORTED BY:
Name:
Position:
Department:

- Do not put the report in the medical record. Send it to the person designated to review it according to your facility's policy.

TRANSFER REPORT

Transfer report done in case of client is transferred from one ward to another ward to receive different level of care. For example: client transferred to recovery room to postoperative ward, when the client no longer requires such intensive services. To facilitate continuity of care transfer report may be given by phone or in person. While giving transfer report, nurse must consider the following points:

- Clients name, age, gender, primary physician, medical diagnosis, surgery required.
- Summary of progress up to the time of transfer.
- Current health status—physical, physiological and psychological.
- Current plan of care.
- Any critical assessment or intervention to be completed shortly after transfer-helps the nurse to establish plan and priority of care.
- Any special precautions such as isolation, etc.
- Need for any special equipments.

The receiving nurse can ask question or clarify explanations about clients status. Sometimes written documentation must include record of information reported. It facilitates the continuity of care.

CONCLUSION

Documentation is the process of communicating in written form about essential facts for the maintenance of history of events over a period of time. An effective health record shows the extent of the health problems' needs and other factors that affect individuals their ability to provide care and what the family believes. What has been done and what to be done now, also can be shown in the records. It also indicates the plans for future visits in order to help the family member to meet the needs. Registers provide indication of the total volume of service and type of cases seen. Clerical assistance may be needed for this. Registers can be of various types such as immunization register, clinic attendance register, family planning register, birth register and death register. Reports can be compiled daily, weekly, monthly, quarterly and annually. Report summarizes the services of the nurse and/or the agency. Reports may be in the form of an analysis of some aspect of a service. These are based on records and registers and so, it is relevant for the nurses to maintain the records regarding their daily case load, service load and activities. Thus, the data can be obtained continuously and for a long period. Records and reports reveal the essential aspects of service in such logical order so that the new staff may be able to maintain continuity of service to individuals, families and communities.

BIBLIOGRAPHY

1. District hospitals-Guidelines for development. WHO. Geneva: HTBS publishers, 1994.
2. Gopalakrishnan, Sunderasan: Material Management, Prentice Hall of India Pvt Ltd, New Delhi, 1979.
3. Gupta S, Kanth S. Hospital Stores Management: An Integrated Approach, 1st Ed. New Delhi: Jaypee Brothers, 2004.
4. Koontz H, Weihrich H. Essentials of Management: An International Perspective, Ist Ed. New Delhi: Tata Mc Graw Hill publishers; 2007.
5. Koontz H, Weihrich H. Management a Global Perspective, 1st Ed. New Delhi: Tata Mc. Graw Hill Publishers; 2001.
6. Kulkarni GR. Managerial accounting for hospitals. Mumbai: Ridhiraj enterprise, 2003.
7. Kumar R, Goel SL. Hospital Administration and Management. Vol 1st ed. New Delhi: Deep and Deep Publications.
8. Wise PS. Leading and Managing in Nursing. 1st Ed. Philadelphia: Mosby Publications, 1995.

REVIEW QUESTIONS

Long Essays

1. Define documentation; enumerate the purpose of recording and reporting.
2. Explain the professional principles of documentation; describe the guidelines for documentation and record keeping.

Short Essays

1. Communication system in the hospital.
2. Types of records and reports used in nursing.
3. Principles of record keeping.
4. Nurses responsibility in recording.
5. Define computerized documentation and explain the advantages of computerized documentation.
6. Describe the methods of recording.
7. Legal issues in recording and reporting.

Short Answers

1. Importance of documentation.
2. Purpose of clinical records.
3. General rules of recording.
4. Standard care plans.
5. Shift report.
6. Incidental report.

MULTIPLE CHOICE QUESTIONS

1. **Documentation is:**
   a. Written communication
   b. Verbal communication
   c. Both (a) and (b)
   d. None of the above
2. **Documentation and reporting are:**
   a. Done for legal purpose
   b. Maintaining consistence of work
   c. Minimizing repetition of work
   d. All of the above
3. **Types of reporting in nursing, *except*:**
   a. Medical report
   b. Shift report
   c. Transfer report
   d. Incident report
4. **Records and reports are important for:**
   a. Decision making
   b. Research and education
   c. Legal issues
   d. All of the above
5. **The following are the characteristics of documents, *except*:**
   a. Transferency
   b. Factual
   c. Completeness
   d. Legible
6. **The advantages of computerized documentation are:**
   a. Systematic approach
   b. Fast communication
   c. Cost effective
   d. All of the above

ANSWERS

1. c   2. d   3. a   4. d   5. a   6. d

CHAPTER 6

Health Assessment

LEARNING OBJECTIVES
- Interview techniques
- Observation techniques
- Purposes of health assessment
- Process of health assessment
  - Health history
  - Physical examination
- Methods: Inspection, palpation, percussion, auscultation, olfaction
- Preparation for examination: Patient and unit
- General assessment
- Assessment of each body system
- Documenting health assessment findings

TERMINOLOGY

- **Assessment:** Diagnostic procedures, history, physical services and tests for the purpose of determining whether or not an eligible Insured is an appropriate candidate for specified healthcare services.
- **Appraisal (assessment):** Appraisal or assessment follows on from the scoping stage of a HIA, where the potential health impacts which have been identified are assessed and evaluated using the available evidence base.
- **Admission assessment:** Comprehensive nursing assessment including patient history, general appearance, physical examination and vital signs completed at the time of admission.
- **Data retrieval:** The collection of patient care data from medical records.
- **Shift assessment:** Concise nursing assessment completed at the commencement of each shift or if patient condition changes at any other time during your shift.
- **Focused assessment:** Detailed nursing assessment of specific body system(s) relating to the presenting problem or current concern(s) of the patient. This may involve one or more body system.
- **Body areas:** Head (including the face); Neck; Chest (including breasts and axillae); Abdomen; genitalia, groin, buttocks; Back (including spine); and each extremity.
- **Organ systems:** Constitutional (vital signs, general appearance), eyes, ear, nose, throat; cardiovascular; gastrointestinal; genitourinary; musculoskeletal; dermatological; neurological; psychiatric; hematological/ lymphatic/immunological.
- **Integumentary:** Both overall body and organ systems should have skin assessments integrated into them. Integument includes skin, hair and nails.
- **Vital signs:** Vital signs, generally described as the measurement of temperature, pulse, respirations and blood pressure, give an immediate picture of a person's current state of health and well being. Normal and abnormal ranges with management guidelines follow for children and adults
- **Auscultation** Use the diaphragm of the stethoscope to auscultate breath sounds.
- **Crackles:** These are high pitched, discontinuous sounds similar to the sound produced by rubbing your hair between your fingers. (Also known as Rales)
- **Wheezes:** These are generally high pitched and "musical" in quality. Stridor is an inspiratory wheeze associated with upper airway obstruction (croup)
- **Rhonchi:** These often have a "snoring" or "gurgling" quality. Any extra sound that is not a crackle or a wheeze is probably rhonchi. Low pitched.

INTRODUCTION

Health assessment is an essential nursing function which provides foundation for quality nursing care and intervention. It helps to identify the strengths of the clients in promoting health. Health assessment also helps to identify client's needs, clinical problems or nursing diagnoses and to evaluate responses of the person to health problems and intervention. An accurate and thorough health assessment reflects the knowledge and skills of a professional nurse. Assessment is a key component of nursing practice, required for planning and provision of patient and family centered care. The registered nurse assesses, plans, implements and evaluates nursing care in collaboration with individuals and the multidisciplinary health care team so as to achieve goals and health outcomes.

DEFINITION

Health assessment is a systematic, deliberative and interactive process by which nurses use critical thinking to collect, validate, analyze and synthesize the collected information in order to make judgment about the health status and life processes of individuals, families and communities.

PURPOSE AND FACTORS AFFECTING HEALTH ASSESSMENT

- To understand the physical and mental well being of the patient.
- To detect disease in its early stage.
- To determine the cause and the extent of disease.
- To understand any changes in the condition of diseases, any improvement or regression.
- To determine the nature of the treatment or nursing care needed for the patient.
- To safeguard the patient and his family by noting the early signs especially in case of a communicable disease.
- To contribute to the medical research.
- To find out whether the person is medically fit or not for a particular task.

Purposes of assessment

- To gather information regarding client's health
- To determine client's normal function
- To organize the collected information
- To confirm hypothesis growing out of the nurse's interview
- To enhance investigation of nursing problems
- To frame nursing diagnosis
- It increases greater managing skill of handling patient's problem
- To identify the health problems
- To identify client's strengths
- To identify need for health teaching

Factors Affecting Health Assessment

- Physical setting.
- Clients personality and behavior
- Communication skill.
- Problem.
- Nurses personality and behavior.
- Nurses knowledge and skill.

PRINCIPLES OF HEALTH ASSESSMENT

In planning and performing health assessment, the nurse needs to consider the following:
- An accurate and timely health assessment provides foundation for nursing care and intervention.
- A comprehensive assessment incorporates information about a client's physiologic, psychosocial, spiritual health, cultural and environmental factors as well as client's developmental status.
- The health assessment process should include data collection, documentation and evaluation of the client's health status and responses to health problems and intervention.
- All documentation should be objective, accurate, clear, concise, specific and current.
- Health assessment is practiced in all healthcare settings whenever there is nurse-client interaction.
- Information gathered from health assessment should be communicated to other health care professionals in order to facilitate collaborative management of clients and for continuity of care.
- Client's confidentiality should be kept.

RESPONSIBILITIES OF NURSE IN HEALTH ASSESSMENT

- The nurse has the responsibility to carry out health assessment on every person under his/her care.
- The nurse should regularly perform focused assessments in response to client needs.
- The nurse needs to obtain client's consent prior to health assessment.
- The nurse should demonstrate a caring attitude, respect and concern for each client when doing a health assessment.
- The nurse has the responsibility in keeping confidentiality about the data being collected from his/her client.
- The nurse obtains information on a client using various techniques and tools, such as history taking, physical

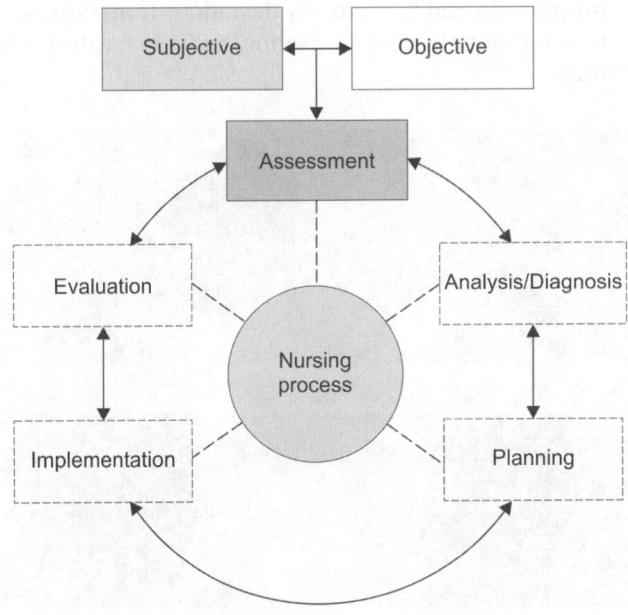

Fig. 6.1: Nursing process steps.

examination, reviewing clients' records and results of diagnostic tests. He/She has to draw inferences from data collected in order to make appropriate and sound clinical judgement.

- The nurse has to acquire specialized skills and competence in collecting accurate and relevant information on the patient's health in performing health assessment in order to make sound clinical decisions.
- The nurse should document the results of health assessment, analyze the data collected, evaluate the client's response to health problems and interventions, and provide feedback to the client as appropriate.
- The nurse should continuously advance their competence in health assessment throughout one's nursing career.
- The nurse who takes up an advanced practice role has the responsibility to prepare himself/herself in order to perform advanced and focused health assessment.

METHODS OF PHYSICAL EXAMINATION

Inspection

Visual examination of the body is called inspection. It is the observation with the naked eyes to determine the structure and functions of the body. Observe the client while facing him or her in the bed or chair. Observe the client's skin color and texture; check for lesions and hair distribution. Look at overall body structure. If the client can be out of bed, observe gait and stance. Note all parts of the body as the examination proceeds. Inspection also evaluates verbal and behavioral responses and mental status.

The following principles should be kept in mind for making accurate inspections:
- Good lighting and exposure are essential.
- Inspect each area for size, shape, color, symmetry and proposition and find out any deviations from normal.
- Use additional lights for examining body cavities, e.g. oral.
- Use sense of olfaction along with visual to detect abnormalities, e.g. bad breath indicates unhygienic mouth conditions. Acidotic smell is significant of diabetic acidosis.

Practice is required to learn inspection.
- **General inspection:** The initial act of physical examination is the inspection of the body as a whole. Most clinicians believe that composite pictures of disease, although composed of many sighs, strike them at a glance; they attempt to teach others perceive likewise. In looking at the patient as a whole, many facts are noted methods in physical examination/inspection. General inspection about motor activity, body builds outstanding anatomic malformation, behavior, speech, nutrition, and appearance of illness.
- **Local inspection:** Focusing observation on a single anatomic region yields hundreds of physical signs. Since only signs perceived by inspection can be illustrated, the myriad of pictures used in books on surgical diagnosis hint the importance of the method in that field. The dermatologist relies almost entirely on the appearance of skin lesions to make a diagnosis.
- Usage more or less confines the term inspection to observation with the unaided eyes. Actually, visual signs are the chief or only rewards in the use of the ophthalmoscope, slit lamp, gonioscope, otoscope, nasoscope, larynogoscope, bronchoscope, gastrocope, thoracoscope, peritoneoscope, cystoscope, anoscope, and sigmoidoscope. The pathologist uses the microscope; the radiologist inspects the fluroscopic screen and photographic films.

Palpation

It is the feeling of the body or a part with the hands to note the size and positions of the organs. In palpation the finger pads and not the finger tips are used.

Obtain information by using the hands and fingers to palpate. A light or deep palpation depends on the area

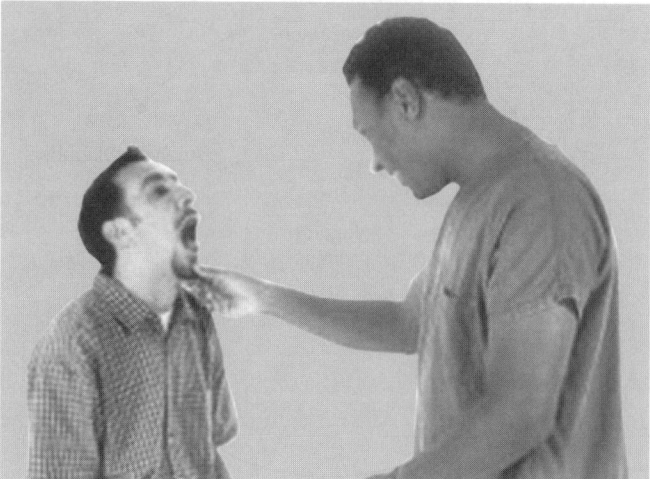

Fig. 6.2: Visual examination.

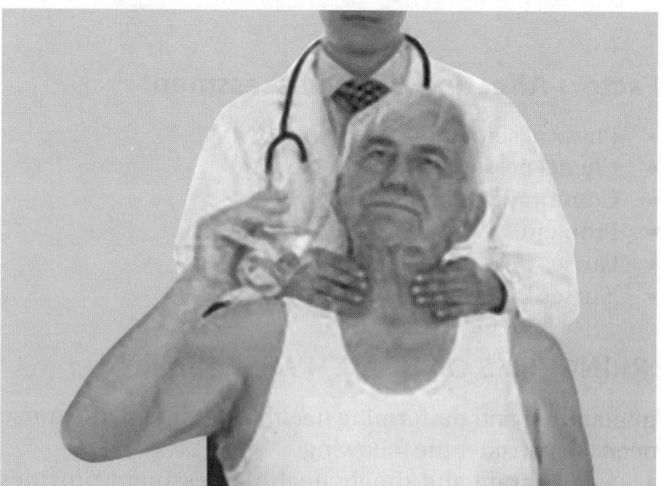

Fig. 6.3: Physical examination: Palpation.

being palpated. The palmar surface of fingers and finger pads are used to determine position of the organs, size and consistency, fluid accumulation, pain, and masses. The ulnar surface of the hand is used to distinguish vibration and temperature. The moisture and warmth of the skin can also be determined during palpation.

The following points are to be kept in mind while doing palpation:

- The client should be relaxed and comfortable. Observe non-verbal signs of discomfort during palpation.
- Palpation to be done with warm hands, short fingernails and a gentle approach.
- Palpation to be done slowly, and gently
- For light palpation the hand is depressed about 1 cm (1/2 inch) and for deeper palpation it should be approximately 2.5 Cms (1 inch).
- Use appropriate parts of the hands for doing various palpations. The usual definition of palpation is the act of feeling by the sense of touch. But this is too limited; when the physician lays his lands upon the patient, he perceives physical signs by his tactile sense, temperature sense, and his kinesthetic sense of position and vibration.

Palpation is widely used in the physical examination especially in the abdomen examination.

- **Sensitive parts of the hand:** Tactile sense. The tips of the fingers are the most sensitive for fine tactile discrimination, and temperature sense. Use the dorsa of the hands or fingers; the skin is much thinner than elsewhere on the hand. Vibratory sense. Palpate with the palmar aspects of the metacarpophalangeal joints rather than with the finger tips to perceive vibrations such as thrills or the precordial cardiac thrust. Probe the superiority for yourself by touching first the fingertip, then the palmar base of your finger, with a vibrating tuning fork. Sense diagnostic mode: Symptoms and signs. Use the grasping fingers, so you perceive with sensations from your joints and muscles.
- **Structures examined by palpation.** Palpation is employed on every part of the body accessible to the examining fingers: all external structures, all structures accessible through the body orifices, the bones, the joints, the muscles, the tendon sheaths, the ligaments, the superficial arteries, thrombosed or thickened veins, superficial nerves, salivary ducts, spermatic cord, solid abdominal viscera, solid contents of hollow viscera, accumulations of body fluids, pus, or blood.
- **Quality elicited by palpation:** Texture. The skin and hair, Moisture. The skin and mucosa. Skin temperature. At various levels of the body. Masses. The size, shape, consistency, mobility, pulsation (expansile or transmitted) precordial cardiac thrust. Crepitus. In bones, joints, tendon sheaths, pleura, subcutaneous tissue. Tenderness. In all accessible tissues. Thrills, over the heart and blood vessels. Vocal fremitus.
- **Special methods of palpation:** Light palpation, Deep palpation, Ballottement, Fluctuation, Fluid wave.

Percussion

It is the examination by tapping with the fingers on the body to determine the condition of the internal organs by the sounds that are produced. It is done by placing a finger of the left hand firmly against a part to be examined and tapping with the fingertips of the right hand. Produces sound waves by using the fingers as a hammer. Place the interphalangeal joint of the middle finger on the skin surface of the nondominant hand. Using the tip of the middle finger of the dominant hand, strike the placed finger. Vibration is produced by the impact of the fingers striking against underlying tissue. Sound or tone of the vibration is determined by body area or organ percussed. Normal lung areas produce a resonance sound; liver sounds are dull and a flat sound is heard over muscle.

Characteristics of sound produced are:

- Resonance: A low pitched and loud sound heard over the normal lung tissues.
- Hyperresonance: Very loud, very low pitch sound longer than resonance and is of booming quality signifies emphysema.
- Tympany: A drum-like sound heard over the air-filled tissues such as gastric air bubble.
- Dull: A medium-pitched sound with a medium duration without resonance heard over solid tissues such as heart. liver
- Flat: A high-pitched sound with a short duration without resonance heard over complete solid tissues such as hand, thigh. In physical diagnosis, percussion is the method of examination in which the surface of the body is struck to emit sounds that vary in quality according to the underlying tissues.

Methods of percussion: The percussion can be done by two methods. These are:

- Direct percussion: Striking the body surface directly with one or two fingers, e.g. ascitic thrill.
- Indirect percussion: Placing the middle finger of the non-dominant hand firmly against the body surface and

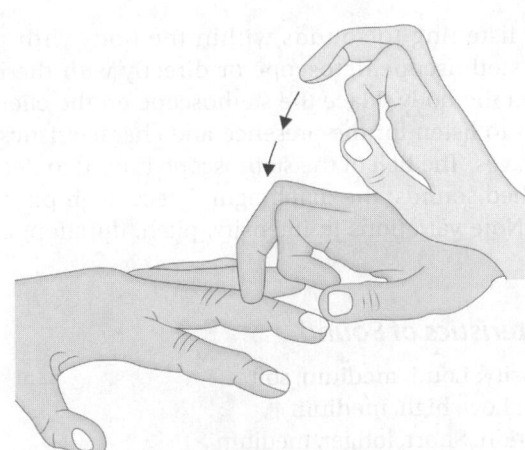

Fig. 6.4: Physical examination: Percussion.

striking the distal joint of non-dominant finger with the middle fingers of the dominant hand.

In the method the left middle finger is laid upon the body surface to serve as a pleximeter; it is struck sharp blow with the tip of the right middle finger, the plexor immediate or direct. The body surface is struck directly with one or more fingers of a hand.

- **Sonorous percussion:** This term is applied to any method of percussion when its purpose is to ascertain the density of the tissue by the sound emitted when struck. Various densities emit sounds given special meanings. The percussion notes may be arranged in sequence according to the density that produces them, from least to most dense: tympany hyperresonance, resonance, impaired resonance, dullness, flatness. Certain steps in normal tissues. Tympany is the sound emitted by percussing the air-filled stomach; resonance is produced by striking the air-filled lungs; flatness results from the thigh. In general the pitch or frequency of the sounds progresses through the series from lowest for tympany to highest for flatness; the duration of the sound ranges in the series from long to short. Sonorous percussion is employed to ascertain the density of the lungs, the pleural space, the pleural layers, and the hollow viscera of the abdomen.
- **Definitive percussion**, where two structures in apposition have greatly contrasting densities, as demonstrated by their percussion notes, mapping of area of greater density furnishes a concept of the size of the structure or the extent of its border. Any method of percussion used for this purpose is termed definitive percussion. Definitive percussion is commonly employed to ascertain the location of the lung bases, the width of the lung apices, the height of fluid in the pleural cavity the width of the mediastinum, the size of the heart, the outline of dense masses in the lungs the size and shape of the liver and spleen, the size of a distended gallbladder and urinary bladder, the level of ascitic fluid.

Auscultation

It is the listening to sounds within the body with the aid of a stethoscope, fetoscope or directly with the ear placed on the body. Place the stethoscope on the client's bare skin to listen for the presence and characteristics of sound waves. The bell of the stethoscope is used to detect low-pitched sounds; the diaphragm detects high-pitched sounds. Note variations in intensity, pitch, duration, and quality.

Characteristics of Sound

- Intensity: Loud, medium, soft.
- Pitch: Low, high, medium
- Duration: Short, longer, medium
- Quality: Booming, hollow, dull, drum like.

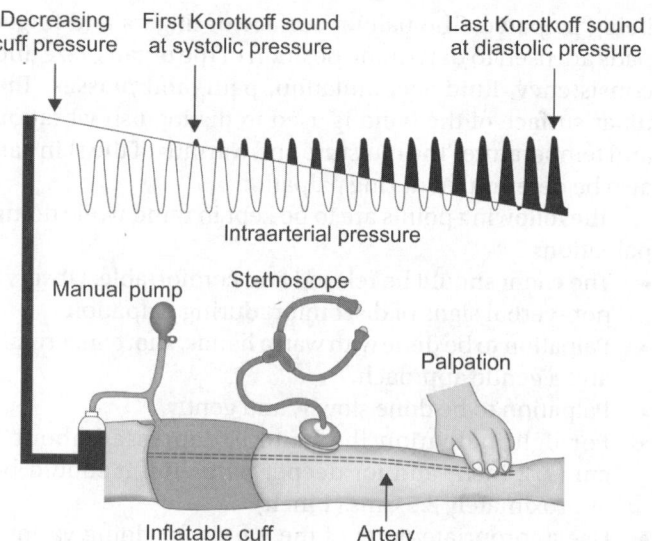

Fig. 6.5: Auscultation method of measuring blood pressure.

Techniques

- Stethoscope is used to block extraneous sounds when assessing the condition of heart, blood vessels, lungs, pleura and intestines.
- Bell/diaphragm after cleaning and warming is placed directly against skin because clothing may interfere with normal sounds.
- Bell used to hear soft pitched sounds like S1, S2 sounds (abnormal vascular sounds, murmur.
- Diaphragm of stethoscope is used to hear high pinched sounds like breath sounds, bowel sounds, normal hear sounds
- By placing diaphragm firmly, stabilize it between index middle finger, listen the characteristics of sound.

Manipulations

It is the moving of a part of the body to note its flexibility. Limitation of movements is discovered by this method.

Testing of Reflexes: The response of the tissues to external stimuli is tested by means of percussion hammer, safety pin, wisp of cotton, hot and cold water, etc.

HEALTH HISTORY

A total client assessment begins with a nursing health history. Using open-ended questions such as "Tell me about . . . ," collect data about past health conditions, current problems, and present needs. The information is obtained through objective (observed) and subjective (stated by client) data collection.

Information obtained from the interview and the physical assessment constitutes the basis for identifying nursing diagnoses and establishing the individualized client care plan. A complete health history includes the following elements:

Health Assessment

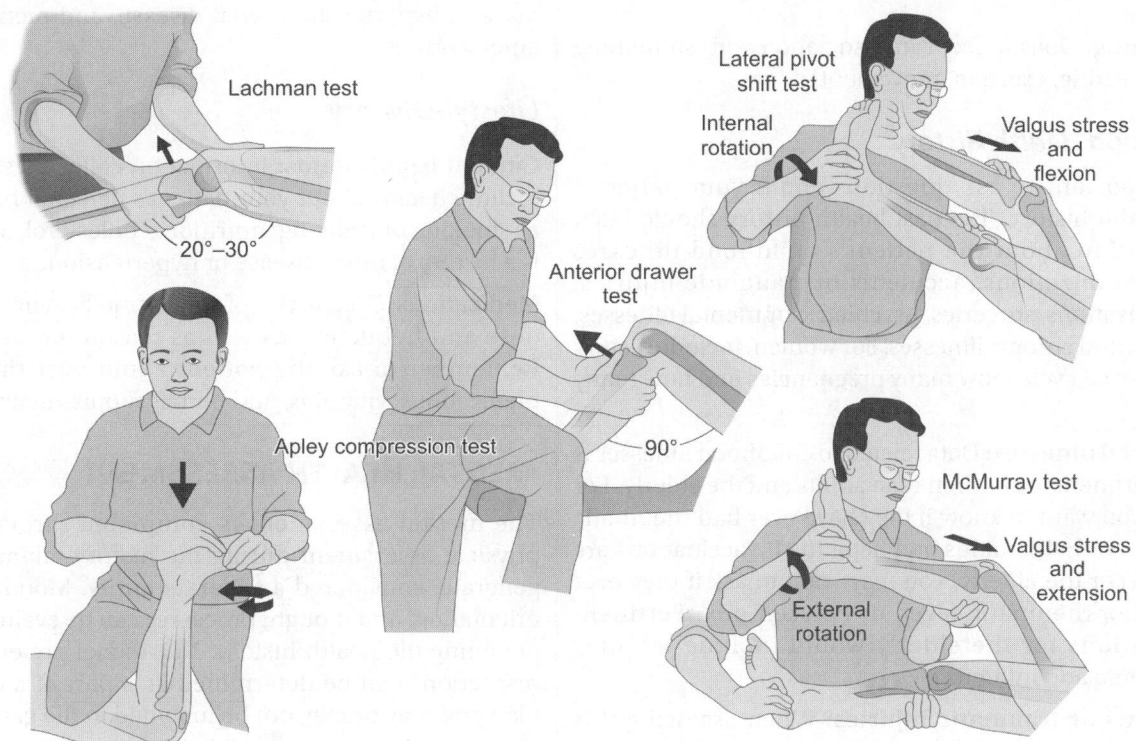

Fig. 6.6: Physical examination: Manipulation technique.

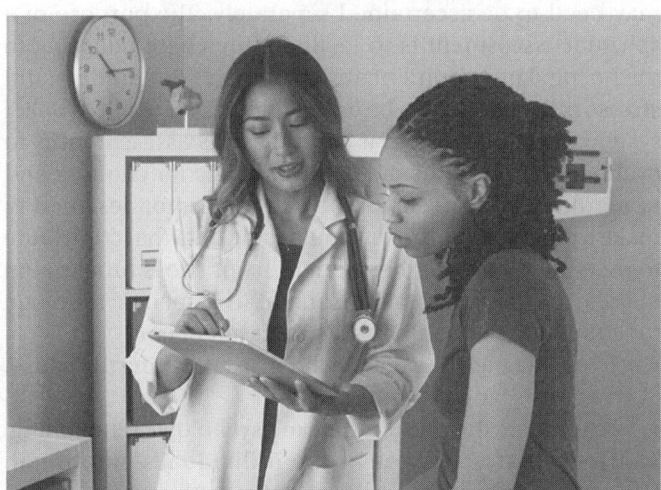

Fig. 6.7: Data collection by using interview technique.

- Biographic information: Age, sex, educational level, marital status, living arrangements.
- Chief complaint: Condition that brought client to health care facility; reason for visit; any recent changes.
- Present health status or illness: Onset of the problem; clinical manifestations, including severity of symptoms; pain characteristics if present.
- Health history: General state of health, past illnesses, surgeries, hospitalizations, allergies, over the counter (otc's) medications, herbal supplements, current medications, and general habits such as smoking, alcohol consumption, or recreational drug use.
- Family history: Age and health status of parents, siblings, and children; cause of death for immediate family members.
- Psychosocial factors, lifestyles: Cultural beliefs that influence health management; religious or spiritual beliefs.
- Nutrition: Dietary habits, preferences, or restrictions.
- Domestic violence: Joint Commission on Accreditation of Healthcare Organizations (JCAHO) requirement.

Present Health Status

Obtaining information about a patient's present health status allows the nurse to investigate current complaints. The mnemonic, PQRST, utilizes a structured format for information gathering, including evaluation of pain, and provides an efficient methodology to communicate with other healthcare providers. Use PQRST to assess each symptom and after any intervention to evaluate any changes or responses to treatment.

PQRST

P = Provocative or Palliative
- What makes the symptom(s) better or worse?

Q = Quality
- Describe the symptom(s).

R = Region or Radiation: Where in the body does the symptom occur? Is there radiation or extension of the symptom(s) to another area of the body?

S = Severity: On a scale of 1-10, (10 being the worst) how bad is the symptom(s)? Another visual scale may be appropriate for patients that are unable to identify with this scale.

T = Timing: Does it occur in association with something else (i.e. eating, exertion, movement)?

Childhood Health History

It is important to ask questions about your patient's past health history. The past health history should elicit information about the patient's childhood illnesses and immunizations, accidents or traumatic injuries, hospitalizations, surgeries, psychiatric or mental illnesses, allergies, and chronic illnesses. For women, include history of menstrual cycle, how many pregnancies and how many births.

Childhood illnesses: Data related to childhood illnesses is more pertinent to children than adults and the elderly. For adults, you want to know if they have ever had rheumatic fever and if their tetanus and hepatitis B vaccinations are current. For the elderly, you may want to ask if they ever had polio, rheumatic fever, or chicken pox. Pertinent vaccinations for the elderly would include tetanus, pneumonia and influenza.

Accidents or traumatic injuries: When assessing this area of the past health history, pay particular attention to patterns of injury, especially in infants, children, women and the elderly

Past Health History

Hospitalizations: Be sure to ask the reason for the hospitalization and the nature of the treatments received while in the hospital such as blood transfusions, surgeries and any follow-up treatments. Remember to include hospitalizations for childbirth

Surgeries: Many surgical procedures are performed on an outpatient basis. Questions regarding surgeries should also be asked in addition to hospitalizations, as patients may not discuss a surgery if there was no associated hospital stay.

Psychiatric or Mental Illnesses: If your patient has a past history of psychiatric or mental illnesses, ask what triggered the illness, if anything, and the course and the progression of the illness. This includes depression and anxiety, as well as diagnosed mental illness

Allergies: Identify what your patient is allergic to (both food and medication), as well as the reaction and response to treatment. It is important to ask about any environmental allergies or sensitivities (such as latex) also

Family History

Family history is important in identifying your patient's risk for certain disease states. Applicable generations with whom to explore health status include grandparents, parents, and the children of your patient. Chronic illnesses or known diseases with genetic components should also be screened for. Chronic illness or disease can include cancer, diabetes, autoimmune disorders, cholesterol, heart disease, hypertension, renal disease, and mental illness, among others.

Lifestyle History

Current health status: Information collected should also include details about your patient's personal habits, such as smoking or drinking, nutrition, cholesterol, and if there is a history of heart disease or hypertension.

Medications: Obtain a list of current medications, including dose and frequency, as well as reason for taking them. Remember to ask the patient about over the counter medications, vitamins, and herbal supplements.

MENTAL HEALTH ASSESSMENT

The mental assessment is completed throughout the physical assessment during the history taking. It is not generally considered a separate entity. Mood, memory, orientation, and thought processes can be evaluated while obtaining the health history. Nutritional preferences and restrictions can be determined as a part of a client care plan and may or may not be included in the general client assessment.

A spiritual assessment can be obtained as a part of the health history, although specific sociocultural beliefs may need to be ascertained separately. The purpose of a spiritual assessment is to facilitate the client adapting to the hospital environment and to help the staff understand stressors the client may be experiencing as a result of belief systems. The purpose of a mental status assessment is to evaluate the present state of psychologic functioning and to monitor safety needs of the client. It is not designed to make a diagnosis; rather it should yield data that contribute to the total picture of the client as he or she is functioning at the time the assessment is made. The specific rationale for completing a mental status assessment is:

- To collect baseline data to aid in establishing the cause, diagnosis, and prognosis.
- To evaluate the present state of psychologic functioning.
- To evaluate changes in the individual's emotional, intellectual, motor, and perceptual responses.
- To determine the client's ability to cope with the present situation.
- To assess the need and availability of support systems.
- To ascertain if some seemingly psychopathologic response is, in fact, a disorder of a sensory organ (i.e. a deaf person appearing hostile, depressed, or suspicious).
- To determine the guidelines of the treatment plan.
- To document altered mental status for legal records.

PREPARATION OF THE PATIENT

- Physical preparation
- Keep the patient clean.
- Shave the part if necessary.

- Keep the patient in a comfortable position which is convenient for the doctor to examine the patient.
- Empty the bladder prior to the examination. Empty the bowels by an enema if required.
- Loosen the garments and change into the hospital dress, if it is the custom.
- Drape the patient with extra sheets and expose only the need areas.
- Avoid unnecessary exposure.

Mental Preparation

- The patient may be quite new to the hospital situation and he may be anxious about his illness.
- He may have false ideas about the medical examination.
- It is the duty of the nurse to allay his anxieties and fears by proper explanations.
- Explain the sequence of the procedure to gain his confidence and co-operation.
- As far as possible a nurse should remain with a female patient during the physical examination.

PREPARATION OF THE ENVIRONMENT

- Maintenance of Privacy
- A separate examination room is needed.
- Keep the doors closed. The relatives are not allowed.
- Drape the patient according to the parts that are exposed.
- Lighting: As far as possible natural light should be available in the examination room, because if a patient is jaundiced, it may not be detected in the artificial light. There should be adequate lighting.
- Comfortable bed or examination table: The patient should be placed comfortably throughout the examination. There should be provision for the maintenance of a suitable position, e.g. a lithotomy position may be maintained when examining the genitalia. To maintain this position, a special examination table with stirrup rods is needed.
- The room should be warm and without draughts.

ADMISSION ASSESSMENT

An admission assessment should be completed by the nurse with a parent or care giver, ideally upon arrival to the ward or preadmission, but must be completed within 24 hours of admission. Admission assessment is to be documented on the nursing admission form. Privacy of the patient needs to be considered all times.

Patient history: History of current illness/injury (i.e. reason for current admission), relevant past history, allergies and reactions, medications, immunization status and family and social history. For neonates and infants consider maternal history, antenatal history, delivery type and complications if any, Apgar score, resuscitation required at delivery and newborn screening tests.

General appearance: Assessment of the patient's overall physical, emotional and behavioral state. Considerations for all patients include: Looks well or unwell, pale or flushed, lethargic or active, agitated or calm, compliant or combative, posture and movement.

Neonate and Infant
- Parent-infant, infant-parent interaction
- Body symmetry, spontaneous position and movement
- Symmetry and positioning of facial features
- Strong cry.

Young Child
- Parent-child, child-parent interaction
- Mood and affect
- Gross and fine motor skills
- Developmental milestones
- Appropriate speech.

Adolescent
- Mood and affect
- Personal hygiene
- Communication.

Vital Signs

Baseline observations are recorded as part of an admission assessment and documented on the patients observation chart.

- **Temperature:** Tympanic temperatures for children older than 6 months. Less than 6 months use digital per axilla.
- **Respiratory rate:** Count the child's breaths for one full minute. Assess any respiratory distress.
- **Heart rate:** Palpate brachial pulse (preferred in neonates) or femoral pulse in infant and radial pulse in older children. To ensure accuracy, count pulse for a full minute.
- **Blood pressure:** Baseline measurement should be obtained for every patient. Selection of the cuff size is an important consideration. A rough guide to appropriate cuff size is to ensure it fits a 2/3 width of upper arm. For neonates without previous hospital admissions do a blood pressure on all 4 limbs.
- **Oxygen saturation:** As clinically indicated.
- **Pain:** FLACC, Faces, numeric scale, Neonatal Pain Assessment Tool. Current pain relief medications/practices.

Additional Measurements

Weight: On admission and/or weekly/daily as clinically indicated.

Height: As clinically indicated.

Head circumference: As clinically indicated.

Blood sugar level (BSL): As clinically indicated.

Physical Assessment

A structured physical examination allows the nurse to obtain a complete assessment of the patient. Observation, inspection, palpation, percussion and auscultation are techniques used to gather information. Clinical judgment should be used to decide on the extent of assessment required. Assessment information includes, but is not limited to:

Airway: Noises, secretions, cough, artificial airway.

Breathing: Bilateral air entry and movement, breath sounds (normal and adventitious), respiratory rate, rhythm, work of breathing: spontaneous/labored/supported/ventilator dependent, any oxygen requirement and delivery mode.

Circulation: Pulses (location, rate, rhythm and strength); peripheral temperature, skin color and moisture, skin turgor, capillary refill time; lip, oral mucosa and nail bed color.

Disability: Use assessment tools such as, Alert Voice Pain Unresponsive score (AVPU) or University Michigan Sedation Score (UMSS), Gross Motor Function Classification System (GMFCS). Identify any aids required such as mobility aids, transfer needs, glasses, hearing aids, prosthetics, orthotics etc. Any abnormal movement or gait.

Focused assessment: Detailed nursing assessment of specific body system(s) relating to the presenting problem or current concern(s) of the patient. This may involve one or more body systems. For example, cardiovascular, respiratory, neurological.

Skin: Color, turgor, lesions, bruising, wounds, pressure injuries.

Input/Nutrition: Appetite, appropriate weight for age, food intolerance, nausea or vomiting, dietary requirements, oral, NG, Gastrostomy, Jejunal, IV, Fluids, Hydration state.

Output/Elimination: Bowel and bladder routine(s), incontinence management, drains and other losses.

Well-being: Mood, emotional state, comfort objects, sleeping habits and outcome, coping strategies, support networks, reaction to admission. Psychosocial assessments e.g. HEADSS

Socio-cultural: Parents/ careers/ guardian, living arrangements, siblings, visiting plans, transport, specific cultural requirements

SHIFT ASSESSMENT

At the commencement of every shift an assessment is completed on every patient and this information is used to develop a plan of care. Initial shift assessment is documented on the patient care plan and further assessments or changes to be documented in the progress notes.

The Shift Assessment includes:

Airway: Noises, secretions, cough, artificial airway.

Breathing: Bilateral air entry and movement, breath sounds, respiratory rate, rhythm, work of breathing, spontaneous/supported/ ventilator dependent, oxygen requirement and delivery mode.

Circulation: Pulses (rate, rhythm and strength); peripheral temperature, color and capillary refill time; skin, lip, oral mucosa and nail bed color.

Disability: Use assessment tools such as, Alert Voice Pain Unconscious scale(AVPU) or University Michigan Sedation Score (UMSS) and record on observation chart. Any aids, mobility or transfer requirements, prosthetics/orthotics required. Blood sugar levels as clinically indicated.

Focused: Assessment of presenting problem(s) or other identified issues, e.g. cardiovascular, respiratory, gastrointestinal, renal, eye, etc.

Pain: FLACC, Faces, numeric scale, Neonatal Pain Assessment Tool.

Hydration/Nutrition: Oral, nasogastric, gastrostomy, jejunal, fasting, breast fed, diet, IV fluids.

Output: Urine, bowels, drains, losses, fluid balance

Risk: Pressure injury risk assessment, falls risk assessment, ID bands.

Wellbeing: Mood, sleeping habits and outcome, coping strategies, reaction to admission.

Social: Family/guardian, discharge plan.

Review the history of the patient recorded in the medical record, however, it may be appropriate to ask questions to add additional details to the history.

FOCUSED ASSESSMENT

A detailed nursing assessment of specific body system(s) relating to the presenting problem or other current concern(s) is required. This may involve one or more body system.

Neurological System

A comprehensive neurological nursing assessment includes neurological observations, cognitive growth and development, fine and gross motor skills, sensory function, seizures and any other concerns. It may not be necessary to perform the entire neurological exam on a patient with no suspicion of neurological disorders. You should perform a complete baseline neurological examination on any patient that has verbalized neurological concerns in their history, or if a noted neurological deficit is discovered. When examining the nervous system, ask the following: Any past history of head injury? (Location, loss of consciousness)

- Do you have frequent or severe headaches? (When, where, how often)
- Any dizziness or vertigo? (Frequency, precipitating factors, gradual or sudden).
- Ever had/or do you have seizures? (When did they start, frequency, course and duration, motor activity

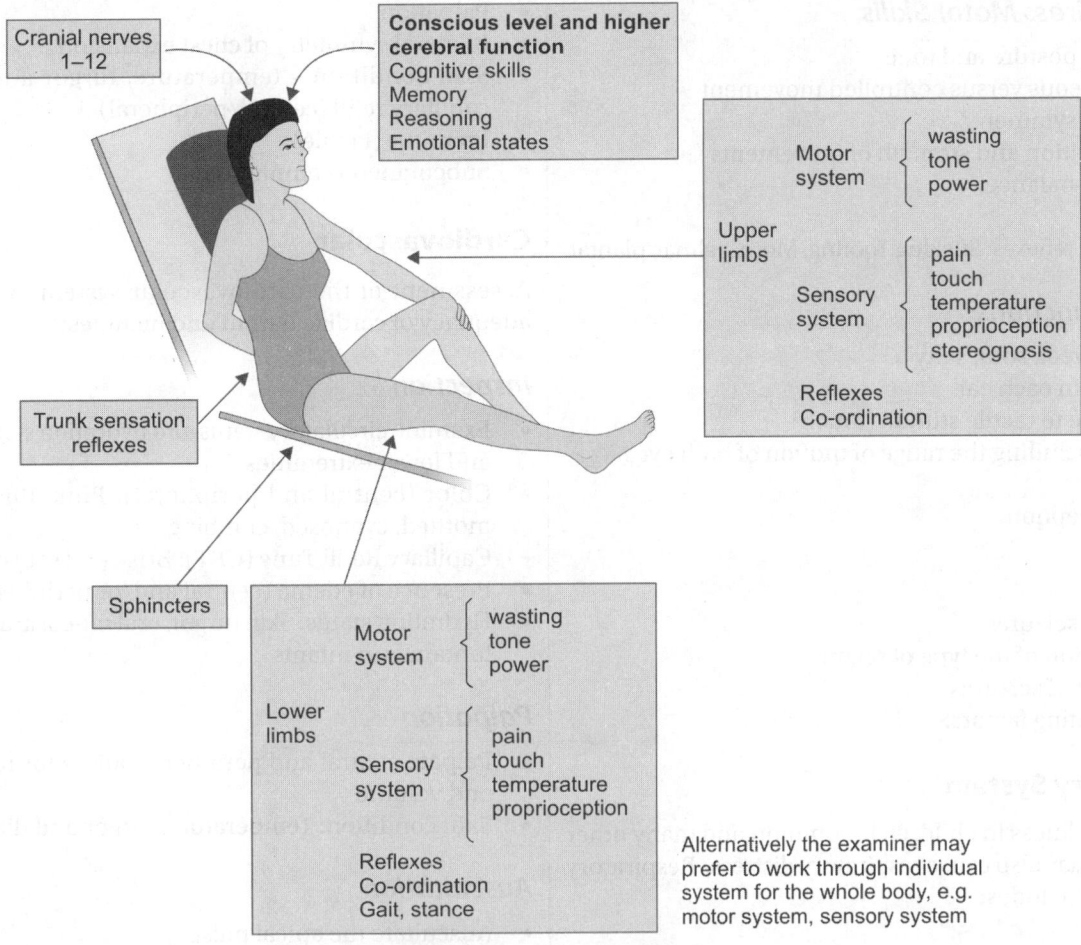

Fig. 6.8: Neurological assessment.

associated with, associated signs, postictal phase, precipitating factors, medications, coping strategies).
- Any difficulty swallowing? (solids or liquids, excessive saliva).
- Any difficulty speaking? (Forming words or actually saying what you intended).
- Do you have any coordination problems? (Describe)
- Do you have any numbness or tingling? (Describe)
- Any significant past neurologic history? (Cerebral vascular accident, spinal cord injuries, neurologic infections, congenital disorders)
- Environmental or occupational hazards? (Insecticides, lead, organic solvents, illicit drugs, alcohol)

Neurological Observations

- Glasgow Coma Scale to assess and interpret the degree of consciousness and is documented on the neurological observation chart
  - Assess the eye opens spontaneously, only when touched or spoken to, only to pain or not at all.
  - Observe the child's best age appropriate verbal response? For infants, an assessment is made of their cry and vocalization.
  - Observe the child's best age appropriate motor response?
- Arm and leg movements, assess right and left and document any differences.
- Pupil size and reaction to light.
- For neonates, check fontanels, check for presence of marks from forceps or vacuum delivery device, or presence of cephalohematoma or caput succedaneum.

Growth and Development

- Observe the head, shape, size and mobility. Head circumference should be measured, over the most prominent bones of the skull (e.g. frontal and occipital bones)
- In neonates and infants palpate fontanels and cranial sutures
- Inspect the spine looking for midline, lumps, dimples, hair or deformities
- Quality of cry or vocalization
- Review the history on attainment of developmental milestones, including progression or onset of regression. Consider attainment of rolling, sitting, crawling, walking, language development, bladder/bowel control, reading, etc.

Fine and Gross Motor Skills
- Observe posture and tone
- Spontaneous versus controlled movement
- Bilateral symmetry
- Coordination and strength of movements
- Gait and balance
- Reflexes
- Neonatal reflexes: Sucking, rooting, Moro, palmar, plantar.

Sensory Functions
- Taste- sweet, sour, salty
- Hearing in each ear
- Response to tactile stimuli (touch)
- Vision including the range of motion of both eyes
- Smell
- Proprioception.

Seizures
- Onset of seizures
- Description of the type of seizure
- Duration of seizures
- Precipitating factors.

Respiratory System

Respiratory illness in children is common and many other conditions may also cause respiratory distress. Respiratory assessment includes:

History
Onset + duration of symptoms: cough/shortness of breath Triggers (dust/aerosol/pollen).

Inspection/Observation
- Observe the overall appearance of the child: Alert, orientated, active/hyperactive/drowsy, irritable
- Color (centrally and peripherally): Pink, flushed, pale, mottled, cyanosed, clubbing
- Respiratory rate, rhythm and depth (shallow, normal or deep)
- Respiratory effort (Work of Breathing WOB): mild, moderate, severe, inspiratory: expiratory ratio, shortness of breath
- Use of accessory muscles (UOAM): Intercostal/subcostal/suprasternal/supraclavicular/substernal retractions, head bob, nasal flaring
- Symmetry and shape of chest
- Tracheal position, tracheal tug
- Audible sounds: vocalization, wheeze, stridor, grunt, cough - productive/paroxysmal
- Monitor for oxygen saturation.

Auscultation
- Listen for absence /equality of breath sounds
- Auscultate lung fields for bilateral adventitious noises, e.g.: wheeze, crackles, etc.
- Palpation
- Bilateral symmetry of chest expansion
- Skin condition – temperature, turgor and moisture capillary refill (central/peripheral)
- Fremitus (tactile)
- Subcutaneous emphysema.

Cardiovascular

Assessment of the cardiovascular system evaluates the adequacy of cardiac output and includes:

Inspection
- Examine circulatory status and hydration status of upper and lower extremities
- Color (central and peripheral): Pink, flushed, pale, mottled, cyanosed, clubbing
- Capillary Refill Time (CRT): Brisk (< 2 sec) or sluggish
- Presence of edema (central and/or peripheral)
- Hydration status: Skin turgor, oral mucosa, and anterior fontanels in infants.

Palpation
- Palpate central and peripheral pulses for rate, rhythm and volume
- Skin condition: Temperature, turgor and diaphoresis.

Auscultation
- Auscultate the apical pulse
- Compare peripheral pulse and apical pulse for consistency (the rate and rhythm should be similar)
- Auscultate the chest for heart sounds and murmurs.

Gastrointestinal

Assessment will include inspection, auscultation and light palpation of the abdomen to identify visible abnormalities; bowel sounds and softness/tenderness. Ensure stomach is not full at time of assessment as this may induce vomiting.

History
- Feeding (type of feed/patterns/difficulties), e.g. TPN, formula feeds, breastfeeding, any allergies/intolerances of feed
- Elimination (frequency, consistency, color, bleeding)
- Pain, cramping, nausea, vomiting (frequency, color, bleeding, consistency).

Previous stoma?
Previous NGT/NJT/PEG/PEJ.

Inspection
- Shape/symmetry of the abdomen (flat, rounded, distended, scaphoid)
- Contour of the abdomen (Smooth, lesions, malformations, any old or new scars)

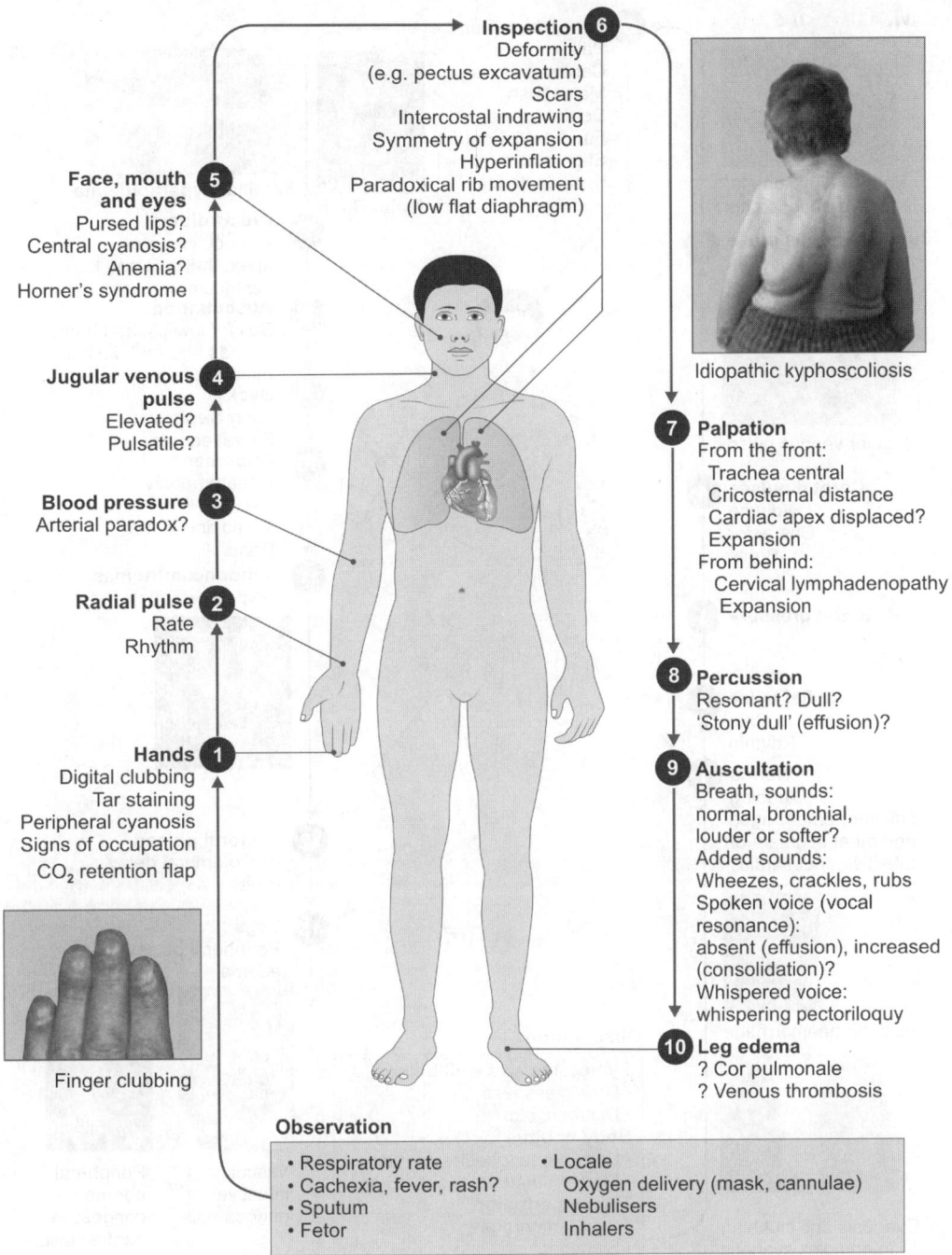

Fig. 6.9: Clinical examination of the respiratory system.

- Distention (mild/moderate/severe – tight/shiny)
- Umbilicus (bulging, scars, piercings) In neonates observe for redness, inflammation, discharge, presence of cord stump
- Inguinal area (bulging, herniation)
- Visible peristalsis
- Presence of NG/NGT/PEG/PEJ (indication)
- Stoma site (dressing regimen/frequency and consistency of output).

Palpation
- Light palpation only to identify
- Guarding
- Tenderness
- Pain (location, characteristics).

Auscultation
- Four quadrants (RUQ, RLQ, LUQ, LLQ) for bowel motility

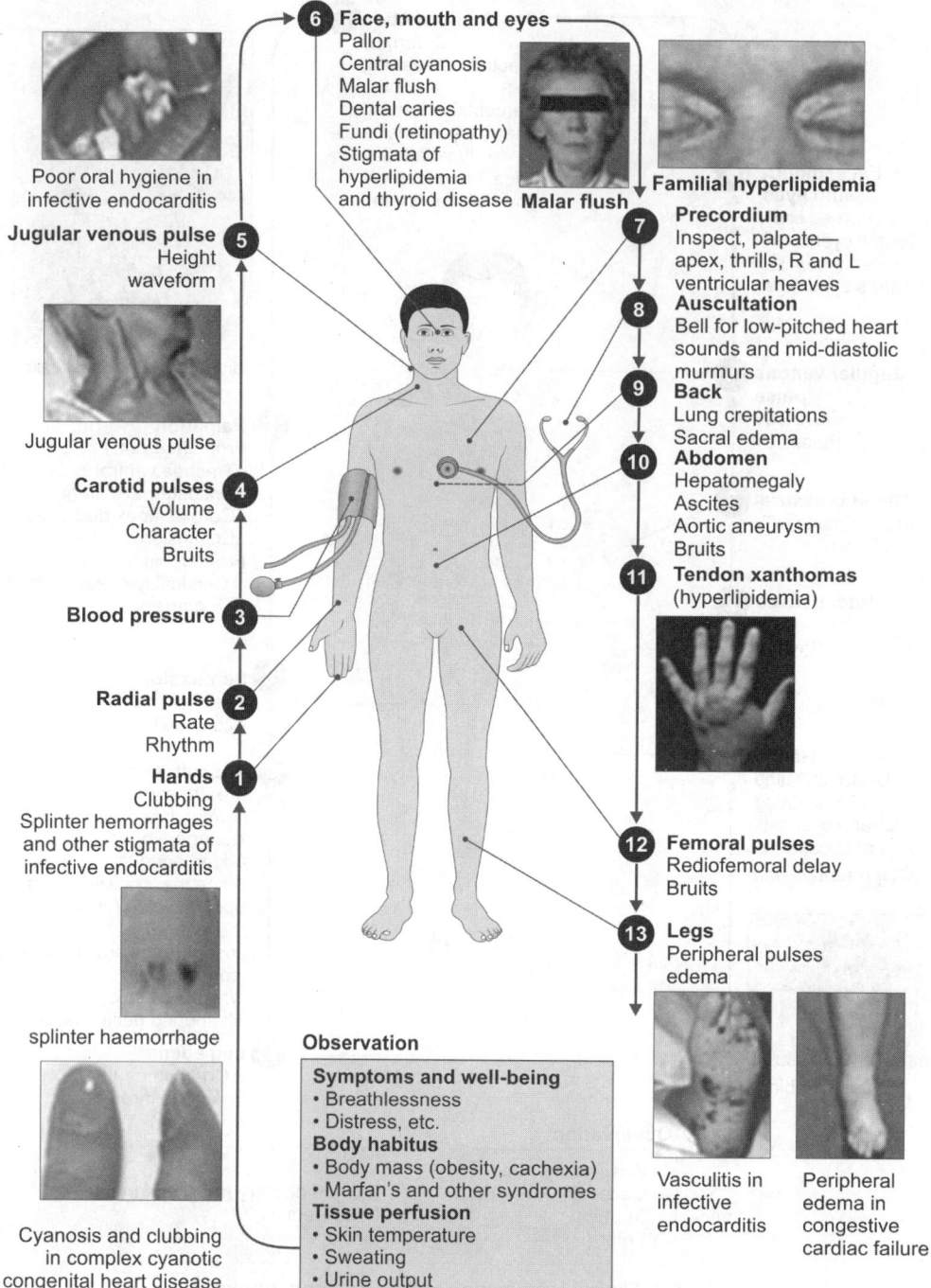

Fig. 6.10: Clinical examination of cardiovascular system.

- Bowel sounds present (frequency/character)
- Absent bowel sounds (one or all quadrants)
- Abdominal girth measurement as clinically indicated.

Renal

- An assessment of the renal system includes all aspects of urinary elimination
- Urinary pattern, incontinence, frequency, urgency, dysuria

- Hydration status including fluid balance, BP and weight
- Growth and feeding, diet or fluid restrictions
- Skin condition: Temperature, turgor and moisture
- Urine output (Normal children <2 yers is between 2-3 mL/kg/hr, >2 years is between 0.5-1 mL/kg/hr)
- Urinalysis (pH, ketones, protein, blood, leukocytes, specific gravity)
- Review blood chemistry results, urea, creatinine, electrolytes, albumin and hemoglobin.

Musculoskeletal

A musculoskeletal assessment can be commenced while observing the infant/child in bed or as they move about their room. Be aware that during periods of rapid growth, children complain of normal muscle aches. Throughout this assessment limbs/joints should be compared bilaterally.

Inspection

- Child's gait and ambulation
- Posture, movement and body symmetry
- Limbs for swelling, redness and obvious deformity
- Joint range of motion: Is it passive or independent? Are limbs moving equally? Is there pain on movement?
- Joints for redness or swelling.

Palpation

- Limbs for muscle mass, tone and strength
- Limbs for pain or tenderness.

Skin

Skin assessment can identify cutaneous problems as well as systemic diseases.

Inspection/Observation

- Color of the skin (pale/flushed, cyanotic, burned tissue).
- Rash: Note the size, color, texture and shape of the lesions (e.g. raised or flat, fluid filled) and the number and distribution (e.g. sparse, numerous, over limbs, etc.), itchy, painful.
- Note which area of the body it covers. Obtain a history of the rash from a parent/career.
- Non-blanchable petechial rash should be reported immediately.
- Bruising/wounds/pressure injuries: Assess any existing wounds
- Treatment Chart, for ongoing wound assessment and management.
- Examine high risk areas regularly, including bony prominences and equipment sites (masks, plasters, tubes, drains, etc.) for pressure injuries (Pressure injury prevention guideline). Report any irregular bruising.
- Nevi/Moles: Observe for size, any irregular borders, variation in colors.
- Larger nevi and changing ones should be reviewed by appropriate medical staff.
- Hair: Observe the condition of the scalp. Cradle cap is most common in newborns and is identified by thick, crusty scales over the scalp. Observe for lice or ticks.

Palpation

- Skin temperature, moisture, turgor, edema, deformities, hematomas and crepitus
- Hair texture for brittleness and moisture.

Eyes

Inspection of the eye should always be performed carefully and only with a compliant child.

Inspection/Observation

- Bilateral symmetry, shape, and placement of eye in relation to the ears
- Bilateral symmetry, size and shape of the pupils, reactivity to light
- Conjunctiva, and eyelids for inflammation, color and discharge
- Color of sclera
- Iris for up slanting/down slanting of palpebral fissures
- Visual acuity, including requirement for glasses or contact lenses
- Visual field
- Presence of tears. Close eyes in unconscious patient to protect cornea from drying and injury.

Ear/Nose/Throat (ENT)

Assessment of throat and mouth is essential as upper respiratory infections, allergies; oral or facial trauma, dental caries and pharyngitis are common in children. This includes a thorough examination of the oral cavity.

Inspection

- Inspect ears for symmetry, shape and position (dysmorphic or malposition ears).
- Observe for any external trauma, obvious cerumen, inflammation, redness or exudate, any obvious discharge, child pulling on ear.
- Inspect nose for symmetry, nasal patency, tenderness, septal deviation, masses or foreign bodies, note the color of the mucosal lining, any swelling, discharge, dryness or bleeding.
- Inspect lips for shape, symmetry, color, dryness, and fissures at the corners of the mouth.
- Inspect teeth for number present, condition, color, alignment, and caries.
- Inspect gingival tissue noting color and condition.
- Observe for bleeding gums, trauma to tongue or oral cavity, and malocclusion.
- Look for excessive fluid/secretions in the mouth.
- Inspect the hard and soft palate for lesions, presence and shape of uvula, size of tonsils, and buccal mucosa for color, exudate, and odor.

Palpation

- Palpate external structures of the ear (tragus, mastoid) for masses, lesions or tenderness.
- Palpate frontal and maxillary sinuses for tenderness in the older child.
  Palpation of the lips, gums, mucosa, palate and tongue may be possible in the compliant or older child, noting lesions, masses or abnormalities.

Evaluation of Assessment

In the evaluation phase of assessment, ensure the information collected is complete, accurate and documented appropriately. The nurse must draw on critical thinking and problem solving skills to make clinical decisions and plan care for the patient being assessed. If any abnormal findings are identified, the nurse must ensure that appropriate action is taken. This may include communicating the findings to the medical team, and the ANUM in charge of the shift. Patients should be continuously assessed for changes in condition while under RCH care and assessments are documented regularly.

PHYSICAL EXAMINATION PROCEDURE

It is a thorough inspection or a detailed study of the entire body or some part of the body to determine the general physical or mental conditions of the body.

Definition

- Physical examination is defined as a complete assessment of patient's physical and mental status.
- A systematic approach to the beside examination of a patient is essential to determine the significance of an abnormal physical finding. It includes five basic methods-namely, inspection, palpation, percussion, auscultation, and olfactory examination.

Competency Skills Required

- **Medically fit:** Medical personal working in hospital must be medically fit, he must have intact all the senses: hearing, viewing, toughing, testing and smelling.
- **Thoroughness:** Physical examination must be done systematically and thoroughly. Thoroughness means collect information by examining all body systems.
- **Knowledge:** Examiner must be confident. He should have up-date knowledge as well as skill in examining client as well as detecting problems.
- **Concentration:** Do the examination with full concentration. Dedication towards work is very important.
- **Accurate technique:** Make sure that accurate technique is used to collect information. Follow all the steps of procedure. It helps in avoiding error in detecting problem.
- **Objectivity:** Avoid personal judgment, bias, clues while examining the client. Make inference based up on findings.

Purpose

- To understand the physical and mental well-being of the patient.
- To detect disease in its early stage.
- To determine the cause and the extent of disease.
- To understand any changes in the condition of diseases, any improvement or regression.
- To determine the nature of the treatment or nursing care needed for the patient.

A comprehensive physical examination should be performed according to age specific preventive health guidelines. American Medical Association clinical practice guidelines recognize the following body areas and organ systems for purpose of the examination:

- **Body areas:** Head (including the face); Neck; Chest (including breasts and axillae); Abdomen; genitalia, groin, buttocks; Back (including spine); and each extremity.
- **Organ systems:** Constitutional (vital signs, general appearance), Eyes, Ear, Nose, Throat; Cardiovascular; Gastrointestinal; Genitourinary; Musculoskeletal; Dermatological; Neurological; Psychiatric; Hematological/lymphatic/immunological.
- **Integumentary:** Both overall body and organ systems should have skin assessments integrated into them. Integument includes skin, hair and nails.

Normal and abnormal findings should be recorded on a health history and physical examination form.

Measurements

Body measurements include length or height, weight, and head circumference for children from birth to 36 months of age. Thereafter, body measurements include height and weight. The assessment of hearing, speech and vision are also measurements of an individual's function in these areas. The Denver Development Screening Test measures an infant's and young child's gross motor, language, fine motor-adaptive and personal-social development milestones. If developmental delay is suspected based on an assessment of a parent's development/behavior concern or if delays are suspected after a screening of development benchmarks, a written referral is to a physician or pediatric nurse practitioner is imperative. A patient's measurements can be compared with a standard, expected, or predictable measurement for age and gender. Deviation from standards helps identify significant conditions requiring close monitoring or referral to a physician or pediatric nurse practitioner. The significance of measurements and actions to take when they deviate from normal expectations are age-specific.

How to Measure Height

- Obtain height by measuring the recumbent length of children less than 2 years of age and children between 2 and 3 who cannot stand unassisted. A measuring board with a stationary headboard and a sliding vertical foot piece is ideal, but a tape measure can also be used.
  - Lay the child flat against the center of the board. The head should be held against the headboard by the parent or an assistant and the knees held so that the

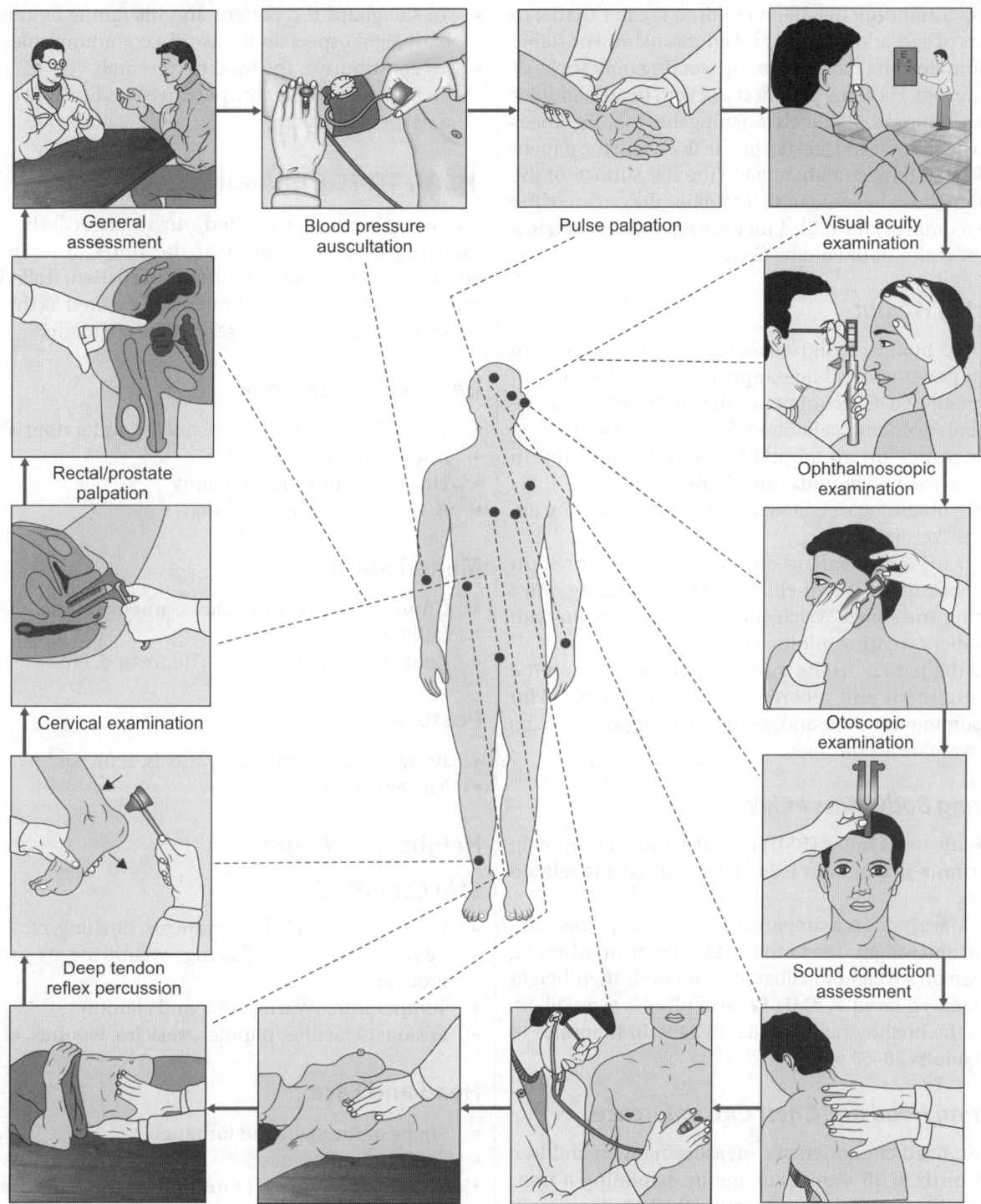

Fig. 6.11: Physical examination techniques.

hips and knees are extended. The foot piece is moved until it is firmly against the child's heels. Read and record the measurement to the nearest 1/8 inch.
- A modified technique in home settings is to lay the child flat and straight where the head should be held by the parent and the knees held so that the hips and knees are extended, mark the flat surface at the top of the head and tip of the heels. Move child and measure the distance between the marks with a tape measure. Read and record the measurement to the nearest 1/8 inch.
- When a recumbent length is obtained for a two-year-old child, it should be plotted on the birth to 36 months growth chart. When a standing height is obtained for a two year old, plot the finding on the 2 year to 18 year chart. After plotting measurements for children on age and gender specific growth charts, evaluate, educate and refer according to findings.

- Obtain a standing height on children greater than 2 to 3 years of age, adolescents, and adults, using a portable stadiometer. The patient is to be wearing only socks or be bare foot. Have the patient stand with head, shoulder blades, buttocks, and heels touching the wall. The knees are to be straight and feet flat on the floor, and the patient is asked to look straight ahead. The flat surface of the stadiometer is lowered until it touches the crown of the head, compress the hair. A measuring rod attached to a weight scale should not be used.

Measuring Weight

- Balance beam or digital scales should be used to weigh patients of all ages. Spring type scales are not acceptable. CDC recommends that all scales should be zero balanced and calibrated. Scales must be checked for accuracy on an annual basis and calibrated in accordance with manufacturer's instructions.
- Prior to obtaining weight measurements, make sure the scale is "zeroed".
- Weigh infants wearing only a dry diaper or light undergarments. Weigh children after removing outer clothing and shoes. Weigh adolescents and adults with the patient wearing minimal clothing.
- Place the patient in the middle of the scale. Read the measurement and record results immediately. Plot measurements on age and gender specific growth charts and evaluate accordingly.

Measuring Body Mass Index

- The body mass index (BMI) is a measure that can help determine if a person is at risk for a weight-related illness.
- Body Mass Index is a simple calculation using a person's height and weight. The formula is BMI = kg/m^2 where kg is a person's weight in kilograms and m^2 is their height in meters squared. A BMI of 25.0 or more is overweight, while the healthy range is 18.5 to 24.9. BMI applies to most adults 18–65 years.

Measuring Head and Chest Circumference

- Obtain head circumference measurement on children from birth to 36 months of age by extending a non-stretchable measuring tape around the broadest part of the child's head. For greatest accuracy, the tape is placed three times, with a reading taken at the right side, at the left side, and at the mid-forehead, and the greatest circumference is plotted. The tape should be pulled to adequately compress the hair.
- Head circumference should be measured each visit.
- Chest: This is measured at the nipple line.
- In a newborn, the head circumference will be about 2 cm larger than the chest circumference. As the child ages, the chest circumference becomes larger than the head circumference.

- To safeguard the patient and his family by noting the early signs especially in case of a communicable disease.
- To contribute to the medical research.
- To find out whether the person is medically fit or not for a particular task.

HEAD TO TOE EXAMINATION

The examination is carried out in an orderly manner focusing upon one area of the body at a time. The observation of the patient starts as the patient walks into the examination room, e.g. a limp may be noted as the patient walks in. The following observations are made:

General Appearance

- Nourishment: Well-nourished or under nourished
- Body build: Thin or obese
- Health: Healthy or unhealthy
- Activity: Active or dull (tired).

Mental Status

- Consciousness: Conscious, unconscious, delirious, talking incoherently
- Look: Anxious or worried, depressed, etc.

Posture

- Body curves: Lordosis, kyphosis, scoliosis
- Movement: Any limp.

Height and Weight

Skin Conditions

- Color: Pallor, jaundice, cyanosis, flushing, etc.
- Texture: Dryness, flaking, wrinkling or excessive moisture
- Temperature: Warm, cold, and clammy
- Lesions: Macules, papules, vesicles, wounds, etc.

Head and Face

- Shape of the skull and fontanel
- Skull circumference
- Scalp: Cleanliness, condition of the hair, drandruff, pediculi, infections like ringworm
- Face: Pale, flushed, puffiness, fatigue, pain, fear, anxiety, enlargement of parotid glands, etc.

Eye

- Eyebrows: Normal or absent
- Eyelashes: Infection, sty
- Eyelids: Edema, lesions, ectropion, entropion
- Eyeballs: Sunken or protruded
- Conjunctiva: Pale, red, purulent
- Sclera: Jaundice

- Cornea and iris: Irregularities and abrasions
- Pupils: Dilated, constricted reaction to light
- Lens: Opaque or transparent
- Fundus: Congestion, hemorrhagic spots
- Eye muscles: Strabismus (squint)
- Vision: Normal, myopia, hypermetropia.

Ears

- External ear: Discharges, cerumen obstructing the ear passage
- Tympanic membrane: Perforations, lesions, bulging
- Hearing: Hearing acuity.

Nose

- External nares: Crusts or discharges
- Nostrils: Inflammation of the mucous membrane, septal deviations.

Mouth and Pharynx

- Lips: Redness, swelling, crusts, cyanosis, angular stomatitis
- Odor of the mouth: Foul smelling
- Teeth: Discoloration and dental caries
- Mucus membrane and gums: Ulceration and bleeding, swelling, pus formation
- Tongue: Pale, dry, lesions, sords, furrows, tongue tie, etc.
- Throat and pharynx: Enlarged tonsils, redness and pus.

Neck

- Lymph nodes: Enlarged, palpable
- Thyroid gland: Enlarged
- Range of motion: Flexion, extension and rotation.

Chest

- Thorax: Shape, symmetry of expansion, posture
- Breathe sounds: Sigh, swish, rustle, wheezing, rales, crepitations, pleural rub, etc.
- Heart: Size and location, cardiac murmurs
- Breasts: Enlarged lymph nodes.

Abdomen

- Observation: Skin rashes, scars, hernia, ascites distension, pregnancy, etc.
- Auscultation: Bowel sounds, fetal heart sounds
- Palpation: Liver margin, palpable spleen, tenderness at the area of appendix, inguinal hernias
- Percussion: Presence of gas, fluid or masses.

Extremities

Movement of joints, tremors, clumbing of fingers, ankle edema, varicose veins, reflexes, etc.

Back

Spina bifida curves.

Genital and Rectum

- Inguinal lymph glands—Enlarged, palpable
- Patency of urinary meatus and rectum (in infants)
- Descent of the testes
- Vaginal discharges
- Presence of sexually transmitted diseases
- Hemorrhoids
- Enlargement of the prostate gland
- Pelvic masses.

Neurological Tests

- Coordination tests
- Reflexes
- Equilibrium tests
- Tests for sensations
- Role of the nurse in the physical examination.

Preparation of the Environment

Maintenance of Privacy

A separate examination room is needed. Keep the doors closed. The relatives are not allowed. Drape the patient according to the parts that are exposed.

Lighting

As far as possible natural light should be available in the examination room, because if a patient is jaundiced, it may not be detected in the artificial light. There should be adequate lighting.

Comfortable Bed or Examination Table

The patient should be placed comfortably throughout the examination. There should be provision for the maintenance of a suitable position, e.g. a lithotomy position may be maintained when examining the genitalia. To maintain this position, a special examination table with stirrup rods is needed.
The room should be warm and without draughts.

Preparation of the Equipment

All the articles needed for the physical examination are kept ready for the examination at hand.
- Sphygmomanometer.
- Stethoscope.
- Fetoscope.
- TPR tray.
- Tongue depressor.
- Pharyngeal retractor.
- Laryngoscope.
- Tape measure.
- Flash light.

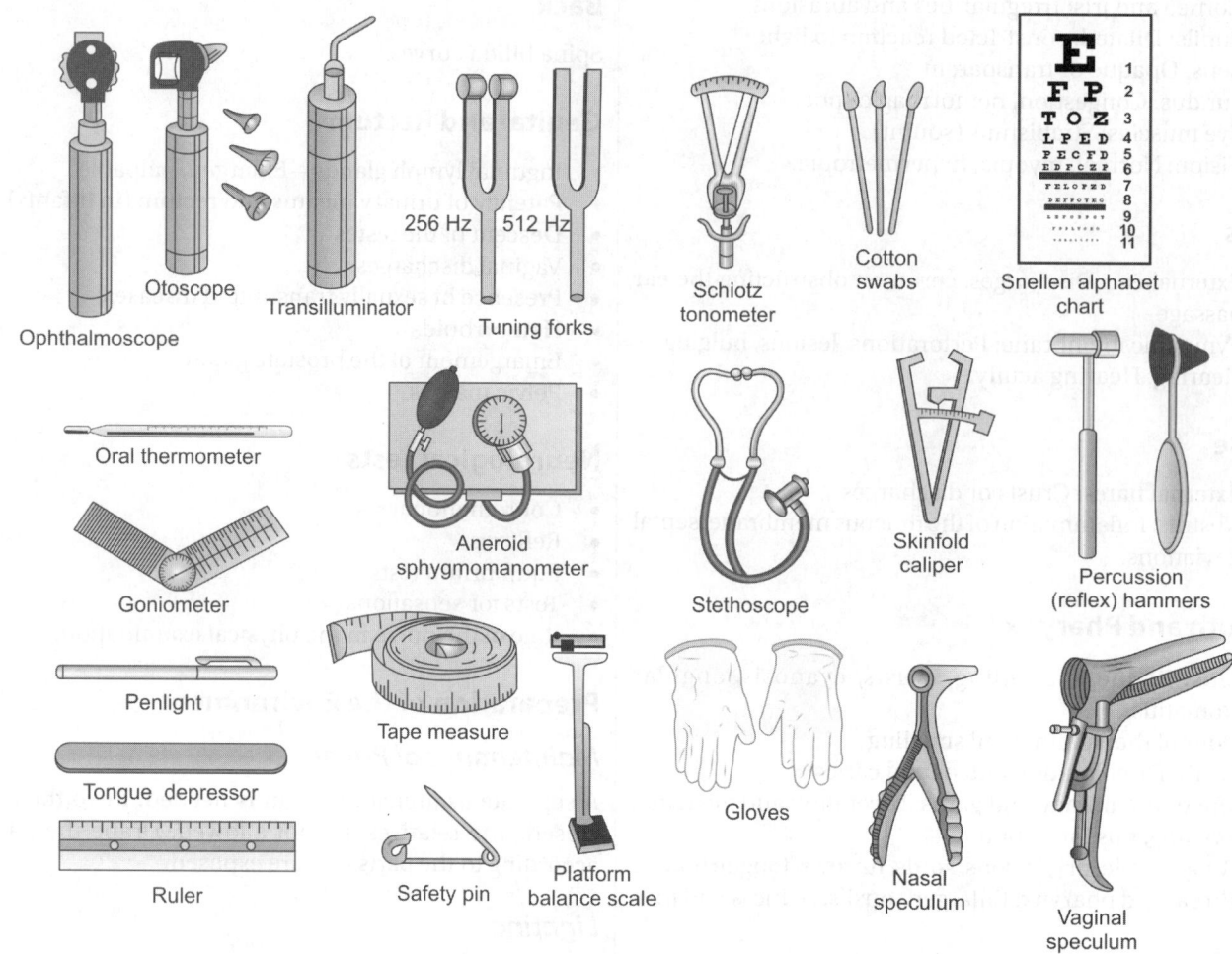

Fig. 6.12: Physical examination instruments.

- Weighing machine.
- Ophthalmoscope.
- Otoscope.
- Tuning fork.
- Nasal speculum.
- Percussion hammer, safety pins.
- Cotton wool, cold and hot water.
- Test tubes.
- Vaginal speculum.
- Protoscope.
- Gloves.
- Sterile specimen bottles, slides.
- Cotton applicators.

Preparation of the Patient

Physical Preparation

- Keep the patient clean.
- Shave the part if necessary.
- Keep the patient in a comfortable position which is convenient for the doctor to examine the patient.
- Empty the bladder prior to the examination. Empty the bowels by an enema if required.
- Loosen the garments and change into the hospital dress, if it is the custom.
- Drape the patient with extra sheets and expose only the need areas.
- Avoid unnecessary exposure.

Mental Preparation

- The patient may be quite new to the hospital situation and he may be anxious about his illness.
- He may have false ideas about the medical examination.
- It is the duty of the nurse to allay his anxieties and fears by proper explanations.
- Explain the sequence of the procedure to gain his confidence and cooperation.
- As far as possible a nurse should remain with a female patient during the physical examination.

Assistance in the Examination

To Take Height and Weight

- To measure the length of the baby who cannot stand, place the baby on a hard surface, with the soles of the feet supported in an upright position.

- The knees are extended and the measurement is taken from the soles of the feet to the vertex of the head.
- The head should be in such a position that the eyes are facing the ceiling.
- After a child can stand, the height can be measured, if the child with the heels back and head against a wall.
- A small flat board held from the top of the head to the wall, will give an accurate measure of the height that is the distance from the floor to the board.
- The weight of a person who can stand is generally measured by a standing scale.
- The patient stands on the platform and the weight is noted on the dial.
- Usually the weight is taken without shoes.
- To take the weight of the baby, a baby weighing scale is used, in which there is a container, where the baby can be laid.
- It is important to weigh a baby unclothed. If weigh with clothes then weigh the clothes separately and subtract this weight from the baby's weight.

To Measure the Skull Circumference

The skull is measured at its greatest diameter from above the eyes to the occipital protuberance.

Examination of the Eyes

- The examination is done in a lying or sitting position.
- The examiner frequently uses a head mirror that reflects light to the patient's face.
- The first examination is one of inspection to determine the movements of the eyes, reaction to light, accommodation to near and far objects.
- For detailed examination of the internal parts of the eye an ophthalmoscope is used.

Examination of the Ears

- The patient may be placed either in a lying or sitting position with the ear to be examined turned towards the examiner.
- Articles used for the examination are a head mirror, ear speculum of various sizes, cotton tipped applicators and autoscope.
- Tuning fork is used to test the hearing.
- A child needs to be carefully restrained.
- Young children sit on their mother's lap with their legs restrained between the mother's knees and their arms held against their back.
- The mother then holds the child's head against the chest.
- Very small infants can be laid on the examination table.

Examination of the Nose, Throat and Mouth

- The patient is usually seated with the head resting against the back of the chair.
- For the examination of the throat, a tongue depressor and a good light are needed.
- For examination of the nose, a nasal speculum and a head mirror are used. Sometimes the autoscope is also used.

Examination of the Neck

The neck needs to be palpated for lymph nodes. In order to assess the thyroid glands, the patient is asked to swallow saliva.

Examination of the Chest

- While examining the anterior chest, the patient is placed in a horizontal recumbent position.
- The chest is examined in several ways.
- It is percussed to determine the presence of fluid or congested areas.
- The physician listens to the sound within the chest by means of a stethoscope.
- To examine the posterior chest, the patient is placed in a sitting position.
- The heart and lungs are examined by percussion and auscultation.
- The breasts are examined by palpation for the presence of lumps or growths.
- The axillae are palpated for enlarged lymph nodes.
- During the examination, the patient's face is turned away from the doctor.

Examination of the Abdomen

- Extremities are inspected, palpated and moved.
- A fine tremor suggestive of hyperthyroidism can be observed, if the patient is asked to hold the arms out in front of him for a few minutes.

ROLE OF NURSE IN HEALTH ASSESSMENT

The professional nurse plays a vital role in the assessment of patient problems. Educational preparation and the clinical setting in part determine the extent to which the nurse participates in the assessment process. For example, a nurse in primary care may perform a comprehensive physical assessment of patients, while a critical care nurse may conduct selected patient assessments to monitor and evaluate current health problems. In either case, nurses are expected to be familiar with and comfortable using physical assessment skills. Today's nurses are sophisticated professionals who require information in order to make clinical decisions. The physical assessment findings provide this information.

RECORDING OF HEALTH ASSESSMENT

Assessment is the first step is the nursing process. In this step, nurse systematically collects verifies, analysis and communicates data about the client's health status. It focuses on gathering the data about a client's state of wellbeing, functional ability, physical status, strengths and responses to actual and potential health problems. Recording of collected data should be done systematically. It saves time, energy and man power by helping the nurse to make right diagnosis and treatment.

CONCLUSION

Health assessment is an important component in health care for proper diagnosis and effective treatment. Health assessment includes the following physical assessment: heat to foot examination, system wise examination, recording height and weight, mental status examination, Laboratory investigation and special investigation. Techniques of physical assessment are inspection, palpation, percussion, manipulation, auscultation and observation

Health assessment of patients falls under the purview of both physicians and nurses. While some nurses practice in extended roles (Advanced Nurse Practitioners), others maintain a more traditional role in the acute care setting. Assessment of patients varies based on both role and setting. A cardiac care nurse will be more familiar with and attuned to cardiac issues. The nursing health assessment is an incredibly valuable tool nurses have in their arsenal of skills. A thorough and skilled assessment allows you, the nurse, to obtain descriptions about your patient's symptoms, how the symptoms developed, and a process to discover any associated physical findings that will aid in the development of differential diagnoses. Assessment uses both subjective and objective data. Subjective assessment factors are those that are reported by the patient. Objective assessment data includes that which is observable and measurable.

BIBLIOGRAPHY

1. Alfaro R. Applying Nursing Diagnosis and Nursing Process: A Step-by-Step Guide, 2nd Ed. Philadelphia: JB Lippincott, 1990.
2. American Nurses Association. Standard of nursing practice. Kansas City, Mo, 1973.
3. Baid H. Patient assessment. The process of conducting a physical assessment: a nursing perspective. British Journal of Nursing 2006;15(13), 710-714.
4. Becker BG, Fendler DJ. Vocational and personal adjustments in practical nursing, 7th Ed. St. Louis: Mosby Year Book, Inc, 1994.
5. Bickley LS, Szilagyi PG, Bates B. Bates' Guide to Physical Examination and History Taking 10th Ed. Philadelphia: Wolters Kluwer Health/Lippincott Williams and Wilkins, 2009.
6. Carpenito LJ. Nursing Diagnosis: Application to Clinical Practice, 4th Ed. Philadelphia, 1992.
7. Carroll-Johnson RM Eds. Classification of nursing diagnoses: Proceedings from the ninth NANDA national conference, Philadelphia: JB Lippincott, 1991.
8. Craven RF, Hirnle CJ. Fundamentals of Nursing: Human Health and Function, Philadelphia: JB Lippincott, 1992.
9. Define health assessment, list out the purpose and factors affecting health assessment.
10. Define physical examination; discuss the competency skills required for doing physical examination?
11. Gettrust KV, Brabec PD. Nursing Diagnosis in Clinical Practice: Guides for Care Planning, Albany, NY: Delmar Publishers, 1992.
12. Hickey PW. Nursing Process Handbook. St. Louis: Mosby Year Book, Inc, 1990.
13. Higginson R, Jones B. Respiratory assessment in critically ill patients: airway and breathing. British Journal of Nursing 2009; 18(8), 456
14. Potter PA, Perry AG. Fundamentals of Nursing Concepts, Process and Practice, 3rd ed. St. Louis: Mosby Year Book, Inc, 1993.
15. Purtilo R. Health Professional and Patient Interaction, 4th ed. Philadelphia: WB Saunders, 1990.

REVIEW QUESTIONS

Short Essays

1. Discuss the methods of physical examination.
2. Describe the characteristics of sound.
3. Techniques used in auscultation.
4. Head to toe examination.
5. Examination of lymph nodes.

Short Answers

1. Direct and indirect percussion.
2. Olfaction.
3. Edema.
4. Examination eyes.
5. Examination of chest.

MULTIPLE CHOICE QUESTIONS

1. **Art of feeling with the hand:**
   a. Palpation
   b. Inspection
   c. Percussion
2. **Recording the observation is called:**
   a. Monitoring
   b. Charting
   c. Documenting
3. **Degree of the heat maintained by the body:**
   a. Saturation
   b. Temperature
   c. Blood pressure
4. **Normal rectal temperature:**
   a. 98.6°F
   b. 99.6°F
   c. 97.6°F
5. **Sudden returned to normal temperature from a very high temperature within a few hours of a day.**
   a. Lysis
   b. Crisis
   c. Fastigium
6. **The body temperature is raised to 105°F is called:**
   a. Hypothermia
   b. Hyperthermia
   c. Hectic fever
7. **Temperature falls in a zigzag manner:**
   a. Lysis
   b. Hypothermia
   c. Hyperthermia

8. **Exchange of gas between atmosphere and blood:**
   a. Pulse
   b. Respiration
   c. Blood pressure
9. **The normal range of blood pressure for an adult:**
   a. 120/80 mm of Hg
   b. 110/70 mm of Hg
   c. 120/90 mm of Hg
10. **Brown color sputum indicates:**
    a. Bronchitis
    b. Bacterial infection
    c. Gangrenous of lung
11. **Coughing out of blood with sputum:**
    a. Hemoptysis
    b. Hematemesis
    c. Epistaxis
12. **The method to produce sound by tapping an area is known as:**
    a. Percussion
    b. Auscultation
    c. Palpation
    d. None of the above
13. **The formula to convert Fahrenheit into Celsius is:**
    a. $C = (F - 32) 5/9$
    b. $C = (F + 32) 9/5$
    c. $C = (F32) 5/9$
    d. $C = (F32) 9/5$
14. **A condition in which the body temperature is higher in the morning than in the evening:**
    a. Inverse fever
    b. Hectic fever
    c. Raise crisis
    d. Rigor
15. **The second stage of rigor is:**
    a. Cold stage
    b. Sweating stage
    c. Hot stage
    d. Warm stage
16. **The degree of compressibility of pulse is known as:**
    a. Strength
    b. Tension
    c. Equality
    d. Volume
17. **The specific gravity of urine is:**
    a. 1.000 to 1.035
    b. 1.010 to 1.035
    c. 1.031 to 1.035
    d. 1.010 to 1.031
18. **Black tarry stool is:**
    a. Hematochezia
    b. Melena
    c. Occult blood
    d. Hematemesis
19. **Greenish color sputum indicates:**
    a. Bacterial infection
    b. Bronchiectasis
    c. Gangrenous condition
    d. Asthma
20. **The pressure when the ventricles are relaxing and the blood pressure at its lowest is:**
    a. Systolic
    b. Diastolic
    c. Pulse pressure
    d. Mean pressure

ANSWERS

1. a	2. c	3. b	4. b	5. b	6. b	7. a	8. b	9. a	10. c	11. a
12. a	13. a	14. a	15. a	16. d	17. a	18. b	19. a	20. b		

CHAPTER 7

Vital Signs

LEARNING OBJECTIVES

Guidelines for taking vital signs

Body temperature:
- Definition, physiology, regulation, factors affecting body temperature
- Assessment of body temperature: Sites, equipment and technique
- Temperature alterations: Hyperthermia, heat cramps, heat exhaustion, heatstroke, hypothermia
- Fever/Pyrexia: Definition, causes, stages, types
- Nursing management
- Hot and cold applications

Pulse:
- Definition, physiology and regulation, characteristics, factors affecting pulse
- Assessment of pulse: Sites, equipment and technique
- Alterations in pulse

Respiration:
- Definition, physiology and regulation, mechanics of breathing, characteristics, factors affecting respiration
- Assessment of respirations: Technique
- Arterial oxygen saturation
- Alterations in respiration

Blood pressure:
- Definition, physiology and regulation, characteristics, factors affecting BP
- Assessment of BP: Sites, equipment and technique, common errors in BP assessment
- Alterations in blood pressure
- Documenting vital signs

TERMINOLOGY

- **Apical pulse:** An apical pulse is a central pulse that is located at the apex of the heart called as point of maximal impulse.
- **Brachial pulse** felt at inner aspects of the biceps muscle of the arm or medially in the antecubital space.
- **Bradycardia:** Heart rate in adult less than 60 beats per minute.
- **Carotid pulse:** At the side of the neck where the carotid artery runs between the trachea and sternocleidomastoid muscle.
- **Cardiac output:** Cardiac output is the volume of blood pumped into the arteries by the heart that equals the result of stroke volume times the heart rate (HR) per minute, e.g. 65 mL × 70 beats per minute = 4.55 L per minute.
- **Dysrhythmia:** A pulse with irregular rhythm is referred as arrhythmia or dysrhythmia.
- **Doppler ultrasound stethoscope:** The electronic device helps to detect pulse rate, volume, rhythm, and to distinguish arterial sound from venous.
- **Femoral:** Where the femoral artery passes alongside of the inguinal ligament.
- **Pulse:** Pulse felt where the femoral artery passes alongside of the inguinal ligament.
- **Pulse deficit:** An apical pulse greater than radial pulse rate indicate that thrust of blood from heart is too weak to be felt at the peripheral site, any difference in apical and radial pulse rate is called pulse deficit.
- **Pulse rhythm:** It is the pattern of the beats and interval between the beats.
- **Pulse volume:** It is also called as the pulse strength or amplitude, refers to force of blood with each beat, it is same with each beat, range from absent to bounding.
- **Pulse pressure:** The difference between diastolic and systolic pressure.
- **Pulse oximeter:** It is a noninvasive device that estimate clients arterial blood oxygen saturation (SaO2) by means of the sensors attached to clients fingers, toe, nose and earlobe.
- **Point of maximum pulse:** The apical pulse in contrast, is a central pulse that is located at the apex of the heart, referred as point of maximum pulse.
- **Posterior tibial:** Pulse felt on the medial surface of the ankle where the posterior tibial artery passes behind the medial malleolus.
- **Posterior dorsa pedal:** Pulse felt on the dorsalis pedis.

- **Radial:** Felt where the radial artery runs along the radial bone, on the thumb of the inner aspect of the wrist.
- **Temporal:** It is site where the temporal artery passes over the temporal bone of the head; site is superior and lateral away from the midline of the eye.
- **Tachycardia:** An excessively fast heart rate over 100 beats per minute.
- **Normothermia:** Body temperature within normal values. Exact normal temperature ranges differ between individuals and can be influenced by some genetic and chronic medical conditions. It is important to ascertain the baseline for individual patients in order to identify abnormal body temperature deviations.
- **Pyrexia:** An elevated body temperature due to an increase in the body temperature's set point. This is usually caused by infection or inflammation. Pyrexia is also known as fever or febrile response. Some causes of fevers do not require medical treatment, whilst other causes need to be identified and treated.
- **Hyperthermia:** An elevated body temperature due to failed thermoregulation. This occurs when the body produces and/or absorbs more heat than it can dissipate.
- **Heat stroke:** A presentation of severe hyperthermia. Thermoregulation is overwhelmed by excessive metabolic production and environmental heat, in combination with impaired heat loss. This is uncommon within an inpatient setting.
- **Low temperature:** A lowered body temperature, where the body loses heat faster than it can produce heat.
- **Hypothermia:** An abnormally low body temperature, where the body temperature drops below a safe level. Both low temperatures and hypothermia can be caused by environmental factors, metabolic complications, disease processes, or can be medically induced.

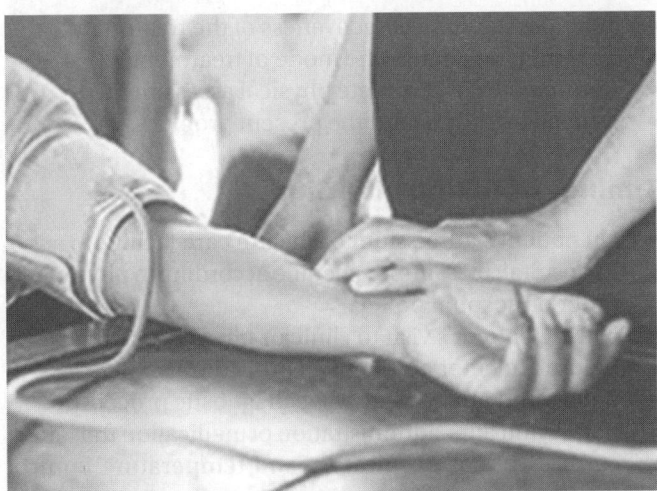

Fig. 7.1: Vital signs measurement technique.

INTRODUCTION

Vital signs include the physiological measurements of temperature, Pulse, BP and respirations. Vital signs are a quick and efficient way of monitoring a patient's condition or identifying problems and evaluating the patient's response to intervening changes. One vital sign can influence characteristics of other vital signs. The basic techniques of inspection, palpation and auscultation are used to determine vital signs. Assessment of vital signs allows the nurse to identify nursing diagnoses, to implement planned intervention and to evaluate success. When the nurse learns the physiological variables influencing vital signs and recognizes the relationship of vital sign changes to other physiological assessment findings, precise determination of the client's health problems can be made.

GUIDELINES FOR ASSESSING VITAL SIGNS

- The nurse caring for the patient is responsible for assessing vital signs. The nurse should obtain the vital signs, interpret their significance and make decisions about interventions.
- Equipment used to measure vital signs must work properly to ensure accurate findings.
- Equipment should be selected based on the client's condition and characteristics.
- The nurse controls or minimizes environmental factors that may affect vital signs.
- The nurse uses an organized, systematic approach when taking vital signs. Each procedure requires a step-by-step approach to ensure accuracy.
- The manner of approach to the patient can alter the vital signs. The nurse should approach the patient in a calm caring manner while taking vital signs.
- Based on patient's condition, the nurse collaborates with the physician to decide the frequency of vital signs assessment.
- The nurse analyzes the results of vital signs measurement. The nurse is often in the best position to assess all clinical finding about a patient.
- The nurse verifies and communicates significant changes in vital signs. The nurse informs the physician of abnormal vital signs.
- Vital signs are documented and communicated to the nurse assuming care of the patient and well of patient.

VITAL SIGNS MEASUREMENT

The vital or cardinal signs are body temperature, pulse respiration and blood pressure. These signs should be looked at in total, to monitor the vital functions of the body. The signs reflect changes in functions that otherwise it might not be observed. Vital signs are the measurements, provided data can be used to determine the patient's usual state of health.

Purpose

- To assess the health-status of an individual.
- To plan and implement the nursing care.

- To understand the effectiveness of the treatment.
- To modify or change the mode of treatment.
- Routine part of complete physical assessment.
- It helps to understand the present problem.

Timings of Taking Vital Signs

- On patient's admission to a health care facility.
- In hospital, on routine schedule according to physician's order or hospital policy.
- During patient's visit to clinic or physician's office.
- Before and after any surgical procedure.
- Before and after any invasive diagnostic procedure.
- Before and after administration of medication that affect cardiovascular, respiratory and temperature control function.
- When the patient's general physical condition changes, e.g. loss of consciousness or increase in intensity of pain.
- Before and after nursing interventions influencing any one of the vital signs, e.g. before ambulating a patient previously on bed rest or before patient performs range of motion exercises.
- Whenever patient reports to nurse any non-specific symptoms of physical distress, e.g. "feeling funny or different."

PRINCIPLES OF VITAL SIGNS

- Vital signs are governed by vital organs and often reveal even the slightest deviation from the normal body functions.
- The changes in the condition of the patient improvement or regression may be detected by the observation of these signs.
- Significant variations in these findings may indicate problems regarding to insufficient consumption.
- Through vital signs, specific information may be obtained that will help in the diagnosis treatment medications and nursing care.
- Patients emotional state may also cause a significant variation in these symptoms.

Methods of Measurement

- Inspection: Inspection means observing with the eye and is associated with light and seeing
- Percussion: Percussion is tapping an area to elicit sounds.
- Auscultation: Auscultation is listening to sounds within the body with a stethoscope.
- Palpation: Palpation is the art of feeling with the hand.

Vital Signs and Normal Values

- Temperature 98.6°F or 37°C in adults.
- Pulse 72 beats/minute in adults.
- Respiration 16 breaths/minute in adults.
- Blood pressure 120/80 mm Hg in adults.

Guidelines for Taking Vital Signs

- The primary nurse caring for the client is the best one to take vital signs, interpret their significance, and make decisions about care.
- Equipment used to measure vital signs must be appropriate and work properly to ensure accurate finding.
- Knowing the normal range for all vital signs helps the nurse to detect abnormalities.
- A client's normal range may differ from the standard range for that age or physical state. Normal values for a client serve as a baseline for comparing in condition over time.
- Know the client's medical history and therapies or medication, for vital sign changes.
- Control or minimize environmental factors that may affect vital signs. Measuring a pulse after client experiences an emotional upset, many yield values that are not clear indicators of the client's current status.
- An organized, systematic approach when taking vital signs ensures, accuracy of findings.

BODY TEMPERATURE: PHYSIOLOGY, REGULATION AND FACTORS AFFECTING BODY TEMPERATURE

Temperature is a Degree of heat maintained by the body. It is the balance between the heats produced and heat lost. Oral temperature: 98.6°F (37°C), Rectal temperature/Tympanic: 99.6°F (37.5°C), Axillary temperature: 97.6°F (36.4°C).

Physiology: Body temperature is of two types: core temperature and the surface temperature. Core temperature is the most important, including deep tissues such as temperature of cranial, thoracic and abdominal cavities. Normal body temperature depends on when, where and in whom it is measured. The body has a regulatory system that keeps the core temperature normal and may vary depending upon the heat produced and the blood flow.

Heat production: Heat is generated in the body's cells through food metabolism. The body converts energy supplied by metabolized nutrients to energy form which can be consumed by body directly. One form of this energy is the thermal energy for regulating body temperature. it is measured in terms of heat. These types of heat liberation is expressed as metabolic rate and measured as BMR. Mostly the heat is produced by deep tissue organ (brain, liver, heart) and skeletal muscles. Skin, subcutaneous tissues and fat of subcutaneous tissues serves as heat insulators for body. When the body heat rises, hypothalamus transmits impulses to reduce the body heat by triggering perspiring, dilating blood vessels and inhabitation of heat production. In case of decreased body heat, hypothalamus spread impulses to stimulate heat production through vasoconstriction (narrowing of blood vessels), muscle shivering and piloeraction.

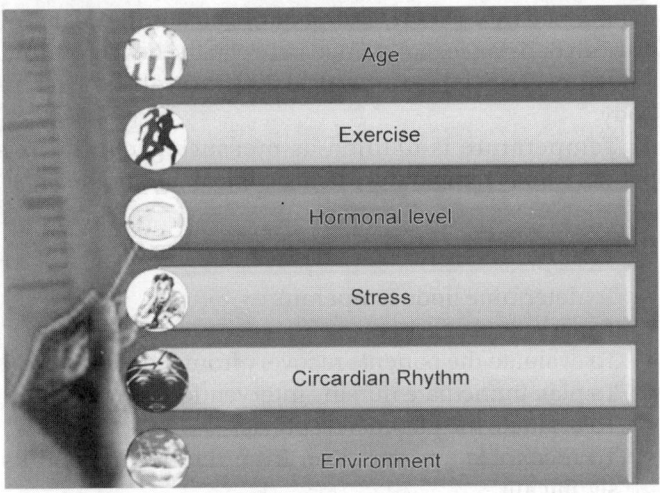

Fig. 7.2: Factors affecting body temperature.

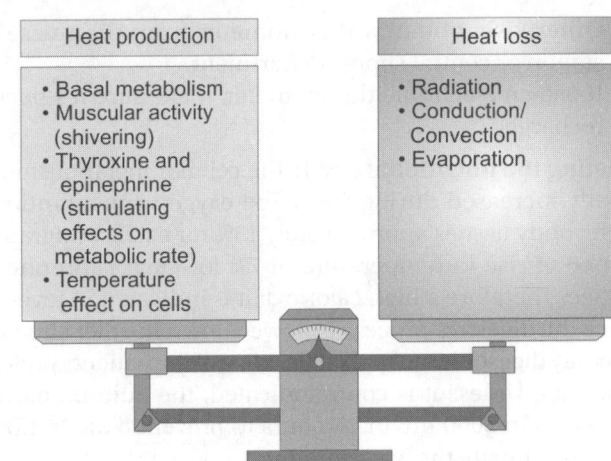

Fig. 7.3: Factors influences heat production.

Regulation of the body temperature: Care of the patients in fevers focuses on reducing the elevated body temperature. When the patient's temperature is moderately elevated, various methods of reducing the temperature be started. The room temperature should be maintained at a comfortable temperature. The room should be well ventilated. The blankets and excess clothing should be removed but prevent the patient from getting draughts. The various methods used for cooling the body are:
- Exposure to cool air an electric fan. Administration of cool drinks.
- Application of cold compress and ice bags.
- Cold sponging and cold packs.
- Cold bath.
- Ice cold lavages and enemas.
- Use of hypothermic blankets or mattresses.

When surface cooling is used treatment is directed at not only cooling the body but also preventing shivering. Shivering must be prevented because it increases metabolic activity, produces heat, increases the oxygen usage markedly, increases circulation, may cause hyperventilation and respiratory alkalosis. It takes longer time to reduce body temperature in a shivering patient

Factors Influences Heat Production

- Metabolism—oxidation of food.
- Muscle activity—exercise.
- Strong emotional excitement, anxiety and nervousness.
- Change in atmospheric temperature.
- Disease condition—bacterial invasion.
- Sympathetic stimulation—Epinephrine and norepinephrine.

Factors Influences Heat Loss

- Sleep: Body temperature is low.
- Fasting: Leads to decreased heat production.
- Illness and lower vitality: Due to depressed nervous system, the heat production is lowered.

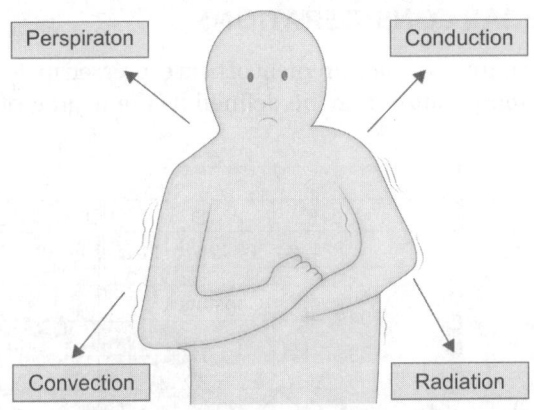

Target cooling rate = 90 watts

Fig. 7.4: Factors influences heat lost.

- Prolonged exposure to cold.
- Use of narcotic drugs.

Body Heat is Lost Through

- **Conduction:** Transfer of heat from body to substance (air, water and cloths) directly in contact.
- **Radiation:** Transfer of heat from body to heat waves which travel through the space.
- **Evaporation:** Transfer to heat from body in form of vapors (liquid is converted into vapors)
- **Convection:** It is transfer of heat from the surface of one subject to the surface, such as skin by movements of heated air or fluid particles.

Preparation of the Equipment

- If a thermometer is included in the admission pack, keep it at the patient's bed side and, on discharge, allow him to take home.

- Otherwise, obtain a thermometer from the nurse's station or central supply department.
- If use an electronic thermometer, make sure it's been recharged.

Meeting the nutritional need: The cellular metabolism is greatly increased during fever. The oxygen consumption in the body tissues approximately 13% for each centigrade degree of rise in temperature of 7% for each Fahrenheit degree. Therefore a high caloric diet is indicated in fevers. Since the digestive process is slowed down the diet should be easily digestible and palatable. Most of the patients prefer fluid diet. Unless it is contraindicated, the fluid intake is increased to 3000 mL in 24 hours to prevent dehydration and to eliminate the waste products.

ASSESSMENT OF BODY TEMPERATURE: SITES, EQUIPMENTS, TECHNIQUES AND SPECIAL CONSIDERATIONS

Temperature is a measurement of heat expressed in degrees. Body temperature may be defined as the degree of heat maintained by the body. Temperature means the degree of warmth or balance maintained between the heat produced (thermo genesis) and heat lost (thermolysis) in the body.

Temperature is defined as measuring/monitoring patient's body temperature using clinical thermometer.

Purpose

- To determine body temperature.
- To assist in diagnosis.
- To evaluate the patients recovery from illness.
- To plan immediate nursing interventions.
- To evaluate the patients response.
- To recognize any variation from the normal and its significant.

Normal Body Temperature for Adults

- Oral: 37°C or 98.6°F
- Rectal: 37.6°C or 99.6°F
- Axillary: 36.4°C or 97.6°F

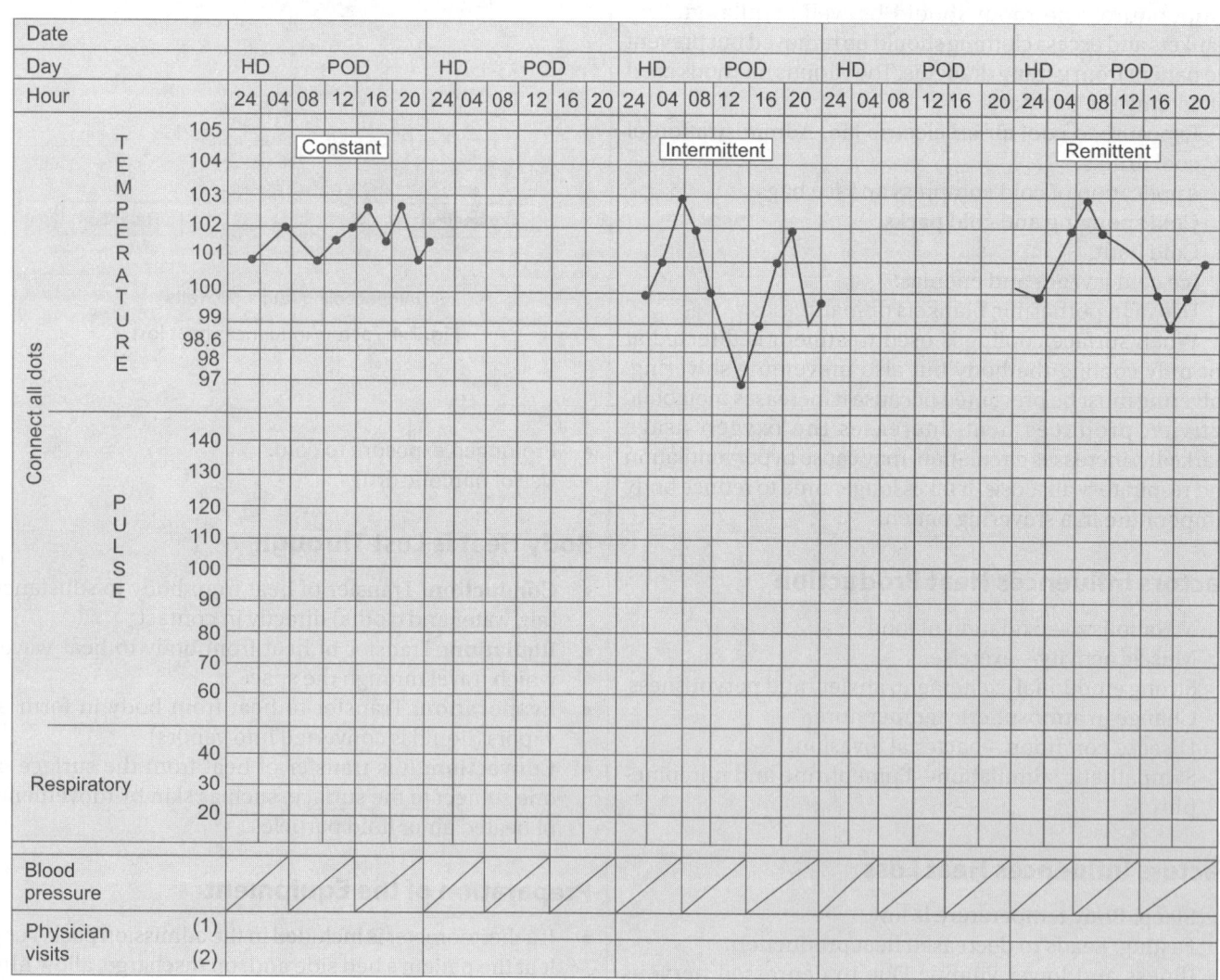

Fig. 7.5: TPR sheet.

Factors Influences Heat Production

- Metabolism: Oxidation of food.
- Muscle activity: Exercise.
- Strong emotion: Excitement, anxiety and nervousness.
- Change in atmospheric temperature.
- Disease condition: Bacterial invasion.
- Sympathetic stimulation: Epinephrine and norepinephrine.

Factors Influences Heat Loss

- Sleep: Body temperature is low.
- Fasting: leads to decreased heat production.
- Illness and lower vitality: Due to depressed nervous system, the heat production is lowered.
- Prolonged exposure to cold.
- Use of narcotic drugs.

Body Heat is Lost Through

- Conduction: Transfer of heat from body to substance (air, water and cloths) directly in contact.
- Radiation: Transfer of heat from body to heat waves which travel through the space.
- Evaporation: Transfer of heat from body in form of vapors (liquid is converted into vapors).
- Convection: It is transfer of heat from the surface of one subject to the surface, such as skin by movements of heated air or fluid particles.

Preparation of the Equipment

- If a thermometer is included in the admission pack, keep it at the patient's bedside and, on discharge, allow him to take home.
- Otherwise, obtain a thermometer from the nurse's station or central supply department.
- If use an electronic thermometer, make sure it has been recharged.

Equipment

- Mercury or electronic thermometer, chemical dot thermometer, or tympanic thermometer.
- Water soluble lubricant or petroleum jelly (for rectal temperature).
- Facial tissue.
- Disposable thermometer sheath or probe cover.
- Alcohol sponge.

Common Sites for Taking Body Temperature

1. Mouth, 2. Axilla, 3. Groin, 4. Vagina, 5. Rectum

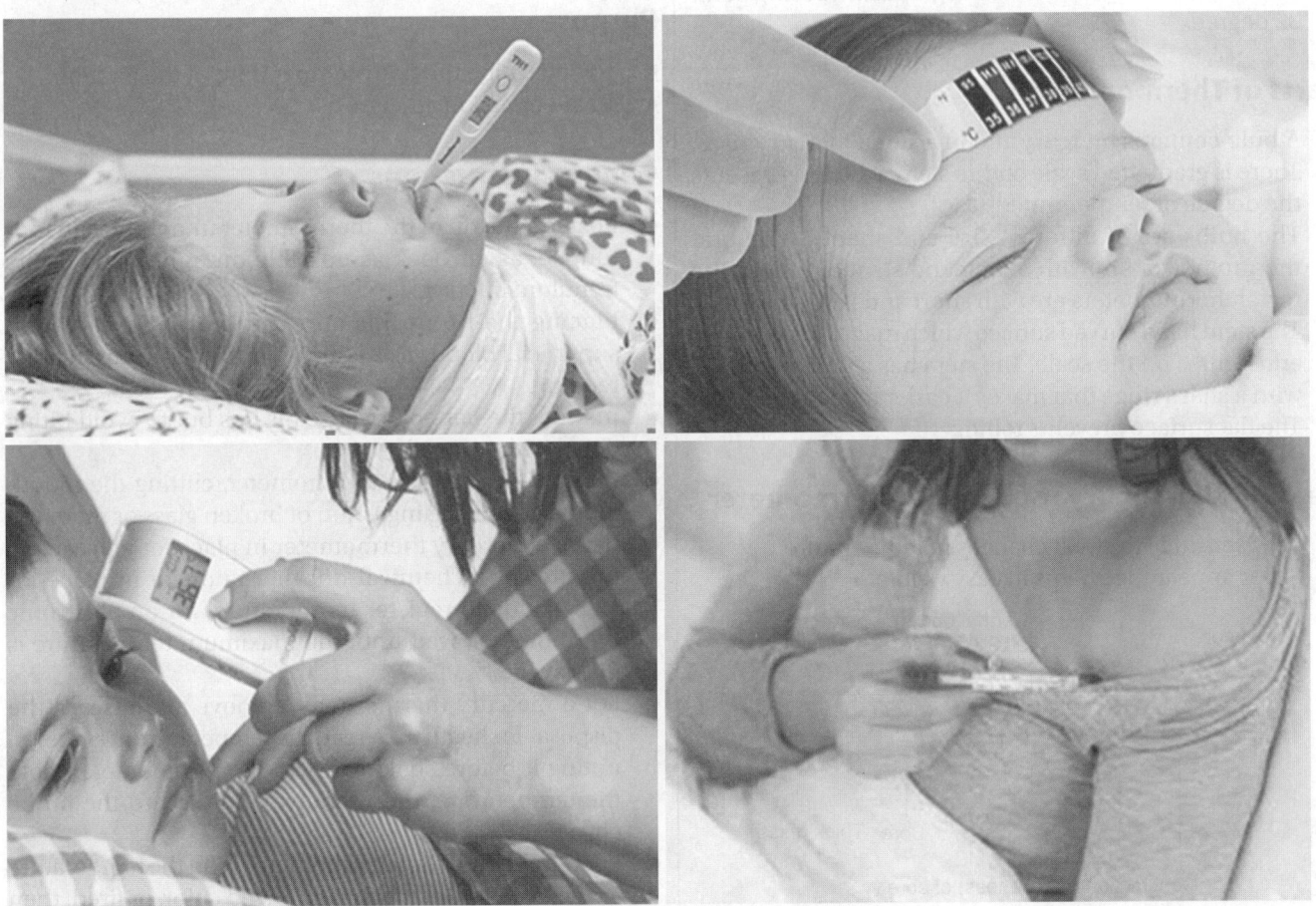

Fig. 7.6: Common sites for taking body temperature.

TYPES OF THERMOMETER

- **The clinical thermometer:** It is an instrument used for measuring temperature of bodily heat or cold in which the mercury remains stationary at registration point until shaken down.
- **Electronic thermometer:** It consists of a battery powered display unit, a thin wire cord and a temperature sensitive probe covered by a disposable plastic sheath to prevent transmission of infection separate probes are available for oral and rectal insertion.
- **Disposable thermometer:** It is a single use thermometer, made of thin plastic strips with chemically impregnated paper, they are used for children to take oral and auxiliary temperature only 45 seconds are needed to record the temperature it is less accurate.
- **Tympanic membrane thermometer:** These are small hand-held devices similar to hodoscopes with disposable speculum. Infrared-sensing electronic and liquid crystal displays. Results are displayed 1 to 2 seconds after placing their speculum in the outer third of the ear canal. It is accurate.

Scales of Thermometer

- Centigrade/Celsius: Boiling point 100 degree and freezing point 0 degree.
- Fahrenheit: Boiling point 212 degree and freezing point 32 degree.

Parts of Thermometer

- A bulb contains mercury and in a stem, mercury rises. There is graduated scale on the stem, which represents the degree of temperature.
- The bulbs are of different size and shapes. The oral thermometers are with a long and slender bulbs. The rectal thermometers are with short and fat bulbs.
- The stem has a curved surface which magnifies the lines and figures on the scale. The stem has a flattened back with a sharp ridge that makes it easier to read the scale. The flat surface prevents rolling.

Reason for Mercury used in the Thermometer

- Very sensitive to small changes in temperature.
- Silver appearance helps in easy visible.

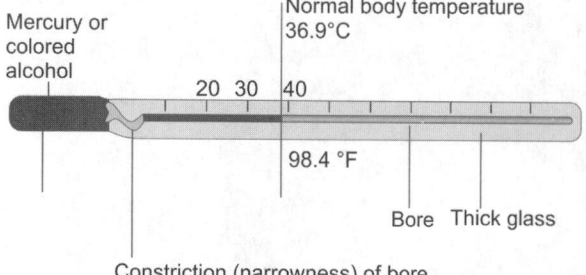

Fig. 7.7: Thermometer (Line diagram).

- Its boiling point is 357°C and freezing point is 39°F.
- The expansion of mercury is uniform.
- Mercury is 13.5 times heavier than water, so small glass tube can be used.

CARE OF THERMOMETER

- Grasp the thermometer securely by the upper end of the stem, never hold it by bulb.
- Shake it down by quick movement of the wrist.
- Move away from articles before shaking the thermometer.
- Be careful that the thermometer will not fall or strike against anything.
- Thermometer is never washed with hot water because heat expands the mercury.
- The used thermometer should be washed with soap and water and should be disinfected with a disinfectant.
- Advantages of using mercury are low price, wide availability reliable accuracy.
- Disadvantages are delay for recording and easy breakability.

ORAL TEMPERATURE

Temperature check by the oral cavity.

Purpose

- To determine the body temperature of the patient.
- To aid in making diagnosis.

General Instructions

- Position the tip of the thermometer under the patient's tongue, as far back as possible on either side of the frenulum linguae.
- Placing the tip in this area, promotes contact with superficial blood vessels and contributes to an accurate reading.
- Instruct the patient to close his lips but to avoid biting down with his teeth.
- Biting can break the thermometer, cutting the mouth or lips or causing ingestion of broken glass or mercury.
- Leave a mercury thermometer in place for at least two minutes or a chemical-dot thermometer in place for 45 seconds to register temperature, for an electronic thermometer, wait until the maximum temperature is displayed.
- For a mercury thermometer, remove and discard the disposable sheath then read the temperature at eye level, noting it before shaking down the thermometer, note the temperature, then remove and discard the probe cover.
- For the chemical dot thermometer, read the temperature as the last dye dot that has changed color, or fired, then discard the thermometer and its dispenser case.

Preliminary Assessment

- Determine the need to measure client's body temperature.
- Assemble equipment.
- Identify the patient, greet the patient and explain the procedure.
- Place the client in comfortable position, assess site most appropriate for temperature measurement.
- Wait 20 to 30 minutes before measuring oral temperature if client has ingested hot or cold liquid or foods.

Equipment

- Oral clinical thermometer.
- Swab in a container.
- Kidney basin or thermometer container.
- Blue pen.
- Watch with second hand.
- Graphic TPR chart (**Fig. 7.5**).
- Paper bag.

Procedure

- Hold the color coded end or system glass thermometer with finger tips.
- If thermometer stored in disinfectant solution, rinse in cold water before using.
- Take swab and wipe thermometer bulb end towards fingers in rotating fashion. Dispose of tissue.

1. Turn on thermometer according to package directions

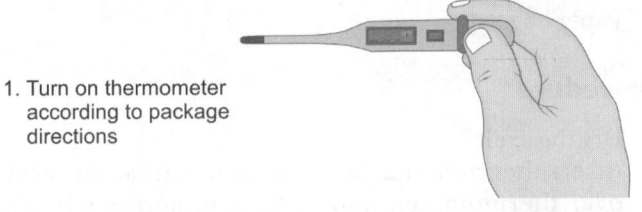

2. Place the tip of the thermometer under one side of tongue toward the back. Close mouth and breathe through nose

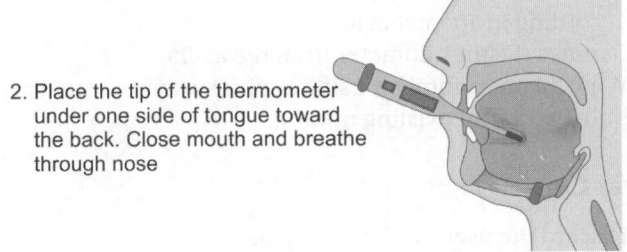

3. Remove the thermometer after you hear the signal (usually a series of beeps) and read the temperature on the screen

A fever is a temperature over 99.5 °F

Fig. 7.8: Oral temperature measurement techniques.

- Read mercury level while holding thermometer horizontally and gently rotating at eye level. If mercury is above desired level, grasp at the tip of thermometer securely and sharply flick wrist down ward. Continue shaking until reading is below 35.5°C.
- Ask client to open mouth and gently place thermometer under tongue in posterior sublingual, lateral to center of lower jaw.
- Ask client to hold thermometer with lips closed. Caution against biting down on thermometer.
- Leave thermometer in place for 2 minutes or according to agency policy.
- Carefully remove thermometer and read at eye level while holding thermometer horizontally.

After Care

- Wipe secretions from thermometer with soft tissue. Wipe in rotating fashion from fingers towards bulb. Dispose of tissue.
- Wash thermometer in lukewarm water, rinse in cool water, dry and replace in container.
- Record the temperature on the chart.
- Wash hands.
- Report any unusual variation to the charge nurse.

Contraindications

- Injuries, inflammation and surgeries of oral cavity.
- Infants, children below 6 years, and patients who cannot retain thermometer in mouth.
- Unconscious, delirious, noncooperative and mentally disturbed patients.
- Patients with mouth breathing, convulsions, oxygen masks, frequent and severe cough.

AXILLARY TEMPERATURE

The temperature is sometimes taken by axilla when it cannot be taken by mouth or contraindicated to check oral temperature.

Purpose

- To determine the body temperature of the patient.
- To aid in making diagnosis.

General Instructions

- Position the patient with the axilla exposed.
- Gently pat the axilla dry with a facial tissue because moisture conducts heat. Avoid harsh rubbing, which generates heat.
- Ask the patient to reach across his chest and grasp his opposite shoulder and to lower his elbow and hold it against his chest. This promotes skin contact with the thermometer.
- Remove a mercury thermometer after 10 minutes; remove an electronic thermometer when it displays

Textbook of Nursing Foundation

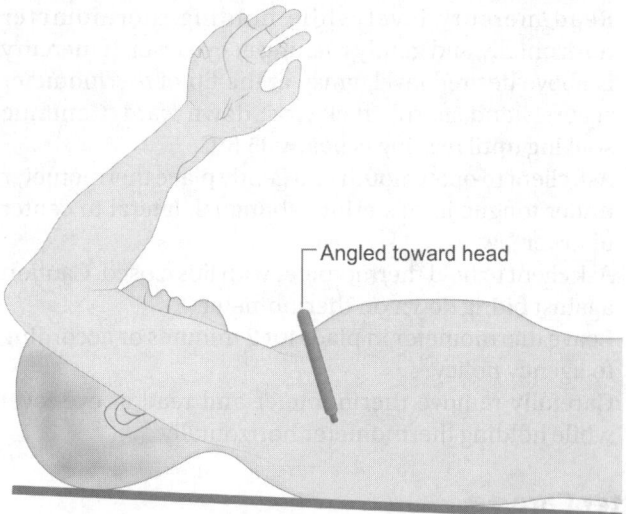

Fig. 7.9: Position of measuring axillary temperature.

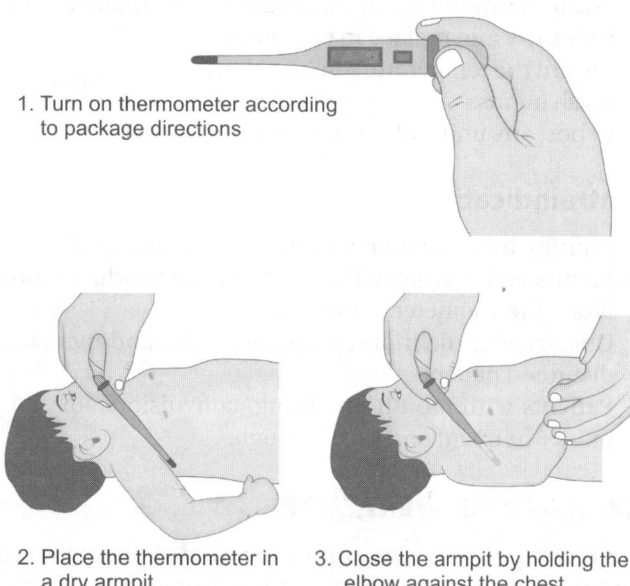

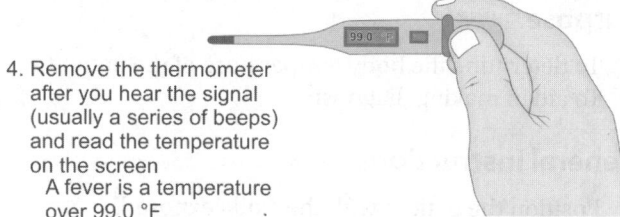

Fig. 7.10: How to measure body temperature: Axillary.

the maximum temperature. Auxiliary temperature takes longer to register than oral or rectal temperature because the thermometer is not closed in a body cavity.
- Grasp the end of the thermometer and remove it from the axilla.

Preliminary Assessment

- Determine the need to measure client's body temperature.
- Assemble equipment.
- Identify the patient, greet the patient and explain the procedure.
- Place the client in comfortable position, assess site most appropriate for temperature measurement.
- Wait 20 to 30 minutes before measuring oral temperature if client has ingested hot or cold liquid or foods.
- Hold the color coded end or system glass thermometer with finger tips.
- If thermometer stored in disinfectant solution, rinse in cold water before using.
- Take swab and wipe thermometer bulb end towards fingers in rotating fashion. Dispose of tissue.
- Read mercury level while holding thermometer horizontally and gently rotating at eye level. If mercury is above desired level, grasp at the tip of thermometer securely and sharply flick wrist downward. Continue shaking until reading is below 35.5° C.

Equipment

- Oral clinical thermometer.
- Swab in a container.
- Kidney basin or thermometer container.
- Blue pen.
- Watch with second hand.
- Graphic TPR chart.
- Paper bag.

Procedure

- Dry the axilla.
- Insert thermometer into center of axilla, low arm over thermometer, and place arm across client's chest.
- Leave the thermometer in place for three minutes or according to apentyeocics.
- Remove the thermometer from the axilla.
- Wipe the thermometer using a spirit swab from stem to bulb use a firm twisting motion.

After Care

- Discard the used swab into the paper bag.
- Read the thermometer holding it horizontally at the eye level, rotates it until the mercury column is seen.
- Place thermometer in the kidney basin.
- Record the temperature on the chart using blue pen and mention axillary.
- Wash hands.
- Report any unusual variations to the charge nurse.
- Recording and reporting. Record temperature on vital sign flow sheet's or nurse's notes. Also record any signs or symptoms of temperature alterations.

RECTAL TEMPERATURE

Rectal temperature measurement is a technique used to measure body temperature by placing a thermometer in the rectum.

Purpose

- To determine body temperature mainly for infants, young children, adult unconscious patient and postoperative patient.
- To aid in making diagnosis.

Indication

- Unconscious patient.
- Neonates.
- Malignant-Hyperthermia.

General Instructions

- Position the patient on his side with his top leg flexed, and drape him to provide privacy. Then fold back the bed linens to expose the anus.
- Squeeze the lubricant onto a facial tissue to prevent contamination of the lubricant supply.
- Lubricate about ½" of the thermometer tip for an infant, 1" for a child for an adult. Lubrication reduces friction and thus eases insertion. This step may be unnecessary when using disposable rectal sheaths because they are prelubricated.
- Lift the patient's upper buttock, and insert the thermometer about 1.3 cm for an infant, 3.8 cm for an adult. Gently direct the thermometer along the rectal wall towards the umbilicus. This will avoid perforating the anus or rectum or breaking the thermometer. It also will help ensure an accurate reading because the thermometer will register hemorrhoid artery temperature instead of fecal temperature.
- Hold the mercury thermometer in place for 2 to 3 minutes or the electronic thermometer until the maximum temperature is displayed. Holding the thermometer prevents damage to rectal tissues caused by displacement or loss of the thermometer. Carefully remove the thermometer, wiping it as necessary. Then wipe the patient's anal area to remove any lubricant or feces.

Preliminary Assessment

- Determine the need to measure client's body temperature.
- Assemble equipment.
- Identify the patient, greet the patient and explain the procedure.
- Place the client in comfortable position, assess site most appropriate for temperature measurement.
- Wait 20 to 30 minutes before measuring oral temperature if client has ingested hot or cold liquid or foods.
- Hold the color coded end or system glass thermometer with finger tips.
- If thermometer stored in disinfectant solution, rinse in cold water before using.
- Take swab and wipe thermometer bulb end towards fingers in rotating fashion. Dispose of tissue.
- Read mercury level while holding thermometer horizontally and gently rotating at eye level. If mercury is above desired level, grasp at the tip of thermometer securely and sharply flick wrist downward. Continue shaking until reading is below 35.5° C.

Equipment

- Oral clinical thermometer.
- Swab in a container.
- Kidney basin or thermometer container.
- Blue pen.
- Watch with second hand.
- Graphic TPR chart.
- Paper bag.

Procedure

- Draw curtain around client's bed or close room door. Assist client to Sims position with upper leg flexed. Move aside bed linen to expose only anal area.
- Squeeze liberal portion of lubricant on tissue. Dip thermometer's bulb end in to lubricant, covering 2.5 to 3.5 cm (1 to 1.5 inches) for adult or 1.2 to 2.5 cm (0.5 to 1.5 inch) for infant.
- With non-dominant hand, separate client's buttocks to expose anus. Ask client to breathe slowly and relax.
- Gently insert thermometer into anus in direction of umbilicus insert 1.2 cm (0.5 inch) for infant and 3.5 cm (1.5 inches) for adult do not force thermometer.

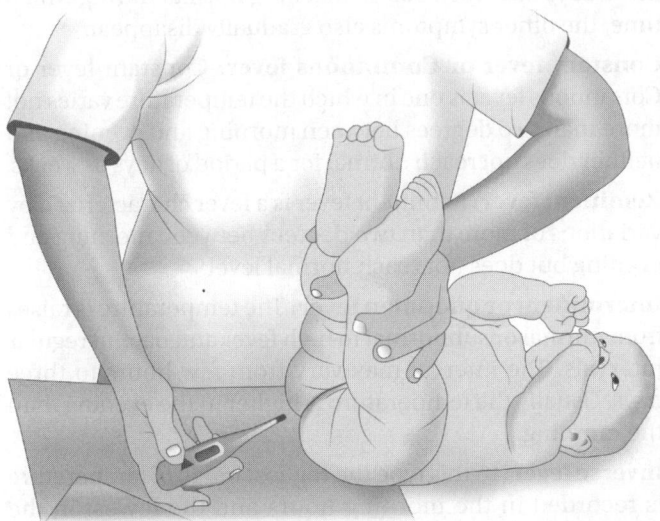

Fig. 7.11: Measurement of rectal temperature.

- If resistance is felt during insertion withdraw thermometer immediately.
- Hold thermometer in place for 2 minutes or according to agency policy.
- Carefully remove thermometer and wipe off secretions with tissue. Wipe in rotating fashion from fingers towards bulb. Dispose of tissue.
- Read thermometer at eye level rotate until scale appears.
- Wipe client's anal area to remove lubricant or feces and discard tissue help client return to comfortable position.

After Care

1. Wipe secretions from thermometer with soft tissue. Wipe in rotating fashion from fingers towards bulb. Dispose of tissue.
- Wash thermometer in lukewarm water, rinse in cool water, dry and replace in container.
- Record the temperature on the chart.
4. Wash hands.
- Report any unusual variation to the charge nurse.

Contraindication

- Injury, inflammation and surgeries of rectum.
- Fecal impaction.
- Chronic diarrhea.
- Patients requiring bowel wash/enema.

FEVER (PYREXIA)

Fever or pyrexia is defined as the rise in body temperature above 99°F (37.2°C). The cause of fever is infections, diseases of the nervous system, certain malignant neoplasms, blood diseases such as leukemia, embolism and thrombosis, heat 'stroke from exposure to hot environment, dehydration, surgical trauma and crushing injuries, skin abnormalities that interfere with heat loss, allergic reactions to foreign proteins and pyrogens, etc. In fever, all the systems of the body are affected. It may vary with the nature of the diseases.

Respiratory system: Shallow and rapid breathing.

Circulatory system: Increased pulse rate and palpitation.

Alimentary system: Dry mouth, coated tongue, loss of appetite, nausea, vomiting, constipation, or diarrhea.

Urinary system: Diminished urinary output, burning micturition, high colored urine.

Nervous system: Headache, restlessness, irritability, insomnia, convulsions, delirium.

Musculoskeletal system: Heavy sweating, hot flushes, goose flush, shivering or rigors.

Integumentary system: Heavy sweating, hot flushes, goose flush, shivering or rigors.

Fever is not a disease but it is a sign. Fever is a protective function of the body, because the rise in temperature prevents the growth of organisms causing the disease. Fever if not too high hastens the destruction of bacteria by increasing phagocytes, and by producing immune bodies. A temperature of 104 to 105°F for several hours will destroy the organisms of syphilis and gonorrhea. The range in the body temperature within which the cells can function efficiently is between 34 to 41°C (94 to 106°F). The central nervous system is extremely sensitive to the temperature variations. Irreversible changes may occur in the nervous system if the body temperature goes above 41°C or below 34°C

Types of Fever

Terms used to describe the types and phases of fever

- **Onset:** Onset or invasion of fever is the period when the body temperature is rising and it may be a sudden or gradual process
- **Fastigium or stadium:** Fastigium or stadium of fever is the period when the body temperature has reached its returning to normal. The fever may subside suddenly (decline by crisis or gradually decline by lysis)
- **Crisis:** Crisis is sudden return to normal temperature from a very high temperature within a few hours or days.
- **True crisis**: The temperature falls suddenly within few hours and touches normal, accompanied by a marked improvement in the patients condition.
- **Subnormal temperature**: When the body temperature falls below normal it is called subnormal temperature. The temperature may vary between 95° to 98°F or 35 to 36.7°C.

Hyperthermia: When the body temperature is raised to 105°F or above it is called hyperthermia.

Hypothermia: If the temperature falls below 95°F or 35°C, the condition is called hypothermia.

False crisis: A sudden fall in temperature not accompanied by an improvement in the general condition is called false crisis. It may be danger signal and not a sign of improvement.

Lysis: The temperature falls in a zigzag manner for two or three days of a week before reaching normal during which time, the other symptoms also gradually disappear.

Constant fever or Continuous fever: Constant fever or Continuous fever is one in which the temperature varies not more than two degrees between morning and evening and neither does not reach normal for a period of days or weeks.

Remittent fever: Remittent fever is a fever characterized by variations of more than two degrees between morning and evening but does not reach normal level.

Intermittent or quotidian fever: The temperature is raises from normal or subnormal to high fever and back at regular intervals. The interval may vary from few hours to three days. Usually the temperature is higher in the evening than the morning.

Inverse fever: In this type the highest range of temperature is recorded in the morning hours and the lowest in the evening which is contrary to that found in the normal course of fever

Hectic fever: When the difference between the high and low point is very great, the fever is called hectic or swinging fever.

Relapsing fever: Relapsing fever is one in which there are brief febrile period followed by one or more days of normal temperature.

Irregular fever: When the fever is entirely irregular in its course, it cannot be classified under any one of the fevers described above and it is called irregular fever.

Rigor: Rigor is sudden severe attack of shivering in which the body temperature rises rapidly to a stage of hyperpyrexia as seen in malaria.

Low pyrexia: In low pyrexia the fever does not rise above 99 to 100°F or 37.2 to 37.8°C.

Moderate pyrexia: The body temperature remains between 100 to 103°F or 37.8 to 39.4°C.

High pyrexia: The temperature remains between 103 to 105°F or 39.4 to 40.6°C.

Hyperpyrexia: The temperature goes above 105°F.

Frequency of taking temperature in the hospital: Frequency of taking temperature is determined by the condition of the patient. For patients who are not seriously ill, it needs to be taken in the morning and evening. The temperature is to be checked every 4 hours or even more frequently for those who are actually ill, who are having high fever, and postoperative patients. If the temperature is taken by rectum or axilla it should be specified in the chart.

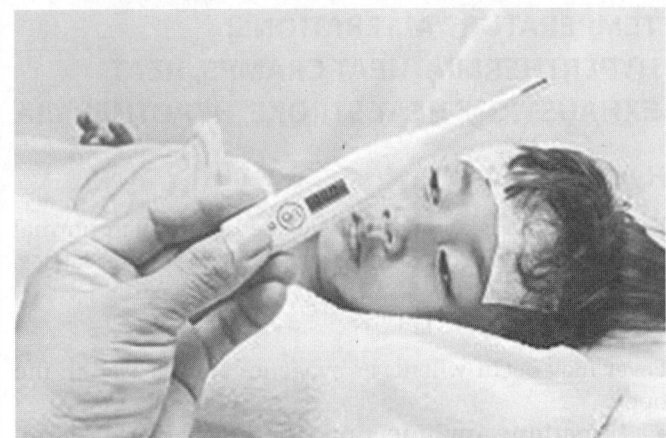

Fig. 10.12: Measurement of fever.

CARE OF FEVER

I. **Regulation of the body temperature:** Care of the patients in fevers focuses on reducing the elevated body temperature. When the patients temperature is moderately elevated, various methods of reducing the temperature be started. The room temperature should be maintained at a comfortable temperature. The room should be well ventilated. The blankets and excess clothing should be removed but prevent the patient from getting draughts. The various method used for cooling the body are:
   – Exposure to cool air an electric fan. Administration of cool drinks
   – Application of cold compress and ice bags
   – Cold sponging and cold packs
   – Cold bath
   – Ice cold lavages and enemas
   – Use of hypothermic blankets or mattresses.

When surface cooling is used treatment is directed at not only cooling the body but also preventing shivering. Shivering must be prevented because it increases metabolic activity, produces heat, increases the oxygen usage markedly, increases circulation may cause hyperventilation and respiratory alkalosis. It takes longer time to reduce body temperature in a shivering patient.

II. **Meeting the nutritional need:** The cellular metabolism is greatly increased during fever. The oxygen consumption in the body tissues approximately 13% for each centigrade degree of rise in temperature of 7 percent for each Fahrenheit degree. Therefore a high caloric diet is indicated in fevers.

Since the digestive process is slowed down the diet should be easily digestible and palatable. Most of the patients prefer fluid diet.

Unless it is contraindicated, the fluid intake is increased to 3000 mL in 24 hours to prevent dehydration and to eliminate the waste products.

Care in rigor: Rigor is characterized by three stages:
- **The first stage or cold stages**: The patient shivers uncontrollably. The skin is cold, face is pinched and pale, and the pulse is feeble and rapid. The temperature rises rapidly to 103°F (39.4°C) or above. In this stage, cover the patient with blankets and apply warmth with hot water bags. Give warm drinks. Protect the patient from falling.
- **The second stage or hot stage:** the skin feels hot and dry and patient feels very thirsty. The shivering stops. The patient may be restless. The temperature may continue to rise during the second stage, remove all the blankets and hot appliances. Cover him only with a thin blanket. Give him cool drinks. Cold compresses are applied to the head to relieve congestion and headache. The temperature is carefully recorded every 10 to 15 minutes. Watch pulse and respirations carefully. If the temperature goes very high (105°F) (40.5°C) cold sponging may be started. Watch for the early signs of sweating.
- **The third stage or stage sweating:** The patient sweats profusely. The temperature falls. The pulse improves. Acute discomforts are diminished. The patient may go into state of shock and collapse if not cared properly.

TEMPERATURE ALTERATIONS: HYPERTHERMIA, HEAT CRAMPS, HEAT EXHAUSTION, HEAT STROKE, HYPOTHERMIA

Hyperthermia

Hyperthermia is a condition elevated more than normal body temperature considered according to various causes.

Causes of Fever

Fever may occur whenever pyogenes are released in the body.
- **Infection:** Any infection whether bacterial, viral, rickettsial, fungal or parasitic give rise to fever.
- **Neoplasms:** Hypernephroma, lymphoproliferative malignancies, carcinoma of pancreas, lung and bone and hepatoma may cause fever.
- **Vascular causes:** Acute myocardial infarction, pulmonary embolism, pontine hemorrhage may also cause fever.
- **Trauma:** A massive crush injury may lead to pyrexia.
- **Immunological diseases:** Diseases like collagen disorders, systemic lupus erythematosus, rheumatoid arthritis, etc. can lead to increase in body temperature. Drug fever and serum sickness are can also cause fever.
- **Endocrine:** Thyrotoxicosis and Addison's disease may raise body temperature. Fever may occur in metabolic disease like gout, acidosis, dehydration, hematological conditions like acute hemolytic crisis. heat stroke and radiation sickness can be accompanied by fever.

Types of Fever

- **Constant or continuous fever:** A continuous fever is one in which the temperature varies not more than two degrees between morning and evening but the temperature does not come to normal during the day.
- **Intermittent fever:** An intermittent fever shows large variations, i.e. the temperature rise from normal to high temperature and comes down at regular intervals. The temperature may vary from few hours to three days.
- **Remittent fever:** In remittent fever, the variation is more than two degree centigrade between morning and evening but fever does not reach normal.
- **Inverse fever:** In this type, highest temperature is in the morning and lowest temperature is in the evening.
- **Relapsing fever:** In this type, there are short febrile periods followed by one or more days of normal temperature.

Stages in the Course of Fever

- **Onset or invasion:** It may be sudden or gradual, according to the disease condition.
- **Fastigium or stadium (height of fever or stage of advance):** Fever remains constant for a few days. Then, it attains a peak level. The highest point is called the fastigium or stadium.

Hyperthermia Clinical Manifestations	
Signs and Symptoms	- Poor appetite
- Flushing	- Vomiting and/or diarrhea
- Skin warm, hot to touch	- Body aches
- Increased metabolic rate	- Fatigue, malaise, weakness
- Skin rash	
- Decreased responsiveness	
- Difficulty concentrating	

- **Defervescence or decline:** It is the period of disappearance of fever.
- **Lysis:** In this, the temperature falls step by step. Temperature comes to normal within 3-4 days or within one week, e.g. in typhoid.
- **Crisis:** In this, the temperature falls suddenly from high fever to normal, e.g. respiratory tract infections.
- **True crisis:** It is associated with improvement of general health of the patient.
- **False crisis:** It is not associated with improvement of general condition.

Severity of Patient with Fever

- Low pyrexia: 99-101° F
- Moderate pyrexia: 101 to 103° F.
- High pyrexia: 103 to 105° F.
- Hyper pyrexia: 105° F and above.

Management of Severe Fever

- Five oral fluids 3 liter per day.
- Give cold sponge to reduce body's surface temperature.
- Give frequent mouth wash and attend to oral hygiene.
- Reduce the external covering on patient's body to promote heat loss through radiation and conduction.
- Do not induce chills.
- Keep clothing and bed linen dry to increase heat loss through conduction and convection.
- Provide cool, circulating air.
- Limit patient's physical activity and provide rest.
- Administer antipyretic medications as per doctor's instruction.
- In severe cases, antipyretic injections are given as per doctor's instruction.
- Check temperature ½ hourly and record to assess the general condition of patient.
- Highest temperature is seen in thyroid crisis. In that case, antithyroid drugs are advised.

Goal and Outcome Criteria

- Patients suffering from balance thermoregulation
- Outcome criteria
- Body temperature in the normal range
- Pulse and respiration in the normal range
- No color change
- No turning

Nursing Management of Hyperthermia

Fever Control

- Monitor temperature at least every 2 hours.
- Monitor in continuous basal temperature.
- 3. Monitor blood pressure, pulse, and respiration.
- Monitor skin color and temperature.
- Monitor level of consciousness.
- Monitor WBC, Hb, Hct.
- Monitor intake and output.
- Give antipyretic.
- Provide treatment to overcome the cause of fever.
- Provide intra venous fluids.
- Compress the patient, on the thigh fold, axilla and neck.
- Increase air circulation.
- Provide treatment to prevent shivering.

Temperature Regulation

- Monitor signs of hyperthermia
- Increase fluid intake and nutrition
- Teach the patient how to prevent fatigue due to heat
- Discuss and clarify the importance of temperature regulation and possible negative effects of cold
- Provide appropriate antipyretic medication as needed
- Use the mattress cool and warm water bath to overcome the interference fit the needs of the body temperature
- Release of excess clothing and covered the patient with only a piece of clothing.

Vital Sign Monitoring

- Monitor blood pressure, pulse, temperature, and respiration
- Record the blood pressure fluctuates
- Monitor the patient's vital signs while standing, sitting and lying
- Auscultation of blood pressure in both arms and compare
- Monitor blood pressure, pulse, and respiration before, during, and after activity
- Monitor the quality of the pulse
- Monitor breathing frequency and cadence
- Monitor the voice of the lungs
- Monitor abnormal breathing patterns
- Monitors temperature, humidity and skin color
- Monitor peripheral cyanosis
- Monitor the availability of a widened pulse pressure, bradycardia, increase in systolic
- Identify the cause of the change in vital signs.

Treating Fever

- Fever usually makes a person feel uncomfortable, and steps may be taken to reduce the fever, by taking age-appropriate medicine, such as paracetamol or ibuprofen, but never aspirin in under-16s.
- Other home care treatments for fever:
- Drink plenty of water or other clear fluid. Iced drinks or ice lollies may have a soothing effect.
- Wear lightweight clothing and don't use blankets and duvets in bed to avoid getting too warm
- Make sure the temperature in the room is comfortable and let fresh air in
- Rest and avoid heavy activity

Subjective Data: "I am not feeling well right now. My head is aching and burning as if the steam comes out of my ears periodically."

Objective Data

- Flushed skin with body temperature of 38.1degreeC per axilla
- Respiratory rate of : 21 breaths per minute
- Pulse rate of: 89 beats per minute
- Unstable blood pressure
- Muscle rigidity; chills
- Profuse diaphoresis

Objectives

Short term goal: Client will be able to resume and maintain normal body temperature after 4 hours.

Long term goal: Client will be free from complications such as irreversible brain or neurologic damage.

Outcome criteria: Client will be able to report and show manifestations that fever is relieved or controlled through verbatim, temperature of 36.8°C per axilla, respiratory rate of 12–18 breaths per minute, pulse rate of 60–75 beats per minute, stable blood pressure, absence of muscular rigidity/chills and profuse diaphoresis after 4 hours of nursing care.

Client will be free from febrile convulsions resulting to brain damage after 1 week of nursing care.

Nursing Interventions

Sl. No.	Nursing action	Rationale
1.	Assess and monitor client's temperature and note for presence of chills/profuse diaphoresis; also note for degree and pattern of occurrence	Temperature 38.9°C–41°C may suggest acute infectious disease process. A sustained fever may be due to pneumonia or typhoid fever while a remittent fever may be due to pulmonary infections; and an intermittent fever may be caused by sepsis or tuberculosis.
2.	Adjust and monitor environmental factors like room temperature and bed linens as indicated.	Room temperature may be accustomed to near normal body temperature and blankets and linens may be adjusted as indicated to regulate temperature of client.

Contd...

Contd...

Sl. No.	Nursing action	Rationale
3.	Apply tepid sponge bath.	It could help in reducing hyperthermia; avoid using alcohol and iced water which may even produce chills and increase client's temperature.
4.	Administer antipyretics as prescribed by the physician.	Antipyretics acts on the hypothalamus, reducing hyperthermia.
5.	Provide cooling blanket as indicated.	It is helpful in reducing increased body temperature especially with temperatures of 39.5°C–40°C.
6.	Encourage client to increase fluid intake.	Water regulates body temperature.
7.	Raise the side rails at all times	To ensure client's safety even without the presence of seizure activity.
8.	Start intravenous normal saline solutions or as indicated.	To replenish fluid losses during shivering chills.
9.	Provide high caloric diet or as indicated by the physician.	To meet the metabolic demand of client.
10.	Educate client of signs and symptoms of hyperthermia and help him identify factors related to occurrence of fever; discuss importance of increased fluid intake to avoid dehydration.	Providing health teachings to client could help client cope with disease condition and could help prevent further complications of hyperthermia.

Heat Stroke or Sun Stroke

This condition is caused by failure of body temperature regulation in the brain. Usually due to high fever or prolonged exposure to heat. Heat stroke may be caused by high temperature in factories or furnaces.

Signs and Symptoms

Headache, dizziness, discomfort, restlessness, Hot and flushed, dry skin, bounding pulse, high temperature above 104°F (40°C), rapid unconsciousness.

First Aid

- Remove the patient to dry and shady place, loosening his collar, and other tight clothings.
- Rise the head and upper part of the body.
- Sprinkle cool water on his body or wrap him in a wet sheet and fan him.
- Keep on taking body temperature every 10 minutes.
- After the body temperature fallen to 102° F wrap him in a dry sheet and keep fan him.
- If the patient is conscious, cool water mixed with salt and glucose for drinking.
- Remove to the hospital.

Heat Exhaustion

It is caused by too high temperature in the atmosphere directly by the sun, or due to hard work and confinement in a close, hot atmosphere like factories etc.

Signs and Symptoms:
- Head ache, dizziness, nausea, vomiting, and sometimes abdominal cramps, or cramps in the limbs.
- Face in pale with cold sweat
- Pulse is weak
- Shallow breathing
- Temperature is normal or slightly raised
- Sometimes there is unconsciousness
- There may be a shock 8.Loss of appetite

First Aid

- Remove the patient to a cool place
- Place him flat on his back
- Loosen his clothing
- Give him plenty of salted water (1/4 liter every ½ hourly)
- Observe the patient

Heat Cramps

These are intermittent, painful contractions of skeleton muscles. These cramps occurs the fluid lost in sweat by drinking water but don't replace sodium. Sodium depletion is responsible for the cramps. Heat cramps usually occur in muscles that have been involved in a strenuous activity. Body temperature is normal and the serum sodium may be normal or low.

First aid:
- Replace the sodium with salt tablets or an electrolyte solution
- Adding salt in the diet will prevent heat cramps

Points to Prevent Heat Injury

- Limiting the strenuous activities in the hot weather
- Stay indoors and wear a minimum of clothing's during heat waves.
- When temperatures are unusually high outdoor activities should be cancelled. 4. Wear clothes that are loose fitting, light in color and cover the body as much as possible when outdoors
- Lose weight if you are obese
- Avoid heavy exercise
- Use measures to improve ventilation and reduce heat by shades
- Cooking should be done in early morning or late evening to avoid heating up the house during the hot part of the day
- Fans and vents over stoves and ovens should be used to help remove heat from the house.

- Eating more salts, but must be accompanied by an increased amount of fluids.
- Drink lot of water, even the person with cardiovascular disease who might otherwise be limiting fluids

Effects of Extreme Cold

Effects of extreme cold are common in person who live or work in a climate where temperature falls below 32°F or are in high altitudes.

Frostbite

Frostbites occurs when the body is exposed to extreme cold temperature.(i.e.) ice crystals forming inside the cell can result in permanent circulatory and tissue damage. Body areas susceptible to frostbite are the ear lobes, tip of the nose, fingers and toes.

Signs and Symptoms

- The exposed part becomes cold, painful and ultimately numb.
- Color first is red, then become white which may later lead to gangrene
- Injured area is white, waxy and firm to touch. Patient uses sensation in the affected area. Nursing action: Gradual warming measures, analgesia, and protection of the injured area.

First Aid

- Remove all wet or tight clothing's from the frost bitten area
- Carry the patient to a closed room without a fire and undress him carefully.
- Remove tight gloves, boots, socks, rings, etc. from the body
- Do not rub the frozen part with snow or anything else
- Put him to bed and cover him snugly with a dry cloth.
- Give him warm drinks
- If face or ear is affected, cover the frozen patch with a gloved hand until normal color and sensation return.
- Sent for a physician immediately.

Important Points to Prevent Cold Injury

- Plan activities carefully to minimize exposure
- Dress for the weather
- Avoid vigorous washing of the face
- Saving the beard until after the day's outing
- Apply protective cream to the face prior to exposure
- Wear several layers of loose warm clothing
- Use hand protection. Mittens are generally more effective than gloves
- Avoid alcohol and cigarettes
- Avoid becoming unduly fatigue
- Do not use snow, ice cold water
- If freezing occurs, avoid thawing the part until refreezing is eliminated as a threat.

RIGOR

Rigor is a sudden attack of intense shivering when the heat regulating center in the brain is disturbed.

It is seen in certain infections like malaria, in allergic reactions after intravenous infusions.

Stages of Rigor

- **Cold stage:** Patient feels chill, extreme shivering and hyperpyrexia. Provide rest and supplementary oxygen, offer hot drinks, provide extra blanket, give more fluids and hot bags can be given for warmth.
- **Hot stage:** Remove extra blanket and hot water bag. Cold sponging and ice-cap compresses can be given.
- **Sweating stage:** Wipe the patient with a wet towel and cover him with a sheet. During all the three stages, take temperature and record it in the chart.

Pathophysiology of Rigors

Shivering is a reflex which occurs when someone feels cold. It is done to raise the body temperature. Hypothalamus in the brain regulates the body temperature and has been likened to internal thermostat. The normal theromstat is set at around 37 degrees. With infection or inflammation, pyrogens, probably cytokines and prostaglandins reset the trigger temperature so that the body feels cold and shaking occurs to raise temperature to the new hypothalamic temperature point.

Other accompanying reflexes that are also body's attempts to raise temperature are including contraction of erector pilae muscles ('goose bumps') and peripheral vasoconstriction. Different pyrogens can be responsible in different conditions. For example, in malaria it is substance hemozoin which causes chills recurring every 3 to 4 days.

Chills are feeling cold after an exposure to a cold environment. Chills mainly occur at the beginning of the infection and are usually associated with fever. A chill with shivering or shaking is rigor. Rigor occurs because the patient's body is effectively shivering in a physiological attempt to increase the body temperature. Rigors are a common accompaniment of high fever.

Management

- Give lots to drink. This helps to prevent a lack of fluid in the body (dehydration). You might find that a child is more willing to have a drink if they are not so irritable. It may help to give some paracetamol and then try again with drinks half an hour or so later.
- Tepid sponging is not recommended because the blood vessels under the skin become narrower if the water is too cold and this may further raise the temperature. People with rigors also find sponging uncomfortable in the shivery phase.

- Cold fans are not recommended for the same reasons, although cooling an over-warm room with adequate ventilation is sensible.
- Children with high temperature (fever) should not be underdressed or over-wrapped.
- Medicines like paracetamol and ibuprofen should not be used for fever unless your child appears distressed:

HOT AND COLD APPLICATIONS

Hot Applications

Moist heat application can be accomplished by a warm bath/shower, hot moist towel or moist heating pad. Heat relaxes the muscles, but can cause an aggravate inflammation. Ice reduces the inflammation, but can cause muscles to tighten; therefore, the process of alternating moist heat and ice is sometimes beneficial. Heat treatment is used as a treatment for many sports related musculoskeletal injuries. There are many forms of heat treatment, with the most effective often depending on the injury in question. Time scale is also an important factor when deciding whether to use heat therapy. The nurse should be aware of contraindications of heat. Most of these are due to the massive increase in blood flow to the area. With conditions such as infection or malignant tumors, heat would increase the risk of spreading the infected or cancerous cells in the much increased blood flow.

Definition: Hot application means the application of an agent warmer than the skin. Heat is applied in either a moist or dry form.

Purpose

- Heat decreases pain.
- To provide comfort.
- To promote circulation.
- To promote suppuration.
- To relax the muscles.
- To promote healing.
- To relieve deep congestion.
- To soften the exudates.
- To stimulate peristalsis.
- To counteract sudden drop in temperature.
- To decrease joint stiffness.
- To relieve bladder distention.

Classifications

Local Heat Applications

Dry heat: Hot water bottles, chemical heating bottles, infrared rays, ultraviolet rays, electric cradles, heating lamps, electric heating pads, and short wave diathermy.

Moist heat: Warm soaks (local baths), hot fermentations (compresses), poultices, stapes, paraffin baths and sitz bath.

General Application

Dry heat: Sun bath, electric cradle and blanket bed.

Moist heat: Steam baths, hot packs, whirlpool bath (full immersion).

Physiological Effects of Hot Applications

- Peripheral vasodilatations.
- Increased capillary permeability.
- Increased local metabolism.
- Increased oxygen consumption.
- Blood-flow is increased.
- Blood viscosity is decreased.
- Lymph flow is increased.
- Motility of leukocytes is increased.
- Muscle tone is decreased.

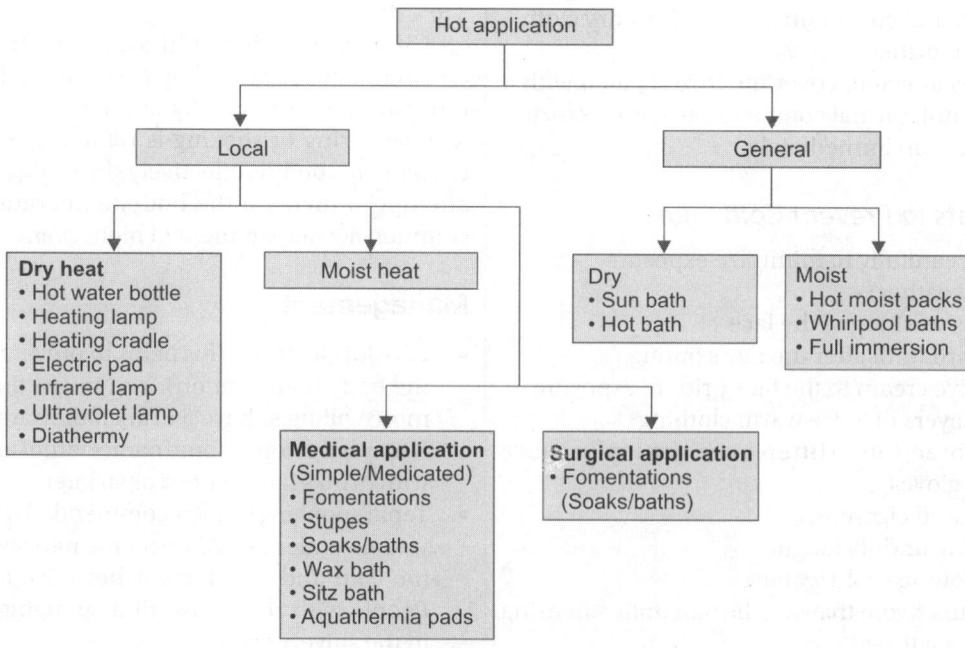

Fig. 7.13: Types of hot application.

Secondary Effect

The primary effect of hot application may last only for 20 to 40 minutes. After this time, the heat application must be discontinued and recovery time of one hour allowed, otherwise secondary effects (vasoconstriction) will take place.

Contraindication to Hot Application

- Heat is not used because heat increases the metabolism.
- Heat is not used for the patients with impaired kidney, heart and lung functions.
- Heat should not be applied to acutely inflamed areas, e.g. acute appendicitis and tooth abscess.
- Heat should not be applied on patient with paralysis weak and debilitated patients.
- Heat should not be applied when there is open wounds and bleeding.
- Heat should not be applied when there is associated with venous or lymphatic diseases.
- Heat should not be applied on patients with metabolic disorder, e.g. patients with diabetes, arteriosclerosis.
- Heat should not be applied on patients with high temperature.

Principles of Hot Application

- Heat causes dilation of blood vessels and increases the blood supply to the area.
- Heat stimulates metabolism and the growth of the new cells and tissues.
- The end organs of the sensory nerves in the skin convey the sensation of heat; the sensations are interpreted in the brain.
- Water is a good conductor of heat.
- The flow of heat is from the hotter area to the less hot area.
- Presence of stream increases the temperature of the hot applications.
- The temperature tolerance varies with individuals and according to the site and area covered.
- Friction produces heat.

Complications of Hot Applications

- Pain
- Burns
- Maceration (with moist heat)
- Redness of the skin
- Edema
- Hyperthermia
- Pallor (secondary effect).

General Instructions

- Protect damaged skin layers. Exposed layers of skin are more sensitive to temperature variations than skin layer.
- Check a patient frequently during hot application, the condition of the skin indicates whether tissue injury is occurring.
- Do not allow a patient to adjust temperature settings.
- Never position a patient in such a way that he cannot move away from the temperature source. This avoids the risk of injuries from temperature exposure.
- Never ignore the complaints of a patient however small they appear to be.

Hot Water Bag

Hot water bag is a common method of applying local dry heat. It used as both a therapeutic and a conform measure.

Hot water bag application is defined as process of applying dry heat by means of a rubber bag on specific part of body.

Purpose

- To provide comfort and warmth.
- To stimulate circulation.
- To relieve pain.
- To relax muscles.
- To promote healing.
- To relieve congestion and inflammation.
- To relieve bladder distension.

Preliminary Assessment

Check

- Doctors order for any specific instructions.
- General condition of the patient.
- Type of application to be used, duration and frequency of treatment.
- Inspect the part for any lesions.
- Presence of any contraindications for the application of heat.
- Self-care ability to follow instruction.
- Articles available in the unit.

Preparation of the Patient and Environment

- Explain the procedure to the patient.
- Provide privacy, if needed.
- Expose only the part that needs treatment.
- Place in a comfortable position.
- Arrange the articles at the bed side.

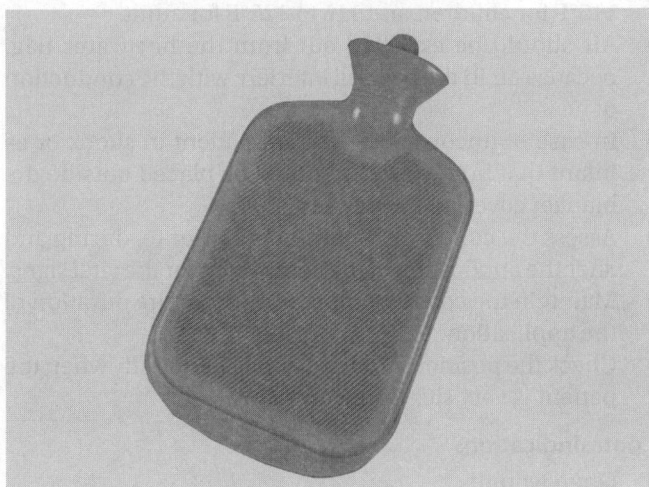

Fig. 7.14: Hot water bag.

Equipment
- Hot water bag with cover.
- Jugs-2.
- Duster-1.
- Towel-1.
- Vaseline or oil.
- Bath thermometer.

Procedure
- Wash hands.
- Check hot water bag for any leakage.
- Check the temperature of water with a bath thermometer.
- The temperature should be 105 to 115° F for children and 115 to 125° F for adults.
- Keep the bag on flat surface.
- Pour hot water into bag until 2/3rd full.
- Expel excess air by permitting water to come to mouth of bag and then close.
- Hold bag upside down to check for leakage.
- Wipe outside with duster put into flannel cover and apply to part.
- Expose only the part that needs treatment and apply it. Apply the hot water bag over the area and cover it with the towel or sheet.
- Provide warmth by covering all non treatment areas with bath blanket or bed covers.
- Remove bag after about 20 to 30 minutes.

After Care
- Dry the area if moist with perspiration.
- Inspect the part for redness.
- Position the patient comfortably on the bed.
- Cover the patient with sheets and remove the drapes if any.
- Empty the bag and hang upside down.
- Replace the articles after cleaning.
- Wash hands.
- Record the procedure in nurse's record sheet.

General Instructions
- The water should not be hot enough to burn the patient.
- The temperature of the water should be between 105 to 115°F for children and 115 to 125°F for adult.
- Air should be expelled out from the hot water bag, because air in the bag will interfere with the conduction of heat.
- In case of unconscious patient, patient in shock or as infant that hot water bag should be placed outside the blanket covering the patient.
- Assess the condition of the patient prior to, during and after the application of the heat, watch for the vital signs.
- Maintain the correct temperature for entire duration of the application.
- Check the position of hot water bag frequently when the patient is very sick or unconscious.

Contraindications
- Open wounds.
- Hypertension.
- Metabolic disorders.
- Impaired kidney, heart and lung functions.
- Acute inflammations.

Infrared Therapy
Infrared radiation is long visible rays of spectrum used therapeutically for production of heat in tissues.

Purpose
- To promote comfort.
- To soften connective tissues.
- To promote healing of bedsores.
- To improve circulation.
- To relieve spasm and pain.
- To promote suppuration.
- To relieve congestion in internal organs.

General Instructions
- The patient and the therapist must wear protective goggles during the procedure.
- Instruct the patient not to touch the lamp, nor to move close to it during procedure.
- Advice the patient not to touch lamp.
- Warn the patient that lamp would become hot after few minutes.
- Advisable for nurse to stand or stay with patient throughout treatment.
- Patient and nurse to avoid facing lamp.
- Keep the patient's skin clean and dry before using infra red lamp.
- It helps in the pigmentation of skin, production of vitamin D and bactericidal activity.
- The duration of treatment is usually 20 minutes.

Preliminary Assessment
- Doctors order for any specific instruction.
- General condition and diagnosis of the patient.
- Self-care ability to follow instructions.
- Type and duration of the treat.
- Articles available in the unit.

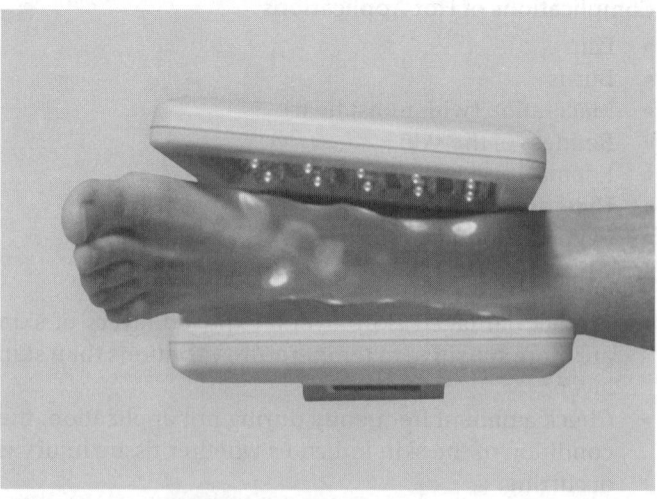

Fig. 7.15: Infrared therapy.

Preparation of the Patient and Environment
- Explain the procedure to the patient.
- Provide privacy if needed.
- Arrange the articles at the bed side.
- Position the patient according to the treatment.
- Expose only the needed part.

Equipment
- Infrared lamp.
- Inch tape.
- Top sheet.
- Goggles.

Procedure
- Wash hands.
- Expose area to which heat is to be applied.
- Drape patient appropriately to avoid exposures.
- Put on goggles to protect patient's eyes.
- Place lamp at a distance 45 cm to 55 cm (18 inches).
- After 5 minutes commencement of treatment.

After Care
- Check the condition of patient's skin for burns, redness and discomfort.
- Position the patient comfortably on the bed.
- Replace the articles.
- Wash hands.
- Record the procedure in nurse's record sheet.

Hot Fomentation

Definition
Hot fomentation is a local moist heat application, over an area by means of two thick pieces of flannel or other soft material, wrung out from boiling water, protected by water, soft covering, wool and bandage.

Hot fomentation is defined as a process of applying moist heat to localized part of body.

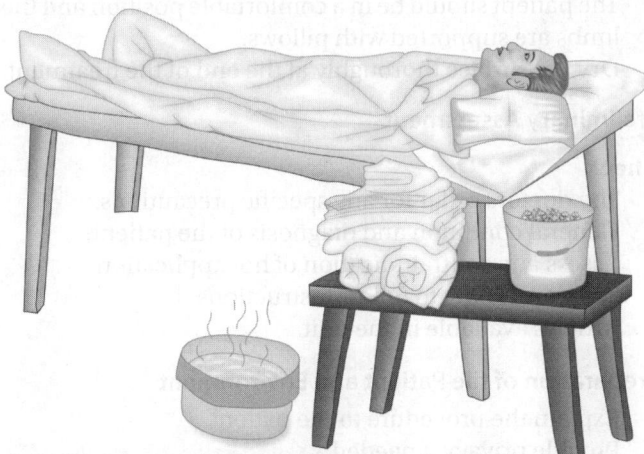

Material necessary for fomentations to chest and back
Hot foot bath, 5 fomentations (1 for back, 2 for chest, 2 in canner, 3 to 5 wool covers, 6 bath towels, basin of ice water for cold compress)

Fig. 7.16: Hot fomentation procedure.

Purpose
- To relieve pain and congestion.
- To relieve inflammation.
- To relieve retention of urine.
- To relieve intestinal and renal colic.
- To stimulate nerve ending to stimulate peristalsis.
- To provide comfort and warmth.
- To relax muscles.
- To promote suppuration.
- To apply sterile compress on wounds.

Classification
- **Simple fomentation:** Boiled or dipped in boiling water is used for fomentation, it is called simple fomentation.
- **Medicated fomentation:** Drug is added to boiled water for fomentations and it is applied to unbroken skin used to relieve tympanites by increasing the peristalsis and relaxing the muscle spasm.
- **Surgical fomentation:** This is a fomentation to broken part of skin like over an open wound. The purpose is to relieve pain and muscle spasm, to reduce swelling and congestion and to accelerate the process of suppuration.

Area of Application
- Whole of the back and sides of axilla are covered to relieve congestion of kidney.
- Joint stiffness or inflammation of the whole joint and some areas above or below the joint are covered.
- In case of stomach pain, the area of application is from xiphisternum to umbilicus and both sides of abdomen.

General Instructions
- Make sure that the skin in intact, not sored or abraded in case of medical fomentation.
- The skin is smeared with little Vaseline/oil before the application of moist heat to prevent scalding.
- The skin is covered with a layer of warm cotton (sterile) in care of open wound until a fresh application is made, if any interval of time elapses between the removal of one and the application of the next.

Preliminary Assessment

Check
- To correct patient.
- The doctors order for specific instruction.
- General condition diagnosis of the patient.
- Inspect the body part for any lesions of the skin.
- Determine the duration and frequency of the treatment.
- Assess the contraindication to the application of heat.
- Self-care ability to follow instructions.
- Articles available in the unit.

Preparation of the Patient and Environment
- Explain the sequence of the patient.
- Provide privacy if needed.
- Arrange the articles at the bedside.
- Drape the part according to the need and expose only the needed part.

- Position the patient comfortable according to the need.
- Place a Mackintosh and towel under the patient to prevent for protection of the bed.
- Expose the area and apply the olive oil, on the part to prevent burns.

Equipment
- A kettle of boiling water.
- Wringer with wringer rods placed in basin.
- Lint or funnel pieces to apply warmth.
- Plates-2 to take the compress to the patient side.

A tray containing:
- Cotton balls in a container to apply the oil.
- Forceps: To hold the cotton balls.
- Olive oil or Vaseline.
- Small mackintosh.
- Water proof cover and cotton pad.
- Abdominal binder and safety pin.
- Paper bag.
- Hot water bag and cover.
- Duster and lotion thermometer.

Procedure
- Wash hands.
- Expose the needed area and observe for any lesions on the skin.
- Place the patient at the edge of the bed near the working side.
- Expose the area and apply Vaseline.
- Place fomentation cloth/pack in wringer. Insert wringer rods and place in basin.
- Check temperature of water (125 to 150° F).
- Pour water on fomentation cloth and wet fully.
- Hold wringer rods with hands and turns in opposite direction to wring out excess water from pad.
- Remove pad by holding one corner over second basin.
- Place flannel Mackintosh over pad.
- Apply bandage/binder depending upon site and secure with pins or adhesive.
- Remove after 10 to 15 minutes.

After Care
- Observe skin for any pallor, extreme redness, pain and discomfort.
- Remove and reapply as needed for better effect.
- After removing, gently dry part.
- Replace the articles after cleaning.
- Wash hands thoroughly.
- Record the procedure in nurse's record sheet.

Soak or Local Bath

A Soak refers to either immersing a body part (e.g. an arm) in a solution or to wrapping a part in gauze dressing and then saturating the dressing with a solution.

Soak may employ wither "Clean technique" or sterile technique. A sterile technique is indicated for any open wounds present on the area.

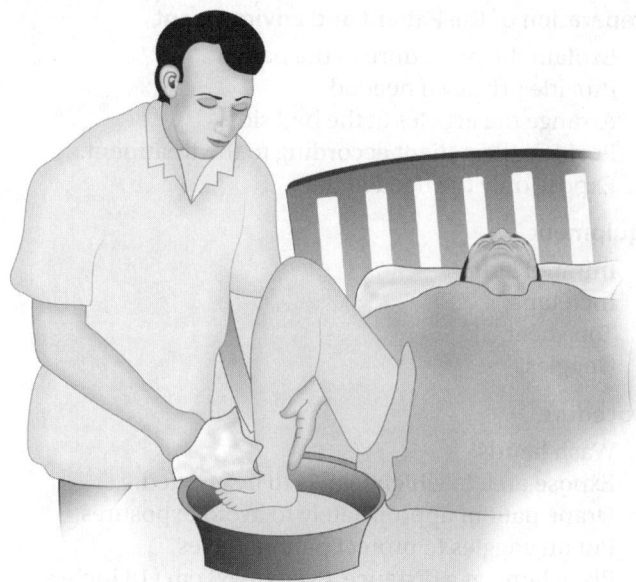

Fig. 7.17: Soak or local bath.

Purpose of Soaks
- To apply heat to hasten suppuration.
- To apply medication.
- To cleanse the wound.
- To relieve edema.
- To relieve muscle spasm.
- To increase circulation.

General Instructions
- The body part to receive the moist heat application is submerged in a basin of warm water at 105 to 110° F (40.5 to 43° C).
- The duration of the treatment is usually 20 minutes.
- Ideally the temperature of the solution should be checked frequently and additional solution added or the solution is replaced in order to maintain the appropriate temperature.
- The patient should be in a comfortable position and the limbs are supported with pillows.
- Dry the surface thoroughly at the end of the treatment.

Preliminary Assessment

Check
- The doctors order for any specific precautions.
- General condition and diagnosis of the patient.
- Assess any contraindication of hot application.
- Self-care ability to follow instructions.
- Articles available in the unit.

Preparation of tile Patient and Environment
- Explain the procedure to the patient.
- Provide privacy if needed.
- Close the window and put off the fan.
- Arrange the articles at the bed side.
- Position the patient comfortably according to the need of the procedure.

Equipment

- Bathtub
- Solution, e.g. normal saline, magnesium sulphate and sterile water.
- Mackintosh
- Extra towel
- Piece of woolen blanket
- Lotion thermometer.

Procedure

- Wash hands.
- Place the Mackintosh to protect bed linen.
- Keep bath tub on the Mackintosh.
- Allow the part to soak for prescribed length of time, usually 15 to 20 minutes.
- Check the temperature of the solution frequently and add additional solution to replace in order to maintain the appropriate temperature.
- Dry the area at the end of the procedure.

After Care

- Remove the bath tub from bed side.
- Observe the part for any skin changes.
- Make the patient comfortable in the bed.
- Replace the articles after cleaning.
- Wash hand.
- Record the procedure in the nurse's record sheet.

Sitz Bath

Sitz bath or hip bath is defined as a bath which is taken in a sitting position. The patient is usually immersed from the midthighs to the hips. Sitz bath is bathing the perineal area in a sitting position. In this the buttocks, thighs and lower trunk are also immersed in water.

Purpose

- To relieve pelvic congestion
- To treat dysmenorrhea
- To relieve pain, after operation, affecting the perineal area.
- To promote drainage of rectal abscess and hemorrhoids.
- To relieve pain following cystoscopy.

General Instructions

- When the patient takes sitz bath care has to be taken to prevent chills, burns and fainting.
- The temperature of the solution or water should be 110 to 115° F or 43 to 46° C.
- The temperature of the water should be checked in between and additional hot water is added as necessary.
- The duration of bath is 15 to 20 minutes.
- Sterile solution, in sterile containers is used for sitz bath. It will reduce the transmission of microorganisms.

Solutions Used for Sitz Bath

- Potassium permanganate 1:5000.
- Boric acid 1 gram to 1 pint.
- Eusol solution.

Sitz bath is Contraindicated During:

- Pregnancy.
- Menstruation.
- Renal inflammation.
- Increased irritability of the genital organs.

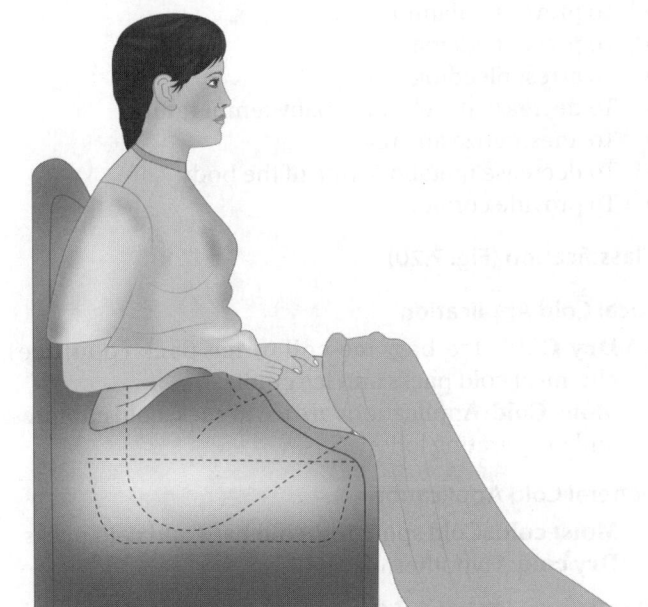

Fig. 7.18: Sitz bath procedures.

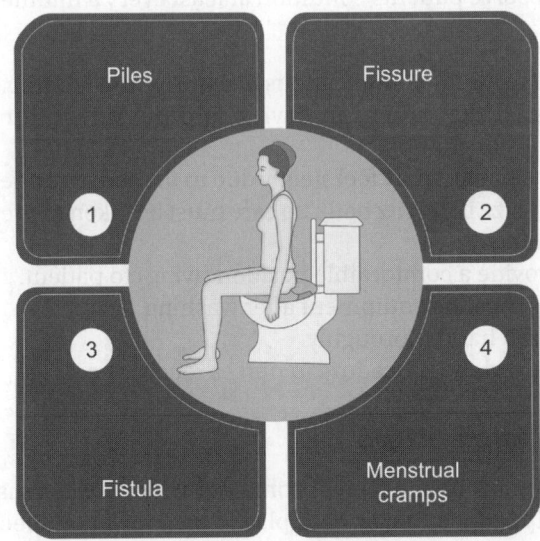

Fig. 7.19: Indications of size bath.

Preliminary Assessment

Check
- Right (correct) patient.
- The doctors order for specific instructions.
- General condition and diagnosis of the patient.
- Type, duration, and medication used for procedure.
- Self-care ability to follow instructions.
- Articles available in the unit.

Preparation of the Patient and Environment
- Explain the procedure to the patient.
- Provide privacy if needed.
- Arrange the articles at the bed side.
- Put off the fan and close the windows.
- Check the temperature of the water with lotion thermometer.
- Position the patient comfortably.

Equipment
1. Basin or bath tub.
2. Bath blanket and safety pins.
3. Bath towel.
4. Lotion thermometer.
5. Mackintosh.
6. Rubber rings.

Procedure
- Hand wash.
- Place bath towel and rubber ring in bottom of tub.
- Fill 1/3 to 1/2 full of water.
- Check the temperature with lotion thermometer.
- Assist patient into the bath tub.
- The initial temperature should be 100° F and gradually increase to 115° F.
- Cover the patient in bath blanket.
- Leave the patient in tub for 10 to 20 minutes.
- Observe patients condition at least every 5 minutes.

After Care
- Observe for complications like burns and fainting.
- Assist the patient in drying and put on clothing to prevent chilling.
- The patient may feel sleepy due to the sedative effect of the size if the sitz bath. So care must be taken to prevent falling.
- Provide a comfortable position (lying) to patient.
- Replace the equipment after washing.
- Wash hand thoroughly.
- Record the procedure in nurses record sheet.

Cold Applications

An ice pack in any type of container which holds crushed or chipped ice. It can be a plastic bag, towel or specially designed ice bag. These tend to cool the underlying tissues more efficiently than commercial chemical or frozen gel packs and remain cold for a longer period. They can be held in place if required by an elastic bandage or specialist wrap.

Primary/Physiological effects	
Hot application	Cold a aplication
Peripheral vasodilatation	Peripheral vasoconstriction
Increased capillary permeability	Decreased capillary permeability
Increased oxygen consumption	Decreased oxygen consumption
Increased local metabolism	Decreased local metabolism
Decreased blood viscosity	Increased blood viscosity
Decreased muscle tone	Decreased muscle tone
Increased blood flow	Decreased blood flow
Increased lymph flow	Decreased lymph flow
Increased motility of leucocytes	Decreased motility of leucocytes

Ice can be used to massage the affected area. Usually cubes are frozen with some form of handle (a simple lollypop stick will suffice) in order to protect the hands of the masseur. This method is most suitable for injured muscles and larger areas. The ice should be stroked up and down the injured muscle. The disadvantage of this type of massage is that the application is phases, that it the ice is in contact with each area only briefly. Following this it is exposed to air temperature which reduces the efficacy of tissue cooling. However, numbing of the area is quite efficient due to the movement of the ice stimulating mechanoreceptors in the muscles.

Definition: Cold application means the application of an agent cooler than the skin. Cold applications are also either moist or dry.

Purpose:
- Cold relieves pain
- To prevent gangrene
- To prevent inflammation
- To prevent edema
- To arrest bleeding
- To decrease the elevated baby temperature
- To anesthetize an area
- To decrease metabolic rate of the body
- To provide comfort.

Classification (Fig. 7.20)

Local Cold Application
- **Dry Cold:** Ice bag, ice collar, ice pack (poultice), chemical cold packs and ice cradle.
- **Moist Cold:** Applications are ice to suck, cold compress and evaporating lotion.

General Cold Application
- **Moist cold:** Cold sponging, cold bath and cold packs.
- **Dry cold:** Hypothermia.

Physiological Effects of Cold Applications

Primary Effects
- Peripheral vasoconstriction
- Decreased capillary permeability

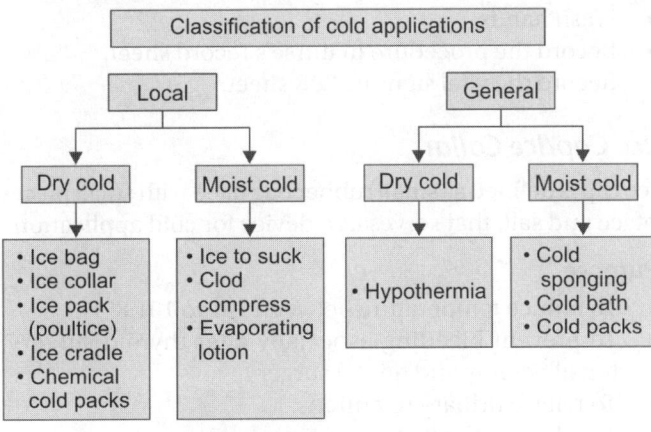

Fig. 7.20: Types of cold application.

- Decreased local metabolism
- Decreased oxygen consumption
- Blood flow is decreased
- Blood viscosity is increased
- Lymph flow is decreased
- Motility of leukocytes is decreased
- Muscle tone is decreased.

Secondary Effects: The primary effect of cold application may last only for 30 minutes to one hour, after this time, a recovery time of one hour must be allowed or secondary effects (vasodilatation) will take place.

Contraindications of Cold Applications

- Cold application should not be applied on patients who are in a state of shock and collapse.
- Cold application should not be applied when there is edema.
- Cold application should not be applied when there is muscle spasm.
- Cold application should not be applied in diseases or disorders associated with impaired circulation.
- Cold application should not be applied when there is decreased sensation.
- Cold application should not be applied when there is infected wound.
- Cold application should not be applied when the patient is having shivering or having a very low temperature.

Principals Involved in Cold Application

- Cold application causes construction of blood vessels and decrease the blood supply to the area.
- Cold application decreases metabolism and the cell activity or growth.
- The end organs of the sensory nerves in the skin convey the sensation of cold; the sensations are interpreted in the brain.
- Woolen materials absorb moisture slowly, but hold moisture longer and colds off less quickly than the cotton materials.
- Moisture left on the skin causes rapid cooling due to evaporation of the moisture.
- Prolonged exposure to moisture increases the skins susceptibility to maceration and skin breakdown.

Complications of Cold Applications

- Pain
- Blisters and skin breakdown
- Maceration (with moist cold)
- Gray-bluish discoloration
- Thrombus formation
- Hypothermia.

General Instructions

- In hyperpyrexia, the temperature of the body should be brought gradually and steadily. Sudden cooling is dangerous to the patient.
- Protect the patient from getting chills. A shivering can raise the temperature, it also allows a patient to catch a cold.
- After the procedure, dry the part gently by patting and not by rubbing to remove the moisture, thereby, to prevent maceration of the skin and further cooling by evaporation.
- Maintain the correct temperature for the entire duration of the application.
- Never ignore the complaints of a patient, however, small they appear to be.

Cold Compress

Cold compress is a local cold moist application made out of folded layers of gauze, lint piece or old soften linen, wring out of cold or ice water or in some evaporating lotion.

Purpose

- To provide comfort.
- To reduce body temperature.
- To reduce inflammation and edema.
- To relieve pain, burning sensation and irritation.
- To anesthetize for short time.
- To control hemorrhage.
- To inhibit bacterial growth and thus prevent suppuration.

General Instructions

- Application of cold compress over the skin helps in conduction of heat.
- Cold application beyond 20 minutes leads to secondary effects.
- Check the temperature every 15 minutes, it helps in detection of any variations in the body temperature.

Preliminary Assessment Check

- The doctor order for any specific instruction.
- General condition and diagnosis of the patient.
- Self-care ability of the patient
- Assess for the need of cold applications.
- Frequency and duration of application for any contraindication of cold application.
- Articles available in the unit.

Preparation of the Patient and Environment
- Explain the procedure to the patients.
- Arrange the articles at the bedside.
- Provide privacy.
- Place the patient in a comfortable position.
- Bring the patient to the edge of the bed.
- Place the mackintosh and towel under the patient to protect the bed.

Equipment
A clean tray containing:
- Bowl with ice water.
- Folded gauze pieces in a bowl.
- Mackintosh and towel.
- Small cotton balls in a bowl.
- Thermometer tray.

Procedure
- Wash hands.
- Pack the ears with cotton balls if compress is to be applied to forehead.
- Take the gauze pieces, immerse it in the water and wring it.
- Make sure that there is no dripping of water and apply it to the part ordered.
- Change it as soon as it becomes warm.
- Check the temperature every 15 minutes.
- Keep a constant watch on the color of the skin. Test the skin for numbness.

After Care
- When the time is over remove the compress.
- Wipe the part and make the patient comfortable.
- Take out the cotton balls from the ears.
- Inspect the part for discoloration or numbness.
- Place the patient in a comfortable position.
- Check the vital signs end of the treatment.
- Replace the articles after cleaning.
- Wash hands.
- Record the procedure in nurse's record sheet.
- Record the vital signs in TPR sheet.

Ice Cap/Ice Collar
Ice cap is defined as small rubber bag filled with small pieces of ice and salt, that serves as a device for cold application.

Purpose
- To reduce temperature between 101 to 101.8° F
- To prevent bleeding especially after thyroid surgery, tonsillectomy and dental surgery.
- To relieve urinary retentions.
- To relieve inflammation.
- To decrease metabolic rate of body.

General Instructions
- Fill the ice bad and ice collar with small pieces of ice and sprinkle sodium chloride.
- The salt lowers the melting point and prevents the ice from melting.
- Check the ice bag for leakage by pouring cold water into it. Empty the water and fill the bag about 1/3 with the ice.
- The ice bag/ice collar is colder than the skin, the ice takes up heat from the body and reduce the body temperature.
- Condensation of moisture collects on the outside of the bag and the flannel cover will absorb this moisture.
- The ice bag is applied for about ½ hour and then it is discontinued for at least one hour to allow for the recovery period.

Preliminary Assessment Check
- Ask the doctor for any specific instructions.
- General condition and diagnosis of the patient.
- Self care ability of the patient.
- Frequency and duration of application.
- For any contraindication of cold application.
- Articles available in the unit.

Fig. 7.21: Cold compress application.

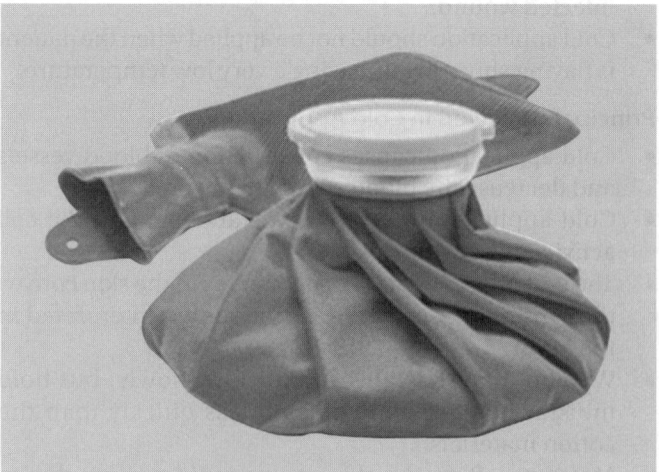

Fig. 7.22: Ice cap.

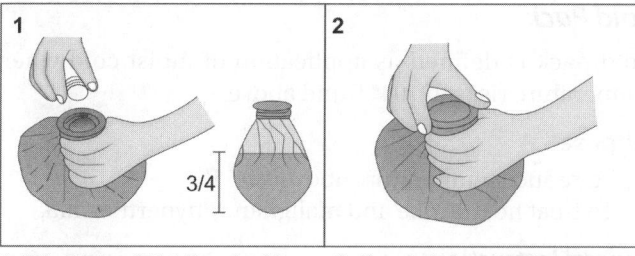

1. Fill with ice 3/4 full and add some water into the ice bag to make it better-fitting
2. Expel air from the ice bag, then cap clockwise until the cap is secured tightly

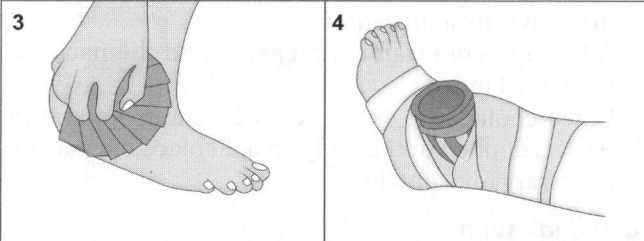

3. Apply the ice bag to desired area
4. You can also fix the ice bag on desired area with bandage for long-time cold compress therapy

Fig. 7.23: Ice cap application procedure steps.

Preparation of the Patient and Environment
- Explain the procedure to the patient.
- Provide privacy if needed.
- Assess the temperature of the patient.
- Position the patient comfortably in the bed.
- Arrange the articles at the bedside.
- Assess the part of body that needs the cold application.

Equipment
A clean tray containing
- Small mackintosh with towel
- Ice cap with ice cubes
- Flannel cover
- Salt
- Thermometer tray
- Duster.

Procedure
- Wash hands
- Fill 2/3rd ice cap with ice cubes and expels air before closing cap.
- Add pinch of salt to ice cubes before closing.
- Check for any leakage.
- Cover bag with flannel cover after drying with duster.
- Placed on desired area.
- Apply for half an hour and then remove.

After Care
- Observe for bluish skin discoloration or mottling.
- Recheck patient's temperature.
- Replace the articles after cleaning.
- Position the patient in a comfortable position.
- Wash hands.
- Record the procedure in the nurse's record sheet and vital signs in TPR sheet.

Tepid Sponge/Cold Sponge

Tepid sponging or cold sponging is a general application of moist cold liquid to cool skin, by evaporation and by the absorption of body heat in the cold water.

Tepid sponge is a process of sponging with tepid water to reduce body temperature by evaporation. The temperature of water used for tepid sponge is 80 to 90° F.

Cold sponge is a moist cold application using ice water when patient's temperature is dangerously raised. The temperature of water used for cold sponge is 60 to 70° F.

Purpose
- Tepid sponge helps to reduce the temperature between 102 and 102.8° F.
- Cold sponge helps to reduce the temperature of above 103° F.
- To stimulate circulation.
- To decrease toxicity.
- Nervousness and delirium.
- To soothe the nerves and promote sleep.

General Instructions
- Cold sponging is used to reduce temperature in a patient with hyperpyrexia (above 103° F).
- Large areas of the body are sponged at one time, permitting the heat of the body to transfer to the cooler solution on the body surface.
- Often wet towels are applied to the neck, axillae, groin and ankles, where the blood circulation is close to the skin surface.
- The vital signs are checked very frequently to detect the early signs of complications.
- The physiological effect of the cold applications are vasoconstriction, decreased blood circulation, decreased capillary permeability, decreased metabolism, decreased blood viscosity, etc.
- The application of moist cold is more effective than the application of dry cold as the moisture distributes the cold to large and deep area.
- There must be a written order for tepid sponge or cold sponge.
- Use long strokes for sponging and avoid circular movements or friction while sponging.
- Keep the hot water bag ready at the foot end of the bed.

Preliminary Assessment Check
- The doctors order for any specific instructions.
- General condition and diagnosis.
- Self-care ability of the patient.
- Assess the duration of application.
- For contraindication to cold application.
- Articles available in the unit.

Preparation of the Patient and Environment
- Explain the sequence of the procedure.
- Provide privacy.
- Check the initial temperature and should be checked after every 15 minutes intervals.
- Position the patient comfortably in the bed.

- Remove the patient gown and place with bath blanket.
- Bring the patient to the edge of the bed.
- Place the long mackintosh and draw sheet under the patient.
- Arrange the articles to the bedside.

Procedure
- Wash hands.
- Mix the water with ice cubes.
- Soak the wash cloths in the ice cold water for sometime.
- Place cold sponge cloths in each axilla and groin.
- Put the face towel under the head, sponge the face and dry with face towel.
- Sponge the neck, right arm from the shoulder to the fingertips for 3 minutes.
- Change sponge cloth when it becomes warm.
- Sponge the left arm, chest and abdomen for 3 minutes.
- Change the water if it becomes dirty and check the temperature.
- Cover the upper half of the body and expose the lower half of the body.
- Sponge the right and left lower limb for 3 minutes.
- Then carefully turn the patient to one side and bring patient to the edge of bed. Sponge the back with long strokes for 3 minutes.
- Dry the part with bath towel and apply spirit on the back.
- Check the temperature at 20 minutes interval and record it in the TPR chart.

Equipment
- A large basin of water (80 to 90° F) for tepid sponging
- Jug with cold water
- Basin with ice pieces
- Bath thermometer
- Mackintosh and draw sheet
- Sponge clothes-6
- Bath towel-1
- Face towel-1
- Thermometer tray
- Ice cap with cover
- Spirit rub
- Bucket

After Care
- Remove the sponge clothes from the axilla and groin. Discard it in kidney tray.
- Dry the body with bath towel.
- Remove the Mackintosh and draw sheet.
- Replace the gown and remove bath blanket.
- Observe for any symptoms of chill or any other abnormality.
- If needed give him hot drinks.
- Position the patient comfortably in the bed.
- Replace the articles after cleaning.
- Wash hands.
- Record the procedure in the nurse's record sheet and vital signs in TPR sheet.

Cold Pack

Cold pack is defined as application of moist cold when temperature rises to 104° F and above.

Purpose
- To reduce temperature above 104° F
- To treat heat stroke and malignancy hyperthermia.

General Instructions
- The pack could be a wash cloth, towel, flannel or a piece of old linen depending up on the size of the body part to receive the application.
- A basin of cold water is prepared and the packs are immersed into it.
- When cooled, the excess water is wrung out and the pack is applied to the body area. Replace the packs as necessary to maintain.

Contraindication
Circulatory disorders like peripheral vascular diseases.

Preliminary Assessment Check
- Check the doctor's order for any specific instructions.
- General condition and diagnosis of the patient.
- Self-care ability of the patient.
- Duration of the treatment.
- Articles available in the unit.

Preparation of the Patient and Environment
- Explain the procedure to the patient.
- Provide privacy.
- Arrange the articles at the bed side.
- Place the patient in comfortable position.
- Place the mackintosh under the patient.

Equipment
- Long mackintosh
- Bed Sheet-2
- Bath towel-6
- Cold compress and ice cap equipment
- Bucket of cold water
- Bath thermometer
- Bowl with crushed ice pieces
- Hot water bag.

Procedure
- Wash hands.
- Pour cold water into basin; add ice cubes to bring temperature to 65° F and wet bath towels.
- Remove top sheet and protect bed with long mackintosh and big sheet.
- Remove patients cloths, cover with wet bath towel from chest to pubic area.
- Place compress on forehead, ice cap on head and hot water bag at feet.
- Wrap hand and legs with wet towel.
- Check the temperature every 15 minutes and replace wet towels.
- Continue procedure for 30 minutes.

After Care
- After completing procedure, remove towels and dry patient thoroughly.
- Remove mackintosh and change wet sheets.
- Dress patient and cover with top sheet.
- Keep patient in a comfortable position.
- Replace the articles after cleaning.
- Wash hands.
- Record the procedure in nurse's record sheet and vital signs in TPR sheet.

PULSE

Pulse is the wave of expansion and recoil occurring in an artery is response to the pumping action of the heart.

Pulse is the heart beat, conveniently felt at the wrist and at any point where an artery passes superficially over the bone.

Pulse is defined as checking rate, rhythm and volume of throbbing of an artery against a bony prominence.

Purpose
- To determine number of heart beats acquiring per minutes create.
- To evaluate amplitude (strength) of pulse.
- To assess the vascular status of limbs.
- To assess response of heart to cardiac medications, activity, blood volume and gas exchange.
- To assess heart's ability to deliver blood to distant area of the body.
- To obtain information about heart rhythm and patterns of beats.

Normal Rate
- Newborn: 140 beats/minute.
- Infant: 120 beats/minute.
- 2–3 years: 100 beats/minute.
- 5–10 years: 90 beats/minute.
- Adults: 70 to 80 beats/minute (average is 72 per minute).
- Old age: May be slower.
- Extremely old age: May be more rapid.

Sites of Taking Pulse
- Radical artery: In front of the wrist
- Brachial artery: Above the elbow
- Carotid artery: Sides of the neck
- Temporal artery: Over the temporal bone
- Facial artery: Above the lower jaw
- Femoral artery: In the groin
- Tibial artery: Below the popliteal fossa.
- Dorsalis pedis artery: On the foot.

Common Sites for Checking Pulse

Sl. No.	Location		Reason for use
1.	Radial	Inner aspect of the wrist on thumb side	Easily accessible
2.	Temporal	Site superior (above) and lateral to (away from the midline) the eye	Used when radial pulse is not accessible. Easily accessible pulse in children
3.	Carotid	At the side of the trachea where the carotid artery runs between the trachea and the sternocleidomastoid muscle	To assess cerebral perfusion
4.	Apical	Left side of the chest in the 4th, 5th, or 6th intercostal space in the midclavicular line	Used to find out discrepancies with radial pulse
5.	Brachial	Medially in the antecubital space	Used to monitor blood pressure and assess for lower arm circulation
6.	Femoral	Below inguinal ligament, midway between symphysis pubis and anterosuperior iliac spine	To assess circulation to lower hip
7.	Popliteal	Medial or lateral to the popliteal fossa with knees slightly flexed	Used to determine circulation to the leg. To take blood pressure in the lower limb
8.	Posterior tibial	On the medial surface of the ankle behind the medial malleolus	To assess circulation to the foot
9.	Dorsalis pedis	Along the dorsum of the foot between extensor tendons of great toe.	To assess circulation to the foot
10.	Ulnar pulse	On the little finger side, outer aspect of the wrist	To assess circulation to ulnar side of hand. To perform Allen's test

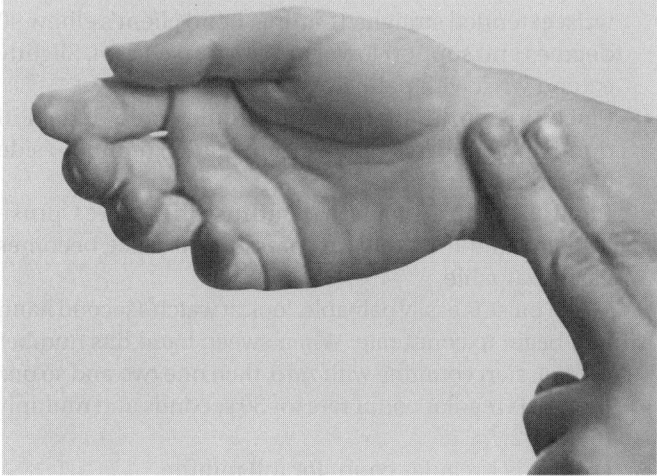

Fig. 7.24: Radial site used for pulse checking.

Factors Affect the Pulse

- Age: Very old have slow pulse rate and children will have faster beat.
- Sex: It is slower in men than in women.
- Stature: It is slower in tall people than in short people.
- Position: The pulse rate is slower than at rest or asleep than in standing position.
- Emotions: Anger or excitement increases the pulse rate temporarily.
- Exercise: It is much faster during exercise.

Characteristics of Pulse

- Rate: Number of beats/minute, corresponds with age (above 100 tachycardia, below 60 bradycardia).
- Rhythm: It is the regularity of beats. The distance between beats (regular).
- Volume: It is the fullness of artery. It is the force of blood felt at each beat (full/large/small).
- Tension: It is the degree of compressibility (High/low).

Abnormal Pulse

- **Rate-tachycardia:** The pulse rate more than 100 beats/minute. It commonly found in patients with fevers. Thyrotoxicosis, organic heart diseases, nervous disorders and intake of drugs like belladonna and alcoholism cause tachycardia.
- **Bradycardia:** Pulse rate less than 60 beats per minute. Caused by opium poisoning heart muscle disorder, cerebral tumors and myxedema.
- **Abnormal rhythms** are intermittent pulse, extra systoles, atrial fibrillation, ventricular fibrillation, sinus arrhythmia.

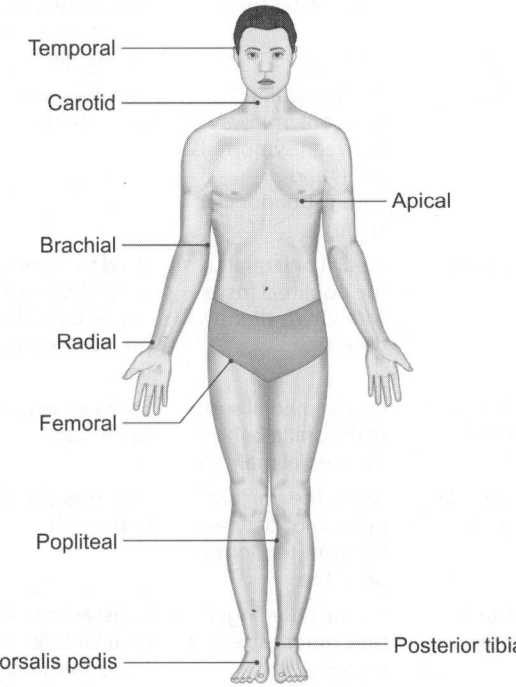

Fig. 7.25: Sites for checking pulse.

- **Abnormal pulse volume causes:** It may be due to low peripheral resistance (as seen in fever, anemia, thyrotoxicosis, hyperkinetic heart syndrome, A-V fistula, Paget's disease, beriberi, liver cirrhosis), increased cardiac output, increased stroke volume (as seen in anxiety, exercise, complete heart block, aortic regurgitation) decreased distensibility of arterial system (as seen in atherosclerosis, hypertension and coarctation of aorta).
- **Water hammer pulse or Corrigan's pulse:** It is a full volume pulse. This type of pulse found in aortic regurgitation. When the blood is forced into the artery, then leaks back in to the ventricle due to the non-closure of the aortic valve.

General Instruction for Taking Pulse

- Count the pulse for one full minute. Especially when there is irregularity.
- Observe rate, rhythm, volume and tension of pulse.
- Pulse should not be taken immediately after exercise, in emotional stress or after a painful treatment.
- Record pulse immediately.
- Choose suitable site for taking pulse.
- Nurse to be aware if patient is on any medication that can interfere with heart rate.
- To check pulse after 10 to 15 minutes, after strenuous physical exercise.
- Notify physician if pulse rate is below < 60/minute or above > 100/minute. Normal and abnormal patterns (missing beats).
- Record in TPR record.

Equipment

1. Watch with second hand.
- Red pen.
- TPR sheet.

Procedure

- Wash hands
- If supine, place client's forearm across lower chest with wrist extended straight. If sitting, bend client's elbow 90 degrees and support lower arm on nurse's arm. Slightly extend wrist with palm down.
- Place tips of the first two or middle three fingers of dominant hand over groove along radial or thumb side of client's.
- Lightly compress against radius obliterates pulse initially, and then releases pressure so pulse becomes easily palpable.
- When pulse is easily palpable, look at watch's second hand and begin to count rate: When sweep hand hits number on dial, start counting with zero, then one two and so on.
- If pulse is regular count rate for 30 seconds and multiply total by 2.
- If pulse is irregular count for full minute.
- Assess regularity and frequency of any dysrhythmia.

- Determine strength of pulse. Note whether thrust of vessel against fingertips is bounding, strong, weak or thread.
- Assist client in returning to comfortable position.

After Care

- Wash hands.
- If pulse is assessed for first time establish as baseline.
- Assess pulse again by having another nurse conduct measurement, if pulse character is abnormal or irregular.
- Record characteristic of pulse in nursing progress sheet or vital sign flow sheet. Also record any accompanying signs and symptoms of pulse alterations.
- Report abnormal findings to the nurse in charge or physician.

RESPIRATION

Respiration monitoring is an involuntary process of inspiration (inhalation) expiration (exhalation) in a patient.

Respiration is the act of breathing in and breathing out. It includes inspiration and expiration. The exchange of gases between the blood and lungs is called external or pulmonary respiration. The exchange of gases between the blood and cell is called internal respiration.

Respiration is the act of breathing. It includes the intake of oxygen and the output of carbon dioxide, i.e. respiration consists of inspiration and expiration.

Purpose

- To determine the respiratory status of the patient
- To determine number of respiration occurring per minute.
- To gather information about rhythm and depth.
- To assess response of patient to any related therapy/medication.

Times of Respiration

- **External respiration:** The exchange of gases between the blood and the air in the lungs is called as external or pulmonary respiration.
- **Internal respiration:** The exchange of gases between the blood and the tissue cells is called as internal or tissue respiration.
- **Regulation of respiration:** It is a rhythmical movements. Respiration are regulated by respiratory center in the brain called medulla oblongata, nerve fibers of the autonomic nervous system and the chemical composition of the blood.

Normal Rates

- At birth: 30 to 40 breaths/minute
- One year: 26 to 30 breaths/minute
- 2 to 5 years: 20 to 26 breaths/minute
- Adolescence: 20 breaths/minute
- Adults: 16 to 20 breaths/minute
- Old age: 10 to 24 breaths/minute

TABLE 7.1: Respiratory rate classification in adult patients.

RR	Range
Eupnea (normal relaxed breathing)	12–20 bpm
Normal range >65 years	12–25 bpm
Normal range >80 years	10–30 bpm
Bradypnea (slow RR)	<12 bpm
Tachypnea (fast RR)	>20 bpm

bpm = breaths per minute; RR = respiratory rate

Factors Influences Respiration

- **Sex:** Female have slightly rapid respiration than the male.
- **Exercise:** Exertion of any type increases the metabolic rate and stimulates respiration
- **Rest and sleep:** During rest and sleep metabolism is decreased so respiration rate is normal or decreased.
- **Emotions:** Sudden stressful condition such as fear and anxiety influences the respiratory rate.
- **Changes in atmospheric pressure:** In high altitudes the content of oxygen in the atmosphere is very low. So rate of respiration is increased and the increased demand of oxygen is fulfilled.

Types of Normal and Abnormal Respiratory Pattern

Type	Description	Location	Characteristics
Vesicular	Soft, low-pitched	Over bronchioles and alveoli; best heard at base of lungs	Best heard on inspiration
Bronchial (tracheal)	"gentle sighing"	One trachea, not normally heard over lung tissue.	Lounder than vesicular sounds, expiratory phase
Broncho-vesicular	Moderately high-pitched "harsh" Moderate intensity	Over bronchioles lateral to the sternum at the first and school? intercostal spaces and between the scapulae	Equal inspiratory and expiratory phases

Characteristics of Commonly Observed Respiratory Patterns

Characteristics of Respiration

- Normal breathing is effortless.
- It is painless, quiet and automatic.
- Normal respiration consists of rhythmical rising and falling of the chest wall.

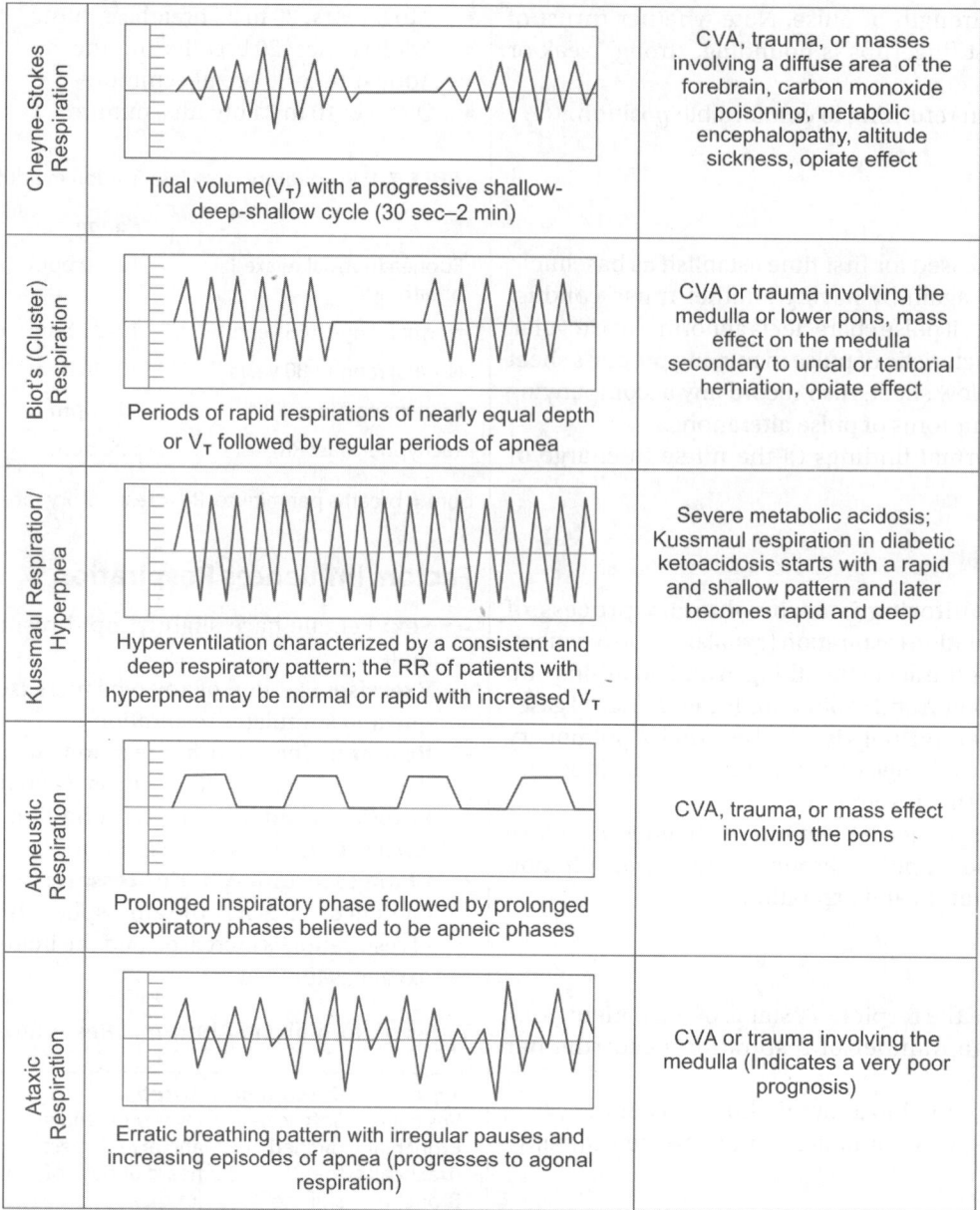

Fig. 7.26: Abnormal respiratory rhythm.

- Respiratory rate in resting adult is 16 to 18 breaths/minute.
- Eupnea: It is regular, even and produces no noise.

Normal Breath Sounds Types

- **Vesicular sound**: Soft, low pitched, gentle sighing. Location: Over bronchioles and alveoli best heard at base of lungs. Characteristics: Best heard on inspiration.
- **Bronchial sound**: Moderately high pitched harsh. Location: Over trachea, not normally heard over lung tissue. Characteristics: Best heard on expiration.
- **Bronchovesicular sound**: Moderate intensity. Location: Over bronchioles lateral to the sternum at the first and second intercostals spaces and between the scapulae.

Adventitious Breath Sounds

- **Rales sound:** Fine crackling sounds, alveolar rales are high pitched bronchial rales are lower pitched. Characteristics: Best heard on inspiration.
- **Rhonchi sound:** Course gurgling, harsh, louder sounds as air passes through bronchi filled with fluid. Characteristics: Best heard on expiration.
- **Wheeze sound:** Squeaky musical sounds often indicative of bronchial constriction. Characteristics: Best heard on expiration.
- **Friction:** Rubbing of the pulmonary and visceral pleura, grating sound. Characteristics: Best heard over the lower anterior and lateral chest.

Abnormal Respirations

- **Stridor respiration:** It is noisy, shrill and vibrating respiration. It is due to obstruction in the upper airway. It is commonly seen in laryngitis and foreign body in the respiratory tract.
- **Wheezing:** Expiration is difficult and louder. It is due to partial obstruction of the smaller bronchi and bronchioles. It is seen in asthma or emphysema.
- **Apnea:** This is a temporary cessation of breathing due to excessive oxygen and lack of carbon dioxide.
- **Dyspnea:** This is forced, difficult or labored breathing. It may be accompanied by pain and cyanosis; it is seen in heart diseases, respiratory diseases, convulsions, etc.
- **Orthopnea:** The patient can breathe only in upright position. Commonly found in congestive cardiac failure.
- **Cheyne-Stokes respiration:** This is respiration which gradually increases in rate and volume until it reaches a climax. Then slowly pause occurs and breathing stops for 5 to 30 seconds and then cycle begins again. It is a periodic breathing usually found in the patients who are near death.
- **Asphyxia:** It is a state of suffocation when the lungs do not get a sufficient supply of fresh air to the vital organs and they are deprived of oxygen.
- **Cyanosis:** It is the blueness or discoloration of the skin and mucous membrane due to lack of oxygen in the tissues.
- **Rale:** An abnormal rattling or bubbling sound caused by the mucus in the air passages as seen in the bronchitis or pneumonia.
- **Kussmauls respiration:** Respiration is abnormally deep but regular, rate is increased. It is seen in diabetic ketoacidosis.
- **Biot's respiration:** It is shallow breathing interrupted by irregular periods of apnea, seen in central nervous system disorders.

General Instruction

- Patient to be unaware of the nurse counting respiration.
- Inform to physician in case of bradypnea, tachypnea or other abnormal respiratory patterns noticed.
- Maintain half hourly checking of respiration and pulse when indicated.

Preliminary Assessment

- Determine the need to assess client's respiration.
- If client has been active, wait 5 or 10 minutes before assessing respiration.
- Assess respirations as first vital sign in infant or child.
- Assess respiration after pulse measurement in adult.
- Be sure client is in a comfortable position, preferably sitting.
- Be sure client's chest movement is visible. If necessary, remove bed lines or gown.

Equipment

- Wrist watches with second hand or digital display.
- Pen and flow sheet or record form.
- TPR chart.

Procedure

- Place client's arm in relaxed a position across the abdomen or lower chest.
- Observe complete respiratory cycle (one inspiration and one expiration).
- After cycle is observed, look at watch's second hand and begin to count rate, when sweep hand hits number on dial, begins time frame, counting one with first full respiratory cycle. If rhythm is regular in adult, count number of respirations in 30 seconds and multiply by 2. In infant or young child count respirations for full minute. If adult has irregular rhythm or abnormally slow or fast rate, count for one full minute.
- Note depth of respirations. This can be assessed subjectively by observing degree of chest wall movement while counting rate.
- Note rhythm of ventilatory cycle. Normal breathing is regular and uninterrupted. Infants breathe less regularly. Young child may breathe slowly and then suddenly breath fastens.
- Replace client's gown and cover with bed lines.

After Care

- Wash hands.
- Compare client's respirations with previous baseline and normal respiratory rate for age group.
- Record any accompanying signs and symptoms of respiratory alterations in nurse's notes or flow sheet.

ALTERATIONS IN RESPIRATION

- **Bradypnea:** The respiratory is abnormally slow (less than 12 breaths per minute). Occurs in coma due to cerebral hemorrhage or large doses of sedatives.
- **Tachypnea:** The respiratory rate is abnormally rapid (greater than 20 breaths per minute).
- **Apnea:** Respirations cease for several seconds.
- **Respiratory arrest:** Persistent cessation of respiration.
- **Hyperventilation:** Rate and depth of respirations increase.
- **Hypoventilation:** Rate is abnormally low and depth is shallow. Shallow respiration occurs in diseases of the lung such as pneumonia and pleurisy.
- **Sighing or air hunger:** Indicates a need for more oxygen. Occurs in severe hemorrhage, diabetic coma or due to stimulation of respiratory center by excess of acid.
- **Wheezing:** Sound made during expiration may be due to obstruction in the lower respiratory tract as in the case of asthma.

- **Stertorous breathing:** Noisy snoring inspiration occurs in unconscious patients which may be due to the tongue slipping back. Peculiar hissing respiration occurs in uremic coma.
- **Stridor:** It is noisy inspiration due to the obstruction of upper respiratory tract. This noise may be harsh, grating or whistling sound.
- **Orthopnea:** Inability to breath easily unless in an upright position.
- **Dyspnea:** Difficult breathing. If it is during inspiration it is due to laryngeal obstruction; if it is during expiration it is due to asthma.
- **Cheyne-Stokes or periodic breathing:** Alternative periods of hyperpnea, occurring in a rhythmical cycle. It is important to note this phenomenon as this is a serious sign.
- **Asphyxia:** Occurs due to lack of oxygen supplied to the cells. This is found in drowning patients or persons who have inhaled poisonous gases (coal gas).

BLOOD PRESSURE

Blood pressure may be defined as the force exerted by blood against the walls of the vessels in which it is contained. Differences in blood pressure between different areas of the circulation provide the driving force that keeps the blood moving through the body.

Purpose

- To obtain baseline date for diagnosis and treatment.
- To compare with subsequent changes that may occur during care of patient.
- To assist in evaluating status of patient's blood volume, cardiac output and vascular system.
- To evaluate patients response to change in physical condition as a result of treatment with fluids or medications.

Indication

- To determine baseline, blood pressure recording and monitor fluctuation.
- To aid in the diagnostic disease.
- To aid in the assessment of cardiovascular system.

Types of Pressure

- **Systolic pressure:** is the highest degree of pressure exerted by the blood against the arterial wall as the left ventricle contracts and forces the blood from it into the aorta.
- **Diastolic pressure:** is the lowest degree of pressure when the heart is in its resting period just before contraction of the left ventricle.
- Pulse pressure is the difference between systolic and diastolic blood pressure. It is measured in millimeters of mercury (mm Hg). It represents the force that the heart generates each time it contracts. Resting blood pressure is normally approximately 120/80 mm Hg, which yields a pulse pressure of approximately 40 mm Hg.
- Normal venous pressure on an average person in a recumbent position is 40 to 110 mm of water. Venous pressure is a valuable index in determining the efficiency of heart muscles.

Scientific Principles

- Exercise, emotion, anxiety, fear, tension and worry cause a temporary rise in blood pressure.
- The brachial artery in superficial in the antecubital area which is convenient place for taking BP.
- A noisy environment and parallax error interfere with correct reading on manometer.
- A twisted cuff may produce unequal pressure and can cause inaccurate reading.
- Accurate reading is possible only when the stethoscope is directly over the artery.

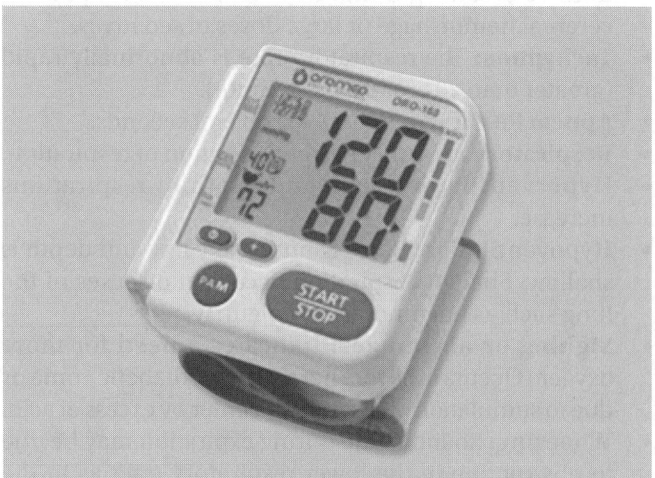

Fig. 7.27: Blood pressure monitor device.

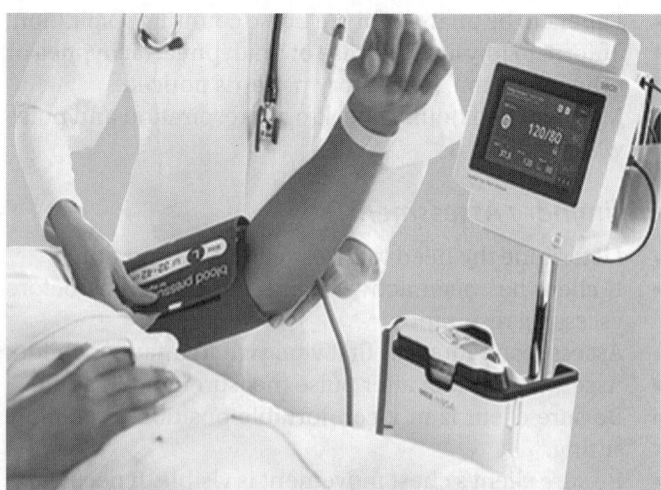

Fig. 7.28: Blood pressure cuff application technique.

- Airtight system of cuff and tubing facilitates accurate reading.
- Sufficient pressure in the cuff obliterates the flow of blood through the brachial artery.

Factors Influencing Blood Pressure

- Age: Adult's blood pressure tends to increase with advancing age.
  The older adult's blood pressure is 140-160/80-90 mm Hg.
- Stress: Anxiety, fear, pain, emotional stress increases blood pressure.
- Medication: Narcotic and analgesics lower blood pressure.
- Diurnal variation: It is lowest in early morning and higher in late evening
- Sex: In men, it is higher than in female.
- Exercise: It will increase blood pressure.
- Bleeding: It causes low blood pressure.

Blood Pressure Systolic–Diastolic

- Newborn 30-50 mm Hg 10 mm Hg
- Infant 70-90 mm Hg 50 mm Hg

Preliminary Assessment

- Identify the patient.
- Check the diagnosis, reason for taking BP schedule frequency of obtaining blood pressure.
- Previous measurement and range of blood pressure.
- Physical and mental state of the patient. Blood pressure taking, on a patient who is angry, anxious or in pain or a crying child.
- Assess the arm on which the blood pressure can be taken. Do not take blood pressure reading on a patient's arm if:
  - The arm has an intravenous infusion on it.
  - The arm is injured or diseased.
  - The arm has a shunt or fistula for the renal dialysis.
  - On the same side of the body where a female patient had a radical mastectomy.

Preparation of the Article

- Sphygmomanometer.
- Stethoscope.
- Piece of paper.

Preparation of the Patient

- Explain the procedure to the patient to gain the confidence and cooperation of the patient.
- Place the patient in a comfortable position either lying down with the arm resting on the bed or sitting with the arm supported on the table at heart level to ensure accurate reading.
- Patient should be resting at least 5 to 10 minutes prior to taking blood pressure.

Procedure

- Wash hands.
- Take the equipment to the bedside.
- Apply deflated cuff evenly with rubber bladder over the brachial artery, the lower edge being 2 inch above the antecubital fossa. The two tubes turning towards the palm.
- Palpate the brachial artery with the fingertips. Place the bell of the stethoscope on the brachial pulse. The stethoscope must hang freely from the ears.
- Close the valve on the pump by turning the knob clockwise. Pump up air in the cuff until the sphygmomanometer registers about 20 mm above the point at which the radial pulsation disappears.
- Open the valve slowly by turning the knob anti-clockwise. Permit the air to escape very slowly. Note the number on the manometer where sound first begins. This is the systolic pressure.
- Continue to release the pressure slowly. The sound become louder and clearer. Note the point on the manometer where the sound ceases. This is the diastolic pressure.
- Allow the air to escape and the mercury to fall zero. Wait for one minute with the cuff deflated.
- Repeat the procedure if there is any doubts about the reading.
- Do not take blood pressure more than three times in succession on reading the same arm.

After Care

- Remove the cuff by rolling it and replace it in the box.
- Assist the patient to cover the arm which was exposed.
- Take the apparatus to the duty room and keep it safely in the cupboard.
- Wash hands.
- Record the readings immediately, with the date and time.

ALTERATION IN BLOOD PRESSURE

Hypertension

Elevated or high blood pressure is known as hypertension. Hypertension is a major factor causing deaths from strokes and myocardial infarction (Heart arrest).

Causes of Hypertension

- Family history of hypertension
- Obesity
- Cigarette smoking
- Alcohol consumption

- High blood cholesterol level
- Continued exposure to stress
- Old age.

Treatment
- Early diagnosis
- Long-term follow up care and therapy.

Hypotension

When the systolic pressure falls to 90 mm Hg or below, that condition is known as hypotension.

Causes of Hypotension
- Dilatation of the arteries.
- Loss of blood, due to hemorrhage.
- Failure of heart muscle to pump adequately Heart attack.

Signs and Symptoms of Hypotension
- Pallor.
- Skin mottling.
- Cold and clammy
- Increased heart rate.
- Decreased urine output.

Monitoring BP

Purposes
- To aid in the diagnosis of the patient's condition
- To guide in his treatment.
- To evaluate the patient's progress.

General Instructions
- See that the patient is relaxed and in a comfortable position.
- Help to take blood pressure for patients with the following conditions.
  - New patients
  - Pre- and postoperative patients
  - Antenatal and postnatal patients
  - Patients with shock and hemorrhage
  - Patients with cardiac conditions and hypertension
  - Patients with neurological disorders.
- Record pulse along with blood pressure.
- Blood pressure is taken at the same arm, same time, same posture daily.

Equipment
- Sphygmomanometer.
- Stethoscope.
- Pen.

Guidelines
- The sphygmomanometers generally used in clinical setting are mercury type and aneroid type. The mercury type sphygmomanometers are more reliable than the aneroid type sphygmomanometers. The aneroid sphygmomanometers give blood pressure reading on dial indicator.
- Systolic pressure is increased in pressure induced by systolic contraction and diastolic pressure is decrease in pressure induced by diastolic relaxation of the left ventricle of heart.
- Never take blood pressure when the patient is excited, exhausted and just after exercise, smoking or meals.
- Allow the patient to rest for five minutes before taking blood pressure.
- Do not use the extremity that is injured, diseased, paralyzed, receiving intravenous infusion or when a female patient is with radical mastectomy on the same side.
- When the arm cannot be used to measure the blood pressure, the thigh can be used being a good alternative site.
- Always take the blood pressure reading on the same side and in the same position to maintain consistency.
- Place the site (arm or leg) about the level of heart while taking blood pressure.
- The apparatus should be in working order. The cuff should be of appropriate size (12-14 cm for arm and 18-20 cm for thigh) and deflated before wrapping around the patient's site.
- While taking blood pressure, certain sounds are heard in sequence. These are called as Korotkoff sounds and are described as under.
  - **Tapping:** The faint clear sounds that gradually become louder, the first tapping sound may be followed by an absence of sound (auscultatory gap) and indicates systolic pressure reading.
  - **Murmuring:** The low swishing sounds that increase with cuff deflation.
  - **Knocking:** The crisp, clear sounds that occur with each heart beat.
  - **Muffling:** Abrupt change of sound indicates first diastolic pressure reading.
  - **No sounds:** The sound disappears and indicates second diastolic pressure reading.
- When deflating the cuff to take the readings, deflate the cuff to 0. Do not stop in between and start inflating again as this gives a false reading.
- Note the variations in blood pressure.

CONCLUSION

Vital signs include the physiological measurements of temperature, pulse, BP and respirations. Vital signs are a quick and efficient way of monitoring a patient's condition or identifying problems and evaluating the patient's response to intervening changes. One vital sign can influence characteristics of other vital signs. The basic techniques of inspection palpation and auscultation are used to determine vital signs. Assessment of vital signs allows the nurse to identify nursing diagnosis, to implement planned intervention and to evaluate success.

When the nurse learns the physiological variables influencing vital signs and recognizes the relationship of vital sign changes to other physiological assessment findings, precise determination of the client's health problems can be made.

BIBLIOGRAPHY

1. Alice L. Price. The Art, Science and Spirit of Nursing, Philadelphia: W.B. Saunders Company, 3rd ed, 1968.
2. Dickinson, Edward C, Limmer, Daniel, O'Keefe, Michael F., edn. Emergency Care, 10th Ed. Upper Saddle River, N.J: Pearson/Prentice Hall, 2005.
3. Kozier, Barbara B, Du Gas, Beverly Witter. Fundamentals of Patient Care: A Comprehensive Approach to Nursing; W.B. Saunders Company, 1967.
4. McClosky JC, Grace HK. Current Issues in Nursing, 4th Ed. St. Louis: Mosby Year Book, Inc., 1994.
5. Mitchell PR, Grippando GM. Nursing Perspectives and Issues, 5th Ed. Albany, New York: Delmar Publishers, Inc., 1993.
6. Mower W, Myers G, Nicklin E, Kearin K, Baraff L, Sachs C. Pulse oximetry as a fifth vital sign in emergency geriatric assessment. Acad Emerg Med 1998;5(9).
7. Potter P, Perry A. Fundamentals of Nursing - Concepts, Process and Practice; Mosby Year Book; 3rd Edition, 1993.
8. Shafer, Kathleen, et. al. Medical-Surgical Nursing; 6th Ed; Saint Louis; C.V. Mosby Co, 1975.
9. Shakuntala Sharma 'Birpuri'. Principles and Practice of Nursing. Jaypee Brothers Medical Publishers (P) Ltd., New Delhi, 1997.
10. Sr. Nancy. Principles and Practice of Nursing; Vol. 1, 3rd Edition; N. R. Brothers. Indore, 1992.
11. Studenski S, Perera S, Wallace D, et al. Physical performance measures in the clinical setting. J Am Geriatr Soc 2003;51(9).
12. Taylor C, Lillis C, LeMone P. Fundamentals of Nursing: The Art and Science of Nursing Care, Philadelphia: JB. Lippincott, 1993.
13. Thresvamma CP. Fundamentals of Nursing, Procedure Manual for General Nursing Course, P. C. Mathew, Kottayam, Kerala, 1992.
14. Virginia Henderson. Principles and Practice of Nursing, New York, MacMillan Publishing Co, 1970.

REVIEW QUESTIONS

Long Essays

1. What are the factors that influence body temperature?
2. State about the altered temperature status.
3. What are the abnormal breathing patterns?
4. Write about the physiology of blood pressure.
5. Explain about measuring blood pressure.

Short Essays

1. How is the body temperature regulated?
2. How will you manage hyperthermia?
3. Write about heat stroke.
4. What are the factors that influence pulse rate?
5. What are the purposes of monitoring pulse rate?
6. Write the factors that influence blood pressure.

Short Answers

1. Define pulse.
2. Define blood pressure.
3. What do you mean by body temperature?
4. What are the sites for assessing body temperature? What are the types of thermometer?
5. What is respiration?

MULTIPLE CHOICE QUESTIONS

1. **Temperature of deep tissues:**
   a. Hypothermia
   b. Normal temperature
   c. Hyperthermia
   d. Core temperature
2. **Body temperature is controlled by:**
   a. Hypothalamus
   b. Pituitary glands
   c. Thalamus
   d. All of the above
3. **Abnormally elevated heart rate above 100 beats per minute in adults:**
   a. Tachycardia
   b. Abnormal rhythm
   c. Bradycardia
   d. None of the above
4. **Condition where there is normal rate and depth of ventilation:**
   a. Tachypnea
   b. Eupnea
   c. Bradypnea
   d. Apnea
5. **Causes of hypotension:**
   a. Blood loss
   b. Heart failure
   c. Dilation of arteries
   d. All of the above

ANSWERS

1. d   2. a   3. a   4. b   5. d

CHAPTER 8
Equipment and Linen

LEARNING OBJECTIVES
- Types: Disposables and reusable
- Linen, rubber goods, glassware, metal, plastics, furniture
- Introduction: Indent, maintenance, inventory

TERMINOLOGY

Medical device: An article, instrument, apparatus or machine that is used in the prevention, diagnosis or treatment of illness or disease, or for detecting, measuring, restoring, correcting or modifying the structure or function of the body for some health purposes.

Medical equipment: Medical equipment is used for the specific purposes of diagnosis and treatment of disease or rehabilitation following disease or injury; it can be used either alone or in combination with any accessory, consumable, or other piece of medical equipment.

Safety inspections: These are performed to ensure the device is electrically and mechanically safe. These inspections may also include checks for radiation safety or dangerous gas or chemical pollutants.

Inspection: Inspection refers to scheduled activities necessary to ensure a piece of medical equipment is functioning correctly.

Complication: A medical condition that arises during a course of treatment and is expected to increase the length of stay by at least one day for most patients

Comorbid condition: A medical condition that, along with the principal diagnosis, exists at admission and is expected to increase hospital length of stay by at least one day for most patients.

Comorbidity: A pre-existing condition on admission that will, because of its presence with a specific diagnosis, prolong the length of stay by at least one day in 75% of the patients.

Clinical practice guidelines: General procedures and suggestions about what constitutes an acceptable range of practices for particular diseases or conditions. These guidelines are usually developed by a consensus of doctors in a given field, such as radiology or cardiology.

Quality: Defined as a measure of the degree to which delivered health services meet established professional standards and judgments of value to the consumer.

Quality assurance (QA): Activities and programs intended to assure the quality of care in a defined medical setting. Such programs include peer or utilization review components to identify and remedy deficiencies in quality. The program must have a mechanism for assessing its effectiveness and may measure care against pre-established standards.

Quality improvement (QI): The more commonly used term in healthcare, replacing Quality Assurance. QI implies that concurrent systems are used to continuously improve quality, rather than reacting when certain baseline statistical thresholds are crossed.

INTRODUCTION

Machinery and equipment are essential and basic tools for hospital services, used on an everyday basis for patient care. Handling materials and equipment are very important responsibility of the nurse working in the hospital. Patient care equipment is defined as powered equipment intended for use in treatment, diagnosis, monitoring, life sustaining or resuscitating functions. Examples of this equipment are defibrillators, patient monitors, infusion devices, patient

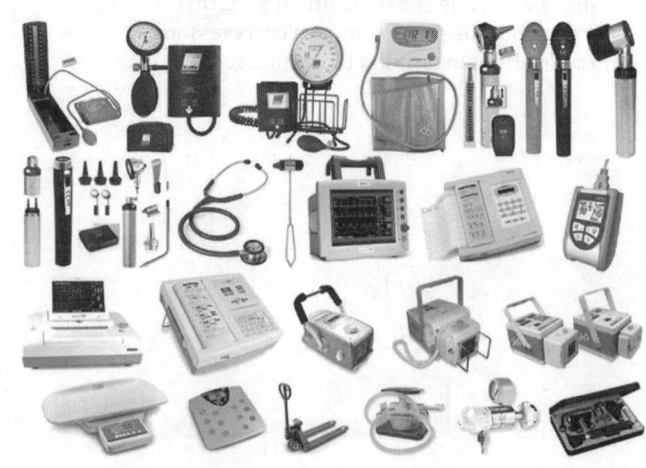

Fig. 8.1: Machinery and equipment used in patient care.

imaging equipment, diagnostic laboratory equipment, beds, etc.

Examples of items that are NOT considered patient care equipment are cart washers, radios, addressographs, etc.

DEFINITION

Equipment maintenance is any process used to keep equipment in reliable working order. It may include routine upkeep as well as corrective repair work. Equipment may include for daily use in the hospital for patient care or diagnostic and treatment purposes.

CONCEPT OF EQUIPMENT MAINTENANCE

Material management is concerned with providing the drugs, supplies and equipment needed by health personnel to deliver health services. The right drugs, supplies and equipment must be at the right place, at the right time and in the right quantity in order that health personnel deliver health services. Without proper material, health personnel cannot work effectively, they feel frustrated and the community lacks confidence in the health services and unless appropriate materials are provided in proper time and are required quantity, productivity of personnel will not be up to expectation.

The nurse needs to demonstrate the knowledge and skills of safe use of equipment in order to:
- Inspect equipment for safety hazards (e.g. frayed electrical cords, loose/missing parts)
- Teach client about the safe use of equipment needed for health care
- Facilitate the appropriate and safe use of equipment
- Remove malfunctioning equipment from client care area and report the problem to appropriate personnel.

GENERAL PRINCIPLES OF INSTRUMENT CARE

- All objects to be disinfected or sterilized should first be thoroughly cleaned to remove all organic matter (blood and tissue) and other residue.
- All items used in patient care shall be kept clean and in proper working condition.

Inventory control involves:
- Maintenance of stores record
- Physical control of materials
- Preservation of materials
- Minimization of obsolescence
- Reconciliation of stocks with book figures

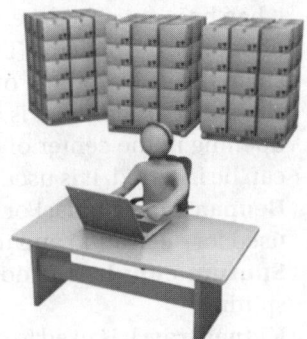

Fig. 8.2: Inventory control measures.

- All medical instruments and other items used for patient care must be cleaned and disinfected or sterilized before use on another patient.
- Excessive moisture on electrical components can cause damage to certain instruments. Disinfectants and cleaners sprayed directly onto electrical devices may cause them to short circuit. This can also happen with excessively wet cleaning cloths.
- Refer to the manufacturer's instructions for use of the appropriate type of disinfectant and the best method of cleaning and sterilizing each piece of medical instrument.
- Ethyl or isopropyl alcohol (70%-90%) is used for chemical disinfection.
- For routine cleaning of most of the items, an ammonium germicidal detergent is available.
- Cleaning and decontamination should begin as soon as possible after use as blood and body fluids can cause pitting of instruments and if left to dry can be difficult to remove.
- When transport to the decontamination area is going to be delayed, soiled instruments should be moistened with a wet towel or enzymatic solution.
- Decontamination and packaging should not be performed in patient care areas.
- Perform periodic calibration of the equipment and the equipment that are faulty should be sent to the Biomedical Engineering Department.

CLEANING AND DISINFECTION OF EQUIPMENT MAINTENANCE

- Soap and water are used are cleaning. Soap emulsifies the fat and lowers the surface tension of the water. The water acts as good solvent.
- Friction aids in mechanical cleansing. Use brush when cleansing a grooved surface. Dusting should be done with a firm and even stroke.
- Abrasives are harmful to the painted and polished surface.
- Aluminous materials (e.g., body discharges) are coagulated by the heat. So it should be removed with cold water.
- Bacteria grows in dark, moist and unclean places.
- Exposure to sunlight destroys some bacteria.
- Disinfection by chemicals depends upon the cleanliness of the article, the straight of the disinfectants and the length of the exposure.
- Effective sterilization depends upon the cleanliness of the article, the degree of heat and the length of exposure.
- Heat, chemicals, abrasive and solvents are harmful to some materials.
- Choosing the correct and simplest method of cleaning, saves time, material and energy.
- Equipment suitable for the purpose for which it is used and in good condition, conveniently located are arranged, saves time, material and energy.
- The cleaning articles are stored in a place meant only for that purpose.

INSPECTING EQUIPMENT FOR SAFETY HAZARDS

- Equipment safety and the safe use of equipment is dependent upon both user safety and equipment safety.
- User safety can be insured when all users of equipment, including nurses, are instructed on proper use and all pieces of equipment are then deemed and validated as competent to correctly and safely use a piece of equipment PRIOR to using it without direct supervision and guidance.
- User safety is also insured when the health care provider asks for the assistance of another and their reinstruction when they believe that they are not competent to use a specific piece of equipment as well as when they inspect the equipment prior to using it with a patient.
- Some of the safety inspection components include the inspection of the piece of equipment for frayed cords, malfunctioning, missing and/or loose parts, and documented evidence of preventive maintenance and safety inspections by those who perform these tasks.
- All equipment that is even possibly unsafe or questionably safe must be immediately taken out of service and sent to the department that is responsible for insuring its safety.
- All health care facilities have established protocols and procedures for the safe use of equipment which include staff education, competency validation, preventive maintenance, and safety inspections.
- Most health care facilities prohibit the patient's use of their own equipment like a radio, television or electric razor; others permit it but only after it has been inspected and deemed safe by personnel who have the knowledge and skills to do so. These personnel do not include nurses. This inspection is typically done by the maintenance or equipment department.

TEACHING THE CLIENT ABOUT SAFE USE OF EQUIPMENT

- Clients, in addition to staff, must be educated about the safe use of equipment, particularly when they are performing self care in the home using medical equipment.
- Safe and effective equipment such as electrical oxygen supplementation therapy and continuous passive motion devices, in addition to nonelectrical equipment such as walkers, canes and other mobility aids, must be safe and deemed safe prior to use.
- The rubber tips on a walker, cane and crutches should be inspected often. All tips that are uneven or worn out must be replaced immediately; preventive maintenance is done by replacing all tips at least once a month even when they are not worn out.
- Clients, in addition to staff, must also be educated about the safe use of equipment, particularly when they are performing self care in the home.

TYPES OF MATERIALS USED IN HOSPITAL

Hospitals need to be prepared ready at all the times in order to provide comprehensive treatment for patients, there is a standard set of equipment that all hospitals should have ready. This list of medical equipment can often be refurbished as well as new, allowing hospitals to afford to carry reserves for these key pieces.

- Self care equipment (for patient's daily life)
- Electronic equipment (ECG monitor, ventilator, etc)
- Diagnostic equipment (tools used to test)
- Surgical equipment (stainless steel tools, OT tools)
- Acute care equipment (dressing materials, etc)
- Storage and transport equipment.

Disposable Equipment

- Items used only once
- Discarded after use
- New items for each patient.

Reusable Equipment

- Items and equipment used for very long time
- These are cleaned, disinfected and sterilized before and after each use
- More care should be given to reusable items than disposable items.

PATIENT CARE EQUIPMENT

- **Cot or bedstead:** The hospital beds are made up of metal, simple in design, light and easily moveable, easy to clean, and strong durable with hard rubber castors. Some bed will have side rails to prevent the patient from falling.
- **Over bed table or cardiac table:** Generally this is used for patients suffering from cardiac diseases to lean and rest forward when he has breathing difficulty. It can also use for eating, reading, and writing and for placing articles for self care.
- **Bedside locker:** It is used to store the patient personal articles.
- **Bedside table:** It can be used for taking the meals and other purposes.
- **Chair and stool:** The chair can be used for the patients when he is out of bed, i.e. while changing the bed linens or bathing the patients. The workers and visitors should sit on the chair and not on the patient's bed.
- **Bedside commode:** It is a chair or wheelchair that has opening in the center of a seat under which a bedpan can be inserted. It is used for defecation and urination.
- **Bedpan and urinals:** For a bedridden patient, these are used for defecation and urination.
- **Sputum cup:** It is used to collect the sputum and spitting.
- **Kidney tray:** It is used to collect vomits, body fluids and soiled dressings.

Equipment and Linen

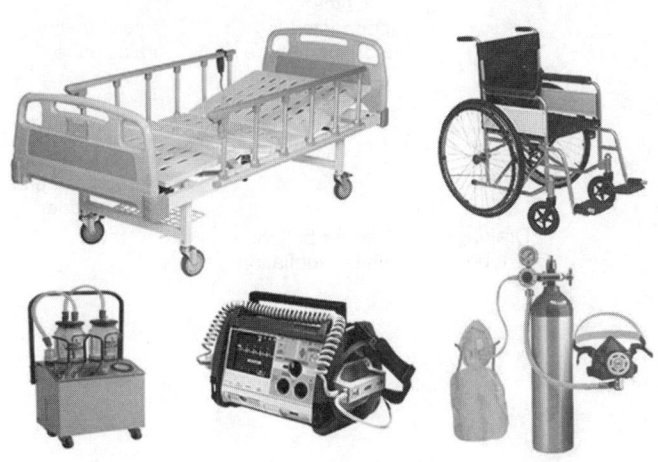

Fig. 8.3: Patient care equipment.

- **Water flask and drinking glasses:** The water flask is filled with drinking water and is given to the patients within his reach.
- **Plate, spoon, fork, knifes, etc:** These are used to serve the meals for the patient and is kept in-patients unit.
- **Call signal:** A bell is kept near the patient to call the nurse in their need.
- **Toilet articles:** Soap with soap dish, toothbrush and toothpaste, mouthwash, comb, etc. are kept in-patients unit. Bucket, mug, basin, etc. are kept in bathroom.
- **Waste basket:** It is used to collect the rubbish.
- **Bedding and bed linens:** The mattress and pillows should be firm, thick and smooth and all should have a washable cover. It gives support to the patients. Bed sheets are made up of strong cotton material, which is used to protect the mattress from soiling and to cover the patients; Draw mackintosh and draw sheet, extents from the patient shoulder to below knee, made up of rubber or plastic material, which is used to protect the mattress and bottom sheet from soiling.

MONITORING EQUIPMENT USED

- **Cardiac or heart monitors:** Cardiac monitors are used to monitor the electrical activity of the heart. The monitor looks like a computer screen with lines, or tracings, moving across the screen. The monitor has electrodes that are attached to the patient's chest with sticky pads.
- **Pulse oximeter:** A pulse oximeter allows the critical care team to monitor the saturation of oxygen in the blood. It looks like a clothespin and is attached to a patient's finger, or it may be smaller and clipped onto the earlobe.
- **Swan-Ganz catheter:** A Swan-Ganz, or pulmonary artery catheter, is used to measure the amount of fluid filling the heart as well as to determine how the heart is functioning. It is inserted through the large vessels of the neck or upper chest and threaded into the heart.
- **Arterial lines (a-lines):** Arterial lines are used for continuous monitoring of blood pressure. Catheters are inserted into an artery, usually in the wrist or, less often, in the bend of the elbow (should not be the brachial artery) or groin. Arterial lines produce a tracing on a monitor that is similar to that of a heart monitor but with a different waveform. Arterial lines can also be used for drawing blood thus eliminating the need for repeated venipunctures (a surgical puncture of a vein for withdrawing blood).

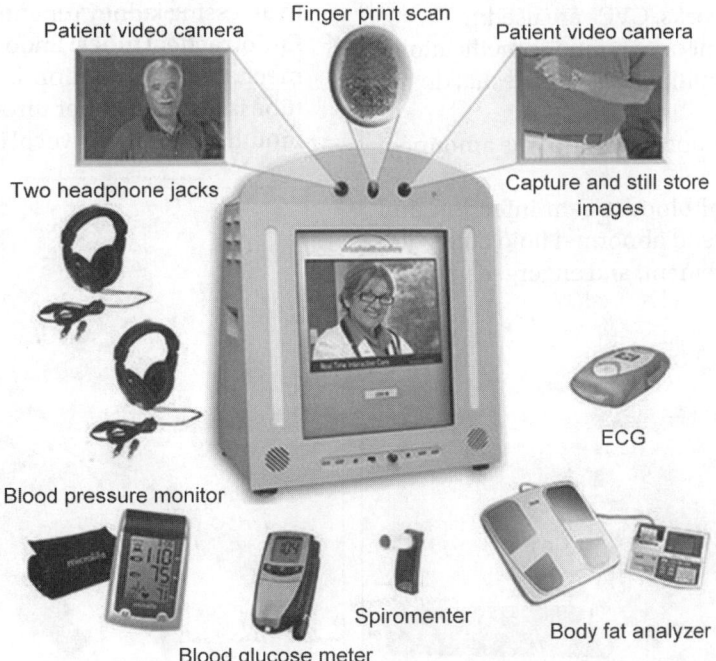

Fig. 8.4: Patient monitoring devices.

- **Acute care physiologic monitoring system:** Comprehensive patient monitoring systems that can be configured to continuously measure and display a number of parameters via electrodes and sensors that are connected to the patient. These may include the electrical activity of the heart via an EKG, respiration rate (breathing), blood pressure, body temperature, cardiac output, and amount of oxygen and carbon dioxide in the blood. Each patient bed in an ICU has a physiologic monitor that measure these body activities. All monitors are networked to a central nurses' station.
- **Intracranial pressure monitor:** It measures the pressure of fluid in the brain in patients with head trauma or other conditions affecting the brain (such as tumors, edema, or hemorrhage). These devices warn of elevated pressure and record or display pressure trends. Intracranial pressure monitoring may be a capability included in a physiologic monitor.
- **Apnea monitor:** It continuously monitors breathing via electrodes or sensors placed on the patient. An apnea monitor detects cessation of breathing in infants and adults at risk of respiratory failure, displays respiration parameters, and triggers an alarm if a certain amount of time passes without a patient's breath being detected. Apnea monitoring may be a capability included in a physiologic monitor.

TUBES AND CATHETERS USED IN HOSPITAL

- **Central venous catheter (CVC):** This type of catheter is a soft, pliable tube that is inserted into a large vessel (vein) in the neck (internal jugular vein), in the upper chest (subclavian vein), or in the groin area (femoral vein). Patients are sedated and receive a local anesthetic prior to insertion. Sutures secure the CVC, which can be left in place for days or weeks. CVCs are used:
  - To administer frequent or continuous medication.
  - To administer large multiple IV products that do not fit in one line.
  - To measure central venous pressure (the amount of fluid in the vessels).

  CVCs carry some risk of bloodstream infection and thrombosis (tenderness and abnormal fluid collection in tissues, impaired movement, and engorged veins).

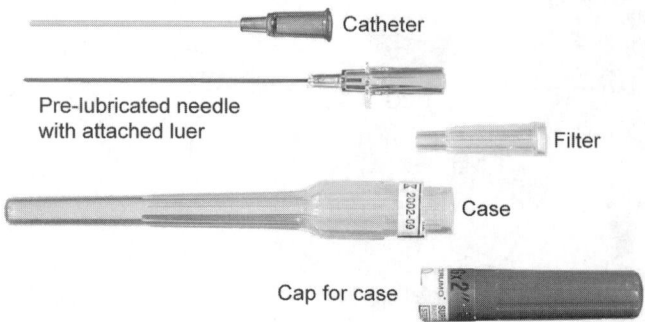

Fig. 8.5: Needles and catheters used in therapeutic procedures.

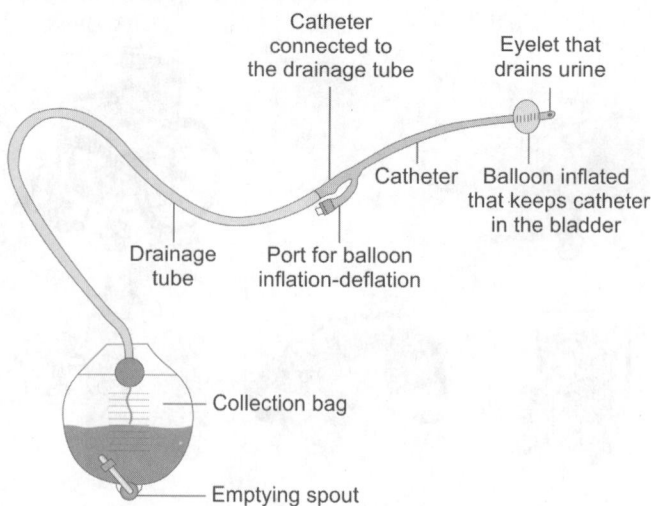

Fig. 8.6: Catheters and drainage tubes.

- **Intravenous (IV):** An IV is a plastic catheter (tube) that is inserted into the veins (peripheral IV) or a larger size catheter inserted into the larger veins of the neck. Fluids, medications, nutrition preparations, and blood products are administered through IV catheters. Patients in ICU often have multiple IVs.
- **Chest tubes:** Chest tubes are inserted through the chest wall into the space around the lung to drain fluid or air that has accumulated and prevent the lung from being able to expand.
- **Urinary catheter:** Urinary catheters, often referred to as Foley catheters, are inserted through the urethra into the bladder. Once in the bladder the catheter is kept in place by a balloon, which is inflated, at the end of the catheter. Urinary catheters continuously drain the bladder and allow for accurate measurement of urinary output, which is extremely important in fluid management and in assessing kidney function.
- **Endotracheal tubes:** Endotracheal tubes are used when mechanical ventilation is necessary. The soft plastic tube is inserted either through the nose or through the mouth, between the vocal cords and into the trachea. A

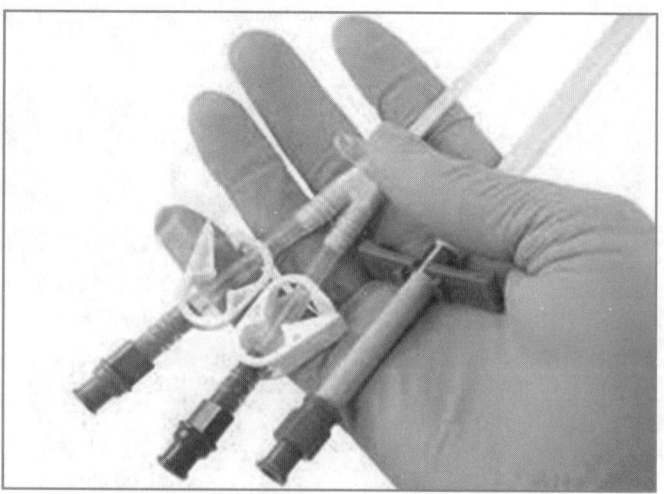

Fig. 8.7: Dialysis catheters and shunt tubes.

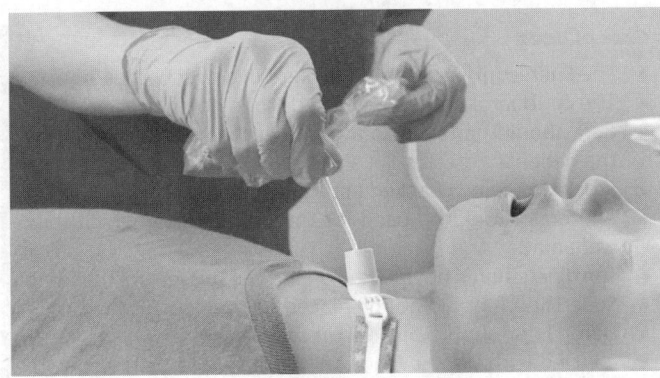

Fig. 8.8: Tracheostomy tubes and suction catheters.

small soft balloon at the end of the tube in the trachea is inflated to prevent air from escaping, thus allowing adequate ventilation by the respirator. The process of having the ET tube inserted is referred to as intubation. Patients who are intubated are unable to speak, so it is important to try to ask yes or no questions to which they can respond by shaking or nodding their head. Some patients may be able to communicate by writing. Most often patients who are intubated require sedation and may not be responsive at all.

LIFE SUPPORT AND EMERGENCY EQUIPMENT

Intensive care equipment for life support and emergency resuscitation includes the following:

- **Ventilator** (also called a respirator)—assists with or controls pulmonary ventilation in patients who cannot breathe on their own. Ventilators consist of a flexible breathing circuit, gas supply, heating/humidification mechanism, monitors, and alarms. They are microprocessor-controlled and programmable, and regulate the volume, pressure, and flow of patient respiration. Ventilator monitors and alarms may interface with a central monitoring system or information system.
- **Infusion pump:** Device that delivers fluids intravenously or epidurally through a catheter. Infusion pumps employ automatic, programmable pumping mechanisms to deliver continuous anesthesia, drugs, and blood infusions to the patient. The pump is hung on an intravenous pole placed next to the patient's bed.
- **Crash cart:** Also called a resuscitation or code cart. This is a portable cart containing emergency resuscitation equipment for patients who are "coding." That is, their vital signs are in a dangerous range. The emergency equipment includes a defibrillator, airway intubation devices, a resuscitation bag/mask, and medication box. Crash carts are strategically located in the ICU for immediate availability for when a patient experiences cardiorespiratory failure.
- **Intraaortic balloon pump:** A device that helps reduce the heart's workload and helps blood flow to the coronary arteries for patients with unstable angina, myocardial infarction (heart attack), or patients awaiting organ transplants. Intraaortic balloon pumps use a balloon placed in the patient's aorta. The balloon is on the end of a catheter that is connected to the pump's console, which displays heart rate, pressure, and electrocardiogram (ECG) readings. The patient's ECG is used to time the inflation and dilatation of the balloon.
- **Neonatal intensive care equipment:** Neonatal intensive care (NIC) units have specialized equipment to care for babies who are unwell, and those born prematurely (before week 37 of pregnancy). Babies in intensive care are placed in incubators, which are clear, enclosed cots that control the baby's body temperature and protect them from infection. The incubators have hand-sized holes to allow the intensive care doctors and nurses to gain access to your baby. Babies in intensive care are monitored and treated in much the same way as adults. Your babies body temperature may be monitored using a small sensor on their skin. The level of oxygen in their blood can also be measured using a clip attached to their hand or foot.
- **Diagnostic equipment:** The use of diagnostic equipment is also required in the ICU. Mobile X-ray units are used

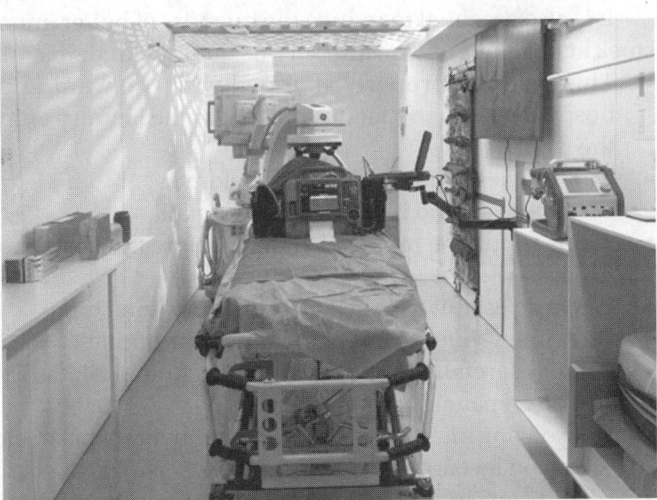

Fig. 8.9: Life saving equipment.

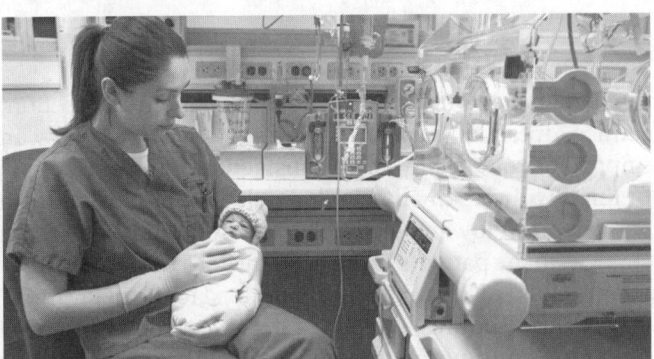

Fig. 8.10: Neonatal intensive care unit equipment.

for bedside radiography, particularly of the chest. Mobile X-ray units use a battery-operated generator that powers an X-ray tube. Handheld, portable clinical laboratory devices, or point-of-care analyzers, are used for blood analysis at the bedside. A small amount of whole blood is required, and blood chemistry parameters can be provided much faster than if samples were sent to the central laboratory.

General Principles for Cleaning Shared Patient Care Equipment

The following principles apply to all equipment used in the assessment and delivery of patient care:
- Any reusable equipment that comes into contact with non-intact skin must be cleaned before it is reused on another patient
- All non-dedicated (shared) equipment and accessories that come into contact with a patient or a patient's environment must be cleaned that uses or transfers the item of clinical equipment between patients
- All equipment must be cleaned immediately if it becomes visibly soiled
- Equipment should be able to readily cleanable, i.e. smooth impervious surfaces such as metal, plastic, vinyl and laminate
- The application of tape on shared patient care equipment is discouraged as it does not allow appropriate cleaning and leaves residue
- All HCWs must comply with Standard and Additional Precautions appropriate for the task
- Appropriate risk assessments, including a review of available manufacturers guidelines, must be carried out prior to the decontamination of equipment with the correct detergent/disinfectant
- Only approved healthcare facility cleaning products to be used and be suitable to the cleaning process required
- Cleaning is still required if a cover has been used, e.g. temperature probe cover
- Additional cleaning may be required in an outbreak situation. Procedures will be determined in consultation with the health service Infection Prevention and Control Clinical Nurse Consultant or delegate.

CARE OF LINEN

Linen management plays a great role in patient satisfaction, reduces infection rate and operation costs and plays an important role in physician satisfaction. Efficient supply of linen without any defect and delay in time becomes a good support towards delivering timely quality healthcare services to the patients. If the hospital does not have proper supply chain of linen, then this may lead to the delay in OT and ICU procedures, patient care services, delay in CSSD operations and ultimately the entire hospital operations suffer.

> **Care of linen**
> - The linen cupboard should be kept in perfect order
> - The cupboards should be locked when not in use
> - Care should be taken to avoid linen being taken home by the patients
> - Stock should be checked at regular intervals
> - All items should be used for the purposes for which they were made
> - Torn linen should not be used on the bed but sent for mending
> - Soiled linen should not be placed on the floor
> - Damp linen should be dried immediately
> - If soiled with urine or motion, these should be rinsed with cold water
> - Remove the strain, where straining is unavoidable old linen should be used
> - The infected linens should be disinfected first.
> - Use mackintosh wherever it is necessary to economize the use of linen.

Shortage of linen leaves patients dissatisfied. Sometimes, even surgeries get cancelled due to shortage of operation theater linen. Also, due to uncertainty in arriving at correct stock, new linen is purchased which results in increasing costs. "In order to overcome the above problems, it is imperative to have a linen management system that automatically tracks soiled and clean linen items continuously through the entire linen cycle.

> **Types of linen**
> The linen that is mostly used in hospitals include:
> - Bed sheets
> - Pillow covers
> - Blankets
> - Towels
> - Patient gowns
> - Surgical gowns
> - Curtains
> - Aprons
> - Door mats
> - Linen hampers
> - Hot water bag covers and other cloth items

It is also essential to reduce the quantity of buffer linen stock at hospitals and ensure service quality standards.
- This must be properly stamped with the ward and hospital names so that it is not lost in the laundry or in the ward.
- New articles should be washed before use.
- Torn linen should be put aside for repair.
- Stains should be removed at once before they become fixed.
- Wet articles must not be left in the dirty linen bin.
- Dirty linen should be sent to laundry promptly.
- Linen is carefully sorted, on its return from the laundry and discrepancies reported.
- Stock-taking must be accurate and frequent so that track is kept on lost articles.
- Dirty linen is sorted and account is written when sending to laundry.

> **Ganga ganesh gives tips before starting inventory for successful linen management:**
> - Knowing and listing every linen items used in the hospital
> - Knowing where the linen can be found Cupboards, beds, soiled linen chute room, laundry, new linen store, etc.)
> - Taking the service of employees in the inventory process to recognize linen by sight
> - Stop the flow of linen. Ensure all soiled linen chutes are sealed prior to the beginning of the inventory
> - Arrange to take inventory on a day/hen occupancy is at its lowest and at the quietest time of the day- often between 12 am and 6 am: since movement or linen is least
> - Make sure the printed inventory papers are in stock
> - Inventory should not be taking more than two-three hours. More employees to be used to quicken the process
> - If the laundry service is outsourced, ensure the laundry register is updated and there is no pending stock which has been sent for rewash.

CARE OF RUBBER GOODS

Rubber goods in common use are aircushion mackintoshes, hot water bottles, ice caps, ice collars, rubber tubes, catheters, rectal tubes, gloves and rubber bed. The nurse should make all efforts to prolong the life of the rubber goods. They should be purchased only after nature and durability have been investigated.

Purpose

- To prevent spread of infection
- To clean the article and prepare for re-use
- To remove stains
- To preserve life of articles.

Different rubber goods used in the hospital:
- Mackintosh- long and draw
- Rubber tubes- gavages, lavage, rectal, flatus, etc.
- Hot water bottle, ice-cap, ice-collars, air-cushion
- Gloves
- Mouthpiece of Ambu-bag
- Pillows- air and water mattresses
- Aquathermia pads
- Rubber bulb used in Asepto syringe and breast pump.

Care of rubber articles:
- Rubber goods get destroy with heat. Do not use hot water to clean sunlight for drying or keep near radiator. Hard rubber tubes and catheters can be boiled
- Hydrocarbons like kerosene, benzene, oils can destroy; hence do not use such things on rubber for cleaning.
- Do not fold rubber sheets; instead roll them with paper or thin cloth lining after powdering them.
- Do not stick pins on rubber goods as they can cut through and cause leakage.
- It is preferable to store rubber goods in wood cupboards instead of metallic ones.
- Always dry rubber goods after cleaning them in shade as heat destroys them.
- Do not use clamps for longer periods on rubber tubes or catheters.
- Time period of the use of a hot water bottle, water flow pads, ice-collar caps should not be more than 15-20 minutes.

> **Care of rubber gloves**
> - It is desired that the wearer of the gloves should wash them on their hands just before they are removed to prevent adherence of blood.
> - After removing from the hands, they are washed with soap and cold water, first on the outside then invert and repeat on the inside.
> - Rinse well with water both inside and outside.
> - Holes and tears are discovered by submerging the glove filled with air in the water. Separate the torn gloves.

> **Principles of care**
> - Natural and synthetic rubber deteriorate with age, exposure to heat, light, moistures and by chemicals.
> - They should not be folded. Avoid exposure to sunlight.
> - Rubber good should never be dried by artificial heat, nor by contact with the radiator or stove.
> - It should be free from grease and acids.

Care of Rubber Articles after Use

- All mackintoshes and rubber articles should be washed in warm soapy water, rinsed and carbonized with 1 in 20 carbolic lotions. Dry thoroughly in a cool place and French chalk powder is sprinkled and either rolled or hung up, never folded. Dry heat and hot sun destroy rubber. Sun causes it to blister. Turpentine will do this too.
- Two rubber surfaces should not come together but must be separated. In the case of hot water bottle, the surfaces are separated by air.
- Mackintoshes in the store cupboard should be examined weekly. If the air is moist, the mackintosh may become sticky.
- Kinking the rubber tubing is ruinous.
- Excessive steam causes rubber gloves to become hard.
- Ointments spoil rubber.
- Excessive boiling makes rubber limp and overstretched.
- Rubber articles should be stored in the dark.

> **The rubber goods in common use are:**
> - Mackintosh
> - Aircushions
> - Hot water bottles
> - Ice caps
> - Rubber tubes and catheters
> - Gloves
> - Rubber beds/air beds/air mattress.

I. Mackintoshes:
- Decontaminate by immersing in a tub of 0.5% chlorine/sodium hypochlorite/chlorhexidine solution.
- Spread the mackintosh on a flat surface and wet it by pouring water on it.
- Use a piece of clean cloth or a plastic scrubber to apply soap and wash away the soap using water.
- Repeat the above process on the other surface.
- Dry it in a shade on a dry horizontal surface by exposing both the surface to air.
- When dry, powder it lightly with dusting powder and roll it with a paper lining on it.

II. Rubber tube and catheters:
- The rubber tube upside down under running water to led the stream of water run through it.
- Use swab stick to remove any organic matter blocking the tip of the tube and eye of the catheter, if needed. Ensure patency.
- Use soap and water clean the dirt and grease on the surface of the catheter or tube.
- Hang the tubes and catheters to dry in a cool/shaded place.
- After drying separate same sized catheters and tubes.
- Power the outer surface using dusting powder; coil the tube by securing the tip into broader end.
- Wrap individual tube and catheter using a piece of thin cloth and boil for five minutes or autoclave.

> **Care of air cushion and rubber bed/air mattress**
> - To clean the air cushion and air bed, don't pour water into them. It is sufficient to clean the outside.
> - During cleaning it should not be filled with air, as air filled items can crack easily by pressure.
> - The valves of the air cushions or air beds should never be immersed in water, as it makes them rusted and damage the item.
> - Store them after slightly inflating them to avoid the sticking of two surfaces.

III. Hot water bottle; ice cap; air cushion:
- Remove the outer cloth cover of each item after use. Decontaminate the air cushion cover.
- Empty the container, e.g. Water from the bottle, ice cubes from the cap and collar
- Deflate the air cushion. Clean the outside of the air cushion with soap and water as it may be soiled with fecal matter or urine.
- Wipe the outer surface of the hot water bottle, ice cap and collar using a piece of clean damp cloth.
- Hang them upside down for drip.
- Blow some air into each of the above mentioned rubber items and close the cap/valve.
- Check each rubber item for leakage of air or water as the cause may be before storing and after each use so as not to cause any harm to the client.
- Store in a cool dry place.
- Send for laundry and store separately in linen.

IV. Gloves:
- It is desired that wearer of the gloves should wash them on their hands just before they are removed to prevent adherence of blood and other organic materials.
- After removing from the hands, they are washed with soap and cold water, first on the outside, then invert and repeat on the inside.
- Rinse well with water both inside outside as described above.
- Holes and tears are discovered by submerging the glove filled with air in the water. If there are holes the bubbles will pass up through the water. Separate torn gloves.
- When both sides are dried, they are powered inside and outside and packed in pairs of the same size, right and left gloves in glove wrapper.
- The torn gloves are patched or vulcanized and may be reused.
- Steam under pressure is the best method of sterilizing gloves. The pressure is kept minimum to prevent melting of the gloves.

V. Ambu bag and face mask:
- Wipe the bag and rubber part the face mask using a piece of clean damp cloth.
- Disinfect using a cotton ball soaked in pure savlon or methylated spirit or 70% alcohol.

CARE OF ENAMEL WARE

The articles commonly used are bedpans, urinals, kidney trays, sputum cups, feeding cups, and trays. The polishing on the enamel is eroded by heat, mercuric salts, acids, alkalis and by chemicals. They are subjected to chipping if dropped on the floor or handled carelessly. Scraping with sharp instruments also result in chipping.

General Principles of Care

- One should avoid mishandling and banging of enamel as they can be chipped off and become unsafe for use.
- Do not boil for longer periods and rapidly cool them, as enamel cannot withstand heat.
- It is preferable not to use enamel items for surgical procedures.
- Wash enamel ware soon after use especially when some antiseptic agents are used in them. Enamel ware can get stained and damaged with strong acids, alkalis and dyes.
- **Care of bedpans:**
  - Before emptying the bedpan, inspect the contents. If there is cotton, they are removed by using a forceps kept for that purpose only.
  - Empty the bedpan into a lavatory pan, care being taken to avoid soiling the sides of the basin.

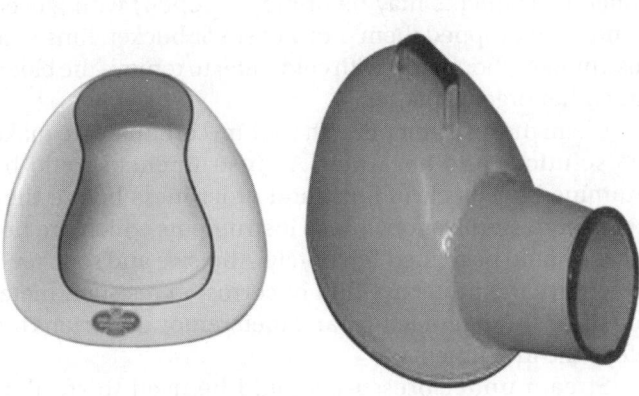

Fig. 8.11: Enamel bed pan and urinal.

> **Care of the bedpans**
> - Before emptying the bedpans, inspect the contents. If there are cotton sponges or sanitary pads should be removed by using a forceps.
> - Empty the bedpan to a lavatory pan
> - Rinse the bedpan with cold water under force - use vim or other cleansing powder to remove the stains and rinse the pan well under the cold running water.
> - Wash with soap and warm water using a brush.
> - To disinfectant the bedpans, soak them in Lysol 1:40 for 1 hour.
> - Bedpans may be placed in direct sun light for few hours to deodorize and to disinfect.
> - Keep them dry for the next use on the bedpan rack.

- Rinse the bedpan with cold water under force.
- Wash with soap and warm water using a brush. Vim may also used to remove the stains. Rinse it well.
- To disinfect the bedpans, soak them in Lysol 1:40 for one hour or they are sterilized in bedpan sterilizers.
- Bedpans may be placed in direct sunlight for few hours to deodorize and to disinfect.
- Keep them dry for the next use on the bedpan rack.
- **Care of urinals:** The urinals should not be left standing for a longer time with urine because a deposit will for on the inside, which is almost impossible to remove. Cleaning and disinfection are done as for the bedpans.
- **Care of sputum cups:** The urinal should may be emptied into the lavatory pan, care being taken not to soil the sides of the pan. Infectious sputum should be rendered harmless by boiling or disinfection by chemicals or it may be disposed by burning. Cleaning and disinfection of the sputum cup is done as for the bedpans. Before the sputum cups are given to the patients, add a small quantity of antiseptic lotion, maintain purpose of which is to prevent the sputum sticking to the sides.

CARE OF STAINLESS STEEL INSTRUMENTS

Stainless steel utensils are suitable for almost every other purpose, because they are easily cleaned, heat resistant and

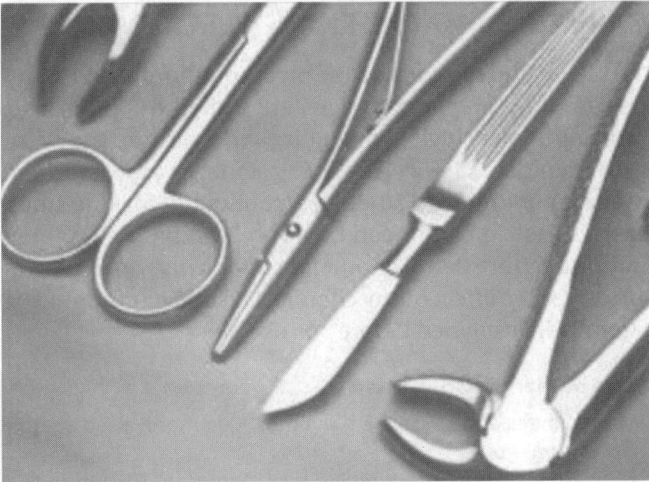

Fig. 8.12: Stainless steel instruments.

unbreakable. When storing, these utensils are to be kept dry, lest the water on them leaves a mark on it.

List of Stainless Steel Instruments

- Forceps, e.g. artery forceps, thumb forceps, Alice, mosquito, kochker's, towel clips, sponge holding, cheatles, etc.
- Different needles, e.g. needles used in IM, IV, SC, injections; biopsy needles (liver, kidney, etc.).

> **Principles of care of stainless steed instruments**
> - All stainless steel items are heat resistant, anticorrosive and long lasting but expensive. So should be handled carefully.
> - Don't boil stainless steel items repeatedly as they become dull
> - They can be sterilized using chemicals and autoclaving
> - Always use gloves while cleaning soiled instruments
> - Dry the instruments properly before storing as the left water cause markings.

- Different scopes, e.g. blades of laryngoscope, bronchoscope, protoscope.
- Sharp instruments, e.g. surgical blades, different scissors, razors, etc.
- Miscellaneous: Spatulas, tongue depressors, tracheal airway, tube clamps, tracheotomy tubes, mouth gag, dilators, tonometer plate, etc.

General Principles of Stainless Steel Instruments Care

- All stainless steel items are heat resistant anticorrosive and long lasting but expensive, hence they should be handled well.
- Do not boil stainless steel items repeatedly as they get dull
- They can be easily sterilized using chemicals and by autoclaving
- Always use gloves while cleaning and washing soiled/contaminated instruments.

CARE OF SURGICAL SHARP INSTRUMENTS

The knives and scissors are the most commonly used sharp instruments. The sharp edges are dulled by rough use, exposing them to high temperature and moisture. The sharp instruments are sterilized by hot air sterilizer, exposing them to a temperature of 160 degree centigrade for one hour. Chemical disinfection can be done by submerging them fully under pure dettol or other disinfectants which are not corrosive. The effect of any chemical disinfectant should be carefully investigated before it is used.

> **Care of sharp instruments**
> - The knifes and scissors are the most commonly used sharp instruments.
> - Sharp instruments are dulled by rough usage, exposing to high temperature and moisture.
> - Sharp instruments are sterilized by hot air sterilizer exposing into a temperature of 160°C for an hour.
> - Chemical disinfections can be done by submerging them fully under pure dettol or other disinfectants.

Steps of Cleaning Sharp Instruments

- Immerse the sharp instruments in a 0.5% chlorine solution or in 2% glutaraldehyde for 20-30 minutes. Add anti-rust agent, e.g. sodium nitrate 0.1%, if available.
- Remove from the disinfectant solution, rinse in sterile water stream, wipe dry, using a dry piece of sterile cloth.
- Store in an appropriate container.

Care of Needles

- Decontaminate all types of needles attached to syringe and flush with 0.5 % chlorine solution/chlorhexidine/sodium hypochloride immediately after use.
- Discard the disposal injection needles with the syringe either in a puncture-resistant container or destroy the needle still attached to the syringe in needle destroyer.
- Send the puncture-resistant container for incineration.
- Send stainless steel needles for autoclaving packed with syringes.
- Remove cannula/stylet of centesis and biopsy needles.
- Flush biopsy needles with a 0.5% chlorine solution, wash with soapy water and rinse in running water.
- Dry them pack and send for autoclaving.

> **Care of needles**
> - Decontaminate all types of needles attached to syringe and flushed with 0.5% chlorine/chlorhexidine or hypochlorite solution
> - Destroy the needle still attached to syringe with the needle destructor and throw into the puncture proof container.
> - Send the puncture proof container for incineration

Care of Other Instruments

A wide variety of instruments are used in the operation theater which may be dangerously contaminated. The soiled instruments may be unhinged (open) with gloved hands and dropped them into a basin or bucket. Rinse the instruments thoroughly with cold water to remove the blood and other organic matter.

Clean the instruments with sodium carbonate (to make 2% solution) and hot water. All instruments should be examined for its cleanliness and orderliness before they are sent to sterilization. Those instruments which are not clean should be treated separately. Abrasive and soap tend to remove the protective film of corrosion resistant metal put on by the manufacturer and their removal shortens the life of the instruments.

Stream under pressure should be used to sterilize instruments whenever possible. When the stream under pressure is not available, boiling water is the best agency for sterilizing instruments. The longer the boiling period, the likelihood that all organisms will be killed.

CARE OF FIBEROPTICS WITH CAMERA ITEM

The fiberoptics with camera items are gastroscope, endoscope, and bronchoscope.

Purposes

- To prevent spread of infection
- To prevent damage to the camera
- To prevent and prolong life of scope.

General Principles

- All fiberoptic scopes are expensive items and require careful handling. These scopes are used in diagnostic labs, radiology department and operation theaters. The scopes are flexible and damaged by heat.
- Detach camera from the scope
- Remove obturator from the scope dwelling it in a piece of dry clean cloth to clean the scope properly.

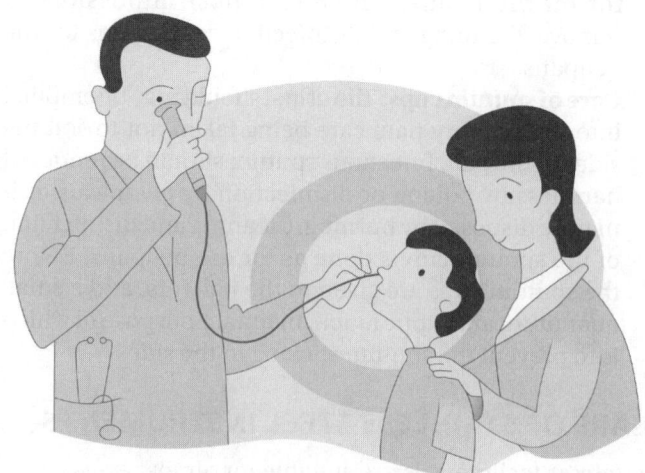

Fig. 8.13: Endoscopic fiberoptic instruments.

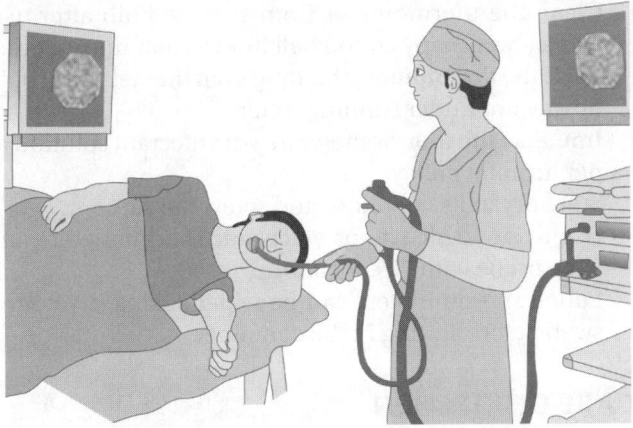

Fig. 8.14: Endoscopic unit and equipment.

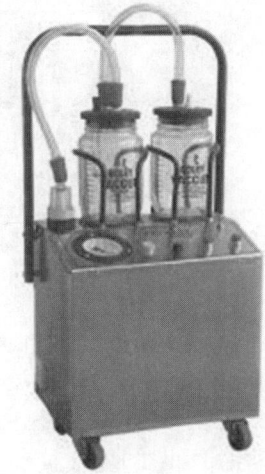

Fig. 8.15: Portable suction apparatus.

- Wipe off the fiberoptic using a gauze pad soaked in 2% glutaraldehyde to disinfect.
- Hang the scope and obturator in the cupboard or in the supply container of the company to avoid damage.

Care of Laryngoscope

- Wipe off saliva from the blade of the laryngoscope, using a dry piece of clean gauze.
- Detach the blade separate and immerse it in a 2% glutaraldehyde solution for 20-30 minutes.
- Remove the blade from the laryngoscope and store in the leather bag in a resuscitation trolley.

Care of Protoscope and Bronchoscope

- Pull out obturator from the scope
- Immerse both obturator and speculum in a 0.5% chlorine solution minimum for ten minutes.
- Discard the chlorine solution and remove both the items from the container.
- Rinse in cold water and then wash in soapy stream.
- Pack and send the scope for autoclaving.

CARE OF SUCTION MACHINE

- Wear clean gloves before handling the jars.
- Add the sodium hypochlorite solution in a sufficient amount to decontaminate the contents.
- Disconnect the tubes, immerse fully in the sodium hypochloride solution for ten minutes.
- Flush the tubing in soapy water and rinse in plain water jet or stream.
- Wash the jars with detergent or liquid soap and rinse thoroughly.
- Keep jars inverted at a dry, safe place to remove residual water completely.
- Empty the contents of glass jars into sewage and flash with plain water.
- Dry and wrap the jars in their cloth and proper pack for autoclaving.
- Ensure intact wiring of the electronic cord with proper earthing.
- Wipe the cord with a piece of clean dry cloth daily.
- Use oil/grease of wheels.
- Wipe the body, handle and glass cover of the pressure gauze with disinfectants.
- Avoid using disinfectants in the jar but if the contents are hazardous then decontaminated before discarding the contents into sewage.
- Change the jar and tubing when a client requires suction for more than 24 hours.
- Keep the jars and tubes disconnected when the machine is not in use.
- Periodically send the machine to workshop for checking of the pump, change of filter tubing and lid, valve and washer and electronic connections.
- Attach fresh suction catheter to the tubing each time the machine is used.
- Use distilled/boiled water in the receiving waste jar.
- Empty the jars daily, irrespective of the amount of fluids aspirated.

CARE OF REFRIGERATOR

- Defrost and empty the contents every week (frost-forming refrigerators).
- Let all the frost melt. Do not use sharp instruments to remove the frost.
- Clean with mild soap solutions inside and outside, clean wipe in plain water.
- Empty and clean frost-free refrigerators once in two weeks
- Return unused/partially used blood products to blood bank or laboratory.
- Discard any unsent blood samples.
- Do not keep milk, food items and drinking water in the refrigerator with pathological products.

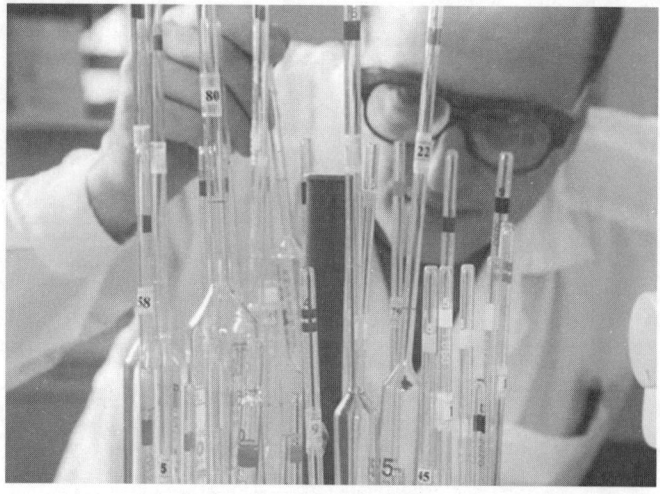

Fig. 8.16: Pipets and glass tubes used in laboratory.

- Put on the power supply and turn the thermostat knob to full. Wait for half an hour. Replace the contents in the refrigerator.
- Do not open the refrigerator door frequently and unnecessarily.
- Avoid keeping the refrigerator door open for more than 30 minutes.
- Keep the refrigerator at a cool dry place away from the walls.

CARE OF GLASS INSTRUMENTS

When buying glassware, it is important to select a hard glass that is resistant to heat and mechanical shock. Facilitate cleaning; the glassware should have a hard smooth surface. Ground glass is very susceptible to erosion by water or steam. Therefore, it should be sterilized with dry heat. Brush and abrasives of all sort are to be avoided in cleaning glass as they cause streaking. Immediate rinsing under cold running water to remove organic matter from the glass articles is essential in prolonging their usefulness.

The glassware used for the parenteral therapy should be rinsed with freshly distilled water. If the distilled water leaves an unbroken film on the surface, it shows that the glass is clean. If any grease is present, the film will be broken and droplets will form. Exposure of the glass to sudden variations of temperature is likely to cause crack in the glass. When sterilizing glass containers, they are to be kept inverted in the autoclave.

Purpose

- To prevent spread of infection
- To prepare for safe re-use.
- To prevent damage to the item and to prolong its life.

Care of Thermometer

- Remove the thermometer from antiseptic solution and wipe it dry from bulb to stem with a dry cotton ball before using.
- Clean the thermometer from stem to bulb after use, using a wet soapy cotton ball in a circular movement.
- Raise the thermometer holding from the stem with bulb downward under running water.
- Immerse the thermometer in a disinfectant solution as per hospital policy.
- Store dry in its container and screw the cap.
- Use disposal sleeve for electronic thermometers and wipe probe with 70% alcohol.
- Lotion thermometers can be wiped, using dry cotton swab before storing in the container.

CARE OF KITCHEN

- Food cupboard is cleaned daily. Each article should have a definite place.
- Sinks must not be allowed to become blocked. Waste food should be placed in the rubbish bin and removed daily. The bin should be emptied and cleaned daily.
- Both bucket and rubbish bin should have tightly fitting lids which should be properly replaced.
- Should the sinks become blocked, simple measures may be tried to unblock it. A label should be placed on the sink with "out of use" on it.
- Food must not be left exposed in the kitchen. Milk must always be kept covered.

DISINFECTING WARD EQUIPMENT

- **Linen and bandages:** Receive into a bucket at bedside containing disinfectant lotion-carbolic lotion 1:40. Keep for 4 hours.
- Pus, urine, stools, vomit and sputum are disinfected before disposal in carbolic lotion 1:20 for 2 hours.
- Immerse receptacles in phenyl lotion 1:20 for 2 hours. Rinse them before use.
- **Infected furniture and mackintosh:** Mop with carbolic lotion 1:20 before routine cleansing.
- **Infected blankets, pillows and mattresses:** In most hospitals these are submitted to steam sterilization, e.g. 25 lbs. pressure at 260° F for ½ an hour.
- **Crockery and glassware when it is inconvenient to boil:** These may be immersed in carbolic lotion 1:20 for 2 hours. Wash thoroughly before use.

CARE OF THE SANITARY ANNEXES

A. **Care of the sanitary annexes** is considered to important and the steps are:
   - This is cleaned thoroughly daily, tidied at frequent intervals and well ventilated.
   - Insides and outsides of the sinks are cleaned.
   - Bedpans and urinals are washed with hot soapy water.
   - Bedpans and urinals are stored in large tanks containing a suitable cheap disinfectant, which is changed daily.

- Ventilated cupboards may be provided for bedpan storage.
- Enamelware is washed daily and stains removed before they become fixed.
- The sanitary annexe should have the following:
  - Lavatory brush and mop.
  - A bucket with a tightly fitting lid to receive dressings prior to their removal to the incinerator.
  - Soil linen box.

B. Care of the flush out
- This is cleaned daily.
- Frequent flushing is required.
- The lavatory brush is stored in a disinfectant, which is changed daily.

C. Care of the bath room
Walls and floors of bath room should be washed daily.

HOSPITAL FURNITURES

Hospital furniture includes things like medication carts, tables and chairs. This type of furniture includes items in private and public hospital rooms, emergency rooms, waiting rooms and private areas for staff. The type of hospital furniture in a room is typically determined by the use of the room, and is made to be functional for both the patient and the physician.

A common type of furniture designed for a hospital room is an adjustable hospital bed. Overbid tables are often placed over the side of the bed, and are often used for dining. Nearly all hospital furniture in a patient room will include a bedside stand with storage compartments for holding medication and supplies. Many maternity patient rooms are furnished with baby cribs allowing mother and newborn to stay together.

Not all hospital furniture is designed for patient rooms. Seating for a hospital waiting room typically consists of couches and chairs. Some waiting rooms are furnished with metal folding chairs, although wood chairs with padded seats are more commonly used. In addition, it's common to find wood shelves or tables for holding magazines and other reading material.

Hospital furniture for patient rooms and emergency rooms may also include privacy screen dividers. As the name suggests, a privacy screen allows discretion and privacy for patients. The screen is typically set on a metal frame. Cloth panels are also used for privacy screens.

STERILIZATION TECHNIQUES

Sterilization is the process by which an object becomes free from all the microorganisms. By sterilization, pathogenic organisms are destroyed.

Sterilization is a process by which the pathogens as well as spores and viruses are destroyed.

Sterilization is the process by which an article, a surface or a medium from all microorganism, both in vegetative and sporing states are sterilized by removing or killing them.

Purpose

- To render the supplies/articles free from pathogens.
- To make complete destruction of microorganisms.
- To sterilize instruments and equipment used in the surgical practice.

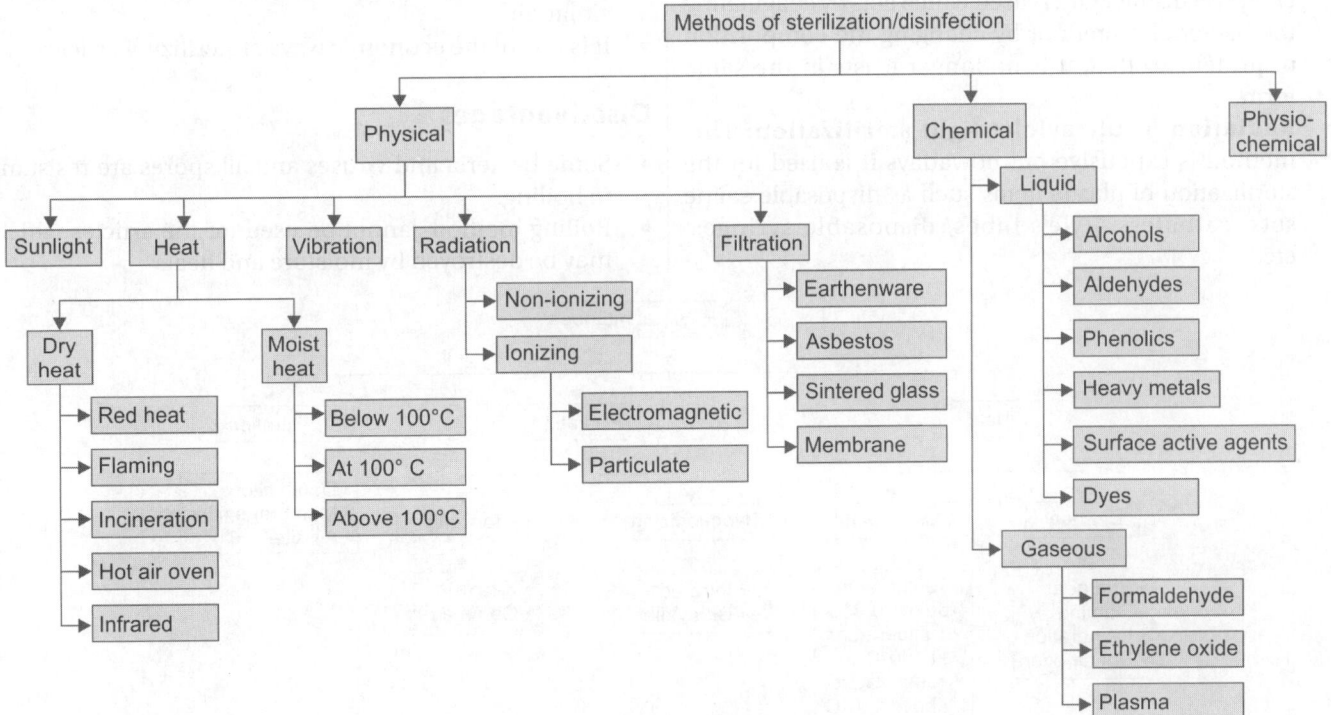

Fig. 8.17: Methods of sterilization.

- To keep the articles in such a condition that they are ready for use at any time.
- For the safety of the patients.

Scientific Principles

- Dust and dirt harbors microorganisms which adversely affect the well-being of patients and retards recovery.
- Proper care of articles prolong its life ensures their utility and provides a neat and finished appearance to promote a feeling of comfort.
- Selection of appropriate simple methods of sterilization saves energy, time and material.
- Water is a universal solvent and so produces surface tension.
- Friction helps in removing dirt and microorganisms from surface.
- Unpleasant odor, sight and noise are disturbing the patient.

Methods of Sterilization

- **Natural method of sterilization**-This method is used to sterilize contaminated linen and bedpans. Direct sunlight will have an affect on acid-fast microorganism. Place the linen or bedpans in direct sunlight for 6 hours for two consecutive days.
- **Physical method of sterilization:** Heat kills all types of bacteria. Boiling is the most commonly used method but spore forming bacteria and acids viruses are not killed by boiling.
- **Chemical method of sterilization:** It is also called as cold sterilization or disinfection by the disinfectants. A chemical disinfectant is used which acts by coagulating the bacterial protein or by changing the composition of protein so that, it is no longer exists in the same form.
- **Radiation or ultraviolet light sterilization:** This method is expensive but nowadays it is used for the sterilization of plastic items such as disposable saline sets, catheters, Ryle's tubes, disposable syringes, etc.

PHYSICAL METHODS OF STERILIZATION

Boiling is the most commonly used method in day-to-day working. Heat is the safest and most useful agent for sterilizing in hospitals. Heat kills all types of bacteria. Methods of applying heat for sterilization are exposure to steam under pressure any heat, boiling, etc.

Boiling (Moist Heating)

Boiling an instrument/article immersed fully in boiling water (100°C) for 10 minutes will kill most of the pathogenic organisms.

General Instructions

- The articles should be clean.
- The articles should be fully immersed in water.
- Close the sterilizer lid tightly.
- Note the time after the water has started to boil.
- Boil it for 7 to 10 minutes.
- Remove the articles with chattel forceps.

Precautions

- Do not pick articles in between, when the boiling is in process.
- Do not boil sharp instruments such as scissors, knives, needles, etc. because boiling blunt them.

Advantages

- Boiling can be used in the home environment and other situation.
- It is one of the economic ways of sterilizing articles.

Disadvantages

- Some bacteria and viruses and all spores are resistant to boiling.
- Boiling method cannot be used for the articles which may be destroyed by moisture and heat.

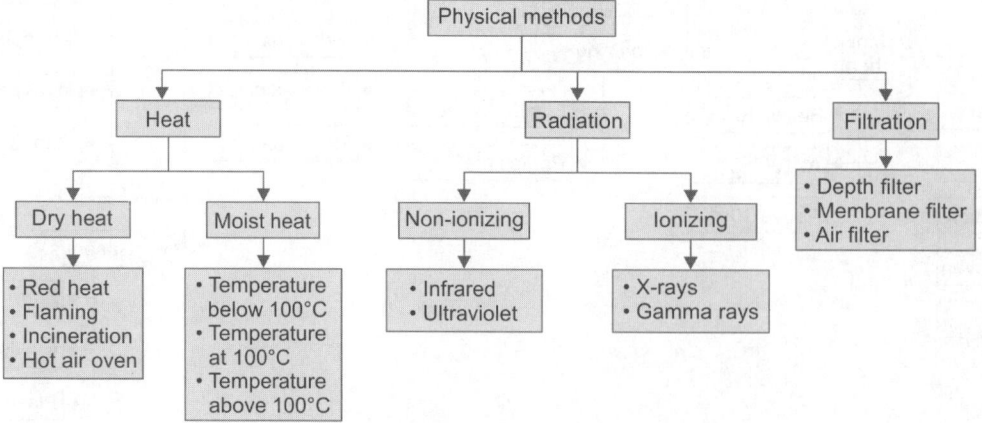

Fig. 8.18: Physical methods of sterilization.

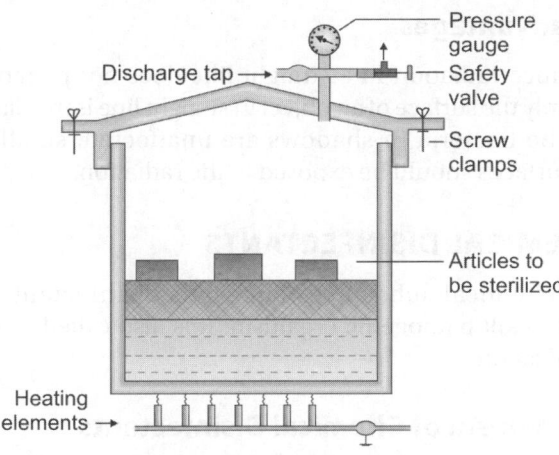

Fig. 8.19: Autoclave machine.

Autoclaving

Autoclaving is the most common method used for sterilizing surgical instruments. It accomplishes sterilization dependably without damage to most of the instrument. It is the best, safest and effective method of sterilization. It destroys the spore forming microorganisms. In this method high temperature, pressure and humidity is used to destroy the bacteria.

Mechanism of Autoclave

- In autoclaving the sterilization is done by steam under pressure. In an autoclave, water boils and its vapor pressure equals that of the surrounding atmosphere.
- When pressure increases inside a closed vessel, the temperature at which boils also increases. Saturated steam has better penetrating power.
- When steam comes into contact with a cooler surface, it condenses into water and given up its latent heat to that surface.
  - Temperature: 121°C
  - Pressure: 15 pounds per square inch (PSI)
  - Time: 15 to 45 minutes.

Instruments Used for Sterilization

- Surgical instruments
- Syringes and needles
- Linen including gowns
- Masks
- Abdominal swabs and dressing.

General Instructions

- All articles must be clean and dry.
- The wrapper and container should allow penetration of the steam into the article.
- The drum should not be too full nor the contents arranged too compactly.
- Cans and jars must be opened and turned to their sides so that steam can penetrate the contents.
- The temperature and pressure of the steam must be 121°C and 1.05 kg/cm^2. So that it will kill all types of microorganisms.
- The destruction of bacteria depends upon the length of time the articles are exposed to steam under pressure. The minimum time is 30 minutes.
- While operating an autoclave, all the air in the chamber must be driven out and replaced by steam.
- When the autoclaving is over, wait for half an hour to dry the materials

HOT AIR OVEN

High temperature and comparatively long exposure times are required for hot air oven. Various types of powders, glass materials, etc. are sterilized by this method.

Mechanism of Hot Air Oven

- It works on the principle of sterilization by dry heat.
  - Temperature: 160°C
  - Time: One hour
- Articles sterilized include glassware, forceps, scissors, scalpels, syringes, liquid paraffin and dusting powder.

Advantages

- All types of microorganisms including spores are killed by this method.
- It is the safest method of sterilization.

Disadvantage

- It is costly method of sterilization.

General Instructions

- Glassware should be perfectly dry before placing in the oven.
- Oven must be allowed to cool down for 2 hours before door is opened after sterilization.

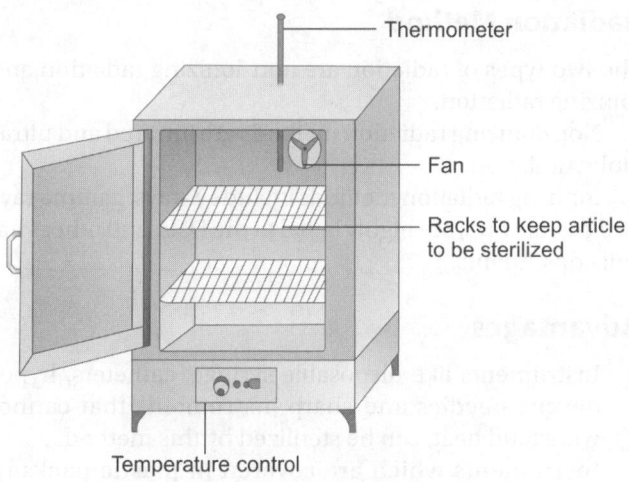

Fig. 8.20: Hot air oven.

- It should not be overloaded.
- Articles should be arranged in such a manner that free circulation of air is possible.

RADIATION METHOD OF STERILIZATION

Radiation or ultraviolet light sterilization: This method is expensive but nowadays it is used for the sterilization of plastic items such as disposable saline set, catheter, Ryle's tubes, etc.

Gas sterilization: Ethylene oxide gas is employed as a sterilizing agent in especially designed chambers in which temperature and humidity can be controlled and from which air can be evacuated.

An exposure period of 3 to 6 hours is needed. Other gases employed for sterilization are formaldehyde and beta propiolactone.

Articles Sterilized

- Surgical instruments with optical lenses.
- Tubing and plastic parts of heart-lung machines.
- Ventilator tubes.
- Disposable syringes.
- Pillows and mattresses.

Advantages

- Exposure to formaldehyde gas under conditions of controlled humidity, temperature and the time exposure will destroy all vegetative forms of bacteria, viruses and most of the spores.
- The best results can be obtained with high concentration of gas humidity above 60% and temperature not less than 180° C.

Disadvantages

- Ethylene oxide has a pungent smell.
- It is an irritant to eye, mucous membrane and skin.

Radiation Method

The two types of radiation are non-ionizing radiation and ionizing radiation.

Non-ionizing radiation methods are infrared and ultraviolet radiation.

Ionizing radiation methods include X-rays, gamma rays and cosmic rays, are highly lethal to the DNA and other vital cell constituents.

Advantages

- Instruments like disposable syringe, catheters, hypodermic needles and sharp instruments that cannot withstand heat, can be sterilized by this method.
- Instruments which are covered in plastic packs or aluminum foils can be sterilized by this method.

Disadvantages

- Since radiation in a straight line does not penetrate, only the surface of an object in straight line is irradiated.
- The bacteria in shadows are unaffected, so all the surfaces should be exposed to the radiation.

CHEMICAL DISINFECTANTS

The chemical substances known as disinfectants are used to kill pathogenic organism. It is also called as cold sterilization.

Mechanism of Chemical Disinfectants

A chemical disinfectant acts by coagulating the bacterial protein or by changing the composition of protein so that it is no longer exist in the same form (**Fig. 8.19**).

Commonly Used Disinfectants

- Phenol
- Lysol
- Formalin
- Dettol
- Alcohol.

Choice of Disinfectant

- The strength of the solution
- Type of bacteria to be killed
- Type of articles
- Length of exposure
- The articles should be fully immersed in the lotion.

Advantages

- This method is used to sterilize instruments which are damaged by heat and metallic objects prone to corrosion.
- It is an easy method.

Disadvantages

- A disinfectant cannot destroy the spores.
- Disinfectants are used in injuries to skin and the articles.

General Instruction

- The disinfectant chosen should destroy the pathogens.
- It should be used in correct strength.
- The article should be fully submerged it.
- The article should be kept in the disinfectant for sufficient time.
- The disinfectant should not be injurious to the skin and the article.
- The disinfectant should be cheap.
- Before dipping the article into the disinfectant, clean it properly to free it from organic material.

TABLE. 8.1: Distinfectant: Mechanism and uses.

Chemical agent	Mechanism	Uses
• Alcohols, Ethanol, Isopropanol	Denaturation of bacterial proteins	Skin antiseptics, surface decontamination of incubators and cabinet interiors, disinfection of clinical thermometers
• Aldehydes, Formaldehyde, Glutaraldehyde	Inactivation of bacterial proteins	Preservation of biological specimens, destroying anthrax spores in wool, fumigation. Cold Sterilant and fixative, surface decontamination, disinfection of hospital instruments, equipment, glassware
• Biguanides, Chlorhexidine	Damage plasma membranes	Skin and mucous membrane disinfectant
• Dyes: Aniline dyes, Malachite green, Acridine dyes Acriflavine, Proflavine	React with acid groups in cell, impair DNA and destroy reproductive capacity	Selective agents in culture media, e.g. LJ media, Skin antiseptic
• Beta propiolactone	Damage DNA, RNA and alkylation	Fumigation, sterilization of biological products
• Halogen chlorine, e.g. Sodium hypochlorite, chloramines, hypochlorous acid, iodine, e.g. Tincture iodine, povidone iodine	Oxidizing agent, Protein denaturation	Surface decontamination, emergency spills, clean-up disinfectant. Antiseptics, decontamination, instrument disinfection
• Metallic salts Silver, e.g. Sliver nitrate, Mercury e.g. Merthiolate, mercurochrome	Combine with sulphhydryl groups, coagulate proteins and inactivate enzymes	Antiseptic to prevent against gonorrheal infection in infants, Antiseptic on wounds
• Phenolic compounds Phenol, Cresol	Damage to cell membranes, inactivation of proteins, oxidases and dehydrogenases	Disinfectant in hospitals
• Peroxides Hydrogen peroxide	Oxidizing agent	Disinfectant
• Quaternary ammonium compounds Zephiran, Triclosan	Surface active agents (cationic detergent)	Surface decontaminant and disinfecting equipment
• Surfactants Soaps and detergent, Sodium lauryl sulphate, Benzalkonium chloride, Cetrimide	Disruption of cell membrane	Detergents and wetting agents

CONCLUSION

Today health care organizations are used high tech disposal items used in various diagnostic and therapeutic procedures. Every department of the hospital uses various items of different makes and materials, out of which many of the items are common like rubber, glass, plastic and enamel. Treatment and maintenance of health of the patient/clients largely depends on the practice of the personal involved in their care. In the office or clinical setting, the nurse must able to identify medical or surgical instruments by their design and function. Medical instruments are used for treatment, assessment and examination purposes. Medical and surgical instruments are made to be either reused or disposed of depending on the instruments use and the manufacture's recommendations. They must be able to name or identify and know the proper use and care of the instruments used for clinic or office procedures. Most can be identified for the use by carefully examining the instrument and its parts; instruments are so especially designed that configurations will usually give clues to their uses.

BIBLIOGRAPHY

1. Harkness-Hoodd, G, Dinched, JR. Total Patient Care: Foundations and Practice of Adult Health Nursing, 8th Ed. St. Louis: Mosby-Year Book, Inc., 1992.
2. Kozier B, Erb G, Olivieri R. Fundamentals of Nursing: Concepts and Process.
3. Kurzen CR. Contemporary Practical/Vocational Nursing, 2nd Ed. Philadelphia: J.B. Lippincott, 1992.
4. Potter PA, Perry AG. Fundamentals of Nursing Concepts, Process and Practice, 3rd ed. St. Louis: Mosby-Year Book, Inc., 1993.
5. Taylor C, Lillis C, LeMone P. Fundamentals of Nursing: The Art and Science of Nursing Care. Philadelphia: J.B. Lippincott, 1993.
6. Timby BK, Lewis LW. Fundamental Skills and Concepts in Patient Care, 5th Ed. Philadelphia: J.B. Lippincott, Co., 1992.

REVIEW QUESTIONS

Long Essays

1. Discuss the equipment used in patient care unit.
2. Enumerate the principles of instrument maintenance.

Short Essays

1. Explain the care of linen.
2. Enumerate the principles of care of rubber goods.
3. Care of enamel wear in the hospital.
4. Discuss the care of stainless steel equipment.
5. Care of fiber optic items.

Short Answers

1. Purpose of mackintosh.
2. Care of bedpans.
3. Care of needles.
4. Care of suction machine.
5. Care of glass instruments.

MULTIPLE CHOICE QUESTIONS

1. **Patient care equipment is defined as powered equipment intended for:**
   a. Use in treatment
   b. Diagnosis and monitoring
   c. Life sustaining or resuscitating functions
   d. All of the above
2. **Disposable equipment are handled by following, *except*:**
   a. Items used only once
   b. Discarded after use
   c. Wash and re-use
   d. New items for each patient
3. **Commonly used disinfectants in the hospital are mentioned below, *except*:**
   a. Phenol
   b. Soap and water
   c. Lysol
   d. Dettol
4. **A chemical disinfectant acts by ——————— the bacterial protein or by changing the composition of protein so that it does no longer exist in the same form:**
   a. Coagulating
   b. Killing
   c. Binding
   d. Preventing
5. **High temperature and comparatively long exposure times are required for:**
   a. Sharps instruments
   b. Hot air oven
   c. Enamel wears
   d. Surgical instruments

ANSWERS

1. d   2. c   3. b   4. a   5. b

CHAPTER 9
Infection Control in Clinical Setting

LEARNING OBJECTIVES

- Nature of infection
- Chain of infection
- Types of infection
- Stages of infection
- Factors increasing susceptibility to infection
- Body defenses against infection: Inflammatory response and immune response
- Health care associated infection (nosocomial infection), introductory concept of asepsis: Medical and surgical asepsis, precautions
- Hand hygiene (hand washing and use of hand rub)
- Use of personal protective equipment (PPE)
- Standard precautions: Biomedical waste management—types of hospital waste, waste segregation and hazards

TERMINOLOGY

Allergen: An antigen, a substance capable of inducing allergy or specific hypersensitivity.

Allergic contact dermatitis: A type IV or delayed-hypersensitivity reaction resulting from contact with a chemical allergen (e.g. poison ivy, certain components of patient care gloves), generally localized to the contact area. Reactions occur slowly over 12-48 hours.

Antibody: A protein found in the blood that is produced in response to foreign substances (e.g. bacteria or viruses) invading the body. Antibodies protect the body from disease by binding to these organisms and destroying them.

Antigen: A foreign substance, usually protein or carbohydrate substance (as a toxin or enzyme) capable of stimulating an immune response, usually the production of antibodies.

Antimicrobial soap: A soap (i.e. detergent) containing an antiseptic agent.

Antiseptic: A germicide that is used on skin or living tissue for the purpose of inhibiting or destroying microorganisms. Examples include alcohols, chlorhexidine, chlorine, hexachlorophene, iodine, chloroxylenol (PCMX), quaternary ammonium compounds, and triclosan.

Antiseptic hand wash: Washing hands with water and soap or detergents containing an antiseptic agent.

Antiseptic hand rub: The process of applying an antiseptic hand-rub product to all surfaces of the hands to reduce the number of microorganisms present.

Asepsis: Prevention from contamination with microorganisms. Includes sterile conditions on tissues, on materials, and in rooms, as obtained by excluding, removing, or killing organisms.

Bioburden: The microbiological load (i.e. number of viable organisms in or on the object or surface) or organic material on a surface or object prior to decontamination, or sterilization, also known as "bioload" or "microbial load."

Biological indicator: A device to monitor the sterilization process that consists of standardized population bacterial spores known to be resistant to the mode of sterilization being monitored. Biological indicators indicate that all the parameters necessary for sterilization were present.

Blood borne pathogens: Disease-producing microorganisms spread by contact with blood or other body fluids contaminated with blood from an infected person.

Blood borne pathogens standard: A standard developed, promulgated, and enforced by the Occupational Safety and Health Administration (OSHA) directing employers to protect employees from occupational exposure to blood and other potentially infectious material.

Chemical sterilant: Chemicals used for the purpose of destroying all forms of microbial life including bacterial spores.

Cleaning: The removal of visible soil, organic and inorganic contamination from a device or surface, using either the physical action of scrubbing with a surfactant or detergent and water or an energy-based process (e.g. ultrasonic cleaners) with appropriate chemical agents.

Contaminated: State of having been in contact with microorganisms. As used in health care, it generally refers to microorganisms capable of producing disease or infection.

Control biological indicator: A biological indicator from the same lot as a test indicator that is left unexposed to the sterilization cycle and then incubated to verify the viability of the test indicator. The control indicator should yield positive results for bacterial growth.

Direct Contact Transmission: Physical transfer of microorganisms between a susceptible host and an infected or colonized person.

Disinfectant: A chemical agent used on inanimate objects (i.e. nonliving) (e.g. floors, walls, sinks) to destroy virtually all recognized pathogenic microorganisms, but not necessarily all microbial forms (e.g. bacterial endospores).

Disinfection: The destruction of pathogenic and other kinds of microorganisms by physical or chemical means. Disinfection is less lethal than sterilization, because it destroys most recognized pathogenic microorganisms, but not necessarily all microbial forms, such as bacterial spores. Disinfection does not ensure the margin of safety associated with sterilization processes.

Endotoxin: The lipopolysaccharide of gram negative bacteria, the toxic character of which reside in the lipid protein. Endotoxins can produce pyrogenic reactions in persons exposed to their bacterial component.

Hand hygiene: A general term that applies to hand washing, antiseptic hand wash, antiseptic hand rub, and surgical hand antisepsis.

Healthcare-associated infection: Any infection associated with a medical or surgical intervention. The term "healthcare-associated" replaces "nosocomial," which is limited to adverse infectious outcomes occurring in hospitals.

Immunity: Protection against a disease. Immunity is indicated by the presence of antibodies in the blood and can usually be determined with a laboratory test.

Immunization: The process by which a person becomes immune, or protected, against a disease. This term is often used interchangeably with vaccination or inoculation. However, the term "vaccination" is defined as the injection of a killed or weakened infectious organism in order to prevent the disease. Thus, vaccination, by inoculation with a vaccine, does not always result in immunity.

Vaccine: A product that produces immunity therefore protecting the body from the disease. Vaccines are administered through needle injections, by mouth and by aerosol.

Ventilation: The process of supplying and removing air by natural or mechanical means to and from any space; such air may be conditioned.

ACRONYMS AND ABBREVIATIONS

Abbreviation	Expansion
ACIP	Advisory Committee on Immunization Practices
ADA	Americans with Disabilities Act
CDC	Centers for Disease Control and Prevention
CMS	Centers for Medicare and Medicaid Services
CoP	Conditions of Participation

Contd...

Contd...

Abbreviation	Expansion
EHR	Electronic Health Record
FDA	Food and Drug Administration
FMLA	Family and Medical Leave Act (of 1993)
HCO	Healthcare Organization
HCP	Healthcare Personnel
HICPAC	Healthcare Infection Control Practices Advisory Committee
HIPPA	Health Insurance Portability and Accountability Act
HIV	Human Immunodeficiency Virus
IIS	Immunization Information Systems
IPC	Infection Prevention and Control
NHSN	National Healthcare Safety Network
NIOSH	National Institute for Occupational Safety and Health
OHS	Occupational Health Services
OSHA	Occupational Safety and Health Administration
PPE	Personal Protective Equipment
PPME	Pre-Placement Medical Evaluation
SESIP	Sharps with Engineered Sharps Injury Protection
TB	Tuberculosis

INTRODUCTION

Infection control is the discipline concerned with preventing Nosocomial or healthcare-associated infection, a practical (rather than academic) sub-discipline of epidemiology. It is an essential, though often under recognized and under supported, part of the infrastructure of health care. Infection control and hospital epidemiology are akin to public health practice, practiced within the confines of a particular health-care delivery system rather than directed at society as a whole.

Infection control addresses factors related to the spread of infections within the healthcare setting (whether patient-to-patient, from patients to staff and from staff to patients, or among staff), including prevention (via hand hygiene/hand washing, cleaning/disinfection/sterilization, vaccination, surveillance), monitoring/investigation of demonstrated or suspected spread of infection within a particular healthcare setting (surveillance and outbreak investigation), and management (interruption of outbreaks). It is on this basis that the common title being adopted within health care is "infection prevention and control".

INFECTION CONTROL: NATURE OF INFECTION, CHAIN OF INFECTION AND TRANSMISSION

Infection prevention and control measures aim to ensure the protection of those who might be vulnerable to acquiring an infection both in the general community and

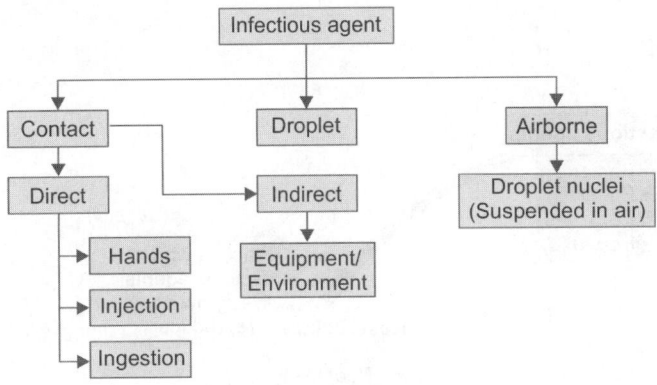

Fig. 9.1: Infectious agent.

Types of Infection

Sl. No.	Type	Definition/description	Example
1.	Primary	Initial infection with a parasite	*Shigella dysenteriae*
2.	Secondary	Primary infection lowers the resistance of the host and later gets infection with another microorganism	Bacterial pneumonia following viral lung infection
3.	Reinfection	Subsequent infection with the same parasite in the same host	Dysentery
4.	Cross	Patient suffering from a disease and new infection is set up from another source	Cold
5.	Nosocomial	Cross infection occurring in hospitals	Pneumonia
6.	Iatrogenic or physician induced	Infection is acquired during therapeutic or investigative procedures	Cold
7.	Focal	Infection at localized sites like appendix and tonsils, general effects are produced	Tonsillitis
8.	Subclinical	Clinical symptoms of an infection are not apparent	Asymptomatic gonorrhea in women and men
9.	Local	Invading microorganisms are limited to a relatively small area of the body	Boils and abscesses
10.	Systemic	Microorganisms or their products are spread throughout the body by blood or lymph	Measles
11.	Mixed	Two or more microbes infecting same tissues	Anaerobic abscess (*E. coli* and *B. fragilis*)
12.	Acute	Have a short duration	Pharyngitis
13.	Chronic	Have a long duration	Tuberculosis
14.	Pyrogenic	Pus forming	Streptococcal infections
15.	Fulminating	Occur suddenly and with severe intensity	Cerebrospinal meningitis
16.	Latent	Parasite after infection remains in a latent or hidden form and produces clinical diseases when the host resistance is lowered	Typhoid fever

while receiving care due to health problems, in a range of settings. The basic principle of infection prevention and control is hygiene.

Goals

- The mission of the WHO Infection Prevention and Control in Health Care initiative is to assist Member States in reducing dissemination of infections associated with healthcare, by assisting with the assessment, planning, implementation and evaluation of national infection control policies.
- The ultimate goal is to assist Member States to endorse quality promotion of health care which is safe for patients, health care workers, others in the health care setting and the environment, and to accomplish these goals in a cost-effective manner.

Objectives

- Develop a cross-sectional, multidisciplinary WHO initiative for Prevention and Control of infections associated with healthcare.
- Provide support to help prevent spread of infectious diseases through evidence-based infection control measures in health care settings.
- Provide support for infection control preparedness and response to public health emergencies of potential international concern.

Infection and Infection Process

The invasion and multiplication of microorganisms such as bacteria, viruses, and parasites those are not normally present within the body. An infection may cause no symptoms and be subclinical, or it may cause symptoms and be clinically apparent. An infection may remain localized, or it may spread through the blood or lymphatic vessels to become systemic (bodywide). Microorganisms that live naturally in the body are not considered infections. For example, bacteria that normally live within the mouth and intestine are not infections.

Infection process: An infection is an invasion of the body by pathogens, or microorganism capable of producing disease. The development of an infection occurs in a cyclical process

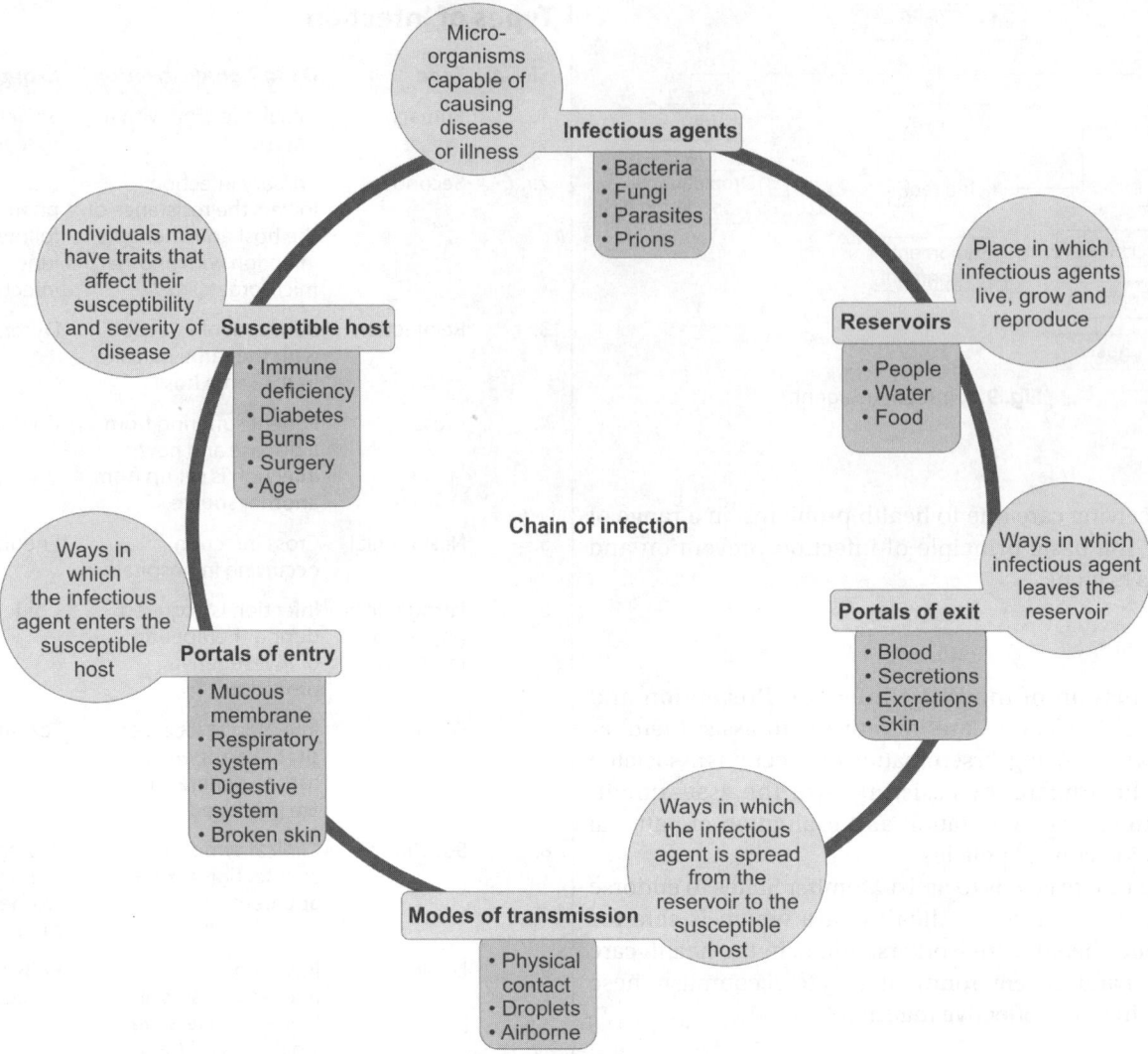

Fig. 9.2: Chain of infection.

that depends on the following six elements. An infection will develop if this cyclical chain remains intact. To prevent the spread of microorganism, the cycle must be interrupted. Nurses use respective practices to break the chain, so that infection will not occur.

Infection agent: The pathogenic organisms include bacteria, viruses, fungi and protozoa and more prevalent agents that are capable of causing infection.

Reservoir: The reservoir for growth and multiplication of microorganism is the natural habitat of the organism. The possible reservoir that supports organism pathogenic to humans includes other human (e.g. TB, syphilis, HIV, HBV), animals (Rabies-dog), food (*Cl. botulinum*), water, milk and inanimate object, e.g. soil, gas gangrene, tetanus).

Portal of exist: The exit from the reservoir is the point of escape for the organism. The organism cannot extend its influence unless it moves away from its original source. There usually a primary exist route for each type of organism. In human common escape routes are as follows:
- Skin and mucous membrane, e.g. *S. aureus*, cause yellowish drainage. *P. aeruginosa* causes greenish drainage.
- Respiratory tract, e.g. *Mycobacterium tuberculosis* causes tuberculosis.
- Genitourinary tract
- GI tract.
- Reproductive tract, e.g. STDs, HIV.
- Blood-serum hepatitis.

Modes of Disease Transmission

Communicable disease may be transmitted from the reservoir or source of infection to a susceptible individual in many different ways, depending upon the infections agent, portal entry and the local ecological conditions.
- **Direct contact:** Infection may be transmitted by direct contact from skin to skin, mucosa to mucosa or mucosa to skin of the same or another person. For example

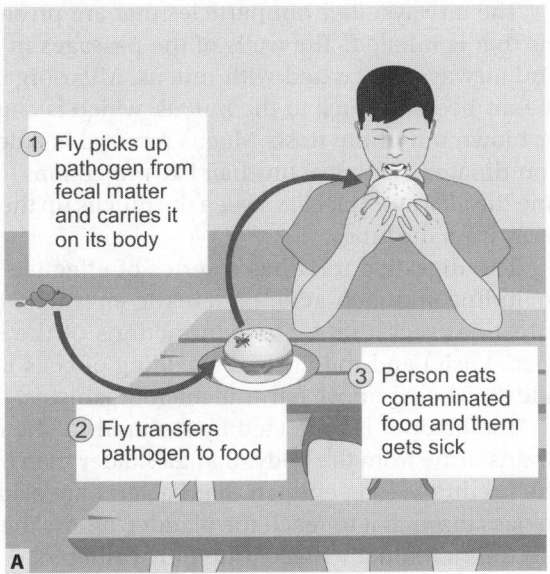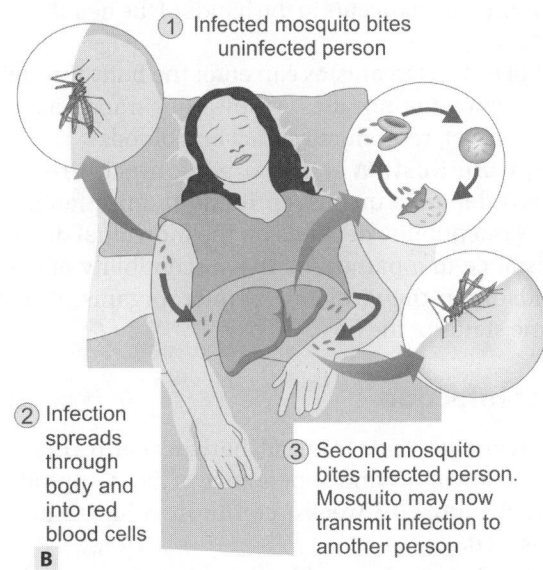

Fig. 9.3: Disease transmission by house fly and mosquitoes.

during touching, kissing, sexual intercourse (STD, AIDS, leprosy, skin infections) and scratching through fingers.
- **Droplet infection:** Droplet infection occurs due to contact transmission by infections agents contained in most respiratory secretions. The microorganisms from nasopharyngeal secretions during coughing, sneezing or speaking and spitting, talking into the surrounding atmosphere (for example respiratory infections, TB, meningitis, etc.).
- **Contact with soil:** Infectious agents (microorganisms) are present in soil can cause disease, when the host comes in the contact with soil (for example hookworm, tetanus, etc.).
- **Inoculation into skin or mucosa:** The disease agent may be inoculated directly into the skin or mucosa. Transmission of infection (syringe/needle) as infection after dog bite.
- **Transplacental (vertical):** Transmission of infectious agent can occur transplacentally.

Chain of infection

An infection will develop if this chain remains intact. Nurses use infection prevention and control practices to break the chain so that infection will not develop.
I. **Infectious agent:** Microorganisms include bacteria, viruses, fungi and protozoa. They are the common infectious agents. The potential for microorganisms or parasites to cause disease depends on the following factors:
   - Sufficient number of organisms
   - Virulence or ability to produce disease
   - Ability to enter and survive to the host
   - Susceptibility of host.
II. **Reservoir:** A reservoir is where a pathogen can survive. Skin of patients, carriers, animals, food, water insects, and inanimate objects are common reservoirs of infection.
III. **Portal of exist:** Microorganisms can enter through a variety of sites such as skin and mucous membrane, respiratory tract, urinary tract, gastrointestinal tract, reproductive tract and blood.
IV. **Modes of transmission:** Direct contact or indirect contact with infected source, contaminated air, water, blood, food, flies, mosquito are the common modes of transmission to infection. Major mode of transmission

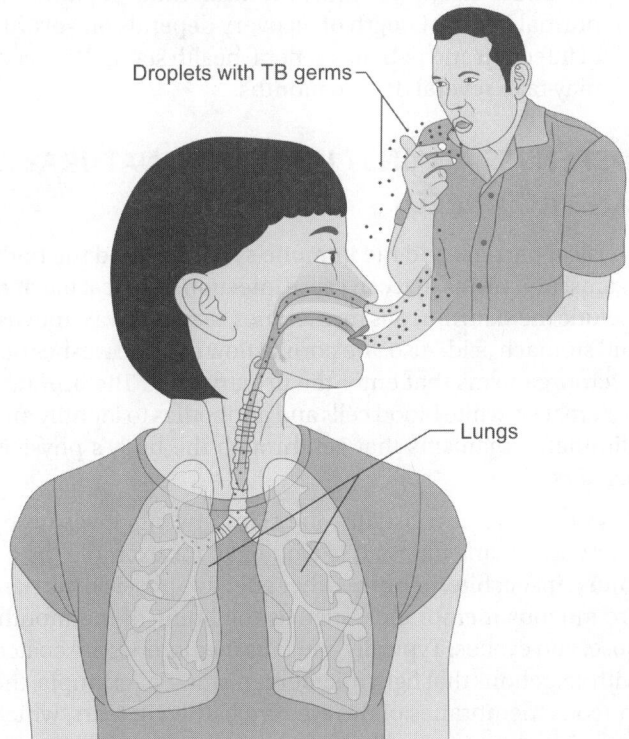

Fig. 9.4: Transmission of infection by respiratory route.

of microorganisms occurs in the hands of the health care providers.

V. **Portal of entry:** Organisms can enter the body through skin, mucous membranes, respiratory tract, gastrointestinal tract, reproductive tract and blood.

VI. **Susceptible host:** Whether a person acquires an infection depends on susceptibility to an infectious agent. Susceptibility depends on the individual degree of resistance to a pathogen. The susceptibility of host depends upon the virulence of microorganisms and immune status of the host.

Course of Infection

I. **Incubation period:** Interval between entrance of pathogen into body and appearance of first symptoms, e.g. chickenpox 2-3 weeks, common cold 1-2 days, mumps 18 days.

II. **Prodromal stage:** Interval from onset of non-specific signs and symptoms (malaise, low-grade fever, fatigue) to more specific symptoms. During this time, microorganisms grow and multiply and patient is more capable of spreading disease to others.

III. **Illness stage:** Interval when patient manifests signs and symptoms specific to a particular disease, e.g. **common cold** - Sore throat, sinus, congestion, rhinitis, **Mumps** - earache, high fever, parotid and salivary gland swelling. The severity of patient's illness depends on the extent of infection, the pathogenicity of the microorganisms and susceptibility of individuals.

IV. **Convalescence:** Interval when acute symptoms of infection disappear until the individual regains his normal health. Length of recovery depends on severity of infection and patient's general health status. Recovery may take several days to months.

DEFENSES AGAINST INFECTION: NATURAL AND ACQUIRED

Physical barriers and the immune system defend the body against organisms that can cause infection. Physical barriers include the skin, mucous membranes, tears, earwax, mucus, and stomach acid. Also, the normal flow of urine washes out microorganisms that enter the urinary tract. The immune system uses white blood cells and antibodies to identify and eliminate organisms that get through the body's physical barriers

Physical barriers: Usually, the skin prevents invasion by microorganisms unless it is damaged, for example, by an injury, insect bite, or burn. Other effective physical barriers are mucous membranes, such as the lining of the mouth, nose, and eyelids. Typically, mucous membranes are coated with secretions that fight microorganisms. For example, the mucous membranes of the eyes are bathed in tears, which contain an enzyme called lysozyme that attacks bacteria and helps protect the eyes from infection

The airways filter out particles that are present in the air that is inhaled. The walls of the passages in the nose and airways are coated with mucus. Microorganisms in the air become stuck to the mucus, which is coughed up or blown out of the nose. Mucus removal is aided by the coordinated beating of tiny hair like projections (cilia) that line the airways. The cilia sweep the mucus up the airways, away from the lungs.

The digestive tract has a series of effective barriers, including stomach acid, pancreatic enzymes, bile, and intestinal secretions. The contractions of the intestine (peristalsis) and the normal shedding of cells lining the intestine help remove harmful microorganisms.

The bladder is protected by the urethra, the tube that drains urine from the body. In males older than 6 months, the urethra is long enough that bacteria are seldom able to pass through it to reach the bladder, unless the bacteria are unintentionally placed there by catheters or surgical instruments. In females, the urethra is shorter, occasionally allowing external bacteria to pass into the bladder. In both sexes, when the bladder empties, it flushes out any bacteria that reach it.

The blood: The body also defends against infection by increasing the number of certain types of white blood cells (neutrophils and monocytes), which engulf and destroy invading microorganisms. The increase can occur within several hours, largely because white blood cells are released from the bone marrow, where they are made. The number of neutrophils increases first, sometimes with an increase in immature forms of neutrophils. If an infection persists, the number of monocytes increases. The blood carries white blood cells to sites of infection. The number of eosinophils, another type of white blood cell, increases in allergic reactions and many parasitic infections, but usually not in bacterial infections. However, certain infections, such as typhoid fever, viral infections, and bacterial infections that overwhelm the immune system, can lead to a decrease in the white blood cell count.

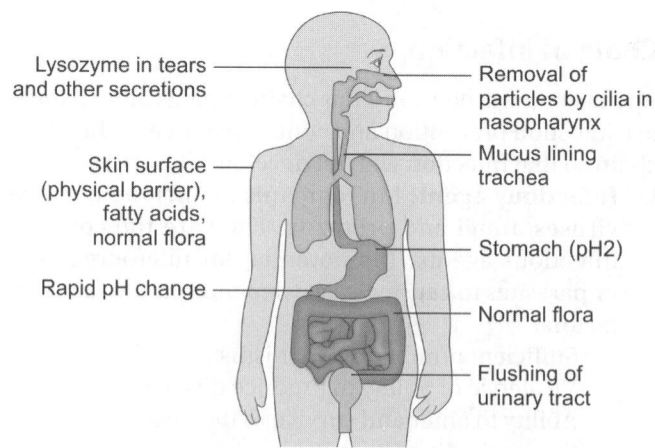

Fig. 9.5: Normal protective mechanism.

Inflammation: Any injury, including an invasion by microorganisms, causes inflammation in the affected area. Inflammation, a complex reaction, results from many different conditions. The damaged tissue releases substances that cause inflammation and that direct the immune system to do the following:
- Wall off the area
- Attack and kill any invaders
- Dispose of dead and damaged tissue
- Begin the process of repair.

However, inflammation may not be able to overcome large numbers of microorganisms. During inflammation, the blood supply increases. An infected area near the surface of the body becomes red and warm. The walls of blood vessels become more porous, allowing fluid and white blood cells to pass into the affected tissue.

The increase in fluid causes the inflamed tissue to swell. The white blood cells attack the invading microorganisms and release substances that continue the process of inflammation. Other substances trigger clotting in the tiny vessels (capillaries) in the inflamed area, which delays the spread of the infecting microorganisms and their toxins. Many of the substances produced during inflammation stimulate the nerves, causing pain. Reactions to the substances released during inflammation include the chills, fever, and muscle aches that commonly accompany infection

Immune response: When an infection develops, the immune system responds by producing several substances and agents that are designed to attack the specific invading microorganisms. For example, the immune system may produce killer T cells (a type of white blood cell) that can recognize and kill the invading microorganism. Also, the immune system produces antibodies that target the specific invading microorganism. Antibodies attach to and immobilize microorganisms-killing them outright or helping neutrophils target and kill them.

The immune system also includes other proteins and chemicals that assist antibodies and T cells in their work. Among them are chemicals that alert phagocytes to the site of the infection. The complement system, a group of proteins that normally float freely in the blood, move toward infections, where they combine to help destroy microorganisms and foreign particles. They do this by changing the surface of bacteria or other microorganisms, causing them to die.

Enzyme is a protein that helps speed up a chemical reaction in the body.

Antigens are substances that are recognized as a threat by the body's immune system, which triggers the formation of specific antibodies against the substance.

Bone marrow is the soft tissue inside bones where blood cells are made.

Lymphatic system is a system that contains lymph nodes and a network of channels that carry fluid and cells of the immune system through the body.

Immunity is the condition of being protected against an infectious disease. Immunity often develops after a germ is introduced to the body. One type of immunity occurs when the body makes special protein molecules called antibodies to fight the disease-causing germ. The next time that germ enters the body; the antibodies quickly attack it, usually preventing the germ from causing disease.

Fever: Body temperature increases as a protective response to infection and injury. An elevated body temperature (fever) enhances the body's defense mechanisms, although it can cause discomfort. A part of the brain called the hypothalamus controls body temperature. Fever results from an actual resetting of the hypothalamus's thermostat. The body raises its temperature to a higher level by moving (shunting) blood from the skin surface to the interior of the body, thus reducing heat loss. Shivering

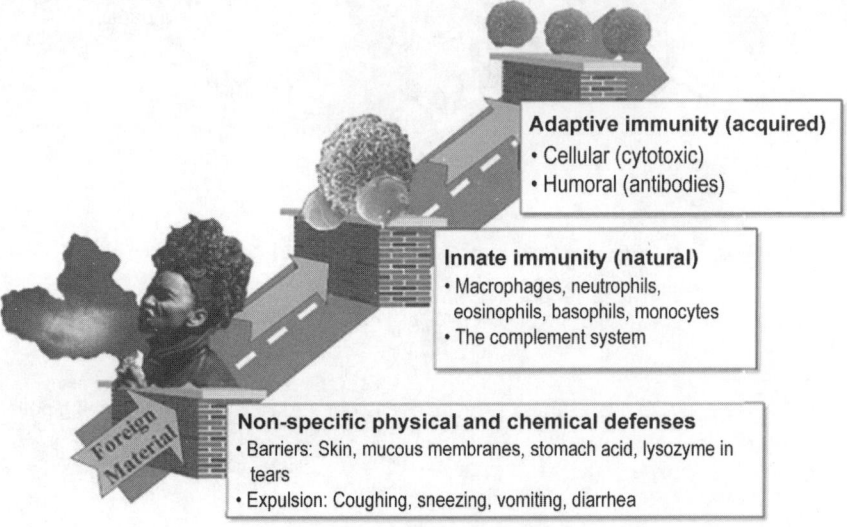

Fig. 9.6: Barriers to invasion.

(chills) may occur to increase heat production through muscle contraction. The body's efforts to conserve and produce heat continue until blood reaches the hypothalamus at the new, higher temperature. The new, higher temperature is then maintained. Later, when the thermostat is reset to its normal level, the body eliminates excess heat through sweating and shunting of blood to the skin.

HOSPITAL–ACQUIRED INFECTION/ NOSOCOMIAL INFECTION

Nosocomial infections are infections which occur as a result of treatment in a hospital, but secondary to the patient's original condition. Infections are considered Nosocomial if they first appear 48 hours or more after hospital admission or within 30 days after discharge. Nosocomial comes from the Greek word 'nosokomeion' meaning hospital (nosos- disease, komeo to take care of). This type of infection is also known as a hospital-acquired infection or more genetically healthcare-associated infections). Most common Nosocomial infections are Ventilator associated pneumonia, *Staphylococcus aureus*, Methicillin-resistant *Staphylococcus aureus*, *Pseudomonas aeruginosa*, *Acinetobacter baumannii*, *Stenotrophomonas maltophilia*, *Clostridium difficile*. Tuberculosis, urinary tract infection, hospital-acquired pneumonia, gastroenteritis.

Definition

The terms hospital-acquired infection, hospital-associated infection, hospital infection or Nosocomial infection (nosocomion, meaning hospital) is defined as infection developing in patients after admission to the hospital, which was neither present nor in the incubation period at the time of hospitalization. Such infections may become evident during their stay in the hospital or, sometimes, after their discharge.

Causes of Nosocomial Infection

Nosocomial infections are commonly transmitted when health care providers become complacent and do not practice correct hygiene regularly. Also, increased use of outpatient treatment in recent decades means that a greater percentage of people who are hospitalized today are likely to be seriously ill with more weakened immune systems than in the past. Moreover, some medical procedures bypass the body's natural protective barriers. Since medical staff moves from patient-to-patient, the staff themselves serves as a means for spreading pathogens.

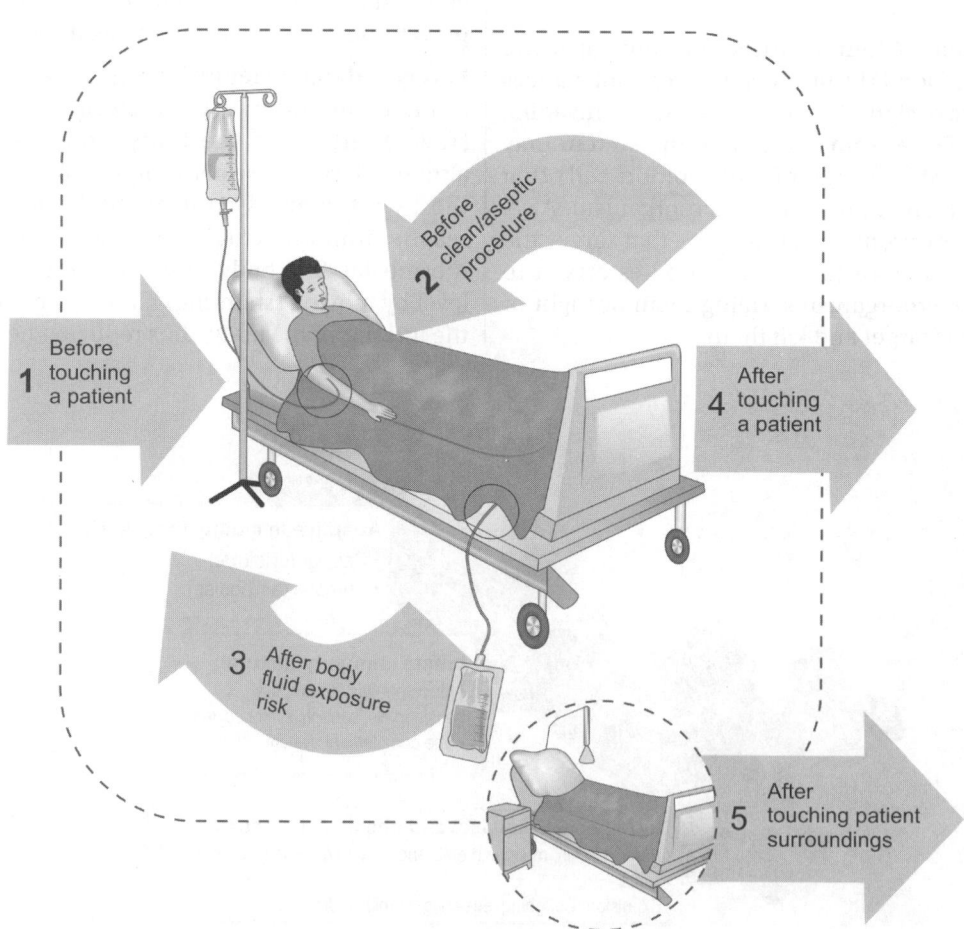

Fig. 9.7: Hand washing prevents disease transmission.

Sources of Infection

- **Exogenous:** Hospital-infection is mostly exogenous from another patient or member of the staff or from the environment in the hospital. Patients and hospital personnel suffering from infection, or asymptomatic carrier are the most important sources. Environmental sources include inanimate objects, air, water and food in the hospital. Inanimate objects in the hospital are medical equipment (endoscopes, cystoscopes, catheters, etc.), bedpans, surfaces contaminated by patients secretions, excretions, blood and body fluids.
- **Endogenous:** Patients own flora may invade the patient's tissue during some surgical operation or instrumental manipulations.

Nosocomial infections	Clinical features	Laboratory features
UTI	Fever Lower abdominal pain, change in urine characteristics	Leukocytosis Positive urine culture 5 (10 CFU of a single organism per mL of urine)
Pneumonia	Fever Pleuritic chest pain Decreased intensity of breath sounds Presence or increase in rales	Leukocytosis Sputum for Gram stain Positive sputum culture Positive chest X-ray
Blood infections	Unexplained fever with chills and rigor pain, tenderness or purulent drainage at the site of insertion of IV access or CVP catheter	Leukocytosis Positive blood culture Positive CVP catheter culture (after catheter removal)
Skin and soft tissue infections	Pain, swelling, tenderness or inflammation and warmth of skin Purulent drainage from skin Fever	Smear for Gram stain Positive swab culture Leukocytosis
Gastroenteritis	Increased frequency of stools Change in consistency of stools Fever Dehydration	Leukocytosis Positive stool culture
Meningitis	Fever Altered sensorium Headache Neck stiffness Vomiting	Leukocytosis CSF-cell count, cell type, culture, sugar, protein

Types of Nosocomial Infection

Almost any microorganism can, on occasion, cause hospital acquired infection but those that survive in the hospital environment for long periods and develop resistance to antibiotics and disinfectants are particularly important. *Staph. aureus* strains, resistant to multiple antibiotics spread globally in the 1950's and 1960's, colonizing hospitals and continue to be very common agents in Nosocomial infection. In recent decades, *E. coli*, Klebsiella, Enterobacter and Proteus have become the most important hospital pathogens, particularly because of dissemination among them of R factor conferring multiple drug resistance.

Pseudomonas aeruginosa and other Pseudomonas species have always been important hospital pathogens because of their intrinsic resistance to most antibiotics and ability to survive and even multiply in disinfectants solutions.

Tetanus spores can survive in dust and may sometimes contaminate items used in hospitals. Hospital tetanus is usually due to faulty sterilization techniques or other lapses in asepsis. HIV and hepatitis B and C viruses are transmitted by contaminated blood or blood products. Screening of blood donors has reduced the risk to a large extent. However, HIV escapes detection during the window period. Reasons why Nosocomial infections are so common include:

- Hospitals house large numbers of people who are sick and those immune systems are often in a weakened state.
- Increased use of outpatient treatment means that people who are in the hospital are sick on average.
- Medical staff moves from patient-to-patient, providing a way for pathogens to spread.
- Many medical procedures bypass the body's natural protective barriers.
- Routine use of antimicrobial agents in hospitals creates selection pressure for the emergence of resistant strains. Thorough hand washing and/or use of alcohol rubs by all medical personnel before each patient contact is one of the most effective ways to combat Nosocomial infections. More careful use of antimicrobial agents, such as antibiotics, is also considered vital.

Modes of Transmission

There are four main routes of transmission of infection:
1. **Contact**
   It is the principal route of transmission of nosocomial pathogens.
   - **Hands or clothing:** The hands of hospital staff are an important vehicle of spread of infection. There is adequate scope of transmission of microorganisms from one person to another by contact of hands and clothing's of attendants.
   S. aureus and *S. pyogenes* are two important pathogens spread by hand contact.
   - **Inanimate objects:** Certain instruments (endoscope, bronchoscope, cystoscope), if not properly disinfected, may transmit pathogenic organisms' e.g. *Pseudomonas aeruginosa*.
2. **Airborne**
   - **Droplets:** Droplets of respiratory infection is transmitted by inhalation.

- **Dust:** Dust from bedding, floors, exudates dispersed from a wound during dressing and from skin by natural shedding of skin scales (measles, staphylococcal sepsis), may contribute in spread of infections, e.g. *Pseudomonas aeruginosa, S. aureus.*
- **Aerosols:** Aerosols produced by nebulizers, humidifiers and air conditioning apparatus transmit certain pathogens to the respiratory tract.

3. **Oral route**

   Hospital food may contain antibiotic-resistant bacteria (*Pseudomonas aeruginosa, E. coli,* Kiebsiella spp. and others), which may colonies the intestine and later cause infection in susceptible patients.

4. **Parenteral route**

   With the introduction of disposable syringes and needles, transmission of infection by parenteral route has been infrequent. However, certain infections may be transmitted by blood transfusion or tissue donation, contaminated blood products (factor VIII) and contaminated infusion fluids. (Hepatitis B and HIV are two viruses which may be transmitted in this way).

5. **Common hospital-acquired infections**
   - **Urinary tract infection:** This is usually associated with catheterization or instrumentation of urethra, bladder or kidneys. Infection can be prevented by strict asepsis during catheterization.
   - **Respiratory infection:** Aspiration in unconscious patients and pulmonary ventilation may lead to Nosocomial pneumonia.
   - **Wound and skin sepsis:** The incidence of postoperative infection is higher in elderly patients. Most wound infections manifest within a week of surgery.
   - **Gastrointestinal infections:** Food poisoning and neonatal septicemia in hospitals have been reported.
   - **Burns:** *S. aureus, Pseudomonas aeruginosa* and *S. pyogenes* are responsible for hospital-acquired infections in cases of burns.
   - **Bacteremia and septicemia:** These may be consequences of infection at any site but are generally caused by infected intravenous cannulae. Infection can be prevented by proper skin toilet before 'cut-down'. Intravenous rehydration in diarrhea should be replaced by oral fluids as early as possible.

Diagnosis and control: Hospital-acquired infection may occur sporadically or as outbreaks. Diagnosis is by the routine bacteriological methods such as direct smear examination, culture and sensitivity testing. This requires the samples from possible sources of infection such as hospital personnel, inanimate objects, water, air or food. Typing of isolate (phage typing, bacteriocin typing, biotyping or antibiogram) may indicate a causal connection. Control of hospital infection should be a permanent ongoing activity. Examples of sources of hospital outbreaks are nasal carriage of staphylococci in hospital staff or Pseudomonas growing in lotions. Carriers should be suitably treated. The cause of infection may be a defective autoclave; therefore, sterilization techniques have to be tested.

Types of Hospital-associated Infections

Type of Infections and Causative Microorganisms

Sl. No.	Type	Causative microorganisms
1.	Urinary tract infections	Klebsiella, Proteus, Serratia, Pseudomonas, *Escherichia coli*, Staphylococci, Enterococci, *Candida albicans*.
2.	Respiratory infection	Staphylococcus aureus, Escherichia coli, Streptococcus pneumoniae, Klebsiella, Enterobacter, Serratia Proteus, Acinetobacter, *Pseudomonas aeruginosa*.
3.	Gastrointestinal infection	Salmonella, shigella, viruses
4.	Eye infection	*Pseudomonas aeruginosa, Staphylococcus aureus*
5.	Wound infection	*Staphylocous aureus, Escherichia coli, Pseudomonas aeruginosa*.
6.	Other infection	Proteus, acinetobacter, hepatitis B virus, human immunodeficiency viruses.

Transmission of Nosocomial Infection

Microorganisms are transmitted in hospitals by several routes, and the same microorganism be transmitted by more than one route. There are five main routes of transmission-Contact, droplet, airborne, common vehicle, and vector borne.

- **Contact transmission,** the most important and frequent mode of transmission of nosocomial infections, is divided into two subgroups: Direct-contact transmission and indirect-contact transmission.
- **Direct-contact transmission** involves a direct body surface-to-body surface contact and physical transfer of microorganisms between susceptible host and an infected or colonized person, such as occurs when a person turns a patient, gives a patient a bath, or performs other patient – care activities that require direct personal contact. Direct-contact transmission also can occur between two patients, with one serving as the source of the infectious microorganisms and the other as a susceptible host.
- **Indirect-contact transmission** involves contact of a susceptible host with a contaminated intermediate object, usually inanimate, such as contaminated instruments, needles or dressing, or contaminated gloves that are not changed between patients. Additionally, the improper use of saline flush syringes, vials, and bags have been implicated in disease transmission even when healthcare workers had access to gloves, disposable needles, intravenous devices and flushes.
- **Droplet transmission** occurs when droplets are produced from the source person mainly during

coughing, sneezing, and talking and during the performance of certain procedures such as bronchoscope. Transmission occurs when droplets containing germs from the infected person are propelled a short distance through the air and deposited on the host's body.

- **Airborne transmission** occurs by dissemination of either airborne droplet nuclei (small-particle residue [5 mm or smaller in size] of evaporated droplets containing microorganisms that remain suspended in the air for long periods of time) or dust particles containing the infectious agent. Microorganisms carried in this manner can be dispersed widely by air currents and may become inhaled by a susceptible host within the same room or over a longer distance from the source patient, depending on environmental factors; therefore, special air handling and ventilation are required to prevent airborne transmission. Microorganisms transmitted by airborne transmission include *Mycobacterium tuberculosis* and the rubella and varicella viruses.
- **Common vehicle transmission** applies to microorganisms transmitted to the host by contaminated items such as food, water, medications, devices and equipment.
- **Vector borne transmission** occurs when vectors such as mosquitoes, flies, rats transmit microorganisms.

Prevention

- **Isolation:** Isolation precautions are designed to prevent transmission of microorganisms by common routes in hospitals. Because agent and host factors are more difficult to control, interruption of transfer of microorganisms is directed primarily at transmission.
- **Hand washing and gloving:** Hand washing frequently is called the single most important measure to reduce the risks of transmitting microorganisms from one person to another or from one site to another on the same patient. Washing hands as promptly and thoroughly as possible between patients contacts and after contact with blood, body fluids, secretions, excretions and equipment or articles contaminated by them is an important component of infection control and isolation precautions.

Although hand washing may seem like a simple process, it is often performed incorrectly. Health care settings must continually remind practitioners and visitors for the proper procedure in washing their hands. All visitors must follow the same procedures as hospital staff to adequately control the spread of infections. An addition to hand washing, gloves play an important role in reducing the risks of transmission of microorganisms. Gloves are worn for three important reasons in hospitals.

First, gloves are worn to provide a protective barrier and to prevent gross contamination of the hands when touching blood, body fluids, secretions, excretions, mucous membranes and nonintact skin; the wearing of gloves in specified circumstances to reduce the risk of exposures to blood borne pathogens. Second, gloves are worn to reduce the likelihood that microorganisms present on the hands of personnel will be transmitted to patient during invasive or other patient care procedures that involves touching a patient's mucous membranes and non intact skin. Third, gloves are worn to reduce the likelihood that hands of personnel contaminated with microorganisms from a patient or a fomite can transmit these microorganisms to another patient. In this situation, gloves must be changed between patient contacts and hands should be washed after gloves are removed.

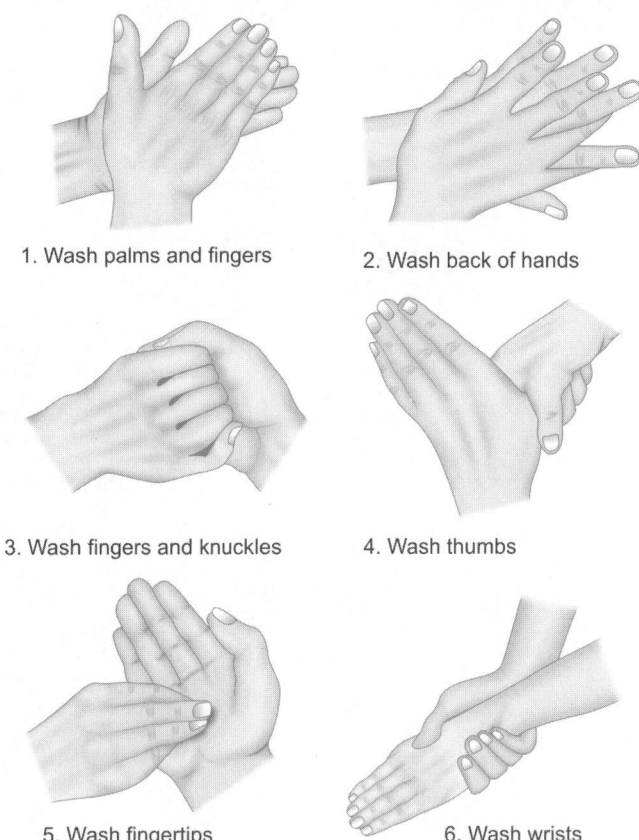

Fig. 9.8: Hand washing technique.

Wearing gloves does not replace the need for hand washing, because gloves may have small, nonapparent defects or may be torn during use, and hands can become contaminated during removal of gloves. Failure to change gloves between patient contacts is an infection control hazard. Examples of nosocomial infections include Methicill in Resistant *Staphylococcus aureus* (MRSA).

Aprons: Wearing an apron during patient care reduces the risk of infection. The apron should either be disposable or be used only when caring for a specific patient.

Mitigation: The most effective way of controlling nosocomial infection is to strategically implementing quality assurance/quality control measures to the health care sectors and evidence-based management can be a feasible approach.

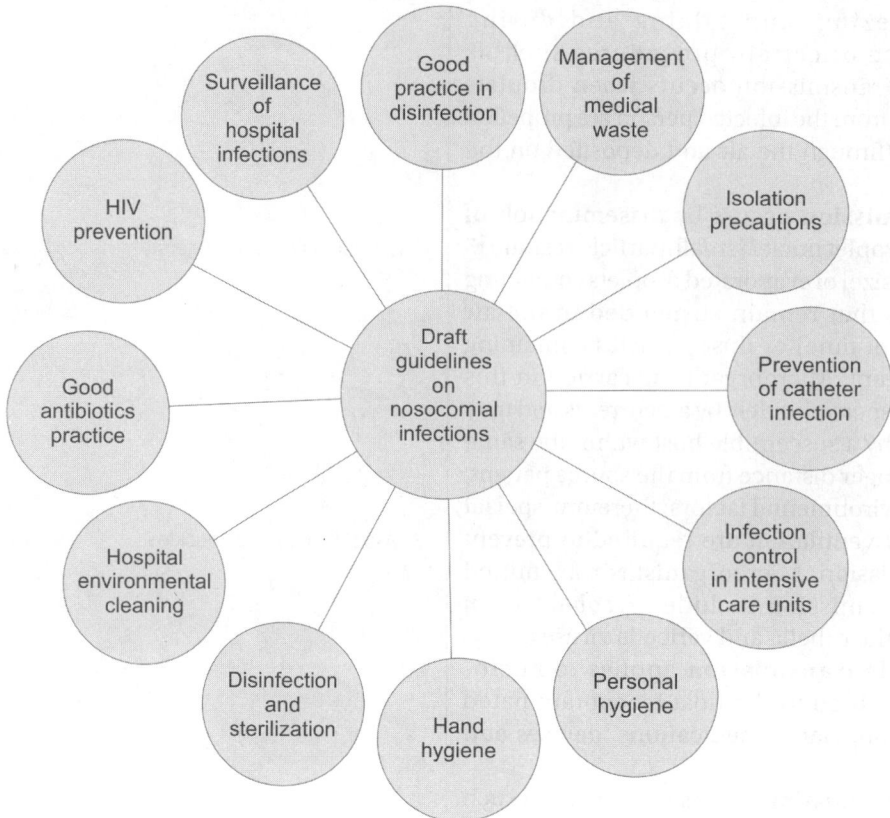

Fig. 9.9: Nosocomial infection preventive measures.

The hospital-acquired infections can be prevented by following means:
- Administration of antibiotic therapy to the carrier staff or source patient to destroy the pathogenic agents.
- Proper sterilization and disinfection of the inanimate objects should be done. This helps to control the source of infection.
- Disinfection of excreta and infected material is necessary to control the exit point of infection.
- Transmission of infection can be controlled by regular washing of hands, disinfection of equipment and change of working clothes.
- The use of sterile dressings, surgical gloves, face-masks and IV fluids further contribute in control of infection.
- Preoperative disinfection of the patient's skin.
- Rational antibiotic prophylaxis.
- Proper investigation of hospital-acquired infection and the treatment of such cases.

Infection control policy: Every hospital must have an effective hospital-acquired infection control committee (HAICC) which should be responsible for the control of hospital-acquired infection (HAT). The committee should be chaired by medical superintendent and should have a microbiologist as infection control officer and heads of all clinical departments, blood bank. Microbiologist, medical record officer, chief of nursing services and infection control sister as members. Chief of all the supportive services (OT, dietetics, laundry, housekeeping, etc.) should be included as invited members.

BARRIER NURSING

Barrier nursing is a set of stringent infection control techniques used in nursing. The aim of barrier nursing is to protect medical staff against infection by patients, particularly those with highly infectious diseases. Reverse barrier nursing is similar, but concentrates on the reverse: protecting vulnerable patients, such as those with weakened immune systems, against infection by medical staff.

Definition

- **Isolation nursing:** Isolation nursing is carried out by placing the patient in a single room or side room.
- **Barrier nursing:** This occurs when a patient(s) is kept in a bay and extra precautions are implemented to prevent spread of the germ.

Barrier techniques infection control
- Aseptic technique
- Isolation
- Safer handling of sharps
- Linen handling and disposal
- Waste disposal
- Handling biological spills
- Environmental cleaning
- Risk assessment
- Staff health

Effective Barrier Nursing

In an ideal world, a patient requiring barrier nursing should be housed away from other patients in an isolation ward. However, not all practices have the luxury of such facilities, which can make effective barrier nursing more difficult—though not impossible—to achieve. The following points should be adhered to.

- **Equipment should be for the sole use of that patient:** Disposable bedding and even food bowls should be considered to minimize the transportation of contaminated equipment.
- **Protective clothing should also be disposable:** Over gowns or overalls are preferable to aprons, as they provide complete, all-round cover. Gowns with loops for fingers allow the placement of gloves over the top, similar to the closed-gloving method, which ensures the personnel's skin is not exposed to contamination. Protective clothing should also be water repellent to prevent strike-through to clothing.
- **A limited number of staff should be responsible** for nursing an isolated patient. Isolating patients can cause them distress, so ensuring the same staff member cares for an individual has the added advantage of building trust, as well as minimizing cross-contamination.
- **Hospital equipment**, such as fluid pumps, thermometers and stethoscopes, should also be reserved for the duration of the patient's treatment. Such items should be thoroughly decontaminated after use.
- **Consider the use of a designated trolley for transporting patients in isolation:** They should only be moved when absolutely necessary. Designated toilet areas should be away from usual toilet areas.
- **Owner visitation should be discouraged**, but this needs to be balanced with the patient's well-being. If visits are permitted, the owner must comply with infection control policies.
- **Ensure your isolation area is well stocked** with its own consumables and cleaning products. However, don't overstock, as you will need to dispose of everything once the patient is moved from isolation – this could become costly.
- **The NHS recommends** barrier nursing for a further 48 hours after a patient is asymptomatic if they have had vomiting or diarrhea.
- **And finally... wash hands.** Although gloves and protective equipment will provide a barrier to bacterial contamination, they should be classed as nothing more than a second skin. Observational studies have shown that not removing gloves and touching inanimate objects, such as door handles and telephones, can contribute to bacterial spread. Nothing substitutes good hand washing – even wearing gloves

Patient considerations invasive devices, such as intravenous catheters, urinary catheters, feeding tubes and chest and wound drains, are potential routes for infection. All invasive devices should be closed systems – for example, intravenous catheters should be appropriately bunged and dressed when not in use, and urinary catheters should be attached to a urinary bag. To minimize the risk of infection, all devices should be removed as soon as possible. Patients most at risk of HAIs include those that have:

- A weakened immune system
- Open wounds
- Any invasive device
- A severe skin condition
- Had recent surgery
- Frequently been given antibiotics.

Protective Clothing

- Staff will wear protective clothing for example gloves, apron and mask (if required) in order to reduce the risk of passing the infection/germ to other patients.
- The type of clothing that staff wear will depend upon what type of care they are carrying out and how the infection is spread.
- If the infection is likely to be spread by breathing in the germs that are causing the infection then staff will wear masks.
- It is very unlikely that visitors will need to wear any protective clothing such as apron or gloves. If they do then nursing staff will advise.

Isolation Ward

In hospitals and other medical facilities, an **isolation ward** is a separate ward used to isolate patients suffering from infectious diseases. Several wards for individual patients are usually placed together in an **isolation unit**.

Isolation room in hospital

- Isolation rooms create barriers between people and germs
- These type of isolations help to prevent the spread of germs in the Hospitals
- Anybody who visits in a Hospital patients who has Isolation sign outside their door should stop at the nurse's station before entering the patients room
- Concise information is placed on the door of isolation room at eye level.

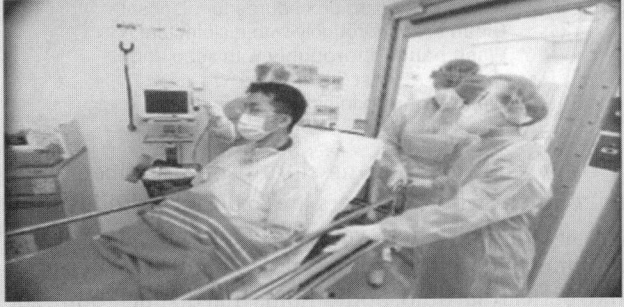

Fig. 9.10: Isolation room.

Design: In an isolation unit, several measures must be implemented in order to reduce the spread of infection. The units are generally placed away from the main hospital, and staff often only works in that unit. In some hospitals, the unit is placed in a separate building. Ventilation is important to reduce the transmission of airborne spores, and the most severely affected patients are placed in separate wards. However, in some circumstances, especially in areas experiencing a major epidemic, make shift isolation wards can be constructed.

Uses: Isolation wards are used to isolate patients who pose a risk of passing a potentially harmful infection on to others. Such infections can range in severity widely, from diseases such as influenza to Ebola, although more precautions are generally taken with diseases of a higher mortality rate. Outside major hospitals, isolation wards can be set up to control infection in crowded places, or those lacking substantial medical facilities. Many major passenger ships contain separate wards which can be converted for use in isolating patients

UNIVERSAL PRECAUTIONS: STANDARDS AND SAFETY PECAUTIONS

Universal precautions refers to the practice of avoiding contact with patients' bodily fluids, by means of the wearing of nonporous such as medical gloves, goggles, and face shields. Medical instruments, especially scalpels and hypodermic needles should be handled carefully and disposed of properly in a sharps container. Pathogens fall into two broad categories, blood borne (carried in the body fluids) and air borne. Standard universal precautions cover both types.

> **Universal precautions**
>
> In order avoid discrimination, treat all bodily fluids and fecal matter as though they may be infected and observe the following precautions:
>
> 1. **Use barrier protection:** Cover up any open wounds or sores before proceeding
> 2. **Wear gloves** when handling bodily fluids or contaminated materials and other waste
> 3. **Wear a face mask/gown**
> 4. **Use caution** when handling sharp objects, needles, and waste
> 5. **Discard contaminated materials** Follow biohazard procedures for disposal
> 6. **Clean area** thoroughly with disinfectant
> 7. **Wash hands thoroughly** with soap and waterfor at least 20 seconds
> 8. **Wash clothing** in hot water

Universal precautions should be practiced in any environment where workers are exposed to bodily fluids, such as: blood, semen, vaginal secretions, synovial fluid, amniotic fluid, cerebrospinal fluid, pleural fluid, peritoneal fluid, pericardial fluid, bodily fluids that do not require such precautions include: feces, nasal secretions, urine, vomitus, perspiration, sputum, saliva.

Universal precautions are the infection control techniques that were recommended following the AIDS outbreak in the 1980s. Essentially it means the every patient is treated as if they are infected and therefore precautions are taken to minimize risk. Essentially, universal precautions are good hygiene habits such as washing and the use of gloves and other barriers correct sharps handling and aseptic techniques.

Conditions Indicating Additional Precautions

- Disease with airborne transmission (e.g. tuberculosis)
- Disease with droplet transmission (e.g. mumps, rubella, influenza, pertussis)
- Transmission by direct or indirect contact with dried skin (e.g. colonization with MRSA) or contaminated surfaces.
- Or any combination of the above.
  Universal precautions are recommended not only for doctors, nurses and patients, but for health care support workers. Some support workers, most notably laundry and housekeeping staff, may be required to come into contact with patients or bodily fluids.

Protective clothing may include but is not limited to:
- Barrier gowns
- Gloves
- Eyewear (goggles or glasses)
- Hair nets
- Shoe coverings.

Body Substance Isolation

Body substance isolation is a practice of isolating all body substances (blood, urine, feces, tears, etc.) of individuals undergoing medical treatment, particularly emergency medical treatment of those who might be infected with illnesses such as HIV, or hepatitis so as to reduce as much as possible the chances of transmitting these illnesses. BSI is similar in nature to universal precautions, but goes further in isolating substances not currently known to carry HIV.

Types of body substance isolation include: Hospital gowns, medical gloves, shoe covers, surgical mask, and safety glasses.

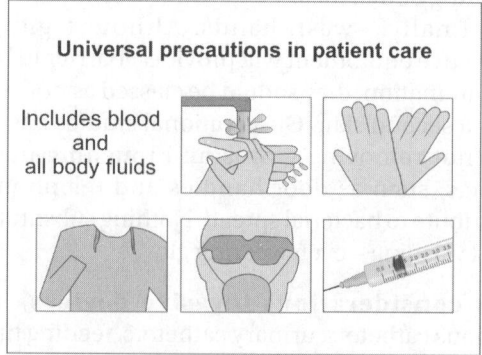

Fig. 9.11: Universal precautions in patient care.

Standard Universal Precautions

- **Barrier protection** should be used at all times to prevent skin and mucous membrane contamination with blood, body fluids containing visible blood, or other body fluids (cerebrospinal, synovial, pleural, peritonea, pericardial, and amniotic fluids, semen and vaginal secretions). Barrier protection should be used with ALL tissues. The type of barrier protection used should be appropriate for the type of procedures being performed and the type of exposure anticipates. Examples of barrier protection include disposable, lab coats, gloves, and eye and face protection.
- **Gloves** are to be worn when there is potential for hand or skin contact with blood, other potentially infectious material, or items and surfaces contaminated with these materials.
- **Wear face protection** (face shield) during procedures that are likely to generate droplet of blood or body fluid to prevent exposure to mucous membranes of the mouth, nose and eyes.
- **Wear protective body clothing** when there is a potential for splashing of blood or body fluids.
- **Never try to pipette** by mouth. Use mechanic pipetting devices instead.
- **Wash hands** or other skin surface, thoroughly and immediately if contaminate with blood, body fluids containing visible blood or other body fluids to which universe precautions apply.
- **Wash hands** immediately after gloves are removed.
- **Avoid accidental injuries** that can be cause by needles, scalpel blades, laboratory instruments, etc. when performing procedures, cleaning instruments, handling sharp instruments, and disposing of used needles, pipettes, etc.
- **Used needles, disposable syringes**, scalpel blades, pipettes, and other sharp items are to be places in puncture resistant containers marked with a biohazard symbol for disposal.

ASEPSIS

Dictionary meaning of asepsis is the state of being free of pathogenic microorganisms. It is the process of removing pathogenic microorganisms or protecting against infection by such organisms.

Definition: Asepsis is the practice to reduce or eliminate contaminants (such as bacteria, viruses, fungi and parasites) from entering the operative field in surgery or medicine to prevent infection. Ideally, a field is "sterile"-Free of contaminants (freedom from infection)—a situation that is difficult to attain.

However, sterility is only a means to the goal of elimination of infection.

- Absence of microorganisms in the environment to reduce the risk of infection.
- Asepsis is the absence of germs or pathogens.

Definition of Aseptic Techniques: Aseptic technique is the effort to keep principles of asepsis:

Asepsis is defined as preventing exposure to microorganisms and prevention of infection. Three things that are extremely important in achieving asepsis are the reduction of time, trauma and trash. Client as free from hospital microorganisms as possible.

- Time of surgical procedure is an important factor, as the longer a procedure takes the greater possibility of the contamination and therefore infection.
- Trauma that is sustained by the tissue as a result of rough handling, drying out upon exposure to room air, excessive dead space, implants or foreign bodies or non-optimal temperatures will contribute to infections.
- Trash refers to contamination by bacteria or foreign matter. It may be possible to follow slightly different procedures for achieving asepsis when performing surgery on small patients such as rodents, birds, reptiles and amphibians. Typically, surgical times are short, incisions are small and the amount of tissue trauma is minimal. These all minimize the risk of infection.

Essential Components of Maintaining Asepsis in a Hospital Include

- Hand washing.
- Utilizing gloves, gown and mask as indicated.
- Cleaning equipment.
- Handling linens in ways that prevent germs from spreading.

Types of Asepsis

The two types of aseptic techniques the nurse practices are medical and surgical asepsis.

- Medical asepsis or clean technique includes procedure used to reduce the number of microorganisms and prevent their spread. Changing a client's bed linen daily or when soiled, hand washing are examples of medical asepsis.
- Surgical asepsis or sterile technique includes procedures used to eliminate microorganisms from an area. Sterilization destroys all microorganisms and their spores. Sterile technique is practiced in Operation Theater and areas where sterile instruments are used. The techniques used in maintaining surgical asepsis are more rigid than those performed in medical asepsis.

Guidelines for maintaining medical asepsis:

- Thorough hand washing is basic technique for infection control.
- Know about the client's susceptibility to infection, e.g. Age, nutritional status, stress, etc.
- Recognize the causative factors and initiate measures to prevent onset and spread of infection.
- Never use aseptic techniques haphazardly.

What is aseptic technique?

- Bacteria are everywhere, and some are good for us while others are harmful.
- Bacteria, viruses, and other microorganisms that cause disease are called pathogens. To protect patients from harmful bacteria and other pathogens during medical procedures, health care providers use aseptic technique.
- Aseptic technique means using practices and procedures to prevent contamination from pathogens.
- It involves applying the strictest rules to minimize the risk of infection. Healthcare workers use aseptic technique in surgery rooms, clinics, outpatient care centers, and other health care settings

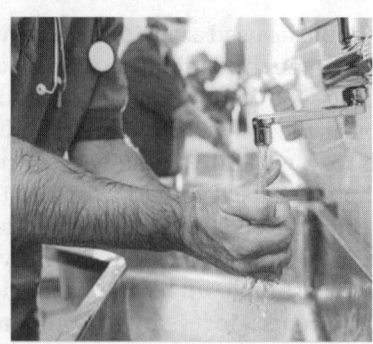

Fig. 9.12: Aseptic technique.

- Protect health workers from exposure to infectious agents.
- Aware of the body sites where nosocomial infections can occur.

Medical hand washing: The most important technique in preventing and controlling transmission of pathogens is hand washing. Hand washing is a vigorous, brief rubbing together of all surfaces of hands lathered in soap, followed by rinsing under a stream of water. Its main purpose is to remove soiled microorganisms from the hands and to reduce total microbial counts over time.

Gamer and Favero (1985) recommended that nurses wash hands in the following situations:
- Before contact with clients who are susceptible to infection.
- After caring for a client.
- After touching organic material.
- Before performing invasive procedures such as administration of injections, etc.
- Before and after handling dressings or touching open wounds.
- After handling contaminated equipment.
- Between contacts with clients in high risk units.
- After removal of sterile and nonsterile gloves.

The ideal duration of hand washing is not known. The Centers for Disease Control and Public Health Service note that washing time of 10 to 15 seconds will remove transient microorganisms from the skin. If hands are more soiled, more time may be required.

SURGICAL ASEPSIS

Surgical asepsis or aseptic technique is designed to eliminate all microorganisms, including spores and pathogens, from an object and to protect an area from microorganisms. Surgical asepsis or aseptic technique is designed to eliminate all microorganisms, including spores and pathogens, from an object and to protect an area from microorganisms.

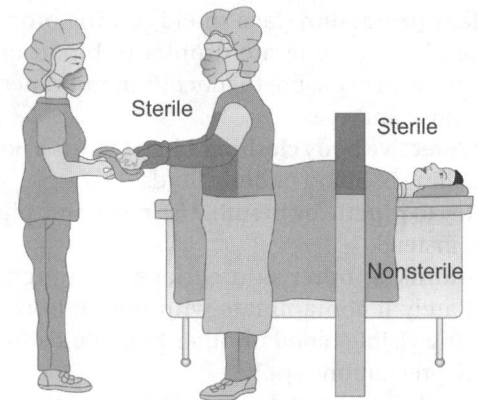

Fig. 9.13: Surgical aseptic technique practiced in operation theater.

Principles of Surgical Asepsis

- A sterile object remains sterile when touched only by another sterile object. This principle guides the nurse in placement of sterile objects and how to handle them.
- Only sterile objects may be placed on a sterile field. All items are properly sterilized before use.
- An object held below a person's waist is contaminated. Nurses never turn their backs on a sterile tray.
- A sterile object becomes contaminated by prolonged exposure to air. Nurse should avoid activities that create air currents such as excessive movements.
- When a sterile surface comes in contact with a wet contaminated surface the sterile object becomes contaminated by capillary action.
- Fluid flaws in the direction of gravity and sterile object becomes contaminated if gravity causes a contaminated liquid to flow over the object surface.
- The edge of a sterile field or container is considered to be contaminated.

Surgical Hand Washing/Scrub

- Articles: Soap/antiseptic detergent
- Running warm water

- Nail brush in antiseptic lotion
- Towels
- Mask and cap

Surgical asepsis is used to keep objects sterile or completely free from all microorganisms. It aims at the elimination of both pathogenic and non-pathogenic microorganisms.

Principles in surgical asepsis

Principles	Rationale
Always face the sterile field Do not turn back or side on a sterile field	Sterile objects which are out of vision are considered questionable and their sterility cannot be guaranteed.
Keep sterile equipment above your waist level or above table level.	Waist level and table level are considered margins of safety and will promote maximum visibility of the sterile field.
Do not speak, sneeze and cough over a sterile field.	To prevent or droplet infection.
Never reach across sterile field	When a nonsterile object is held above a sterile object, gravity causes microorganisms to fall into the sterile field.

Surgical Aseptic Procedures

- **Theater dress**: All persons entering the operation theater must change into theater clothing, and should wear antistatic shoes. There is special dress for doctors, nurses and other theater staff. Cotton is the material used for these dresses. It allows both, circulation of air over the body, and evaporation from the skin.
- **Mask**: It should be worn by nurses within the aqua theater.
- **Theater headwear**: All the staff working in the actual theater must ensure that their hair is completely covered. A wide range of attractive and practical headwear is now available in a variety of colors designs. Where large numbers of staff are employed, it may be useful to use different colors or patterns to denote grades. Disposable hats are popular because they are light weight and comfortable to wear and they do not interfere with hearing.
- **Gowning**: The gown will be prepared on a sterile towel by the circulator. Disposable hand towels can be included in the gown pack. The various steps to be taken in this connection are:
  - Pick up one towel so that it remains folded in half, length-wise.
  - Use one end of the towel to dry one hand, starting with fingers.
  - Use the other end of the towel to dry the arm, using a slower circular motion. Never return to an area which has been dried.

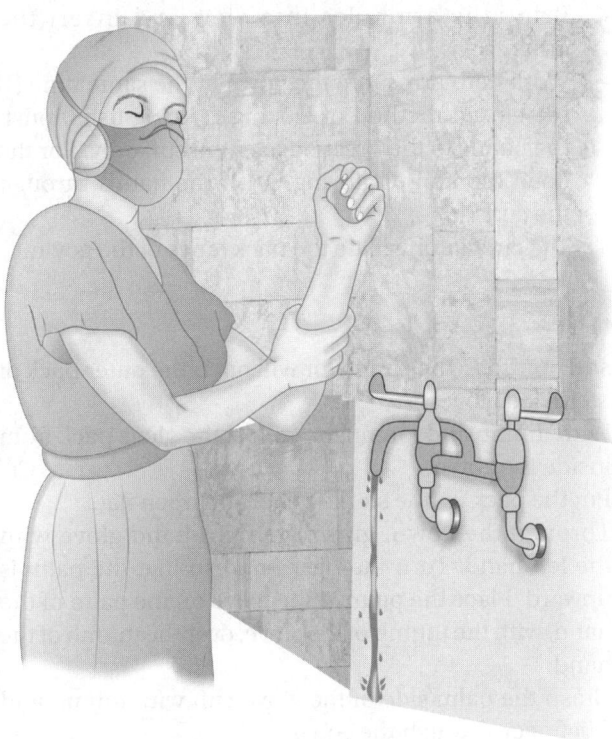

Fig. 9.14: Surgical hand washing.

Hand washing prior to Surgery: The firsthand-wish of the day should last for five minutes or as long as it takes to ensure that hands are both clean and disinfected.

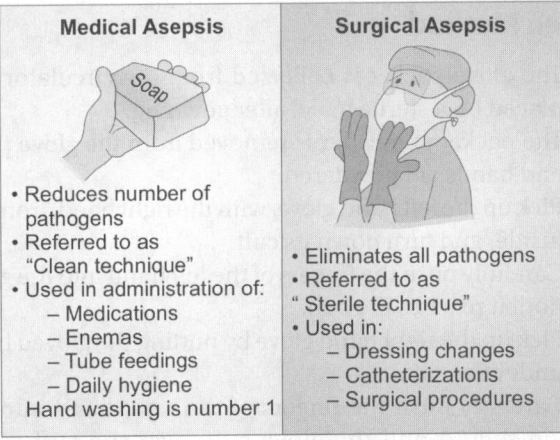

Fig. 9.15: Difference between medical and surgical asepsis.

- Repeat the procedure for the other hand.
- Discard the used towel.
- Pick up the gown firmly. It should be packed inside out to avoid the risk of touching the outside with the ungloved hand.
- Find the top of the gown. It is useful to have an indicator on gowns. This can be a colored tab or a mark, denoting the top.

- Hold the gown securely as it unfolds.
- Bring the armholes into view and insert the arms.
- Work both arms into the gown at the same time (If the closed method of gloving is being used, push the hands to the inner edge of the cuff only. For the open method of gloving, push the hands through the cuffs).
- The circulator will tie the back tapes of the gown.

Gloving

Closed method: The circulator will open the outer pack of the sterilized gloves.

- With thumb and forefinger, collect the glove pack from inside the gown.
- Put the pack on the sterile towel and open flat.
- Through the gown, grasp the right-hand glove with the left hand. Turn the right hand so that the palm is upward. Place the palm of the glove on the palm of the hand, with the thumb of the glove, over the thumb of the hand.
- Grasp the palm side of the glove cuff with thumb and forefinger, through the gown.
- With the left hand, still inside the cuff grasp the top cuff of the glove and pull it over the fingers.
- Push the fingers into the glove. Grasp the sleeve and glove, and pull on.
- Repeat the procedure for the left hand.
- Gloves can now be adjusted.

Open Method

- The glove packet is collected from the circulator and placed on a sterile towel after gowning.
- The packet of powder is removed from the glove pack, and hands are powdered.
- Pick up the left hand glove, with the right hand, from the inside, and turn down its cuff.
- Carefully push the fingers of the left hand into the glove until it reaches the cuff.
- Pick up the right hand glove by putting the gloved hand under the cuff.
- Carefully push the fingers of the right hand into the glove, and pull the glove cuff, over the cuff of the gown.
- Now pull the cuff of the left hand glove completely, over the gown cuff, of the left hand.

TRANSMISSION-BASED PRECAUTIONS

Transmission-based precautions are extra steps to follow for illnesses that are caused by certain germs. Transmission-based precautions are followed in addition to standard precautions. Some infections require more than one type of transmission-based precaution.

Disease-specific isolation recommendations

Standard Precautions
- CMV
- HIV
- Hepatitis B and C
- Aspergillosis

Contact Precautions
- MRSA (mask if respiratory infection)
- VRE
- Adenovirus
- Diarrhea
- C. difficile
- Rotavirus
- *E Coli* 0157
- Enterovirus
- Salmonella
- Shigella
- Hepatitis A
- Herpes zoster (shingles, localized)
- Herpes simplex
- Parainfluenza (mask if coughing)
- RSV (mask if productive cough)
- Lice
- Scabies
- Chickenpox (symptomatic, until all lesions crusted and dried)

Droplet Precautions
- Pertussis
- Influenza A or B
- MRSA (respiratory infection)
- *Neisseria meningitidis* (suspected or confirmed)
- Coxsackie
- Bacterial meningitis (for 24 hours after effective antibiotic therapy
- RSV (droplet and contact)
- Mumps
- Rubella

Airborne Precautions
- Chickenpox
- Disseminated herpes zoster (shingles)
- Measles

N-95 Mask:
- Tuberculosis
- SARS
- Avian influenza

Fig. 9.16: Disease-specific isolation recommendations.

Follow transmission-based precautions when an illness is first suspected. Stop taking these precautions only when that illness has been treated or ruled-out and the room has been cleaned. Patients should stay in their rooms as much as possible while these precautions are in place. They may need to wear masks when they leave their rooms.

Airborne precautions may be needed for germs that are so small they can float in the air and travel long distances.

- Airborne precautions help keep staff, visitors, and other patients from breathing in these germs and getting sick.
- Germs that warrant airborne precautions include chickenpox, measles and tuberculosis bacteria.
- Patients who have these germs should be in special rooms where the air is gently sucked out and not allowed to flow into the hallway. This is called a negative pressure room.
- Anyone who goes into the room should put on a well-fitted respirator mask before they enter.

Contact precautions may be needed for germs that are spread by touching.

- Contact precautions help keep staff and visitors from spreading the germs after touching a patient or an object the patient has touched.

- Some of the germs that contact precautions protect from are **C. difficile** and norovirus. These germs can cause serious infection in the intestines.
- Anyone entering the room—who may touch the patient or objects in the room—should wear a gown and gloves.

Droplet precautions are used to prevent contact with mucus and other secretions from the nose and sinuses, throat, airways, and lungs.
- When a patient talks, sneezes, or coughs, droplets that contain germs can travel about 3 feet.
- Illnesses that require droplet precautions include influenza (flu), pertussis (whooping cough), and mumps.
- Anyone who goes into the room should wear a surgical mask.

ROLE OF THE NURSE IN INFECTION CONTROL

The roles and responsibilities of the nurses in infection control are as follows:
- Providing staff education on infection control
- Reviewing infection control policies and procedures
- Reviewing client medical records and laboratory reports to recommend appropriate isolation procedures
- Screening client record for community acquired infection
- Consulting with employer health departments concerning recommendation to prevent and control the spread of infections among personnel such as tuberculosis testing
- Gathering statistics regarding the epidemiology of nosocomial infections
- Notifying public health department of incidences of communicable diseases
- Conferring with all hospital departments to investigate unusual events or clusters of infection
- Educating clients and families
- Identifying infection control problems with equipment
- Checking microorganism sensitivity to antibiotics in use and reminding medical staff of resistance.

Teaching about infection control: Clients should be taught to use basic principles of asepsis at home and in public facilities. Teaching about medical aspects and infection control is a challenging nursing responsibility. The following are examples of medical aseptic practices used in home:
- Wash hands before preparing food and before eating
- Prepare food at temperature sufficiently high to ensure that they are safe to eat
- Use care with cutting boards and utensils and wash hands, before and after handling raw meat
- Keep food refrigerated, especially those containing mayonnaise
- Wash raw fruits and vegetables before serving them
- Use pasteurized milk
- Wash hands after using the bathroom
- Use individual personal care items, such as wash cloths, towels, tooth brushes.

Observe infection prevention in public facilities by following these guidelines:
- Wash hands after using any public bathroom
- Use paper towels or hot air dryers in restroom
- Use individually wrapped drinking straws
- Use tongs to lift food from common service trays in caterings food stores, and salad bars. The community reinforces medical aseptic practices in several ways which includes the following:
    - Use of sterilized combs and brushes in barber and beauty shops
    - Examination of food handlers for evidence of disease
    - Enforcement of frequent hand washing by food handlers.

Gowning for Isolation

The use of gowns in isolation is important primarily to protect clothing from getting soiled while administering patient care. The gown also prevents contact with infections microorganisms that could have exited from the patient. Donning, and isolation gown, is indicated when caring for patients with diseases characterized by heavy drainage, infectious and acute diarrhea and other gastrointestinal disorders, respiratory disorder, skin wounds or burns and urinary disorders.

The supply needed for gowning for isolation is as 'isolation gown'. Isolation gowns open at the back with ties at the neck and the waist. This keeps the gown securely closed, protecting the back of the uniforms, as well as the fronts. The gown should be long enough to cover the uniform and have long sleeves with cuffs for added protection.

The nurse gowns for isolation for the following reasons:
- To prevent the nurse from contracting an infection from patients
- To prevent medical personnel from contaminating the patient who has a disease affecting the immune system.

Donning Gloves

Nurses or health care personnel wear/don gloves if there is any possibility of contact with infectious material. Nurses

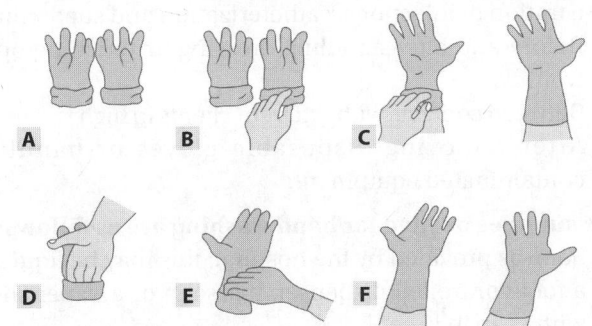

Figs. 9.17A to F: Gloving technique.

wear gloves for all types of patient care for the following reasons:
- To protect the nurse and the nurses family from disease
- To protect the patient from the nurse, who may be considered a contaminator to the patient
- To protect the personnel from contact with the infectious microorganism.

The supply needed for donning gloves is a 'pair of gloves'.

Donning a Mask

A mask should be worn for the following purposes:
- To prevent the wearer from inhaling microorganism that travel on airborne droplets for short distances or that remain suspended in the air for longer periods
- To prevent inhaling pathogens if resistance is reduced or if being transported to another area (patient use)
- To discourage that wearer from touching the mouth, nose, or eye and from transmitting infection material.

Double Bagging

A single bag is adequate if the contaminated articles can be placed in the bag without contamination of the outside of the bag. Double bagging is recommended when it is impossible to keep the outer surface of the single bag, free from contamination. The second bag should be labeled for color coded to alert nursing personnel's and to prevent contamination of housekeeping personnel's when handling contaminated material. Double bag can be used for safe removal of any article from room.

Double bagging has purposes, i.e. to prevent spread of microorganism to the surrounding area and to prevent potential accidental exposure of personnel to contaminated article. The supplies and equipment needed for double bagging are as follows:
- Single isolation bag
- Special color coded bag
- Holder for isolation bag
- Isolation gown, mask and clean gloves
- Holder for laundry bags

Isolation Technique

The type of isolation technique followed will depend on transmissibility of the pathogen. The use of environmental barriers will keep pathogens in a confined care, i.e. private room, isolation room, closed door, protective gown, masks and gloves and shoe covers. The nurse follows isolation technique to prevent the transmission of infection from microorganisms by preventing pathogens from leaving the room of the infected patient or from entering the room of a highly susceptible patient.

The supplies and equipment needed for isolation technique are as follows:
- Isolation gown, masks, gloves
- Clean linen
- Single and double isolation bags
- Paper towels
- Running water
- Soap with dispenser
- Holder for isolation bag and laundry bag.

Medical Hand Washing

Hand washing is a vigorous, brief rubbing together of all surfaces of hands lathered in soap, followed by rinsing under a stream of water. The purpose is to remove soil and transient organisms from the hands and to reduce total microbial counts over time. It is the most important preventive technique for interrupting the infection process.

Hand washing is the single most important means for preventing the spread of infections. It is frequently, however, incorrectly or inadequately done in an attempt to save time. Unfortunately, this may cause increased infections and longer patient hospitalization at increased cost. Contaminated hands are a prime cause of cross infection. The need for hand washing depends on the type, intensity, duration and sequence of activity. Hand washing of nurses recommended the following situations:

- Upon arising at the clinical unit prior to beginning a period of duty. This will serve to decrease the microorganism transported to the hospital from external environment. Nurses also wash their hands prior to leaving the area for rest and meal break in order to decrease of microorganism to other areas of the hospital and to themselves.
- Before contact with clients who are susceptible to infections, e.g. newborn infants, clients with leukemia, organ transplant recipients and HIV +ve cases, in order to prevent the spread of microorganisms.
- After caring for infected clients.
- Prior to performing any clean duties such as preparing medications, handling food trays, assembling equipment or selecting clean linen.
- After touching organic material, i.e. after performing any duties involving contaminated articles such as bedpans, surgical dressings, soiled tissues or dirty linen.
- Before performing invasive procedures such as administration of injections, catheterization and suctioning.
- Before and after handling dressing or touching open wounds.
- Between contacts with different clients in high risk units.
- After removing disposable gloves or handling contaminated equipment.

The supplies needed for hand washing are as follows:
- Soap as provided by the hospital; this may be liquid in a foot controlled dispenser, bar soap or a paper sheet with soap in it
- Stick or brush for cleaning fingernails.

TRANSPORTATION OF INFECTIOUS PATIENTS

Limiting the movement and transport of patients infected with virulent or epidemiologically important microorganisms and ensuring that such patients leave their rooms only for essential purposes reduces opportunities for transmission of microorganisms in hospitals.

When patient transport is necessary, it is important that 1. Appropriate barriers (e.g. masks, impervious dressings) are worn or used by the patient to reduce the opportunity for transmission of pertinent microorganisms to other patients, personnel, and visitors and to reduce contamination of the environment; 2. Personnel in the area to which the patient is to be taken are notified of the impending arrival of the patient and of the precautions to be used to reduce the risk of transmission of infectious microorganisms; and, 3. Patients are informed of ways by which they can assist in preventing the transmission of their infectious microorganisms to others

Patients on precautions should not be taken out of their isolation rooms for nonessential purposes. When it becomes necessary to transport the patient to another area of the hospital, appropriate barriers to prevent disease transmission should be utilized such as masks, gowns and gloves. These barriers should remain in place for the entire period the patient is out of the isolation room. Before transporting a patient on Airborne Precautions out of the isolation room, see Policy for Transporting Patients on Airborne Precautions.

Infected patient transport within institution

- If patient has airborne or droplet transmitted infection should only leave room, if essential
- Patient should wear mask during transport
- Transport personnel should wear appropriate PPE
- Transport route should avoid populated areas
- Receiving personnel should be aware of what PPE and infection control procedures are needed and when patient is coming
- Protect stretchers or wheelchairs appropriately
- Appropriate hand hygiene should be used

Steps

- Notify Ambassador Services and the area expecting patient that the patient requires isolation precautions.
- Explain transportation procedure to patient.
- Outside room, drape a clean sheet over the stretcher or wheelchair to cover entire area which will come in contact with patient.
- Those accompanying patient must don gown, mask, and gloves as indicated by type of isolation/precaution.
- For patients on Airborne, Contact, or Droplet Precautions, patient's nurse should place mask on patient. Carry a paper bag and specimen cup for disposal of respiratory secretions, if necessary.
- Assist patient onto stretcher or wheelchair. Cover patient with a clean sheet or blanket obtained outside room. If patient must be transported in his bed, wipe exposed areas of bed with a germicide (head and foot of bed, handrails, areas which may be touched during transport). If a child needs to be transported, use an extra (clean) crib if at all possible.
- The front of the patient's chart should be labeled with the appropriate isolation sticker.
- After readying patient for transport, remove any isolation garb which has had direct contact with the patient or patient's environment and don fresh garb.
- Transport patient to other area being careful to not touch elevator buttons, doorknobs, or handles with contaminated gloves. Ask others to push elevator buttons or do so with a part of the body unlikely to have been contaminated during the transport (e.g. an elbow).
- Report to personnel receiving patient that the patient is on isolation, and make sure they know the precautions that are necessary.
- When transportation of patient is completed, discard linen in plastic bag and remove garb as in procedure.
- With clean gloves on, disinfect stretcher, wheelchair or bed (if an extra bed was used) with hospital disinfectant.
- Remove gloves, cleanse hands.

DECONTAMINATION OF EQUIPMENT AND UNIT

The need for decontamination depends on the suspected exposure and in most cases will not be necessary. The goal of decontamination after a potential exposure to a biological agent is to reduce the extent of external contamination of the patient and contain the contamination in order to prevent further spread. Decontamination should only be considered in instances of gross contamination. Decisions regarding the need for decontamination should be made in consultation with state and local health departments.

Decontamination of exposed individuals prior to receiving them in the healthcare facility may be necessary to ensure the safety of patients and staff while providing care. When developing Bioterrorism Readiness Plans, facilities should consider available locations and procedure for patient decontamination prior to facility entry.

Depending on the agent, the likelihood for re-aerosolization or the risk associated with cutaneous exposure, clothing of exposed persons may need to be removed. After removal of contaminated clothing, patients should be instructed (or assisted if necessary) to immediately shower with soap and water. Potentially harmful practices, such as bathing patients with bleach solutions, are unnecessary and should be avoided.

Clean water, saline solution, or commercial ophthalmic solutions are recommended for rinsing eyes. If indicated, after removal at the decontamination site, patient clothing should be handled only by personnel wearing appropriate personal protective equipment, and placed in an impervious bag to prevent further environmental contamination.

PERSONAL PROTECTING EQUIPMENT

The following includes recommendations for patient decontamination when the contaminate is a biological agent. Preferred staff protection for biological decontamination is generally at PPE.

Gloves

- Gloves should be worn when contact with blood or body fluids is anticipated.
- Gloves should be worn when touching environmental surfaces and/or patient care articles likely to be contaminated or soiled with blood or body fluids.
- Gloves should be put on just prior to performing a patient care task that involves contact with blood or body fluids.
- Gloves should be removed immediately, without touching non-contaminated surfaces, as soon as the patient care task is complete.
- When performing multiple procedures on the same patient, gloves should be changed after contact with blood and body fluids that contain high concentrations of microorganisms (e.g. feces, wound drainage or oropharyngeal secretions) and before contact with a clean body site such as non-intact skin and vascular access sites.

Facial Protection

Facial protection should be worn when performing patient care tasks likely to generate splashing or spraying of blood and body fluids onto the mucous membranes of the face. Facial protection may include:
- Disposable, fluid-resistant masks
- Eye shields (goggles with side-shields)
- Face shield

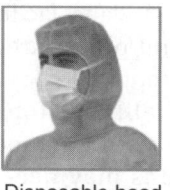
Disposable hood

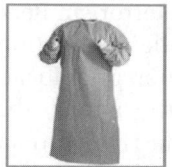
Disposable non-woven gown

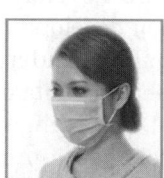
3 Ply mouth mask

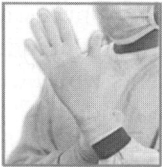
Surgical gloves

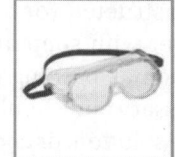
Disposable eye gear

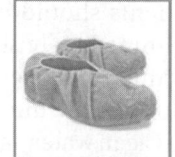
Disposable shoe cover

Fig. 9.18: Types of personal protection equipment (PPE kit).

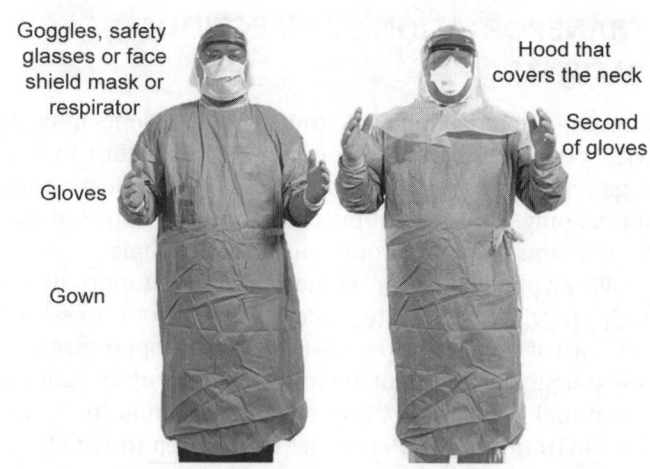

Fig. 9.19: Nurse equipped with personal protective equipment.

Gowns

- Disposable fluid-repelling gowns should be worn to protect skin and clothing when performing procedures likely to generate splashing or spraying of blood and body fluids.
- Plastic aprons may be worn for procedures likely to soil clothing but are unlikely to generate splashing or spraying of blood or body fluids (e.g. cleaning incontinent patients).
- The material composition of the gown should be appropriate to the amount of fluid penetration likely to be encountered.
- Soiled gowns must be removed after patient contact.

BIOMEDICAL WASTE MANAGEMENT

A hospital is an institution which produces many types of waste material. Housekeeping activity generates considerable amount of trash, the visitors and others bring with them food, fruits and other materials which must be in some way disposed off. In addition to waste that is produced in all residential buildings, hospitals generate pathological waste (blood soaked dressings, carcasses and similar waste).

These waste materials must be suitably disposed off immediately lest they putrefy, emit foul smells, act as a source of infection, disease and become a public health hazard. Hospital waste still finds its way to roadside heaps of rubbish, where it mixes with municipal corporation solid waste, rendering it hazardous for the environment and the public. All these years, the management of hospital waste was relegated to the hands of nurses, ward boys, ward ayahs, sweepers and sanitary workers. Now, the 'Hospital waste' also termed as 'Biomedical waste' and the management of biomedical waste shall be the duty of every person who has control over an institution or its premises of an institution generating biomedical waste, which includes a hospital, nursing home, clinic, dispensary, veterinary institution, animal house, pathological laboratory, blood bank by whatever name called to take all steps to ensure that such waste is handled without any adverse effect to human health and the environment.

Infection Control in Clinical Setting

Category	Type of bag/container used	Type of waste	Treatment/disposal options
Yellow	Nonchlorinated plastic bags Separate collection system leading to effluent treatment system	a) Human anatomical waste b) Animal anatomical waste c) Soiled waste d) Expired or discarded medicines e) Chemical waste f) Micro, bio-t and other clinical lab waste g) Chemical liquid	Incineration or plasma pyrolysis or deep burial
Red	Nonchlorinated plastic bags or containers	**Contaminated waste (recyclable)** tubing, bottles, intravenous tubes and sets, catheters, urine bags, syringes (without needles) and gloves.	Auto/micro/hydro and then sent for recycling, not be sent to landfill
White	(Translucent) puncture, leak, tamper proof containers	**Waste sharps including metals**	Auto or dry heat sterilization followed by shredding or mutilation or encapsulation
Blue	Cardboard boxes with blue colored marking	**Glassware**	Disinfection or auto/micro/hydro and then sent for recycling

Nurses are responsible and accountable for professional behavior that involves application of the nursing process and cooperation with appropriate others within current legislation affecting the practice of nursing according to professions code of ethics and practice with the context of the policies and practices of the employing agency and within the customs and values of the society in which the nursing care is being provided. This has direct application to hospital nursing practice, which includes biomedical waste management.

Concept of Waste

As we know that waste constitutes an important part of the environment to which man is continuously exposed, which includes refuse or solid wastes, excreta or night soil and sullage. The term 'refuse' is applied to all solid waste from human habitations that is not covered by the sewers, i.e. all wastes other than sullage (waste water or slop water and comprises all liquid wastes including industrial waste. It includes public refuse (originating from homes, hotels, institutions, street, stables and markets) and industrial refuse. The solid waste originating from homes or domestic refuse consists of garbage, rubbish and ash.

- Garbage is the waste from food during its handling at various stages including preparation, cooking and serving.
- Rubbish comprise of dirt, dust and bits of paper, wood, clothing, glass, rubber, plastic, metal, etc.

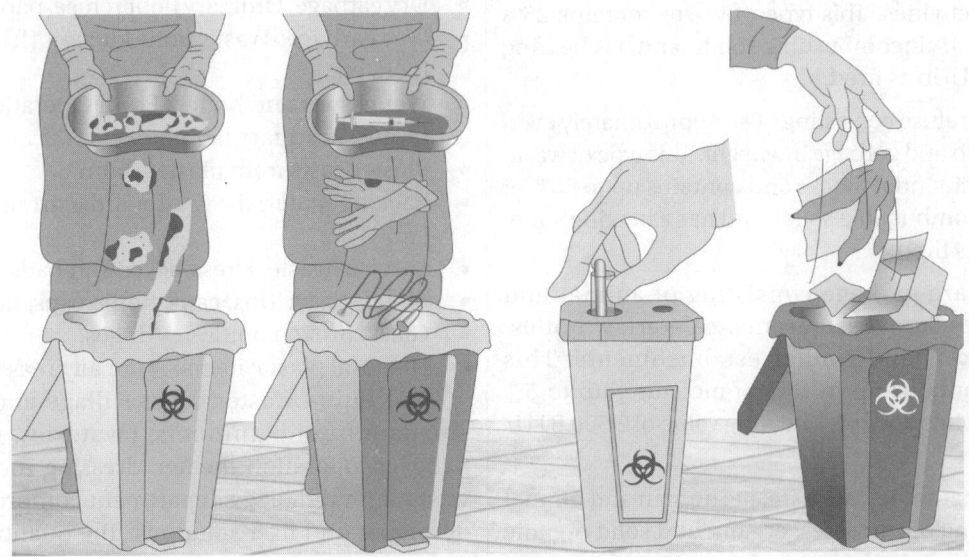

Fig. 9.20: Segregation of hospital waste.

- Ash is the residue after burning of fuel. Different types of wastes impinge upon physical, mental and social health in various ways. For example, solid waste if allowed to accumulate, is a health hazard, because:
  - It decomposes and favors fly breeding (Flies may help to spread certain diseases like diarrheal disease).
  - It attracts rodents (for example, rats may help to spread dengue fever or plague, etc.) and also attracts vermin (e.g. mosquito help to transmit malaria or filaria).
  - The pathogens which may be present in the solid waste, may be conveyed back to man's food through flies and dust; dust may harbor Tubercle bacilli and other micro-organisms which cause diseases accordingly).
  - There is a possibility of water and soil pollution may lead to many infections and infestations (e.g. soil polluted with night soil may be rich in tetanus spores).
- Heaps of refuse present an unsightly appearance and nuisance from bad odors.

Types of Waste

Wastes are divided into following types which include:

Type 0 wastes refers to a waste which is a mixture of highly combustible as paper, cardboard, cartons, wooden boxes and combustible, floor sweeping from commercial, industrial and housekeeping activities. The mixture contains up to 10% weight of plastic bags, coated paper, laminated paper, treated corrugated paper, oily rags and plastic and rubber scraps. This type of waste contains 10% of moisture, 5% incombustible solids and has heating value of 8500 BTU/lb as fired.

Type 1 waste is rubbish consisting of combustible waste such as paper cartons, rags, wood scrap, sawdust, foliage, and floor sweeping from domestic, commercial and industrial activities. This type of waste contains 25% moisture, up to 10% incombustible solids, and has heating value of 6500 BTU/lb as fired.

Type 2 waste is a refuse consisting of an approximately even mixture of rubbish and garbage by weight. This type of waste is common to residential blocks and contains up to 50% of moisture, 7% incombustible solids and has a heating value of 4300 BTU/lb as fired.

Type 3 wastes are garbage consisting of animal and vegetable wastes from restaurants, cafeterias, hotels, hospitals, markets and similar establishments. This type of waste contains up to 70% of moisture, up to 5% incombustible solids and has a heating value of 2,500 BTU/lb as fired.

Type 4 waste is pathological waste, i.e. human and animal remains consisting of carcasses, organs, and solid organic wastes from hospitals, laboratories, abattoirs, animal pounds and similar source containing up to 85% moisture, 5% incombustible solids and having a heating value of 1000 BTU/lb as fired.

Types 5 and 6 wastes are by product waste, gaseous, liquid, semi-liquid, and solid from industrial operations. Calorific value must be determined for the individual material to be destroyed.

Classification of Hospital Waste

Hospital waste can be defined as any discarded, unwanted residual matter arising from the hospital or activities related to the hospital 'Disposal' covers the total process of collecting, handling, packing, storage, transportation and final treatment of wastes. Hospital waste can be classified into two major groups—solid wastes and liquid wastes.

WHO Classification

Waste Categories	Description and Examples
General waste	No risk to human health, e.g. Office paper, wrapper, kitchen waste, general sweeping, etc.
Pathological waste	Human tissue or fluid, e.g. Body parts, blood, body fluid, etc.
Sharps	Sharp waste, e.g. Needle, scalpes, knives, blades, etc.
Infectious waste	Which may transmit bacterial, viral or parasitic disease to human being, waste suspected to contain pathogen, e.g. laboratory culture, tissues (swabs) bandage, etc.
Chemical waste	Laboratory reagent, disinfectants, film developer
Radioactive waste	Unused liquid from radiotherapy or lab research, contaminated glasswares, etc.

The solid wastes of a hospital include the following:
- Dry garbage: Ordinary floor refuse, papers, flowers, fresh
- Wet garbage: Waste from kitchen (fruit peels, leftover food, etc.)
- Wet tissues and bones: From Operation Theater, labor rooms, mortuary laboratory.
- Plaster casts from plaster room.
- Packing materials: Cardboard, cartons, paper packets, etc.
- Surgical waste: Dressing, cotton pads.
- Metal waste: Tins, cans, bottle caps, needles.
- Glass: Broken bottles, syringes.
- Disposal plastic items: From all areas in hospital.

The liquid wastes cover sullage and sewage which emanate from bathrooms, lavatories, toilets, kitchen, pantries, operation theater, dressing room, laundry and waste from radiology department comprising of chemical developer and fixer solutions. The quantity of total liquid waste is estimated at 300 to 400 liters per bed per day.

Biomedical Waste

In daily usage, waste refers to pieces of paper, pieces of cloth, leftover food, portion of commodity, ashes, animals droppings, animals dead bodies including unused articles swept from roads, markets, hospitals, etc. 'Hazardous wastes', refers to waste or parts of waste, according to their physical, chemical components and their infection that could cause sickness, death or possibility of being harmful to health of animals' things and environment if its collection, transportation and disposal are inappropriately managed. Now the term 'Hospital waste' replaced by the term 'biomedical waste'. According to World Health Organization, "Medical Waste" refers to that portion of a health care or research facilities total waste stream that contains potentially infectious agents, hazardous chemicals or radioactive materials, which includes:

- **Solid medical waste:** Wastes such as needles, infusion sets, bandages, anatomical wastes, isolation wastes and all other materials contaminated or potentially contaminated with blood and/or body fluids from medical diagnoses, treatment or research.
- **Liquid medical waste:** Wastes such as blood, body fluids, dialysis solutions, chemical reagents, solvents, acids, heavy metal solutions, film developers, cytotoxic and other pharmaceuticals resulting from medical treatment or research.
- **Isolation waste:** All disposable materials associated with a medical patient or isolated from other patients to prevent transmission of a very infectious disease.
- **Household waste (domestic):** Solid wastes that do not contain solid biomedical waste, household waste originating from medical treatment or research centers include uncontaminated wastes such as office paper and packaging material. According to the Gazette of India "Biomedical Waste" means any waste, which is generated during diagnosis, treatment or immunization of human beings animals or in research activities pertaining there to or in the production or testing of biological and including categories mentioned in Schedule 1 Union Ministry of Environment and Forest, Gazette Notification dated 20 July, 1998 which includes the following:
  - **Category No. 1:** Human anatomical waste: Human tissues, organs, body parts.
  - **Category No. 2:** Animal waste: Animal tissues, organs, body parts, carcasses, bleeding parts, fluids, blood and experimental animals used in research, waste generated by veterinary hospitals or colleges, discharges from hospitals or animal house.
  - **Category No. 3:** Microbiology and biotechnology waste: Waste from laboratory cultures, stocks or specimen of microorganisms live or attenuated, vaccines, human and animal cells culture used, infectious agents from research and industrial laboratories, waste from production of biological toxins, dishes, devices used for transfer of cultures.

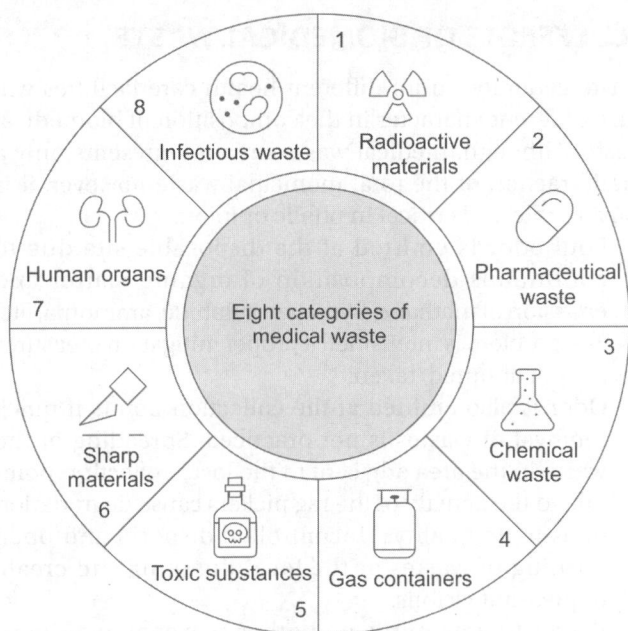

Fig. 9.21: Categories of medical waste.

  - **Category No. 4:** Waste sharps: Needles, syringes, scalpels, blades, glass, etc. that may cause puncture and cuts. This includes both used and unused sharps.
  - **Category No. 5:** Discarded medicine and cytotoxic drugs: Wastes comprising of outdated, contaminated and discarded medicines.
  - **Category No. 6:** Solid waste: Items contaminated with blood and fluids including cotton, dressings, soiled plaster casts, linen beddings, other material contaminated with blood.
  - **Category No. 7:** Solid waste: Wastes generated from disposable items other than the waste sharp such as tubings, catheters, intravenous sets, etc.
  - **Category No. 8:** Liquid waste: Waste generated from laboratory; washing, cleaning, housekeeping, and disinfecting activities.
  - **Category No. 9:** Incineration ash: Ash for incineration of any biomedical waste.
  - **Category No. 10:** Chemical: Use in production of biological, chemicals, used in disinfection as insecticides, etc. Thus, biomedical waste refers to any waste that consists wholly or partly of human tissue or animal tissue, blood and other body fluids, excretions, drugs or other pharmaceutical products including antineoplastic drugs, swabs, dressings, syringes, needles or other sharp instruments being waste which unless rendered safe, may prove hazardous to any person coming in contact with it and any other waste arising from medical, nursing, dental, pharmaceutical or similar practice, investigation including radioactive waste, treatment, care, teaching or research or collection of blood and blood product from transfusion, being waste, which may cause infection to any person coming in contact with it.

ILL EFFECTS OF BIOMEDICAL WASTE

Waste generated from different health care facilities will have different character in the composition of biomedical waste. Although, medical waste stream represents only a small fraction of the total municipal waste however, it is most visible and critical in public opinion.

- Foul odor is emitted at the disposable site due to continuous decomposition of organic matter and emission of methane, hydrogen sulphide, ammonia, etc. The problem is intensified if proper mitigation measures are not adopted/taken.
- Odor is also emitted at the collection points if quick removal of wastes is not practiced. Spreading of the waste in the area adjacent to the local collection point due to the activity of the rag pickers cause degradation of esthetic quality. Uncontrolled disposal and open burning of wastes at the local dumping site create unpleasant visions.
- Domestic rats, birds and other scavenging animals besides being esthetically unpleasant also act as reservoirs for many organs is transmissible to people, including plague, forms of typhus, leptospirosis, trichinosis, psittacosis, and salmonella infection.
- Chemical control of both house flies and rodents is not very effective because of widespread resistance to insecticides. The essential basis of control remains denial of access to food and harborage by covered storage bags and efficient removal of waste.
- Aedes mosquitoes, vectors of dengue fever and yellow fever, breed prolifically in discarded containers that trap rain water. Culex mosquitoes, vectors of filariasis, breed in polluted stagnant water. Such breeding sites often occur where hospital drains are blocked by solid waste.
- Hospital-acquired infections (nosocomial infections) have shown increase in incidence due to mismanagement of hospital wastes, e.g. hospital gangrene, hepatitis B and C, HIV and AIDS, tuberculosis, cholera, diphtheria, etc. and transfusion associated virus.
- Psychological and emotional distress related to the recognizable body parts like amputated limbs, abortus and dead feature thrown with the waste. Waste handlers working at the municipal dumping site refuse to handle waste which has body parts. Injury to the waste handlers leads to infections.

Problems Associated with BMW

Organism	Diseases caused	Related waste item
VIRUSES HIV, Hepatitis B, Hepatitis A,C, Arboviruses, Enteroviruses	AIDS, Infectious Hepatitis, Dengue, Japanese encephalitis, tic-borne fevers, etc.	Infected needles, body fluids, human excreta, soiled linen, blood, body fluids
BACTERIA Salmonella typhi, Vibrio cholerae, Clostridium tetani, Pseudomonas, Streptococcus	Typhoid, Cholera, Tetanus, Wound infections, septicemia, rheumatic fever, endocarditis, skin and soft tissue infections	Human excreta and body fluid in landfills and hospital wards, Sharps such as needles, surgical blades in hospital waste.
PARASITES Wucheraria bancrofti, Plasmodium	Cutaneous leishmaniasis, Kala Azar, Malaria	Human excreta, blood and body fluids in poorly managed sewage system of hospitals.

- It is reported that 60% of all hospital staff sustain injuries from sharps, knowingly or unknowingly during various procedures undertaken in the health care facilities. Hospital personnel working in operation theater are specially prone to needle injuries while suturing. Injury to the professionals like physician, surgeons and nurses may lead to infection such as hepatitis B and HIV infections because they handle the waste during performing surgical or diagnostic procedures. The effects associated with poor hospital waste management include the following:

Health Hazards

- Injuries from sharp to all categories of hospital personnel and waste handlers.
- Nosocomial infections due to poor infection control and poor waste management.
- Risks of infections outside the hospital for waste handlers, scavengers and eventually the general public.
- Risks associated with hazardous chemicals, drugs being handled by persons handling wastes at all levels.
- 'Disposable' being repacked and sold without being even washed.
- Drugs disposed being repacked and sold to unsuspecting buyers.

Environmental hazards: Toxic emissions like dioxins, furan gases carbon, sulphur particles from defective and inefficient incineration:

- Indiscriminate disposal of incinerator ash and residues.
- Leach ate from improper waste residues, leading to contamination of ground water.

At present, most health care workers, managers and administrators are familiar with the risk of disease transmission of blood borne pathogens.

Health Hazards of Various Waste

Waste materials	Potential hazards
Human anatomical waste	Psychological stress
Human anatomical waste, soiled waste, microbial waste, sharps	Infections and disease
Animal wastes	Infectious rabies, Anthrax and other
Sharps, cytotoxic and radioactive drugs, incinerator wastes	Injuries
Chemical, cytotoxic, radioactive, incinerator wastes	Dermatitis, conjunctivitis, bronchitis
Cytotoxic, radioactive drugs and materials, chemical wastes	Cancer, genetic mutation
Cytotoxic and other drugs, liquid and chemical wastes	Poisonings

In summary, the following areas need attention:
- Availability and use of hand washing facilities.
- Identification labeling and disposal of contaminated equipment like used syringes, needles, etc.
- Provision, use, accessibility and condition of PPE as and when required.
- Correct housekeeping practices.
- Establishment and implementation of hepatitis B, C and tetanus vaccination and post-exposure evaluation and follow-up.
- Compliance with hazard communication requirements.
- Proper labels and signs.
- Information and training.
- Record keeping including medical records for employees with occupational exposure, Training records.
- Hepatitis B, C and tetanus vaccination declaration forms.

Biomedical waste contains (or is likely to contain) blood borne pathogens. All workers who handle it are, therefore, at risk of exposure and are subject to the requirements including training, vaccination, protective equipment and clothing.

Air contamination: Most biomedical waste treatment and transport systems under normal operating conditions contaminate air, combustion systems and chemical treatment systems, all carry the potential to release toxic gases, vapors and particulates into the work area. In addition, systems that pre-shared biomedical waste (e.g. chemical, microwave, autoclave and irradiation systems) also carry the potential to release microbial aerosols into the work area. For working with the incinerator system, a respirator should be worn during manual ash clean out or charging of the incinerator.

Heat and fire hazards: All higher temperature thermal systems like boiler, incinerator and autoclave are potential sources of heat and fire at the workplace. Radiant and convective heat can greatly increase temperatures in the work area and may cause worker discomfort, heat stress or serious injury. During unusually warm weather, operators should be encouraged to take frequent short breaks and drink plenty of fluids. Any behavioral or physical symptoms of fatigue should be immediately brought to the attention of the authorities. Although, people usually get used to moderate condition of hot and cold over the course of about two to three weeks, this alone is rarely sufficient protection. Therefore, the amount of radiant and convective heat escaping to the surrounding work area must be reduced.

Eye injury hazards: Fully enclosed safety eye-cover should be routinely worn by all workers handling biomedical waste, especially those working with incinerators. High temperature systems carry the additional hazard of infrared radiation which can cause corneal cataracts and blindness.

Noise: Many biomedical waste treatment systems can be noisy. Noise poses a serious health problem and can cause irreversible hearing loss due to long-term exposure.

Need for biomedical waste management: In recent years, the number of health care facilities both in the Government and private sectors has grown considerably. All these health care facilities generate waste as a result of health care activities. No reliable figures about the quantum of waste generated per person per day are available. However, studies have estimated that the quantum of waste generated from hospitals ranges from 1.5 to 2.5 kg per day per patient. It may be more in specialized health care facilities like dialysis centers. In the west, the quantity of water generated is 4 to 5 kg per day per patient.

Objectives of Biomedical Waste Management

The objectives of the biomedical waste management are grouped as general and specific as given below:

General Objectives
- Reduction of the impact of this waste on the community.
- Reduction of the chances of infection and accidental injury to the workers.
- Reduction of cost of total treatment of waste.

Specific Objectives
- Motivation and sensitization of health care personnel.
- Training of health care personnel.
- Segregation of waste so that each type is treated in a auditable manner and thus minimizing harm.
- Using proper disinfection technology, depending on the type of waste.
- Fixing of responsibility in institutions for biomedical waste disposal and treatment.

ELEMENTS OF BIOMEDICAL WASTE MANAGEMENT

Biomedical waste management (both infectious and noninfectious) should be managed through a pathway composed of six elements, each must be addressed in terms

of personnel and material costs and occupational and safety risks. The six elements are:
1. Separation (segregation)
2. Identification (different colors-coded bags)
3. Handling (collection, measurement, storage, transport)
4. Treatment (off-site and on-site)
5. Waste reduction (by shredding)
6. Disposal.

Separation/Segregation: Good segregation practices will lead to decrease in total biomedical waste. There is a significant impact on cost saving by the implementation of street waste segregation practices. Each category of waste (according to Schedule 1, of the rules) has to be kept segregated in proper container or bag as the case may be. Such container must be sturdy enough to contain the designed maximum volume and weight of the waste without damage. It should be without any puncture or leakage. The container should have a cover, preferably operated by foot, if plastic bags are to be used, they have to be securely fitted within a container in such a manner that they stay in place during opening and closing of the lid and can also be removed without difficulty. The sharps must be multilated by a needle cutter, placed in the department/ward itself before putting them in puncture proof sharp containers. Attempts should be made to designate fixed places for each container that it becomes a part of regular scenario and practice for the concerned medical as well as nursing staff.

Identification: The color coding and type of container for disposal of biomedical wastes will be made according to Schedule II (Biomedical Waste Management and Handling Rules 1998). When a bag or container is sealed, a tag indicating the name of the department, type of waste, its content/composition, the person responsible arid his/her designation, date, shift, time, etc. has to be attached. A water proof marker pen should be used for writing.

Handling: The collection containers for biomedical waste have to be sturdy, leak proof, of adequate size and wheeled; two wheeled bins may be used. The four wheeled containers have two fixed wheels and two castors and they are fitted with wheel locking devices to prevent unwanted rolling. There should be not sharp edges or corners, especially metallic bins. Collection timings and duty chart should be pasted in a prominent place with copies given to the concerned waste collectors and supervisors. For general waste from the office, kitchens, garden, etc. normal wheel barrows may be used.

Separate service corridors for taking waste matter from the storage area to the collection room must be provided. These corridors should not cross the paths used by patients and visitors. The waste has to be taken to the common storage area first, from where it is to be taken to the treatment/disposal facility either within or outside premises, as the case may be. The wheel barrows containing general waste may be sent to a dumper container or further segregated as described under the rules of transportation, of biomedical waste. It is important that the following

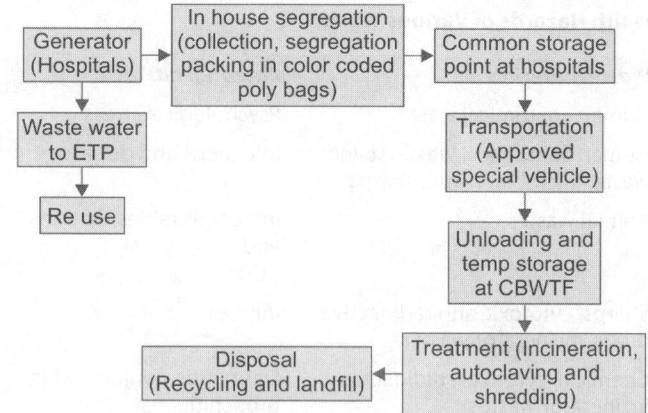

Fig. 9.22: Biomedical waste.

points be observed when transporting the waste within the hospital:
- Containers and bags should always be closed during transport.
- The earth used for this purpose will have smooth surface and be easy to clean, e.g. carts made with fiber glass bodies have smooth surface.
- The carts should be used exclusively for transporting waste.
- The carts should be washed daily with water, detergents and disinfectants.
- The waste bags or containers should never be dragged on the floor.
- The waste should never be transferred from one receptacle to another.
- In particular, the thumb rules while handling BMW are as follows:
  – Direct contact with the wastes must be avoided.
  – Bags should not be overfilled so that they may be closed easily.
  – Bags should not be emptied into other bags.
  Smaller units such as nursing homes, pathological laboratories, etc. do not have many department/units. In this case, intermediate storage is not required. They should install a needle cutter and a small device for cutting, plastic tubing, gloves, etc. and separate steam autoclave/microwave exclusively established for this purpose. Adequate precaution should be taken for occupation and environmental hazards. Staffs, who handle clinical waste bags and containers, should be trained to be aware of the following to avoid injuries and accidents:
- When waste bags/containers are three-fourth full, they should be sealed.
- All bags and containers must conform to the different color coding system. Labeling can be done by writing the information on the bags an outer container.
- Separation of biomedical wastes to be done at source (in different color coding bags).
- Check that waste bags are effectively sealed.

- Origin of the waste is marked on the waste bag or container.
- Bag should be picked up by the neck and placed so that they can be picked up by the neck again for further handling.
- Manual handling of waste bags should be minimized to reduce the black of needle prick injuries.
- Bags should not be clasped against the body and too many bags should not be carried at a time.
- Avoid the bag hitting the body when being carried. Yellow bags and blue/white translucent bags should not be thrown or dragged. Sharp containers should be picked up and carried by the handle provided. The other hand should not be used to support the bottom of the container.
- Clinical waste should be kept only in a specified storage area.
  Staff should know the appropriate cleaning and disinfection procedures in case of accidental spillage and how to report an incident. Simple color coding system for plastic bags. Secure plastic color coded bags before waste handling.
- Poster should wear protective clothing like gloves, overall, etc.
  If the bag is soiled, it should be placed in another clean bag of the same color.
- Under no circumstances should any one insert their hands into any waste container.

Treatment: There are five broad categories of medical waste treatment technologies, which include: Mechanical process, Thermal process, Chemical process, Irradiation process and Biological process.

- **Mechanical process** are used to change the physical form or characteristics of the waste, either to facilitate waste handling or to process the waste in conjunction with other treatment steps. The two primary mechanical processes are compaction and shredding. Compaction involves compressing the waste into containers to reduce its volume. Shredding which also includes granulations, grinding, pulping and the like, is used to break the waste into smaller places. This process is not safe but still can be used accordingly.
- **Thermal process** use heat to decontaminate or destroy medical waste. Most microorganisms are rapidly destroyed at temperature ranging from 120 to 195°F and most living organisms are killed at 212°F. The basic thermal treatment processes are: Autoclave, Hydroclave, and Incineration.
- Chemical process is a chemical treatment, synonymous with chemical disinfection or simply disinfection. Most chemical waste treatment systems use a disinfectant solution in combination with shredding to provide decontamination and disfigurement. However, several systems feature strong chemical reactions which destroy or disintegrate the waste and a few use chemical polymers to encapsulate the waste. This treatment is recommended for waste sharps, solid and liquid waste, as well as chemical wastes. Chemical treatment involves use of at least one percent hypochlorite solution with a minimum contact period of 30 minutes or other equivalent chemical reagents such as phenolic compound, iodine, hexachlorophene, iodine alcohol, or formaldehyde-alcohol, etc. Pre-shredding of the waste is desirable for better contact with the waste material.
- **Irradiation process:** Irradiation is synonymous with electromagnetic or ionizing radiation. Currently, one vendor is developing a process utilizing Cobalt 60 and another vendor is developing a system utilizing an electron beam accelerator unit or electron beam gun for irradiating and sterilizing the medical waste.
- **Biological process:** In the conveyor transports waste to a shredder. The shredder residue is mixed with water and pumped as slurry to a tank containing enzymes where biological reaction takes place. Treated residue is pumped from the tank through a screw press to separate solids. Solid residues are compacted and collected in a bin for disposal. In addition to the above treatment, techniques required for sanitary and secured land filling and nonhazardous and nontoxic may be taken care by composting and control recycling of packaging material.

Disposal: Biomedical waste can be disposed off in several ways as briefed in treatment. After the disposal treatment, the resultant residual waste may be deposited safely in a landfill designated for this purpose. The establishment requires provision for segregated for this purpose. The establishment requires provision for segregated storage (according to rules which can be packed in sealed containers/sturdy bags and handed over to the agency carrying them to the common treatment/disposal facility).

SAFETY AND HEALTH ISSUES IN A NUTSHELL

Personal protective clothing (PPC) and personal protective equipment (PPE) must be available to the staff and its usage ensured.

Personal Protective Clothing

- Gloves:
  - Disposable vinyl gloves in all patient care areas.
  - Latex surgical gloves for operative procedures.
  - Heavy duty thick rubber gloves for waste handlers.
- Masks: Simple, reusable plastic masks to protect health care workers from splashes.
- Aprons: Full sleeved, knee length cotton aprons must be worn at all times.

Personal Protective Equipment

- Footwear: Gumboots for waste handlers. The trousers must remain outside the gumboots.
- Eye shield.

- Apron: A reusable heavy duty, autoclavable rubber apron may be worn where heavy contamination/excessive splashing is expected, e.g. in labor room, operation theater, etc.

General

- Hand washing facility: Soap and water should be available at all time.
- Drinking water: Safe drinking water must be available for waste handlers, working near boilers to prevent dehydration.
- Immunization: Tetanus, hepatitis B.
- Maintenance of health records.

NURSES' ROLE AND RESPONSIBILITY IN BMW

- Disinfect the waste so that it is no longer the source of pathogenic organisms.
- Reduce the bulk in order to reduce requirements for storage and transportation.
- Make waste unrecognizable for esthetic reason.
- Recycling of infectious plastic wastes can be considered only after adequate disinfection/ sterilization, e.g. glass, paper, corrugated cardboard, aluminum, X-ray film, reclaimed silver from X-ray film, plastics (noninfectious components).
- Disposable items like gloves, syringes, etc. should be mutilated after use to prevent illegal packing and reuse.
- Wastes minimization can be done by:
  - Purchase of reusable items made of glass, rubber, metal, etc.
  - Select non-PVC plastic.
  - Strengthen sterilization procedure.
  - Adopt proper procedure and policies of BMW.
  - Establish effective sound recycling policy.
- There should be three types of container available at each point namely for general waste, infected non-sharp waste and infected sharp waste.
- Color coding of bags be done as per rules.
- Needles, syringes other sharp instruments and objects, should be placed in a puncture- resistant plastic/metal container at the work station.
- Needles, syringes and such other should be boiled, hydroclaved/autoclave or chemically disinfected and then disposed.
- Alternatively, transport sharps to a central site for treatment, reused containers if at all only after cleaning and disinfecting.
- 40 percent needle prick injuries are due to resheathing, so do not recap.
- Reusable glass syringes and needles.
  - Aspirate hypochloric solution.
  - Immerse in flat tray for 20 minutes.
  - Rinse with water several times.
- Chemical disinfection prior to disposal is required for sharps, disposable infectious plastics/Rubber, infectious glassware, blood and body fluids, by:
  - Using one percent hypochlorite or equivalent disinfectant. Proper concentration is essential.
  - Ensuring all surfaces come in contact with chemical (including lumen).
  - Contacting time at least 30 minutes.

CONCLUSION

The nurse plays a critical role in preventing and controlling infectious disease. The beginning nursing student participates significantly in the prevention process from the initial introduction to nursing care. An important component in preparing for clinical nursing practice is an understanding of the infection process and prevention techniques. Microbiology and other science courses provide background information about pathogenic organisms. The transfer of these scientific principles to the applied art and science of nursing involves an awareness of the dynamics of the infectious process.

Currently health care workers have an abundance of scientific knowledge about pathogenic organisms and their transmission from one person to another. Methods to control the spread of the micro organisms are standardized in recommendations from the Centers for Disease Control and Prevention (CDC), and the Occupational Safety and Health Administration (OSHA). In nursing, measures to prevent the transmission of infectious microorganisms from patient to patient become a significant component of care. This prevention is achieved through the practice of medical asepsis and standard precautions. Standard precautions include universal precautions and nosocomial infection.

BIBLIOGRAPHY

1. Alice L. Price. The Art, Science and Spirit of Nursing, Philadelphia, WB Saunders Company, 3rd Edition, 1968.
2. Anon, 2003. Scrapping the HI-Tech Myth Computer Waste in India. Published by Toxics Link, 2003.
3. Anon, 2006. Note on E-waste, TNPCB, and Chennai, 2006.
4. Anon, Economic Appraisal, Evaluation 2004-2005.
5. Kozier Barbara B, Du Gas Beverly Witter. Fundamentals of Patient Care: A Comprehensive Approach to Nursing. WB Saunders Company, 1967.
6. Manohar D, Reddy PR, Kotaih B. Characterization of solid waste of a super specialty hospital- a case study. Ind. J Environ. Health. 1998;40(4), 319–326.
7. McClosky JC, Grace HK. Current Issues in Nursing, 4th Ed. St. Louis: Mosby Year Book, Inc., 1994.
8. Mitchell PR, Grippando GM. Nursing Perspectives and Issues, 5th Edition. New York: Delmar Publishers, Inc., 1993.
9. Mondal NC, Saxena, VS Singh. Impact of pollution due to tanneries on groundwater regime. Current Science, 2005; Vol. 88, No. 12: 1988-1994.
10. Notification: Bio-medical Waste (Management and Handling) Rules, 1998. Ministry of Environment and Forests, GOI (E), part 3(ii), New Delhi, 27.07.1998.

11. Potter P, Perry A. Fundamentals of Nursing-Concepts, Process and Practice, 3rd Edition. Mosby Year Book, 1993.
12. Shafer, Kathleen, et. al. Medical-Surgical Nursing, 6th Edition. Saint Louis; CV Mosby Co., 1975.
13. Shakuntala Sharma 'Birpuri'. Principles and Practice of Nursing. Jaypee Brothers Medical Publishers (P) Ltd., New Delhi, 1997.
14. Sr. Nancy, Principles and Practice of Nursing; Vol. 1, 3rd Edition. NR Brothers, Indore, 1992.
15. Taylor C, Lillis C, LeMone P. Fundamentals of Nursing: The Art and Science of Nursing Care. Philadelphia: JB Lippincott, 1993.
16. Thresvamma CP. Fundamentals of Nursing, Procedure Manual for General Nursing Course, PC Mathew, Kottayam, Kerala,1992.
17. Virginia Henderson, Principles and Practice of Nursing, New York, MacMillan Publishing Co., 1970.

REVIEW QUESTIONS

Long Essays

1. Define infection process; explain the modes of infection transmission.
2. Describe the methods of decontamination techniques of hospital equipment and unit.
3. Define surgical asepsis; describe the methods and techniques used.
4. Define personal protective equipment; explain its type's uses and techniques.

Short Essays

1. Explain the chain of infection.
2. Define nosocomial infection, explain the sites and causes of nosocomial infection.
3. Define barrier nursing; explain the nurse role in barrier nursing.
4. Describe the open and closed methods of gloving techniques.
5. Enumerate and explain the transmission based precautions.
6. Explain the steps used in surgical hand washing techniques.
7. Define bio-medical waste management, explain the approaches used for the hospital biomedical waste management.

Short Answers

1. Types of hospital acquired infections.
2. Isolation ward.
3. Isolation system.
4. Hospital waste.
5. Respiratory isolation.

MULTIPLE CHOICE QUESTIONS

1. **Infection control is the discipline concerned with preventing ——————— infection in the hospital:**
   a. Nosocomial infection
   b. Pandemic infections
   c. Epidemic infection
   d. Chronic infection
2. **Infection may be transmitted by direct contact from skin to skin, mucosa to mucosa or mucosa to skin of the same or another person is called:**
   a. Nosocomial infection
   b. Vertical infection
   c. Droplet infection
   d. Horizondal infection
3. **The potential for microorganisms or parasites to cause disease depends on:**
   a. Sufficient number of organisms
   b. Virulence or ability to produce disease
   c. Ability to enter and survive to the host and susceptibility of host
   d. All of the above
4. **The damaged tissue releases substances that cause inflammation and that direct the immune system to do the following, *except*:**
   a. Strengthen the immune system
   b. Attack and kill any invaders
   c. Dispose of dead and damaged tissue
   d. Begin the process of repair
5. **Objectives of biomedical waste management is:**
   a. Reduction of the impact of this waste on the community
   b. Reduction of the chances of infection and accidental injury to the workers
   c. Reduction of cost of total treatment of waste
   d. All of the above

ANSWERS

1. a   2. c   3. d   4. a   5. d

CHAPTER 10

Comfort, Rest and Sleep, and Pain

LEARNING OBJECTIVES

- Comfort:
  - Factors influencing comfort
  - Types of beds and bed making
  - Therapeutic positions
  - Comfort devices
- Sleep and rest:
  - Physiology of sleep
  - Factors affecting sleep
  - Promoting rest and sleep
  - Sleep disorders
- Pain (discomfort):
  - Physiology
  - Common cause of pain
  - Types
  - Assessment
  - Pharmacological and nonpharmacological pain relieving measures
  - Invasive techniques of pain management
  - CAM (Complementary and alternative healing modalities)

TERMINOLOGY

- **Comfort** is defined as the contented enjoyment in physical or mental well-being, freedom from pain or trouble and anxiety.
- **Discomfort** is defined as want of comfort or ease due to client or annoyance.
- **Bed making:** The technique of preparing different types of bed making patients/clients comfortable in his/her suitable position for a particular condition.
- **Fanfold:** Specifically folding the edge of the sheet used in the bed 6-8 inches outward.
- **Mitered corner:** A means of anchoring sheet on mattresses.
- **Toe pleat:** A fold made in the top bed clothes to provide additional space for patients toes.
- **Foot drop:** Plantar flexion of the foot with permanent contracture of the gastronomies (calf) muscle and tendon.
- **Bed cradle:** Is a curved, semicircular made of metal that can be placed over a portion of the patient's body.
- **Hospital bed:** It is usually about 26-28 inches (65-70 cm) above to floor.

INTRODUCTION

Comfort is concerned with rest, with exercise, with the relation of one part of the body to another, with the bed and the whole environment. Comfort is a phase of every procedure as it is an aspect of the total care of the patient. Comfort devices are invented articles which would add to comfort of patient when used in appropriate manner. These devices relieve the discomfort and help in maintaining correct posture. Various comfort devices are used for giving comfort to the patient, such as: pillows, back rest, foot rest, bed block, bed cradles, sand bags, air cushion, rubber and cotton rings, air and water mattress and knee rest.

COMFORT MEASURES

Definition

- Comfort is a state of free from pain and discomfort tension and anxiety.
- Comfort is defined as the contented enjoyment in physical or mental well-being freedom from pain or trouble.
- Discomfort is defined as want of comfort or ease due to pain or annoyance.
- Comfort devices are the mechanical devices to promote comfort to the patient.
- Comfort devices are invented articles which would add to the comfort of the patient when used in the appropriate manner, by relieving the discomfort and helping to maintain correct posture.

Comfort measures
• Provide quiet, clean, uncluttered environment
• Provide warmth or coolness as indicated
• Provide personal hygiene: keep patient clean and dry, linen changes, oral care
• Provide activity as indicated: TV, radio, reading material
• Explain all procedures, Tests, hospital routines
• Facilitate family visits and support
• Check with patient at regular intervals about his comfort/discomfort
• Keep call light within reach and encourage patient to call you if needed

Purpose

- To promote comfort.
- To prevent discomfort.
- To alleviate discomfort.
- To ensure that the patient has rest.
- To assist the patient to obtain an adequate sleep to meet his requirement.
- To maintain correct posture.

Principles Relevant to Comfort

- Definite periods of sleep are an essential component of the circadian rhythm in human being.
- Adequate amounts of sleep are needed for optimal physical and psychosocial functioning of the individual.
- Individual needs for sleep vary with age, growth patterns, health status and individual differences.
- Lack of sufficient sleep impairs a person's physical functioning, his mental alertness and his social relationship.
- Individual habits vary with regard to bed time rituals.
- Sleep pattern may be disturbed by changes in person's normal daily living patterns by social and emotional problems, by physical problems and by minor irritation or discomforts.
- Sleeps at times are almost invariable disturbed by illness.

Factors promoting and inhibiting comfort

Factors promoting	Factors inhibiting
Normal temperature	Too high or too low temperature
Normal humidity	Dry or too humid environment
Safe, clean, quiet and comfortable environment	Unsafe, unpleasant and stressful environment
Comfortable positions	Dirty and soiled bed and linen
Neat and clean bed and linen	Poor ventilation
Good ventilation	Glaring or too dim lighting
Pleasant odors	Unpleasant odors
No fear	Fear
No stress and worry	Stress and worry

Factors Influencing Comfort

- Pain.
- Restriction of movements due to weakness.
- Wrinkled, soiled and wet sheets.
- Delayed or inadequate attention to meet the personal needs.
- Lack of exercise.
- Temperature extremes.
- Too Bright lights and glares.
- Fear and anxiety due to illness.
- Insecurity feeling.
- Lack of sleep.
- Uncomfortable position.
- Indigestion and irregular bowel movements

Causes of Discomfort

- Pain.
- Restriction of movements due to weakness.
- Wrinkled soiled and wet sheets.
- Delayed or inadequate attention to meet the personal needs.
- Lack of exercise.
- Temperature extremes.
- Too bright lights and glares.
- Fear and anxiety due to illness.
- Insecurity feeling.
- Lack of sleep.
- Uncomfortable position.
- Indigestion and irregular bowel movements.

Cause of Discomfort

- Pain
- Restriction of movements due to weakness
- Wrinkled, soiled and wet bed sheets
- Improper arrangement of pillows
- Delayed or inadequate attention to meet the personal need such as cleanliness, elimination, nourishment etc.
- Lack of exercise
- Extreme temperature
- Inadequate ventilation

Factors Promoting Physical Comfort

Immediate Needs

- Morning care.
- Evening care.
- Bedtime care.

BED MAKING

The primary aims of bed making is to provide comfort and safety of the patient, e.g. using pillows for support; preventing bed-sores by means of clean smooth sheets. The morale of the patient is greatly helped by good bed making. It makes economy of time, effort and equipment, e.g. being prepared for an emergency admission; using rubber sheeting to prevent soiling of linen, mattress and pillow. It also gives cleanliness, order and pleasing appearance to patient's unit. The the screens are needed for privacy, a damp duster, fresh linen as necessary, a bed stripper, chair or stool on which to put linen, and a receptacle for soiled linen. If the patient is heavy or ill, get the help of another nurse or the patient's relatives, to support her. The patient should be pleasantly greeted and any conversation should include the patient.

Definition

- Bed making is a systematic way of preparing the appropriate bed based on the condition of the patient, which adopts scientific principles of nursing.

- Bed making is a process of keeping the bed clean, neat and tidy. Also keep ready for admission, transfer, examination, treatment and to promote comfort for the patient.
  - To promote comfort and safety.
  - To give the unit or ward a neat appearance.
  - To promote cleanliness.
  - To save time, material and effort.
  - To prevent pressure sore.
  - To monitor the patient condition.
  - To promote therapeutic relationship.
  - To educate the patient and family.
  - To receive the patient during emergency.

Principles Involved in Bed Making

- Systematic way of doing save time, energy and material.
- Good body mechanics maintains the body alignment and prevents fatigue.
- A safe and comfortable bed will ensure rest, sleep and prevents several complications in bedridden patient, e.g. pressure sore, foot drop, etc.
- Microorganisms are found everywhere on bed, bed sheets, blanket, pillow cover and the articles used by the patient and in the environment.
- Keep the bed and environment clean and neat. It helps to provide physical and mental health.

Purpose of Bed Making

- Simple beds
  - Closed or unoccupied bed.
  - Open bed
  - Occupied bed.
- Special beds
  - Operation bed
  - Cardiac bed
  - Fracture bed
  - Amputation bed.

General Instructions

- Wash hands before and after procedure.
- Do not expose the patient unnecessarily.
- Do not cover the patients face while placing the linen.
- Does not mix clean linen with soiled linen.
- Maintain good body mechanics.
- Make the bed firm, smooth and unwrinkled.
- Practice economy of time, energy and material.
- Nursing principles such as individuality, comfort, safety and good workmanship should be kept in mind during the bed making.
- Inspect the cot, mattress and pillows daily for the purpose of vermin and destroy them if found on the bed.

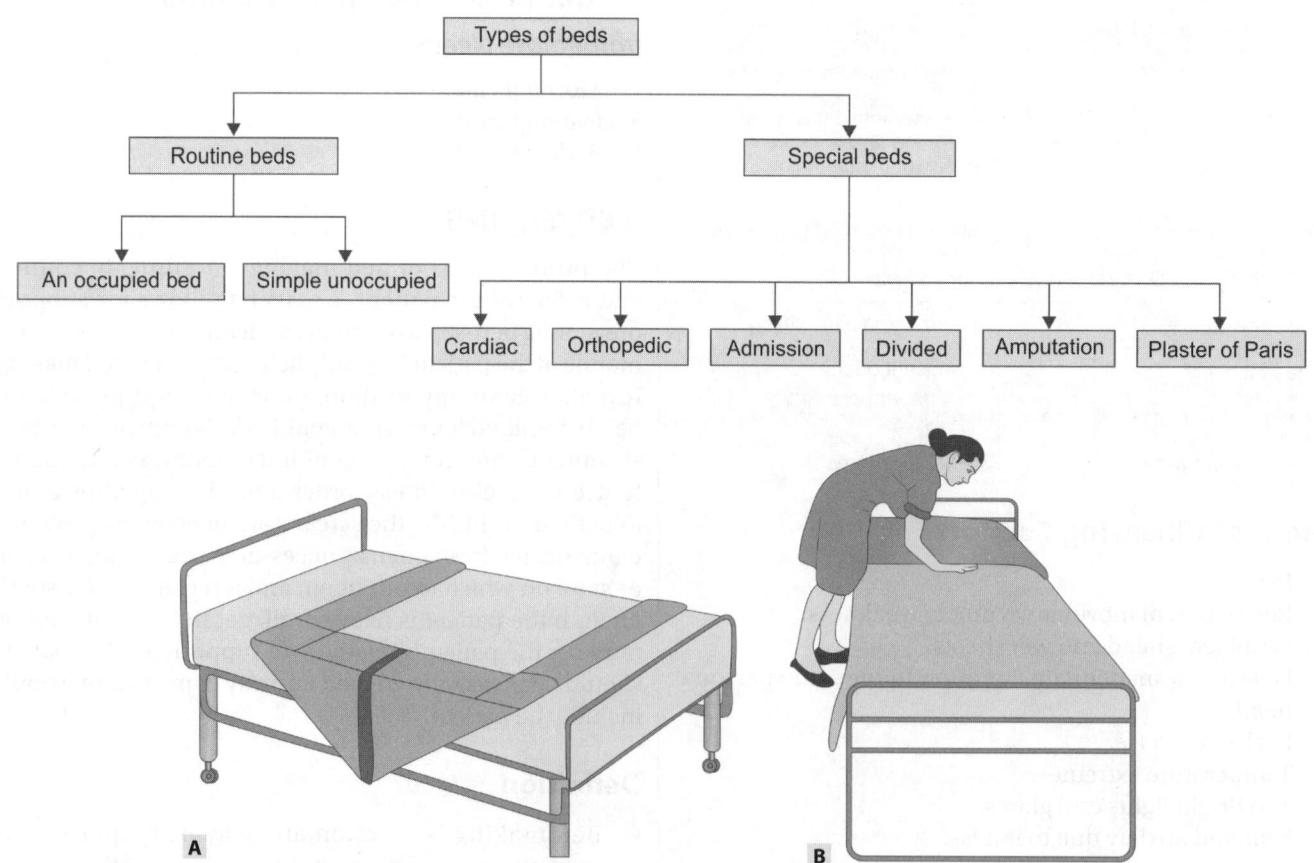

Figs. 10.1A and B: Types of beds and nurses prepared the open bed.

- Always get extra help to make a bed for helpless patient and prevent from falling.
- Make adaptations according to climatic differences, individual needs, customs and habits of the patient.
- The cotton mattress must be turned, aired and made free from lumps and creases.

Preliminary Assessment

Check

- The doctor's order for specific precautions regarding the movement and positioning of the patient.
- Assess the patient's ability for self-care.
- The furniture and linen available in the patients unit.
- The number of clean linen needed.
- Assess the articles needed for the comfort of the patient, e.g. blankets, backrest, etc.

Equipment

Usual articles in the patients unit:
- Bed/cot-Metal rods/Spring wood.
- Mattress-Firm, thick, smooth with washable covers.
- Bed spread/Top sheet.
- Draw mackintosh-Shoulder to below the knees.
- Draw sheet (Cotton) drawn from side-to-side.
- Pillow-Cotton/foam with pillow case.
- Blanket.

Articles Needed for the Complete Change

- Mattress covers.
- Top sheets-Two (Bottom and Top Sheets).
- Draw sheet.
- Pillow cover.
- Counterpane.

Extra Articles

- A bowl with antiseptic solution.
- Duster: Two (One dry duster and another damp duster).
- Laundry bag: To discard the soiled linen.
- Foot stool: To place clean linen.

Procedure

- Explain the procedure.
- Provide privacy if needed and put off the fan.
- Lower the head end if patient condition permits.
- Place the stool at bed end and keep clean linen.

Stripping and Remaking an Open Bed

- Wash hands.
- Place the pillow on the chair.
- Remove the bed spread, blanket and top sheet separately.
- Fold the draw sheet.

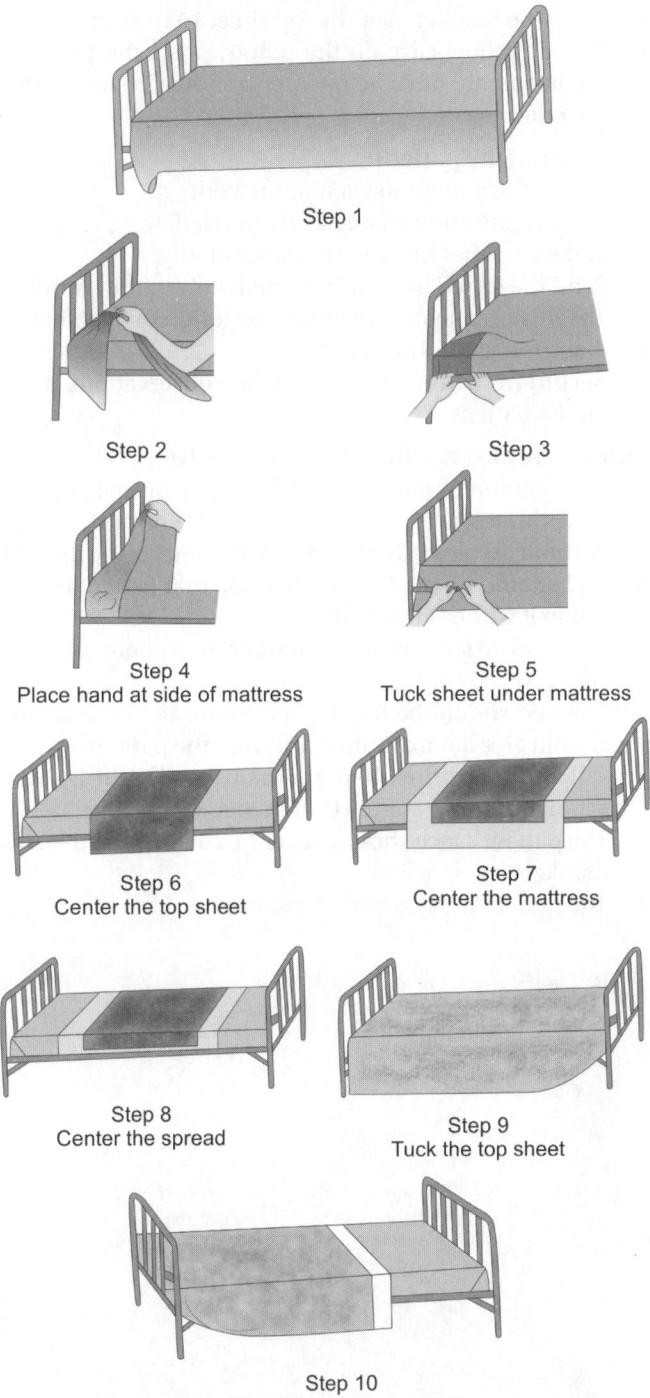

Fig. 10.2: Bed making procedure steps.

- Roll the mackintosh and place it over the chair.
- Remove the bottom sheet folding it into six.
- Remove the mattress cover if soiled.
- Dust the mattress with a dry duster.
- Use damp duster for cleaning the furniture.
- Make a mitered corner. Tuck at the top and foot end. Secure the corner properly.
- Place the clean bottom sheet and tuck at one side of the bed. Go to the opposite side and tuck the sheets in the same manner.

- Place the blanket over the top sheet 15 to 20 cm.
- Put the pillow case on the pillow, place the pillow at the head end, and the open end should be away from the entrance.

Aftercare of the patient:
- Assess the patient to get into the bed.
- Replace the comfort device if any used.
- Make sure that the unit is clean and tidy.
- Send the soiled linen bag immediately to the laundry.
- The duster is soaked in antiseptic lotion to disinfect it.
- Wash the hand thoroughly.
- Record in the nurse's order of any observations made on the patient.

Rules to be observed when making beds:
- All equipments should be collected before starting.
- Two nurses are required and they should work in harmony avoiding jerky movements and jarring the bed.
- Bed should be made in such a way that patient can be put in it without difficulty.
- It should be suitable for treating certain conditions, e.g. shock.
- The bed should be free from crumbs and creases and should give a maximum comfort to the patient.
- Pillows and other bed accessories should be well arranged to give support where necessary.
- The patient's face should never be covered by sheets or blankets.
- The patient must never be exposed.
- Extra assistance should be available and, if necessary, one should be called upon to help lift the patient.
- When pillows are being shaken the nurse should turn away from the patient.
- Any conversation during bed making should not be on personal matters between the nurses.
- The open side of a pillow case should be away from the main door of the ward.
- Always have a dirty linen bin at hand in which to put dirty linen.
- Dirty linen should not be carried across the ward to prevent cross infectoin.
- Allow room for the patient feet for free movement or turning when placing the top sheet over the patient.
- Always wash hands before and after bed making.

UNOCCUPIED BED OR CLOSED BED

A closed bed is an empty bed, in which the top covers are arranged that all linen beneath the spread is fully protected from dust and dirt while waiting for the patient.

An unoccupied bed is an empty bed, and is fully covered with a counterpane to protect it from dust and dirt.

Purpose
- To give a clean comfortable bed.
- To keep bed ready for the admission.
- To keep it ready for any emergency.

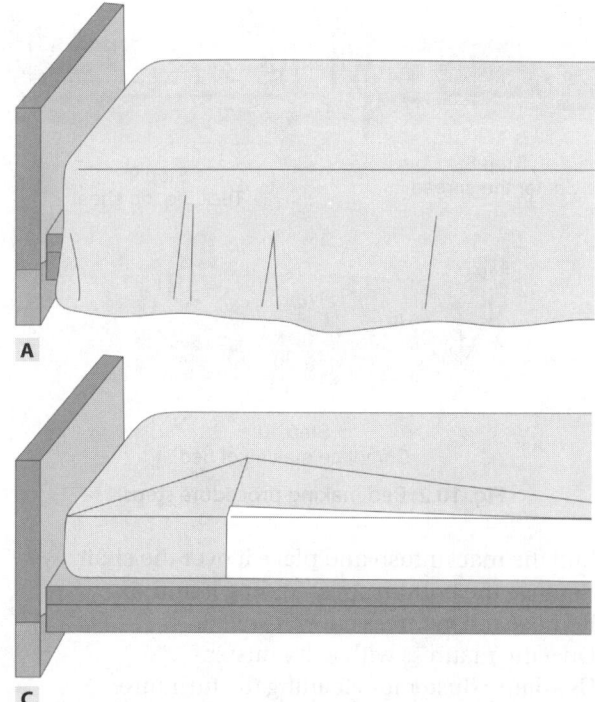
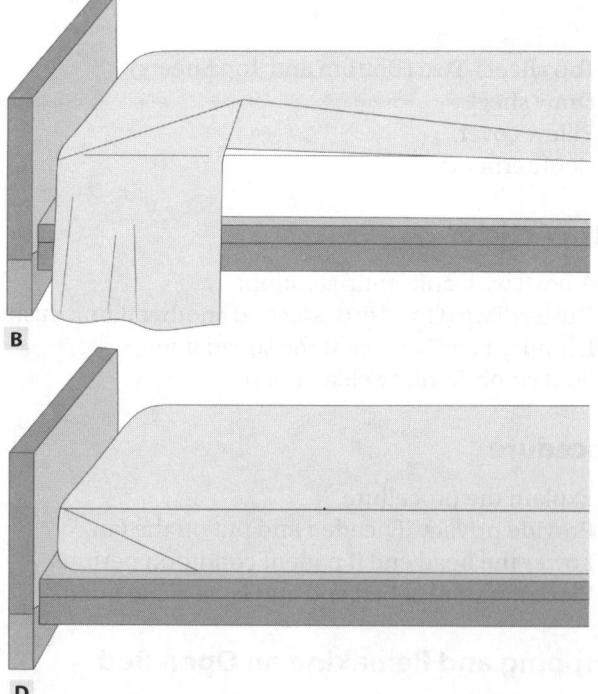

Figs. 10.3A to D: Steps to make a mitered corner: A mitered corner is being made on a flat bottom sheet. (A) The sheet is hanging over the side of the bed. (B) Grasp the edge of the sheet about 12 inches from the foot of the bed and lift it up, forming a triangle. Lay the triangular fold on the top of the bed, and smooth the hanging portion of the sheet against the side of the mattress. (C) Tuck the hanging portion of the sheet underneath the mattress, while holding the triangular fold taut against the top of the bed. (D) Bring the triangular fold back down over the edge of the mattress, and tuck it underneath. This process is the same for the upper corners of the bed and for the top linens.

- To protect the bed from dust and dirt.
- To give the room a neat and tidy appearance.

General Instructions

- Use clean and uniform linen.
- Avoid linen from touching uniform or floor.
- Use principles of body mechanics.
- To prevent wrinkles, pull linen tight as they are tucked.

Equipment

- Chair/stool/trolley-hampers.
- Dusters-2.
- Basin with water/lotion savalon 1:100.
- Mattress protector.
- Mattress with cover.
- Long mackintosh.
- Bed sheets-2.
- Pillow with cover.
- Draw sheet with mackintosh.
- Blankets (if required).
- Bed spread (counterpane).

Procedure

- The nurse should wash her hands.
- Collect all articles on a chair, stool or trolley.
- Remove the bed cloths, by folding one by one.
- Discard the soiled linen in to the hamper or bucket.
- Clean the bed with wet duster.
- Spread bottom bed sheet, spread mattress cover, long mackintosh, draw mackintosh, draw sheet and tuck them on your side.
- Go to the other side and tuck them.
- Spread top sheet to the full length on the mattress.
- Spread blanket over the top sheet.
- Tuck at the foot end by making corners.
- Keep pillow with case and place it at the head end.
- Spread counterpane to the full length by making corners.

Aftercare

- Place the bed in alignment with other beds to add to the esthetic value.
- Lock the bed wheel to prevent moving of bed.
- Place the bed locker on working side of the bed.
- Replace the stool under the bed and remove extra-equipment from the bed side.
- Take the bucket or hamper in to the sluice room.
- Wash and dry duster and basins.
- Wash hands.

OPEN BED

Open bed is a suitable, comfortable and appropriate for hospitalized patient.

Open bed is made as usual and one corner of the linen is folded back to let the patient in. The top linen is fan folded to the foot end of the bed or to one side of the bed.

Purpose

- To provide a clean bed.
- To maintain clean environment.
- To adapt according to comfort needs of patient.

General Instructions

- Nurse should assess the patient's condition for ambulation.
- Nurse should remove watch and wash hands before and after the procedure.
- Switch off the fan before starting bed making.

Procedure

- Assess the patient general condition.
- Explain to patient about the need of bed making.
- Assist the patient to get out of the bed.
- Make the patient to sit comfortably on stool or chair.
- Adjust the bed in flat position to a comfortable height.
- Spread the bed clothes, fold them one by one.

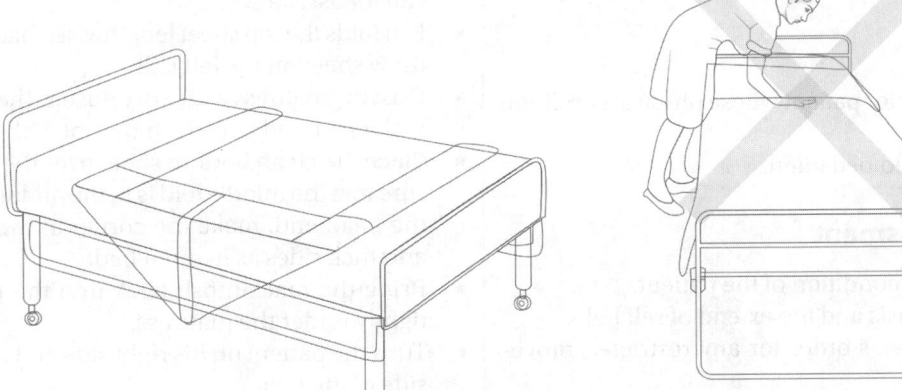

Fig. 10.4: Maintaining body mechanics while preparing the bed.

- Dust the bed with damp duster and mattress with dry duster.
- Clean under surface of mattress and then body of cot. Clean foot end and cot legs.
- Place the mattress cover, bottom sheet and tuck it neatly.
- Make mitered corner with top sheet and also make toe pleat.
- Replace pillow with free ends facing away from entrance of room/door.
- Place the blanket over the top sheet, at the foot of bed.

Types of Toe Pleat

Vertical Pleat: Fold a six inches plea lengthwise in the top clothes from the center to the foot end, at the center of mattress.

Equipment

- Chair/Stool
- Duster
- Basin with water
- Hamper/Dirty linen basket
- Linen to change
- Bucket, if there is soiled linen.

Horizontal Pleat: Fold a two inches pleat across the top clothes at the center of foot of the mattress.

Aftercare

- Assess the patient to get in the bed.
- Position the patient comfortably
- Cover the patient with top sheet neatly.
- Use side rails if needed.
- Clean inside and outside of locker and arrange patient's belonging neatly.
- Replace the equipments.

OCCUPIED BED

Occupied bed is made for a patient who cannot get out of the bed.

Occupied bed is making a comfortable bed when patient is unable to get out of bed. It is usually done by two persons.

Purpose

- To provide comfort for patient whose physical condition confines to bed.
- To change the soiled bed linen.

Preliminary Assessment

- Assess the general condition of the patient.
- Identify the diagnosis and the extend of self help.
- Check the physician's order for any restricted movements.

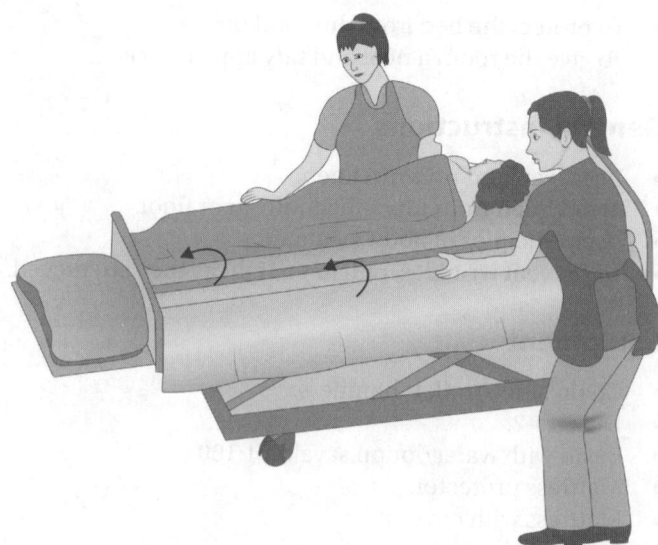

Fig. 10.5: Bed linens are changed for bedridden patients.

- Arrange help from others.
- Collect clean linen to change.

Equipment

- Chair/Stool.
- Duster.
- Basin with disinfectant solution (7% Lysol).
- Hamper/Dirty linen basket.
- Bucket to collect soiled linen.
- Mattress cover, long mackintosh, big sheets, draws sheet and blankets.
- Comfort measure: Back rest, foot rest and extra pillows.
- K-basin, BP apparatus and oxygen access if needed.

Procedure

- Wash hands thoroughly.
- Organize the articles at the bedside in order to use.
- Explain how the patient can assist and the sequence of the procedure.
- Remove all pillows except one loosen the bedding on all sides.
- Turn the patient on his left side. If the patient is very ill, call for assistance.
- Fan folds the top sheet lengthwise, mackintosh and then draw sheet on the left side.
- Dust the mattress with a dry duster. Then lift the mattress with one hand and clean the cot with a damp duster.
- Place the clean bottom sheet over the mattress making sure that the middle fold is in the middle of the bed. Tuck the head end, make the corner at the top and bottom and tuck sides as in open bed.
- Bring the mackintosh back into the place and tuck it tightly under the mattress.
- Turn the patient on his right side and go to the opposite side of the bed.

- Remove the soiled line and put them in the laundry bag. Straighten out the bottom sheet, rubber sheet, draw sheet and tuck them separately and firmly.
- Position patient comfortably. Cover the patient with top sheet up to shoulder level.
- Replace towels and blanket and use side rails if needed.

OPERATION BED

Postoperative bed is prepared to receive patients who had undergone surgical procedure.

Postoperative bed is prepared for a patient who is recovering from the effects of anesthesia following a surgical operation.

Purpose

- To place the patient easily in bed with minimum discomfort.
- To make comfortable and safe bed for the patient who is receiving from anesthesia.
- To prepare to meet any emergency.
- To keep the bed warm in order to provide comfort.
- To avoid wastage of time, energy, and material.
- To promote easy and quick transfer of the patient from the trolley to the bed.
- To protect the mattress and bedding from bleeding, vomiting, drainage and discharges.

Equipment

- All the articles required for simple bed.
- Gauze pieces, narrow mackintosh and sheet.
- Artery forceps.
- Mouth gag, airway and tongue depressor.
- TPR tray, BP apparatus.
- Bed blocks-2.
- Hot water bag with cover.
- IV, stand.
- Kidney tray and paper bag.
- Suction apparatus and oxygen cylinder.

Procedure

- Collect equipments. Arrange fresh folded linen in following order on stool bed (Blanket, towels, sponge, face and bath towels, draw sheet, mackintosh, bottom sheet, long mackintosh, mattress cover).
- Use Lysol 7% to clean mattress and cot, similar as in open bed.
- Cover mattress with fresh cover and tuck firmly.
- Spread long mackintosh length wise from top to bottom covering mattress.
- Spread bottom sheet and tuck neatly.
- Place small mackintosh and a draw sheet at head end of mattress and tuck firmly.
- Tie towels at head end and place blanket at foot and similar to making open bed.
- Top sheet, draw mackintosh and draw sheet will be received along the patient, which should be firmly tucked.
- Place a clean tray with mouth gag, airway, bowl with cotton and gauze pieces, artery forceps, on the bed locker.
- Keep IV stands, basket, K-basin with tissue paper at bedside.
- Depending upon patient's condition, keep articles in postoperative unit.
- Keep extra blanket in postoperative unit.

CARDIAC BED

Cardiac bed is used to help the patient to assume a sitting position, which can afford him greatest amount of comfort with least strain.

Cardiac bed is used for the patients with heart diseases or dyspnea to provide easy breathing for the patient with minimum strain.

Purpose

- To relieve dyspnea.
- To assist recovery of the patient.
- To provide comfort to the patient.
- To prevent complications.

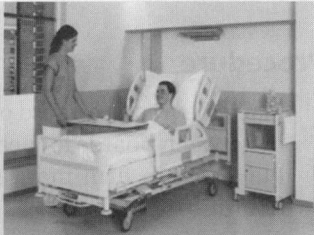

Cardiac bed:
Cardiac bed is made with special arrangements, which are required by a cardiac patient. Cardiac patient's bed is made in a manner to ease the respiration of patient. Bed is provided with extra pillows to be kept on head side of patient to keep the patient in prop up position for better airflow.

There is special cardiac table provided with the patient bed with all equipment available for emergency cardiovascular support, like oxygen masks, nasogastric tubes, etc.

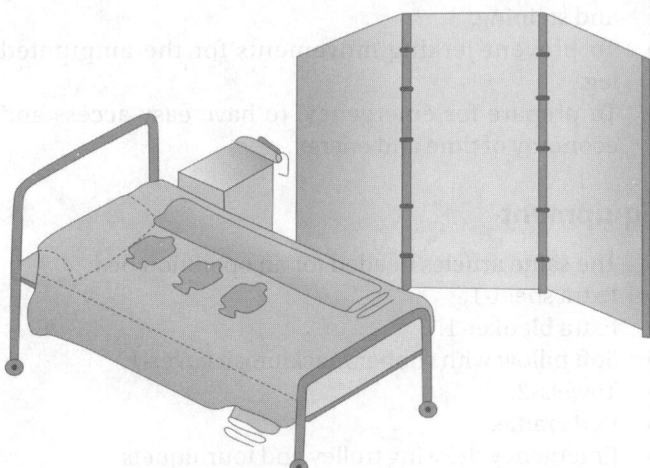

Fig. 10.6: Postoperative bed prepared to receive the patient from operation theater.

Additional Articles Needed

- Additional pillows-1.
- Back rest-1.
- Cardiac table-1.
- Air cushion-1.
- Knee pillow-1.
- Foot rest-1.

Procedure

- Prepare the bed as open bed, with foot rest placed at foot end of the bed.
- Place the back rest at patient's back and arrange pillow in comfortable position.
- Place the cardiac table over the blankets and a pillow over it to allow the patients hands to rest on it.
- Adjust knee pillow, air cushion and make the patient comfortable.

FRACTURE BED

Fracture bed is used for a patient with fracture of the trunk or extremities to provide firm support by the use of firm mattress.

Fracture bed is used for orthopedic patients; fracture board is used under the mattress to provide a firm support for the patient.

Fracture bed is a hard firm bed designed for the patient with fracture particularly of spine, pelvis or femur.

Purpose

- To make the patient comfortable.
- To maintain position.
- To aid immobilizing the fracture.
- To prevent unnecessary pain.
- To give firm, even support to the fractured limbs and back.

Equipment

- All articles required for simple bed.
- Fracture board.
- Sand bags with cover.
- Bed cradle.
- Extra pillows.

Procedure

- Place the fracture board on the cot in such a way that is in between boards for aeration.
- Place a thin firm mattress or pad over the fracture board.
- The bed is prepared as simple open bed.

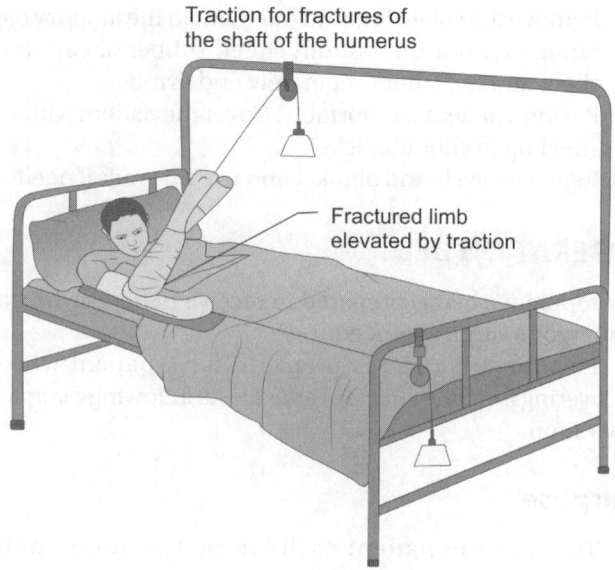

Fig. 10.7: Fracture bed.

- Make the patient comfortable and leave the unit tidy.

AMPUTATION BED

Amputation bed or stump bed or divided bed which is used by the nurse for the patient after amputation of the lower limb, where it is necessary to keep the stump visible and elevated.

Amputation or stump bed is used for the patient whose leg is amputated.

Purpose

- To keep the stump in good position.
- To observe the stump for hemorrhage constantly and apply tourniquet instantly if necessary.
- To give extra warmth.
- To ensure more safety and comfort by preventing soiling and staining.
- To prevent jerking movements for the amputated leg.
- To prepare for emergency, to have easy access and economy of time and energy.

Equipment

- The same articles needed for an operation bed.
- Extra sheet-1.
- Extra blanket-1.
- Soft pillow with rubber mackintosh cover-1.
- Towels-2.
- Bed cradle.
- Emergency dressing trolley and tourniquets.

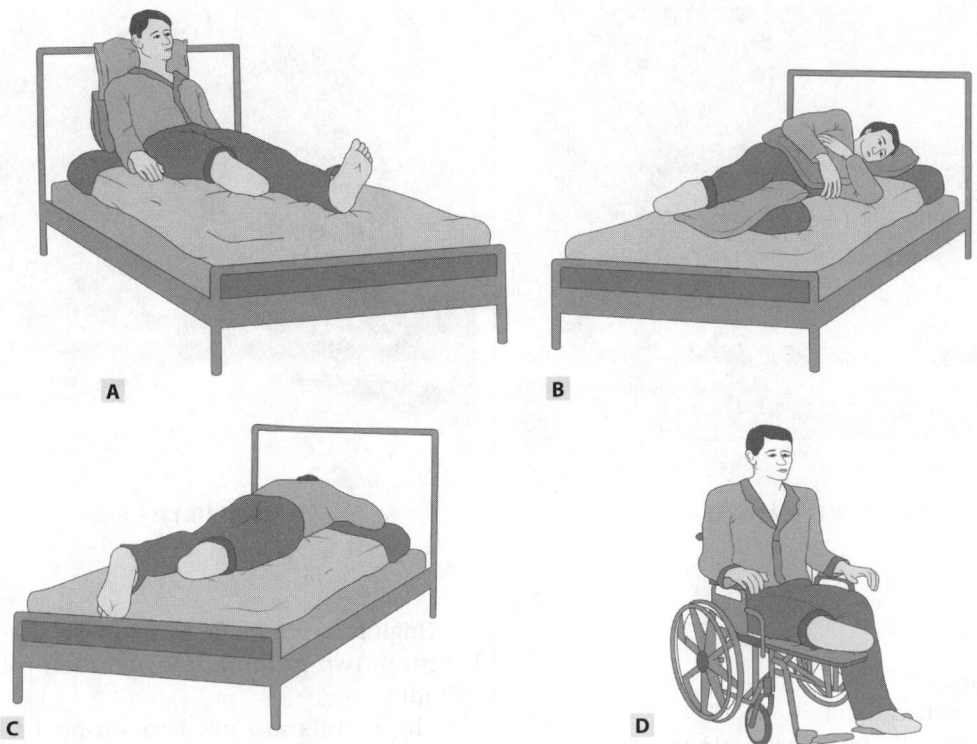

Figs. 10.8A to D: Bed prepared for patients who had undergone amputation.

Procedure

Arrange the articles at the bedside. Place the linen in order to use:
- Prepare the foundation bed as in operation bed.
- To make the lower half, use one sheet and blanket, for upper also, one top sheet and blanket.
- Keep the lower half of the bed overlapped with the upper half as in this way we can easily separate the two halves and observe the stump.
- Elevate the stump over the soft pillow covered with mackintosh.
- Place the sand bags on either side of the stumps to prevent it from jerking, sand bags help and prevent bleeding from jerking.
- Bed cradles are used to take up the weight of the bed linen.
- Cover the patient and make the unit tidy.

COMFORT DEVICES

Mechanical service or comfort devices are invented articles which would add to comfort of patient when used in appropriate manner. These devices relieve the discomfort and help in maintaining correct posture.

Mechanical Devices

- Pillows.
- Back rest.
- Rolls.
- Foot rests/Foot boards.
- Sand bags.
- Air and water mattress.
- Rings.
- Bed cradle.
- Bed blocks.
- Air cushion.

PILLOW

Pillows are used to give comfortable position to the patient. These are most commonly used to support various body parts.

Purpose

- To maintain proper body alignment.
- To support body part in good alignment.
- Help to reduce pressure.
- It can be folded, rolled or tucked firmly against the body to maintain position.
- It is used to support head, neck, arms, legs and parts of the back; adds to the physical comfort.

BACK REST

Back rest is a mechanical device which provides a suitable support and rest for the back of the patient in sitting position.

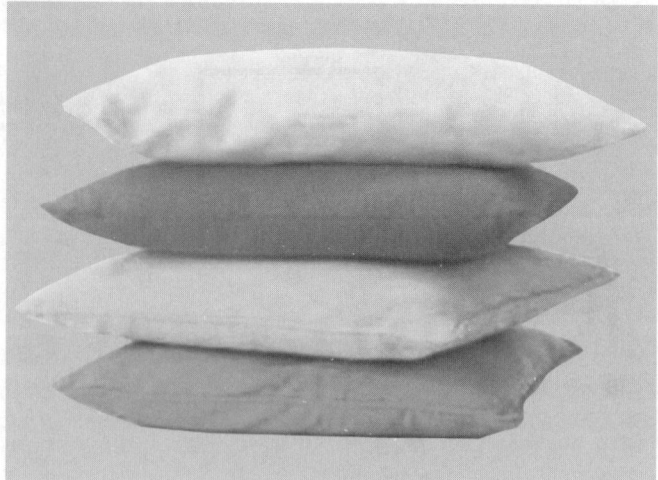

Fig. 10.9: Pillows.

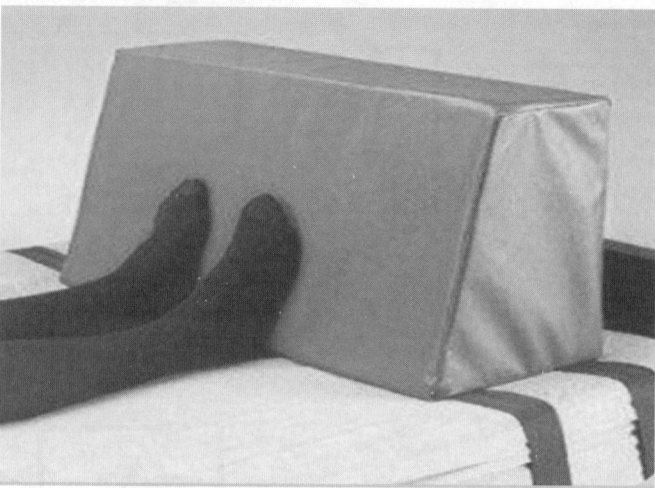

Fig. 10.11: Footboard.

Purpose

- To support back.
- To facilitate easy breathing.
- It is given especially for heart patients and asthma patients.
- This position is used in postoperative period.

ROLLS

Hand rolls are made of cloth that rolled in to a cylinder about four to five inches long and two to three inches in diameter and stuffed firmly.

Purpose

These are used to keep the fingers from being held in a tight fist leading to flexion contracture in patients who are unable to move hands due to paralysis, injury or disease.

Thigh rolls are made by folding a sheet to the desired length of two to three feet and then rolled into a tight cylinder.

Thigh rolls are used to support hips and thighs preventing them from outward rotation and keeping the feet in good alignment in case of paralysis, fracture of femur of hip surgery.

FOOTRESTS

Footrests are the mechanical device used to give rest to feet. Sand bags or foot board may be substituted.

Purpose

- It helps to maintain the normal position of feet.
- It is used for the comfort.
- To prevent foot drop.

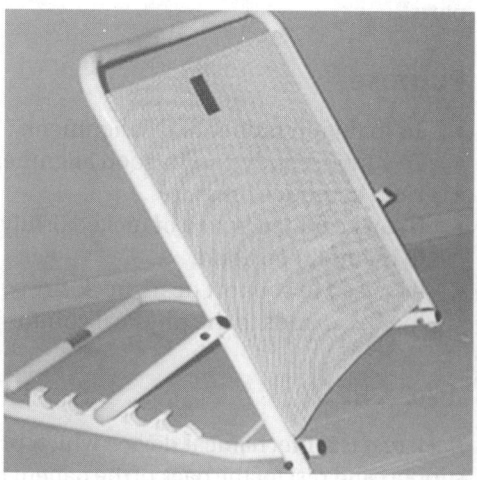
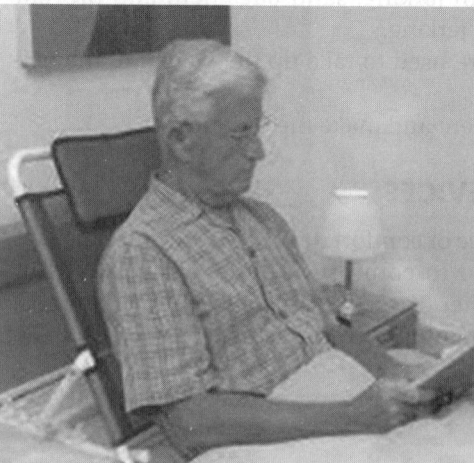

Fig. 10.10: Back rest.

SAND BAGS

Sand bags are canvas, rubber or plastic bags filled with sand and are 1, 5 and 10 lbs in weight. Sand bags are used to immobilize a part.

Purpose

- To relieve discomfort.
- Used to support the body part.
- Used to immobilize the body part.
- Used to support as in fractures bones.
- To prevent foot drop or wrist drop.

AIR AND WATER MATTRESSES

Air and water mattresses are used for very thin or obese patients and for those who are prone to get pressure sores. The principles is that pressure exerted by the body, will be distributed equally in all directions.

Air and water mattresses are plastic mattresses with two sets of chambers. To use them place the mattress on the bed and fill air or water in the compartment. Cover the mattress with light bottom clothes.

Purpose

- To improve circulation.
- To provide comfort.
- To prevent pressure sores.
- Used in very thin or very obese patients.
- Used in chronic bedridden patients.

Caution

Avoid punctures in the mattress with needles, pins or other sharp objects.

RINGS

Air rings are made of rubber. The air ring is inflated about half full tested for leakage, covered and the placed under the patient's hip in such a way that the value is on one side and not in contact with body.

Cotton rings are made wrapped with bandage. These are placed under the bony prominences such as heels and fastened in place if necessary.

Purpose

- Used to lift the hip from bed to prevent bed sores.
- It helps to prevent direct pressure on bony prominence.
- It improves the circulation.

BED CRADLES

Bed cradles vary widely in size and in material. Bed cradles are of wooden, metal or electronic. The bed cradles support and take off the weight of the bedding.

Bed cradle are semicircular in shape made of wood or metal or entirely made of metal tubing or slats.

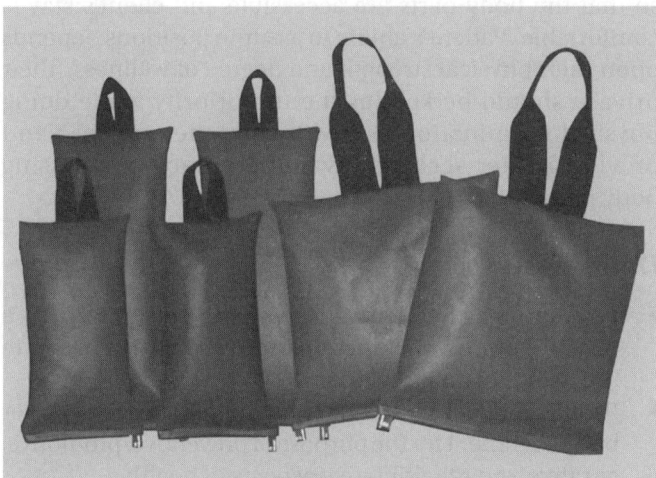

Fig. 10.12: Sand bags.

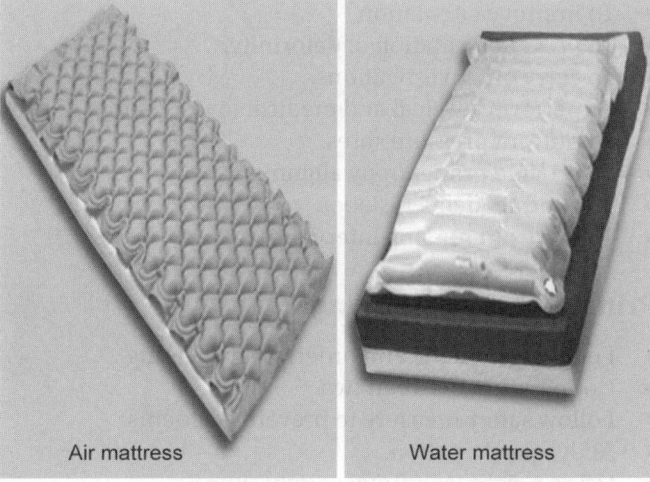

Fig. 10.13: Air and water mattresses.

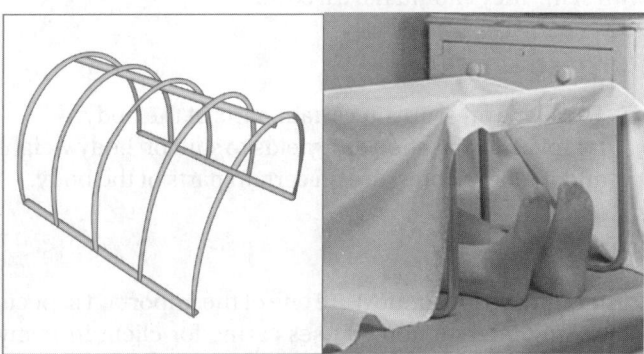

Fig. 10.14: Bed cradle.

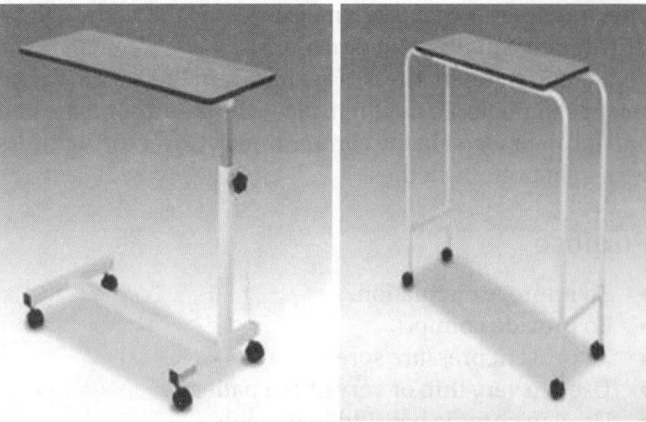

Fig. 10.15: Cardiac tables.

Purpose

- Used to prevent the top cloth is coming in contact with the patients especially in burns patients.
- To apply heat in case of dying plaster casts.
- Electronic bed cradles are used to supply the desired warm in the case of shock.

BED BLOCKS

Bed blocks are made up of wood size, may be high or low. These are placed under the foot of bed for various reasons.

Purpose

- To prevent shock.
- To arrest hemorrhage.
- To retain enema.
- After spinal anesthesia.
- After tonsillectomy.
- To provide traction.
- To position in postural drainage.

AIR CUSHION

Air cushions are round in shape and made up of rubber. These can be inflated with air. These are used to take off the weight of the body.

Air cushion should not be applied directly in contact with skin. They should have a cover.

Purpose

- To relieve pressure on certain parts of the body.
- It provides relaxation as it yields to shift off body weight and it relieves pressure on certain parts of the body.

POSITIONS

Positions used for comfort are one of the important aspects in nursing intervention. Nurses caring for client in many setting and situations can adapt various comfortable

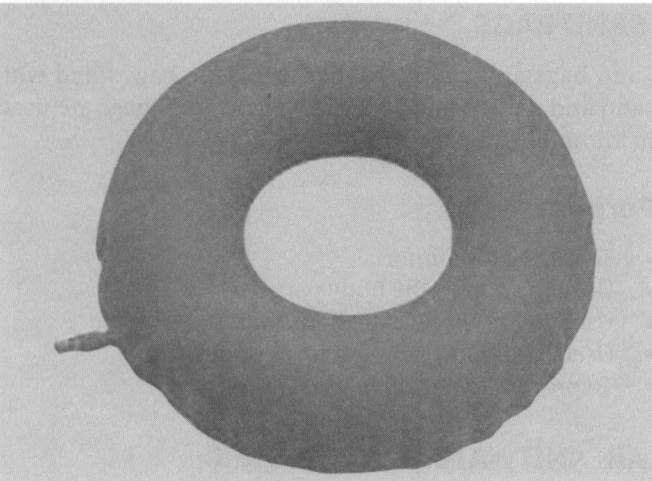

Fig. 10.16: Air cushion.

positions, to provide them a comfortable stay. Moreover, different positions are used for physical examinations so that the body parts are accessible and client's stay is comfortable. Patient's ability to assume positions depends upon their physical strength and degree of wellness. Their privacy should be kept as the top priority while doing physical examination as it will keep them at ease and provide greater accessibility and accuracy in assessing body parts.

Definitions

- Positioning is defined as placing the person in such a way to perform therapeutic interventions to promote the health of an individual.
- Positioning defined as placing the person in a proper body alignment for the purpose of preventive, promotive, curative and rehabilitative aspects of health.

Purpose of Positioning

- To provide comfort to the patient.
- To relieve pressure on various parts.
- To improve circulation.
- To prevent formation of deformity.
- To carry out investigations.
- To perform surgical and medical investigations.
- To prevent pressure sores.
- To provide proper body alignment.
- To conduct delivery/labor.
- To carry out nursing interventions.

Principles of Positioning

- Follow systematic and orderly way of doing.
- Cooperation between two.
- Follow safety measure to prevent accidents.
- Active participation.
- Using a right technique at right time.

Factors Involved in Positioning

- Need of an individual.
- Self-care ability.
- Extend of disability.
- Nature of disease condition.
- Level of consciousness.
- Protocol of the hospital.

Types of Positions Used

- Dorsal position.
- Dorsal recumbent position.
- Lithotomy position.
- Lateral position.
- Prone position.
- Sims' position.
- Knee-chest position.
- Trendelenburg's position.
- Fowler's position.

Types of Patients Need Special Care

- Unconscious patient.
- Infant and children.
- Hemiplegics and paraplegic patients.
- Immediate postoperative patients.
- Orthopedic patients.
- Cardiac patients.

General Instructions

- Maintain good body alignment of the patient at all times.
- Support body parts in good alignment by using supportive devices to promote comfort and prevent muscle strain.
- Avoid prolonged flexion of any one body segment by changing the position at least every two hours.
- Reduce the pressure caused by bodyweight of his or her body or object by changing the position and using protective devices.

Preliminary Assessment

- Check the patient's general condition.
- Check the physicians order for any limited movements.
- Assess the self-care ability of an individual.
- Arrange the comfort devices near the bedside.
- Identify the deformed extremity.
- Support the immobilize area during positioning.
- Identify the rationale before positioning.

Equipment

- Extra man power if needed.
- Extra pillows.
- Sheets and sheet rolls.
- Comfort devices such as back rest, cardiac table, sand bag, etc.

Procedure

- Explain the procedure to the patient.
- Provide privacy.
- Arrange the articles and manpower (if needed)
- Untie the bed sheets.
- Turn/lift/ambulate gently.
- Place and support with extra pillows under pressure points.
- Special care taken at pressure areas.
- Cover the patient with top sheet.
- Hand wash
- Record the time, position and condition of the skin.

SUPINE/DORSAL POSITION

Supine position the patient lies on his back with his head and shoulders are slightly elevated. One pillow is given under the head. His legs should be slightly flexed. A small pillow is placed under his knees.

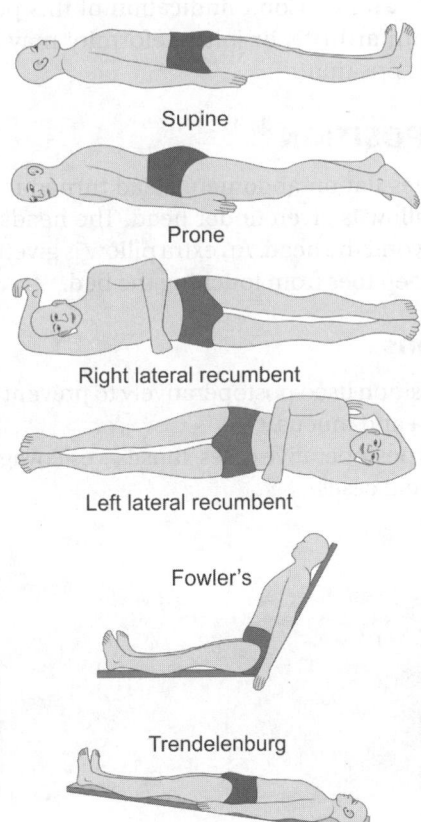

Fig. 10.17: Types of positions.

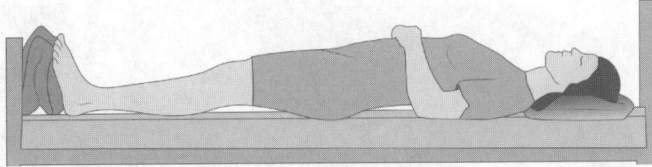

Fig. 10.18: Supine position.

Indications

- The usual position used by the patient.
- Used for examination of the chest and abdomen.

Procedure

- Place the patient on back with one pillow under the head, arms and hands at the sides, knees flexed and separated.
- Place the air ring under the hips and cotton rings or foam pads under the heels to reduce the pressure.
- Align the patient's body in good position.
- Support the body parts in good alignment for comfort when the patient is paralyzed.

Contraindications

- Elderly patients
- Patients with operation on abdomen, breast and thorax.
- Prone to hypostatic pneumonia.
- Patients with long-standing illnesses and neurological conditions.

DORSAL RECUMBENT POSITION

Patient lies on back, knees fully flexed, thighs flexed and externally rotated feet flat on the bed.

Indications

- It is used for catheterization, vaginal douche, vulval, vaginal and rectal examination.
- It is also used for vaginal operations and insertion of tampons.
- Patients who are in the convalescent period.
- Patients with gastric conditions.
- Patients with chest conditions.
- Patients with abdominal or pelvic operations unless erect sitting position is indicated.

Procedure

- Place the patient on back in bed with two or more pillows under the head and one pillow under the knees or maintain his position by elevating the top of bed on blocks.
- Place the air ring under the hips and cotton rings or foam pads under the heels to reduce the pressure.
- Align the patient's body in good position.
- Support the body parts in good alignment for comfort when the patient is paralyzed.

LITHOTOMY POSITION

The patient lies on her back. The legs are separated and thighs are flexed on the abdomen and the legs are on the thighs. The patient's buttocks are kept the edge of the table and legs are supported by stirrups.

Indications

- This position is given during gynecological examinations, treatments, and operations on genitourinary system.
- For delivery of baby.
- For rectal examinations and operations.

Procedure

- Explain the procedure to the patient.
- Provide privacy.
- Position the patient to lie on his back with one pillow under the head.
- Keep the legs well separated and the thighs are well flexed on the abdomen and the legs on the thighs.
- Buttocks are kept on the edge of the table and the legs are supported on stirrups.

Contraindications: Contraindication of this position are patients with arthritis or joint deformity may be unable assume this position.

PRONE POSITION

A patient lies flat on abdomen. Head turned to sideways. One soft pillow is given under head. The heads are at the sides or beyond the head. An extra pillow is given under the ankles to keep toes from touching the bed.

Indications

- This position used postoperatively to prevent aspiration of saliva and mucus.
- Used in postoperative cases, tonsils, vesicovaginal fistula and spinal cases.

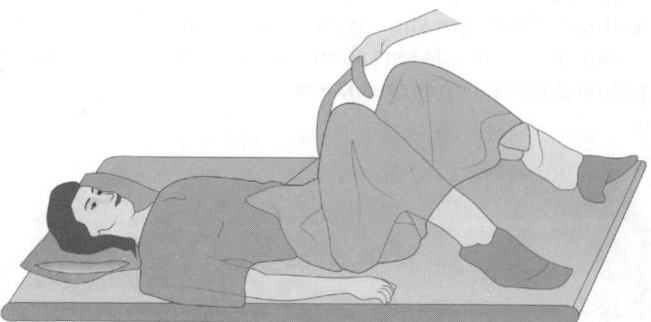

Fig. 10.19: Dorsal recumbent position.

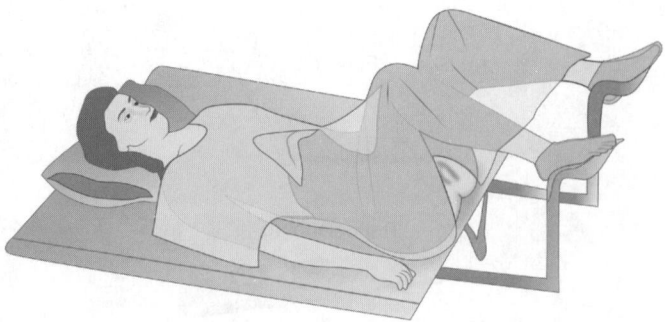

Fig. 10.20: Lithotomy position.

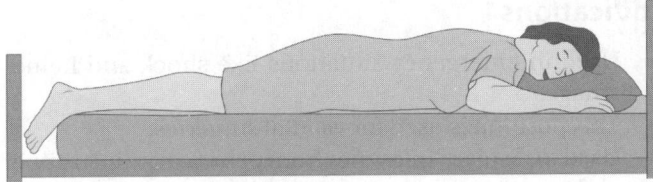

Fig. 10.21: Prone position.

- To prevent bed sores.
- To relieve abdominal distention.
- Used for patients having injuries and burns on back.

Procedure

- Explain the procedure to the patient.
- Provide privacy.
- Place the patient flat on abdomen with one pillow under the head.
- Turn patients head to one side and align the patient in good position.
- Support the body parts in good alignment for comfort.
- Place both arms lies at the sides of the heads.

Contraindications

This position is not well tolerated by the elderly or patients with cardiovascular or respiratory problems.

LATERAL POSITION

Patient lies on left side with legs flexed at thighs. A pillow is kept in front of the abdomen and at the back and one under the upper leg.

Indications

- Lateral position is used for giving back care enemas and colonic irrigation.
- Used for examination of perineum or rectum inserting suppositories.
- For taking rectal temperature.
- For change of position.
- Lateral position is a relaxing position.
- Giving back care.

Procedure

- Explain the procedure to the patient.
- Provide privacy.

- For left lateral position place the patient on left side with buttocks to the edge of bed, both thighs flexed and left arm underneath.
- For right lateral position, place the patient on right side with buttocks to the edge of bed, both thighs flexed and right arm underneath.
- Place air ring under the hips to reduce pressure on trochanters and at the hip joints, the cotton rings or foam pads under the ankles of lower legs to reduce the pressure on ankles.
- Align the patient in good position and make sure the patient is not lying on his arm.
- Support the body parts in good alignment for comfort.

SIMS' POSITION

Sims' position is similar to the lateral position except that the patient's weight is on the anterior aspects of the patient's shoulder girdle and hip. The patient's lower arm is behind him and the upper arm is flexed at the shoulder and elbow.

Indications

- This position is used for unconscious patient.
- It is used for rectal examinations.
- Used for vaginal examinations.
- Used for relaxation in antenatal exercises.

Procedure

- Explain the procedure to the patient.
- Collect articles need at the bed side.
- Provide privacy.
- Place the patient on the side.
- One pillow is placed under the head with the left cheek resting on it.
- The left arm is drawn behind the body and the right arm may be in any position comfortable for the patient.
- The right thigh is flexed against the abdomen.
- The left leg is extended well.
- Cover the patient with top sheet neatly.

Contraindications: Patients with deformities of the hip or knee may be unable to assume this position.

KNEE-CHEST/GENUPECTORAL POSITION

Patient rest on the knees and the chest. The head is turned to one side with one cheek on a pillow. A pillow is placed under the chest. The weight is on the chest and knees.

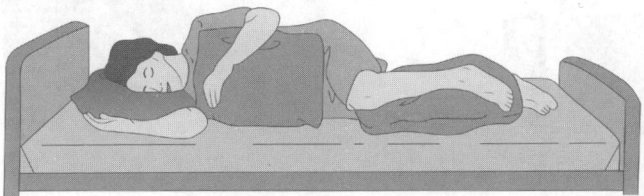

Fig. 10.22: Lateral position.

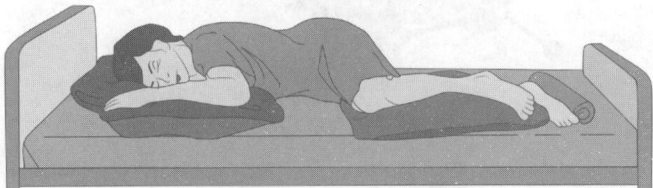

Fig. 10.23: Sims' position.

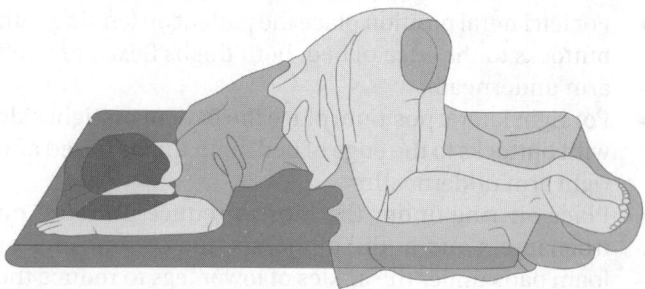

Fig. 10.24: Knee-chest position.

Indications

- This position is used for sigmoidoscopy.
- Used for vaginal and rectal examinations.
- Used in first aid treatment in cord prolapse or retroverted uterus.
- As exercise for postpartum and gynecology patients.

Procedure

- Explain the procedure to the patient.
- Collect the needed articles at the bed side.
- Provide privacy.
- Make the patient rests on the knees and chest.
- The head is turned to one side with the cheek on a pillow.
- The arms should be extended on the bed and flexed at the elbows to support the patient partially.
- The weight should rest on the chest and knees which are flexed so that the thighs are at right angles to the legs.

Contraindications: Patients with cardiovascular and respiratory problems cannot assume this position.

TRENDELENBURG'S POSITION

Trendelenburg's position, the patient lies on his back. The patient's head is low. The foot of the bed is elevated at 45 degree angle. The body is on an inclined place and the legs hang downward over the end of the table.

Indications

- Used in emergency situations like shock and hemorrhage.
- This position is used for vaginal surgeries.
- Used to displace intestines from pelvic cavity in to upper abdomen.
- Used during operations on the pelvic organs.
- To arrest bleeding from lower limb.

Procedure

- Explain the procedure to the patient.
- Arrange the article need at the bed side.
- Provide privacy (If needed).
- Place the patient lied on his back.
- Elevate the foot end at 45 degree angle.
- The body is on an inclined plane with hips higher than the bed.
- The knees are flexed and the legs hang downward over the end of the table.
- The patient is carefully supported to prevent slipping.
- Draping done depends upon the kind of operation to be performed.

FOWLER'S POSITION

Fowler's position is a sitting position in which the head is elevated, at least, a 45 degree angle. Back rest and two pillows are used for the back and head.

Fowler's position the main weight bearing areas of the patient are the heels, sacrum and the posterior aspects of the ileum.

Indications

- To relieve dyspnea.
- To improve circulation.
- To prevent thrombosis.
- Postoperatively to assist drainage from abdominal or pelvic cavity.

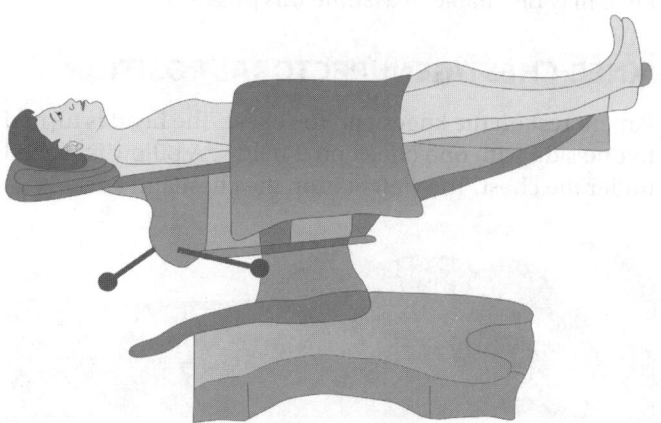

Fig. 10.25: Trendelenburg position.

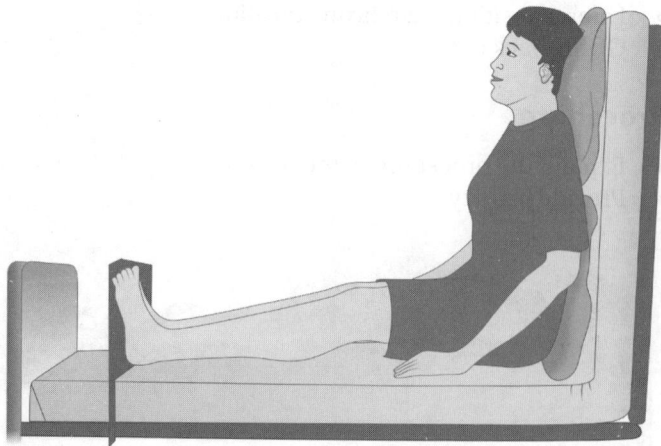

Fig. 10.26: Fowler's position.

- To relax the muscles of the abdomen, back and thighs.
- To relieve tension on the abdominal sutures.
- To promote comfort.
- To localize infection.
- To relieve edema of the chest and abdomen.

Procedure

- Explain the procedure to the patient.
- Arrange the articles needed at the bedside.
- Provide privacy.
- Place the patient in sitting position with arms at the sides and knees raised with pillow.
- Maintain this position; elevate the head of bed to 45-60 degree angle (Semi-fowler) or 60-90 degree angle (High-fowler).
- Elevate the knee rest to an angle of 15 degree or place a small pillow under the knees.

Pain: Nature, Types, Factors Influencing Pain, Assessment and Management

Pain disables people more than any single disease entity. It is probably the most common reason for a person to seek health care. Most medical-surgical problems are associated with pain, resulting either from:

- The disease process
- Diagnostic tests
- Treatment modalities
- Undergoing surgery
- Performed surgery.

List the Three Components of Pain

Pain appears to have three components:

- A stimulus, physical or mental.
- A bodily sensation of hurting.
- The reaction of the person experiencing it.

The nurse spends more time with the clients than any other members of the health care team and therefore has the opportunity to make a significant contribution towards increasing the patient's comfort and relieving pain.

Definition: Pain is a subjective, unpleasant, sensory and emotional experience associated with actual or potential tissue damage. Whatever the patient says it is, it is existing whenever he says it does.

Types of Pain

Acute pain: Acute pain is a very common occurrence. It indicates that some degree of damage has occurred within the body that requires some form of treatment or intervention. Healing may also be accompanied by acute pain. As healing progresses, the pain subsides and gradually disappears. Acute pain is accompanied by muscle tension and anxiety.

Chronic pain: Chronic pain is sometimes defined as pain that lasts for 6 months or longer. An episode of pain may assume the characteristics of chronic pain long before 6 months have elapsed, or some types of pain may remain primarily acute in nature for longer than 6 months. Nevertheless, after 6 months the majority of pain experiences are accompanied by problems associated with chronic pain.

Factors Influencing Pain Perception

Referred pain: Referred pain is felt in areas other than those stimulated. It may occur when stimulation is not perceived in the primary areas. For example, the person having a heart attack may complain only of pain radiating down the left arm when in fact, the tissue damage is occurring in the myocardium.

Referred pain occurs most often with damage or injury to visceral organs, and the pain is referred to cutaneous surfaces.

Psychogenic pain: The term "Psychogenic" has been used to describe pain where no physical pathology has been found or where the pain appears to have a greater psychological basis than a physical one. A caution here is that diagnostic tests are not definitive measures and may not be sophisticated enough to detect pathophysiologic changes. Distinguishing between physical and emotional components of pain is difficult and it is important to remember that all pain is real.

Clinical manifestation of pain: The patient's response to the pain may be any one or a combination of possible reactions. These may include:

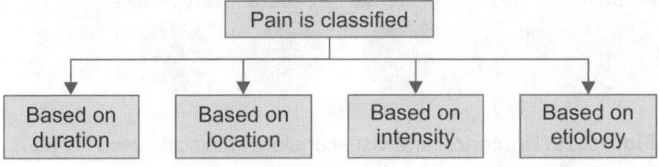

Fig. 10.27: Types of pain.

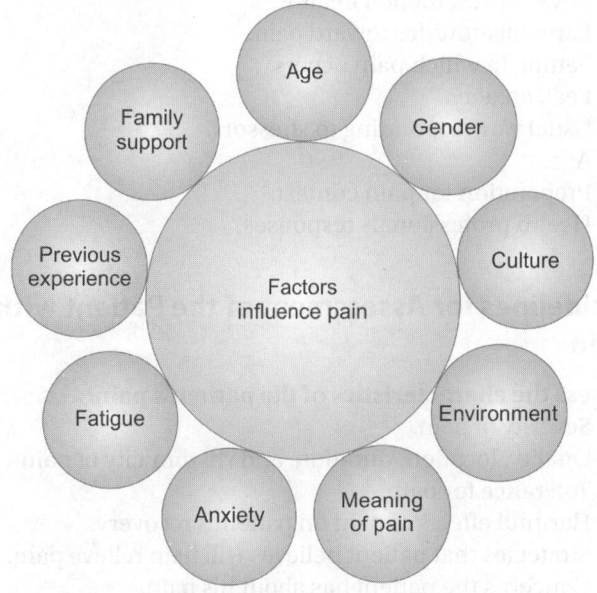

Fig. 10.28: Factors influencing pain perception.

- Physiologic manifestations.
- Verbal statements.
- Vocal behaviors.
- Facial expressions.
- Body movements.
- Physical contact with others.
- Alterations in response to the environment.
- Adaptation of physiological and behavioral response.

These behaviors vary greatly from one person to another and may differ within the same person from one time to the next.

The character (quality) of pain
1. Pricking or cutting pain • A sharp and localized pain. It is of cutaneous origin and is caused by pricking or cutting the skin by a sharp object
2. Burning pain • A less well localized pain. It is usually of cutaneous origin and is caused by burns or inflammations of the skin
3. Aching pain • A dull-aching nature. It is more diffuse and felt coming from deeper tissues, e.g. rheumatic pains
4. Throbbing pain • Is characterized by fluctuation of its intensity with arterial pulsations. It results from localized inflammation in deep tissues, as in abscess formation
5. Colicky pain • Pain results from spasm of plain muscles in the walls of hollow viscera

Factors that Influence Responses to Pain

- Meaning of pain to individual person.
- Degree of pain perception.
- Past experience.
- Cultural values.
- Social expectations.
- Physical and mental health.
- Parental attitudes toward pain.
- Setting in which pain occurs.
- Fear, anxiety.
- Usual way responding to stressors.
- Age.
- Preparation for pain context.
- Health professionals responses.

Guidelines for Assessment of the Patient with Pain

Assess the characteristics of the patient's pain:
- Severity of pain.
- Quality, location, duration, and rhythmicity of pain.
- Tolerance for pain.
- Harmful effects of pain on patient's recovery.
- Strategies that patient believes will help relieve pain.
- Concerns the patient has about his pain.

Pain Assessment
Precipitating/alleviating factors: • What cause the pain? What aggravates it? has medication or treatment worked in past? **Q**uality of pain: • Ask the patient to describe the pain using words like "sharp, dull, stabbing, burning" **R**adiation • Does pain exist in one location or radiate to other areas? **S**everity • Have patient use a descriptive, numeric or visual scale to rate the severity of pain? **T**iming • Is the pain constant or intermittent, when did it begin?

Assess the patient's behavioral responses to the pain experiences:
- Determine if the pain is acute or chronic.
- Observe for the following behavioral responses:
  - Physiologic manifestations (changes in pulse, blood pressure, respiratory rate, etc.)
  - Verbal statements
  - Vocal responses
  - Facial expressions
  - Body movements
  - Alteration in response to the environment
  - Physical contact with others
  - Adaptation of physiological and behavioral responses
  - Effect of pain on ability to communicate and carry out usual activities of daily living.

Assess factors that influence responses to pain:
- Ethnic and cultural factors.
- Previous pain experiences.
- Meaning of the pain experiences.
- Patient's responses to pain relief strategies.

Nursing Diagnosis for Patient with Pain

The nursing diagnoses given to clients experiencing pain are pain (implying acute pain) and chronic pain. When writing the diagnostic statement, the nurse may further specify the type of location of the pain (e.g. postoperative chest, abdominal, back). Biologic factors and precipitating factors, when known, must be part of the diagnostic statement.
- Ineffective airway clearance related to postoperative incisional chest pain.
- Anxiety related to past experience of poor control of pain and to anticipation of pain.

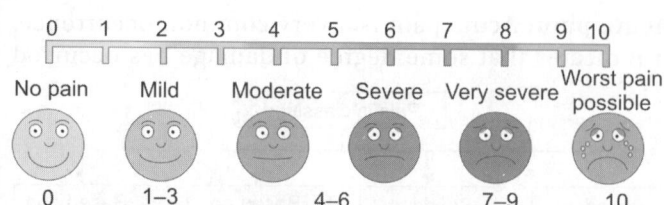

Fig. 10.29: Numerical and visual analog. Pain scale used for pain measurement.

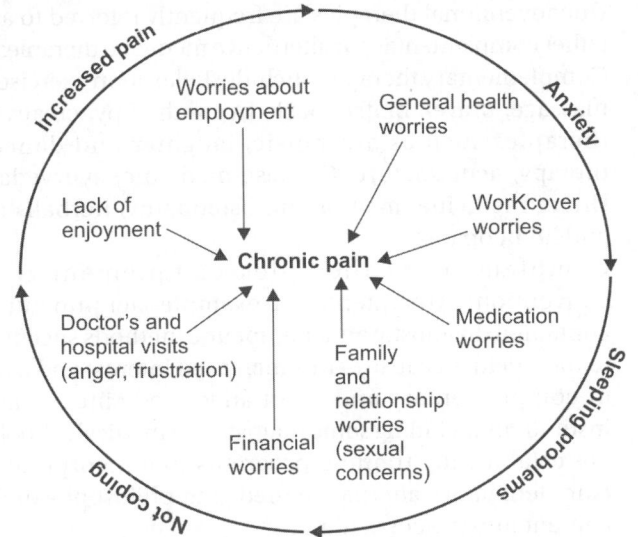

Fig. 10.30: Causes of chronic pain.

- Ineffective breathing pattern related to postoperative abdominal pain.
- Ineffective individual coping related to prolonged continuous back pain, ineffective pain, management and inadequate support systems.
- Fear related to anticipated pain after surgery.
- Altered health maintenance related to chronic pain and fatigue.
- Hopelessness related to ineffective pain management strategies.
- Knowledge deficit (Pain control measures) related to lack of exposure to information resources.
- Impaired physical mobility related to arthritic pain in knee and ankle.
- Self-care deficit: Bathing/hygiene, dressing/grooming, toileting related to pain in the joints.
- Sleep pattern disturbance related to increased pain perception at night.

Planning: The nurse identifies nursing interventions that will assist the client in achieving the overall client goals of preventing, modifying or eliminating pain so that the client is able partially or completely to resume usual daily activities and be able to cope more effectively with the pain experiences. When planning, nurses need to choose appropriate pain relief measures for the client. Nursing interventions may include a variety of pharmacological and non-pharmacological interventions.

Implementation: Pain management is the alleviation of pain or a reduction of pain to a level comfortable that is acceptable to the client. It includes two basic types of nursing interventions.
- Pharmacologic.
- Non-pharmacologic interventions.

Generally speaking, a combination of strategies is available for the client in pain sometimes strategies need to be tried and changed until the client obtains effective pain relief.

General Strategies for Pain Management

- Assess the patient's pain status based on the patient's past experience.
- Incorporate the following factors in the assessment of the patient's pain status:
  - Location/characteristics.
  - Onset.
  - Frequency.
  - Intensity.
  - Quality,
  - Precipitating factors.
  - Effective pain control measures.
  - Pain expression style (verbal, crying, moaning).
  - Impact on quality of life.
  - Effect of sleep/wake pattern.
  - Effect on energy level.
- Apply previous strategies that have controlled pain.
- Explore strategies that have been successful in the past.
- Assess the patient's willingness to incorporate non-pharmaceutical pain control measures.
- Administer medication as per the physician's orders.
- Immobilize or rest affected area.
- Relieve pressure areas with turning or pressure reduction devices such as air-fluidized support systems.
- Suggest and instruct the patient in relaxation techniques, short simple techniques with the nurse directing for acute pain: more complex techniques for chronic pain.

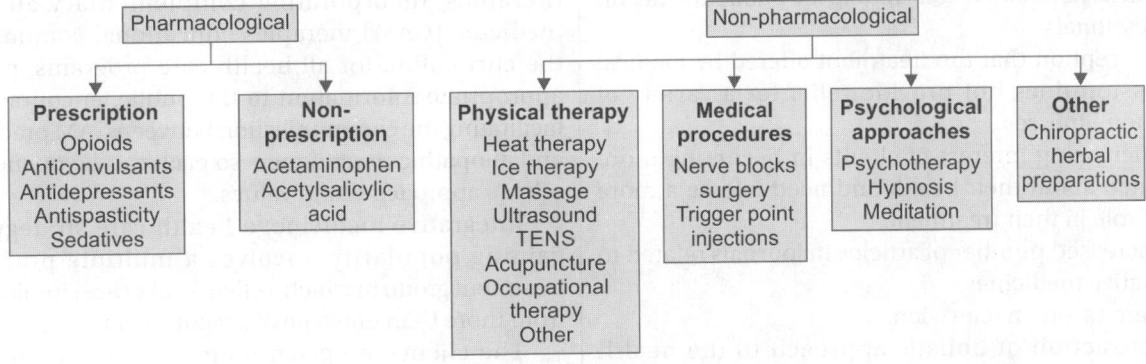

Fig. 10.31: Chronic pain treatment.

- Encourage the patient's attention to proper posture and alignment.
- Provide therapeutic positioning.
- Rest affected area.
- Provide distraction.
- Use hypnotic strategies as prescribed.
- Provide music therapy.
- Use counter stimulation: Pressure, massage, vibration, heat/cold, external analgesics, transcutaneous nerve stimulation.
- Provide a supportive environment.
- Help the patient to identify activities that may enhance pain.
- Discuss strategies to reduce enhancement of pain.
- Discuss strategies to avoid these activities within the patient's lifestyle.
- Provide touch, especially for infants or for disoriented or unresponsive patients.

COMPLEMENTARY/ALTERNATIVE THERAPIES OF HEALTH

Changes in science and medicine have provided the knowledge and technology that have successfully altered the course of many illnesses. Despite the success of allopathic medicine, many conditions such as arthritis, chronic backache, gastrointestinal problems, allergies, headache, insomnia, etc. have been difficult to treat and more clients are exploring alternative methods to relieve their symptoms.

It is estimated that 75% clients referred to practitioners due to health problems such as stress, pain and other health conditions have no known etiology. While allopathic medicine is quite effective in treating numerous physical ailments such as bacterial infections, structural abnormalities, acute emergencies. It is in general less effective in preventing diseases, decreasing stress-induced illnesses, managing chronic disease, and caring for the emotional and spiritual needs of individuals.

USES OF COMPLEMENTARY THERAPY

The use of complementary and alternative medicine is not new to health care, but the last two decades have seen a huge rise in its popularity, both among the public and health care professionals.

- The perception that the treatment offered by medical profession does not provide relief for a variety of common illnesses.
- The increasing interest of clients in becoming more educated about their health and need to take a more active role in their treatment.
- The increased number of articles in journals related to alternative medicines.
- Programs seen on television.
- The attraction of holistic approach to the health care that incorporates the mind, body and spirit.

- Unconventional therapies are frequently referred to as either complementary or alternative medicine therapies.
- Complementary therapies include: Relaxation exercise, massage, prayer, biofeedback, hypnotherapy, creative therapies such as art, music, laughter and dance therapy, acupuncture, Chinese medicine, ayurveda, Unani medicine, meditation, osteopathy, herbalism and homeopathy.
- Complementary therapies complement the conventional treatment. For example, acupuncture contained diagnostic and therapeutic methods specific to their field. Because of this increased interest and use of complementary and alternative medicine, many institutions including some mainstream medical school, are establishing training programs that incorporate complementary alternative medicine philosophy and content into the curriculum.
- Integrative medical programs are being developed that allow health care consumer the opportunity to be treated by a team of providers consisting of both allopathic and complementary practitioners.
- Interest in complementary alternative medicine is also evident from the increased number of articles in medical journals and the development of several journals that specifically focus on complementary and alternative medicines.

NURSES' ROLE IN COMPLEMENTARY THERAPIES

The increased interest in complementary therapies has gone up significantly in the last 15 years. This increased interest comes not only from health care consumers, but also from allopathic physicians who have increased concern that allopathic medicine is not meeting the needs of clients. It is also seen that many allopathic practitioners are reserved about these therapies because of the lack of evidence. There is a group of people who think is just for pampering and cannot see the medical benefit.

Although many professionals are exploring the use of complementary therapies and monitoring research being conducted in this area. Proposals put forth by these groups include assessing the need of the public for complementary therapies, incorporating complementary alternative medicine (CAM) therapies educational components in the curriculum for all health care programs, providing appropriate information to the public, encouraging and facilitating the communication between CAM practitioners and allopathic practitioners so each can be opened to the other's approaches and values.

Integrative medicine, a health care strategy that is gaining popularity, involves a multiple-practitioner treatment group in which a client seeks care simultaneously from more than one type of practitioners.

The clients are given option to choose the kind of practitioner they feel would benefit their particular health problem. Most often clients suffering from chronic health problems get benefit from CAM therapies where traditional allopathic medicine is not treating their problem completely. In Indian scenario, this is not practiced in reality, but this approach of open communication and practice between CAM practitioners and allopathic practitioners could potentially benefit a large number of patients.

INTEGRATIVE APPROACH IN HEALTH CARE

As integrative medicine approach is consistent with the holistic approach, nurses have the potential of becoming essential participants in this type of health care philosophy. Nurses should be knowledgeable of complementary therapies to make recommendations. Nurses should also be able to provide advice to clients regarding when to seek conventional therapy. As nurses work very closely with their clients and are in unique position of becoming familiar with the client's religious and cultural viewpoints and existential issues. They may be able to determine which CAM therapy would be more appropriately aligned with their beliefs and offer recommendations accordingly. It is also important to obtain specific consent from a patient before carrying out any complementary procedure. As it is not part of our mainstream treatment yet, it should never be used on unconscious patients.

Client's interest and participation in complementary therapies is increasing. Therefore it is important for nurses to be knowledgeable of these complementary therapies. It is also important for nurses to keep abreast of the current research being done in this area to provide accurate information not only to the clients, but to other health care professionals also. Many studies related to complementary therapies have involved small number of subjects and were not well controlled. More research studies are needed to validate the effectiveness of complementary therapies.

BIOFEEDBACK

Biofeedback is a rapidly developing scientific field that has grown in physiology, psychology and electronics. Ordinarily, we are unaware of the subtle internal body activities that are part of our everyday lives. Biofeedback uses sensitive electronics to detect and amplify these activities in order to bring them to be aware. By allowing us to observe these activities, biofeedback also allows us to learn to modify them. Since we are immediately aware to the outcome of our attempts, we can gradually learn to produce the results we desire.

Types of Biofeedback

Electromyography (EMG) muscle biofeedback: Electromyography biofeedback measures electrical activity created by muscle contractions. Often use for relaxation training and performance training, stress and pain management.

Thermal or temperature biofeedback: Thermal biofeedback is used to train people to quiet the nervous system arousal mechanisms which produce hand and feet cooling. This is often used for relaxation, stress and pain management and anxiety.

Biofeedback technique: It trains the central nervous system, feedback brain electrical activity, called brainwaves. This is the fastest growing field in biofeedback. Mainly used in depression, anxiety, insomnia, head injury, obsessive compulsive disorder, anger, autism.

Skin conductance level (SCL)/galvanic skin response (GSR)/electro-dermal response (EDR): These are all measures of physiological activity in skin. Part of it is based on sweat gland activity. This measure is very useful for relaxation and stress management. It is very much useful with attention deficit disorders, hyperactivity disorder.

Mechanism of Action

Biofeedback self awareness and regulation techniques teach people to develop greater awareness of their physical and mental behavior. People learn to take greater control and responsibility for their health and as they become more aware of unhealthy symptom perpetuating behaviors, such as tensed muscles, constricted blood vessels (Hypertension), over-reactive nervous system activity, rapid heart rate, respiration or sweat gland activity or upsetting thought.

Biofeedback devices magnify or zoom in on body behaviors, therefore people get more information than their normal sensory awareness provides. The feedback information is combined with coaching, training and sometimes therapeutic interventions aimed at producing more healthy, normalized or more effective functioning.

NON-PHARMACOLOGICAL THERAPIES

- **Distraction:** It is a useful tool for helping alleviate both acute and chronic pain. These techniques work equally well with adults and children. It simply involves diverting the patient's attention away from the sensation of pain towards other thoughts. Some examples of specific techniques involve the following:
  - Encourage the patient to recount a recent exciting or pleasant experience: Encourage the patient to relate information from all the senses, i.e. touch, taste, smell, hearing, and sight. Children can be encouraged to recite rhymes or participate in a game.
  - Music is an excellent distracter and relaxant: The patient need to select music based on personal preferences. Encourage the patient to actively listen. Have the patient close the eyes, concentrate on the music and tap out the rhythm of the music. A study conducted by Ishii et al (1993) demonstrated that music is effective to relieve a pain associated with a compulsory posture and also play a significant role on pain management in palliative therapy.

- Participate in rhythmic singing: Chants, hymns, or simple songs with the strong beat are good to use with both adults and children. Tapping the foot or fingers for emphasis is an additional distracter.
- Rhythmic breathing exercises are another distracter: The patient may do these exercises with eyes closed or focusing on an object. The patient focuses on the breath and silently repeats "In, 2, 3, and 4-Out, 2, 3, and 4". Breathing is to be deep and slow, preferably from the abdomen.
- Laughter therapy for 5-10 minutes enhances the comfort of clients suffering from pain. Cousin 1974, experienced relief from pain for 1 hour following 10 minutes belly laughter.

- **Visualization:** It is a form of distraction that uses images to modify the perception of pain and decrease the intensity of the pain experience. This is a useful strategy with all age groups, practicing it for approximately 20 minutes, 2 to 3 times a day, will improve the effectiveness of the images. One common method of visualization is guided imagery. An imaginary "magic glove" or "magic blanket" may be put in place before a painful procedure such as an intravenous injection.
- **Hypnosis:** The clinical application of hypnosis is usually executed by a registered hypnotherapist. This technique works with all age groups. This technique involves achieving deep relaxation and then listening to or giving oneself positive suggestions. From review of literature, many studies have shown relationship of hypnosis in pain reduction.
- **Massage:** It had a long history of use in the treatment of muscular pain. The effect of massage is similar to heat in that circulation and removal of cellular waste products is enhanced. It is a valuable technique for reducing anxiety and promoting relaxation. Many studies have shown positive effect of massage in promoting relaxation and decreasing pain perception.
- **Relaxation techniques:** Successful reduction of anxiety and fear assists the individual to feel more comfortable and experience a decreased perception of pain.
- **Biofeedback technique:** It is useful for individuals with chronic pain. The individuals learn to control non-conscious physiological responses such as blood pressure and muscle tension through the use of mental images and thought processes.
- **Meditation:** This is a useful relaxation technique for patients with acute and chronic pain. Prior to beginning the meditation the patient selects a soothing word, relax or calm. The patient may close or leave them open to focus on the object. With every breath in, the patient silently says the word that was chosen.

Miller and Perry in quasi-experimental study found that cardiac surgery patients who were taught simple deep breathing relaxation techniques preoperatively had decreased pain perception, decreased vital signs at statistically significant level.

- **Therapeutic touch:** It is a method of directing the energy through the hands. The technique produces a relaxation response and a perception of pain relief. A study conducted in hospital has shown a positive effect of therapeutic touch on the pain perception of patients after the surgery. Turner (1994) studied the effect of therapeutic touch on reducing the pain and infection among hospitalized patients.

NURSES' ROLE IN PAIN MANAGEMENT

The pain perception is multifaceted in that it encompasses an individual's physical, emotional, cognitive and experiential realm. The uniqueness of each patient explains the distinctiveness each one's response to pain and provides the rationale for customized care plan. As nurses are the persons who are providing care to patients round the clock. They are using different approaches for promoting the health and early recovery. As pharmacological and surgical methods of pain management are not free from side effects/complications, nurses should use non-pharmacological methods. While using these nonpharmacological methods, nurses not only relieves the pain perception of client but also promotes psychological wellbeing. With this, patient feels energetic and also feels emotionally satisfied. As many studies conducted in the hospital has shown the positive effect of these methods on promoting the health, nurses should participate actively in using these non-pharmacological methods. Along with this research studies can be conducted.

CONCLUSION

Nurses are supposed to think and act best for the patients and are striving hard to achieve it. Nurse is one who takes care of patient's environment and his treatment plan. Due to the evolution of aroma therapist, the aesthetic side of ward and hospitals are now looked by them. Earlier the massage therapies were done by nurses may be due to specialization and load of work on nurses, this area is handled by them. So now this therapy is gaining momentum as a complementary therapy. It is necessary for nurses to keep abreast of the recent advancements and developments in the field of science. Nurses should acquire the basic understanding of the chemical structure and physical properties of essential oils as well as knowledge of the safe application of a few commonly available oils and plan to use them in their practice.

BIBLIOGRAPHY

1. Alice L. Price. The Art, Science and Spirit of Nursing, 3rd Ed. Philadelphia, WB Saunders Company, 1968.
2. Harkness-Hood G, Dincher JR. Total Patient Care: Foundations and Practice of Adult Health Nursing, 8th Ed. St. Louis: Mosby Year Book, Inc, 1992.
3. Kozier B, Erb G, Olivieri R. Fundamentals of Nursing: Concepts and Process,
4. Kozier Barbara. B, Du Gas, Beverly Witter. Fundamentals of Patient Care: A Comprehensive Approach to Nursing. WB Saunders Company, 1967.

5. Kurzen CR. Contemporary Practical/Vocational Nursing, 2nd Ed. Philadelphia: JB Lippincott, 1992.
6. McClosky JC, Grace HK. Current Issues in Nursing, 4th Ed. St. Louis: Mosby Year Book, Inc., 1994.
7. Mitchell PR, Grippando GM. Nursing Perspectives and Issues, 5th Ed. New York: Delmar Publishers Inc, 1993.
8. Potter PA, Perry AG. Fundamentals of Nursing Concepts, Process and Practice, 3rd Ed. St. Louis: Mosby-Year Book, Inc, 1993.
9. Shafer, Kathleen, et. al. Medical-Surgical Nursing, 6th Ed. Saint Louis: CV Mosby Co, 1975.
10. Shakuntala Sharma 'Birpuri'. Principles and Practice of Nursing. Jaypee Brothers Medical Publishers (P) Ltd., New Delhi, 1997.
11. Sr. Nancy. Principles and Practice of Nursing, Vol. 1, 3 Ed. NR Brothers. Indore, 1992.
12. Taylor C, Lillis C, LeMone P. Fundamentals of Nursing: The Art and Science of Nursing Care, Philadelphia: JB Lippincott, 1993.
13. Taylor C, Lillis C, LeMone P. Fundamentals of Nursing: The Art and Science of Nursing Care. Philadelphia: JB Lippincott, 1993.
14. Thressamma CP. Fundamentals of Nursing, Procedure Manual for General Nursing Course. PC Mathew, Kottayam, Kerala, 1992.
15. Timby BK, Lewis LW. Fundamental Skills and Concepts in Patient Care, 5th Ed. Philadelphia: JB Lippincott, Co, 1992.
16. Virginia Henderson. Principles and Practice of Nursing. New York: MacMillan Publishing Co., 1970.

REVIEW QUESTIONS

Long Essays

1. Define comfort, explain principles relevant to comfort.
2. Define bed making, explain the preparation of unoccupied bad.
3. Define pain; explain the factors influencing pain perception.

Short Essays

1. Explain the principles involved in bed making.
2. Explain postoperative bed.
3. Define comfort devices and explain their types.
4. Define position explain the types, purposes and principles.
5. Describe fowler position.
6. Trendelenburg's position.
7. Nursing diagnosis for patient with pain.
8. Nurses' role in complementary therapies.

Short Answers

1. Factors influencing comfort.
2. Amputation bed.
3. Cardiac bed.
4. Back rest.
5. Bed cradles.
6. Air cushion.
7. Prone position.
8. Knee-chest/genupectoral position.
9. Types of pain.
10. Biofeedback.

MULTIPLE CHOICE QUESTIONS

1. **Factors influencing comfort are the following, *except*:**
   a. Pain and restriction of movements due to weakness
   b. Wrinkled, soiled and wet sheets
   c. Delayed or inadequate attention to meet the personal needs
   d. All of the above
2. **Bed making is a systematic way of preparing the appropriate bed based on the condition of the patient, which adopts _____ of nursing.**
   a. Scientific principles
   b. Moral principles
   c. Ethical principles
   d. Legal principles
3. **An unoccupied bed is an empty bed, and is fully covered with a counterpane to protect it from:**
   a. Infection
   b. Dust and dirt
   c. Insects
   d. Pollution
4. **The purpose of operation bed is:**
   a. To prepare to meet any emergency
   b. To keep the bed warm in order to provide comfort
   c. To avoid wastage of time, energy, and material
   d. All of the above
5. **Factors that influence responses to pain:**
   a. Ethnic and cultural factors
   b. Previous pain experiences
   c. Patient's responses to pain relief strategies
   d. All of the above

ANSWERS

1. d   2. a   3. b   4. d   5. d

CHAPTER 11
Promoting Safety in Health Care Environment

LEARNING OBJECTIVES

- Physical environment: Temperature, humidity, noise, ventilation, light, odor, pest control
- Reduction of physical hazards: Fire, accidents
- Fall risk assessment
- Role of nurse in providing safe and clean environment
- Safety devices: Restraints: Types, purposes, indications, legal implications and consent, application of restraints: skill and practice guidelines
- Other safety devices: Side rails, grab bars, ambu alarms, etc.

TERMINOLOGY

Absolute duty: No defence available against non-compliance with statutory requirement.

Accident: An incident which results in death, injury, loss, or damage.

Accident triangle: Indicates statistical relationship and severity of accident.

Carcinogen: A substance or physical agent that causes cancer.

Carcinogenic: Inherent potential of a substance or physical agent to be a carcinogen.

Fall: A fall is an event which results in a person coming to rest inadvertently on the ground or floor or other lower level.

Anticipated falls: May occur when a patient whose score on a falls risk tool indicates she or he is at risk of falls.

Unanticipated falls: Occur when the cause of the fall is not reflected in the patient's risk factor for falls, conditions exist which cause the fall, yet these are not predictable (e.g. the patient faints suddenly).

Accidental falls: Occur when a patient falls unintentionally, usually as a result of tripping or slipping, as a result of equipment failure or other environmental factors. Patients cannot be identified as being at risk for falls prior to this type of fall.

Risk assessment tool: A conceptual framework that organizes knowledge on the etiology of predicting falls.

Danger: A state or condition in which personal injury and/or asset damage is reasonably foreseeable. The presence of a hazard.

Dependent (failures): Failures of two or more elements of a system where these failures cannot be considered independent (q.v). Common cause and common mode failures are dependent failures.

Dermatitis: Inflammation of the skin. When the condition is due to contact with a substance at work it is called 'occupational' or 'industrial' dermatitis.

Diversity: Performing the same function in a redundant system (q.v) by different means in different elements, including different technologies and/or design and implementation methods.

Error: Mistake; error of judgment leading to action resulting in an accident and its subsequent effects.

Fire precautions: The measures taken and the fire protection features provided in a building (e.g. design, systems, equipment and procedures) to minimize the risk to the occupants from the outbreak of fire.

Fire prevention: The concept of preventing outbreaks of fire, of reducing the risk of fire spreading and of avoiding danger to persons and property from fire.

First aid: The skilled application of accepted principles of treatment on the occurrence of an accident or in the case of sudden illness, using facilities or materials available at the time

Harm: Injury to or death of persons, or damage.

Hazard: A potential source of harm.

Hazardous event: The occurrence of a hazard, generally used in the context of the failure of a safety related system.

Hazan: Hazard analysis.

Hazid: Hazard identification.

Incident: An unplanned, unexpected event which has the potential to lead to an accident although may not do so.

Mistake: A human action that produces an unintended result.

Mitigation: Factors or events which can prevent a hazard escalating to an accident, or can reduce the likelihood or severity of an accident. mitigation can be provided by a number of means including engineered systems, procedures and providence - "good luck".

Narcotic: Agent that depresses brain functions, e.g. organic solvents.

Near miss: An incident, which did not show a visible result, but had the potential to do so.

Negligence: The omission to do something, which a reasonable person, guided upon those considerations which ordinarily regulate the conduct of human affairs would do, or something, which a prudent and reasonable person would not do.

Pollution prevention: Focuses on stopping pollution being produced in the first place, or reducing any waste generation at the source.

Pollution control: Those measures taken to control pollution and wastes after they have been generated or produced.

Toxic: Inherent potential of a substance to cause harm.

Toxin: Substance that causes harm.

INTRODUCTION

A healthy environment is fundamental to life, and attention to the effects of the environment on human health is essential if we are to achieve the goal of health for all. As nurses working in the health care profession we have a responsibility to the people of the world to be an environmental health activist and raise awareness of the health implications of environmental changes, to support policies to reduce health vulnerability and to build capacity to adapt to climate change (WHO, 2005). The nurse's role as an environmental activist. This will be discussed in the context of environmental health advocacy in the home, community and workplace regarding clean water, food and air.

DEFINITION

Patient safety defined as an essential part of nursing care that aims to prevent avoidable errors and patient harm. Patient safety is a feature of a healthcare system and a set of tested ways for improving care.

OBJECTIVE/GOALS OF PATIENT SAFETY

The delivery of safe, high-quality patient care is of utmost importance to nurses. As nursing care spans all areas of care delivery, nurses are well placed to prevent harm to patients and improve the quality and safety of healthcare delivered across all settings. As such, nurses should be central to the design and operation of all health providers' patient safety systems and processes. A panel of patient safety experts—composed of nurses, physicians, pharmacists, risk managers, clinical engineers, and other professionals who have hands-on experience with patient safety issues in a variety of health care settings. Below are the seven key recommendations:

1. Improve the accuracy of patient identification. Use at least two patient identifiers when providing care, treatment, and services. Make sure that the correct patient gets the correct blood when they get a blood transfusion.
2. Improve the effectiveness of communication among caregivers. Report critical results of tests and diagnostic procedures to the right staff person on a timely basis.
3. Improve the safety of using medications. Label all medications, medication containers, and other solutions on and off the sterile field in perioperative and other settings. Record the correct information about each patient's medicines. Compare those medicines to new medicines given to the patient. Make sure the patient knows which medicines to take when they are at home.
4. Reduce the harm associated with clinical alarm systems. Make improvements to ensure that alarms on medical equipment are heard and responded to on time.
5. Reduce the risk of health care-associated infections. Use the hand cleaning guidelines from the CDC, and set goals for improving hand cleaning.
6. Identify safety risks inherent in the patient population. Find out which patients are most likely to try to commit suicide.
7. Conduct a preprocedure verification process. Make sure that the correct surgery is done on the correct patient and at the correct place on the patient's body. Mark the correct place on the patient's body where the surgery is to be done. Pause before the surgery to make sure that a mistake is not being made.

SAFETY IN HEALTH CARE ENVIRONMENT

Patient Safety is a health care discipline that emerged with the evolving complexity in health care systems and the resulting rise of patient harm in health care facilities. It aims to prevent and reduce risks, errors and harm that occur to patients during provision of health care. A cornerstone of the discipline is continuous improvement based on learning from errors and adverse events.

Patient safety is fundamental to delivering quality essential health services. Indeed, there is a clear consensus that quality health services across the world should be effective, safe and people-centered. In addition, to realize the benefits of quality health care, health services must be timely, equitable, integrated and efficient.

To ensure successful implementation of patient safety strategies; clear policies, leadership capacity, data to drive safety improvements, skilled health care professionals and effective involvement of patients in their care, are all needed.

PATIENT SAFETY IN THE HOSPITAL

The patient environment of care plays a vital role in the discipline of patient safety for every hospital. The hospital is safe place for patients and for those that work and of the utmost importance for all health care personnel. Patient safety is dependent upon both the caregiver and the environment in which care is provided.

Practice of patient safety (WHO)
• Be aware of look-a like, sound-a like medication name • Proper patient identification • Explain in detail during patient hand/take-overs • Performance of correct procedure at correct body site • Careful about electrolyte imbalance • Assuring proper treatment during shifting • Avoid catheter and tubing, wrong connections • Single use of injection syringes • Improved hand hygiene to prevent healthcare-associated infections • Practice surgical safety guidelines

Patients (and their families) look for visible, palpable evidence that demonstrates that a hospital is a safe haven and that those who care for them are skilled, involved, and, ultimately, will protect them. In their state of acuity, patients see and hear everything in relationship to themselves, looking and listening for signs and symbols that will offer hope and security as they navigate through the healthcare crisis.

OPTIMUM ENVIRONMENT FOR THE PATIENT

There are a few factors which are considered essential to well-being, are as in **Figure 11.1**.

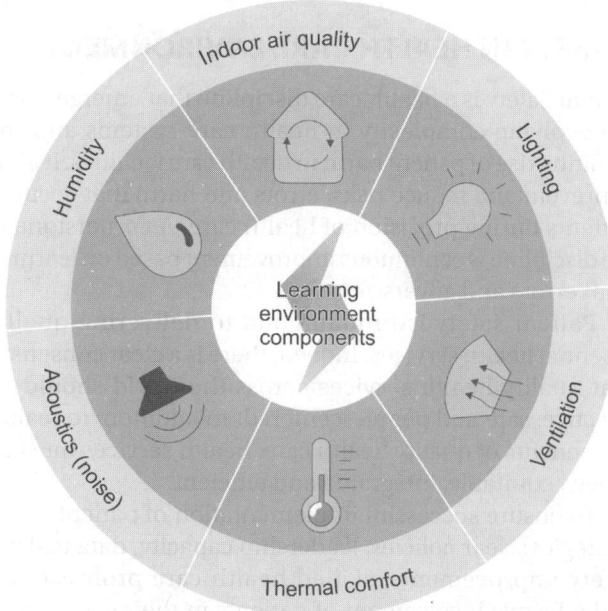

Fig. 11.1: Leaning environment components.

- Adequate lighting during the day and night
- Provision of an atmospheric temperature and humidity that promotes normal body functions
- Sufficient air movement to evaporate sweats and favors vascular changes within the skin
- Atmospheric pressure within man's tolerance
- Provision for disposal of refuse on excreta
- Removal of dust, injurious chemicals and pathogenic bacteria from the atmospheric air
- Reasonable cleanliness of all surface and furnishing that the individual is likely to handle
- A dwelling place free from insects, animal pests, fire hazards, mechanical injuries, electric shocks, radiation and poisons
- Free from disagreeable odors and noises, harmony of town and design in the immediate surroundings, Provision of privacy, etc.

INFLUENCE OF EXTERNAL ENVIRONMENT

Atmospheric temperature: In an ideal temperature, the person does not feel chilly but it should be sufficiently warm enough to cause perspiration. A room temperature ranging from 68 to 72°F (20–22°C) considered comfortable.

Humidity is the amount of moisture in the air. It affects the evaporation of moisture from the skin. A humidity of 40–60% considered comfortable.

Environmental safety
• Adequate light • Adequate ventilation, exhaust fan • Stairs with hand rails • Window-door-closer • Slip preventing floors • Fire extinguishers and fire alarms • Prevent noise pollution • Heavy and fixed beds • No waterlogging in bathrooms • Call system for patients • Adequate no. of bed screens to maintain privacy of the patient

- **Air movement:** Ventilation means movement in the air. The chief purpose of ventilation is to supply fresh air and to maintain a proper humidity. Air in motion increases the radiation of heat from the skin and improves circulation and respiration. The velocity of the air movement should be 15–45 feet/minutes or 1 to 3 miles/hour. Air may keep in motion by opening doors and windows, and by the use of fans and air conditioners. The air movement should not be much to cause draughts.
- **Lighting:** The amount of light is an important factor in comfort. It is provided by natural or artificial light. Avoid direct light on the face and eyes. Prevent glare. Artificial light should not be too strong for reading. Remember it is difficult for a patient to rest when there is excessive light. He will not be able to read and write when there is dim light. The amount of light depends upon the use of light, the kind of work being done. Conditions of the

patient, age of the patient and the time of the day. The patient if conscious, control of a light should have within his reach, which he can control.

- **Noise:** Noise produces irritability, restlessness, fatigue and exhaustion. In an acutely ill patient noise interfere with sleep. On the contrary, a melodious sound induces pleasure. The degree of noise may be reduced by various measures. Noise caused by friction may be reduced by lubrication. Use of rubber tyres and castors for trolleys and wheel chairs reduce the sound when moving furniture. Make echo proof rooms. Avoid dropping object. Loud talking, laughing and heavy walking with shoes with in the hearing of ill persons should be avoided. Whispering is also not good, as it tends to cause apprehension and uncertainty in the patient.
- **Purity of air:** Dust cause significant hazards to patients. Dust in hospital may be laden with microorganisms, which cause infection in addition to irritation of the respiratory tract of precipitating allergic reaction. To control the dust, it is important to avoid those activities that stirrup dust such as dusting and dry duster and sweeping damp dusting and cleaning, folding bed linen and gently shaking them rather than flapping them, restricting the cigarette smoking and above all providing proper ventilation and ample spacing of bed maintains the purity of air.
- **Elimination of unpleasant odors:** Good ventilation, cleanliness, proper disposal of excreta and rubbish are necessary to eliminate unpleasant odors.
- **Water supply and sewage disposal:** There should be provision for safe water supply and disposal of excreta.
- **Esthetic factor:** The environment becomes attractive, it appeals to the series whether we are conscious or not, the design or arrangement of the room contributes to its harmony. Through skillful use of color, the room can be made attractive. Color preferences vary with age, sex and race. Flower vase, picture and curtains add to the pleasant outlook of the room. Esthetic considerations should include freedom of unpleasant sights. Bedpans, urinals, soiled dressings and used linen, etc., should be removed from the sick room immediately.

THERAPEUTIC ENVIRONMENT

A **therapeutic environment** is supportive of each individual and recognizes that people with dementia are particularly vulnerable to chaotic environmental influences. A therapeutic environment should be person-centered—individualized, flexible, and designed to support differing functional levels and approaches to care.

Environment as therapeutic resources: An emerging concept in dementia care is the use of design as a therapeutic tool-recognizing that there is a connection between the environment and how people behave. In this model, homes or buildings used for the care of people with memory impairment and dementia are designed or remodeled to encourage community, maximize safety, support caregivers, cue specific behaviors and abilities, and redirect unwanted behaviors.

Physical environment: Maintaining a positive and healthy physical environment is an important aspect of dementia care. People with dementia rely on environmental cues to support them physically, cognitively, and emotionally. Unfamiliar, chaotic, or disorganized environments are stressful and can cause anxiety, disorientation, and other behavioral problems. It is possible to design a supportive therapeutic environment for people with dementia-whether

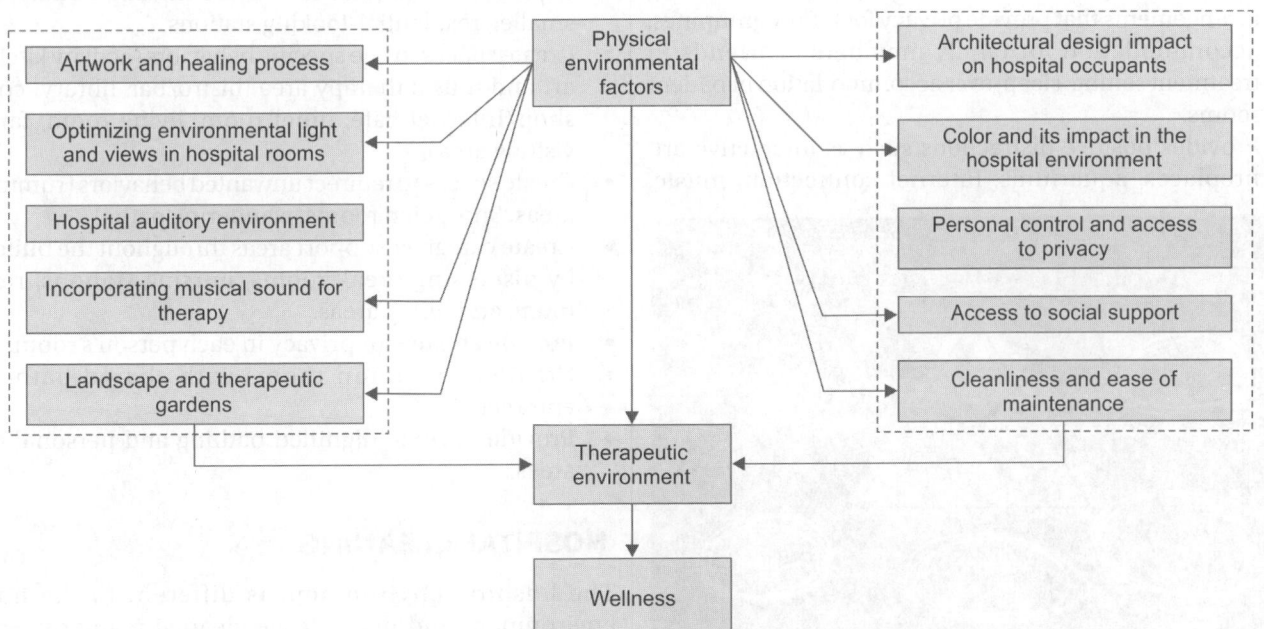

Fig. 11.2: Physical environmental factors.

it is a new facility, the retrofit of an existing building, or a home modification. They assert that physical environment should:
- Provide support for caregivers
- Ensure and maximize safety and security
- Adapt to changing needs
- Support functional abilities through meaningful activity
- Regulate and provide opportunities for positive stimulation
- Maximize awareness and orientation
- Provide opportunities for socialization
- Protect the need for privacy
- Maximize autonomy and control
- Support the continuity of the self, maintain links with their earlier life.

Goals of healing environment: The goal of all healing environments is to engage patients in the conscious process of self-healing and spiritual growth. Spaces are designed to be nurturing and therapeutic and, most important, to reduce stress. This is a research-based approach to design (also known as evidence-based design), aimed at eliminating environmental stressors and putting patients in contact with nature in the treatment setting. According to "The Business Case for Creating a Healing Environment" written by Jain Malkin, the physical setting has the potential to be therapeutic if it achieves the following:
- Eliminates environmental stressors such as noise, glare, lack of privacy and poor air quality.
- Connects patients to nature with views to the outdoors, interior gardens, aquariums, water elements, etc.
- Offers options and choices to enhance feelings of being in control - these may include privacy versus socialization, lighting levels, type of music, seating options, quiet versus 'active' waiting areas.
- Provides opportunities for social support-seating arrangements that provide privacy for family groupings, accommodation for family members or friends in treatment setting; sleep-over accommodation in patient rooms.
- Provides positive distractions such as interactive art, fireplaces, aquariums, Internet connection, music, access to special video programmes with soothing images of nature accompanied by music developed specifically for the healthcare setting.
- Engenders feelings of peace, hope, reflection and spiritual connection and provides opportunities for relaxation, education, humor and whimsy.

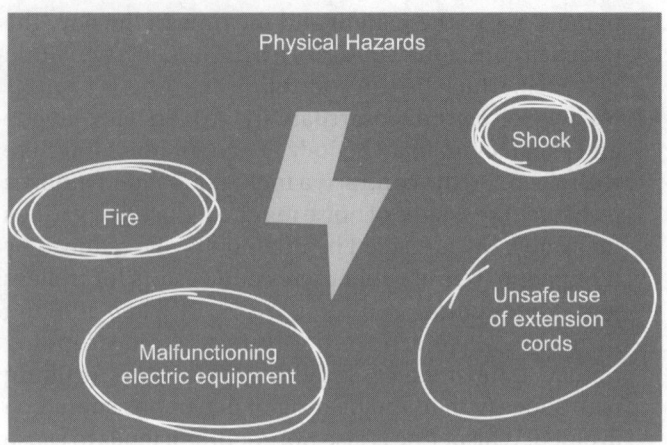

Fig. 11.4: Electrical hazards.

Adopting physical environment: Whatever the situation, the physical environment can be adapted to meet the physiologic and social needs of those with dementia. Campernal and Brummett (2000) use these therapeutic design goals when developing or retrofitting an environment for people with dementia and memory disorders:
- Arrange spaces to resemble a natural community.
- Create continuous circulation routes with looping corridors and areas of interest.
- Include residents in the design of new features such as walking paths and gardens.
- Create safe, purposeful, and accessible outdoor areas.
- Replace institutional, centralized nursing stations with smaller, residential-looking stations.
- Create spaces to cue specific behaviors (activity kitchen, art and music therapy area, bistro/bar, library, coffee shop/Internet café, quiet room, living room, family visiting area).
- Create spaces to redirect unwanted behaviors (rummage areas, Snoezelen rooms, wandering paths)
- Create caregiver support areas throughout the building by dispersing break rooms, nursing stations, rehab room, and utility areas.
- Provide an area for privacy in each person's room.
- Create companion rooms with shared bath and entrance.
- Provide normal, dignified bathing and personal care areas.

HOSPITAL CLEANING

The hospital environment is different to the home environment and needs to be cleaned regularly. Some cleaning can be done daily while others are weekly, monthly

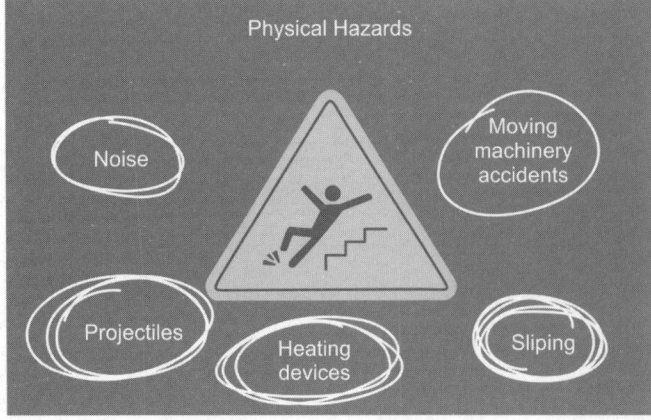

Fig. 11.3: Types of physical hazards.

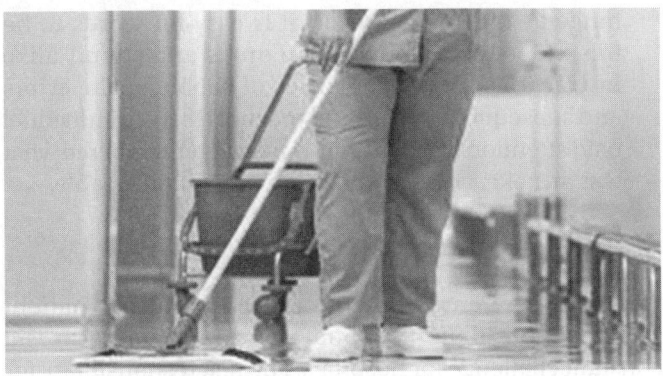

Fig. 11.5: Wet floor can cause accident.

and annually. By cleaning the area we can be sure that we have made every effort to reduce cross contamination and exposure to unknown pathogens (Fig. 11.5). This also ensures that the health care team is working in a safe and clean environment. These cleaning tasks are shared between the nursing and cleaning departments, depending on the size and availability of appropriate staff in each hospital. Cleaning can include:

Daily

- Nursing station bench tops/desk
- Equipment used that day (slit lamps, lens sets and prisms, blood pressure machines, stethoscopes, surgical equipment and recovery anesthetic items, etc.)
- Perioperative work areas: Operating room and anesthetic bays, sterilization room, holding and recovery rooms
- Phones, doors and door handles
- Patient beds and bedside tables
- Floors: brushed and mopped
- Bathroom: toilet, sink, shower, washbowl
- Waste bin washed over
- Plastic or vinyl chairs
- At the end of each day clean out toilet brushes, wash clothes and buckets.
- Dispose of dirty water in a safe manner
- Bottom of your nursing shoes
- Staff kitchen/rest areas.

Weekly

- Equipment such as sterilizers and anesthetic machines (check the manufacture details first)
- Surgical microscope lenses and other ophthalmic viewing devices (with approved cloths)
- Walls and windows.

Monthly

- Dust clean inside cupboards and shelves
- Material based pillows and mattresses
- Bed and trolley wheels (both in the patient stay area and the operating room)

Third Monthly (Quarterly)

- Window curtains
- Privacy curtains dividing patient beds
- Walls and ceilings not usually in reach by the nurses
- Inside nursing staff change areas or lockers
- Chairs made of a fabric material.

Personal Cleaning Tip

The nurse's personal equipment, such as pens, scissors and clip boards, can also harbor contaminants. Wipe down your equipment regularly throughout the day.

REDUCTION OF PHYSICAL HAZARDS: FIRE AND ACCIDENTS

Hazards may occur in mechanical plants, hospital kitchen, laundry and a diagnostic area, etc., people who are vulnerable to hospital hazards are grouped in to 3 categories—1. Patient who is ill, 2. The staff, because of the nature of work, and 3. the visitors, who worried about the patient. Every hospital must formulate one committee who will remain alert and alternative to prevent physical hazards.

Preventive measures for the occurrence of fire:

- Hospital should have and implement the policy related to preventing the hospital hazards.
- Material used for building hospital should be incombustible or flame proof.
- In order to prevent accidental fire, there must be proper selection and installation of equipments.
- Electrical devices, appliances and equipments should be installed, operated and maintained in accordance with manufacturers recommendations.
- Hospital refrigerator which containing flammable liquids must be placed safely.
- Sufficient space should be provided around the mechanical equipment and electrical services. This will ensure safe operation and good maintenance of equipment.
- There should be proper facilities for the handling and disposal of the linen. Adequate space should be available for organizing the routine work in laundry.
- Installation of automatic fire detection and alarm system prevent accidental fire.
- All hospital building should be provided with an internal fire alarm system. Such system will give immediate notice to hospital staff taking necessary actions.
- Every hospital must have effective communication system, this will help in intimating the authorizes to take needy actions.
- All elevators. Lifts have emergency signal system as well as safety devices.
- No smoking signs must be displayed in areas where patient is on oxygen therapy.

FIVE STEPS TO IMPROVE SAFETY

Here are five steps that will improve overall hospital safety and lead to increasing patient satisfaction:

1. **Remove stored equipment from public areas:** A common practice in hospitals is to make hallways a storage area for equipment in waiting. Risks can be high when unforeseen situations happen, such as when a visitor trips over a cart wheel that is protruding into the walkway, or a rushing staff member hurriedly comes around a corner, falling due to IV poles and monitors left in the pathway If there is no alternative, only minimum equipment needed should be tolerated. Good planning and a commitment to safety must drive creative and effective storage options that are far safer than hallways.
2. **Minimize hospital room clutter:** In her Notes on nursing (1860), Florence Nightingale said that nothing in the patient's room should prevent the nurse from seeing dust and dirt for fear of insidious contamination. In the hospital room, this means keeping clutter away, properly storing or removing clothing, meals trays, and basically everything not immediately needed or being used. Maintaining a clean and un-encumbered patient room is essential to keep the patient safe. "Clean" in this case is not only about "cleaning," but, as stated, involves putting away or removing those things that are not serving the immediate patient needs. This may be challenging but should be mandatory. Patients and families will appreciate the need for keeping the room safe and will participate in order to minimize preventable risk.
3. **Eliminate or organize area clutter:** Nursing stations must be well managed so that everything that needs to be seen can be seen. Cluttered desks are layered, often with both essential and non-essential items; if there are layers, much of what is there cannot be seen. Organize the paperwork so that it can be found, but don't let piles of records hide themselves in plain view of everyone else. Trust in the confidentiality of individual medical records is threatened when desks are piled high with patient records or other paperwork.
4. **Assure overall cleanliness of all areas:** What is cluttered does not look clean; what is not clean, looks cluttered. A study in the UK showed hospitals that were perceived to be unclean had a 10% higher rate of infection. Perception confirms the otherwise invisible reality. Stains in carpets, privacy curtains, unkempt bathrooms, lingering meal trays and housekeeping carts tell a tale of sloppiness that cannot be tolerated. This includes public bathrooms as well as patient toileting areas.
5. **Minimize auditory clutter:** Considering unnecessary noise as auditory clutter puts into perspective the risks for patients and staff. Ambient noise in the hospital, regardless of source, has been associated with everything from sleep deprivation to medication errors, from patient falls to breaches in confidentiality. Because the general noise occurs in the same frequency range as the spoken voice, it is easy for words to be misunderstood. Sound-alike drugs and sound-alike instructions spoken into a sea of babble, invite errors and subsequent mistakes in practice. If every individual paid attention to where they were and remembered what was at stake, noise would be far more manageable.

CARE OF PATIENTS UNIT

Improving the environment of care to improve patient safety is more than just about perception; rather it is a constant challenge for hospitals. Further, responsibility for safety resides in each department and individual. From administration to the clinical and nonclinical staff, to housekeeping and volunteers, the shared accountability for patient safety has no boundaries. It demands an open and honest evaluation of the norms, values and current environment of the hospital, prioritizing eliminating or minimizing unnecessary and often inadvertent risks to patients, families and staff. Furthermore, because outcomes are systemic, only the hospitals that commit to being a culture of safety will be successful over the long term. It is requisite that each individual be proactive in addressing patient safety which, in turn, will result in better patient and staff outcomes.

It is the duty of the nurse to ensure that the patient's unit is kept clean and tidy at all times. She should learn all the cleaning skills in order to teach others and should willingly clean where necessary. The patient and his relatives are also taught to keep the unit clean and tidy.

General cleaning of ward and equipments:
- Sweep and mop the floor at least twice a day.
- Clean the floor with antiseptic solution.
- Keep the unit well ventilated and do not close the top ventilating windows.
- Dust the walls and roof from time to time in order to remove cobwebs.
- Clean the windows and doors regularly.

Furniture

- **Bed steads:** Dust every day while making the bed. Carbolize or wash with soap and water and dry well after discharge of the patients.
- **Lockers:** Dust every morning and evening when tiding the ward. Keep the bed side locker always clean and neat.
- **Cupboards:** Keep clean and tidy. Arrange the supplies after drying absolutely. Use naphthalene balls to protect.
- **Bed cradles, back-rests, over bed tables, chairs and stools** are to be cleaned every day. Iron furniture is cleaned with a dry duster to prevent rusting.
- **Bathrooms:** Scrub and wash the floors every day. Avoid stagnation of water on the floors. Dispose the waste material properly in dustbins.
- **Lavatories:** Check the flushing system is in working condition. Clean it with cleaning powder using a brush.

scrub and wash the floors daily. Teach the patients and relatives regarding the proper use of lavatory.
- **Wash basins:** Clean them twice a day with cleaning power using a brush. Remove the spots with some spot removing agent. Pour boiling water down the wash basin drains every day.
- **Cabinet for sanitary wares:** Keep the racks clean, neat and tidy. Store the sanitary wares in racks neat and tidy and ready for use.

Vermin and Insects

- Clean the patient's unit regularly. Eliminate all the breeding places. Keep garbage well covered and dispose of all refuse as soon as properly.
- Store food properly. Use fly screens on windows and doors.

FURNISHING PATIENT'S UNIT (FIG. 11.6)

- **Cot or bedstead:** The hospital beds are made-up of metal, simple in design, light and easily moveable, easy to clean, strong, durable with hard rubber castors. Some bed will have side rails to prevent the patient from falling.
- **Over bed table or cardiac table:** Generally, this is used for patients suffering from cardiac diseases to lean and rest forward when he has breathing difficulty. It can also use for eating, reading, and writing and for placing articles for self care.
- **Bedside locker:** It is used to store the patient personal articles.
- **Bedside table:** It can be used for taking meals and other purposes.
- **Chair and stool:** The chair can be used for the patients when he is out of bed, i.e. while changing the bed linens or bathing the patients. The workers and visitors should sit on the chair and not on the patient's bed.
- **Bedside commode:** It is a chair or wheel chair that has opening in the center of a seat under which a bedpan can be inserted. It is used for defecation and urination.
- **Bedpan and urinals:** For a bedridden patient, these are used for defecation and urination.
- **Sputum cup:** It is used to collect the sputum and spitting.
- **Kidney tray:** It is used to collect vomits, body fluids and soiled dressings.
- **Water flask and drinking glasses:** The water flask is filled with drinking water and is given to the patients within his reach.
- **Plate, spoon, fork, knifes, etc:** These are used to serve the meals for the patient and is kept inpatients unit.
- **Call signal:** A bell is kept near the patient to call the nurse in his or her need.
- **Toilet articles:** Soap with soap dish, toothbrush and toothpaste, mouthwash, comb, etc. are kept in patient's unit. Bucket, mug, basin, etc. are kept in bathroom.
- **Waste basket:** It is used to collect the rubbish.

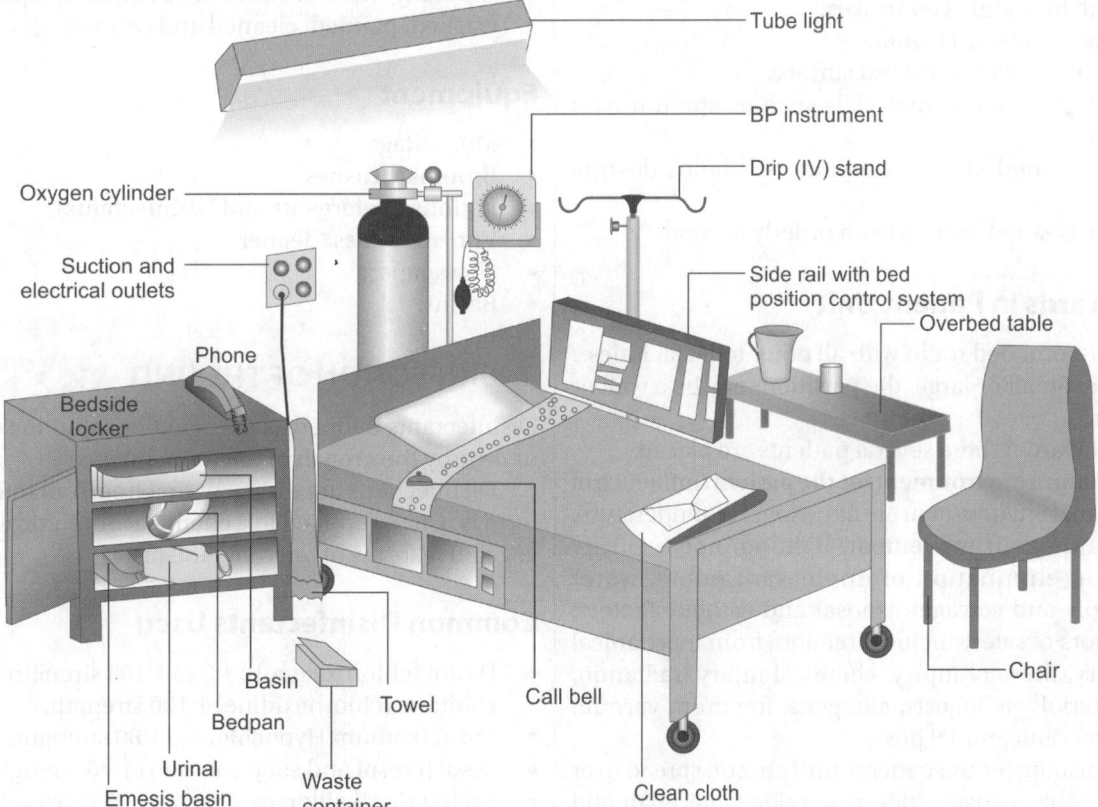

Fig. 11.6: Patient's unit.

- **Bedding and bed linens:** The mattress and pillows should be firm, thick and smooth, and all should have a washable cover. It gives support to the patients. Bed sheets are made up of strong cotton material which is used to protect the mattress from soiling and to cover the patients.

Draw mackintosh and draw sheet, extends from the patient shoulder to below knee, made up of rubber or plastic material, which is used to protect the mattress and bottom sheet from soiling. Sometimes Kelley's pads used in the place of a mackintosh.

Definition: Care of patient unit is defined as keeping the patient's unit clean, neat, and tidy. To provide maximum comfort to the patient. Patient's unit is the area furnished and equipped according to the need to give adequate care to the patient.

Purpose of the Unit Care

- To provide comfort to patient.
- To prevent cross infection.
- To keep the unit clean and neat.
- To keep the unit away from microorganisms.
- To keep the articles ready for use.
- To prolong the life of the articles.

Principles of Good Housekeeping

- Wear gloves before cleaning the unit.
- Use a damp dusting
- Dust with firm and even strokes.
- Use disinfectant for cleaning.
- Use a brush to clean grooved surface.
- Remove albuminous materials such as sputum with cold water.
- Expose cleaned area to sunlight as it helps destroy bacteria.
- Keep the cleaned articles in an orderly fashion.

Type of Wards in Patient Unit

- Private Room: Bed room with all other toilet facilities.
- Cubicles: Small or large, the partition may be a wall or curtains.
- General Ward: Where several patients are placed
  - **Optimum environment for the patient:** Influence of external environment are atmospheric temperature, humidity, air movement, lighting, noise, purity of air, elimination of unpleasant odors, water supply and sewage disposal and esthetic factors. Factors of safety include freedom from mechanical injury, thermal injury, chemical injury, radiation, bacteriologic ingests, allergens, free from vermin, insects and animal pests.
    Furnishing for the patients unit are cot, spread over bed, table, bedside locker, bed side table, chair and stool, bedside commode, bedpans and urinals, sputum cup, kidney trays, water flasks and drinking glasses, plate, spoon, fork, knives and toilet articles.
  - **Carliolization:** It is a process of disinfecting the whole external environment of the patient and rendering it free from pathogenic organisms.

Principles of Cleanliness

- Plan your work for cleanliness, to avoid waste of your energy and time.
- Do dusting after sweeping.
- Dust with a clean duster.
- Use a damp dusting for collecting dust.
- Soap and water or phenol 1:60.
- Dusting should be done from top to bottom.
- Dusting should be done with firm and even stroke.
- Use covered dustbin to collect the dust and waste material.
- Growth of bacteria is high in dark, moist and unclean places. So care should be taken while cleaning the congested places.
- Use brush when cleaning grooved surfaces.
- Replace all the equipments used for cleaning.
- Wash hands after dusting.

Types of Cleaning

- Daily Cleaning: Two to three times a day (floor, articles, furniture, dustbin and cupboards).
- Weekly: Roof, walls, ceiling fans, cobwebs.
- Annually: The ward should be emptied, repaired, white washed, painted, cleaned and washed.

Equipment

- Mops/Rags
- Brooms/Brushes
- Lotions (Detergents and Disinfectants)
- Vim and Glass Cleaner
- Newspapers
- Basins.

DISINFECTION OF THE UNIT

Disinfectants defined as the agent or solutions used to kill or destroy the growth of microorganisms.

Disinfectants are the agent that free from infection. The term is usually applied to a chemical or physical agent kills vegetative forms of microorganisms.

Common Disinfectants Used

- Dettol (chloroxylenol): 1:2 to 1:100 strength.
- Hibitane (chlorhexidine) 1:100 strength.
- Eusol (sodium Hypochlorite) 1:80 strength.
- Lysol (cresol and soap solution) 1:40 strength.
- Savlon (0.3% chlorcexidine and 3% cetrimide) 1:20.
- Phenol (carbolic acid) 1:10 to 1:20 strength.

- Formalin (formaldehyde) 50 g/1 liter of water.
- Betadine (iodine) 1:40 Strength.
- H_2O_2 (liberates O_2) 1:80 Strength.

Dilution formula: The volume of stock solution to be used. Formula = Strength of lotion required/strength of stock solution × volume of solution required.

Responsibilities of Nursing Personnel

- To delegate the responsibilities to other.
- To supervise the ward cleanliness.
- To provide adequate supplies for cleaning.
- To make the patients environment safe.
- To replace or repair the damaged article.
- To keep the environment pleasant to promote comfort of the patient.
- To maintain the unit attractive and free from physical, chemical and biological hazards.

Environment Setting

- Atmospheric temperature of 20–22°C is considered comfortable.
- Humidity of 40–60% is more suitable.
- The room should be well ventilated.
- Adequate and artificial light should be provided.
- Noise should be minimum as it interferes with the rest and sleep of the patient.
- Damp dusting is done to maintain the purity of air.
- Eliminate unpleasant odors by maintaining proper cleanliness.
- Provide provision for good water supply.
- Sewage system must be in working order.
- Keep the ward neat and make necessary arrangements.

SAFETY DEVICES: RESTRAINTS

Restraints are used to restrict the movements of the sick baby in the bed. The restraints should select the appropriate, safe and comfortable one. However, the use of restraints should be restricted to the minimum.

Purposes

- Children may need to be restrained for some diagnostic therapeutic procedures or during physical examination and also in order to protect the child from injury.
- Restraints maintain the child's safety and protect him from injury. It also facilitates examination and minimizes the child's discomfort.

Principles of restraints:

- Restraints should be individualized and afford as much dignity to the patient as the situation allows.
- Any restraint should be human and professionally administered.
- Protocols to ensure patient safety should be developed to address observation and treatment during the period of restraint and periodic assessment as to the need and means of restraint.
- The use of restraints should be carefully documented. Such documentation should include the reasons for and means of restraint and the periodic assessment of the restrained patient.
- The method of restraint should be the least restrictive necessary for the protection of the patient and others.
- Patient restraint or seclusion requires comprehensive patient assessment, and the emergency physician's principal legal and ethical responsibility is to patients who present to be seen and treated in the emergency department.
- The use of restraints should conform to applicable laws, rules, regulations, and accreditation standards.

Objectives for Restraints

- To avoid clients from falling
- To prevent interruption of therapy.
- To prevent confused or combative client from removing any life supportive equipments.
- To reduce the risk of injury to others.

General Instructions

- Explain the need for application and type of restraints.
- Need should be made to understand the family and friends of the client
- Restraints should be used with great care.
- Assistance should be taken.
- Allow freedom to move.
- Circulation must not be occluded by restraints.
- Pad the bony prominences.
- While appling restraints, see that the normal body positions can be assumed.
- Untie the restraints at least every 4 hours.
- Client with restraints should be visited at least every 3o-60 minutes.
- Do not apply linen restraints with a regular knot.
- Fasten restraint to bed frame and not to side-rails.
- Never use restraints over an IV site.
- While removing, remove one restraint at a time.
- Skin folds should be clean and dry prior to application of restrain.
- Ensure that there are no wrinkles in restraint.

Types of Restraints

- **Mummy device:** Mummy device involves securing a sheet or blanket around the child's body in such a way that his arms are held to his sides and his leg space movements are restricted **(Fig. 11.7)**.

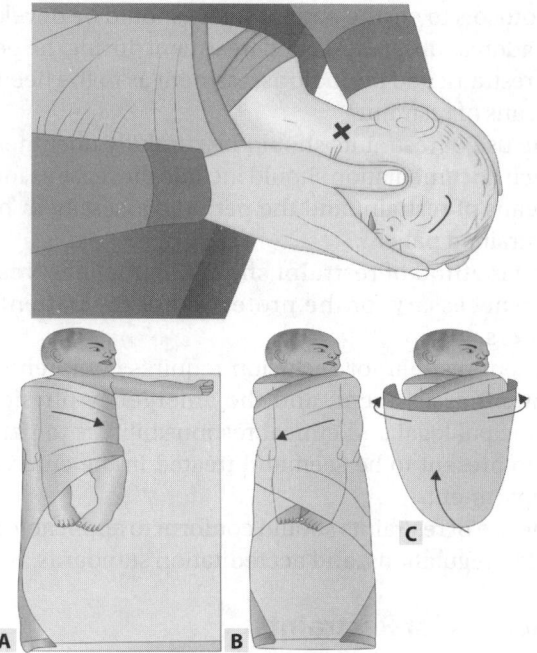

Fig. 11.7: Mummification procedure.

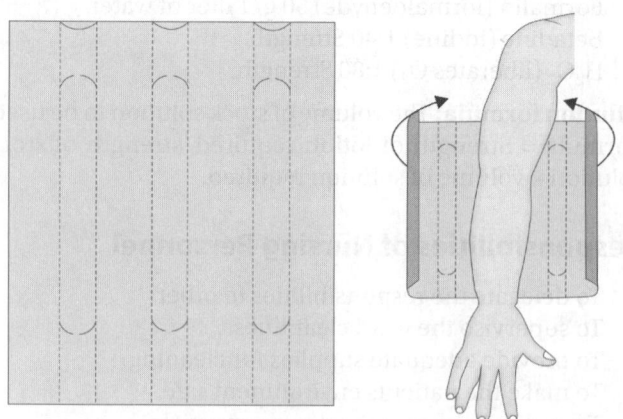

Fig. 11.8: Elbow restraint.

Purposes of mummy restraints are examination or treatment of the head and neck, e.g. ENT examination or scalp venipuncture.

Procedure: The child is placed in an open blanket which is adjusted in such a way that one edge is under the child's neck and another extends beyond its feet. The child's arms are placed by the sides.

- **Elbow restraints** are used to prevent the infant from flexing his elbow so that he is unable to remove the nasogastric tube or scalp vein **(Fig. 11.8)**.

    Purposes of elbow restraints are may be useful in cases after operation on head, face, scalp infusion, to secure transanastomotic nasogastric tubes and to prevent scratching in case of skin disorder.

    Procedure: Elbow is extended, padded and bandaged with a wooden spatula placed on the anterior or flexor aspect.

- **Jacket restraint:** Jacket restraint is used to prevent the child from climbing out of the crib or chair.

    Procedure: The jacket is put on the child keeping the laces at the back, so that child can not touch them. The long tapes on the jacket are fixed to the understructure of the crib.

- **Clove-Hitch restraint:** Clove-Hitch restraint is used to immobilize the arm or leg. It is prepared from a piece of gauze or soft cloth or crepe bandage **(Fig. 11.9)**.

    Procedure: The wrist or ankle is placed in the loops of the device. The ends of the device are pulled to make it firm and tied to the cot frame. It should be tight enough to prevent slipping off the hand or foot.

- **The crib-net restraint** is used to prevent the child from climbing over the side rails. It is applied over the crib and on the sides of the crib.

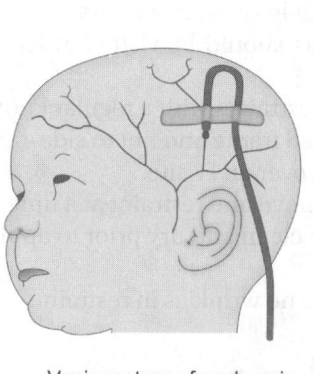
Venipuncture of scalp vein

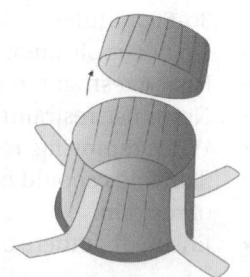
Paper cup taped over venipuncture site for protection. A clear plastic cup may also be used

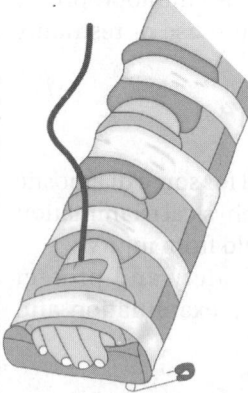
Restraint of arm when hand is site of infusion

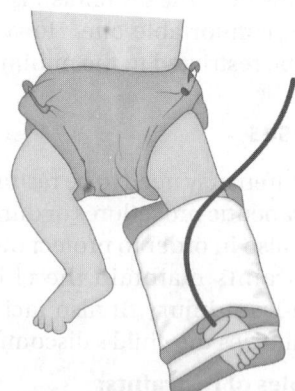
Infant's leg taped to sandbag for immobilization (IV site should be visible)

Fig. 11.9: Clove-Hitch restraint.

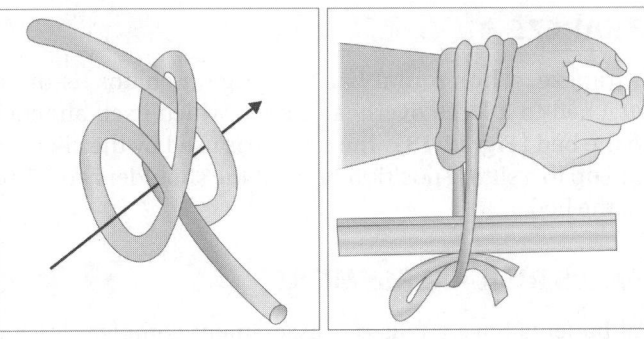

Fig. 11.10: Restraint with hand.

- Asphyxia or aspiration pneumonia.
- Development of other complications: inability to client to escape from injury or accidents.
- Psychic injury—client may feel that he is punished.
- Strangling and death.

Procedure: The crib net restraint should be fixed to the cot frame, so that the side rails can be lowered when necessary without removing the net. When the rails are up, the child can stand in the crib but cannot climb over the side-rails.

- **Restraint with hand:** Restraint with hands provides bodily contact and a feeling of security. It is useful for infants and restraining for certain procedures **(Fig. 11.10)**.

  Purposes of restraint with hands—positioning for femoral venipuncture and restraining for lumbar puncture.

  Procedure: Femoral venipuncture—the infant placed on his back and his legs spread apart in a frog like fashion. Lumbar puncture—Infant placed on lateral side, the knees and neck is in a flexed position.

- **Safety belts:** It is made of electrically non-conductive materials. These are frequently used on stretchers and operation tables in order to prevent the client from falling.

Hazards of Restrains

- Tissue damage under restraints due to constant friction.
- Damage to other parts of body, e.g., dislocation.
- Development of pressure sores.
- Ischemia or nerve damage.
- Food drop or wrist drop.

SIDE RAILS (FIGS. 11.12A TO C)

Side rails are safety measures that come under category of environmental control. These are attached to both sides of the bed to prevent the client from getting out or falling out of the bed. Side rails must be kept raised on beds of all clients who have altered level of consciousness.

Objectives

- To prevent the client from getting out of bed.
- To prevent the client from falling out of bed.
- To observe the client.
- To prevent the type of injury.

Uses of Side Rails

- Client with altered level of consciousness.
- The elderly clients.
- The debilitated clients.
- Children.

Side rails (safety rails) are bed rails that not only prevent clients from falling out of bed, but also help the client to change position while in bed.

Potential Benefits of Bed Rails

- Aiding in turning and repositioning within the bed.
- Providing a hand-hold for getting into or out of bed.
- Providing a feeling of comfort and security.
- Reducing the risk of patients falling out of bed when being transported.
- Providing easy access to bed controls and personal care items.

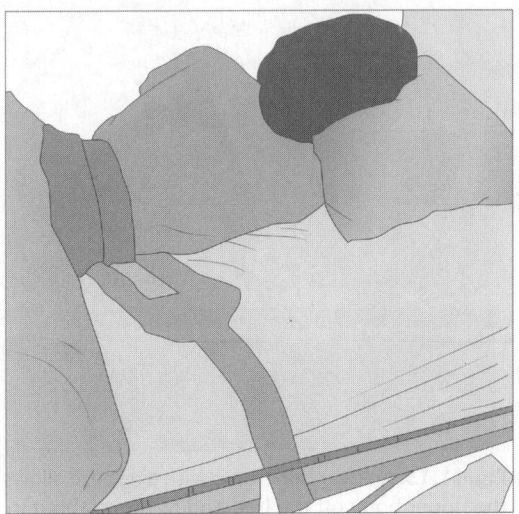
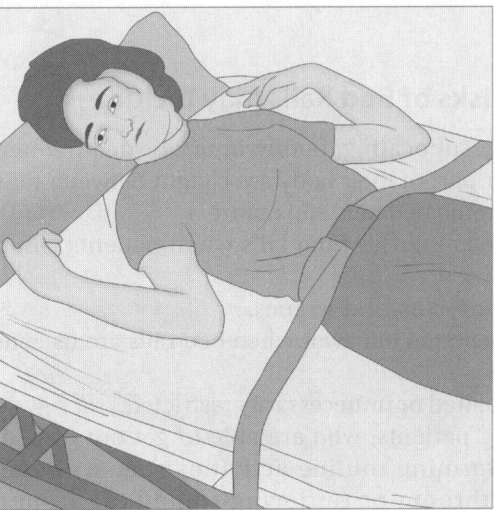

Fig. 11.11: Waist restraint.

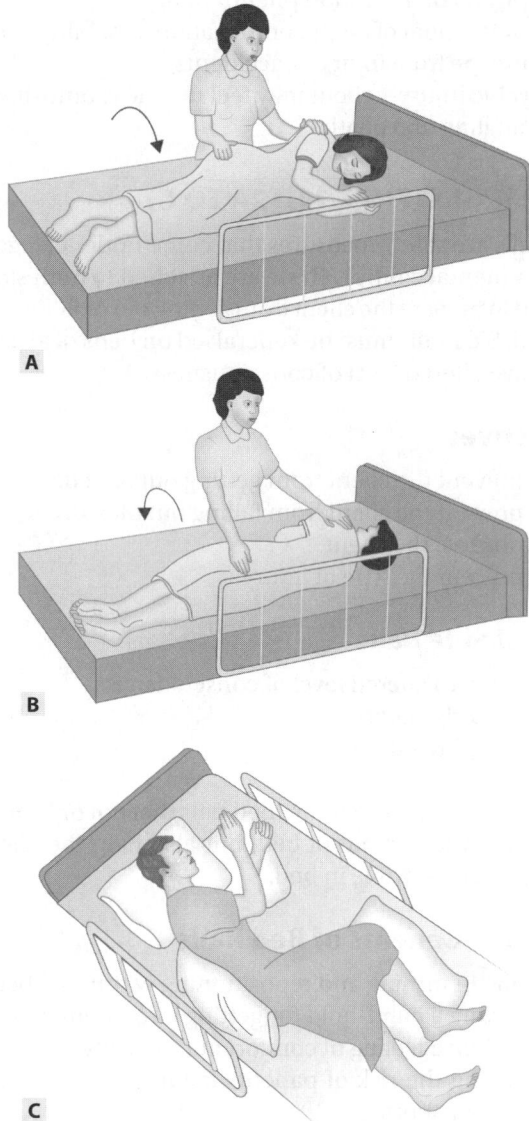

Figs. 11.12A to C: Side rails: (A) Nurse stands on right side while turning; (B) Assisting to turn; (C) Side rails kept on both sides after the procedure.

Potential Risks of Bed Rails May Include

- Strangling, suffocating, bodily injury or death when patients or part of their body are caught between rails or between the bed rails and mattress.
- More serious injuries from falls when patients climb over rails.
- Skin bruising, cuts, and scrapes.
- Inducing agitated behavior when bed rails are used as a restraint.
- Feeling isolated or unnecessarily restricted.
- Preventing patients, who are able to get out of bed, from performing routine activities such as going to the bathroom or retrieving something from a closet.

TRAPEZE

A trapeze, a horizontal bar hanging on chains, is often attached to a large overhead frame, which itself attaches to the bed **(Fig. 11.13)**. The trapeze is used by the client to pull up to a sitting position or to lift the shoulders and hips off the bed.

FALLS RISK ASSESSMENT

All patients have a falls risk assessment completed using the Little Schmidy **Falls Risk Assessment Tool** completed at the following stages:
- On admission or as soon as after the admission
- Daily or when a patient's condition changes
- When the patient is transferred from one ward/department to another
- Following a fall incident.

The falls risk assessment score is documented in the Primary Assessment flow sheet in the EMR. The falls risk assessment tool does not replace clinical judgment, if a patient does not present with a high risk score but is thought to be high risk by medical or nursing staff, allied health, parents or carers extra precautions to protect such patients should be documented and auctioned.

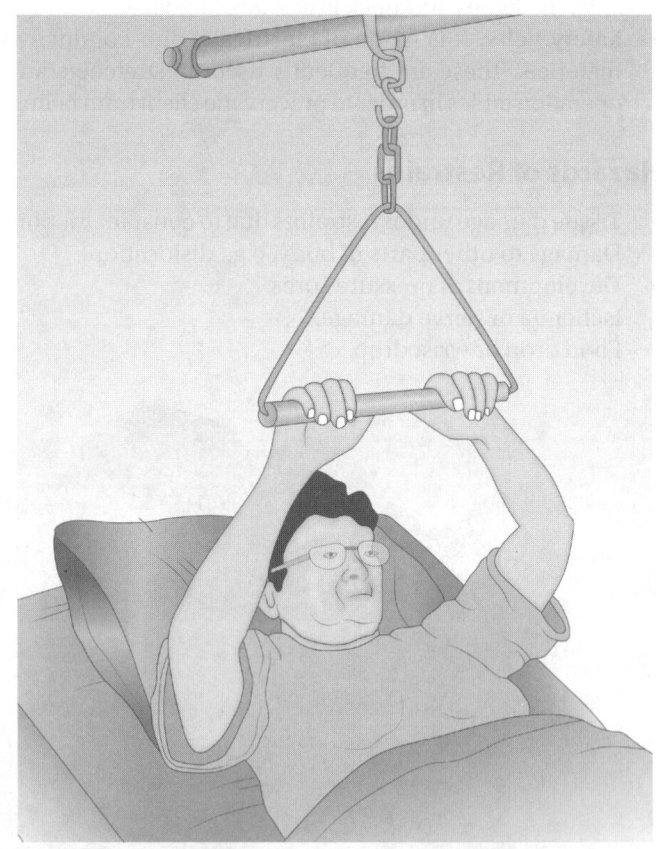

Fig. 11.13: An over bed frame with a trapeze allows the client to lift the upper body off the bed and to move about in bed. It can also be used for bed exercises.

Reference Guide
Little Schmidy Falls Risk Assessment

- Document the appropriate score in the Patient Care Record or relevant MR
- Patient risk score should be assessed 1. Daily, 2. When the patient condition changes, 3. When transferred to a new department/unit, and 4. Following a fall incident
- Interventions and actions should be documented on Falls Plan or in Progress Notes

Falls Risk Assessment		Score	
Mobility			
	Completely immobile	0	Select one score per section
	Ambulant with no gait disturbance	0	
	Ambulate or transfer with assistive device	1	
	Ambulate with unsteady gait and no assistive device	1	
Mental state			
	Coma/unresponsive	0	
	Developmentally appropriate and alert	0	
	Developmentally delayed	1	
	Disorientated	2	
Toileting			
	Nappies	0	
	Independent	0	
	Needs assistance with toileting	1	
	Independent with urinary frequency or diarrhea	1	
History of Falls			
	No	0	
	Yes before admission	1	
	Yes during admission	2	
Medication			
	Anticonvulsants, opioids, diuretics, sedatives, bowels prep	1	
Action			
Falls score is equal to or greater than 3 or based on patient's diagnosis or patient's condition warrants falls prevention program 1. Commence Falls High Risk Management Plan (refer to Falls Prevention Clinical Guidelines) 2. Discuss prevention strategies with parents/carers and ensure a copy of Falls safety in hospital—kids health information is given			

Factors Influencing Risk

- **Environmental issues:** Are a common cause of falls, some examples of previous incidents at the RCH have included inappropriate use of cot side or side rails, equipment clutter, wet floors, nurse call buttons out of patient reach or the use of faulty equipment. By implementing the standard safety measures listed above these risks can be greatly reduced.
- **Age:** RCH incident data identified the adolescent group (10-17 years) have the highest risk of falls in hospital closely followed by the toddler group (1-2 years). The developmental stage and ambulation capabilities are key potential fall risk factors
- **Medical diagnosis:** Various medical conditions may increase a child's risk of falling. Some high risk diagnosis includes drop seizures, severe ataxia, epilepsy surgery or patients who have had a craniectomy, for these patients' soft helmets may be considered.
- **Mental state:** Altered mental state is the most commonly identified risk factor for falling and is perhaps the most difficult to manage in terms of minimizing the risk of falling. Use of a High/Low bed should be considered for those with significant neurological impairment, such as post-traumatic amnesia (PTA).
- Mobility: Impaired mobility and orthopedic restrictions are key potential fall risk factors, interventions, such as non-slip footwear, supervising or assisting with transfers can reduce risk.
- **Elimination:** Special toileting needs are a factor for increased risk of falling. Simple strategies, such as regularly checking patients and toileting patients regularly will help minimize risk.
- **Bed rest:** The majority of falls occur at the patient's bedside, interventions, such as ensuring the bed is in a low position, the brakes are locked, appropriate use of bed rails and ensuring patients can reach necessary items will reduce the risk of falling.

- **Medications:** Use of medications such as Barbiturates, Phenothiazines, Sedatives, Hypnotics, Antidepressants, Laxatives and Diuretics may increase the risk of falls. Care should be taken to check the patient regularly following administration and inform the parents/carers of possible associated side effects.
- **Length of stay:** RCH incident data shows that most of our patients who fall do so in the first 5 days of admission and have had previous admissions to hospital
- **History of falls:** Patients who have a history of falls in hospital or at home have an increased risk of falling again, appropriate precautions should be implemented.

PATIENT FALL PREVENTION AND ASSESSMENT

Falls are the most common cause of pediatric injury leading to emergency department visits. It is widely acknowledged that children are at risk of falls in the community and with many education programs supporting prevention, it is important that this education is reflected in the hospital environment. Children fall as they grow, develop coordination and new skills, and are often unaware of their limitations. Therefore one could conclude that all children are at some risk of falling.

Aim: The nursing staff and the multidisciplinary team of the importance of maintaining a safe environment for all patients; assist with identifying patients who are high risk of fall; provide the tools to educate families and carers of the potential risk of falls and outline strategies to develop individualized management plans of care to reduce risk for high risk patients.

Maintaining a Safe Environment for All Patients

All pediatric patients are considered at risk of falling and simple prevention strategies should be put in place to ensure the risk of injury is minimized.
- Patients are nursed in an appropriate bed; children 2 years and under should be nursed in a cot
- Orientate all patients, parents/carers to room and ward

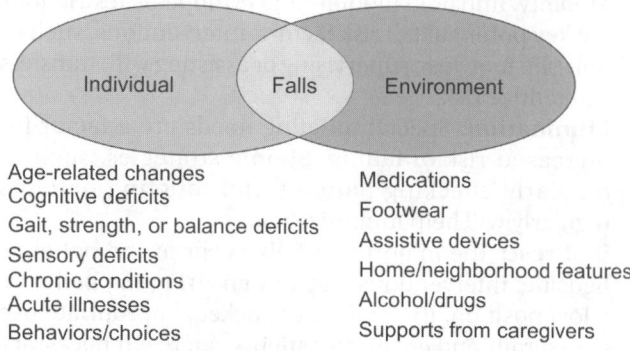

Fig. 11.14: Factors affect fall.

- Keep beds in low position with brakes on and bed ends in place
- Side rails and cot sides are raised for appropriate age and patient groups
- Appropriate non-slip footwear for ambulating patients
- Nurse call within reach; educate patients and families on its functionality
- Maintain adequate lighting in child's room; low level lighting at night
- Keep floors clear of clutter including equipment and toys
- Secure and supervise all children with a safety belt or harness in wheelchairs, highchairs, strollers, infant seats and any specialist seating (e.g., Tumbleforms)
- Children on trolleys are always under the immediate and direct supervision of a staff member or a caregiver
- Infants in an incubator have portholes securely fastened and door closed unless directly attended
- Hourly rounding will support the provision of proactive care such as the need for assistance to the bathroom
- Assist unsteady patients with ambulation; refer to physiotherapy notes where available
- Place necessary items a patient may need within reach (drinking water, phone, etc.)
- Patients who have received sedation or general anesthetic may be unsteady and require supervision
- Ensure equipment is well maintained and serviced appropriately (such as wheelchairs and commodes).

Educating families and carers: Half of falls incidents within the RCH occur when a parent or carer is present. Whilst most parents are aware of maintaining a safe environment for their children in the home environment, many are unaware of the environmental risks when in hospital due to being in an unfamiliar environment accompanied with increased levels of anxiety related to hospital admission.

The hospitalization of children provides an opportunity to reinforce parent/carer information and education concerning normal psychological and motor development of small children, which is related to falls risks and other hazards both inside and outside hospital.

Parents/carers should be encouraged to:
- Reinforce hospital orientation with their child
- Provide non-slip footwear for their child whilst in hospital—no mobilizing in socks
- Maintain physical contact with infant when cot sides are down, when bathing or weighing their infant
- Assist their child to the toilet when appropriate
- Use bed rails or cot sides where appropriate when leaving child's bedside, even for short periods
- Inform nursing staff when their child is unattended
- Keep infant or child in a suitable bed.

Management

- Standard safety measures should be put in place for all patients regardless of the risk identified.

- Falls score equal to or greater than 3 necessitates the implementation of a falls high risk management plan which is located in the Primary Assessment flow sheet within the EMR.
- For all patients identified as high risk, i.e. those with a falls risk score of 3 or greater; a Falls High Risk Management Plan must be commenced. The plan will be developed in collaboration with the child's parent or carer and will be specific to the patient's individual needs.
- The plan will remain in use until the patient's falls risk score changes. If the falls risk score alters a new plan will be implemented as the patient's needs may have changed.
- Patient risk should continue to be assessed daily, once the patient's risk score is less than 3 and the patient's risk of falling is reduced, a management plan is no longer required; however it is important that a safe environment is always maintained.
- A physiotherapist can advise as to how to safely support the patient during positioning, transfers, standing, walking and use of mobility aids.
- An occupational therapist can ensure safe setup of the ward bedroom, bathroom and toilet to minimize falls risks and recommend management techniques/assistive equipment for self-care tasks.

In the Event of the Occurrence of a Fall

- Ensure patient safety
- Provide immediate supportive action for the child
- Conduct a physical examination, measure and document vital signs
- Commence neurological observation if the child's head was the first point of impact
- Do not move the patient until injuries are identified
- Notify appropriate medical staff
- Ensure safe transfer back to bed, consider using a hoist if necessary.

Documentation of a Fall Event

- Record the incident in the EMR, including: description of event (location, activity occurring, time, who was present), assessment findings, interventions and patient outcomes, notification of the incident to the parent.
- Report the incident through the hospital incident reporting system, VHIMs. All falls, including near misses should be reported. The information from reported falls is used to gain insight of the causes of falls for patients at the RCH and continuously improve the local falls prevention program
- The Medical staff/AUM or NUM to inform the parents if they are not present that:

A fall has occurred:
a. What factors contributed to the fall?
b. Outcome of post-fall assessment
c. What additional protective measures have been put in place?

COMMON ERRORS IN PATIENT SAFETY

Every year, millions of patients suffer injuries or die because of unsafe and poor-quality health care. Many medical practices and risks associated with health care are emerging as major challenges for patient safety and contribute significantly to the burden of harm due to unsafe care. Below are some of the patient safety situations causing most concern.

Medication errors are a leading cause of injury and avoidable harm in healthcare systems: globally, the cost associated with medication errors has been estimated at US$ 42 billion annually.

Health care-associated infections occur in 7 and 10 out of every 100 hospitalized patients in high-income countries and low- and middle-income countries respectively.

Unsafe surgical care procedures cause complications in up to 25% of patients. Almost 7 million surgical patients suffer significant complications annually, 1 million of whom die during or immediately following surgery.

Unsafe injections practices in health care settings can transmit infections, including HIV and hepatitis B and C, and pose direct danger to patients and health care workers; they account for a burden of harm estimated at 9.2 million years of life lost to disability and death worldwide (known as Disability Adjusted Life Years (DALYs).

Diagnostic errors occur in about 5% of adults in outpatient care settings, more than half of which have the potential to cause severe harm. Most people will suffer a diagnostic error in their lifetime.

Unsafe transfusion practices expose patients to the risk of adverse transfusion reactions and the transmission of infections. Data on adverse transfusion reactions from a group of 21 countries show an average incidence of 8.7 serious reactions per 100,000 distributed blood components.

Radiation errors involve overexposure to radiation and cases of wrong-patient and wrong-site identification. A review of 30 years of published data on safety in radiotherapy estimates that the overall incidence of errors is around 15 per 10,000 treatment courses.

Sepsis is frequently not diagnosed early enough to save a patient's life. Because these infections are often resistant to antibiotics, they can rapidly lead to deteriorating clinical conditions, affecting an estimated 31 million people worldwide and causing over 5 million deaths per year.

Venous thromboembolism (blood clots) is one of the most common and preventable causes of patient harm, contributing to one third of the complications attributed to hospitalization. Annually, there are an estimated 3.9 million cases in high-income countries and 6 million cases in low- and middle-income countries.

Prevention of Accidents in Hospital

- Hospital should have and implement the policy related to preventing the hospital hazards.

- Nurse must be aware of the hospital policy as well as have sound knowledge base. She must be able to recognize circumstances that may lead to accidents.
- Equipments used in hospital must be quiet, durable, simple to operate and easily repairable.
- While give care to client, nurse must ensure the safe working place, she must make use of good body mechanics.
- Report regarding accidents should be given to the safety committee of hospital in instituting the preventive measures.
- No slippery material should be used in floors, floors should be washed and polished timely clean and spillage from floor immediately in order to prevent slipping.
- Other safety measures can be taken to avoid accidents in hospital. These are the use of side rails, restraints, belt, etc.

Medical errors may occur in different health care settings, and those that happen in hospitals can have serious consequences. The Agency for Healthcare Research and Quality, which has sponsored hundreds of patient safety research and implementation projects, offers these 10 evidence-based tips to prevent adverse events from occurring in the hospital.

Prevent central line-associated blood stream infections: Be vigilant preventing central line-associated blood stream infections by taking five steps every time a central venous catheter is inserted: wash your hands, use full-barrier precautions, clean the skin with chlorhexidine, avoid femoral lines, and remove unnecessary lines. Taking these steps consistently reduced this type of deadly health care-associated infection to zero in a study at more than 100 large and small hospitals.

Re-engineer hospital discharges: Reduce potentially preventable readmissions by assigning a staff member to work closely with patients and other staff to reconcile medications and schedule necessary follow-up medical appointments. Create a simple, easy-to-understand discharge plan for each patient that contains a medication schedule, a record of all upcoming medical appointments, and names and phone numbers of whom to call if a problem arises.

Prevent venous thromboembolism: Eliminate hospital-acquired venous thromboembolism (VTE), the most common cause of preventable hospital deaths, by using an evidence-based guide to create a VTE protocol. This free guide explains how to take essential first steps, lay out the evidence and identify best practices, analyze care delivery, track performance with metrics, layer interventions, and continue to improve.

Educate patients about using blood thinners safely: Patients who have had surgery often leave the hospital with a new prescription for a blood thinner, such as warfarin brand name: Coumadin®, to keep them from developing dangerous blood clots. However, if used incorrectly, blood thinners can cause uncontrollable bleeding and are among the top causes of adverse drug events. A free 10-minute patient education video and companion 24-page booklet, both in English and Spanish, help patients understand what to expect when taking these medicines.

Limit shift durations for medical residents and other hospital staff if possible: Evidence shows that acute and chronically fatigued medical residents are more likely to make mistakes. Ensure that residents get ample sleep and adhere to 80-hour workweek limits. Residents who work 30-hour shifts should only treat patients for up to 16 hours and should have a 5-hour protected sleep period between 10 p.m. and 8 a.m.

Consider working with a Patient Safety Organization: Report and share patient safety information with Patient Safety Organizations (PSOs) to help others avoid preventable errors. By providing both privilege and confidentiality, PSOs create a secure environment where clinicians and health care organizations can use common formats to collect, aggregate, and analyze data that can improve quality by identifying and reducing the risks and hazards associated with patient care.

Use good hospital design principles: Follow evidence-based principles for hospital design to improve patient safety and quality. Prevent patient falls by providing well-designed patient rooms and bathrooms and creating decentralized nurses' stations that allow easy access to patients. Reduce infections by offering single bed rooms, improving air filtration systems, and providing multiple convenient locations for hand washing. Prevent medication errors by offering pharmacists well-lit, quiet, private spaces so they can fill prescriptions without distractions.

Measure hospital's patient safety culture: Survey hospital staff to assess your facility's patient safety culture. AHRQ's free Hospital Survey on Patient Safety Culture and related materials are designed to provide tools for improving the patient safety culture, evaluating the impact of interventions, and tracking changes over time. If the health system includes nursing homes or ambulatory care medical groups, share culture surveys customized for those settings.

Build better teams and rapid response systems: Train hospital staff to communicate effectively as a team. A free, customizable toolkit called Team STEPPS™, which stands for Team Strategies and Tools to Enhance Performance and Patient Safety, provides evidence-based techniques for promoting effective communication and other teamwork skills among staff in various units or as part of rapid response teams. Materials can be tailored to any health care setting, from emergency departments to ambulatory clinics.

ROLE OF NURSE IN SAFE AND CLEAN ENVIRONMENT

Nurses have an important role to play in general environmental management in the workplace. This management have reviewed the theoretical and historical foundations of environmental issues in nursing, showcasing our former and current nursing leaders who have led the way in addressing environmental conditions in health care facilities, and noting that today there is an even greater need to practice nursing in an environmentally responsible manner. This has provided an overview of issues within the scope of everyday practice for nurses. It has also pointed to ways in which nurses can work to prevent the entry, into health care facilities, of materials that can be environmentally hazardous, and identified environmental problems related to solid, biohazardous and hazardous chemical wastes.

CONCLUSION

Patient safety is the cornerstone of high-quality health care. Much of the work defining patient safety and practices that prevent harm have focused on negative outcomes of care, such as mortality and morbidity. Nurses are critical to the surveillance and coordination that reduce such adverse outcomes. Much work remains to be done in evaluating the impact of nursing care on positive quality indicators, such as appropriate self-care and other measures of improved health status.

BIBLIOGRAPHY

1. Aspden P, Corrigan J, Wolcott J, et al. (Eds). Patient Safety: achieving a New Standard for Care. Washington, DC: National Academies Press, 2004.
2. Austin D. Predicting and Preventing Falls in the Hospital, Science of Caring, University of Science California San Francisco, 2017.
3. Ayliffe GAJ, Collins BJ, Lowbury EJ, et al. Ward floors and other surfaces as reservoirs of hospital infection. Journal of Hygiene (Cambs) 1967;365:515-36.
4. Clancy CM, Farquhar MB, Sharp BA. Patient safety in nursing practice. J Nurs Care Qual. 2005;20(3):193-7.
5. Collins BJ. The hospital environment: how clean should a hospital be? Journal of Hospital Infection 1988;11(suppl A):53-6.
6. Cooper CL, Nolt JD. Development of an evidence-based fall prevention program. Journal of Nursing Care Quality, 2007; 22(2):107-12 Clinical Excellence Commission. (2014), Falls Prevention, Health, New South Wales Government.
7. Franck LS, Gay CL, Cooper B, et al. The Little Schimdy Pediatric Hospital Fall Risk Assessment Index: A diagnostic accuracy study. International Journal of Nursing Studies, March 2017;68:51-9.
8. Hill-Rodriguez D, Messmer PR, Williams PD, et al. The Humpty Dumpty Falls Scale: A Case-Control Study. Journal for Specialist in Paediatric Nursing. 2009;14(1):22-32.
9. Maki DG, Alvarado CJ, Hassemer CA, et al. Relation of the inanimate environment to endemic nosocomial infections. New England Journal of Medicine 1982;307:1562.
10. Patient safety—Global action on patient safety. Report by the Director-General. Geneva: World Health Organization; 2019 (https://apps.who.int/gb/ebwha/pdf_files/WHA72/A72_26-en.pdf, accessed 23 July 2019).

REVIEW QUESTIONS

Long Essays

1. Define patient safety; explain objective/goals of patient safety.
2. Define therapeutic environment, explain nurses role.
3. Patient fall prevention and assessment.

Short Essays

1. Safety in health care environment.
2. Influence of external environment.
3. Hospital cleaning.
4. Reduction of physical hazards: fire and accidents.
5. Care of patients unit.
6. Disinfection of the unit.
7. Safety devices: restraints.
8. Common errors in patient safety.
9. Role of nurse in safe and clean environment.

Short Answers

1. Optimum environment for the patient.
2. Atmospheric temperature.
3. Purpose of the unit care.
4. Principles of good housekeeping.
5. Prevention of accidents in hospital.
6. Side rails.
7. Hazards of restrains.
8. Trapeze.

MULTIPLE CHOICE QUESTIONS

1. **A human action that produces an unintended result:**
   a. Mistake
   b. Hazard
   c. Danger
   d. Accident
2. **Preventive measures for the occurrence of fire:**
   a. Hospital should have and implement the policy related to preventing the hospital hazards.
   b. Material used for building hospital should be incombustible or flame proof.
   c. In order to prevent accidental fire, there must be proper selection and installation of equipments.
   d. All of the above
3. **General cleaning of ward and equipments includes the following, *except*:**
   a. Sweep and mop the floor at least twice a day
   b. Painting the walls
   c. Clean the floor with antiseptic solution
   d. Keep the unit well ventilated and do not close the top ventilating windows
4. **Common disinfectants used in the hospital is:**
   a. Dettol (chloroxylenol): 1:2 to 1:100 strength.
   b. Eusol (sodium Hypochlorite) 1:80 strength.
   c. Lysol (cresol and soap solution) 1:40 strength.
   d. All of the above
5. **The objectives for restraints includes all, *except*:**
   a. To avoid clients from falling
   b. To prevent confused or combative client from removing any life supportive equipments
   c. To punish the patient
   d. To reduce the risk of injury to others

ANSWERS

1. a   2. d   3. b   4. d   5. c

CHAPTER 12

Hospital Admission and Discharge

LEARNING OBJECTIVES

- Admission to the hospital unit and preparation of unit
  - Admission bed
  - Admission procedure
  - Medicolegal issues
  - Roles and responsibilities of the nurse
- **Discharge from the hospital**
  - Types: Planned discharge, LAMA and abscond, referrals and transfers
- Discharge planning
- Discharge procedure
- Medicolegal issues
- Roles and responsibilities of the nurse
- Care of the unit after discharge

INTRODUCTION

Admission to hospital can be a traumatic experience with anxiety and fear for anyone. The nurse is one of the most important person that client meet in hospital. The duration and severity of illness influence his/her reaction to admission procedure. The entrance of a patient into a health care agency such as a hospital or a private clinic is termed as admission. A patient enters the hospital by himself or he may be brought to the hospital by his relatives, friends, neighbors or others. Mentally ill patients, persons, who have tried to commit suicide and accident patients, are admitted through a legal process.

ADMISSION TO HOSPITAL UNIT

Admission is defined as allowing a patient to stay in hospital for observation, investigation, treatment and care **(Fig. 12.1)**.

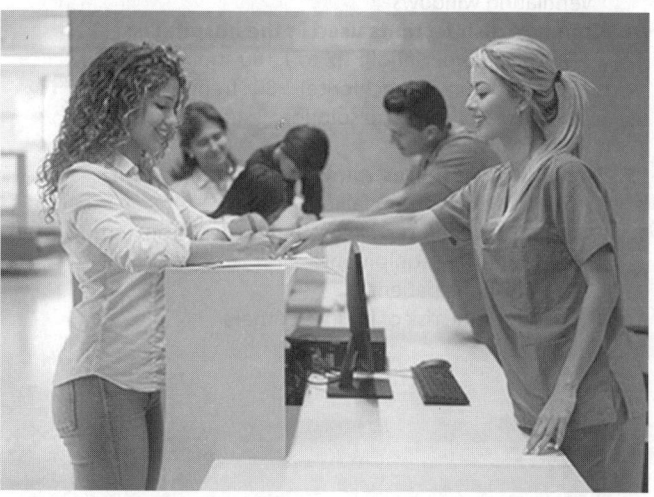

Fig. 12.1: Orientation for newly admitted patient.

Admission is the entry of a patient into a hospital ward for therapeutic or diagnostic purposes.

Purpose

- To establish guidelines regarding admission of patients.
- To make the patient feel welcome, comfortable and at ease.
- To acquire vital information regarding the patient.
- To assess the patient from which a nursing care plan can be initiated and implemented.

Principles Involved

- Sudden change or strangeness on the environment produces fear and anxiety.
- Entering the hospital is a threat to one's personal identity.
- People have diversity of habits and modes of behavior.
- Illness can be novel experience for the patient and brings stress on his physical and mental health.

Need for Hospital Admission

All ill person enters the hospital to get his disorder cured when a healthy individual gets admitted into a hospital for a day or for investigations and observations and in order to find whether he is suffering from any illness which has not been manifested by any external signs and symptoms. Patients, who have become seriously ill suddenly, come the hospital without having had any time to settle their family work affairs. Hence, they are not only worried and anxious about the illness, but also are upset about various other problems affect their family. Nurses must understand their physical and mental problems and be very kind and understanding.

General Instructions

- To receive the patient and help him to adjust to the hospital environment.
- To welcome and establish a positive initial relationship with the patient and relatives.
- To obtain the needed identifying data concerning the patient.
- To provide immediate care, safety and comfort.
- To collaborate with patient in planning and providing comprehensive care.
- To observe, report signs and symptoms and general condition of the patient.
- To secure safety of the patient and his belongings.

Types of Admission

Emergency admission: Means the patients are admitted in acute conditions requiring immediate treatment, e.g. patient with accidents, poisonings, burns and heart attacks.

- As soon as the patient arrives to the emergency room or rings the bell, welcome the patient with compassion and love, allow one of the nearest relatives to be with the patient.
- According to the patient's condition, provide wheelchair or a Bed trolley.
- Make him/her comfortable on the bed, provide privacy and cover the patient always with a bed sheet.
- Take a brief history of his/her complaints and if the patient is not able, make the same from the caretaker (attendant).
- Check vital signs and call the doctor on duty to see the patient.
- Carry out the doctors prescriptions accurately.
- Allow only one caretaker to be near the patient and send to medical record department to prepare the patient folder. See that all the details are entered including fathers name (even if he is deceased).
- If admission is required, ask the doctor to give admission form and ask the caretaker to perform the formalities. The patient should be shifted to the ward as early as possible, after giving the initial care.
- Emergency nurse shift the patient to the ward, however if the emergency is busy, request the particular ward to come and take the patient.
- No patient should be sent out without any treatment.

Routine admission: The patients are admitted for investigation and medical or surgical treatment is given accordingly, e.g. patients with hypertensions, diabetes and bronchitis.

General Instructions

- Nurses should make every effort to be friendly and courteous with the patient.
- Make proper observations of the patient's condition, record and report.
- Orient the patient and his relatives to hospital and ward policies.
- Observe policies in dealing with medicolegal cases.
- Deal with the patients belonging very carefully communicable diseases.
- Insolate the patient if suffering from communicable diseases.
- The nurse should recognize the various needs of the patient and meet them without delay.
- The needs to understand the fears and anxieties of patient and help to overcome.
- The nurse should find out the likes and dislikes of the patient and include the patient in his plan of care.
- The nurse should address the patient by their name and proper title.
- Patient's valuables and clothes should hand over to the relatives with proper recording.

Equipment

- Admission bed
- Thermometer tray, BP apparatus and stethoscope
- Equipments used for physical examination such as weighing machine, inch tape and other articles.
- Admission slips.
- Patients case sheet, doctors, nurses and progress notes.
- Investigation forms: Blood, X-ray, urine, stool and sputum.
- Bath tray if needed.
- Completely record in a file.

Procedure (Fig. 12.2)

- Greet the patient and his relatives and introduce yourself to them.
- Receive the patient cordially and seat comfortable.
- Introduce him to other person in the ward.
- Complete the admission record.
- Collect history and carry out simple physical examination.
- Carry out the prescribed treatment and keep a record.

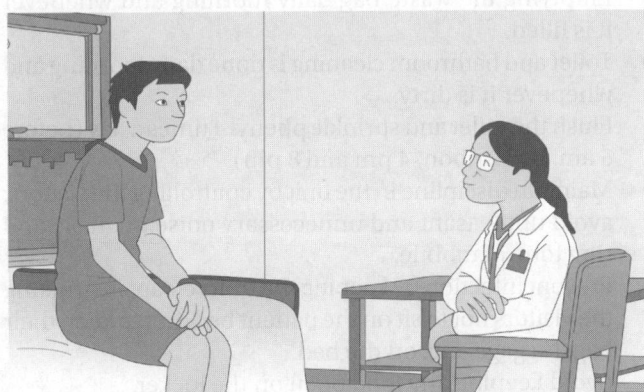

Fig. 12.2: Health assessment.

- Help the patient to maintain personal hygiene and change into hospital clothes.
- Orient the patient to the ward: Toilet, bath room, drinking water supply, nurse's station and treatment room.
- Handover the patients valuable to his relatives.
- Issue visitor pass.
- Encourage patient to take hospital diet especially when therapeutic diet is ordered.
- Obtain local address or telephone number, relatives lodge room and document in admission record.

UNIT AND ITS PREPARATION

It is the duty of the nurse to ensure that the patients unit is kept clean and tidy at all times. She should learn all the cleaning skills in order to teach others and should willingly clean where necessary. The patient and his relatives are also taught to keep the unit clean and tidy.

Objectives

- To make the patient safe and comfortable.
- To teach the patient the importance of cleanliness, orderliness, ventilation and brightness.
- To make everything convenient for the patient.

Requirements in Patients Unit

- Patient cot with mattress, pillow and needed bed linen.
- Table/bedside locker on the right of the patient.
- Stool/chair.
- Fan, light and windows.
- Wash basin, toilet and bedroom near to the patients unit.

Daily Care of Patients Unit

- Daily morning bed making.
- Daily dusting of the entire unit with 2% cresol. Ask the caretaker to empty the locker, clean it and teach them to rearrange their things in order.
- Arrange the unit with only what is required for the patient.
- Sweeping, swabbing the unit is done in the morning.
- Emptying the waste bag daily morning and whenever it is filled.
- Toilet and bathroom cleaning is done daily morning and whenever it is dirty.
- Flush the toilet and sprinkle phenyl 4 times a day (before 6 am, by 12 noon, 4 pm and 8 pm)
- Maintain discipline in the unit by controlling the visitors, avoid unpleasant and unnecessary noise of music and ring tone of mobile.
- Prevent infection by keeping the units clean, instructing the visitors not to sit on the patient bed, not to keep their bag, luggage, etc. on the bed.
- Avoid keeping any food open on the locker.
- Ward sweeping is done twice a day.
- Swabbing the ward, once a day and whenever required.
- Swabbing the verandah and common places three times a day.
- Rearranging the bed in the noon by 3 pm and early morning before 6 am
- Provide safe drinking water for the patient.
- Often visit the patient unit for any timely needed.

ADMISSION PROCEDURE

Admission means allowing a client to stay in the hospital for observation, investigations and treatment of disease he is suffering from.

Types of Admission

- **Emergency admission:** Clients are admitted in acute conditions requiring immediate treatment, e.g. client with heart attack, accidents, poisoning, etc.
- **Routine admission:** Clients are admitted for investigations and planned treatments and surgeries, e.g. client with hypertension, diabetes, bronchitis, etc.
- Transfer from one ward to another.

General Instructions

- Nurses should make every effort to be friendly and courteous with the patient.
- Make proper observations of the patient's condition, record and report.
- Orient the patient and his relatives to hospital and ward policies.
- Observe policies in dealing with medicolegal cases.
- Deal with the patients belonging very carefully communicable diseases.
- Insolate the patient if suffering from communicable diseases.
- The nurse should recognize the various needs of the patient and meet them without delay.
- The needs to understand the fears and anxieties of patient and help to overcome.
- The nurse should find out the likes and dislikes of the patient and include the patient in his plan of care.
- The nurse should address the patient by their name and proper title.
- Patient's valuables and cloths should handover to the relatives with proper recording.

Equipment

- Admission bed
- Thermometer tray, BP apparatus and stethoscope
- Equipments used for physical examination such as weighing machine, inch tape and other articles.
- Admission slips.
- Patients case sheet, doctors, nurses and progress notes.

- Investigation forms—blood, X-ray, urine, stool and sputum.
- Bath tray, if needed.
- Completely record in a file.

Procedure

- Greet the patient and his relatives and introduce yourself to them.
- Receive the patient cordially and seat comfortable.
- Introduce him to other person in the ward.
- Complete the admission record.
- Collect history and carry out simple physical examination.
- Carry out the prescribed treatment and keep a record.
- Help the patient to maintain personal hygiene and change into hospital clothes.
- Orient the patient to the ward—toilet, bath room, drinking water supply, nurse's station and treatment room.
- Handover the patients valuable to his relatives.
- Issue visitor pass.
- Encourage patient to take hospital diet especially when therapeutic diet is ordered.
- Obtain local address or telephone number, relatives lodge room and document in admission record.

SPECIAL CONSIDERATIONS

Orientation to the Ward

- The patient who is not very ill, are allowed to move about can be taken round the ward.
- Introduce the other patients to him and vice versa, and also with the nursing personnel working in the ward.
- Orient the patient to the whole ward, duty room, toilet rooms, and the unit prepared for him.
- After making the patient to be seated comfortably explained the hospital policies, procedures, and routines to the patients and his relatives. Tell him what is expected from him.
- Explain to him the time for meals serving, the doctors visit, visiting time the prayer service, if any and other hospitals routines.

Care of Belongings

- It is always good policy to discourage patients to keep valuable things and money with them.
- Send the valuables to home through relatives. If he does not have anyone with him, enter the description of items in the register and send the valuables to the office for safe custody.
- Get the patient's signature or thumb impression in the register. However, inform the patient that he will get back his valuables on discharge.
- It is important that you take care of the patient's clothing, should see that the clothing are cleaned and stored away with proper label or send them home for a fresh set of clean clothes. However, encourage patients to use hospital clothing.
- If a patient is suffering from infectious disease, see that the clothing are disinfected and cleaned before they are sent home or stored away.

MEDICOLEGAL ISSUES

A medicolegal case (MLC) is a patient who is admitted to the hospital with some unnatural pathology and has to be taken care of in concurrence with the police and/or court.

- The following are the cases to registered as medicolegal cases: Assault, fall from height, road traffic accident, rape, suspected brought dead, murder, alcohol intoxication, burns, poison consumption, self-inflicted, suicidal attempt, hanging and drowning.
- Police intimation has to be written by the CMO with correct name, address, age; diagnosis and identification mark and send to the particular police station of the area through hospital driver with a register.
- Seal as MLC on the case as well as on the folder before shifting to the ward.
- Do not give any records or investigation reports of hospital to the patient and relatives.

> **Admission and discharge**
> - Whenever a medicolegal case is admitted or discharged, the same should be intimated to the nearest police station at the earliest.
> - It is always better to inform the police through the casualty of the hospital where the medicolegal register is usually maintained and necessary entries can be made in it.
> - While discharging or referring the patient, care should be taken to see that he receives the Discharge Card/Referral Letter, complete with the summary of admission, the treatment given in the hospital and the instructions to the patient to be followed after discharge.
> - Failure to do so renders the doctor liable for "negligence" and "deficiency of service".

- Keep under strict custody all the records and reports of such patients.
- If the patient wants to go as LAMA (left against medical advice) obtain his/her signature on the record but reports should not be given. Send the intimation to the police station against as LAMA with details where they are going, whether hospital or home.
- In case of death, police intimation should be sent and the body should be handed over to the police and take the signature, name and designation of the police in detail.
- Enter all the details in the death register and write in red ink as MLC.
- Postmortem for MLC cases is a must. Information should be given to the forensic department as soon as

the patient dies, brief them regarding the time of death and place from which the police has to come.
- The police have to come before postmortem and do mortuaro (Marger) inquest which takes about one to two hours. So before the doctor's arrival this procedure can be performed. During the martuaro the forensic department attendant has to assist the police.
- The police have to take over the body by signing on the admission record and take his PC number/designation and name. 12.If the MLC body is brought from outside, the police has to give a written requisition along with the body, which has to be preserved carefully.
- After the postmortem the police will hand over body to the party.
- In case of women's death before 11 years of marriage and the case is MLC the taluks magistrate (Tahsildar) has to be informed and postmortem has to be done in his presence (which will be arranged by the police). There should be two doctors out of which one should be a lady doctor.
- The dead body must be sent out for postmortem if the forensic doctor is not available or as per the wish of police. The death summary has to be given to the police (Xerox copies of history and doctors sheet can be given if death summary is not ready)

Brought Dead to Emergency (Fig. 12.3)

- Examination should be done from head to toe for any abrasions, cuts, wounds, strangulation marks or any unusual smell.
- Declaration of death and giving death certificate is left to the doctor's discretion.
- If it is known case, treated earlier in the hospital, the doctor can decide whether to give death certificate after examination of the body.
- Be kind and informative to bystanders regarding autopsy, sending police intimation, speak to them very politely. If the cause of death is not known postmortem should be done.

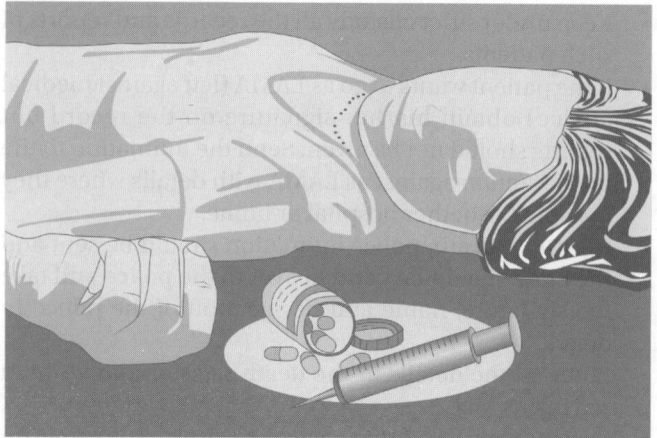

Fig. 12.3: Patient brought unconscious to hospital.

Types of Clients, which are Categorized as MLC in a Hospital

- Road traffic accident (RTA)
- Injuries inflicted during brawls/fights, shooting, bomb blasts, etc.
- Suicide
- Homicide
- Burns
- Poisoning
- Rape victim
- Assault.

Role of Nurse in Medicolegal Cases

- Obtain complete history from patient or significant other(s).
- Inform the police officer/constable on duty in the hospital and the Chief Medical Officer (CMO).
- When it is made an MLC, then record it on the patient's case sheet with red ink right hand top corner.
- Do not give any statement about patient's condition to police, magistrate or media. Only a doctor is to give information.
- When a patient has to be discharged, inform the police officer/constable on duty in hospital and/or the CMO, after clearance from others, then only discharge.
- If an MLC patient absconds inform the CMO and the treating doctor, immediately
- No MLC patient can go LAMA.
- Document the care given to the patients timely, accurately and duly sign the nurse's notes.
- Records and all documents pertaining to patient and his care, during his stay in the hospital, must be kept safely, should be handed over to the authorized person as designated by the hospital authority.
- In case of death of an MLC, the body is not to be handed over to the relatives. It needs to be accurately labeled and sent to the mortuary. CMO and/or police officer should be informed simultaneously. Appropriate authority must be informed.

PATIENT'S BILL OF RIGHTS

Patient's rights are among the most important of the issues involved in biomedical ethics influencing almost every aspect of the professional's ethical considerations. The American hospital association (AHA) has recognized the importance of patient's rights and published a patient's Bill of Rights. Patient awareness of individual rights and needs and availability of the various imaging techniques provides both opportunities and complications for the imaging professional.

Nurses are not all levels of health care, but they are primary functionaries and the largest component of health manpower. Nurses while rendering care in a politically oriented health under the Consumer Protection

Act are increasingly facing ethical issues. Nursing ethics are the professional standard of conduct practiced by nurse practitioners related to or in accordance with approved moral behavior in rendering health care services. In 1973, the American Hospital Association adopted Patient's Bill of Rights as national policy statement and distributed it to its members in the health care organizations throughout the nation. There are twelve rights summarized below:

1. The patient has a right to a considerate and respectful care.
2. The patient has a right to obtain complete and concerned information concerning the diagnosis, treatment and prognosis from his physician for the patient's expected understanding.

Patients have the right to
- Be treated for the life-threatening, chronic disease of addiction with honesty, respect and dignity.
- Know what to expect from treatment, and the likelihood of success.
- Be treated by licensed and certified professionals.
- Evidence-based treatment.
- Be treated for co-occurring behavioral health conditions simultaneously.
- An individualized, outcomes-driven treatment plan.
- Remain in treatment as long as necessary.
- Support, education and treatment for their families and loved ones.
- A treatment setting that is safe and ethical.

3. The patient has a right to receive the necessary information from his physician regarding the treatment and the procedures involved in it.
4. The patient has a right to refuse the treatment to the extent permitted by the law and to be informed about the medical consequences of his action.
5. The patient has a right to privacy concerning his own medical care program.
6. The patient has a right to expect all communications and records pertaining to his care should be treated as confidential.
7. The patient has a right to expect within the capacity a hospital must make reasonable response to the request made by the patient for services.
8. The patient has a right to obtain information as to any relationship of his hospital to other health care institution a care is concerned.
9. The patient has a right to be advised if the hospital proposes to engage him in or perform human experimentation affecting his treatment.
10. The patient has a right to expect reasonable continuity of care.
11. The patient has a right to examine and receive an explanation of his hospital bills regardless of the source of payment.
12. The patient has a right to know what hospital rules and regulations apply to his conduct as a patient.

ROLE AND RESPONSIBILITIES OF NURSE IN ADMISSION

A nurse has an important role to play in the reception the patient to the hospital. The following are the purposes of this procedure:
- Prepare the patient both physically and mentally for his stay in the hospital.
- To help the patient to be comfortable and to provide him with a clean and safe environment.
- To give a good impression of the hospital and its service so that the patient will fully cooperate with the treatment and nursing care. A patient may be coming to hospital for the first time. He leaves his familiar home surrounding and his loved ones and comes to an unknown place and to unknown people.

Any change in human life is anxiety producing and is viewed with fear. Added to this, his physical condition gives him fear and anxiety. Hence, it is the nurse's duty

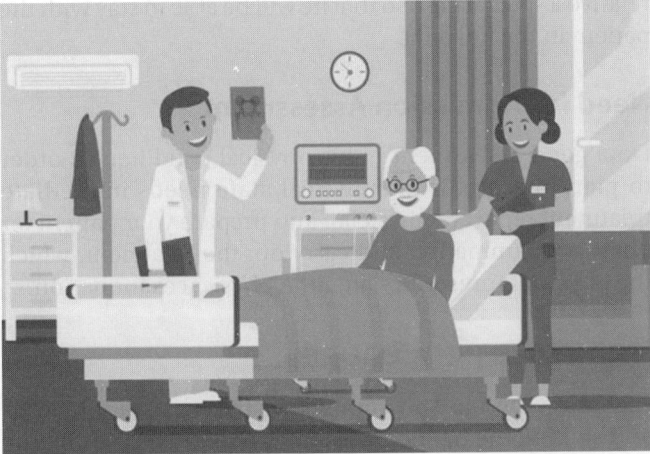

Fig. 12.4: Orienting the patient during admission.

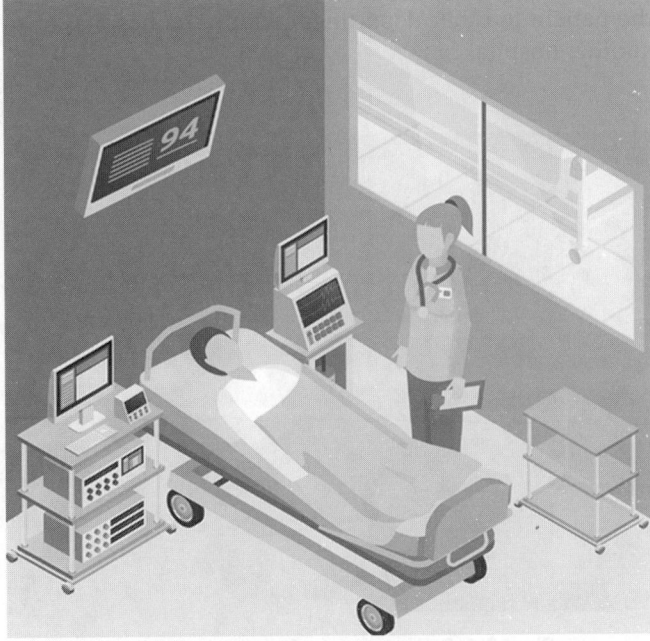

Fig. 12.5: Care of patient in emergency department.

to receive the patient, kindly sympathetically and with an understanding of his illness. If he is admitted, he is given a diet sheet and sent to the ward. If he is too ill and needs immediate attention he is given emergency treatment and then transported to the ward (**Fig. 12.6**).

As soon as the patient comes to the ward, receive him, his relatives and his friends as if you are receiving your guests into your home. Ask them to be seated while you prepare the bed ready for the patient. If the patient is in a serious condition, the ward nurse is informed in advance about the arrival of the patient, so that the patient does not have to wait till the bed is made ready.

Need for Orientation to Place and Person

Inform the patient and his relatives about the hospital routine, the hospital rules, the general set up of the ward and the personnel working in the ward. Inform the patient's relatives about the time of visiting hours and supply them with visiting passes. If the patient is seriously ill give the relative a special pass so that he will be able to stay with the patient in the hospital.

Need for Admission Assessment

Do a good assessment of his physical condition in order to plan his care. If his physical state needs immediate treatment report to physician and prepare your patient for physical examination and carry out the treatment, which the physician prescribes after the physical examination.

TRANSFER PROCEDURE

Preparing the patient, completing the necessary records and shifting the patient to another department within the hospital or to another hospital. Transfer/referral is the preparation of a patient and the referral records to the shift the patient to other department within the hospital or to another hospital.

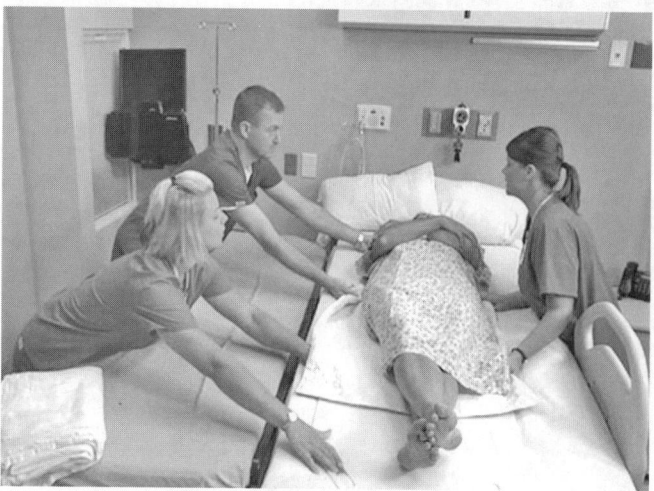

Fig. 12.6: Patient transfer from bed to trolley.

Definition

Transfer is defined as preparing patient, completing necessary records and shifting patient to another department within the hospital or to another hospital/home.

Purpose

- To obtain necessary diagnostic tests and procedure.
- To provide treatment and nursing care.
- To provide specialized care.
- To place most appropriate utilization or available personnel and services.
- To match intensity of nursing care, based on patients level of needs and problems.

Types of Transfer of the Patient

- **Internal transfer:** To transfer the patient in a unit that provides special care or care suited to his needs, e.g. from general ward to ICU.
- **External transfer:** To transfer the patient from one hospital to other hospital for the purpose of special care, e.g. from general hospital to specialized hospital-cancer centre.

Preliminary Assessment

- Assess the method for transport, inform receiving nurse.
- Maintain patient's physical well being during transport to new nursing unit.
- Provide verbal report about patient's condition to the receiving unit nurse.
- Be sure all documentation including care plan is completed.
- Assist patient's arrival to the new unit.
- Announce patient's arrival to the new unit.
- Transport patient to a new room and assist in transfer to bed.
- Handover to receiving nurse.

Equipment

- Wheelchair/stretcher
- Identification labels
- Patients belongings
- X-rays.

Investigation Reports

Patient records and file.

Procedure

Transfer to another hospital/department:
- Check the doctor's order for transfer of patient
- Inform the patients and relatives
- Inform to the ward sister where the patient needs to be transferred

- Check the chart for complete recording of vital sings, nursing care and treatment given
- Collect patients X-ray, medicine and other belongings
- Cancel the hospital diet or transfer
- Assist the relative to collect other belongings
- Make arrangement to settle the due bills if going to another hospital
- Record time, mode of transfer and general condition of the patient
- Assist in transferring sick patient to wheel chair/stretcher and accompany patient to new area
- Handover patient documents, belonging and report verbally to the in charge nurse/and sister
- Collect the ward articles
- Inform to the concern person/department regarding transfer of the patient
- Clean unit thoroughly and keep ready for next patient.

DISCHARGE PLANNING

Discharge planning is the development of an individualized discharge plan for the patient prior to leaving the hospital, to ensure that patients are discharged at an appropriate time and with provision of adequate post-discharge services. Discharge planning strategy highlights the key elements of engaging the patient and family in discharge planning: Include the patient and family as full partners in the discharge planning process,

Discuss with the patient and family five key areas to prevent problems at home:
- Describe what life at home will be like
- Review medications
- Highlight warning signs and problems
- Explain test results
- Make follow-up appointments

Educate the patient and family in plain language about the patient's condition, the discharge process, and next steps at every opportunity throughout the hospital stay Assess how well doctors and nurses explain the diagnosis, condition, and next steps in the patient's care to the patient and family and use teach back. Listen to and honor the patient and family's goals, preferences, observations, and concerns.

DISCHARGE FROM HOSPITAL

Discharge is preparation of patient to leave hospital and to return to own environment. Patient is prepared for discharge when he is admitted in the hospital. He should be prepared physically and mentally to leave the hospital or ward.

Discharge planning is the plan evolved before a patient is transferred from one environment to another. This process involves the patient, family, friends, and the hospital and community health care teams.

Discharge planning is an integral part of the continuity of nursing care for patients throughout their hospital stay.

Purpose

- To ensure continuity of care to patient after discharge.
- To assist patient to complete hospital formalities before returning home.
- To assist patient to return to a state of optimal independent living.
- To assist the patient in discharge process.
- To acknowledge patients right in deciding to leave hospital.

Reasons for Discharge

- Cured
- Transfer to other hospital
- Discharged at request
- Discharged against medical advice
- Death.

Discharge to Home

The discharge to home or another hospital or another unit within the hospital is initiated by the doctor who advises the patient that he is well enough to leave the hospital or requires treatment in another unit within the hospital or in an another hospital.

Discharge to Another Hospital or Another Unit within the Hospital (Referral)

When a patient or family is not satisfied with the treatment or care given and wants to leave the hospital against the medical advice in such cases the patient or the relative is asked to sign a statement that he is going or taking the patient on his own will and responsibility.

Discharge Against Medical Advice

Patient leaves the hospital against the medical officer's advice, when a patient escapes from the hospital without the knowledge of the hospital staff and without signing the said statement he is treated as absconded in the records.

TYPES: PLANNED DISCHARGE, LAMA, ABSCOND, REFERRALS AND TRANSFER

Planned Hospital Discharge

Discharge from the hospital is the point at which the patient leaves the hospital and either returns home or is transferred to another facility such as one for rehabilitation or to a nursing home. Discharge involves the medical instructions that the patient will need to fully recover. Discharge planning is a service that considers the patient's needs after the hospital stay, and may involve several different services such as visiting nursing care, physical therapy.

LAMA

LAMA has been defined in the broadest terms as any patient who insists upon leaving against the expressed advice of the treating team. Escape (absence without leave, absconding, or elopement), whereby the patient leaves the hospital without notification by escaping from an involuntary unit or walking out of a voluntary unit, also has been considered by some clinicians and researchers to be a form of discharge against medical advice. Others do not regard escape as a form of discharge against medical advice because the essential element of physician's expressed advice against leaving is lacking in this situation.

Abscond

Absconding-patients leaving the ward/hospital without permission.

DISCHARGE PROCEDURE

Inform the patient and the relatives a day or two before the discharge. Get the discharge slip prepared after checking the vital signs and examining the patient. The nurse should see that the patient's personal hygiene is maintained; he is dressed in home clothes and has taken meals. Handover the patient's belongings and any valuable, which have been kept safely, to the patient or the relative under proper receipt. Complete the unit admission and discharge registered case sheet and other records. Handover the case sheet and other records medical record department under proper receipt. Inform the hospital authorities about the discharge if the patient is medicolegal. Handover the discharge slip to the patient or relative and explain about the treatment and the diet to be taken at home, follow-up visit and inform to bring the discharge slip on every visits, any special advices pertaining to condition. See that the patient receives all the medicines as per discharge slip. Check the hospital things before the patient leaves the ward. Place the patient in the wheelchair or stretcher according to the patient's condition until he leaves the hospital. Immediately after the patient leaves, reorganize the patient unit.

General Instruction

Prepare patient and family during hospitalization with adequate information in relation to probable date of discharge, approximate in patient bill and relevant home care.

Preliminary Assessment

Check

- The doctor's written order for discharge.
- Inform patient and relative about discharge.
- Document relevant discharge information.

Departments to be informed

- Drug return to pharmacy department
- Diet cancellation
- Oxygen/ventilator charges summary
- Accounts department
- Billing section.

Procedure

- Check doctors written order for discharge.
- Inform patient and relatives about discharge.
- Document relevant discharge information.
- Make sure all the fees are included such as special investigations, special matters or devices, doctors or surgeon's fees and narcotic drugs used (if any).
- Obtain discharge prescription after retaining the medicines to be continued for that day and after discharge. Send all other continued for that day and after discharge. Send all other medicines for refunding (include ward replacement).
- Send chart to billing section with relevant information.
- One bill is ready and chart is received back in ward, ensure that bill is settled. Check the cashier's signature in the discharge bill.
- Help the patient to obtain discharge summary, medical certificate and drugs.
- Ensure that patient is instructed regarding medication follow up, out patient visit, etc.
- Accompany the patient up to transport near exit gate.

After Discharge

- Record time date and condition of the patient at departure.
- Send chart to medical record department and inform to the concern departments.
- After the patient has gone, the bed should be washed, blankets kept in sunlight, mackintosh washed and dried.
- The room and all utensils should be cleaned and kept ready for next use.
- In case of infected cases, utensils should be disinfected and then cleaned. The linen should be disinfected and then send to laundry.
- When discharging the medicolegal cases, the patient's dead body should be handed over to the police, before that concerning police station should be informed about the patient's discharge/death.
- Patient or dead body is handed over to the police and asks the police to sign with date and time.

Discharge Teaching Goals

- Understand his illness.
- Complies with his drug therapy.
- Carefully follows his diet.
- Manages his activity level.
- Understands his treatments.
- Recognizes his need for rest.

- Knows about possible complications.
- Knows when to seek follow-up care.

Role and Responsibilities of the Nurse

- Inform the patient and the relatives a day or two before the discharge.
- Get the discharge slip prepared after checking the vital signs and examining the patient.
- The nurses should see that the patient's personal hygiene is maintained; he is dressed in home clothes and has taken meals.
- Handover the patient's belongings and any valuables, which have been kept safely, to the patient or the relative under proper receipt.
- Complete the unit admission and discharge registers, case sheet and other records.
- Handover the case sheet and other records to medical record department under proper receipt.
- Inform the hospital authorities about the discharge if the patient is medicolegal.
- Handover the discharge slip to the patient or relative and explain about:
  - the treatment and the diet to be taken at home
  - follow-up visits and inform to bring the discharge slip on every visits
  - any special advices pertaining to condition
- See that the patient receives all the medicines as per discharge slip.
- Check the hospital things before the patient leaves the ward.
- Care of unit after discharge.

CARE OF UNIT AFTER DISCHARGE

- The sanitation of the bed, bedside cabinet, and general area of the patient care unit with a detergent/germicidal agent after the patient is discharged or transferred from the nursing care unit.
- Performed at every patient care unit before the area is prepared for the next patient.

Reasons for Terminal Cleaning of the Patient Care Unit

- Prevention of the spread of microorganisms.
- Removal of encrusted secretions from framework or bedside rails.
- Removal of residue of body wastes from the mattress.
- Deodorizing of the bed frame, mattress, and pillow.

Guidelines for Terminal Cleaning

- Review wards standing order procedures for specific procedures.
- Use only authorized disinfectant/detergent or germicidal solution for cleaning.
- Check to ensure the bedside cabinet is cleared of any valuables belonging to the patient.
- Check bed linens for personal items (dentures, contact lenses, money, jewelry, etc.) belonging to the patient.
- Prevent spread of microorganisms by carefully removing linen from the bed.
- Use caution when cleaning the under frame and bedsprings.
- Replace any torn mattress or pillow covers.
- Allow the mattress and pillow to air-dry thoroughly before remaking the bed.

Rules for Use of Disposal or Non-reusable Items

- Do not attempt to reuse (for another patient) or resterilize disposables.
- Sterile disposables are considered sterile providing the wrapper is not broken or torn or the expiration date has not passed.
- Sterile disposables with torn or broken wrappers must be discarded.
  - Use disposables for the specific purpose(s) for which they were designed.
  - Follow manufacturer's directions when using disposables.

CONCLUSION

The nurse should welcome him or her as a guest whom she is glad to see, and should be quick to notice whether she is able to walk or whether she should be carried to the ward or admitting room. As soon as possible after admission, give the patient a bath. Comb her hair, clean the finger and toe nails and trim them if necessary. Before the relatives go home, see that there is an arrangement for food and drink for the patient, and for any personal articles that need to be brought from home. During discharge the patient and the relatives should be informed in advance so that suitable arrangements can be made. Clothing and any personal possessions are returned to the patient or the relations. She is informed if and when she is required to attend the out-patients department or special clinic. The patient should be given her out-patient number receipt for hospital bill paid and any medications ordered to take at home.

BIBLIOGRAPHY

1. Alice L. Price. The Art, Science and Spirit of Nursing, Philadelphia: WB Saunders Company, 3rd Edition, 1968.
2. Kozier, Barbara. B and Du Gas, Beverly Witter. Fundamentals of Patient Care: A Comprehensive Approach to Nursing. WB Saunders Company, 1967.
3. McClosky JC, Grace HK. Current issues in nursing, 4th Edition. St. Louis: Mosby Year Book, Inc., 1994.
4. Mitchell PR, Grippando GM. Nursing Perspectives and Issues, 5th Edition. Albany, New York: Delmar Publishers, Inc., 1993.

5. Potter P, Perry A. Fundamentals of Nursing—Concepts, Process and Practice. Mosby Year Book; 3rd Edition, 1993.
6. Shafer, Kathleen, et. al. Medical-Surgical Nursing, 6th Edition. Saint Louis: CV Mosby Co., 1975.
7. Shakuntala Sharma 'Birpuri'. Principles and Practice of Nursing. Jaypee Brothers Medical Publishers (P) Ltd., New Delhi, 1997.
8. Sr. Nancy. Principles and Practice of Nursing, Vol. 1, 3rd ed. N. R. Brothers. Indore, 1992.
9. Taylor C, Lillis C, LeMone P. Fundamentals of Nursing: The Art and Science of Nursing Care. Philadelphia: JB Lippincott, 1993.
10. Thresvamma CP. "Fundamentals of Nursing", Procedure Manual for General Nursing Course, P. C. Mathew, Kottayam, Kerala, 1992.
11. Virginia Henderson. Principles and Practice of Nursing. New York: MacMillan Publishing Co., 1970.

REVIEW QUESTIONS

Long Essays

1. Discuss in detail about admission procedure and roles and responsibilities of a nurse in admission.
2. Explain the purpose and types of discharge and enumerate the role and responsibilities of a nurse?
3. Discuss the purpose, types and need of transferring the patient?

Short Essays

1. Explain emergency admission procedure.
2. Describe the unit preparation for a new patient.
3. Discuss the Medcolegal issues in admission.
4. How will you care the unit after discharge?
5. What is the importance of discharge planning?

Short Answers

1. Define admission.
2. What is the purpose of admission?
3. What are the types of discharge?
4. List out the principles followed in admission.
5. Discuss care of belongings.

MULTIPLE CHOICE QUESTIONS

1. **Emergency admission means the patient admitted in case of:**
   a. Routine examination
   b. For treatment
   c. Acute condition
   d. None of the above
2. **Ethical consideration involves:**
   a. Respects and justice
   b. Beneficence
   c. Fidelity
   d. All of the above
3. **LAMA stands for:**
   a. Left against medical advice
   b. Leave application for medical advice
   c. Limited access to medical advice
   d. None of the above
4. **Types of clients, which are categorized as MLC in a Hospital:**
   a. Road traffic accident (RTA)
   b. Injuries inflicted during brawls/fights, shooting, bomb blasts, etc.
   c. Suicide
   d. All of the above
5. **Reasons for terminal cleaning of the patient care unit:**
   a. Prevention of the spread of microorganisms.
   b. Removal of encrusted secretions from framework or bedside rails.
   c. Removal of residue of body wastes from the mattress.
   d. All of the above.

ANSWERS

1. c   2. d   3. a   4. d   5. d

CHAPTER 13

Mobility and Immobility

LEARNING OBJECTIVES

- Elements of normal movement, alignment and posture, joint mobility, balance, coordinated movement
- Principles of body mechanics
- Factors affecting body alignment and activity
- Exercise: Types and benefits
- Effects of immobility
- Maintenance of normal body alignment and activity
- Alteration in body alignment and mobility
- Nursing interventions for impaired body alignment and mobility: Assessment, types, devices used, method
- Range of motion exercises
- Muscle strengthening exercises
- Maintaining body alignment: Positions
- Moving
- Lifting
- Transferring
- Walking
- Assisting clients with ambulation
- Care of patients with immobility using nursing process approach
- Care of patients with casts and splints

TERMINOLOGY

- **Immobility** is inability to move a body part or the whole body. Immobilization can be prescribed or unavoidable restriction of movement.
- **Joint mobility:** A joint is the functional unit of the musculoskeletal system. The bone of the skeleton articulate at the joints. Most of the skeletal muscles attach to the two bones at the joint. Muscles are therefore called flexors, extensors and internal rotators.
- **Range of motion:** The range of motion of a joint is the maximum movement that is possible for that joint.
- **Degrees of immobility:** The unconscious patient is often completely immobilized immobility is sometimes called partial, as in a patient with a fractured leg.
- **Tone:** A state of resting muscle activity, which can be influenced by many external factors (e.g. temperature, anxiety, wellness and pain).
- **Flexion:** The state of being bent. The cervical spine is flexed when the chin is moved toward the chest.
- **Extension:** The state of being in a straight line. The cervical spine is extended when the head is held straight.
- **Hyperextension:** The state of exaggerated extension. The cervical spine is hyperextended when the person looks overhead, toward the ceiling.
- **Abduction:** Lateral movement of a body part away from the midline of the body. The arm is abducted when it is held away from the body.
- **Adduction:** Lateral movement of a body part toward the midline of the body. The arm is adducted when it is moved from an outstretched position toward the body.
- **Rotation:** Turning of a body part around an axis. The head is rotated when moved from side to side to indicate "no."
- **Circumduction:** Rotating an extremity in a complete circle. Circumduction is a Combination of abduction, adduction, extension, and flexion.
- **Supination:** The palm or sole is rotated in an upward position.
- **Pronation:** The palm or sole is rotated in a downward position.
- **Traction:** Traction, simply defined, is a physical pulling force that exerts pulling on the bodily part. Traction is used for the external fixation of a fracture. It is used to maintain anatomically correct alignment, reduce pain and decrease muscle spasms.
- **Splints:** The primary purposes of splinting for limb fractures are to protect soft tissue from further damage, to reduce the client's pain, to reduce the possibility of a fat embolism, and to minimize painful muscular spasms.
- **Braces:** Braces are applied to various parts of the body to provide support and alignment of the part. Some commonly used braces are neck braces, back braces, and elbow braces.
- **Casts:** It is a shell, frequently made from plaster that encases a limb to stabilize and hold anatomical structures—most often a broken bone in place until healing is confirmed.

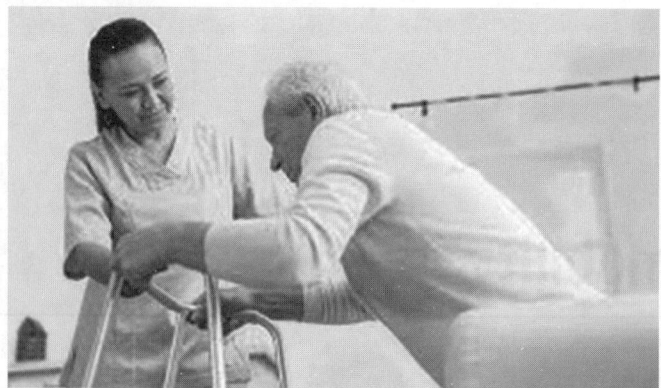

Fig. 13.1: Nurse assist for patients mobility.

INTRODUCTION

Physical exercise is any bodily activity that enhances or maintains physical fitness and overall health. Physical fitness is a general state of good health as a result of nutrition and exercise. Our bodies are made for activity. Movement is one of the definitions of life. The human body is endowed for it in terms of strength, agility, flexibility, and precision. To remain in good health with a sound circulatory and respiratory system, we must all exercise regularly.

The main factors involved are age, body type and level of health. For example, older people have to take special precaution to avoid sudden, jarring movements that could impose excessive strain. Therefore, they would benefit most from gentler forms of exercise such as leisurely swimming or yoga. People who want to lose weight may need prolonged steady types of exercise such as golf, swimming, or walking; which do not put extreme burden on the joints. Conditions, such as, high blood pressure or obesity may prevent vigorous physical exercise. For other problems resulting in restricted mobility and stiffness, flexibility exercises are advisable.

DEFINITION

- **Normal movement** may be considered as a skill acquired through learning (or development) for the purpose of achieving the most efficient and economical movement or performance of a given task and is specific to the individual.
- **Posture** can simply be defined as a 'position' or 'arrested movement'. It considers the position of the body and its relationship to whatever is supporting it (i.e. a chair, the floor, a table that's being leaned on).

BASIC ELEMENTS OF NORMAL MOVEMENT

Our ability to move contributes to our self worth as well as our well-being. Mobility is necessary for all aspects of life. As we become less mobile in later stages of life results into health problems. Factors that contribute to immobility, especially in the hospital, including a greater length of stay in hospital, the more severe the illness is going to be and an emotional and physical toll on the individual.

Alignment and posture helps to optimize on being able to stand or move. Alignment: Look at them from anterior view and look at shoulders and hips they should be aligned. Lateral and side view is plum line. Look at earlobe, shoulder, hip, anterior part of knee and the posterior part of their heel.

Posture: Erect lordosis, kyphosis or scoliosis.

Joint mobility: Some joints has a wide range of movement. Shoulder joint is a ball and socket joint as well as hip joint. Some joints are saddle joints in hands with limited flexibility compared to ball and socket. Joint mobility is affected by genetics, age, and disease processes and how physically active we are in our lifetime.

Coordinated movement is influenced by cerebral cortex, which initiates voluntary movement. And cerebrum in back of head is in charge of coordinating motor activity and the basal ganglia maintain posture as well.

BENEFITS OF EXERCISE

Prevents muscle atrophy and prevents osteoporosis

Musculoskeletal system: Helps with our bone density. Maintain size, tone of muscle. Exercise nourishes joints and maintains ROM and stability so we can continue to use muscles as we age.

CV system: Exercise decreases risk of CVA as well as ACS (acute coronary syndrome). With respiratory system, it improves gas exchange and helps immune system to function better.

Respiratory system: When exercising we do deep breathing. We get increased pressure in abdominal cavity which helps return lymph fluid back to lymph nodes and circulation.

GI system: Increases GI tract tone. We have less likely to have constipation and impaction.

Metabolic system: Exercise decreases triglycerides, cholesterol and hemoglobin A1c levels. When we exercise, we have glucose 4 transporters inside of our cells. When we exercise the gluc 4 transporter cells go to outside of cells and bring glucose inside of our cell without insulin. This is extremely important especially with patient with diabetes. They need to exercise. They need these gluc 4 transport cells to normalize blood sugar.

GU system: Increased blood flow to kidney and increased elimination of waste products with better efficiency.

Immune system: Increased lymph flow during the time we are exercising and increases resistance to viruses and also exercise helps to decrease formation of malignant cells. All of us have malignant cells in our body but immune system takes care of them so they don't wreak havoc on our system.

Psycho neurological: When we exercise we have increased endorphins and elevate our mood. We breathe heavier so we have increased oxygen. This creates euphoria effect. Exercise decreases stress, decreases anxiety and improves sleep.

Cognitive function: Improved decision-making and increased attention span when we are resting.

MOBILITY

Mobility defined as the ability to move freely, easily, rhythmically and purposefully in the environment. The ability to move also influences persons self-esteem depends on a sense of independence and a feeling of usefulness.

Structure and Functions

- **Joint mobility:** A joint is the functional unit of the musculoskeletal system. The bone of the skeleton articulate at the joints. Most of the skeletal muscles attach to the two bones at the joint. Muscles are therefore called flexors, extensors and internal rotators.
- **Range of motion:** The range of motion of a joint is the maximum movement that is possible for that joint.
- **Degrees of immobility:** The unconscious patient is often completely immobilized immobility is sometimes called partial, as in a patient with a fractured leg.

FACTORS AFFECTING MOBILITY

- **Age:** It greatly affects activity levels and general mobility. Generally as people grow older they slow down.
- **Energy level:** Energy level varies greatly among individuals. An individual demonstrates different energy level at different times.
- **Lifestyle:** People learn early in life often from families, the value of activity in relation to health. Some people of activity in relation to health. Some people participate in physical activity regularly in an effort to maintain or improve their health.
- **Fear and pain:** The mobility can also be limited because of fear or pain, a patient recovering from surgery may be reluctant to move for fear of opening the incision or because of the pain experienced with movement.
- **Disability:** A disability is a persistent mental or physical weakness that prevents a person from caring out the normal activities of life.
- **Therapeutic modalities:** Sometimes movement is limited to treat medical problems. Restrictive devices such as caste, braces and splints may be used to immobilize certain areas of body parts to promote healing.
- **Affective disorders:** Severe affective disorders can hinder mobility, depression and catatonic states result in limited mobility, not because of physical impairment but because the person lacks the desire to move.
- **Trauma:** Trauma often results in accidental injury to joints, tendons, ligaments, muscles or bones. Such damage can be minor, affecting body alignment and mobility to short time. Severe trauma can also cause extensive damage to the spinal cord or brain.
- **Chronic health problems:** Chronic health conditions often decreases mobility because such disorder limit the oxygen and nutrients delivered to the muscles. The substances are important for muscle contraction and movement.
- **Skeleton-muscular defects:** Any impairment of skeleton-muscular system can affect the body alignment and joint mobility, skeletal strength and body movements. Demineralization of bone, as in osteoporosis increase risk of fracture. Rheumatoid arthritis limits mobility because movement causes pain.
- **Neuromuscular defects:** Any disease that impairs the ability of nervous system to control muscular movement and coordination hinder functional mobility.
- **Congenital problems:** Congenital problems usually affect normal musculoskeletal or neurological development. Some problems such as congenital dysplasia can be corrected with treatment. Others such as spina bifida or cerebral palsy cannot be cured, so treatment is aimed at promoting the greater degree of functional mobility and preventing complications.

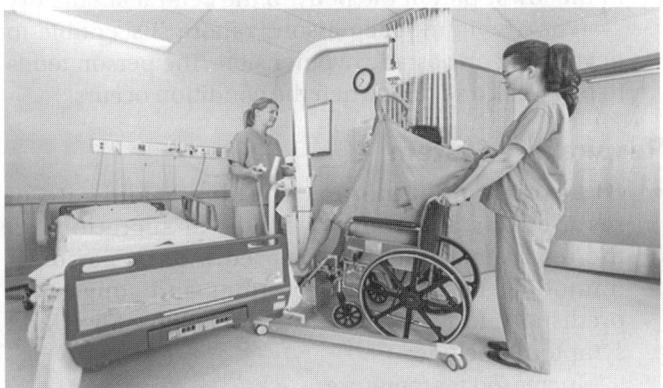

Fig. 13.2: Patient transfer from wheelchair to bed.

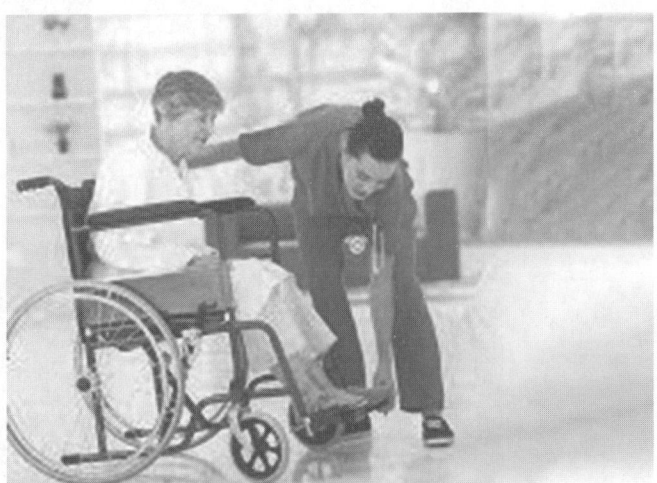

Fig. 13.3: Nurse assist patient to sit in wheelchair.

Patients at High Risk of Immobility

- Poorly nourished.
- Decreased sensitivity to pain, temperature or pressure.
- Patients have existing problems with cardiovascular system.
- Patients have existing problems with respiratory system.
- Patients have existing problems with neuromuscular system.
- Unconscious patients.

Nurses Responsibility in Assessing Mobility

- **Range of motion:** When assessing joint movement, asks the patient to move selected body parts. When a patient moves a joint the nurse should assess the degree of movement, joint swelling or redness, muscle development tolerance, and discomfort report the patient.
- **Gait:** It is the manner or style of walking. Assessing gait can provide data concerning the patients balance and coordination, posture, safety and ability to walk without assistance.
- **Exercise and activity tolerance:** By determining an appropriate activity level for a patient, the nurse can predict whether a patient has the strength to participate in activities that require similar expenditure of energy.

Physical Complications of Immobility

- Hypostatic pneumonia.
- Pulmonary embolism.
- Thrombophlebitis.
- Orthostatic hypotension.
- Pressure ulcers or pressure areas.
- Decreased peristalsis with constipation and fecal impaction.
- Urinary stasis with renal calculi formation.
- Contractures and muscle atrophy.
- Altered fluid and electrolyte status.

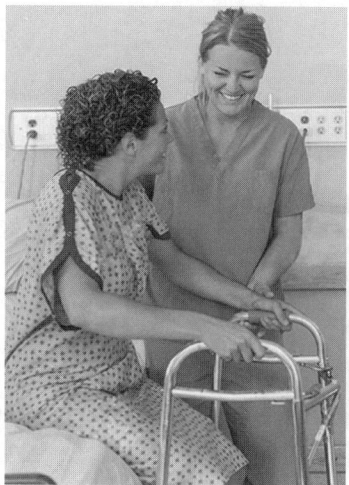

Fig. 13.4: Nurse assist to use walker.

Effects of Exercise

- **Cardiovascular system:** Increased cardiac output, strengthening cardiac muscle, decreased resting heart rate and improved venous return.
- **Pulmonary system:** Increased respiratory rate and depth, improved alveolar ventilation, decreased work of breathing and improved diaphragmatic excursion.
- **Metabolic system:** Increased basal metabolic rate, increased use of glucose and fatty acids, increased triglyceride breakdown, increased gastric motility and increased production of body heat.
- **Musculoskeletal system:** Improved muscle tone, increased joint mobility, improved muscle tolerance to physical exercise, possible increase in muscle mass and reduced bone loss.
- **Psychological factors:** Improved tolerance to stress, reports of feeling better and reports of decrease in illness.

EFFECTS OF MOBILITY

Cardiovascular System

- Venous stasis caused by prolonged inactivity that restricts or slows venous circulation. Muscular activity, especially in the legs, helps move blood toward the central circulatory system.
- Increased cardiac workload due to increased viscosity from dehydration and decreased venous return. The heart works more when the body is resting, probably because there is less resistance offered by the blood vessels and because there is a change in the distribution of blood in the immobile person. The result is that the heart rate, cardiac output, and stroke volume increase.
- Thrombus and embolus formation caused by slow flowing blood, which may begin clotting within hours, and an increased rate in the coagulation of blood. During periods of immobility, calcium leaves bones and enters the blood, where it has an influence on blood coagulation.
- Orthostatic hypotension probably due to a decrease in the neurovascular reflexes, which normally causes vasoconstriction, and to a loss of muscle tone. The result is that blood pools and does not squeeze from veins in the lower part of the body to the central circulatory system. The immobile person is more susceptible to developing orthostatic hypotension. The person tends to feel weak and faint when the condition occurs.

Respiratory System

- **Hypostatic pneumonia:** The depth and rate of respirations and the movement of secretions in the respiratory tract is decreased when a person is immobile. The pooling secretions and congestion predispose to respiratory tract infections. Signs and symptoms include:
  - Increased temperature.
  - Thick copious secretions.

- Cough.
- Increased pulse.
- Confusion, irritability, or disorientation.
- Sharp chest pain.
- Dyspnea.
- **Atelectasis:** When areas of lung tissue are not used over a period of time, incomplete expansion or collapse of lung tissue may occur.
- **Impaired coughing:** Impairment of coughing mechanism may be due to the patient's position in bed decreasing chest cage expansion.

Musculoskeletal System

- **Muscle atrophy:** Disuse leads to decreased muscle size, tone, and strength.
- **Contracture:** Decreased joint movement leads to permanent shortening of muscle tissue, resistant to stretching. The strong flexor muscles pull tight, causing a contraction of the extremity or a permanent position of flexion.
- **Ankylosis:** Consolidation and immobility of a joint in a particular position due to contracture.
- **Osteoporosis:** Lack of stress on the bone causes an increase in calcium absorption, weakening the bone.

Nervous System

- Altered sensation caused by prolonged pressure and continual stimulation of nerves. Usually pain is felt at first and then sensation is altered, and the patient no longer senses the pain.
- Peripheral nerve palsy.

Gastrointestinal System

- Disturbance in appetite caused by the slowing of gastrointestinal tract, secondary immobility, and decreased activity resulting in anorexia.
- Altered digestion and utilization of nutrients resulting in constipation.
- Altered protein metabolism.

Integumentary System

Risk of skin breakdown, which leads to necrosis and ulceration of tissues, especially on bony areas.

Urinary System

- Renal calculi (kidney stones) caused by stagnation of urine in the renal pelvis and the high levels of urinary calcium.
- Urinary tract infections caused by urinary stasis that favors the growth of bacteria.
- Decreased bladder muscle tone resulting in urinary retention.

Metabolism

- Increased risk of electrolyte imbalance. An absence of weight on the skeleton and immobility causes protein to be broken down faster than it is made, resulting in a negative nitrogen balance.
- Decreased metabolic rate.
- Altered exchange of nutrients and gases.

Psychosocial Functioning

- Decrease in self-concept and increase in sense of powerlessness due to inability to move purposefully and dependence on someone for assistance with simple self-care activities.
- Body image distortions (depends on diagnosis).
- Decrease in sensory stimulation due to lack of activity, and altered sleep-wake pattern.
- Increased risk of depression, which may cause the patient to become apathetic, possibly because of

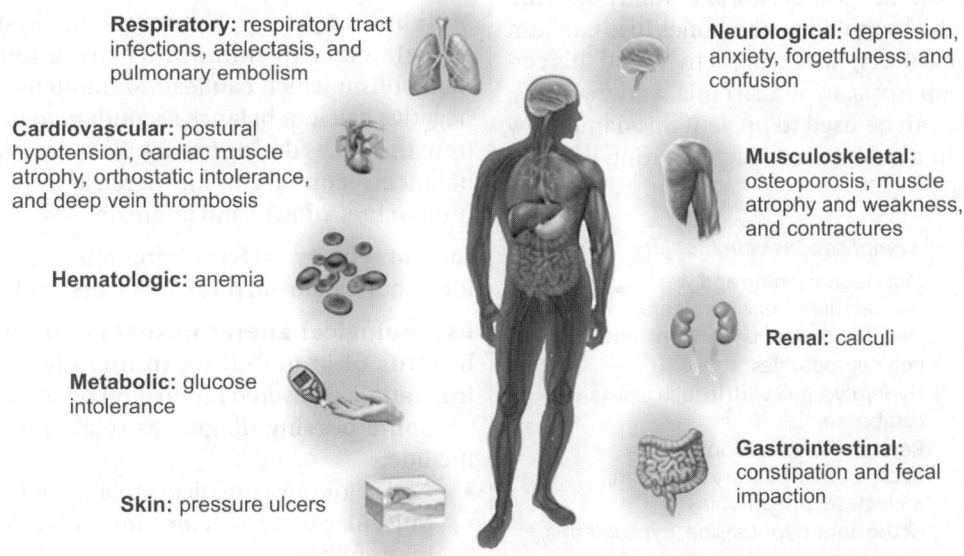

Fig. 13.5: System wise complications of immobility.

decreased sensory stimulation; or the patient may exhibit altered thought processes.
- Decreased social interaction.

COMPLICATIONS OF IMMOBILITY

The hazards or complications of immobility, such as skin breakdown, pressure ulcers, contractures, muscular weakness, muscular atrophy, disuse osteoporosis, renal calculi, urinary stasis, urinary retention, urinary incontinence, urinary tract infections, atelectasis, pneumonia, decreased respiratory vital capacity, venous stasis, venous insufficiency, orthostatic hypotension, decreased cardiac reserve, edema, emboli, thrombophlebitis, constipation and the loss of calcium from the bones, are highly costly in terms of health care dollars and in terms of client suffering. Many of these costly complications of immobility can, and should be, prevented whenever possible.

Immobility and complete bed rest can lead to life threatening physical and psychological complications and consequences. Members of the nursing care team and other health care professionals like physical therapists must, therefore, promote client mobility and prevent immobility whenever possible. Immobility can adversely affect all physiological bodily systems.

The complications and hazards associated with immobility and according to body system are described below:

Urinary system: As the result of immobility, the urinary system can be adversely affected with urinary retention, urinary stasis, renal calculi, urinary incontinence and urinary tract infections.

Gastrointestinal system: Constipation, impaction and difficult to evacuate feces can occur as the result of immobility and the lack of exercise that is needed to promote normal bowel functioning. These bowel alterations are further confounded when the client is not getting adequate fluid intake.

Musculoskeletal system: The muscles, joints and bones are adversely affected by immobility. The bones lose calcium as a result of the lack of weight bearing activity and this can lead to disuse osteoporosis, hypercalcemia, and fractures. At times a tilt table can be used to prevent this damage by placing the client in a position of weight bearing to avoid these complications.

The joints are affected with stiffness, pain, impaired range of motion and contractures including foot drop which is a plantar flexion contracture. Some of these joint disorders can be prevented with frequent and proper positioning of the client in correct bodily alignment, the provision of range of motion exercises to all joints several times a day, and the use of devices like a hand roll and a bed board to prevent contractures of the hands and feet, respectively.

Muscles are adversely affected with weakness and atrophy as the result of immobility. These hazards of immobility can be prevented with range of motion exercises and in bed exercises such as isotonic, isometric and isokinetic muscular exercises.

Respiratory system: Some adverse respiratory system effects relating to immobility include the thickening of respiratory secretions, the pooling of respiratory secretions and an increased inability of the client to mobilize and expectorate these secretions, all of which can lead to atelectasis, hypostatic pneumonia, and respiratory tract infections. Immobility can also lead to shallow, ineffective respirations, decreased respiratory movement, and a decrease in terms of the client's vital capacity.

Some of these complications of immobility can be prevented with respiratory hygiene measures such as deep breathing, coughing, postural drainage, percussion and vibration.

Circulatory system: The circulatory system is jeopardized by immobility; some of these respiratory complications and risks include venous stasis, venous dilation, decreased blood pressure, edema, embolus formation, thrombophlebitis and orthostatic hypotension which is a risk factor that is often associated with client falls.

Some of these complications can be prevented with leg exercises, the use of sequential compression devices or antiembolism stockings, and the initiation of falls risk prevention measures when an immobilized client is adversely affected with orthostatic hypotension.

Metabolic System: The metabolic system alterations associated with immobility are a decreased rate of metabolism which can lead to unintended weight gain, a negative calcium balance secondary to the loss of calcium from the bones during immobilization, a negative nitrogen balance secondary to an increase in terms of catabolic protein breakdown, and anorexia.

Integumentary system: Immobility places clients at risk for skin breakdown, pressure ulcers, and poor skin turgor.

Psychological alterations: Some of the psychological hazards of immobility can include apathy, isolation, frustration, a lowered mood, and depression.

Some nursing diagnoses related to immobility can include:
- At risk for pressure ulcers related to immobility
- Muscular weakness and muscular atrophy related to immobility
- At risk for venous stasis and emboli related to immobility

Body System	Complications of Immobility
Musculoskeletal	Muscle shortening and wasting, joint contractures, bone demineralization
Gastrointestinal	Decreased motility; constipation, ileus
Neurologic	Polyneuropathies
Endocrine	Hyperglycemia with insulin resistance; catabolism
Respiratory	Retention of secretions, decreased respiratory excursion; atelectasis, pneumonia
Cardiovascular	Orthostatic hypotension, hypovolemia, deep vein thrombosis, embolization
Integumentary	Pressure ulcer

- At risk for altered and impaired respiratory functioning related to immobility
- At risk for falls related to orthostatic hypotension secondary to immobility
- At risk for osteoporosis and fractures related to the loss of calcium from the bones secondary to the lack of weight bearing activity
- Plantar flexion contracture related to immobility
- Apathy related to immobility
- Loss of complete range of motion related to immobility.

PROVIDING CARE TO CLIENTS WITH IMMOBILITY

The interventions for immobility according to system that can be adversely affected with immobility, in addition to the constant monitoring of the client, assessments and reassessments for these hazards, include:

Urinary system: Maintain adequate fluid intake, measure, document and monitor the client's intake and output to insure an adequate fluid balance status.

Gastrointestinal system: Maintain an adequate fluid intake, encourage a high fiber diet, encourage out of bed activity including ambulation unless it is contraindicated, and the administration of treatments such as stool softeners, fiber additives, enemas, and laxatives, as ordered.

Musculoskeletal system: Range of motion exercises to all bodily parts, muscle strengthening exercises including isotonic, isometric and isokinetic exercises, aids to assist in positioning the client in correct bodily alignment, and early weight bearing activity.

Respiratory system: Encouraging the client to perform deep breathing and coughing, and the provision of postural drainage, percussion, inspiratory respiratory exercises and vibration.

Circulatory system: Active or passive range of motion, positioning, mobilization, leg exercises, the use of sequential compression devices or antiembolism stockings, and the initiation of falls risk prevention measures when an immobilized client is adversely affected with orthostatic hypotension.

Metabolic system: The encouragement and provision of a healthy diet with ample protein.

Integumentary system: Maintain good nutrition, encourage fluids, turn and position every two hours and maintain clean and dry skin without any pressure, friction or shearing.

Psychological alterations: Providing an adequate amount of stimulation, encourage visits and other diversions.

NURSING MANAGEMENT

History: The nurse collect history from the patient regarding the causative factors of immobility, such as intrapersonal factors including psychological factors (e.g., depression, fear of falling or getting hurt, motivation); physical changes (cardiovascular, neurological, and musculoskeletal disorders, and associated pain).

Physical Examination

Alignment: Do this when they are standing. Anterior view: Shoulder, hips aligned. Side view: looks at PLUM line. Joints: inspect them, palpate to see warmth, tenderness, deformity, crepitation (sound you hear with movement) **Movement:** ask if they need assistance to move. Are they alert. Good balance. **Coordination:** Put them at side of bed and are they able to maintain weight and trunk. If they maintain weight of trunk they should be able to stand and maintain weight.

Muscle Mass

Activity tolerance: Determines strength and endurance. We can do a BP, heart rate, strength of heart rate, respiratory depth, rhythm and rate before we exercise and watch them during exercise and after exercise. If patient complains of SOB or dizziness or symptoms when exercising in hospital walking. Then stop that activity.

Nursing Diagnoses

These are related to decreased mobility or decreased/altered level of consciousness
- Activity intolerance
- Impaired physical mobility
- Sedentary lifestyle
- Fear of falling ineffective
- Coping low self-esteem
- Powerlessness
- Risk for fall
- Self-care deficit
- Risk for infection
- Risk for injury
- Risk for disturbed sleep pattern.

Planning

Activity: Plan according to activity for tolerance. Eat in chair for meals and ambulate in hospital.

Body positioning: Keep them properly aligned. Use body supports. Put something in hands so they won't curl up.

Bowel elimination: Evacuate bowels every 24 hours with or without any type of aid.

Fall prevention: Educate them. "Please do not get out of bed without assistance." Give clear instructions on fall prevention. Call bell, keep bed in low position and hourly rounding. Be careful with patient with room away from nursing station and altered level of consciousness and impulsiveness.

Physiological and cognitive consequences: Focus on their strengths. Be positive "Yesterday you did this and now you can do this" Don't worry about 20 years ago they can run marathon. Be positive and focus on what they can do and set goals that are achievable. Joint movement: Do passive range of motion to prevent stiff joints leading contractures.

Mobility: Enhance it- goal is to get out of bed tid. Whatever goal is for mobility, try to obtain it.

Respiratory status: Prevent atelectasis or pneumonia, teach them deep breathing, doing pursed lip breathing. Using the incentive spirometer with them. Turning them every 2 hours to prevent secretions. These are all nursing interventions. Do not need physician to be able to do these.

Self care: Promote independence. Do not do things for them if they can do to these themselves.

Sleep: At least do 7 hours of sleep. Limit naps during the day. Plan some type of activities. Plan the sleeping pill with them. Sometimes that decreases anxiety as well. If patient requests sleeping pill at 9:30, make sure to let them know you will give it at that time to decrease their anxiety.

Stress level: Talk to them, what are their concerns? Do they need back rub. How are they doing with their hospitalization?

Weight control: Maintain healthy BMI 18.5 to 24.9 kg/m^2.

Implementing

Maintain or promote body alignment and mobility: Max for most nurses to lift is 35 pounds. Make sure you get help if you are lifting more than that. Make sure bed is at waist level. Use back to lift.

Wide support: Shoulder and feet must be at the same width or wider than shoulders are.

Position clients appropriately: Eliminate pressure from bony prominences. Make sure the angel slides, chucks and linens don't have any wrinkles on them. Do not have patients lay on their gown. Pull the gown from underneath them. This all creates pressure to skin. Patients head of bed must be up 30° with tube feedings or respiratory problems. Anything else, their head should be down because when head is up there is more pressure on sacral coxy area, which makes that area break down. Also float heels- pillow is not on heels so heels float and good arm support as well.

Moving and turning clients in bed: Make sure wheels locked on bed. Max inflate the bed is better to slide and turn patient. It is easier to move patient when the bed is inflated to firm, but make sure to adjust it back and not keep it as inflated when you leave them. Do not drag them. Use those turn sheets. Some patients must be log rolled because of cervical or back injuries.

Transferring clients: Let patients know you are going to move them from one place to another. Say to patients who are altered "You are not going to fall" because a lot of patients have a fear of falling. So make sure to have enough staff, you get a transfer board if needed, bed needs to be at right height and try to lift and not drag patients.

ROM exercises: Great if active ROM. If they need passive range of motion, move the joint until the point of slight resistance, you must stop. Stop if complaining of pain. Do 3-5 reps a day, ideally twice a day (once on day shift, the other on night shift).

Ambulating clients: Good trunk support (must be able to hold themselves up in bed without side rails. If they can do that, then the next step is to get up and ambulate them. If they do not have good trunkal support then you need physical therapy and it is out of the nurse's hands because we want to make sure the patients are moving safe and can support their own weight.

Prevent complications of immobility: Move to prevent complications.

BODY MECHANICS

Body mechanics is coordinate effort of the musculoskeletal and nervous system. Body mechanics maintains proper balance, posture and body alignment during lifting, bending, moving and performing activities of daily living. Body mechanics of the efficient use of the body as a machine. As a means of locomotion it is directly related to the function of bones. Joints muscles, nerves and brains to maintain posture balance.

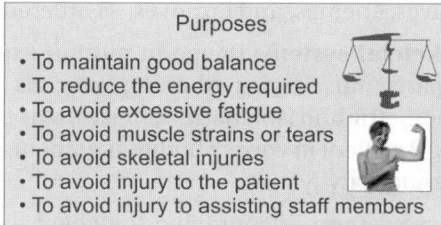

Meaning of body mechanics: Knowledge of a client's body and how it moves is important. Knowledge of your own body and what happens to it when you care for clients with altered mobility is also important. Before you lift or move a client, determine the causes and consequences of the client's illness and implement the use of Safe Patient Handling and Management Algorithms to determine the appropriate client moving/transfer protocols. These guidelines also indicate the equipment needed for safe client transfer/moving, or the need for the lift team. This knowledge enables you to move the client without causing additional discomfort.

Objectives

- To prevent fatigue.
- To prevent deformities such as kyphosis, lordosis and scoliosis.
- To promote physiological function of the body.
- To reduce the expenditure of energy.
- To maintain the balance of the body. Without undue strain on the body parts.
- To contribute to ones beauty.

Elements of Body Mechanics

- **Body alignment:** It refers to the condition of joints, tendons and muscles in various body positions, correct body alignment reduced strain.
- **Balance:** Balance a body in correct alignment is balanced and objects are balanced when its center of gravity is close to its base of support. Good posture helps in body balance.
- **Coordination:** Coordinated body movements use the weight and friction correctly. It enhance the nurses ability to lift, transfer and position patients.
- **Regulation of movement:** Use leverage of bones, tendons, muscles and joints in moving. Muscles, as a group, work together to stabilize and support body weight when a person is sitting or standing.

Rules of Good Mechanics

- Maintain anatomical position in all activities.
- Use the longest and strongest muscles of the extremities to provide the energy needed in the strenuous activities.
- Keep the object close to the body to prevent unnecessary strain on the muscles.
- Use the weight of the body to pull or push an object by keeping the body, above the object.
- Keep works close the body.
- Flex the knees to come close to the object instead of bending the back.
- Place the feet apart to provide a wide base of support.
- Slide, roll or push an object rather than lifting it in order to reduce the energy needed to lift the weight against the pull of gravity.

Assessment of Body Alignment

- **Standing position:** Head extended, normal curves of back reduced to minimum, chin in and back, chest most forward part, shoulder slightly abducted, elbows slightly flexed, wrist extended and fingers flexed. Abdomen flat and relaxed buttocks contracted, thighs extended and slightly abducted, knees slightly flexed and feet pointing straight ahead. Parallel about 3 inches apart and at right angles to legs.
- **Sitting position:** Head should be erect with chin in and back also keep the curves of back normal with chest most forward part and shoulders abducted, elbows flexed and supported, wrists extended. Fingers flexed, abdomen flat and relaxed, thighs flexed at right angles to trunk, knees flexed at right angles to thighs, feet flexed at right angles to legs and supported on floor or by some other means.

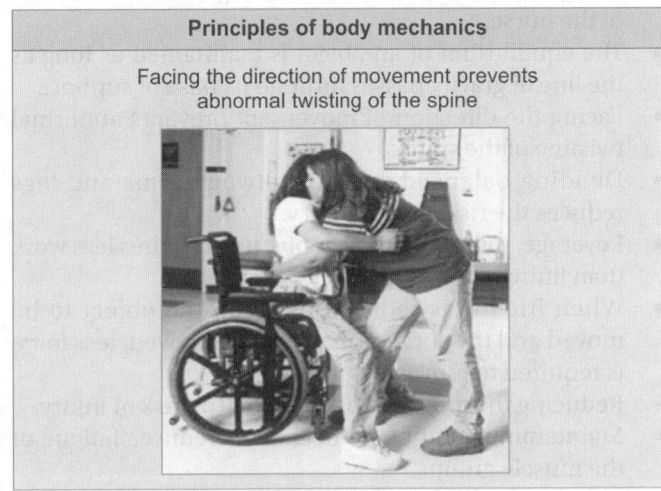

Principles of body mechanics

Facing the direction of movement prevents abnormal twisting of the spine

- **Postural abnormalities:** Torticolis, lordosis, kyphosis, kypholordosis, scoliosis, congenital hip dysplasia, knock knees, bow legs, club foot, foot drop and pigeon toes.

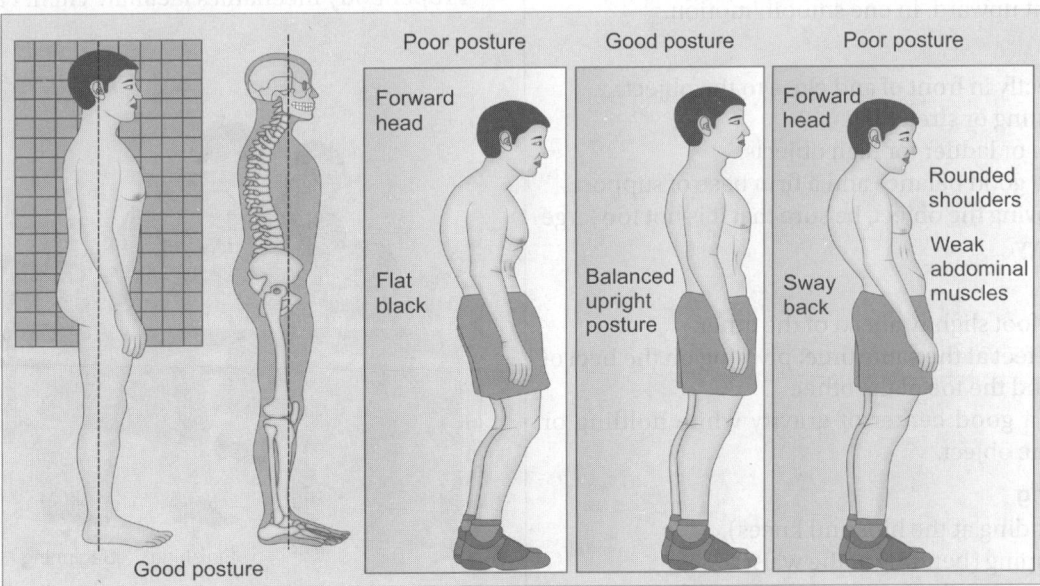

Fig. 13.6: Comparison of good posture and poor posture.

Body Mechanics for Health Care Workers

- When planning to move the patient arrange for adequate help. Use mechanical aids if help is unavailable.
- Encourage patient to help as much as possible.
- Keep back, neck, pelvis and feet aligned. Avoid twisting.
- Person with the heaviest load coordinates efforts of the team involved by counting to three.
- Set (tighten) abdominal and gluteal muscles in preparation for move.

Principles of Body Mechanics

- The wider the base of support, the greater the stability of the nurse.
- The lower the center of gravity the greater the stability of the nurse.
- The equilibrium of an object is maintained as long as the line of gravity passes through its base of support.
- Facing the direction of movement prevents abnormal twisting of the spine.
- Dividing balanced activity between arms and legs reduces the risk of back injury.
- Leverage, rolling, turning or pivoting requires less work than lifting.
- When friction is reduced between the object to be moved and the surface on which it is moved, less force is required to move it.
- Reducing the force of work reduces the risk of injury.
- Maintaining good body mechanics reduces fatigue of the muscle groups.
- Alternating periods of rest and activity helps to reduce fatigue.

Techniques of Body Mechanics

Lifting
- Use the stronger leg muscles for lifting.
- Bend at the knees and hips; keep your back straight.
- Lift straight upward, in one smooth motion.

Reaching
- Stand directly in front of and close to the object.
- Avoid twisting or stretching.
- Use a stool or ladder for high objects.
- Maintain a good balance and a firm base of support.
- Before moving the object, be sure that it is not too large or too heavy.

Pivoting
- Place one foot slightly ahead of the other.
- Turn both feet at the same time, pivoting on the heel of one foot and the toe of the other.
- Maintain a good center of gravity while holding or carrying the object.

Avoid Stooping
- Squat (bending at the hips and knees).
- Avoid stooping (bending at the waist).
- Use your leg muscles to return to an upright position.

NURSING PROCESS IN BODY MECHANICS

Assessment: Data Base
- Evaluate personnel's knowledge of the principles of body mechanics.
- Evaluate personnel's knowledge of how to use correct muscle groups for specific activities.
- Assess knowledge and correct any misinformation about body alignment and how to maintain it with each position.
- Assess knowledge of physical science and application to balance and body alignment.
- Assess the competency of spinal cord and associated musculature.
- Assess the muscle mass of the long, thick, and strong muscles of the shoulders and thighs.

Planning: Objectives
- To promote proper body mechanics while caring for clients
- To maintain good posture, thereby promoting optimum musculoskeletal balance
- To provide knowledge of the musculoskeletal system, body alignment, and balance in order to assist the nurse in caring for clients
- To correct body mechanics, promote health, enhance appearance, and assist body function.

Implementation: Procedures
- Applying body mechanics
- Maintaining proper body alignment
- Using coordinated movements
- Using basic principles.

Evaluation: Expected Outcomes
- Correct body mechanics are used when preparing for and providing client care
- Injuries are prevented to both the nurse and the client
- Proper body mechanics facilitate client care.

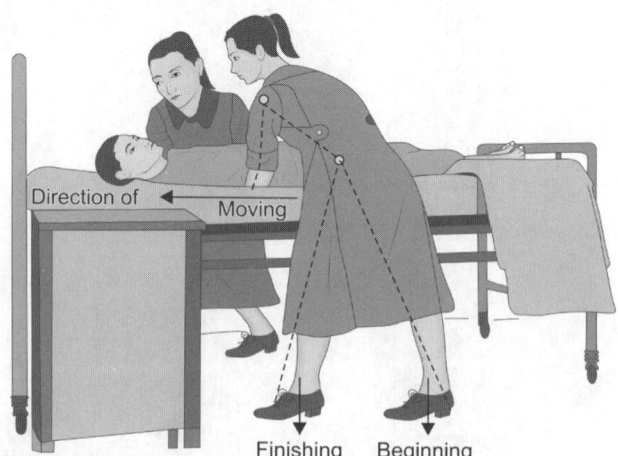

Fig. 13.7: Correct body mechanics while moving the patient.

- Clients and nurses are not injured when nursing care is provided.
- Center of gravity is maintained when lifting objects.

The two concepts of body mechanics and patient mobility are directly related to one another. Nursing personnel must learn and practice proper principles of body mechanics to prevent injury to themselves and injury to their patients. When assisting patients in mobility, nurses must be constantly aware of their own body mechanics. Most injuries occur when nursing personnel perform tasks that require repetitive movements, uncomfortable posture, and exertion to assist patients in activities such as feeding, dressing, bathing, toileting, repositioning, and ambulation.

RANGE OF MOTION EXERCISE

Range of motion exercise help to prevent contractures and joint stiffness by moving the entire patient's joints through their complete range of motion is not very appropriate.

Purpose

- To stimulate circulation.
- To restore normal motion for joints.
- To maintain muscle strength.
- To restore coordination.
- To prevent contractures.
- To facilitate comfort.

Types of Range of Motions

- Passive: No assistance from the patient.
- Active: Patient does without assistance.
- Active assisted: Patient needs some assistance to perform motion.

Preliminary Assessment Check

- The doctors order for any specific instructions such as position, movements, etc.
- Assess the general condition and diagnosis of the patient.
- Self-care ability of the patient.
- Mental status to follow instructions.

Preparation of the Patient and Environment

- Explain the sequence of the procedure.
- Provide privacy.
- Adjust the height of the bed if possible.
- Place the patient in comfortable position.

Procedure

- Wash hands thoroughly.
- Support the extremity or the part to be moved above and below joint.
- Do not hold the joint.

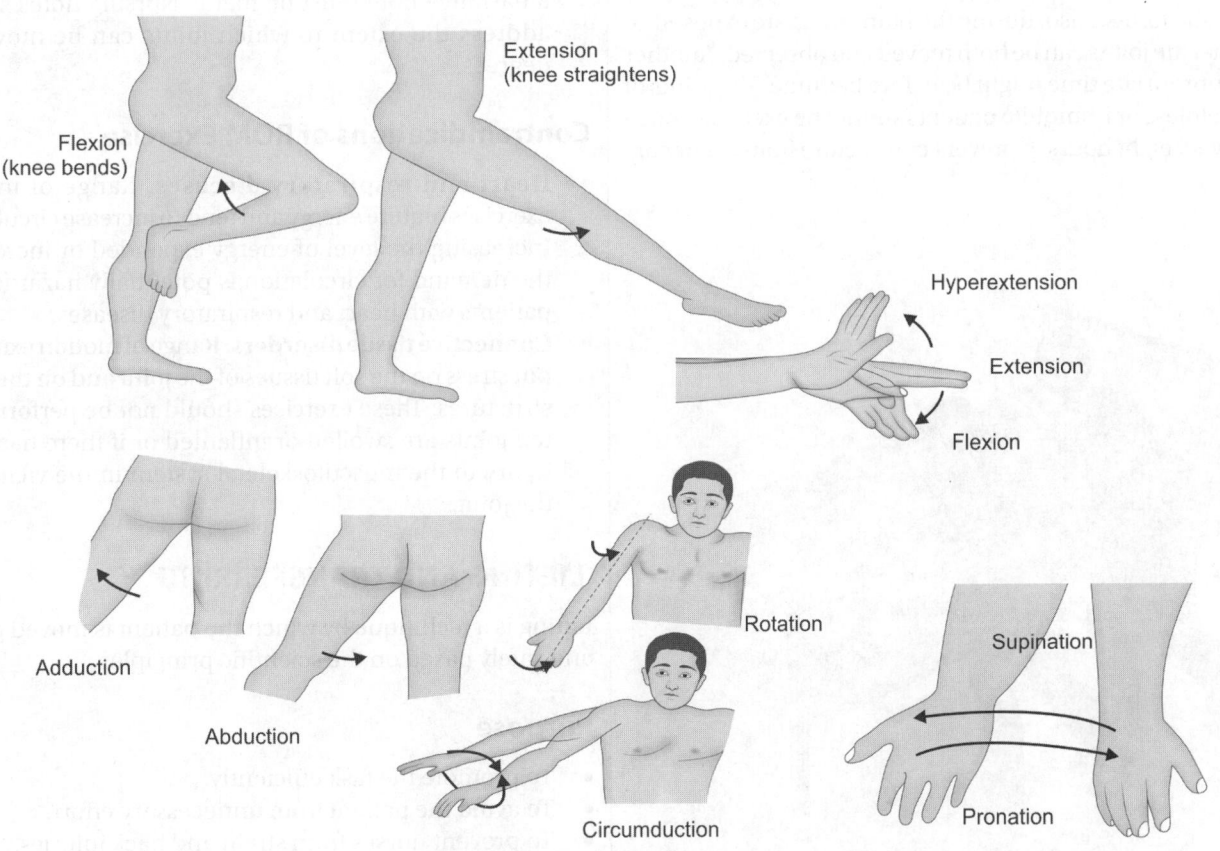

Fig. 13.8: Range of motion exercises.

- Move joint through full range of motion.
- Perform all movements smoothly and slowly.
- If pain or strong resistance is present do not force movement.
- Perform each movement three times during exercise periods per day.
- Exercise period may be incorporated to an activity such as bed bath.
- Move all joints of the body during the exercise period.

After Care

- When the exercise is completed, adjust the patient to a comfortable position.
- Place side rails properly to promote safety.
- Wash hands thoroughly.
- Record the procedure in the nurse's record sheet.

Guidelines for Range of Motion Exercise

- Plan when range of motion exercises should be done. Plan whether exercises will be passive, active-assistive, or active. Involve the patient in planning the program of exercises and other activities because he/she will be more apt to do the exercises voluntarily.
- Expect the patient's heart rate and respiratory rate to increase during exercise.
- Range-of-motion exercises should be done at least twice a day. During the bath is one appropriate time. The warm bath water relaxes the muscles and decreases spasticity of the joints. Also, during the bath, areas are exposed so that the joints can be both moved and observed. Another appropriate time might be before bedtime. The joints of helpless or immobile patients should be exercised once every eight hours to prevent contracture from occurring.
- Joints are exercised sequentially, starting with the neck and moving down. Put each joint needing exercise through the range of motion procedure a minimum of three times, and preferably five times. Avoid overexerting the patient; do not continue the exercises to the point that the patient develops fatigue. Some exercises may need to be delayed until the patient's condition improves.
- Start gradually and move slowly using smooth and rhythmic movements appropriate for the patient's condition.
- Support the extremity when giving passive exercise to the joints of the arm or leg.
- Stretch the muscles and keep the joint flexible.
- Move each joint until there is resistance, but never force a joint to the point of pain.
- Keep friction at a minimum to avoid injuring the skin.
- Return the joint to its neutral position.
- Use passive exercises as required, however, encourage active exercises when the patient is able to do so.

Documentation

- **Evaluation:** Evaluate the patient in terms of fatigue, joint discomfort, and joint mobility.
- **Record keeping:.** Range of motion is often placed on a flow sheet. If a flow sheet is not used, an entry should be made in the Nursing Progress Notes using a narrative format. If there is any adverse response to the exercises, a narrative note must be made. Nursing notes should address the extent to which joints can be moved in degrees.

Contraindications of ROM Exercise

- **Heart and respiratory diseases.** Range of motion exercises require energy and tend to increase circulation. Increasing the level of energy expended or increasing the demand for circulation is potentially hazardous to patients with heart and respiratory diseases.
- **Connective tissue disorders.** Range of motion exercises put stress on the soft tissues of the joint and on the bony structures. These exercises should not be performed if the joints are swollen or inflamed or if there has been injury to the musculoskeletal system in the vicinity of the joint.

LIFTING AND TRANSFERRING

Lifting is a technique by which the patient is moved gently and safely based on the scientific principles.

Purpose

- To promote the task efficiently.
- To avoid the patient from unnecessary effort.
- To prevent nurses from strain and back injuries.
- To promote comfort to the patient.

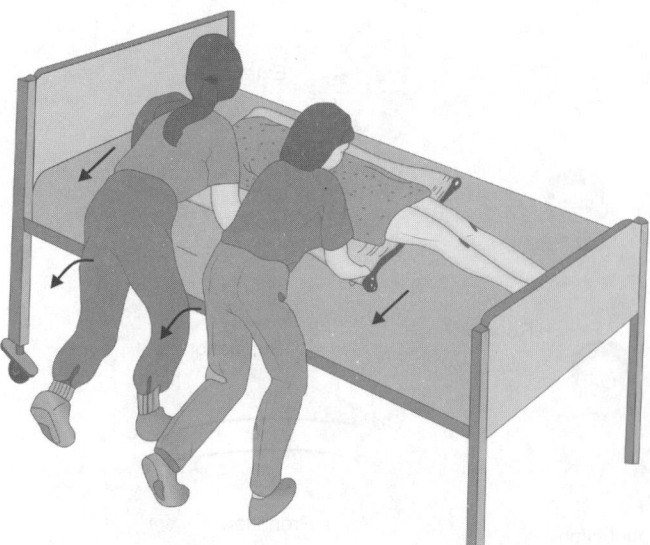

Fig. 13.9: Position changing from supine to right lateral.

Lifting Criteria

- **Position of weight:** The weight of the object to be lifted should be as close to the lifter as possible.
  Position the object in such a manner utilizes the lifting force of the nurse because the object to be lifted is in the same place as the nurse.
- **Height of the object:** The best height for lifting an object vertically is slightly above the level of the middle finger of a person with the arm hanging at the side.
- **Maximum weight:** Weight of the object should not be more than 35% of the nurse's body weight.
- **Body position:** It varies with different lifting tasks.

General Principles of Lifters and Moving

- **Position yourself:** Correct foot position is essential to maintain balance.
- **Keep you straight:** A straight back helps maintain even pressure on the bones in the spinal column, reducing the chance of injury.
- **Lift with leg muscles:** Leg muscles are much stronger than lower muscles. Lift with your legs, you can avoid strain on back muscles and lift more weight.
- **Select a suitable grasp:** Using the correct grip minimize the strain on lifters because they do not have to make muscles over-work to maintain their hold.
- **Tuck you chin:** The act of tucking the chin may reduce the need for spinal muscles to contract, so there is less chance of muscle strain in the back.
- **Use rocking movements:** Rocking on object builds momentum which can aid the lifting process.

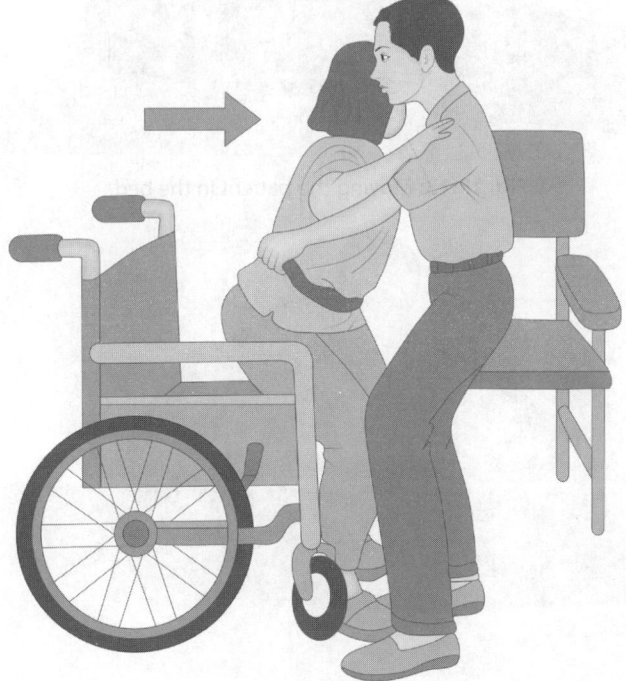

Fig. 13.10: Assisting the patient to shift from wheelchair to sitting chair.

- **Hold the load close:** If you hold the load as close to you as possible, you will cut down on the stress exerted on your arms and back.
- **Don't twist or bend:** Moving your feet instead of your upper body can help balance the load and minimize the strain in your back and abdominal muscles.

General Instructions

- Plan the movement of the patient ahead of time and be sure the path is clear.
- Flex the knees and hip joints but keep the trunk as vertical as possible.
- Keep the patient as close to the body as possible.
- Avoid jerking and twisting during the lift.
- Heavy patients should be moved in bed by sliding them rather than lifting them.
- Assistance should be requested when lifting or moving heavy patients.
- The height of the bed should be adjusted before lifting or moving.
- The patient is moved to the edge of the bed before he is lifted from the bed.
- In order to co-ordinate the movements of the workers and to maintain the patient's body in correct alignment throughout.
- Unless contraindicated, encourage the patient to use his abilities as much as possible.
- Observe the patient for symptoms of orthostatic hypotension such as fainting, dizziness, sweating, etc.
- Always lock the wheels of the bed and stretcher prior to transferring a patient to increase the maximum static friction between the wheels and the floor.

Nurses Responsibility in Lifting and Moving

- Evaluate the situation.
- Explain to the patient exactly what you are going to do.
- Provide equipment (e.g. ladder) which may help the patient assist in the move.
- Adjust the chair, stretcher, etc. to the bed level or vice versa and lower any hand drill or side rail.
- Hold the patient close-This will help keep your balance strain on your arms and back.
- Keep your feet apart, this will provide a stable base.
- Use gentle rocking movements to assist the initial movement of the patient.
- When working with others, make sure everyone knows what to do in advance and move at the same time.

Preliminary Assessment Check

- Doctors order for specific precautions.
- General condition and diagnosis of the patient.
- Level of consciousness
- Self-care ability
- Mental status to follow instructions

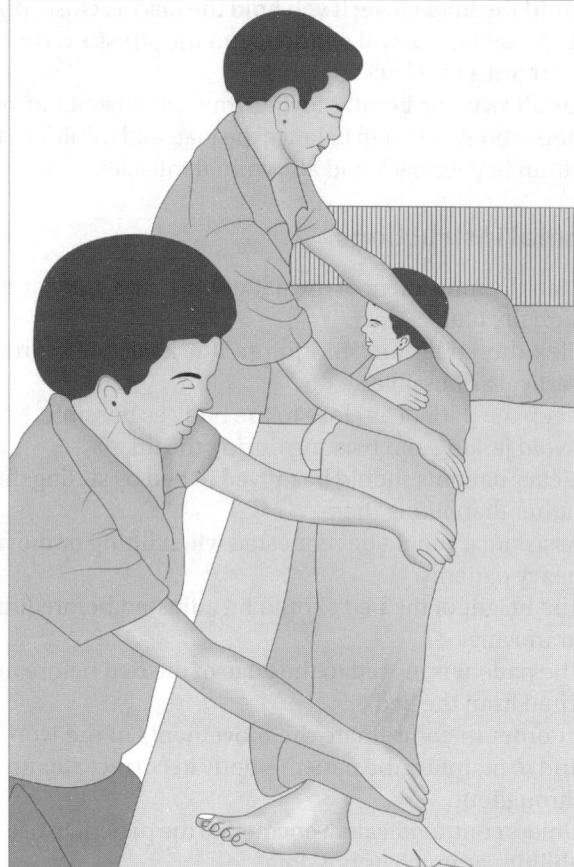

Fig. 13.11: Changing position from side to side.

- Presence of tubes and lines, e.g. IV line Foley's catheter, etc.
- Number of personnel required to move the patient safely.
- Articles available in the patients unit, e.g. stretcher, IV poles, clamps for disconnecting tubes, etc.

Preparation of the Patient and Environment

- Explain the sequence of the procedure.
- Provide privacy.
- Adjust the bed to the working height.
- Provide bedpan/urinal if needed.
- Arrange the articles at the bed side.
- Remove all comfort devices used for the patient.
- Clamp the catheter to prevent back flow of urine during the transfer.
- Clamp the nasogastric tube and other tubes if any.
- Place the foot stool if needed.
- Encourage the patient assist if possible.

Procedure

Moving the Patient in Bed (to side)

- Wash hands and dry it.
- Place the bed in flat position.
- Place the patient in supine position.
- The nurses place their arms on bed sliding them under the patients head, shoulders, chest, hips and legs.
- Wait for the leader signal by counting 1, 2, 3.
- When the leader counts 3, move the patient to the side of the bed using a right angle pull maneuver.

Assisting the Patient to Sit on the Side of Bed

- Wash hands and dry it.
- Place the patient in supine position.
  - Flex the knee gently (left leg only).

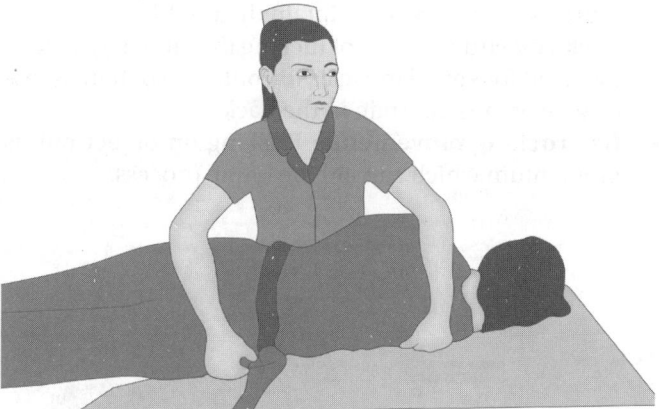

Fig. 13.13: Moving the patient in the bed.

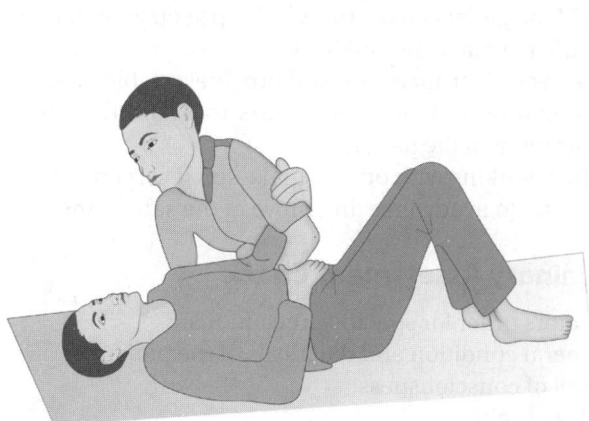
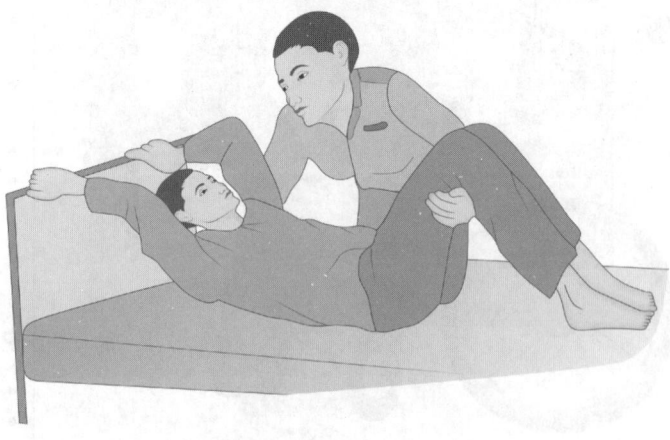

Fig. 13.12: Patient lifting technique.

- Support one hand at the shoulder and other in the hip.
- Turn gently to right side of the patient.
- Assess the patient to slide heels off the edge of mattress.
- Simultaneously raise his or her head and trunk by pushing the mattress with the fist of the left hand and grasping the edge of the mattress.
- Then roll upward on elbow till he/she reaches a sitting position.
- Assist the patient to place both arms extended backwards with palms supporting on the mattress and both feet flat on floor to maintain sitting position.

Shifting the Patient from Bed to Stretcher
- Position the stretcher at right angle to head or foot of the bed.
- Call helpers and position them at the bedside.
- Move the patient to the edge of the bed.
- At the count of '1' the nurses slide their arms under the patient to support the body sections of the patient.
- At the count of '2' the nurses stand with the back erect holding the patient's near to their body as possible.
- On the count of '3' the nurses take one step backward and pivot on their heels towards the stretcher.
- At the count of '4' move to the side of the stretcher and stand with a wide base and flexed knees ready to lower the patient into the stretcher.
- At the count of '5' the nurses lower the patient to the stretcher in a back lying position.

Assisting the Patient from Bed to Chair or Wheelchair
- Place the wheelchair or armchair at the right side of the bed.
- Wheels should be locked.
- Helps the patient to sit on the right side of the bed.
- The nurse stands in front of the patient, facing the patient.

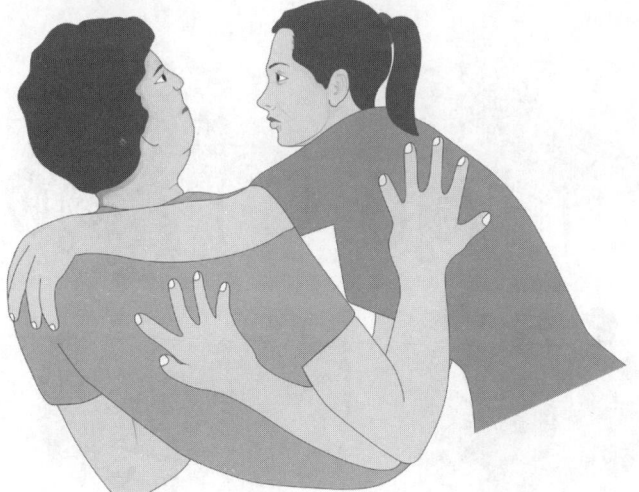

Fig. 13.14: Nurse assisting patient to sit.

- Tell the patient to slide his buttocks close to the edge of the bed by shifting his weight alternately from right to left buttock till his feet placed on the floor in a forward-backward wide based position.
- One foot placed at the back of the other, slightly under the bed.
- Tell the patient to stand on command by simultaneously leaning forward, pushing with the foot placed at the back as he straightens his legs.
- The patient stands upright by balancing himself on the armchair, side rails or mattress.
- Tell the patient to place his left arm on the farm arm of the chair or wheelchair and pivot on the heel of his feet and bringing the buttocks towards the wheelchair.
- Ask the patient to step back to the wheelchair until he is close enough to touch the seat and grasp the other arm of the chair with his right hand.
- Tell the patient to lean forward and lower his buttocks slowly to the seat by bending knees and elbows.
- Observe for correct sitting posture. Reserve the procedure to return the patient from wheelchair to the bed.

After Care
- Make sure that the patient is in a correct alignment and is comfortable.
- Replace the pillows and other comfort devices as needed.
- Raise the side rails if necessary for the safety of the patient.
- The nurse should remain with the patient in front of him when the patient assumes a sitting or standing position.
- Tidy up the unit.
- Wash hands thoroughly
- Record the procedure in the nurse's record.

LOG ROLLING
- Logrolling is a technique used to turn a patient whose body must at all times be kept in a straight alignment (like a log).
- This technique is used for the patient who has a spinal injury.
- Logrolling is used for the patient who must be turned in one movement, without twisting.
- Logrolling requires two people, or if the patient is large, three people.

Technique
- Wash your hands.
- Approach and identify the patient (by checking the identification band) and explain the procedure (using simple terms and pointing out the benefits).

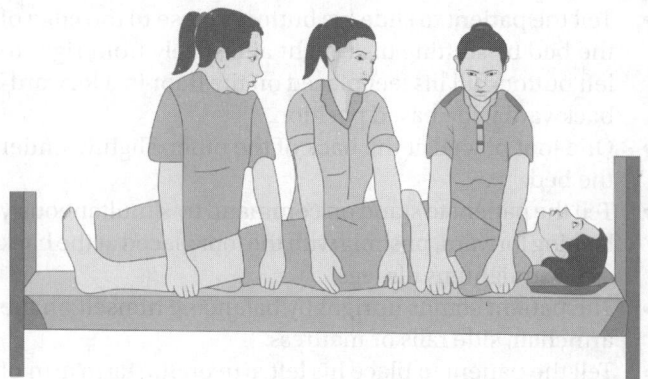

Fig. 13.15: Log rolling technique.

- Provide privacy.
- Position the bed.
  - The bed should be in the flat position at a comfortable working height.
  - Lower the side rail on the side of the body at which you are working.
- Position yourself with your feet apart and your knees flexed close to the side of the bed.
- Fold the patient's arms across his chest.
- Place your arms under the patient so that a major portion of the patient's weight is centered between your arms. The arm of one nurse should support the patient's head and neck.

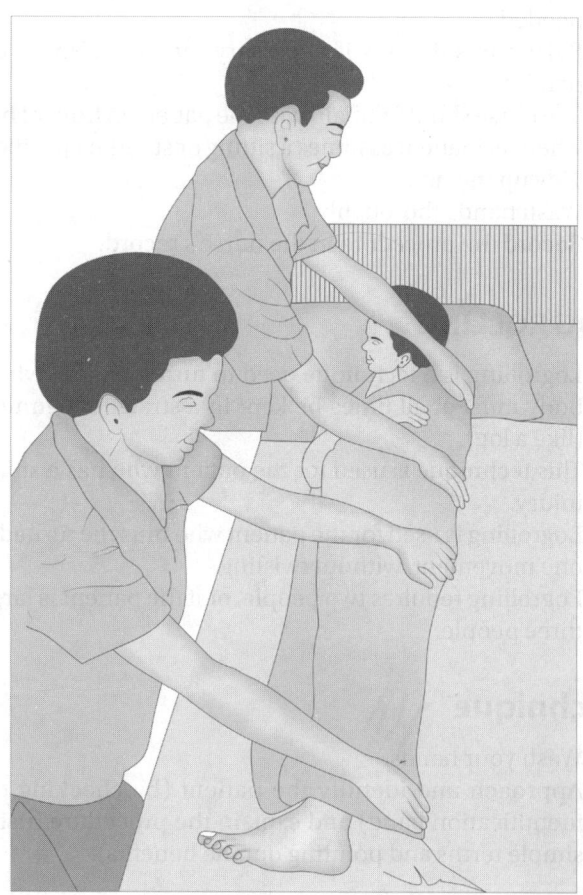

Fig. 13.16: Turning from side to side.

- On the count of three, move the patient to the side of the bed, rocking backward on your heels and keeping the patient's body in correct alignment.
- Raise the side rail on that side of the bed.
- Move to the other side of the bed.
- Place a pillow under the patient's head and another between his legs.
- Position the patient's near arm toward you.
- Grasp the far side of the patient's body with your hands evenly distributed from the shoulder to the thigh.
- On the count of three, roll the patient to a lateral position, rocking backward onto your heels.
- Place pillows in front of and behind the patient's trunk to support his alignment in the lateral position.
- Provide for the patient's comfort and safety.
  - 1 Position the call bell.
  - 2 Place personal items within reach.
  - 3 Be sure the side rails are up and secure.
- Report and record as appropriate.

TRANSFERRING PATIENT FROM BED TO WHEELCHAIR

Transfer of a partially dependent patient from bed to wheelchair.

Purposes

- Enhance the wellbeing of a patient.
- To transfer to other departments for investigation like: X-ray, ultrasonography, electroencephalography, etc.
- Improves self image and ability to move around.

Procedure

- Explain the purpose of use of wheelchair.
- Assess the patient's ability to move.

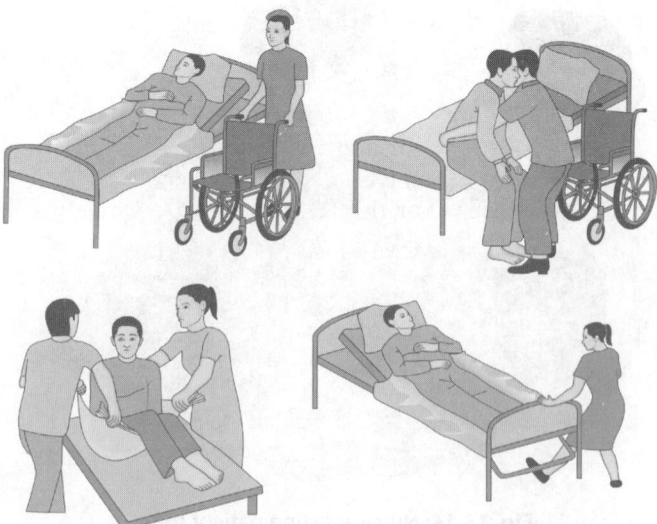

Fig. 13.17: Lifting and transferring: Transferring from bed to wheelchair.

- Place the wheelchair at the right side of the patient and lock it.
- Raise the bed to the level of wheelchair.
- Elevate the head end of the bed, slide down the rails.
- Provide privacy; take assistance from male, female orderlies.
- Help the patient to stand in front of the wheelchair.
- Lift up foot rest and assist to sit on the chair.
- In case of chronic hemiplegic, one nurse stands behind the patient, slide hands under axillae and holds at the chest level.
- Other nurse/nurse orderlies stands in front of the patient holds his legs and simultaneously lift the patient to the wheelchair by counting 1,2,3.
- Provide extra pillow at the back, keep his / her arms on the chair arms and feet on the foot rest.
- Make patient comfortable by helping to sit straight.
- Fasten him/her with a seat belt to prevent falling forward.
- Unlock the breaks and gently transfer for the purpose.

TRANSFER FROM WHEELCHAIR TO BED

Patients who are weak, very ill and with fracture of legs are transferred from the outpatient department to the ward by wheelchair.

Procedure

- Explain the technique of sliding from the wheelchair to the bed, if the patient is able to move by himself.
- Keep the wheelchair with the middle close to the bed and lock the wheelchair.
- Ask for the MNO / FNO assistance. One has to be at the back side and one in the front of the patient lifting the patient's knees and thighs up.
- Nurse should count 1, 2, and 3 then both simultaneously lift the patient from the wheel chair on to the middle of the bed.
- Slowly help the patient to lie down by giving support to the head and back and place the legs on bed.
- Place the patient in correct body alignment and make comfortable by giving extra pillows.

TRANSFER FROM BED TO STRETCHER AND STRETCHER TO BED

A bedridden patient may need to be transferred from stretcher to bed, from bed to stretcher for several reasons. Minimum 5 persons are required.

Indications

- Patients with spinal injury.
- Patients after surgery.
- Patients with CVA and unconscious.
- Patients with multiple injuries/orthopedic problems.

Procedure

- Check the doctor's order.
- Keep the stretcher ready with necessary articles.
- Explain the procedure and purpose to the patient.
- Provide privacy.
- Keep the stretcher parallel to the bed. Lower the side rails and lock the wheels of the bed and stretcher.
- Loosen the draw sheet on both sides of the bed.
- If there is a roller keep it under the back of the patient and roll into the stretcher on count 1,2,3 taking care of the head. Place the arms across his chest.
- If the roller is not available, middle person hold the draw mackintosh, one hold the head, another hold the legs and lift the patient from the bed to the stretcher on count of 1,2, 3.
- Remove the roller, slide up the side rails of the stretcher.
- Cover the patient and fasten belts safety across the patient's chest and waist.
- Adjust head of the stretcher according to the patient's condition.
- Place a pillow under the head and provide other comfortable measures.
- Unlock the wheels and move the stretcher for the specific purpose.
- Check the vital signs and observe for any complications.
- Record and report the procedure.

PLASTER CASTS

A cast is an immobilizing device, made of plaster bandages, fiber glass or a thermolabile plastic material.

Purposes of a Cast

- To immobilize and hold bone fragments in reduction.
- To apply uniform compression on soft tissues.
- Prevention of deformities.
- Correction of deformities.

Types of Casts

The condition, being treated, influences the type and thickness of the cast applied. Generally speaking, the joints, proximal to the area to be immobilized, are included in the cast.

- **Short arm cast:** It extends from below the elbow to the proximal palm crease.
- **Gauntlet cast:** It extends from below the elbow to the proximal palm crease, including the thumb (thumb spica).
- **Long arm cast:** It extends from the upper level of the axillary fold to the proximal palm crease. The elbow usually is immobilized.
- **Short leg cast:** It extends from below the knee to the base of toes.

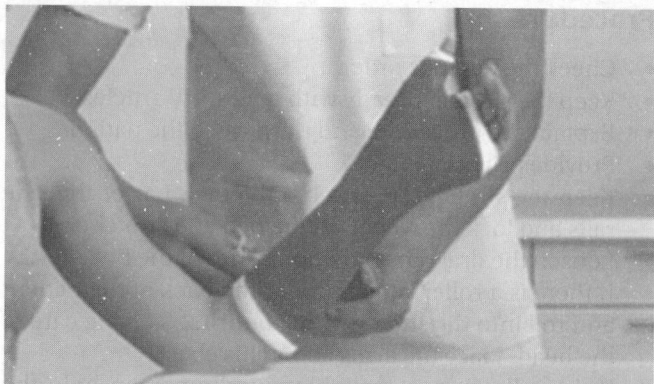

Fig. 13.18: Plaster cast application.

- **Long leg cast:** It extends from the junction of the upper and the middle third of the thigh to the base of the toes; the foot is at a right angle in a neutral position.
- **Walking cast:** It is a short or long leg cast with a walking device.
- **Body cast:** It incorporates a position of the trunk and one or two extremities.
- **Shoulder spica cast:** It is a body jacket that encloses the trunk and the shoulder and elbow.

Casting Material (Plaster of Paris)

- Plaster of Paris (anhydrous calcium sulphate) is a chalky white powder made by a process that removes water from gypsum.
- In the process of making plaster of paris, crystals of gypsum are broken up and heat is applied to remove water from the crystals.
- A chemical process of rehydration occurs when plaster of paris is placed in water.
- The exothermic reaction that takes place, during this recrystallization, or, setting period, generates heat which can be felt in the newly applied cast.
- Plaster of paris bandages come in individually wrapped pre-controls of crinoline, impregnated with plaster.
- The bandages are available in varying widths from 2" to 8". Plaster is available in various setting speeds, extra fast (2 to 4 minutes), fast (5 to 8 minutes) and slow (10 to 18 minutes).
- The strength of a completed cast is determined by the number of layers of plaster used. Usually, a cast consists of 5 to 7 layers of plaster bandages in unreinforced areas.
- Plaster of Paris splints of varying sizes are also available.

CAST APPLICATION

- Prior to the application of the cast, the patient should be informed that he will feel warm under the plaster, but the application of cast is not painful.
- The patient is draped to prevent the plaster from smearing on those parts of the body that are not being cast.
- The part to be cast is cleansed with soap and water, and dried. Padding with cotton is placed over the area on the bony prominences.
- Orthopedic cast padding is used.

Trimming the Cast

- After application, the plaster is cleaned from the patient's skin with a damp towel from the area around the cast.
- The cast is trimmed with a cast knife. Any complaint by the patient of painful areas under the plaster should be reported and investigated.

Drying a Cast

- A cast should be exposed to circulating air, so that it will dry. It should be covered.
- The patient should be kept under a fan. After a cast has cooled and it starts to harden, the arm or leg in the cast is elevated above the level of the heart to reduce swelling.
- The cast should not be allowed to rest on hard surfaces or sharp edges that can cause a dent in the cast, and, subsequently, pressure sores.

Immediate Cast-care following Application: Immediate care is needed to avoid complications. Mainly two types of complications occur:
- Constriction of circulation.
- Pressure on tissues and bony parts.

Constriction of circulation: Surgery on trauma causes swelling due to hemorrhage and edema. If circulation is restricted, gangrenous neurosis will occur. Signs of circulatory impairments are noted by assessing the toes and fingers of a leg and arm after cast. They should be pink in color, warm to touch and easily moved. Unrelieved pain, swelling, blanding or discoloration, tingling, numbness, inability to move fingers and toes or any temperature changes must be reported immediately.

If constriction of circulation is suspected, the cast may be bivalved to reduce pressure or a window may be cut in the cast.

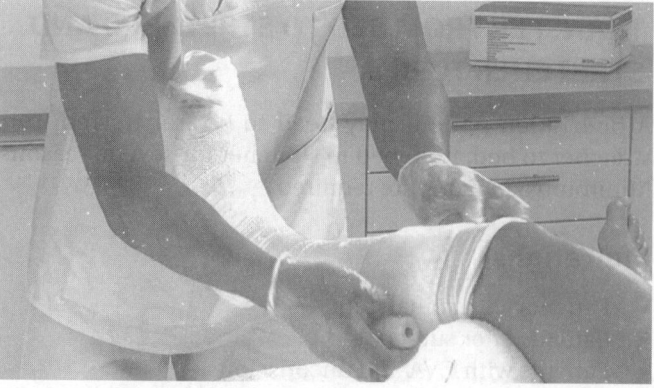

Fig. 13.19: Cast applied on lower extremity.

Pressure on Tissues or Bony Parts

- Any cast that exerts pressure on tissues may cause neurosis, pressure sores, nerve paralysis or paralysis.
- Severe pain over bony prominences is a warning sign of an impending pressure sore.
- If the pain disappears, it indicates ulceration. So, watch for pain over the pressure points. In case of pain, no analgesics are advised but localize the exact site of pain.
- When a patient is moved from side to side in a large cast, three people are required while moving. Use the palms of the hand to lift the patient.

Skin and Hygienic Care

- Skin around the edges of the cast must be inspected frequently for signs of irritation. Use a flash light. Accessible skin should be massaged with an emollient.

> **Procedure for application of cast**
> - Assess client's health status (not be diabetic/malnourished).
> - Explain the procedure to client and start IV line as advised.
> - Immobilize the part by applying splint to affected part and provide position on bed.
> - Assess the affected part for rashes, breakdown and bruising.
> - Provide skin care before the cast/slab application (if it is open/ compound fracture then prepare client for surgery).

- Pressure areas develop over any bony prominences. A common site of pressure, from a large cast, is the buttocks. When the patient is turned on his abdomen, the exposed skin can be washed carefully and massaged with fingers; remove the plaster crumbs from inside and massage the area. No inserters should be used to scratch the inside of the cast.
- The area of the cast around the perineum needs to be protected from excretions. When the cast is dry, the perineum is covered with a towel and the perineal area of the cast sprayed.

Nursing Care of Patient with a Plaster Cast

Although a patient with an arm or leg cast is much more self-reliant than a patient in a body or spica cast, it is a nursing responsibility to monitor all patients and assist as needed. Nursing management includes the following actions to assess the effectiveness of the cast.

- Check the edges of the cast and all skin areas where the cast edges may cause pressure. If there are signs of edema or circulatory impairment, notify the charge nurse or physician immediately.
- Slip your fingers under the cast edges to detect any plaster crumbs or other foreign material.
- Move the skin back and forth gently to stimulate circulation
- Lean down and smell the cast to detect odors indicating tissue damage. A musty or moldy odor at the surface of the cast may be the first indication that necrosis from pressure has developed underneath.
- Check the integrity of the cast by looking for cracks, breaks, and soft spots
- The casted body part must be examined and assessed frequently in order to prevent complications.
- Assess the casted part by checking the following.
  - Assess circulation by performing the blanching test and comparing the skin temperature and blanching reaction of the affected limb to that of the unaffected limb.
  - Assess the presence of sensation in the affected limb by touching exposed areas of skin and instructing the patient to describe what he felt.
  - Assess the motor ability of the affected limb by having the patient wiggle his fingers or toes.
- Patient education will do much to prevent complications. Instruct the patient to do the following.
  - Avoid resting cast on hard surfaces or sharp edges that may dent the cast and cause pressure sores.
  - Never use a pen or other foreign object to "scratch" inside the cast. This may cause skin damage and infection.
  - Report any danger signs like pale, cold fingers or toes, tingling, numbness, increased pain, pressure spots, odor, or feeling that the cast has become too tight to the nursing staff immediately
  - Report any damage to the cast such as cracks, breaks, or soft spots.
  - Never attempt to remove or alter the cast.
- After a leg cast is applied, prevent or alleviate swelling by elevating the extremity above the level of the heart.
- If the patient has an arm cast, instruct him to make and release a tight fist.
- Encourage the patient to wiggle his fingers and toes frequently.

CONCLUSION

Mobility is defined as the "ability to move freely, easily, rhythmically, and purposefully in the environment. It is an essential part of living. People must be able to move to protect themselves from trauma and to meet their basic needs. Mobility is vital to independence; a fully immobilized person is "as vulnerable and dependent as an infant". The risk factors associated with immobility are client deconditioning, a cognitive impairment, spasticity, poor cardiac functioning and poor tolerance for activity, inadequate muscular strength, impaired balance, improper bodily posture and alignment, an impaired gait, pain, the use of sedating medications, joint pain and stiffness in addition to other skeletal problems, obesity, and neurological impairments in addition to a physiological health problem that mandates that the client be on complete bed rest.

BIBLIOGRAPHY

1. Bowling A. Measuring health: A review of quality of life Measurement Scales. 3rd ed. Maidenhead: Open University Press, 2004.
2. Brown CJ, Williams B, Woodbury LL, et al. Barriers to mobility during hospitalization from perspectives of older patients and their nurses and physicians. J Hosp Med. 2007; 2(5):305–13.
3. Corcoran, P. Use it or lose it-the hazards of bed rest and inactivity. West J Med. 1991;154(5):536-8.
4. Creditor MC. Hazards of hospitalization of the elderly. Ann Intern Med. 1993;118:219–23.
5. Hodgson CL, Berney S, Harrold M, et al. Clinical review: early patient mobilization in the ICU. Crit Care. 2013;17(1):207.
6. Kuys S, Dolecka U, Guard A. Activity level of hospital medical patients: an observational study. Arch Gerontol Geriatr. 2012;55:417–21.
7. Markey DW. Brown RJ. An interdisciplinary approach to addressing patient activity and mobility in the medical-surgical patient. J Nurs Care Qual. 2002;16(4):1–12.
8. Needham D. Mobilizing patients in the intensive care unit: improving neuromuscular weakness and physical function. JAMA. 2008;300:1685–90.
9. Padula CA, Hughes C, Baumhover L. Impact of a nurse-driven mobility protocol on functional decline in hospitalized older adults. J Nurs Care Qual. 2009;24(4):325–31.
10. Tucker D, Molsberger SC, Clark A. Walking for wellness: a collaborative program to maintain mobility in hospitalized older adults. Geriatr Nurs. 2004;25:242–5.

REVIEW QUESTIONS

Long Essays

1. Define mobility, explain the benefits of exercises.
2. Describe the effects of mobility on various system on the body.
3. Define body mechanics, explain the nursing process in body mechanics.

Short Essays

1. Basic elements of normal movements.
2. Factors affecting mobility.
3. Complications of immobility.
4. Providing care to clients with immobility.
5. Range of motion exercises.
6. Log rolling.
7. Transferring the patient from bed to wheelchair.

Short Answers

1. Complications of immobility.
2. Elements of body mechanics.
3. Rules of good mechanics.
4. Lifting and transferring.
5. Types of casts.

MULTIPLE CHOICE QUESTIONS

1. **Benifits of exercise in prevention of complications are the following, *except*:**
   a. Muscle atrophy
   b. Osteoporosis
   c. Diabetes
   d. Contractures
2. **Physical complications of immobility is:**
   a. Hypostatic pneumonia
   b. Pulmonary embolism
   c. Thrombophlebitis
   d. All of the above
3. **Body mechanics is coordinate effort of the musculoskeletal and ----------- system.**
   a. Endocrine system
   b. Nervous system
   c. Renal system
   d. Cardiac system
4. **Range of motion exercise help to prevent contractures and joint stiffness by moving the entire patient's ---------**
   a. Joints
   b. Bones
   c. Muscles
   d. Ligaments
5. **------------- is a technique used to turn a patient whose body must at all times be kept in a straight alignment.**
   a. Log rolling
   b. Position changing
   c. Transferring
   d. Lifting

ANSWERS

1. c 2. d 3. b 4. a 5. a

CHAPTER 14
Patient Education

LEARNING OBJECTIVES
- Patient teaching: Importance, purposes, process
- Integrating nursing process in patient teaching

INTRODUCTION

Nurses' patient education is important for building patients' knowledge, understanding, and preparedness for self-management. Managers reorganized patient education routines and structures, generally due to economic constraints. Nurses' pedagogical competence development was unclear, and practice-based experiences of patient education were considered very important whereas theoretical pedagogical knowledge was considered less important. Managers' support for nurses' practical- and theoretical-based pedagogical competence development needs to be strengthened.

The ultimate goal of patient educational programs is to achieve long-lasting changes in behavior by providing patients with the knowledge to allow them to make autonomous decisions to take ownership of their care as much as possible and improve their own outcomes. Patient education is an integral part of the nursing process, and nephrology nurses can use this process to assess, plan, implement, and evaluate an effective and individualized patient education program.

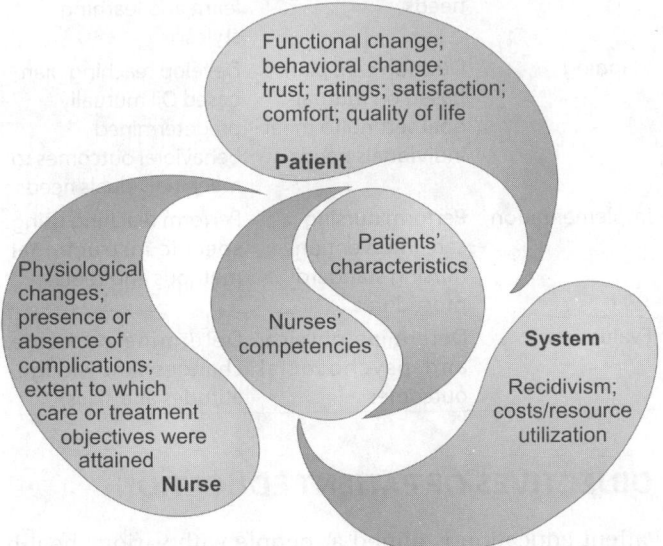

Fig. 14.1: Components of patient education.

CONCEPT OF PATIENT EDUCATION

Education on health issues is necessary for a patient's physical and mental health. Everybody finds themselves in situations where they require special knowledge and skills in order to meet their basic needs and sustain their lives. One such situation relates to loss of health and hospitalization

All patients have the right to be educated on maintaining their health, disease prevention, and health promotion. Health promotion is the process of advancing knowledge, influencing attitudes, and determining relevant solutions so that people can make informed choices, change their behavior, and subsequently attain a desirable level of physical and mental health and improve their social and physical environment.

Effective patient education starts from the time patients are admitted to the hospital and continues until they are discharged. Nurses should take advantage of any appropriate opportunity throughout a patient's stay to teach the patient about self-care. The self-care instruction may include teaching patients how to inject insulin, bathe an infant or change a colostomy pouching system.

DEFINITION

Patient education is the process by which health professionals and others impart information to patients and their caregivers that will alter their health behaviors or improve their health status.

THERAPEUTIC PATIENT EDUCATION

The concept of therapeutic patient education and health care providers tends to talk to patients about their disease rather than train them in the daily management of their condition.
- Therapeutic patient education is designed therefore to train patients in the skills of self-managing or adapting treatment to their particular chronic disease, and in coping processes and skills.
- It should also contribute to reducing the cost of long-term care to patients and to society.

- It is essential to the efficient self-management and to the quality of care of all long-term diseases or conditions, though acutely ill patients should not be excluded from its benefits.
- Therapeutic patient education is education managed by health care providers trained in the education of patients, and designed to enable a patient (or a group of patients and families) to manage the treatment of their condition and prevent avoidable complications, while maintaining or improving quality of life. Its principal purpose is to produce a therapeutic effect additional to that of all other interventions (pharmacological, physical therapy, etc.).

VALUE OF PATIENT EDUCATION

- Improved understanding of medical condition, diagnosis, disease, or disability.
- Improved understanding of methods and means to manage multiple aspects of medical condition.
- Improved self-advocacy in deciding to act both independently from medical providers and in interdependence with them.
- Increased compliance: Effective communication and patient education increases patient motivation to comply.
- Patient outcomes: Patients more likely to respond well to their treatment plan: fewer complications.
- Informed consent: Patients feel you've provided the information they need.
- Utilization: More effective use of medical services – fewer unnecessary phone calls and visits.
- Satisfaction and referrals: Patients more likely to stay with your practice and refer other patients.
- Risk management: Lower risk of malpractice when patients have realistic expectations.

Planning: Teaching Process

Examples of writing goals under different learning domains:

Cognitive	Affective	Psychomotor
• The client will give 5 examples of side effects of Lasix • The client will describe 3 indications of Lasix • The client will state how he plans to always have the drug available (... with 100% accuracy) (... by ... the end of the teaching session; before discharge, etc.)	• The client will share his/her feelings related to taking Lasix for hypertension • The client will share his/her intentions to make needed changes in lifestyle including seeking help from health professional when needed	• The client will practice new health-related behaviors regarding using of Lasix for example: Checking blood pressure and heart rate regularly • Weighing self-daily and monitoring intake and output

COMPETENCIES OF HEALTH EDUCATOR

Competencies expected of health care providers in therapeutic patient education Health care providers should be able, individually and in teams, to:
- adapt their professional behavior to patients and their disease (acute/chronic)
- Adapt their professional behavior to patients, individually, and in their families and groups
- Adapt constantly their roles and actions to those of the health care and the education teams with whom they cooperate
- Communicate empathetically with patients
- Recognize the needs of patients
- Take account of the patients' emotional state, their experience and their representations of the disease and its treatment
- Help patients to learn
- Educate patients in managing their treatment and in using the available health, social and economic resources
- Help patients to manage their way of life
- Educate and advise patients on the management of crises and of factors that interfere with the normal management of their condition
- Select patient-education tools
- Use and integrate these tools in the care of patients and in the patients' learning process (contract with patients)
- Take account in therapeutic patient education of the educational, psychological and social dimensions of long-term care
- Evaluate patient education for its therapeutic effects (clinical, biological, psychological, educational, social, economic) and make the indicated adjustments
- Periodically evaluate and improve the educational performance of health care providers.

Domain	Nursing Process	Education Process
Assessment	Appraise physical and psychosocial needs	Determine learning needs, readiness to learn and learning styles
Planning	Develop care plan based on mutual goal setting to meet individuals needs	Develop teaching plan based Oil mutually predetermined behavioral outcomes to meet individuals needs
Implementation	Perform nursing care interventions nursing standard procedures	Perform teaching using specific instructional methods and tools
Evaluation	Determine physical and psychosocial outcomes	Determine outcome changes (knowledge, atitudes and skills)

OBJECTIVES OF PATIENT EDUCATION

Patient education is aimed at people with various health conditions to help improve their understanding of their health status through interactive communication between patient and healthcare provider enabling knowledge and self-care skills to be improved. Healthcare providers can then encourage patients to participate in decisions-making about their care which enables them to take increasing control of their own condition. This increases the likelihood of patients following and adhering to their care plan as they themselves are able to integrate effective self-management into their daily lives.

Health care providers trained in those educational skills may contribute to:
- Improved quality of life, as well as longer life, of their long-term care patients
- Improved quality of care in general (as acutely ill patients should also benefit from those educational skills)
- Lower medical, personal and social costs, and ultimately lower global costs.

NEED OF PATIENT EDUCATION

Patient education improves the knowledge, skills, and motivation of patients about maintaining and improving their health. Patient education is known to improve patient satisfaction and quality of life, reduce the incidence of complications, cost of treatment, and rate of readmission, reinforce healthy behaviors and reduce unhealthy behaviors, reduce patient anxiety, decrease the effect of symptoms, shorten the hospital stay time, increase the participation in health care programs, and improve the patient autonomy in daily activities.

BENEFITS OF PATIENT EDUCATION

- Improved health outcomes
- Improved understanding of condition
- Increased use of cognitive coping strategies
- Increased motivation
- Improved quality of life
- Improved long-term outcomes
- Improved feelings of well-being
- Satisfaction.

- Empowers patients to take an active role
- Less time off work
- Greater independence
- Increased self-efficacy
- Increased self-management
- Increased life-expectancy
- Reduces complications
- Fewer sleep problems
- Fewer hospital admissions
- Overall better healthcare experience
- Decreased tiredness, stress, anxiety and depression.

Benefits of Providing Patient Education

- Healthcare professional satisfaction
- Effective use of resources
- Reduced burden on tax payers
- Fewer appointments required
- Fewer hospital admissions
- Shorter stays in hospital
- Fewer out-patient visits.

IMPORTANCE OF PATIENT EDUCATION

Patient education is a significant part of a nurse's job. Education empowers patients to improve their health status. When patients are involved in their care, they are more likely to engage in interventions that may increase their chances for positive outcomes. The benefits of patient education include:
- Prevention of medical conditions such as obesity, diabetes or heart disease.
- Patients who are informed about what to expect during a procedure and throughout the recovery process.
- Decreasing the possibility of complications by teaching patients about medications, lifestyle modifications and self-monitoring devices like a glucose meter or blood pressure monitor.
- Reduction in the number of patients readmitted to the hospital.
- Retaining independence by learning self-sufficiency.

Care plan	Discharge letter or patient report	A clinical report leaflet	Patient education
- Assessment(s) - Aim - Expected outcomes of care (goals/ objectives) - Planned interventions - Nursing record of care given - Evaluation of care	- Diagnosis - History of illness - Summary of medical, nursing and paramedical care - Arrangements for ongoing care - Patient's and/or carer's understanding of the situation - Further needs - Contacts for information or support	- Topic - Aim - Literature review - Methodology - Findings - Discussion - Recommendations for practice/further research - References - Appendices	- Health problem or illness - Explanation of cause, signs and symptoms - When to "act" and seek medical advice - Investigations and procedures people commonly undergo - Common medical treatments - Commonly asked questions - Self-help - Contacts

PRINCIPLES OF PATIENT EDUCATION

Patient-centered care is the practice of caring for patients (and their families) in ways that are meaningful and valuable to the individual patient. It includes listening to, informing and involving patients in their care. The IOM (Institute of Medicine) defines patient-centered care as: "Providing care that is respectful of, and responsive to, individual patient preferences, needs and values, and ensuring that patient values guide all clinical decisions."[1]

Eight Principles of Patient-centered Care

Using a wide range of focus groups — recently discharged patients, family members, physicians and non-physician hospital staff—combined with a review of pertinent literature, researchers

1. **Respect for patients' values, preferences and expressed needs:** Involve patients in decision-making, recognizing they are individuals with their own unique values and preferences. Treat patients with dignity, respect and sensitivity to his/her cultural values and autonomy.
2. **Coordination and integration of care:** During focus groups, patients expressed feeling vulnerable and powerless in the face of illness. Proper coordination of care can alleviate those feelings. Patients identified three areas in which care coordination can reduce feelings of vulnerability:
   - Coordination of clinical care
   - Coordination of ancillary and support services
   - Coordination of front-line patient care.
3. **Information and education:** In interviews, patients expressed their worries that they were not being completely informed about their condition or prognosis. To counter this fear, hospitals can focus on three kinds of communication:
   i. Information on clinical status, progress and prognosis
   ii. Information on processes of care
   iii. Information to facilitate autonomy, self-care and health promotion
4. **Physical comfort:** The level of physical comfort patients report has a significant impact on their experience. Three areas were reported as particularly important to patients:
   i. Pain management
   ii. Assistance with activities and daily living needs
   iii. Hospital surroundings and environment.
5. **Emotional support and alleviation of fear and anxiety:** Fear and anxiety associated with illness can be as debilitating as the physical effects. Caregivers should pay particular attention to:
   - Anxiety over physical status, treatment and prognosis
   - Anxiety over the impact of the illness on themselves and family
   - Anxiety over the financial impact of illness.

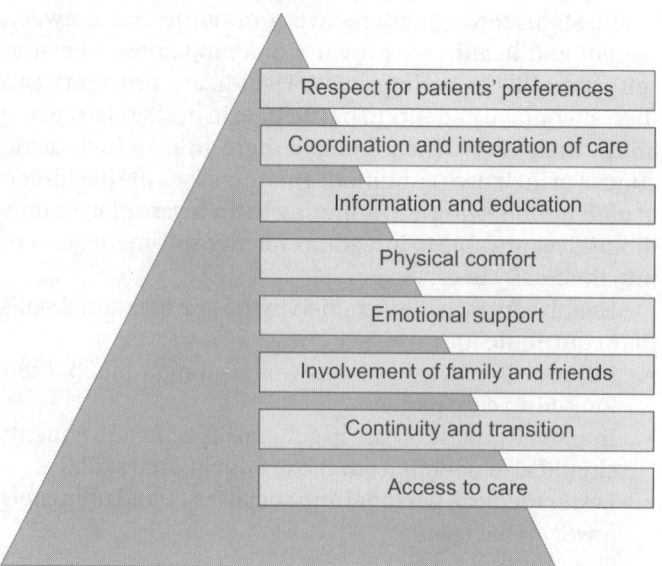

Fig. 14.2: Picker's eight principles of patient-centred care.

6. **Involvement of family and friends:** This principle addresses the role of family and friends in the patient experience. Family dimensions of patient-centered care were identified as follows:
   - Providing accommodations for family and friends
   - Involving family and close friends in decision making
   - Supporting family members as caregivers
   - Recognizing the needs of family and friends.
7. **Continuity and transition:** Patients expressed concern about their ability to care for themselves after discharge. Meeting patient needs in this area requires the following:
   - Understandable, detailed information regarding medications, physical limitations, dietary needs, etc.
   - Coordinate and plan ongoing treatment and services after discharge
   - Provide information regarding access to clinical, social, physical and financial support on a continuing basis.
8. **Access to care:** Patients need to know they can access care when it is needed. Focusing mainly on ambulatory care, the following areas were of importance to the patient:
   - Access to the location of hospitals, clinics and physician offices
   - Availability of transportation
   - Ease of scheduling appointments
   - Availability of appointments when needed
   - Accessibility to specialists or specialty services when a referral is made
   - Clear instructions provided on when and how to get referrals.

At a global level, there is a seismic shift in thinking about empowering patients to take an active role in their care plan. At one view we see first-hand how technology can help transform healthcare facilities and help them realize their ambitions to engage patients and significantly improve outcomes.

ELEMENTS OF AN EDUCATIONAL PROGRAM

The following educational elements should be provided for in the planning of an educational program for health care providers in therapeutic patient education:
- Establish, with learners, guidelines for organizing their own learning
- Guide learners in the selection of relevant health or service problems and objectives
- Assign to each problem adequate learning time
- Contract with learners the criteria of certifying evaluation
- Provide learners with valid self-evaluation
- Instruments select relevant learning sites
- Provide learning resources
- Adjust the programme on the basis of continuous assessment
- Ensure a system of program accreditation.

EFFECTIVE PATIENT TEACHING STRATEGIES

Below are 10 strategies to help nurses incorporate teaching into their daily practice.
1. **Start right away:** Teaching should really begin at the time of admission. During assessment, planning and diagnosing, nurses should identify the needs and problems of the patient and his or her family, as well as their education level.
2. **Document the teaching process:** It is important to document your teaching from admission through discharge, as it can impact evaluation and reimbursement, as well as help newer nurses learn effective strategies. Good documentation can help maintain care continuity when the patient's care is transitioned from one nurse to the next.
3. **Set goals together:** From the beginning, the nurse and patient should decide together on goals and objectives, ensuring that each person understands the goals and why achieving the goals is important. Be sure to continually evaluate and reformulate goals and objectives as patient care progresses.
4. **Emphasize necessary strategies:** In the inpatient setting, many patients fear losing their independence. Patients will be motivated to learn what is necessary for them to care for themselves. Nurses should therefore emphasize these strategies.
5. **Timing is everything:** Choose a mutually agreed upon time to teach. Look for a time that is good for both you and the patient. For example, patients that have just heard their diagnosis may need time to process that information before they are open to learning. Also, look for a time when you will not be interrupted and the patient will not be distracted by visitors, meal time, etc.

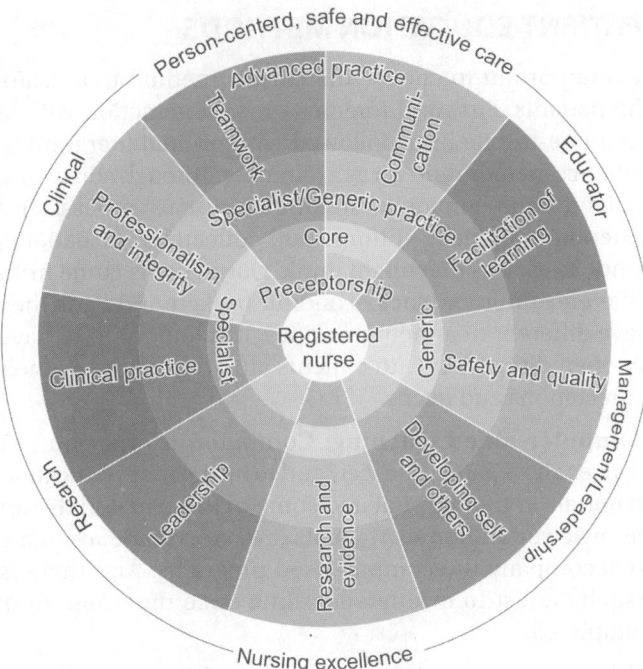

Fig. 14.3: Role of nurse in patient education.

6. **Know what they already know:** Nurses do not want to spend time going over something that the patient already knows. That time is better spent educating or coaching the patient in other ways. If the patient already knows why they need to take a medication, but they don't always do it, perhaps the teaching time is better spent on motivating the patient to care for themselves.
7. **Consider education level and literacy:** Not all patients can understand complex medical terms and some may not be able to read. Other patients may be very well-educated and be familiar with medical terminology. Others may have limited English proficiency, so a medical interpreter will be needed. Tailor your teaching to each patient's level of understanding, to be the most effective.
8. **Seeing and hearing is believing:** Customize your teaching to the patient's physical abilities. If a patient can't hear well, they may not digest verbal instructions. Those that are vision-impaired won't be able to read patient handouts.
9. **Break it up:** Look for those ideal teaching moments where you can impart small bits of education and engage the patient by evaluating his or her understanding. Doing this in small increments helps you and the patient. It's much easier to fit in a small teaching moment while you're in the patient's room than it is to spend a big chunk of time on discharge day. And, the patient doesn't have to digest all of the information at once.
10. **Consider costs and income:** Keep your recommendations practical, especially for patients on a fixed income.

PATIENT EDUCATION METHODS

It is important to choose the correct method to educate the patients. First and foremost, most interaction will be on a one-to-one basis followed with printed literature to enhance memory and act as a reminder. Through education, patients can be made aware of their disease process and potential treatment options. But, educating our patients is not as easy as one might think. Our patients come from different ethnic and socioeconomic backgrounds; and they have different treatment priorities. It is important to have an open discussion with patients and to get to know their expectations and needs.

Computer-aided teaching: Computer or other output devices allow patients to view and to hear patient education materials in the hospital and some of these materials can be reviewed at home. Manuals are often made available to accompany the computerised programs. And there is usually a test to evaluate learning once the program is completed.

Video education: Video education is very similar to computer-based training. But, it is more difficult to evaluate learning. A written post-test could be used after the video is reviewed. But, it is important with both of these media to consider the patients' educational level, language, and hearing/seeing abilities.

Demonstration: Demonstration is another effective patient-teaching technique. Patients can be showed how to complete a task or how a process works in a one-on-one setting, and then they can do the task more effectively at home. However, in an acute care setting this might be more difficult to do. The pace is much faster, but case managers or patient care assistants can be used to assist the nurse if needed. And, demonstration does ensure that patients fully understand the teaching, and it allows them to get feedback and ask questions in a safe arena.

Written material: Written material seems so easy and routine. But, it can be effective. For instance, material with pictures can offer instructions or explanations. Written material related to prescribed medicines is also a necessity. And, it can offer instructions in a step by step fashion. Once again, it is important to evaluate the patients' literacy level, language, and sight before handing out routine teaching materials.

Discharge instructions: At the time of discharge, patients can be equipped with a set of instructions with follow-up appointments, medication teaching, and phone numbers. Many discharge instructions can easily be printed using PHR and EMR software systems. These instructions usually give phone numbers (of whom to call with questions) and follow-up appointment instructions.

Discharge prescriptions: Prescriptions for discharge medications are usually included in these instructions. It is important to verify that the patient knows the names, the purpose, and the dosage instructions for these medications. If needed, verify with the case manager that the patient can afford these medications; and if needed, call them into their pharmacy before discharge.

There are countless methods of educational materials including:
- Leaflets/Booklets
- Posters
- Flipcharts
- Models—anatomical and diagrammatic
- Apps—phone/Ipad
- Electronic media
- Focus groups
- One-to-one meetings
- Websites
- The Expert Patients Programme.

EVALUATING PATIENT LEARNING

Effective patient teaching also requires evaluation and documentation. Learning can be evaluated in the following ways:

- **Asking questions:** Simply ask questions to see whether there is information that needs reinforcing.
- **Observe return demonstration:** Watch the patient perform a task (i.e. self inject insulin) to see if the technique is correct.
- **Assess the data:** Ask the patient to record his blood pressure, blood glucose, or weight at home. And, review the records at the next visit. These records will demonstrate how effective the current treatments have been.
- **Talk with the patient/family:** At the next visit, or before discharge, talk with the family to see how the patient has been doing, or before they leave the hospital, engage in open dialogue about barriers or concerns. This is very similar to the idea of "asking questions", but both methods are useful.

BARRIERS IN PATIENT EDUCATION

Nurses and nurse midwives have historically considered patient education one of their most important responsibilities. Increasingly, however, appropriate and comprehensive patient education has become more difficult to accomplish. Patient education is a dynamic and continuous process that should be implemented during the entire time of hospital stay and even afterward.

Psychological Barrier

- Emotional disturbance
- Fear
- Level of intelligent
- Ego.

Environmental Barrier

- Lack of ventilation
- Lack of privacy
- Over crowding.

Cultural Barrier

- Level of knowledge and understanding
- Customs
- Beliefs
- Religion
- Language.

Receiving information doesnot guarantee learning. That is because **external** barriers to learning, such as environmental and sociocultural factors, as well as internal barriers to learning, including psychological and physiological factors, can influence a person's learning experience and ability.

Sociocultural factors include language barriers. If you are educating a foreign patient that doesn't really understand English very well, they might be willing to learn but simply would not be able to. Other sociocultural barriers include a person's value system. Some cultures may not value advice from a particular person or about a particular topic. A person's educational background is an important barrier to learning as well.

Internal barriers include psychological and physiological factors. Psychological barriers include things like:

- Fear
- Anger
- Anxiety
- Depression.

Nursing instructors and curriculum planners should ensure more emphasis on patient education at the initial semesters of nursing education curriculum and make sure that it is included in the evaluation of students. Hospital officials should provide a dedicated education environment with suitable facilities, tools, and atmosphere for patient education. Also, special education programs need to be developed for less educated patients.

Some of the barriers were related to the poor academic performance of nursing students. It was found that many patients may not be prepared to receive an education because of age, illiteracy, or cultural and social barriers. Hospital officials can appoint a nurse as the person responsible for providing patient education at appropriate times. Clinical nursing instructors should give a higher priority to patient education and consider using it as a student evaluation criterion in order to encourage more participation on the part of students. Also, patient education practice should be performed in all wards of hospitals by the entire medical staff and a training environment should be provided for this purpose.

TIPS TO IMPROVE PATIENT EDUCATION

Preventing re-hospitalization is a huge responsibility, especially in consideration of costly penalties that are levied for early readmissions. To accomplish this, nurses need to constantly improve patient teaching and education prior to discharge. Some of the things nurses can do to advance patient education include:

- Delegate more responsibilities to support staff and be more focused on patient education.
- Begin educating patients with every encounter from admission.
- Find out what the patient already knows. Correct any misinformation.
- Feed patients information in layman's terms. Utilize visual aids as often as possible.
- Question their understanding of the care, and plan for the next lesson.
- Use returns demonstration when administering care. Involve the patient from the very first treatment.
- Ask the patient to tell you how they would explain (step-by-step) their disease or treatment to their loved one.
- Make sure the patient understands the medications as you administer them. Make sure they understand how and when to refill medications.
- Provide patients with information about signs and symptoms of their.

NURSES' ROLE IN PATIENT EDUCATION

Patient education is a significant part of a nurse's job. Education empowers patients to improve their health status. When patients are involved in their care, they are more likely to engage in interventions that may increase their chances for positive outcomes. The benefits of patient education include:

- Prevention of medical conditions such as obesity, diabetes or heart disease.
- Patients who are informed about what to expect during a procedure and throughout the recovery process.
- Decreasing the possibility of complications by teaching patients about medications, lifestyle modifications and self-monitoring devices like a glucose meter or blood pressure monitor.
- Reduction in the number of patients readmitted to the hospital.
- Retaining independence by learning self-sufficiency.

CONCLUSION

Many patients lack knowledge about healthcare. Nurses must assess their patients to pinpoint the best way to educate them about their health and determine how much they already know about their medical condition. They need to build a rapport with patients by asking questions to zero in on concerns. Nurses may have to adjust their teaching strategies to fit the patient's preferences. Many patients want detailed information, though some may request only a checklist. Effective patient education starts from the time patients are admitted to the hospital and continues until they are discharged. Nurses should take advantage of any appropriate opportunity throughout a patient's stay to teach the patient about self-care. The self-care instruction may include teaching patients how to inject insulin, bathe an infant or change a colostomy pouching system. Without proper education, patients may go home and resume unhealthy habits or ignore the management of their medical condition.

BIBLIOGRAPHY

1. Cross S. The Role of Practice Nurses in Educating Patients to Self-care, 2011.
2. Duffy FD. Counseling for behavior change. In: Goldman L, Schafer AI (eds). Goldman-Cecil Medicine, 25th Edition. Philadelphia, PA: Elsevier Saunders; 2016.
3. Education for Health: A Manual on Health Education in Primary Health Care. Geneva, Switzerland: WHO Publications, 1988.
4. Edwardson SR. Patient education in heart failure. Heart Lung. 2007;36(4):244-52.
5. Falvo DR. Communicating effectively in patient teaching: enhancing patient adherence. In: Falvo DR (ed). Effective Patient Education: A Guide to Increased Adherence, 4th Edition. Sudbury, MA: Jones and Bartlett, 2010.
6. Ghorob A. Health coaching: teaching patients how to fish. Fam Pract Manag. 2013;20(3):40-2.
7. Kiger AM. Teaching for Health, 3rd Edition. London: Elsevier Ltd, 2004.
8. Miller WR, Rollnick S. Motivational Interviewing - Helping People Change, 3rd Edition. London: The Guilford Press, 2013.
9. Naidoo J, Wills J. Developing Practice for Public Health and Health Promotion. 3rd ed. London: Elsevier Ltd., 2011.
10. Noohi E, Abbaszadeh A. Process of patient education and Orem's self care theory, an integrative model curriculum: a qualitative study. J Qual Res Health Sci. 2017;5(4):419-31.
11. Office for National Statistics. Internet Access - Households and Individuals, 2013.
12. Rankin SH, Duffy Stallings K, London F. Patient Education in Health and Illness. 5th ed. Philadelphia: Lippincott Williams and Wilkins, 2005.
13. Russell SS. An Overview of Adult Learning Processes, 2006.
14. Wilson PM, Kendall S, Brooks F. The Expert Patients Programme: a paradox of patient empowerment and medical dominance. Blackwell Publishing Ltd., 2007. Available

REVIEW QUESTIONS

Long Essays

1. Define patient education, discuss therapeutic patient education in detail.
2. Explain the principles of patient education.
3. Describe the patient education methods.

Short Essays

1. Values of patient education.
2. Competencies of health educator.
3. Importance of patient education.
4. Elements of an educational program.
5. Effective patient teaching strategies.
6. Barriers in patient education.
7. Nurses' role in patient education.

Short Answers

1. Teaching process.
2. Objectives of patient education.
3. Need of patient education.
4. Benefits of patient education.
5. Tips to improve patient education.

MULTIPLE CHOICE QUESTIONS

1. All patients have the right to be educated on maintaining their health
   a. Disease prevention
   b. Health promotion
   c. Both a and b
   d. None of the above
2. Health promotion is the process of --------
   a. Advancing knowledge
   b. Influencing attitudes, and
   c. Determining relevant solutions
   d. All of the above
3. Therapeutic patient education is designed therefore to train patients in the skills of ---------
   a. Self-managing or adapting treatment to their particular chronic disease
   b. Coping processes and skills
   c. Both a and b
   d. None of the above
4. Environmental barrier in patient teaching is:
   a. Lack of ventilation
   b. Lack of privacy
   c. Over crowding
   d. All of the above
5. Psychological barriers include the following, *except*:
   a. Fear
   b. Anger
   c. Pain
   d. Anxiety

ANSWERS

1. c   2. d   3. c   4. d   5. c

CHAPTER 15

Hygiene

LEARNING OBJECTIVES

- Factors influencing hygienic practice
- Hygienic care: Indications and purposes, effects of neglected care
  - Care of the skin (bath, feet and nail, hair care)
  - Care of pressure points
  - Assessment of pressure ulcers using Braden scale and Norton scale
- Pressure ulcers—causes, stages and manifestations, care and prevention
- Perineal care/menstrual care
- Oral care, care of eyes, ears and nose including assistive devices (eye glasses, contact lens, dentures, hearing aid)

TERMINOLOGY

- **Hygiene:** Hygiene is defined as the science and art which is associated with the prevention and promotion of health. Hygiene is science of health, which includes all the factors contributing to healthful living.
- **Habits:** Habits are the highly automated and self executed behavior of man. Habits can be related to physical activities or mental like those related to paying attention or thinking.
- **Personal hygiene:** Personal hygiene implies to those principles of physical cleanliness and mental health, which are practiced by a person at individual level.
- **Sexual health:** Sexual health is an integration of the somatic, emotional, intellectual and social aspects of sexual being, in ways that positively enrich and enhance the personality, communication and love.
- **Mental health:** Mental health is defined as the capacity in an individual to form harmonious relations with others and to participate in or contribute constructively to the changes in his social and physical environment.
- **School hygiene:** School hygiene or school health is a branch of community health to facilitate optimum health to schoolchildren. It also includes prevention of diseases, early diagnosis.
- **Attitude:** It is a mental structure or framework that includes motivational, perceptual, emotional and cognitive reactions. It also manifests the individual concepts, thoughts or imaginations, which direct his behavior towards a specific direction.
- **Adjustment:** It can be defined in the form of social process in which a person is able to develop the tendency of cooperation in his environment.
- **Health behaviors:** It includes all those activities and actions adopted by man as a protection against diseases. The concept of health behavior includes rules of personal health, good health habits and taking preventive steps against diseases.
- **Menstrual hygiene:** Menstrual discharge is a normal physiological process. Menstrual hygiene describes the basic elements of hygiene during menstruation to promote feeling of well being and prevention of diseases. This hygiene practices includes daily bath, keeping the genital organs clean and dry, placing a clean sanitary pads and taking proper nutrition and rest.

INTRODUCTION

The word hygiene has evolved from the Greek term "Hygia" which means "Goodness of Health". Hygiene is the science of health and includes all factors which contribute to healthful living. Hygiene is the science of health and its preservation; it also refers to practices that are conducive to good health. Good personal hygiene is important to a person's general health.

DEFINITION

- Hygiene defined as "the science and art which is associated with the preservation and promotion of health".
- Hygiene defined as that "science of health, which includes all the factors contributing to the healthful living".

TYPES OF HYGIENE

- **Social hygiene:** Social medicine has replaced the word social hygiene, its objective to study man as a social animal in its total environment. The scope of social medicine includes science of social structure and functions, social pathology and social treatment, etc.

- **Industrial hygiene:** Occupational health, which has broader meaning. Its scope is extended up to the health of labor working in all types of occupation and different aspects of health.
- **School hygiene:** School hygiene or school health is an important branch of community health, which facilitating optimum health to school children.
- **Preventive medicine:** Nowadays, a broader term community medicine is used. Preventive medicine plays primary role in immunization as specific protection and general methods of improvement in health.
- **Personal hygiene:** Personal hygiene or personal health implies to those principles of physical cleanliness and mental health. Personal hygiene is not only limited to taking care of body and keeping it clean, rather the mental and spiritual aspects are also an integral part of it.

FACTORS INFLUENCING HYGIENE PRACTICES

- **Personal preferences:** Each individual has his own desires and preferences about when to bathe, shave, and perform hair care. Same way each individual select different products according to the personal preferences, needs and financial resources. The nurse assists the client in delivering individualized care to the client.

Factors influencing hygiene	
Social practices Ethnic, social, and family influences on hygiene patterns	**Personal preferences** Dictate hygiene practices
Body image A person's subjective concept of his or her body appearance	**Socioeconomic status** Influences the type and extent of hygiene practices used
Knowledge base and environment The person's level of knowledge and climatic conditions	**Psychological factors** Mental and psychological issues

- **Social practices:** Social groups influence hygiene practices and preferences. During childhood, hygiene practices are influenced by family customs and as children enter their adolescent years, hygiene practices may be influenced by the peer group behavior. During the adult years, work groups and friends shape the expectations of people and in the older adults hygiene practices may change because of living conditions and available resources.
- **Socioeconomic status:** The type and extent of hygiene practices are influenced by a person's economic resources. The nurse determines which products/supplies, the client can afford.
- **Health belief and motivation:** Knowledge regarding the importance of hygiene for well-being influences hygiene practices. Only knowledge is not enough. The client must be motivated to maintain self-care.
- **Cultural beliefs:** A client's cultural beliefs and personal values influence hygiene care.
- **Physical condition:** Certain type of physical limitations or disabilities often lacks the physical energy to perform hygiene care, e.g. a client with traction or who has an intravenous line, will need assistance for hygiene maintenance.

PERSONAL HYGIENE

Personal hygiene has a significant role in every society. Every culture develops and maintains its standards and methods of maintaining personal cleanliness. Habits are formed for performing actions to keep the body clean and functioning normally.

Personal hygiene includes all those personal factors which influence the health and well being of an individual. It consists of the body regarding bathing and washing, care of hair, nails and feet, mouth cleanliness and care of the teeth, care of the nose and ears, clothing, postures, exercises, recreation, rest and relaxation, sleep habits and nutrition.

Personal hygiene is necessarily maintained for a person's comfort and well-being. A variety of personal and sociocultural factors influence the client's hygiene practices. The nurse determines a client's ability to perform self-care and provides hygienic care according to the client's needs and preferences. While providing hygiene, the nurse must preserve as much client's independence as possible, ensure privacy, convey respect and foster the client's physical comfort.

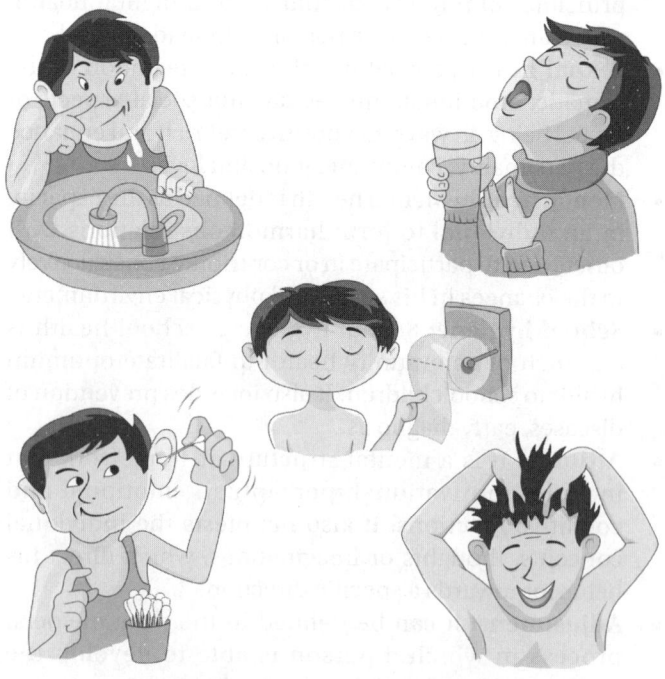

Fig. 15.1: Activities of daily living.

Definition

Personal hygiene defined as that "the healthy practices and lifestyle helps in the maintenance and promotion of individual health physically, emotionally, socially and spiritually".

Purposes of Personal Hygiene and Protect from Disease

- To prevent illness.
- To promote good health.
- To improve the standard of health.
- To maintain quality life of an individual.
- To promote mental well being.
- To promote socially and spiritually health.
- To improve the self esteem in the society.
- To maintain resistance and prevent from infection.

Principles of Personal Hygiene

- Hygiene practices are learnt.
- Changes occur throughout the life span, it also affects the health care practices.
- Individual differences exit from one individual to other.
- Health practices of people vary with cultural values and personal values.
- Health practices directly influences the physical, mental, social and spiritual health of an individual.
- Good health practices prevent entry of microorganism into the body.
- Nature acts as a first line of defence on human health natural light and ventilation.

Components of a Good Personal Hygiene Program

Good personal hygiene includes:
- Maintaining personal cleanliness
- Wearing proper work attire
- Following hygienic hand practices
- Avoiding unsanitary habits and actions
- Maintaining good health
- Reporting illnesses

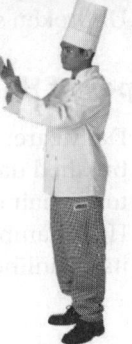

Factors Influences on Personal Hygiene

- **Social practices:** Social groups influence including the type of personal care. During childhood, hygiene is influenced by family customs.
- **Personal preferences:** Each person has individual desires and preferences about when to bath, shave and perform hair care. Individual selects different products according to personal preferences, needs and financial resources.
- **Body language:** An individual general holds for the person. Body image is a person's subjective concept of his or her physical appearance. These images can change frequently. When individual undergo surgery, illness or a change in functional status, body image can change dramatically.
- **Socio economic status:** A person's economic resources influence the type and extent of hygiene practices used. Socioeconomic status may influence his or her ability to regularly maintain hygiene.

Factors affecting personal hygiene

- Social practices
- Personal preferences
- Body image
- Socioeconomic status
- Health beliefs and motivation
- Cultural variables

- **Health beliefs and motivation:** Knowledge about importance of hygiene and its implications for well-being influences hygiene practices. However, knowledge alone is not enough. The individual also must be motivated to maintain self-care.
- **Cultural variables:** An individual's cultural beliefs and personal values hygiene care. People from diverse cultural background follow different self-care practices. Culturally maintaining cleanliness may not hold the same importance for some ethnic groups as it does for others.
- **Physical condition:** The nurse quickly learns that clients with certain types of physical limitations or disabilities often lack of physical energy and dexterity to perform hygienic care. A client in traction or a cast or who has an intravenous line or other device connected to the body will need assistance with hygiene.

Importance of Personal Hygiene

- Maintenance of physical hygiene in a state of health is a personal value and individual responsibility.
- Personal hygiene helps maintenance of physical and psychological homeostasis.
- Personal hygiene helps to promote individuals comfort, safety, and well being.
- A clean mouth and teeth aids to the patients a feeling of self-approval.
- Healthy hygienic practices and technique, which provides economy of time, material and energy.
- Stimulation of circulation by massage and brushing is essential to maintain the hair healthy.
- Keeping the scalp clean by brushing and shampooing will help to relieve from dandruff.
- Moving the body joints in their whole range of movement helps to prevent muscle contraction and improve circulation.
- Good personal hygiene is essential during sickness as well as in health.

Nurses Role in Personal Hygiene

- Direct provision of hygienic care provides the nurse with an ideal opportunity for daily assessment of the patient's physical and emotional state.
- The process of daily bathing, oral hygiene, care of the hair, nails and massage forms a vital part of the nurse-patient interaction.
- The nurse should assess the needs of patients and identifying related nursing problems.
- The nurse needs to collect further information about the patient's identified problems.
- The nurse needs to develop an appropriate nursing care plan in terms of the data collected and relevant nursing principles.
- The nurse has to implement the nursing care plan to provide optimum quality of nursing care for individual patients.
- The nurse has to evaluate the success of the nursing care plan and adjusting it to meet the patient's changing needs.
- The nurse also participates in carrying out the physician's orders and refers to the physician pertinent observations and information about the patient.
- The nurse has to motivate the patient to resume independence and responsibility for care as the condition permits.
- The nurse must apply knowledge of pathophysiology to provide good preventive hygienic care. The nurse has to integrate knowledge of anatomy, physiology and pathology during hygienic care.

HEAD TO TOE CARE

Oral hygiene means the cleanliness of the mouth oral hygiene includes measure to prevent the spread of disease from the mouth and increase the comfort.

Objectives

- To keep the mouth and teeth in good condition.
- To prevent the mucous membrane from becoming dry and cracked.
- To prevent sores which resulting in ulceration.
- To prevent bacterial in the mouth from causing local and general infections.
- Emollients help to soften the dry mucous membrane to prevent cracking.

Complication of Neglected Oral Hygiene

Local complication: Offensive breath, glossitis, pyorrhea, sores and crust, root abscess, adenitis, tonsillitis, otitis media, parotitis, sinusitis and dental caries.

General complications: Loss of appetite, joint disease, inhalation pneumonia, rheumatism and heart disease.

Care of Hair

Care of hair is part of the personal hygiene. It is another way of helping the patient feel good about him and maintain a good mental attitude.

Objectives

- To maintain cleanliness of the scalp and hair
- To prevent matting of hair.
- To promote comfort and to stimulate circulation of the scalp.
- It gives an opportunity of observation of the scalp and hair.
- It maintains a glossy and healthy appearance of hair and gives satisfaction to the patient.

Scientific Principles

- Well combed and attend hair provide comfort to the patient and make appearance more attractive.
- Neglected hair and scalp contain dirt and microorganism and also produce infection of the scalp.
- Unbroken skin acts as a barrier to infection.

Types of Hair Care

- Daily care: The hair should be thoroughly combed and brushed daily. A woman usually needs more attention to the hair due to its length.
- Hair shampoo: shampooing the hair in order to maintain its cleanliness.

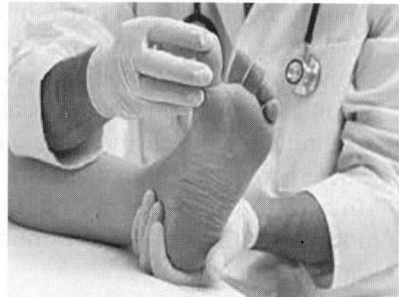 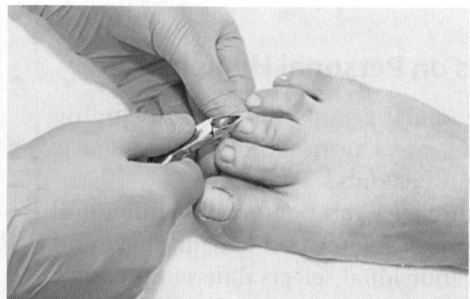

Fig. 15.2: Care of toe and nails.

- Treatment of hair: Pediculosis treatment-it is the treatment given with DDT 5 percent or carbolic lotion 1:40. applied thoroughly on the scalp and it is left for overnight, and the next day a thorough bath is given and the linen is changed.

Problems of Neglected Hair Care

Neglected hair care cause sticky and heavy and acquires a sour, unpleasant odor, which may be quite distressing the patient. Pediculosis is associated with poor hygiene, crowded living condition and exposure to other individuals. The people with pediculosis complaints of severe itching of the scalp and scratch the head continuously giving rise to abscess formation. The lice are blood suckers and cause anemia. They also spread disease, e.g. typhus fever, relapsing fever, trench fever.

Care of the Eyes, Nose, and Ears

The eyes, nose and ears are important organs which require no special care in daily life. Hygienic care of these organs is always done as part of the general bathing procedure. Hygienic are of the eyes, ears and nose prevents infection and helps to maintain their functions.

Essential Steps in Eye, Ear and Nose

- Eyes are cleaned from the inner to the outer canthus.
- During a bath, each eye is cleaned with a separate portion of the wash cloth.
- Excessive accumulation of secretions make patient sniff or blow the nose.
- The patients who cannot remove secretions needs assistance to clear the congestion and protect from nasal mucosa.
- Babies and small children a wisp of cotton moistened with warm water or oil, introduced into the anterior nares and rotated gently, cleanses the nostrils.

Common Problems of Neglected Care

Poor eye, ear causes debris may accumulate behind the ear and in the anterior aspect of the external ear. This can lead to ulceration of the skin. Collection of cerumen or ear wax, in the external auditory canal cause difficulty in hearing.

ORAL HYGIENE

Oral hygiene means maintaining the cleanliness of the mouth. Oral hygiene includes measures to prevent the spread of disease from the mouth and increase the comfort of the patient.

It is important because mouth is the portal entry of food and digestion starts from mouth. So, the entry of any pathogen in mouth directly affects health.

Purpose

- To prevent and treat mouth infections.
- To keep the mouth fresh and clean.
- To prevent the mucous membrane from becoming dry and cracked.
- To prevent dental carries and tooth decay.
- To prevent sores which resulting in ulceration.
- To stimulate salivation and increase appetite.
- To prevent infection of parotid glands.
- To prevent complications such as stomatitis, glossitis, pyorrhea and parotitis, etc.
- To stimulate circulation in gums thus maintaining health firmness.
- To maintain oral hygiene among bedridden patients.

The Patient Who may Require Frequent Mouth Care

- Unconscious patients.
- Helpless patient.
- Patient with higher pyrexia.
- Malnourished and dehydrated patients.
- Patients who are not taking oral feeds.
- Patients having local diseases of mouth.
- Paraplegic patients.
- Patients having a local disease of mouth.
- Postoperative patients.

Scientific Principles

- Any new treatment or exposure to unfamiliar situation produces fear and anxiety.
- Food particles left in the mouth promote the growth of microorganism.
- Soap which is constituent of most dentifrice has a low surface tension and spreads readily and penetrates in between teeth.
- Cold water reduces friction and hot water destroys dentures.
- Cough reflex is depressed in unconscious patients.
- Giving mouth care provides opportunity to observe the condition of mouth and teeth..
- Knowledge about the technique of keeping the mouth healthy helps in practicing it and maintains.
- A clean mouth and teeth aids to the patient a feeling of self-approval.
- Emollient helps to soften the dry mucous membrane to prevent cracking.
- Patients comfort and safety may be enhanced by practice of good techniques, which provide economy of time, material and energy.

Solutions Commonly Used for Mouth Wash

- Potassium permanganate ($KMnO_4$) 1:5000 (1 crystal to a glass of water).

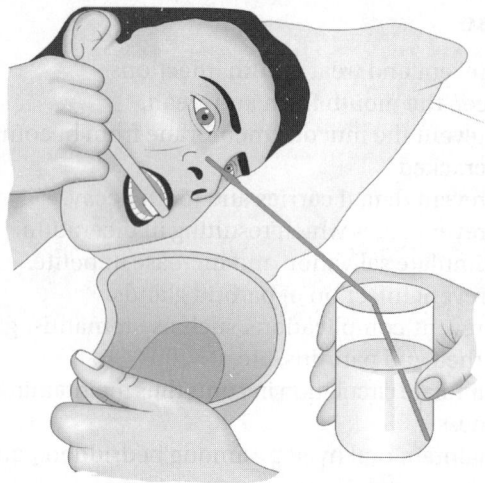

Fig. 15.3: Assisted oral care for bedridden patient.

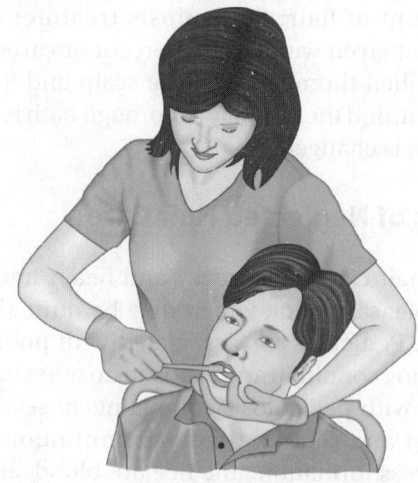

Fig. 15.5: Partially assisted oral care by the nurse.

- Sodium chloride—1 teaspoon to a pint of water
- Potassium chloride—4–6%
- Hydrogen peroxide (H_2O_2) 1:8 solution.

Dentifrices Used

- Glycerin with lime juice equal parts.
- Sodium bicarbonate paste.
- Reliable tooth paste or powder.

Emollient Used Commonly

- Cream or butter.
- White vaseline.
- Liquid paraffin.
- Glycerin borax
- Olive oil.

Preliminary Assessment of the Patient and Environment

- Identify the patient and observe the general condition of the patient.
- Check the condition of the mouth.
- Assess the ability of the patient to cooperate.
- Prepare the patient for acceptance and realization.
- Assess the status of health habits.
- Decide the type of dentifrice and emollient to be used.
- Assess the frequency of mouth care needed.

- Note the precautions to be observed while moving the patient.
- Articles available in the unit.
- Make sure about any drink to be given after mouth care if advisable.

Equipment

A tray containing of:
- Mackintosh and towel.
- Small jug with warm water.
- Feeding cup.
- Small cups—2.
- Artery forceps—1.
- Dissecting forceps—1.

A small container containing of:
- Paper bag.
- Kidney tray.
- Choose one of the solutions for mouthwash.
- Choose one of the emollients.
- Gauze piece.
- Face towel—1.

Procedure

- Bring patient to edge of bed.
- Position pillow according to comfort of patient.
- Place small mackintosh with face towel on patient's chest.

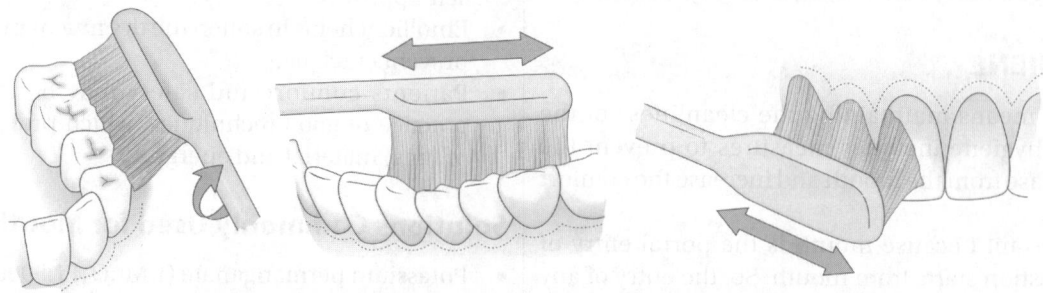

Fig. 15.4: Care of dentures.

For unconscious

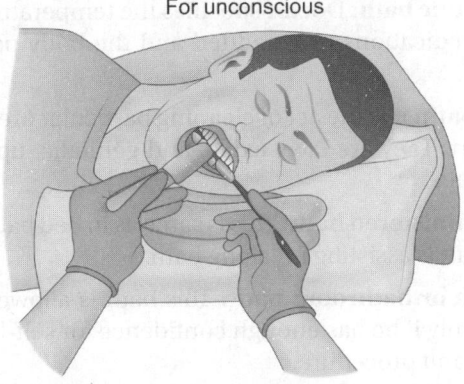

Fig. 15.6: Oral care for an unconscious patient.

- Place K-basin close to chin of patient.
- Raise head end of the bed to 45°.
- Pour antiseptic solution in to cup.
- Soak gauze piece in solution and squeeze out excess solution by using artery clamp.
- Use same clamp to clean patient's mouth (avoid mixing of clamps).
- Clean using up and down movements from gums to crown, clean oral cavity from proximal to distal, outer to inner aspect.
- Discard used cotton balls into K-basin.
- Provide tumbler of water and instruct the patient to gargle mouth, Position K-basin so that spillage is avoided.
- Clean tongue from inner to outer aspect.
- Provide water to rinse mouth and dry face with towel.
- Lubricate lips using swab stick.
- Rinse the used articles and replace equipment.
- Document time, solution used, condition of oral cavity, abnormalities noticed and patient's response.

Complication of Neglected Mouth Care

Local Complications

- Parotitis-Inflammation of the parotid glands.
- Stomatitis-Inflammation of the mucus membrane of the mouth.
- Gingivitis-Inflammation of the gums.
- Glossitis-Inflammation of the tongue.
- Dental carries-Forms cavity in the teeth.
- Root abscess-Pus formation in the root of the teeth.
- Periodontal diseases-It is also known as pyorrhea or pus formation in the sockets of teeth.
- Bleeding gums-Deficiency of vitamins C and use a hard brushing of the teeth.

Complication Neighboring Structure

- Parotitis-Inflammation of the parotid gland.
- Rhinitis-Inflammation of sinus cavity.
- Otitis media-Inflammation of middle ear.
- Tonsillitis-Inflammation of the tonsils.
- Adenitis-Inflammation of the adenoids.

Systemic Complication

- Anorexia-Loss of appetite.
- Bacterial endocarditis-Inflammation of the endocardium.
- Gastritis-Inflammation of the stomach.
- Nephritis-Inflammation of the kidneys.
- Rheumatic arthritis-Inflammation of the joints.

Recording and Reporting

- Record the procedure with date, time and condition of the mouth, teeth, etc. on nurse's record.

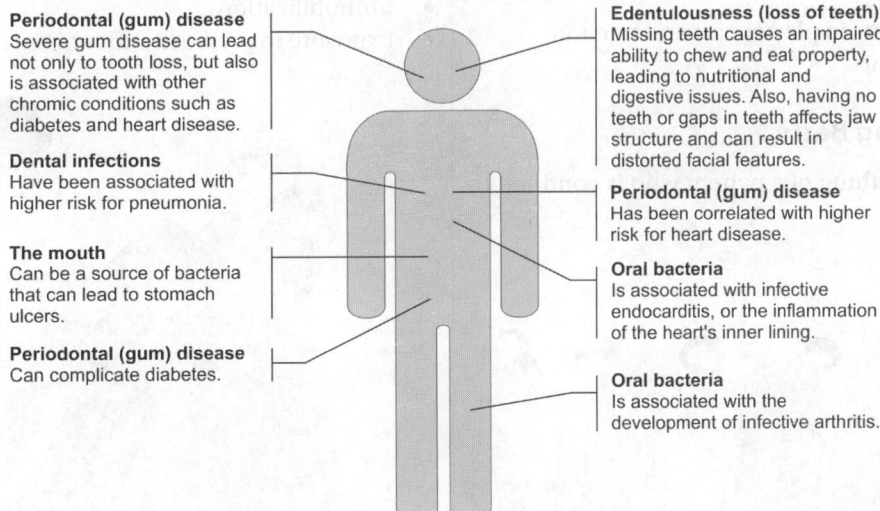

Fig. 15.7: Complications of neglected mouth care.

- Report and record any abnormal condition to the ward sister and physician.
- Give health education to the patient and relatives on oral hygiene.

BED BATH

Bed bath means bathing a patient who is confined to bed and cannot have the physical and mental capability of self-bathing.

Bath is the act of cleaning the body. Baths are given for therapeutic purposes.

Purpose

- To cleanse body of dirt, debris and perspiration.
- To refresh.
- To stimulate circulation.
- To provide comfort and relaxation.
- To enhance self-concept.
- To provide tactile stimulation.
- To facilitate head to be assessment.
- To regulate body temperature.
- To induce sleep.
- To prevent pressure sore.
- To remove toxic substances from body surface.
- To maintain an effective nurse-patient relationship.
- To give health instruction to patient.
- To remove unpleasant odors due to perspiration.
- To relieve fatigue.
- To prevent contractures by giving exercises.
- To minimize the skin irritation.

Types of Patients Needing Bed Bath

- Unconscious or semiconscious patients.
- Postoperative patients.
- Patients with strict bed rest.
- Paraplegic patients.
- Orthopedic patients in plaster cast and traction.
- Seriously ill patients.

Types of Cleansing Bath

Bed bath: It is the bathing of a patient who is confined to bed.

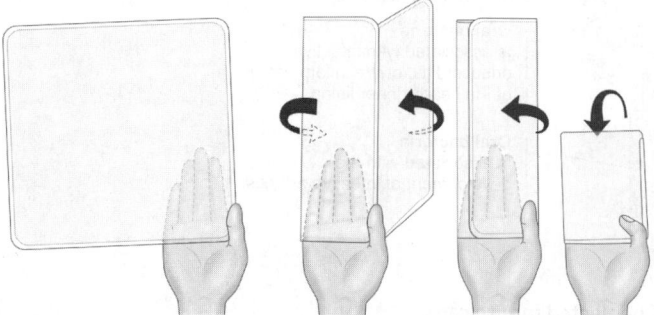

Fig. 15.8: Technique of folding the sponge cloth.

Therapeutic bath: Doctor specifies the temperature of the water, medications to be added and the body part to be treated.

Partial bath: It is the act of cleaning particular areas in the body part. They are face, axilla, and genitalia, upper and lower limbs.

Self-administered bath: This is same as in bed bath except the patient is assisting in taking bath.

Tub bath or bathroom bath: This bath is allowed to the patient only if he has enough confidence for self-help and to withstand procedure.

Scientific Principles

- Heat is conveyed to the body by convection.
- The tolerance of heat is different in different persons.
- The skin is sometimes irritated by the chemical composition of certain soaps.
- Moving the joints through their full range of movement helps prevent loss of muscle tone and improves circulation.
- Long smooth strokes on the arms and legs that are directed from the distal end to proximal increases the rate of venous flow.
- Healthy unbroken skin is a defense against harmful agents and assures resistance to injuries to a certain extent.
- Hygiene practices vary in society according to the socioeconomic standard and culture of the individual.
- Practice of food technique save time, energy material and adds to the comfort of the patient.
- Sensory receptors in the skin are sensitive to heat, pain touch and pressure.

Factors Affecting the Skin

- Impaired self-care.
- Immobilization.
- Exposure to pressure and moisture.

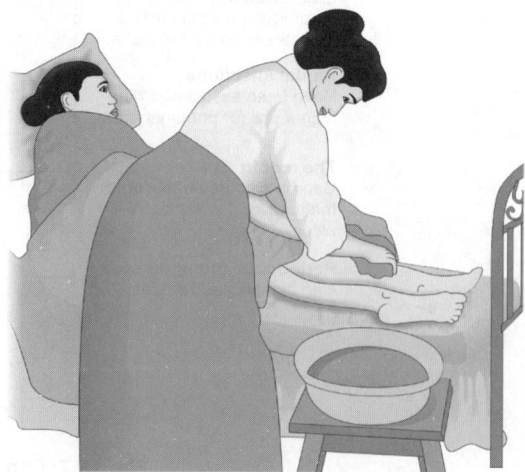

Fig. 15.9: Care of lower extremities.

- Vascular insufficiency.
- Reduced sensation.
- Nutritional alterations.
- Constrictive external devices.

General Instructions

- Explain the procedure to the patient.
- Maintain privacy of the patient.
- Put off the fans and close the windows and doors to avoid chill.
- Do not give bath immediately after the lunch.
- Cleaning is to be done from the cleanest area to the less clean area.
- The temperature of the water should be 110° F to 115° F.
- A thorough inspection of the skin and back is necessary to find our early signs of pressure sore.
- Use soap which contains less alkali.
- Special attention must be given to the creases and folds and bony prominences between fingers and toes and public region.
- Remove the soap completely to avoid the drying effect of the soap on the skin.
- Do not touch the body with wet hands it is unpleasant to the patient.
- Creams or oils used to prevent drying or excoriation of the skin.
- The nurse should maintain good posture and balances of the body during bed bath.

Baths

- Type of bath depends on the patient's condition and ability to help.
- **Complete bed bath (CBB)**
  - Health assistant bathes all parts of the body; which includes oral bygiene
- **Partial bed bath (PB)**
  - Health assistant bathes some parts of body and also gathers supplies needed by the patient
- **Tub bath or shower**
  - Assistant helps by providing towels and supplies, preparing tub or shower area

Preliminary Assessment

- Identify the patient and assess the need.
- Check doctors order for any specific precautions.
- Assess the general condition of the patient.
- Assess the patient's ability of self-help.
- Assess the patient's mental status to follow directions.
- Check the patient's preference for soap, powder, etc.
- Check whether the patient has taken the meal in the previous one hour.
- Find out the available articles in the unit.
- Provide privacy avoid draught and maintain proper light.
- Teach the patient and relatives about personal hygiene.

Preparation of the Patient and Environment

- Explain the sequence of the procedure to the patient.
- Close the windows and doors to prevent draughts put off the fan.
- Arrange the necessary articles at the bedside.
- Maintain the room temperature which will be must comfortable for patient.
- Adjust the height of the bed to the comfortable work of the nurse.
- Bring the patient to the edge of the bed and towards the nurse to prevent overreaching.
- Provide privacy by means of curtains.
- Offer bed pan or urinals if necessary.
- Keep the patient flat if the condition permits remove extra pillows and back rest.
- Remove the personal clothing and cover the patient with the bath blankets.

Equipment

- Basins—2 (big land small 1).
- Soap and soap dish.
- Wash cloth—2.
- Bath towel—2.
- Face towel—1.
- Bath blanket of sheet—1.
- Surgical spirit and powder.
- Nail cutter.
- Comb and oil.
- Kidney tray or paper bag.
- Jugs—2.
- Bucket—1.
- Clean bed linen.
- Clean dress to patient.
- Bucket or a laundry bag.
- Bath thermometer—1.

Procedure

- Explain the procedure.
- Remove the patients dress, cover with bath sheet while removing top sheet and dress.
- Mix hot and cold water in basin half full and check the temperature on the back of your hand.
- Spread face towel around neck.
- Wet sponge towel and form mitten around gingers after removing excess water.
- Clean body in following order:

Face

- Wet and apply soap to forehead, face, over and behind ear and neck.
- Clean eyes from inner to outer canthus.

- Rinses sponge towel and allow patient to wipe face.
- Dry with face towel, replace at head end of bed.

Arms

- Place towel lengthwise under the farthest arm if there is IV do not disturb it.
- Take soapy bath mitt and soap the arm and axilla.
- Massage the pressure areas.
- Place the hand in basin of water to wash.
- Rinse and dry well, paying attention to skin under breast.
- Recover with towel.

Chest

- Avoid unnecessary exposure.
- Cover chest with towel and turn bath sheet down to abdomen.
- Wet chest and apply soap in rotatory movement, paying attention to skin creases.
- Remove soap thoroughly by wiping from neck to check.
- Dry with bath towel.

Abdomen

- Fold top sheet up to suprapubic region cover the chest with bath towel.
- Wet and clean abdomen with soap.
- Clean umbilicus and dry with bath towel.
- Cover the patient with top sheet and remove towels.

Back

- Turn the patient on side or left lateral position. Close to edge of bed, with back towards nurse.
- Expose back including buttocks, spread bath towel on bed, close the patients back.
- Wet the area and apply soap with rotatory movements clean and remove soap and dry the area.
- Give massage by applying firm pressure with palms and fingers from sacrum to shoulder in sequence, covering whole back.
- Help the patient to return to supine position.

Legs

- Uncover the farthest leg and place towel under leg.
- Apply soap to the leg and give special attention to the groin.
- Massage the pressure points.
- Place foot in basin of water to wash.
- Rinse and dry well, paying special attention in between the toes.
- Repeat the procedures on the near leg.

Pubic Region

- Clean pubic region with wet large rag piece (for helpless patient).
- Permit patient to clean if so desired.
- Discard rag pieces into large K-basin.
- Give perineal care for helpless patient.

Aftercare

- Provide clean gown and paijama.
- Replace articles after cleaning.
- Discard dirty water in sluice room.
- Clean the bed linen if needed.
- Offer a hot drink (coffee or tea) if permitted.
- Position the patient for comfortable and proper alignment.
- Cut short the finger nails and toe nails.
- Comb the hair and arrange the hair.
- Hand wash.
- Record the procedure in the nurse's record with time, date, type and abnormalities noticed.

CARE OF EYES, NOSE AND EARS

Hygienic care of eyes, ears and nose prevent infection and helps to maintain their functions. Hygienic care of these organs is always done as part of the general bathing procedure.

Purpose

- To maintain the cleanliness of eye, ear and nose.
- To prevent infection.
- To keep the organ in normal functioning.
- To prevent obstruction.

Factors Affecting

- Systemic disease condition (diabetes and hypertension).
- Acute illness (viral or bacterial infection).
- Trauma (blow or foreign bodies).
- Medication (ototoxic drugs).

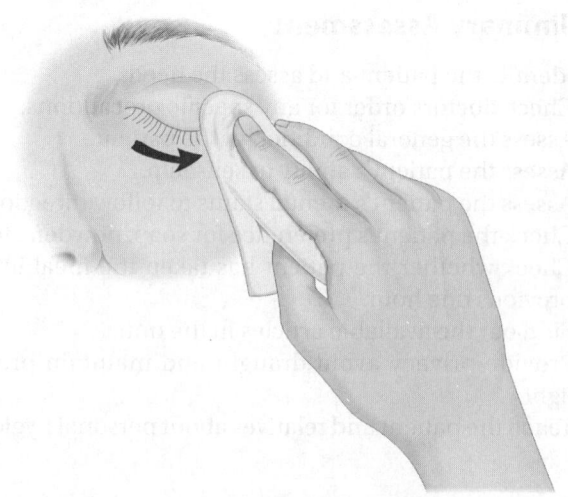

Fig. 15.10: Care of eyes.

- Allergic substances.
- Congenital anomalies.

Common Problems

Eye: Conjunctivitis (burning, itching, red-watery and painful eyes with increased secretions) cataracts, glaucoma, strabismus, and squint.

Ear: Otitis media, impact cerument and foreign bodies.

Nose: Mechanical irritation and obstruction.

General Instructions

Eye

- Unconscious patients are at risk for eye injury. Daily swabbing of eye with wet sterile cotton is important.
- Cleaning is done from the inner canthus of eye to the outer canthus of the eye.
- Use normal saline to remove the crust.
- During bath, each eye is cleaned with a separate portion of the wash cloth.
- When sterile procedure is required, each eye cleaned with separate swabs, swabbing each once only.

Ear

- Do not use pins or slides to clean ears. Only use clean buds to clean ears.
- Poor hygiene of ear, debris may accumulate behind the ear and in the anterior aspect of the external ear.

Nose

- Observation of nose for signs of discharge, lesions, edema and deformity is required.
- External crusted secretions can be removed with a wet wash cloth or a cotton applicator moistened with oil, normal saline or water.
- Foreign bodies and small children a wisp of cotton moistened with water or oil, introduced into the anterior flares, and rotated gently cleanses the nostrils.

Preliminary Assessment

Check

- Patients diagnosis.
- Doctors order for specific instructions.
- Assess the general condition.
- Self-care ability.
- Articles available in the unit.

Preparation of the Patient and Environment

- Explain the procedure.
- Arrange the articles at the bedsides.
- Place the patient in flat if the condition permits.
- Protect the pillow and the bed with a Mackintosh and towel under the head.

Procedure

- Wash the hand to prevent cross infection.
- Pour sterile saline into the bowl and wet the cotton balls.
- Stand in front of the patient.
- Clean the eyes with the sterile swabs.
  - Squeeze the excessive water from the swab in the saline bowl.
  - No pressure on the eyeball.
  - Gently wipe the lids from the inner to the outer canthus.
  - One swab for one swabbing.
  - Separate swabs for each eye.
- When the eyes are clean, stop the procedure, wipe the face with the face towel.

Aftercare

- Instill any medications that are ordered.
- Remove the mackintosh and towel from under the patient head.
- Adjust the position of the patient.
- Replace the articles to the utility room.
- Wash hand thoroughly.
- Record and report the procedure in the nurse's record.

CARE OF HANDS, FEET AND NAILS

Hands are more contaminated area and soaking in water enables the nurse to clean them thoroughly.

Feet are considered to be the least clean area. Placing the foot in the water and cleaning facilitates through cleaning.

Care nail is done by cut short finger nails and the toe nails. To prevent skin injury and injection.

Purpose

- To keep clean.
- To prevent skin injury (% scratching).
- To prevent infection.
- To promote comfort.
- To improve grooming.
- To promote self-esteem.
- To detect or examine the abnormalities.
- To prevent worm infestations.

Factors Affecting the Care

- Infection and injury.
- Vascular insufficiency.
- Systemic disease condition.
- Poor health practices.
- Sociocultural back ground.

Examination Includes

Examination of all skin surfaces, areas between fingers and between toes, shape, size and number of fingers and toes.

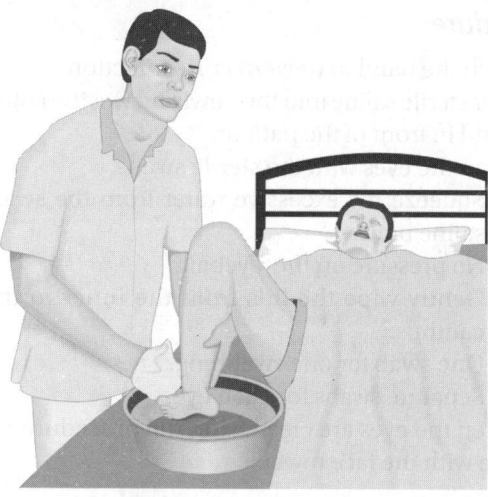

Fig. 15.11: Care of feet.

The condition of the nails such as nail plate, nail color the lunula, shape, thickness, texture, angle and then tissues around the nails.

Common Problems

- Calculus: Thickened position of epidermis. It is painless.
- Corns: Keratosis caused by friction and pressure from shoes.
- Plantar warts: Fungal lesions on sole of foot.
- Ingrown nails: It occurs due to improper nail trimming.
- Athletics foot: Tinea pedis—fungal infection of foot.
- Rams horn nails: long curved nails.
- Paraonychia: Inflammation of tissues surrounds nails.

Special Foot Care

- Clean the feet daily in lukewarm water using soap.
- Dry the feet and the part between toes.
- Do not cut corns or calculus.
- Wear shoes with porous uppers.
- If dryness is noted along the feet, use olive oil or lanolin and rub gently into the skin.
- Avoid wearing elastic stocking.
- Inspect the feet the soles, the heels and the area between toes daily.
- Wear clean socks and stockings daily.
- Do not walk bare foot.
- Wear shoes or chapels, especially designed soft ones.
- Exercise lower extremities to improve circulation.
- Avoid burns to feet by hot water or hot water bag.
- Treat minor injuries immediately under strict aseptic techniques.
- Consult doctor for even minor injuries.

Equipment

- Clean basin—2 with warm water.
- Large tray—1.
- Basin to dip foot or hand—1.
- Sponge cloths.
- Towel—1.
- Nail clipper—1.
- Mackintosh and towel—1.
- Over bed table—1.
- Bath thermometer—1.

Procedure

- Collect all articles and place near the bed side to save time and energy.
- Explain the procedure to allay fear and anxiety.
- Wash hand to prevent cross-infection.
- Provide privacy by screening.
- Take the warm water 100–110° F in a basin.
- Wash the hands first and then feet with soap and water and dry it with clean towel.
- Soak the nails in the warm water and apply soap.
- Brush the nails and place between fingers and toes and clean it with water.
- Remove the water basin and dry the areas with towel.
- Cut short the nails and collect it in the K-basin or paper bag.
- Use wet cotton balls or gauze pieces to clean the tips of the nails.

Aftercare

- Place the patients hand, feet comfortably.
- Replace the articles and equipment.
- Discard the dirty water in sluice room.
- Wash the articles used and keep ready for the next use.
- Wash hands.
- Record and report the date, time, procedure and abnormalities noted in the nurse's record.

BACK CARE/BACK MASSAGE/BACK RUB

Back care means cleaning and massaging back, paying special attention to pressure points.

Back massage provides comfort pleases and relaxes the patient; thereby it facilitates the physical stimulation to the skin and the emotional relaxation.

Back rub means attending the back and pressure points of body with special care it is often called as back care or back massage **(Fig. 15.12)**.

Purpose

- To give comfort to the patient.
- To stimulate blood circulation.
- To promote rest and sleep.
- To prevent pressure sores.
- To assess the skin condition.
- To relax and relieve tension in tissues and muscles.
- To refresh patient and relieve fatigue.

Hygiene

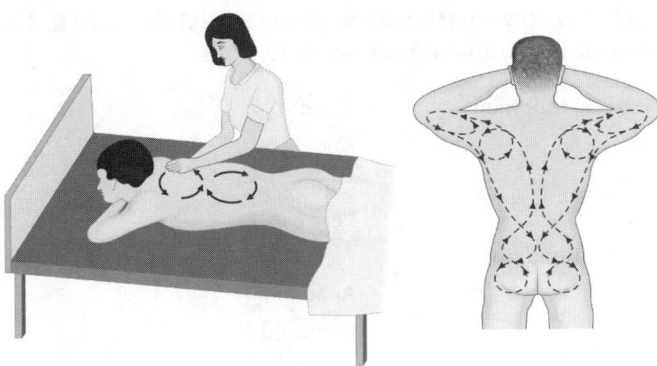

Fig. 15.12: Back rub/back massage.

General Instructions

- Back care given as a part of morning care and evening care.
- Pressure points are attended more frequently and the position is changed.
- When the skin is greasy, moist, thin about to break or patient is in continent or edematous used spirit or powder to reduce friction.
- When the skin is dry, use oil for back rub. Spirit toughens the skin and powder reduces friction oil lubricates the skin and, hence, reduces friction.
- When giving back rub, use more pressure on upward strokes towards the head and less pressure on the downward stokes.
- Back rub may be contraindicated in patients susceptible to clotting disorders.

Equipment

A tray containing of
- A basin of warm water.
- Sponge cloths-2
- Soap and towel.
- Surgical spirit or back-rub lotion and powder.
- Mackintosh and towel.
- Kidney tray and paper bag.

Procedure

- Wash hands and explain the procedure.
- Screen the patient and explain the procedure.
- Turn the patient on his side.
- Turn back top bedding and expose only required part.
- Spread towel close to the patients back to protect bed linen.
- Wash back thoroughly from cervical spine to the coccyx.
- Apply soap in the same manner. Run hands firmly and slowly up the back on either side of the vertebral column up the neck and down across the shoulders.
- Pour some spirit in to hand applies firmly in a circular motion repeat until back is thoroughly rubbed with it.
- Wash off soap and dry thoroughly with towel.

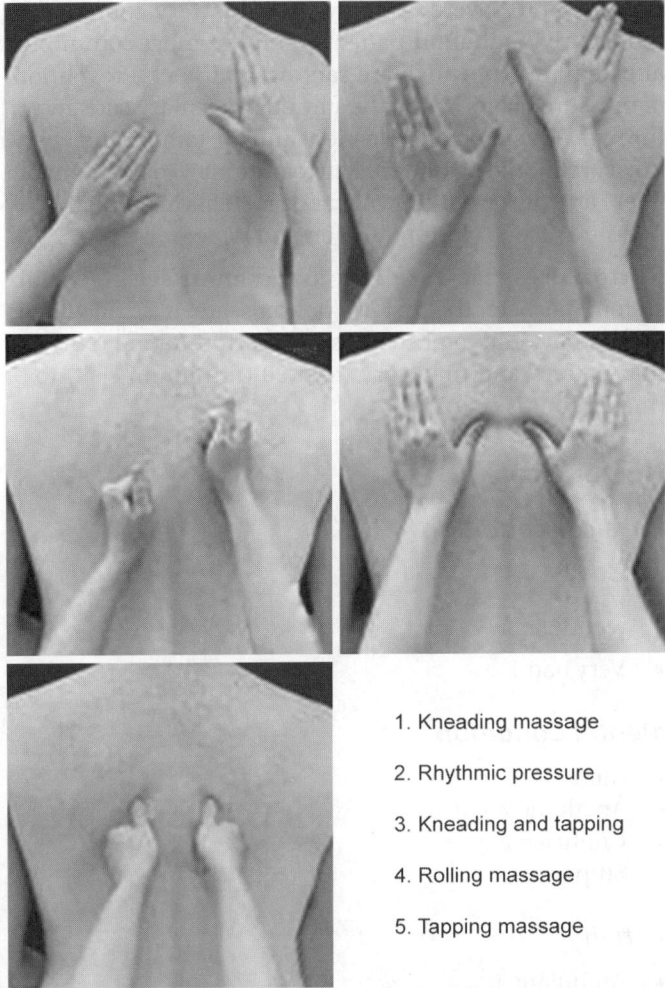

1. Kneading massage
2. Rhythmic pressure
3. Kneading and tapping
4. Rolling massage
5. Tapping massage

Fig. 15.13: Steps of back rub techniques.

- The back must be rubbed three to five minutes especially over pressure points.
- Apply talcum powder on the back on dry skin.
- Remove the towel.
- Cover the patient with top bedding.

Aftercare

- Make the patient comfortable.
- Remove the screen and equipment.
- Clean the articles with soap and water and keep ready for next use.
- Wash hands.
- Record the date, time treatment and observation made on nurse's record.

ASSESSMENT OF PRESSURE ULCERS USING BRADEN SCALE AND NORTON SCALE

Pressure ulcer (decubitus, bedsore) is defined as localized injury to the skin or underlying tissue over a bony prominence as a result of pressure with friction and shear. Clinical presentation can vary from simple reactive hyperemia to severe osteomyelitis. It is very common in the elderly bedbound patients, and the most commonly affected body portions are sacrum and heel. Prevention of pressure ulcers should be started by primary care givers through education of the patient and the family, and every measure should be undertaken to prevent its development. There are three well-known scaling systems in prediction of pressure ulcers: Norton, Braden and Water low.

Norton pressure sore risk assessment scale scoring system has been the first evaluation scale. It is still widely used today. The total score is the Norton Rating (NR) for that patient and may vary from 20 (minimum risk) to 5 (maximum risk).

Norton Scale

Physical Condition

- Good 4
- Fair 3
- Poor 2
- Very bad 1

Mental Condition

- Alert 4
- Apathetic 3
- Confused 2
- Stuporous 1

Activity

- Ambulant 4
- Walks with help 3
- Chair bound 2
- Bedfast 1

Mobility

- Full 4
- Slightly impaired 3
- Very limited 2
- Immobile 1

Incontinence

- None 4
- Occasional 3
- Usually urinary 2
- Urinary and fecal 1

Braden Scale Risk Factors

- Sensory/perception
- Moisture
- Activity
- Mobility
- Nutrition
- Friction/shear

NR below 9: Very High Risk, 10 to 13: High Risk, 14 to 17: Medium risk, above 18: Low risk.

Psysical condition	Good	4
	Fair	3
	Poor	2
	Very bad	1
Mental condition	Alert	4
	Apathetic	3
	Confused	2
	Stuporous	1
Activity	Ambulant	4
	Walks with help	3
	Chairbound	2
	Bedfast	1
Mobility	Full	4
	Slightly impaired	3
	Very limited	2
	Immobile	1
Incontinence	None	4
	Occasional	3
	Usually urinary	2
	Urinary and fecal	1
Greater than 18	Low risk	
Between 18 and 14	Medium risk	
Between 14 and 10	High risk	
Lesser than 10	Very high risk	

Another rating system getting more and more popularity is Braden Scale, more recent and precise than the Norton scale, which evaluates factors such as sensory perception, skin wetness and nutrition status.

Braden Scale

Sensory Perception

- No impairment 4
- Slightly limited 3
- Very limited 2
- Completely limited 1

Moisture

- Rarely moist 4
- Occasionally moist 3
- Very moist 2
- Constantly moist 1

Activity

- Walks frequently 4
- Walks occasionally 3
- Chairfast 2
- Bedfast 1

Mobility
- No limitation 4
- Slightly limited 3
- Very limited 2
- Completely immobile 1

Nutrition
- Excellent 4
- Adequate 3
- Probably inadequate 2
- Very poor 1

Friction and shear
- No apparent problem 3
- Potential problem 2
- Problem 1

Braden score greater than 18: Low risk, between 18 and 14: Medium risk, between 14 and 10: High risk, lesser than 10: Very high risk

Weight/Size relationship:	Skin type and visual aspect of risk areas:	Sex/Age:	Special risk
0. Standard	0. Health	1. Male	Tissue malnutrition:
1. Above standards	1. Frail	2. Female	8. Terminal/cachexia
2. Obese	1. Dry	1. 14–49 years	5. Cardiac insufficiency
3. Below standards	2. Edematous	2. 50–64 years	6. Peripheral vascular insufficiency
	1. Cold and hemid	3. 65–74 years	2. Anemia
	2. Alterations in color	4. 75–80 years	1. Smoker
	3. Wounded	5. Over 81 years	
Continence:	**Mobility:**	**Appetite:**	**Neurological deficit:**
0. Complete, urine catheter	0. Complete	0. Normal	5. Diabetes, paraplegic, ACV
1. Ocasional incontinence	1. Restless	1. Scarce/feeding tube	**Surgery:**
2. Urine catheter fecal incontinence	2. Apathy	2. Liquid intravenous	5. Orthopedic surgery below waist
	3. Restricted	3. Anorexia/Absolute diet	5. Over 2 hours in surgery
3. Double incontinence	4. Inert		**Medication:**
	5. On chair		4. Steroids, cytotoxics, antiinflammatory drugs in elevated dosage

Scoring: Over 10 points: at risk. Over 16 points: high risk, Over 20 points: very high risk.
Source: Waterlow."

Braden scale: How to Score Risk Factors
- Score risk factors from 1 to 4 except—score friction/shear from 1 to 3.
- Risk factor score of 1 is the lowest level of functioning.
- If a category falls between two numbers, choose the lower score.

How to Interpret Braden Score
- Total score ranges from 6 to 23.
- Lower Braden score indicates higher level of risk for pressure ulcer development.
- In most cases, a score of 18 or less indicates at-risk status. Tailor this number to fit your hospital or unit.
- Low subscale score indicates risk from that factor. Address all deficits in care planning.

Limits of Risk Scores
Some assessment tools include a scoring system to predict pressure ulcer risk:
- No tool has perfect predictability.
- Even patients with a low risk score may need intervention.
- If you base a patient's individualized care plan on the risk score alone, the care plan will not be tailored to all of his or her risk factors.
- Instead, use a comprehensive approach to risk assessment to identify pressure ulcer risk factors.

Lastly, Waterlow scale evaluates multiple factors, and has the risk of over-assessment. Pressure ulcer aspect has been discussed adequately amongst nurses. However, the treating surgeons should also be well aware of the various risk factors and the risk assessment scales.

CARE OF PRESSURE POINTS/BEDSORE

A bed sore or pressure sore decubitus ulcer is an ulcer occurring on the skin of any bedridden patient, particularly over bony prominences or where two skin surfaces press against each other.

Bed sore is the term applied to the local gangrene or ulcer caused by certain conditions associated with the confinement of bed. Due to constant pressure circulation becomes slow and finally death of tissues occurs.

Purpose
- To improve circulation.
- To facilitate healing.
- To prevent infection.
- To prevent further damage.
- To treat bedsores.

Cause of Pressure Sores

- **Direct or immediate cause:** The pressure is caused by the weight of the body continuously remaining in one position, splints, casts and bandages.
- **Friction:** Friction of the skin with rough bedding causes injury to the skin. The friction is caused by wrinkles in the bed cloths, cramps of food in the bed, chipped or rough bed pans and hard surfaces of plaster casts and splints.
- **Moisture:** The skin contact with moisture for a prolong period can lead maceration of the skin.
- **Pressure of pathogenic organisms** due to unhygienic condition pathogenic organic multiplies and infection settles on the skin.

Predisposing Factors

- Patient with long term illness, fracture patients.
- Patients with spinal injury.
- Paralysis and limited movements.
- Emaciated and malnourished patients.
- Elderly with circulatory problems.
- Obese patients.
- Edematous patients.
- Patients with incontinence.
- Diabetic patients with ulcers (diabetic foot).

Common Sites Liable to get Bed Sore

- **In supine position:** Occiput, scapula, sacral region, hips and elbow.
- **In side lying position:** Ears, acromian process of shoulder, ribs, greater trochanter of hips medial and lateral condyles of knee and maleolus of ankle joint..
- **In prone position:** Ears cheeks acromian process, breast in female genitalia, knees and toes.

Clinical Manifestation of Pressure Sore

- Redness, heat, tenderness, and discomfort in the area.
- The area becomes cold to touch and insensitive.
- Local edema.
- Later, the area becomes blue, purple of mottled.

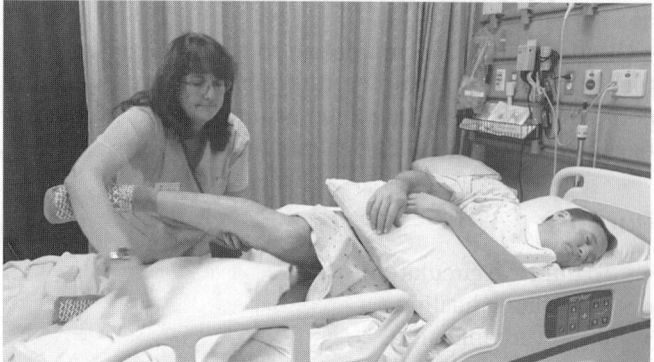

Fig. 15.14: Position changing every 2 hours for unconscious patient.

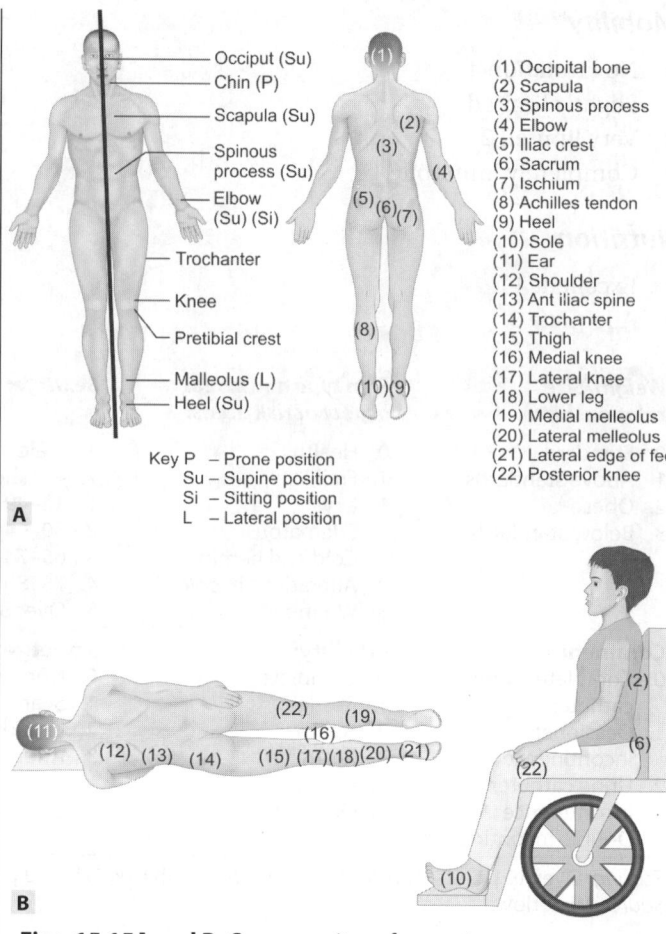

Figs. 15.15A and B: Common sites of occurring pressures sores.

- Due to continued pressure that circulation is cut off, the gangrene develops and affected area is sloughed.

Preventive Measure of Bed Sore

- Confirm the high risk patients and daily examination for the signs and symptoms.
- Relieve pressure by using special mattress, beds and comfort devices.
- Change position and giving back care four times a day for all bedridden patients.
- Loosening tight bandages and restraints.
- Avoid friction by providing smooth, firm and wrinkle free bed, keep the bottom clothes free from crumbs and foreign bodies.
- Prevent moisture by changing linen when, it is wet or soiled. Giving back care to patients immediately following micturation and defecation.
- Avoid mechanical or physical injury to the skin from improper fitting of prosthesis or from burns caused by excessively hot or cold applications.
- Use a bed cradle to lift the weight of bed linen off the patient to enable him or her to move in bed freely.
- Supply well balanced diet and adequate fluids to maintain general health of the patient.

Stages/Degree of Pressure Sore Based on

Clinical Manifestations

First degree: The skin is red, tender, inflamed and painful.

Second degree: The skin is blue or mottled insensitive, circulation cut off, gangrene develops and epidermis breaks.

Third degree: Suppuration and sloughing occurs which may burrow right down to the bones.

Curative Measures Based on Degrees of Pressure Sore

First degree: Detect the early signs and symptoms of bedsore and report them to the sister in charge and the doctor. Carry out all the preventive measure with special care to prevent extension of bedsore and further occurrence of pressure sores. While giving back care/massage, do not over the reddened or inflamed area itself but start just outside the affected area and move outwards in a circle using circular motion.

Second degree: If the pressure sore is blue or mottled insensitive, circulation cut, off gangrene develops or epidermis breaks.

The treatment included
- Inform and report to the ward sister and physician.
- Prevent the ulcerated area from infection.
- Use normal saline for cleaning the area.
- Sloughing is more; use hydrogen peroxide solution also for cleaning, cut off the slough.
- Apply heat for healing of the wound. Use 100 watt electric bulb for l0 mts.
- Apply zinc oxide ointment on the surface of the wound.

Third degree: If the bed sore is suppuration and sloughing occurs which may burrow right down to the bones.
- Inform and report to the ward sister and physician.
- To treat infection, apply soframycine ointment locally and give systematic antibiotics after culture and sensitivity.
- Provide nutritious diet (high in protein and vitamins) sunlight and fresh air.
- If slough is present, clean the wound with hydrogen peroxide twice daily if the slough is loose, it may be cut off.
- If there is delay in wound healing, skin grafting can be done.

Aftercare

- Place the patient in comfortable position.
- Use proper and adequate comfort devices.
- Change the patient's position at frequent intervals.
- Remove the articles from the bedside and replace it in a proper place.
- Hand washing.
- Recording and reporting-date time, type of pressure sore and treatment in the nurses record.

CARE OF HAIR

Care of hair means maintaining cleanliness of hair, i.e. free from dandruff, dirt, nits, lice, flakes, dryness and irritation.

Purpose

- To keep hair clean and healthy.
- To promote growth of hair.
- To have a neat and tidy appearance.
- To prevent itching, infection, dandruff, lice, flakes, dryness and irritation.
- To prevent loss of hair.
- To prevent accumulation of dirt.
- To stimulate circulation.
- To prevent tangles.
- To promote comfort.
- To have a sense of well-being.

Three Aspects of Hair Care

- Daily care by brushing and combing.
- Head bath in order to maintain to cleanliness.
- Treatment of hair for lice infestation.

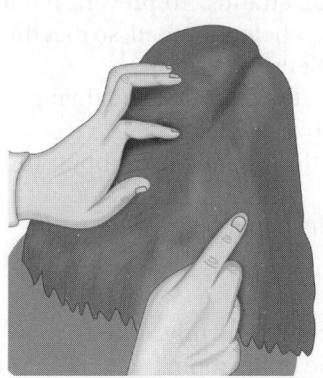 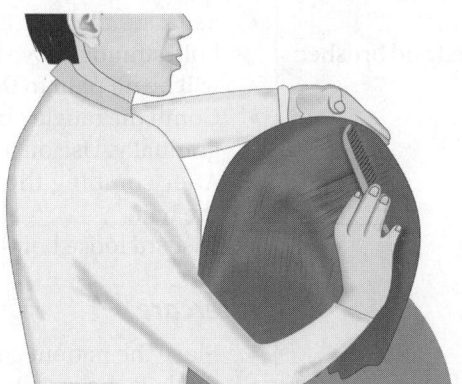 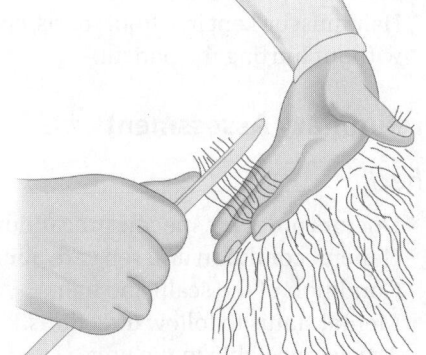

Fig. 15.16: Hair care.

Factors Influence on Hair

- General health of a person.
- A well balanced diet.
- Light and fresh air.
- Daily practices (hair wash and combing).
- Hair brushing and massage.
- Endocrine disorder.

Factors Affecting Hair

- Altered level of consciousness.
- Physical weakness or disease condition.
- Immobility and ageing.
- Insect bite and infestations.
- Accumulated secretions.
- Hormonal changes.
- Physical and emotional stress.
- Poor health practices.
- Effects on drug.

Common Hair Scalp Problems

- Dandruff: Sealing of scalp accompanied by itching.
- Pediculosis: Lice infestation.
- Alopecia: Hair loss.
- Tangled and matted hair.
- Dryness.
- Flakes.
- Irritation.

HAIR COMBING

The hair can be combed and washed in the morning so that the patient can feel refreshed and appear well groomed before starting daily activities.

General Instructions

- Hair needs to be brushed daily in order to be healthy.
- Long hair should be combed at least once a day to prevent if from matting.
- Teeth of the comb should be dull to prevent scratching of the scalp.
- Hair must be kept free from snarls, combed and brushed without hurting the patient.

Preliminary Assessment

Check

- Doctors order for specific precautions.
- General condition and self care ability.
- Condition of the scalp and hair.
- Mental status to follow directions.
- Articles available in the unit.

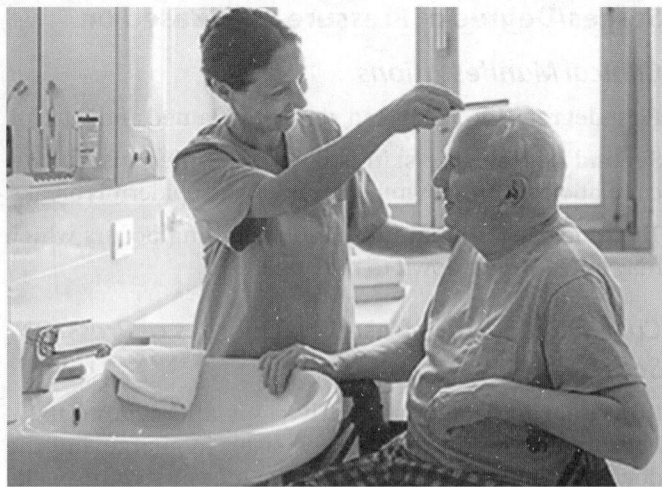

Fig. 15.17: Maintain grooming by combing.

Preparation of the Patient and Environment

- Explain the procedure.
- Arrange the article at the bedside.
- Provide privacy and adequate light.
- Make the patient to sit on a bedside chair or stool.
- Protect the bottom sheet and pillow case with a towel.
- Protect the nurse's uniform by wearing aprons.

Equipment

- Clean comb.
- Mackintosh and towel.
- Coconut oil in a container.
- Kidney tray and paper bag.
- Kidney tray with carbolic lotion 1:20 to destroy the lice and to disinfect the comb.

Procedure

- Wash hands and take required articles at bedside.
- If possible as patient to sit on a stool otherwise side-lying or Fowler's position.
- Place the Mackintosh under the head of the patient.
- Each half of the hair is treated separately without causing strain on the patient.
- Separate the hair in small strands. To prevent pulling hold strands above the part being combed, so that there will be no pain to the patient.
- Comb the tangle out from the ends first and then go up gradually. Use oil to remove tangles.
- After combing the hair thoroughly, use ribben to tie the hair.
- Discard loose hair into the paper bag.

Aftercare

- Place the patient comfortable and tidy.
- Replace the articles to the utility room.

- Wash hands thoroughly.
- Record and report the procedure in nurse's record sheet.

HAIR WASH/BED SHAMPOO

Hair wash/Bed shampoo is a special care of the hair may be required for patients who are in bed for a prolonged period of time.

Shampooing the hair should be performed whenever the hair and scalp are dirty.

Purpose

- To keep hair and scalp clean and healthy.
- To promotes sense of comfort and self-esteem.
- To complete the treatment of pediculi.

General Instructions

- The patients are given hair wash at least once a week for bedridden patients.
- Avoid hair wash for patients who have just taken meals at least for an hour.
- Avoid exposure and chilling by keeping the patient covered with top clothes.
- If the patients are very sick, note pulse before and after the hair wash.
- Do not let the patient exert and try to avoid exertion to the patient as far as possible.

Preliminary Assessment

Check

- Doctors order for specific precautions.
- General condition for the patient.
- Self-care ability.
- Patients preference for soap, shampoo, oil, etc.
- Patients mental state to follow instructions.
- Availabilities of ward article.

Preparation of the Patient and Environment

- Explain the procedure.
- Arrange the articles at the bedside.
- Provide privacy.
- Position the patient (flat) comfortably to the edge of the bed (if condition permits).
- Remove the extra pillows and back rest.
- Make an improvised through (Kelley's pad) and place it under the hand to facilitate the drainage of water in to receptacle.
- Place the bucket on the low stool close to the side of the bed. The distal end of the Mackintosh (trough) is received in to it.
- Plug the ear with cotton balls.

Equipment

- A tray contains bath towels—2.
- Face towel—1.
- Long Mackintosh—1.
- Cotton swabs—2.
- Liquid soap or shampoo.
- Hair comb.
- Kidney tray.
- Paper bag and news paper.
- Bucket—1.
- Mug—1.
- Jugs—2 (hot and cold water).
- Safety pins.

Procedure

- Wash hands thoroughly.
- Provide privacy and remove extra pillows and blanket.
- Unless contraindicated move the patients head and shoulder to the edge of the bed.

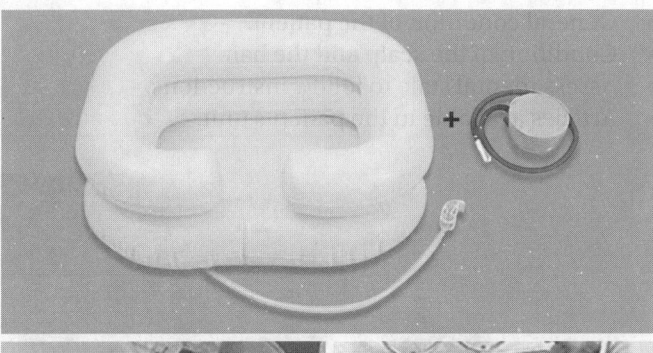
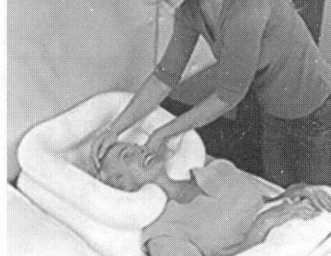
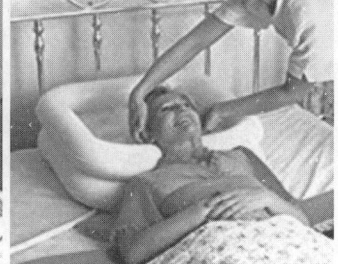

Fig. 15.18: Hair washing for bed ridden patient.

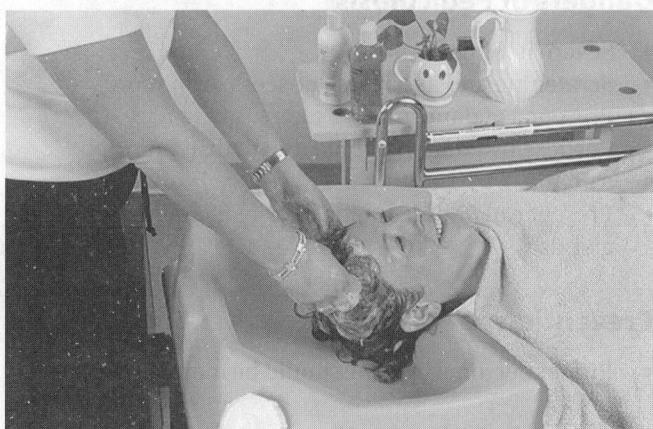

Fig. 15.19: Hair shampoo in technique.

- Place the Mackintosh under patients shoulder keeping the head down Mackintosh should form a trough to carry dirt water into the bucket.
- Plug the ears with cotton balls.
- Place towel around patients shoulder and pin securely at the neck.
- Mix hot and cold water at 100°F and wet the hair.
- Apply soap solution, rubbing well into scalp using the tips of fingers.
- Rinse it thoroughly and repeat the same until the hair is clean. Squeeze off water from the hair.
- Dry with towel, dry the face with face towel removes the trough and place it in basin. Discard the cotton swabs used in the ears into the paper bag.

Aftercare

- Place the patient in comfortable position.
- Dry the hair, comb and arrange hair when completely dry.
- Change linen if wet.
- Replace the articles into utility room.
- Wash hands thoroughly.
- Record and reporting the procedure in nurses record street.

PEDICULOSIS TREATMENT

Pediculosis is defined as the state of being infected with lice. Pediculi or lice is a small blood sucking parasite.

It is associated with poor personal hygiene. It can be acquired in overcrowded, unsanitary conditions and exposure to infected persons.

Purpose

- To destroy pediculi and nits.
- To prevent its transmission to other.
- To promote comfort.
- To promote sense of well being.

Dangers of Pediculosis

- Severe itching.
- Scratching and as a result, abscess formation.
- Presence of dandruff.
- Restlessness and insomnia due to discomfort.
- Anemia.
- Presence of nodules at the back of head due to infected glands.

Prevention of Pediculosis

- Proper personal hygiene should be maintained by every person.
- Daily hair combing and frequently washing it.
- If the patient complains of itching or scratches the head, examine hair and scalp thoroughly.

Medications Used for Pediculosis Treatment

- DDT powder one part to nine part of talcum powder.
- Kerosene mixed with equal parts of sweet oil destroys both lice and nits.
- Carbolic lotion 1:40.
- Readily available lysol.
- Preparations containing gamma benzene hexachloride available in the market and can be used according to the instruction on the label.

Types of Pediculi

- Pediculus capitis: Which infest the head.
- Pediculus corporis: Which infest the body and is found with its flits in the clothing.
- Pediculus pubis: This infests the axillary and pubic hair, the eyebrows and sometimes the eyelashes.

General Instructions

- The parasiticides are applied thoroughly on the scalp (to the body if necessary) and is left for overnight.
- On the next day a thorough bath is given and the linen is changed.
- The linen should be thoroughly disinfected to remove the lice from the cloths.
- Since the parasiticides are not effective against the nits (eggs) the procedure is repeated after a week.

Preliminary Assessment

Check

- Doctors order for specific precautions.
- General condition of the patient.
- Condition of the scalp and the hair.
- Assess mental stale to follow instructions.
- Articles available in the patients unit.

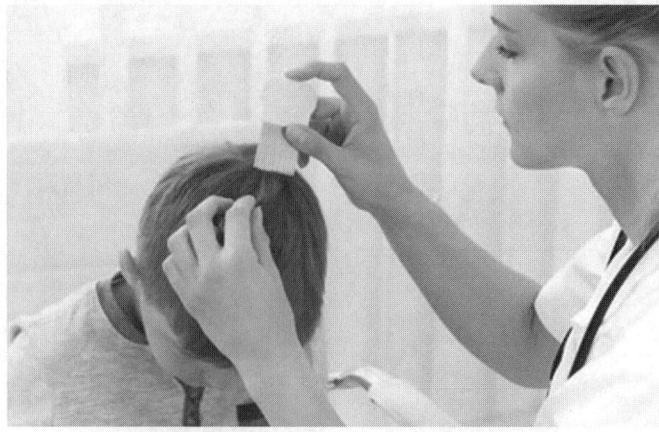

Fig. 15.20: Pediculosis treatment.

Equipment

A tray containing:
- Mackintosh—1.
- Bath towels—2.
- Wash cloth—1.
- A cap, a triangular bandage or a towel folded diagonally.
- Safety pins.
- Kidney tray with disinfectant, e.g. carbolic acid 1:40.
- Paper bag.
- Hair comb.
- Cotton swabs or gauze piece in a container.
- Vaseline.
- Gown mask and cap.
- Bucket with antiseptic solution, e.g. carbolic acid 5 percent.

Preparation of the Patient and the Unit

- Explain the sequence of procedure.
- Provide privacy by means of screens.
- Arrange the articles conveniently on the bedside.
- Place the patient flat if the condition permits.
- Bring the patients head and shoulder to the edge of the bed.
- Protect the pillow and bed with a mackintosh and a towel.
- Protect the patient's eyes with a clean damp wash cloth.
- Put off the fan to prevent the parasiticide spilling over the face during its application.
- Loosen the hair and comb out the tangles.

Procedure

- Wash hands thoroughly.
- Put on gown, mask and cap.
- Part the hair into small sections and apply the parasiticide on the hair and scalp, rubbing gently.
- In long hairs, the medicine is to be applied along the whole length of the hair.
- Roll up the long hair to the top of the head and cover the head with cap or triangular bandage or by a towel folded diagonally secure it with pins.

Note: The treatment is done in the evening and left over night.

Aftercare

- Remove the Mackintosh and towels from under the patients head.
- Tidy up the bed; place the patient in a comfortable position.
- Remove the gown, mask and cap and put them into the antiseptic lotion.
- Replace the articles in their proper place after clean and disinfect.
- Record and report the procedure in the nurses record sheet.
- The hair is washed in the following morning.
- Comb the hair with a fine toothed comb.
- Repeat the procedure after one week because the nits are not affected by the parasiticides.
- Disinfect all the articles that have come in contact with the hair by immersing them in carbolic acid 1:20 for one hour before washing.

CARE OF THE PERINEUM

Perineal care defined as clean the perineum from the cleanest to the less clean area, the urethral orifice to the anal orifice.

Perineal care includes the external genitalia and surrounding area. During perineal care, clean the area around the urinary meatus before cleaning the area around the anus.

Purpose

- To prevent sepsis.
- To remove discharges and prevent bad odor.
- To relieve itching.
- To promote healing of stitches.
- To promote comfort.

Perineum Care for Special Group of Patients

- Unable to do self-care or bedridden patients.
- After surgery on the genitourinary system.
- Patients with indwelling catheters.
- Patients with excessive vaginal discharges.
- Postpartum patients.
- Incontinence of urine and stool.
- Genitourinary tract infections.

Preliminary Assessment

Check

- Doctors order for any specific instruction.
- Assess the condition of the perineal skin-itching, irritation, ulcers, edema, drainage, etc.
- Assess the need and frequency of care.
- Assess the self-care ability of the patient.
- Mental state to follow instructions.
- Articles available in the patients unit.

Preparation of the Patient and the Environment

- Explain the sequence of the procedure.
- Provide privacy.
- Arranged the needed articles at the bed side.
- Place the Mackintosh under the buttocks, over the draw sheet.
- Place a clean bedpan on the bed on your working side.
- Unite the pads-if any, and observe the discharges its color, odor, amount, etc.

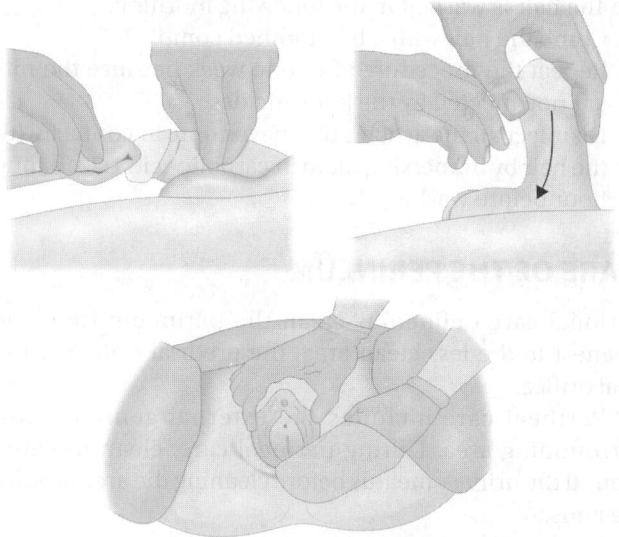

Fig. 15.21: Perineal care.

Equipment

A tray containing
- Mackintosh.
- A jug with warm water or antiseptic solution.
- Wet cotton balls or rag pieces in a bowl.
- Gauze or rag pieces in a container.
- Long artery forceps in the kidney tray.
- Paper bag.
- Clean (personal and bed linen) dressing pads, etc. as needed.
- Soap, soap dish, towel and wash cloth of the patient is able to do himself.
- Bed pan.

Procedure

- Wash hands thoroughly to prevent cross infection.
- Pour water over the perineum to wash off the discharges from the perineal area **(Fig. 15.21)**.
- Hold the swabs with forceps and clean from above downwards towards the anal canal.
  - Use one swab for one swabbing.
  - Clean the perineum from the mid line outward in the following order: The vulva, the labia minora on both sides, inside of the labia majora on both sides and the outside of the labia majora on both sides (start cleaning from more clean area to less clean area).
  - Clean the perineal region and the anus thoroughly
- Remove the bed pan by supporting the hip. Turn the patient to one side and dry the buttocks with a dry rag pieces.

Aftercare

- Apply the medicine and pad if necessary.
- Remove the Mackintosh if an extra one is used.
- Change the linen if necessary.
- Provide comfortable position to the patient.
- Clean the articles and replace it in a proper place.
- Wash hands thoroughly.
- Record and report the procedure in a nurses record sheet.

CLOTHING

In choosing clothes, the followings points should be considered durability, comfort and cheapness. Moreover they should be easily washable, attractive in appearance and simple. The choice of materials for clothes is important. Light weight, loosely woven materials are bad conductors of heat and so are used to conserve the body heat.

Cotton is good in warm weather as it easily absorbs perspiration and quickly dries, so cooling the body. It is reasonably inexpensive and easy to wash. The choice of colors for clothing is important. White and light colors are cool whereas darker colors particularly red and black are warm.

The design of clothes is also important. They should be well fitting easy to put on and take off.

Any necessary elastic should be sufficiently wide to be comfortable and not too tight. Underclothing should be frequently changed. Boys and girls as they grow older should learn to choose their own clothes, should be allowed to develop their own styles and use colors to suit their own personalities.

The most effective teaching is done by teachers and parents who should set a good example. Damp clothes whether wet from rain or perspiration should be changed immediately to prevent excessive chilling of the body.

CARE OF DENTURES

Care of dentures of artificial teeth is the responsibility of the nurse to guard against offending patient, by helping them to take care of their mouth.

Equipment Needed

- Soft bristled tooth brush.
- Denture tooth brush.

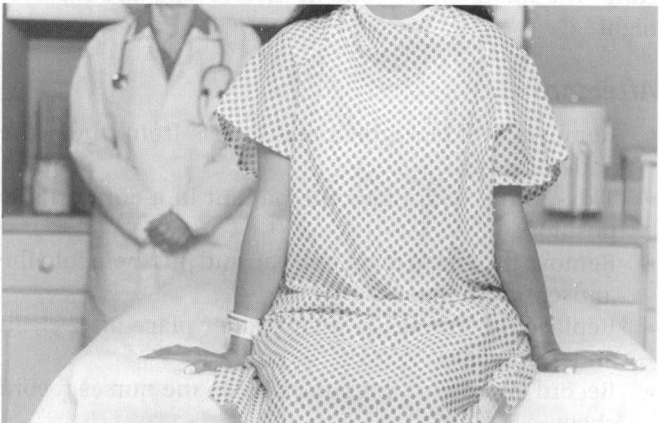

Fig. 15.22: Proving hospital gown to the patient.

- Dentifrice.
- Warm and cold water in glasses.
- Gauze pieces.
- Wash cloth.
- Plastic denture cup.
- Gloves.
- Basin.

Procedure

- Explain and secure the cooperation of the patient.
- Remove the denture and inspect the oral cavity for abnormalities if any.
- Wash hands and keep the articles near the bed side sink.
- Take a basin and fill half of it with water.
- Put on gloves to reduce transmission of infection.
- Ask the patient to remove dentures and place them in the basin.
- Brush the dentures. Use back and front motion. Clean inside and outside by brushing.
- Rinse dentures thoroughly in running water.
- Return them to the patient to keep them in a denture cup in cold water.
- With a soft bristled tooth brush the gum with tooth paste as well as the palate of tongue also.
- Rinse the mouth thoroughly with cold water.
- Wipe the face and make the patient comfortable.
- Replace the used articles and record the procedure.

Precautions

- In cleaning dentures, they should be held firmly as water reduces friction between the teeth and finger. They are liable to slip and fall down.
- Denture should be dipped in cold water to prevent friction.
- Hot water may destroy dentures, dentures are expensive and maybe difficult to replace if broken or lost.
- Privacy should be maintained.

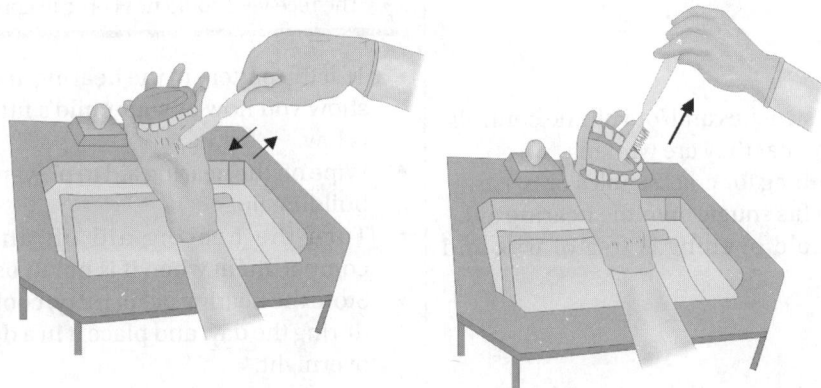

Fig. 15.23: Dentures cleaning procedure.

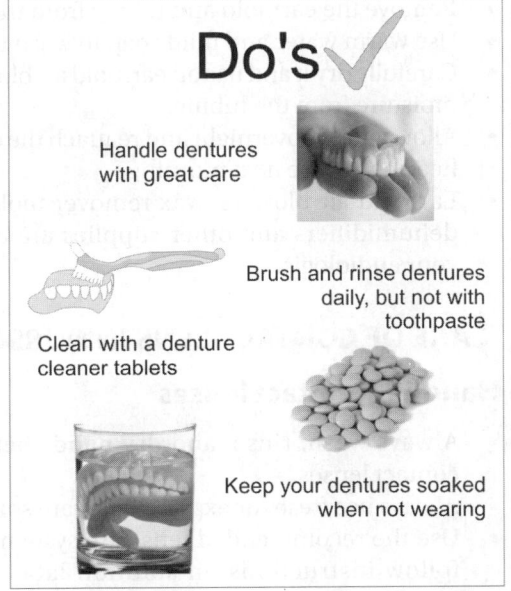
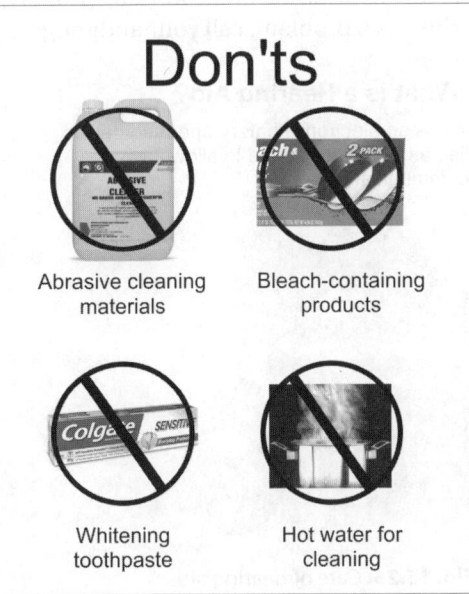

Fig. 15.24: Do's and don'ts in denture care.

- Discourage the use of brushed with hard bristles because they cause grooves in dentures.
- If the patient is capable of self-care, arrange the articles within the easy reach of the patient.
- Encourage the patients to wear the denture during the day. This will improve the eating technique, speech appearance and contour of the mouth.
- Seriously ill patient or a patient who is under anesthesia or an unconscious patient, the denture is removed for fear of dislodging the denture and blocking the respiratory passage.
- When dentures are removed from the patient's mouth, they should be stored in a labeled container to prevent lost and breakage.

CARE OF HEARING AID IN NURSING

Hearing aids are delicate instruments that need attention to ensure good operation. Before you put the hearing aid on your child, you should give it a quick visual inspection and listening check. Here is a checklist you should follow every day:

Visual Inspection

- If the hearing aid has switches and/or volume controls, check them to be sure that they are working.
- Check the earmold tubing for cracks, holes or twists.
- Make sure the tubing fits snugly onto the hearing aid.
- Make sure the earmold opening is free of wax and moisture.

Listening Check

A parent or caregiver must listen to the hearing aid every day before putting the hearing aid in the child's ear. Listen for static or crackling sounds. By doing this daily check, you will notice right away if the hearing aid is not working properly. If you think that there is a problem, call your audiologist.

What is a Hearing Aid?

- A hearing aid is an electronic, batery-operated device that amplifies and changes sound to allow for improved communication

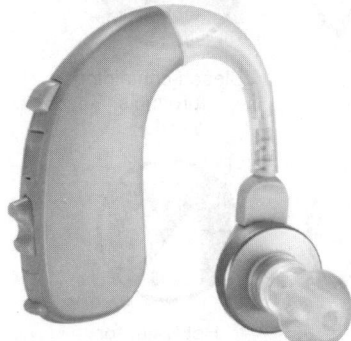

Fig. 15.25: Care of hearing aids.

Cleaning Hearing Aids and Earmolds

To keep your child's hearing aids and earmolds working well, you must keep them clean and store them safely.

Daily Care

- Wipe off the earmold with a soft tissue or cloth each time it is removed from the ear.
- Check the opening for earwax build-up. If wax is present, gently remove it with a pipe cleaner, tooth pick or wax tool. Do not poke the earmold with sharp objects. Keeping the earmold clean will usually prevent wax from building up.

Care and maintenance of hearing aids
- Prevent it from falling down
- Don't spill liquids on the hearing aids
- The hearing aids should be fitted well
- Cords should not be twisted or knotted
- Protect it from dust, dirt and heat
- Remove the battery from hearing aids when it is not in use
- The receiver should not come in contact with water

- Test the battery in the hearing aid (your audiologist will show you how at your child's fitting) and change it if it is low.
- Wipe off the hearing aid to prevent dirt or moisture from building up.
- Turn the hearing aid off and open the battery compartment when it is not in use.
- Store the hearing aid in a dry, cool place when not in use during the day, and place it in a dry-aid or dehumidifier overnight.

Weekly or as Needed Care

- Wash the earmold when needed.
- Remove the earmold and tubing from the hearing aid.
- Use warm water and mild soap to wash the earmold.
- Carefully dry it and use an earmold air blower to remove moisture from the tubing.
- Allow it to dry overnight and reattach the earmold to the hearing aid the next morning,
- Earmold air blowers, wax remover tools, hearing aid dehumidifiers and other supplies are available from your audiologist.

CARE OF CONTACT LENS IN NURSING

Handling contact lenses

- Always wash, rinse, and dry hands before handling contact lenses.
- Always use fresh, unexpired lens care solutions.
- Use the recommended lens care system and carefully follow instructions on solution labeling. Different

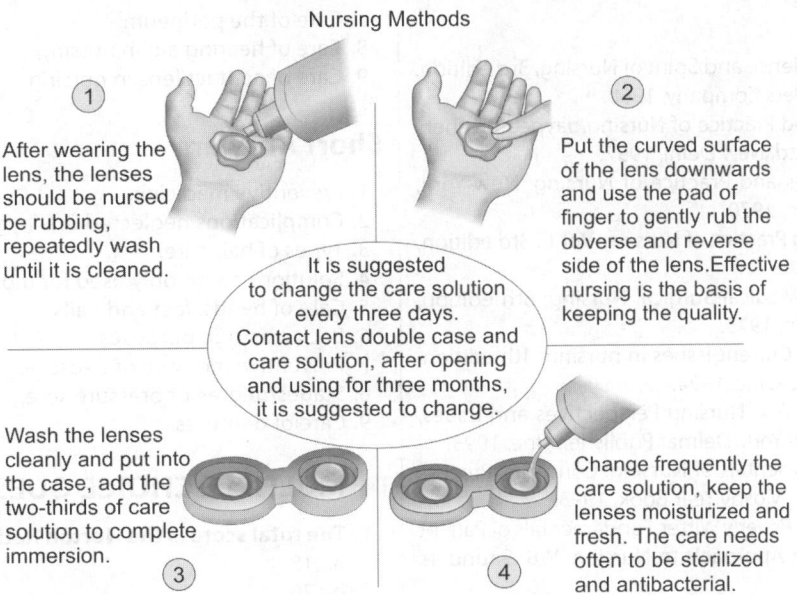

Fig. 15.26: Care of contact lens.

solutions cannot always be used together, and not all solutions are safe for use with all lenses. Do not alternate or mix lens care systems unless indicated on solution labeling.
- Always remove, clean, rinse, enzyme and disinfect your lenses according to the schedule prescribed by your eye care professional. The use of an enzyme or any cleaning solution does not substitute for disinfection.
- Do not use saliva or anything other than the recommended solutions for lubricating or rewetting your lenses. Do not put lenses in your mouth.
- Lenses prescribed in a frequent replacement program should be thrown away after the expiration of the wearing period prescribed by your eye care professional.
- Never rinse your lenses in water from the tap. There are two reasons for this:
  1. Tap water contains many impurities that can contaminate or damage your lenses and may lead to eye infection or injury.
  2. You might lose the lens down the drain.
- Clean one lens first (always the same lens first to avoid mix-ups), rinse the lens thoroughly with recommended saline or disinfecting solution to remove the cleaning solution, mucus, and film from the lens surface. Follow the instructions provided in the cleaning solution labeling. Put that lens into the correct chamber of the lens storage case. Then repeat the procedure for the second lens.
- After cleaning, and rinsing, disinfect lenses using the system recommended by your eye care professional. Follow the instructions provided in the disinfection solution labeling.
- To store lenses, disinfect and leave them in the closed/unopened case until ready to wear. If lenses are not to be used immediately after disinfection, you should consult the labeling of the storage solution for information on lens storage.
- After removing your lenses from the lens case, empty and rinse the lens storage case with solution(s) recommended by the lens case manufacturer; then allow the lens case to air dry. When the case is used again, refill it with fresh storage solution. Replace lens case at regular intervals.

CONCLUSION

Personal hygiene includes all those personal factors which influence the health and well-being of an individual. It consists of the body regarding bathing and washing, care of hair, nails and feet, mouth cleanliness and care of the teeth, care of the nose and ears, clothing, postures, exercises, recreation, rest and relaxation, sleep habits and nutrition. The nurse has to implement the nursing care plan to provide optimum quality of nursing care for the individual patients. The nurse must apply knowledge of pathophysiology to provide good preventive hygienic care. The nurse has to integrate knowledge of anatomy, physiology and pathology during hygienic care.

BIBLIOGRAPHY

1. Price Alice L. The Art, Science and Spirit of Nursing, 3rd edition. Philadelphia. WB Saunders Company, 1968.
2. Birpuri SS. Principles and Practice of Nursing. Jaypee Brothers Medical Publishers (P) Ltd, New Delhi, 1997.
3. Henderson V. Principles and Practice of Nursing. New York, MacMillan Publishing Co, 1970.
4. Sr. Nancy. Principles and Practice of Nursing; Vol 1., 3rd edition, NR Brothers. Indore, 1992.
5. Shafer Kathleen, et al. Medical-Surgical Nursing; 6th edition, Saint Louis. CV Mosby Co, 1975.
6. McClosky JC, Grace HK. Current issues in nursing, 4th edition. St Louis: Mosby Year Book, Inc, 1994.
7. Mitchell PR, Grippando GM. Nursing Perspectives and Issues, 5th edition. Albany, New York: Delmar Publishers, Inc, 1993.
8. Potter P, Perry A. Fundamentals of Nursing: Concepts, Process and Practice 3rd edition. Mosby Year Book, 1993.
9. Kozier Barbara B, Du Gas, Beverly Witter. Fundamentals of Patient Care: A Comprehensive Approach to Nursing; WB. Saunders Company; 1967.
10. Taylor C, Lillis C, LeMone P. Fundamentals of Nursing: The Art and Science of Nursing Care. Philadelphia: J.B. Lippincott, 1993.

REVIEW QUESTIONS

Long Essays

1. Define hygiene; explain the factors and types of hygiene.
2. Define personal hygiene; explain the principles and factors influences of personal hygiene.
3. Define bed bath; explain the purpose, principles and procedure.

Short Essays

1. Importance of personal hygiene.
2. Care of the eyes, nose, and ears.
3. Assessment of pressure ulcers using Norton scale.
4. Care of pressure points/bedsore.
5. Hair wash/bed shampoo.
6. Pediculosis treatment.
7. Care of the perineum.
8. Care of hearing aid in nursing.
9. Care of contact lens in nursing.

Short Answers

1. Preventive medicine.
2. Complications neglected oral hygiene.
3. Types of hair care.
4. Solutions commonly used for mouth wash.
5. Care of hands, feet and nails.
6. Back massage purposes.
7. Preventive measure of bedsore.
8. Stages/degree of pressure sore.
9. Care of dentures.

MULTIPLE CHOICE QUESTIONS

1. **The total score is the Norton Rating (NR) is:**
   a. 15
   b. 20
   c. 25
   d. 30
2. **Cause of pressure sores are the following, *except*:**
   a. Fracture
   b. Friction
   c. Moisture
   d. Pressure of pathogenic organisms
3. **Purpose of bed shampoo is:**
   a. To keep hair and scalp clean and healthy
   b. To promotes sense of comfort and self-esteem
   c. To complete the treatment of pediculi
   d. All of the above
4. **Dangers of pediculosis is:**
   a. Severe itching
   b. Scratching and as a result, abscess formation
   c. Presence of dandruff
   d. All of the above
5. **Purpose of perineal care includes the following, *except*:**
   a. To prevent sepsis
   b. To promote sex
   c. To remove discharges and prevent bad odor
   d. To relieve itching

ANSWERS

1. b   2. a   3. d   4. d   5. b

CHAPTER 16
Nursing Process

LEARNING OBJECTIVES

- Critical thinking competencies, attitudes for critical thinking, levels of critical thinking in nursing
- Nursing process overview
- **Assessment:**
  - Collection of data—types, sources, and methods
  - Organizing data
  - Validating data
  - Documenting data
- **Nursing diagnosis**
  - Identification of client problems, risks and strengths;
  - Nursing diagnosis statement—parts, types, formulating
  - Guidelines for formulating nursing diagnosis,
- NANDA approved diagnosis
- Difference between medical and nursing diagnosis
- **Planning:** The planning stage is where goals and outcomes are formulated that directly impact patient care. These patient-specific goals and the attainment of such assist in ensuring a positive outcome. Nursing care plans are essential in this phase of goal setting. Care plans provide a course of direction for personalized care tailored to an individual's unique needs.
- **Implementation:**
  - Process of implementing the plan of care
  - Types of care—direct and indirect
- **Evaluation:** Evaluation process, documentation and reporting

TERMINOLOGY

Nursing process: Nursing process is a systematic, rational method of planning and providing individualized nursing care.

Nursing diagnosis: A nursing diagnosis is a clinical judgment concerning a human response to health conditions/life processes, or vulnerability for that response, by an individual, family, group or community. A nursing diagnosis provides the basis for selection of nursing interventions to achieve outcomes for which the nurse has accountability.

Problem-focused nursing diagnosis: A clinical judgment concerning an undesirable human response to health conditions/life processes that exists in an individual, family, group, or community.

Syndrome: A clinical judgment concerning a specific cluster of nursing diagnoses that occur together, and are best addressed together and through similar interventions.

Actual: identifies an occurring health problem.

Potential: identifies a high risk health problem.

Wellness: focused on promoting or enhancing a patient's level of wellness.

Evaluation: Assessing the client's response to nursing interventions and then comparing the response to the goals or outcome criteria written in the planning phase.

Planning: Planning expected outcomes to resolve or minimize the identified problems of the client. In collaboration with the client, the nurse develops specific nursing intervention for each nursing diagnosis.

INTRODUCTION

Nurses face an endless variety of situations involving client's family members, health care staff, and peers. Each situation poses new experiences and problems involving client's care, different approaches to resolving problems, and different results as to whether approaches were successful. In every clinical situation it is important for a nurse to think critically and make sound judgments so that clients ultimately receive the very best nursing care. Critical thinking is not a simple step-by-step, linear process that can be learned overnight. It is a process acquired only through hard work, commitment, and an active curiosity toward learning. Ideally, critical thinking becomes a habit of mind, a part of each nurse's character.

CRITICAL THINKING AND NURSING JUDGEMENT

Critical thinking is the art of thinking about your thinking while you're thinking in order to make your thinking better: more clear, more accurate, or more defensible. It includes five modes of thinking: total recall, habits, inquiry, new ideas and creativity. Critical thinking helps the nurse to find options for solving client's problems. Both the nurse and the client need to be effective thinkers so that they can find the problems accurately and set realistic outcomes. By using critical thinking they can plan, implement and evaluate quality care.

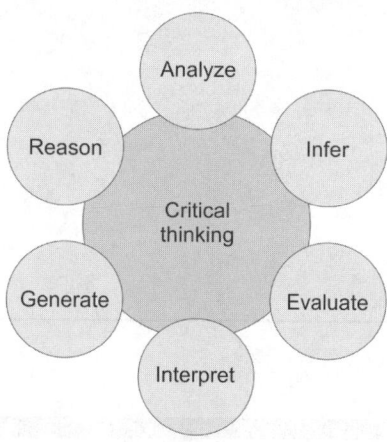

Fig. 16.1: Critical thinking steps.

Definition of Critical Thinking

- Norris (1989) defined "Critical thinking as reasonable and reflective thinking that is focused upon deciding what do believe or do".
- Miller and Malcom, "Critical thinking is a cognitive process that involves weighing the accuracy and logic of evidence-an understanding of the nature of valid inferences, abstractixons and generalizations".

Meaning of Critical Thinking

- Critical thinking is a form of judgment, specifically purposeful and reflective judgment. Using critical thinking one makes a decision or solves the problem of judging what to believe or what to do, but does so in a reflective way.
- Critical thinking gives due consideration to the evidence, the context of judgment, the relevant criteria for making that judgment well, the applicable methods or techniques for forming that judgment, and the applicable theoretical constructs for understanding the nature of the problem and the question at hand.
- These elements also happen to be the key defining characteristics of professional fields and academic disciplines. This is why critical thinking can occur within a given subject field (by reference to its specific set of permissible questions, evidence sources, criteria, etc.) and across subject fields in all those spaces where human beings need to interact and make decisions, solve problems, and figure out what to believe and what to do.
- Within the framework of scientific skepticism, the process of critical thinking involves acquiring information and evaluating it to reach a well-justified conclusion or answer. Part of critical thinking comprises informal logic.

In a seminal study on critical thinking and education in 1941, Edward Glaser defines critical thinking as follows.

COMPONENTS OF CRITICAL THINKING

Brookfield (1987) identified four components of critical thinking:
1. Indemnifying and challenging consumptions.
2. Becoming aware of the importance of context in creating meaning.
3. Imaging and exploring alternatives.
4. Cultivating a reflective skepticism.

Now day's health care consumers know their rights and want to take an active part in deciding what they need and the type of care they will require. This change consumer orientation requires nurses to recognize and develop critical thinking skills that utilize logical or analytical and creative approaches to solving problems. Critical thinking skills that integrate these approaches will provide practitioners with expertise in flexible, individualized and situation specific problems solving.

IMPORTANCE OF CRITICAL THINKING

The ability to think critically, as conceived in this volume, involves three things—(1) an attitude of being disposed to consider in a thoughtful way the problems and subjects that come within the range of one's experiences, (2) knowledge of the methods of logical inquiry and reasoning, and (3) some skill in applying those methods.

Critical thinking calls for a persistent effort to examine any belief or supposed form of knowledge in the light of the evidence that supports it and the further conclusions to which it tends. It also generally requires ability to recognize problems, to find workable means for meeting those problems, to gather and marshal pertinent information, to recognize unstated assumptions and values, to comprehend and use language with accuracy, clarity, and discrimination, to interpret data, to appraise evidence and evaluate arguments, to recognize the existence (or nonexistence)

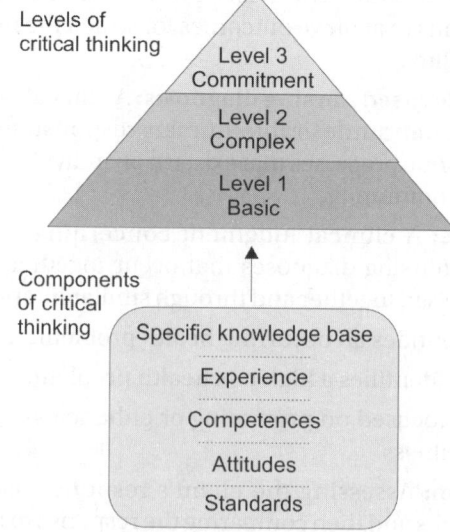

Fig. 16.2: Levels of critical thinking.

of logical relationships between propositions, to draw warranted conclusions and generalizations, to put to test the conclusions and generalizations at which one arrives, to reconstruct one's patterns of beliefs on the basis of wider experience, and to render accurate judgments about specific things and qualities in everyday life.

CRITICAL THINKING IN NURSING

Healthcare consumers of the modern day know their rights and want to take an active consumer orientation, require nurses to develop critical thinking skills that utilize logical and intuitive approaches to solve problems. Critical thinking is an essential quality in patient care management. Critical thinking is a special acquired skill used to generate, apply, analyze, synthesize and evaluate information is crucial for nursing professionals. The need for this skill is determined by nursing, commitment to the care of the total person, nursing's contact with persons of varying sociocultural and religious backgrounds, and the recognition that nursing is both an art and a science.

Nursing care management requires a range of intellectual, interpersonal and technical competencies to be effective. Critical care thinking approach avoids nursing care based upon imitation or tradition and enables nurse to provide a more sensitive and comprehensive nursing care. Critical thinking is a process and cognitive skill that we apply to identify and define a problem and opportunities for improvement. Critical thinking helps us to generate, examine and evaluate decisions. The capacity for critical thinking and decision making by its members is a prerequisites for a profession which claims autonomy.

SPECIAL SKILLS REQUIRED FOR CRITICAL THINKING

- Coming to understand that the smallest unit of "meaning" is not the *claim* or *sentence* or belief, but the argument.

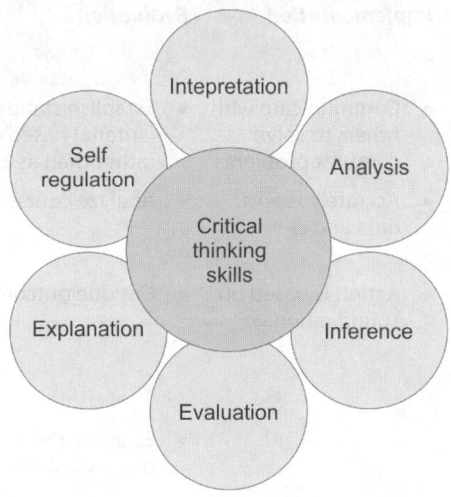

Fig. 16.3: Skills required for critical thinking.

- Recognizing the thesis.
- Recognizing the argument.
- Recognizing and assessing the logic of the argument.
- Practicing negative criticism which is to show or discover that some part of the argument is mistaken or otherwise inadequate.
- Practicing positive criticism which is not simply to agree. Rather, it can be to shore up some part of the argument that is weak.
- Positive criticism may also be to anticipate the most serious objections which are likely to be raised and to build a defense against them within the rules of critical thinking.
- Understanding and using the distinction between theme (or topic) and thesis (or main belief).
- Understanding and using the concept of a "prima facia" claim.
- Understanding and using a counter-argument.
- Understanding and using a paradigm case.
- Understanding, recognizing and using the distinction between chronological order and logical order.
- Understanding and using the distinction between the "context of discovery" the "context of proof".

CHARACTERISTICS OF GOOD CRITICAL THINKER

Raymond S. Nickerson (1987), an authority on critical thinking, characterizes a good critical thinker in terms of knowledge, abilities, attitudes, and habitual ways of behaving. Here are some of the characteristics of such a thinker:

- Uses evidence skillfully and impartially.
- Organizes thoughts and articulates them concisely and coherently.
- Distinguishers between logically valid and invalid inferences.
- Suspends judgment in the absence of sufficient evidence to support a decision.
- Understands the difference between reasoning and rationalizing.
- Attempts to anticipate the probable consequences of alternative actions.
- Understands the idea of degrees of belief.
- Sees similarities and analogies that are not superficially apparent.
- Can learn independently and has an abiding interest in doing so.
- Applies problem-solving techniques in domains other than those in which learned.
- Can structure informally represent problems in such a way that formal techniques, such as mathematics, can be used to solve them.
- Can strip a verbal argument of irrelevancies and phrase it in its essential terms.

- Habitually questions one's own views and attempts to understand both the assumptions that is critical to those views and the implications of the views.
- Is sensitive to the difference between the validity of a belief and the intensity with which it is held.

Characteristics of Critical Thinkers	
Habitually inquisitive well-informed trustful of reason open-minded flexible fair-minded in evaluation honest in facing personal biases prudent in making judgments	Willing to reconsider clear about issues orderly in complex matters diligent in seeking relevant information reasonable in the selection of criteria focused in inquiry persistent in seeking results that are as precise as the subject and the circumstances of inquiry permit

- Is aware of the fact that one's understanding is always limited, often much more so than would be apparent to one with a noninquiring attitude.
- Recognizes the fallibility of one's own opinions, the probability of bias in those opinions, and the danger of weighting evidence according to personal preferences.

CRITICAL THINKING THROUGH NURSING PRACTICE

A clinical nurse has to possess analytical skill and decision making abilities. While assessing a patient or clinical situation a nurse must be able to ask the right questions, probe into matter, be perceptually aware of verbal and nonverbal cues and make sense of information received. The nurse must also be able to make clinical nursing judgments by categorizing, organizing and analyzing the pieces of information collected through nursing assessment. The nursing process demands the nurse to think critically to analyze human responses to problems.

Nursing process	Critical thinking
Assessment	• Observing • Distinguishing important from unimportant data • Validating data • Organizing data • Categorizing data
Analysis/diagnosis	• Finding patterns and relationships • Making inferences • Stating the problem • Suspending judgment
Planning	• Generalizing • Transferring knowledge from one situation to another • Developing evaluative criteria • Hypothesizing
Implementation	• Applying knowledge • Testing hypotheses
Evaluation	• Deciding whether hypotheses are correct • Making criterion-based evaluations and judgments

Critical thinking as applied to nursing process implies: exploring and acquiring information about nursing concerns, apprising the collected data, analyzing the relationships among the data, and interfering conclusions about the patient's needs from the data. Decisions must be flexible to modify or adapt the planned nursing intervention after evaluation. An important process demands the nurse to think critically to analyze human responses to problems. Critical thinking as applied to nursing process implies: exploring and acquiring information about nursing concerns, apprising the collected data, analyzing the relationships among the data, and interring conclusions about the patient's need from the data. Decisions must be flexible to modify or adapt the planned nursing intervention after evaluation.

TABLE 16.1: Application of critical thinking to nursing proces.

Assessment	Diagnosis	Outcome identification and planning	Implementation	Evaluation
• Gather patient data	• Develop well thought out conclusion	• Explore alternative actions	• Communicate with others to solve complex problems	• Establish standards (criteria) based on logic rather than assumptions
• Interpret data	• Seek reasons and principles that justify nursing judgments	• Collaborate with others	• Accrately report data and clues	• Analyze course of action
• Keep an open mind by questioning assumptions about data	• Test conclusions against criteria	• Examine assumptions • Reframe problems in order to generate solutions	• Action is based on sound rationale	• Critique outcomes
• Thinking about what information to collect	• Suspend judgment when data is insufficient	• Generate ideas and possible solutions		• Evaluate the soundness of conclusions
• Making conclusions based on the data	• Differentiate essential and trivial data			

An important process that enhances nurse's cognitive competencies is reflection. Nursing is a practice orientated profession. Nursing knowledge grows not only out of the theoretical search but also out of every day practice. In order to promote evidence-based nurses have to closely observe their practices and reflect on them for suitability to the situation. However the current clinical nursing situation hardly provides nurses with opportunity for reflection. Neither do nurses hold regular clinical meeting to discuss practices, identify problems and generate ideas to improve the situation. The primacy of critical thinking in nursing rests upon decision making in nursing practice while delegating nursing care activities. In addition to this, models of care such as consumer focused care and organizational models such as shared governance require nurses to think critically and collaborate. To collaborate effectively, the nurse practitioner must evaluate a variety of perspectives, and contribute to generating new ideas and solutions.

Critical Thinking Attitudes and Applications in Nursing Practice

Critical thinking is a reasoning process by which individuals reflect on analyze their own thoughts, actions, and knowledge. To be a good critical thinking requires dedication and a desire to grow intellectually. A nurse learns that foe each client cared for, there is a large source of scientific knowledge and practice based information to consider.

The depth of nursing knowledge coupled with knowledge of each client's unique clinical situation makes it challenging to provide the most appropriate plan of care for a client. As a beginning nurse, it is important to learn the steps of the nursing process and to incorporate the elements of elements of critical thinking. For example, while assessing a client's plan, a nurse must consider all symptoms, analyze his or her interpretation of the source, analyze the relevance of the pain to the client's clinical situation, choose interventions, and evaluate the consequences of treatment choices.

Critical thinking is ongoing with information being analyzed from many sources. If one places the nursing process within the context of the critical thinking model, one is able to see two processes occurring together. As the nurse engages in nursing process for the care of a client, he or she is also synthesizing critical thinking knowledge, experience, standards and attitudes. The nurse who is assessing a client's pain does not focus only on what the client reports about the pain and what the nurse is able to observe and measure.

Critical Thinking in Clinical Application

- **Confidence:** Learn how to introduce yourself to a client. Speak with conviction when you being a treatment or procedure. Do not lead a client to think that you are certain of being able to perform care safely. Always be prepared before performing a nursing activity.
- **Thinking independently:** Read the nursing literature, especially when there are different views on the same subject. Talk with colleagues and share ideas about nursing interventions.
- **Fairness:** Listen to both sides in any discussion. If a client or family member complains about a colleague, listen to the story and then speak with the colleague as well. Weigh all facts.
- **Responsibility and authority:** Ask for help if you are uncertain about an aspect of client care. Report any problems immediately. Follow standards of practice in your care.
- **Risk taking:** If your knowledge causes you to question a physician's order, do so. Be willing to recommend alternative approaches to nursing care when colleagues are having little successes with clients.
- **Discipline:** Be thorough in whatever you do. Use known scientific and practice-based criteria for activities such as assessment and evaluation. Take time to be thorough, and manage your time effectively.
- **Perseverance:** Be wary of any easy answer. If colleagues give you information about a client, and some fact seems to be missing, so clarify information or talk to the client directly. If problems of the same type continue to occur on a nursing division, bring colleagues together, look for a pattern, and find a solution.
- **Creativity:** Look for different approaches if intervention is not working. A client may need a different positioning technique or a different instructional approach that will suit his or her unique needs.
- **Curiosity:** Always ask why. A clinical sign or symptom can indicate a variety of problems. Explore and learn more about the client so as to make appropriate clinical judgments.
- **Integrity:** Recognize when your opinion may conflict with those of a client; review your position, and decide how best to produced to reach mutually beneficial outcomes. Do not compromise nursing standards or honesty in delivering nursing care.
- **Humility:** Recognize when you need more information to make a decision.

When you are newly assigned to a clinical division and you are unfamiliar with the clients, asked to be oriented to the area. Ask RNs regularly assigned to the area for assistance. Read the professional journals regularly to keep update on new approaches to care.

LEVELS OF CRITICAL THINKING IN NURSING

Critical thinking involves the use of a group of interconnected skills to analyze, creatively integrate, and evaluate what you read and hear. To become a critical thinker you must be able to decide whether an author's opinions are true or false, whether he or she has adequately defended those ideas, whether certain recommendations are practical, as well as whether particular solutions will be effective. Critical thinking involves the use of a kind of thinking called reasoning, in which we construct and/or evaluate reasons to support beliefs. Critical thinking also involves reflection- the examination and evaluation of our own and others' thoughts and ideas. Finally critical thinking is practical. Actions are more rational if they are based on beliefs that we take to be justified. Critical thinking then, is the careful, deliberate determination of whether we should accept, reject or suspend judgment about the truth of a claim or a recommendation to act in a certain way.

Step 1: Knowledge: In terms of critical thinking, the basic level of acquisition of knowledge requires that you be able to identify what is being said: the topic, the issue, the thesis, and the main points.

Step 2: Comprehension: Comprehension means understanding the material read, heard or seen. In comprehending, you make the new knowledge that you have acquired your own by relating it to what you already know. The better you are involved with the information, the better you will comprehend it. As always, the primary test of whether you have comprehended something is whether you can put what you have read or heard into your own words.

Step 3: Application: Application requires that you know what you have read, heard, or seen, that you comprehend it, and that you carry out some task to apply what you comprehend to an actual situation.

Step 4: Analysis: Analysis involves breaking what you read or hear into its component parts, in order to make clear how the ideas are ordered, related, or connected to other ideas. Analysis deals with both form and content.

Step 5: Synthesis: Synthesis involves the ability to put together the parts you analyzed with other information to create something original.

Step 6: Evaluation: Evaluation occurs once we have understood and analyzed what is said or written and the reasons offered to support it. Then we can appraise this information in order to decide whether you can give or withhold belief, and whether or not to take a particular action.

NURSING PROCESS OVERVIEW: APPLICATION IN PRACTICE

The nursing process is a problem solving approach used by nurses to meet the needs of the patient. It is a deliberative method that relies on the use of cognitive, interpersonal and psychomotor skills. The nursing process is the systematic, rational method of planning and providing nursing care. Its goal is to identify a client's health status, actual or potential health care problems, to establish plans to meet the individual needs and to deliver specific nursing interventions to meet those needs. The nursing process is cyclical, that is the component of the nursing process follows a logical sequence, but more that one component may be involved at any given time. The nursing process provides a framework for accountability in nursing.

Definition

- The Nursing process is cyclical, that is the component of the nursing process follows a logical sequence, but more than one component may be involved at any given time. The nursing process provides a framework for accountability in nursing.
- The Nursing process can be defined as an orderly, systematic way of identifying the clients(patient) problems, making plans to solve them, initiating the plans or assigning others to implement it and evaluating the extent to which the plan was effective in resolving the problems identified.
- Nursing Process: An evolving procedure consisting of five components by which a person's health status and needs are identified (assessment and diagnosis), plans are developed (planning), care is delivered (implementation), and outcomes are evaluated (evaluation) as the physical, social, and emotional problems of the person are resolved and/or new problems are identified.

Meaning of Nursing Process

The nursing process is cyclical, that is the component of the nursing process follows a logical sequence, but more than one component may be involved at any given time. The nursing process provides a framework for accountability in nursing. The nursing process can be defined as an orderly, systematic way of identifying the clients (patient) problems, making plans to solve them, initiating the

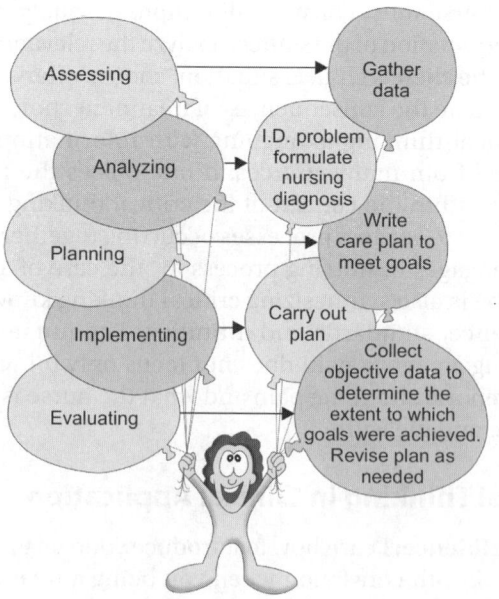

Fig. 16.4: Nursing process steps.

plans or assigning others to implement it and evaluating the extent to which the plan was effective in resolving the problems identified.

Purpose of Nursing Process

Primary purpose of nursing process is to help the nurse to manage each patients nursing care intellectually, scientifically and judiciously. Other purposes are:
- To help the patient in maintaining health.
- To protect client from illness.
- To identify clients health status.
- To identify client's actual and potential health problems.
- To determine priorities.
- To initiate/establish plan for meeting the identified needs.
- To deliver the specific nursing interventions.
- To evaluate effectiveness of care provided.
- To promote recovery from illness.
- To promote return to a state of maximum functioning.

Characteristics of Nursing Process

- Problem oriented process.
- Universally accepted process.
- Cyclic and dynamic process.
- Inter-personal and collaborative process.
- It involves creativity and designing.
- Goal oriented process
- Open and flexible
- Client oriented and individualized approach.
- Systematic and planned approach.
- Emphasis on feedback.

Advantages of Nursing Process

When used effectively, the nursing process offers many advantages:
- Nursing process patient-centered, helping to ensure that your patient's health problems and his response to them are the focus of care.
- It enables you to individualize care for each patient.
- It promotes the patient's participation in their care, encourages independence and concordance and gives the patient a greater sense of control – important factors in a positive health outcome.
- It improves communication by providing you and other nurses with a summary of the patient's recognized problems or needs.
- It promotes accountability for nursing activities, which in turn promotes quality assurance.
- It promotes critical thinking, decision-making and problem-solving.
- It is outcome-focused and encourages the evaluation of results.
- It minimizes errors and omissions in care planning.

STEPS IN THE NURSING PROCESS

The nursing process consists of five steps or components. These five steps of the nursing process are assessment, nursing diagnosis, planning, implementation and evaluation. The scientific nursing activities and responsibilities are associated with each steps of the nursing process.

Assessment: It is collecting, verifying and organizing data about the client's health status. Data about physical, emotional, developmental, social, cultural, intellectual and spiritual aspects of the client's are obtained from a variety of sources and are the basis for actions and decisions taken at a subsequent phases.

Nursing diagnosis: It is a process of making a clinical judgment about a client's potential or actual health problem. Nursing diagnosis is the statement of the judgment. In this phase, the nurse sorts, clusters the data and analyzes, what are the actual and potential health problems for which the client needs nursing assistance and what may be the contributing factors to this problem?

Planning: It involves a series of steps in which the nurse and client set priorities, formulate goals or expected outcomes and establish a written care plan for nursing interventions. The plan to resolve or minimize the identified problems of the client and to coordinate the care provided by all the health team members.

Implementation: It is putting the nursing care plan into action. During the implementation phase, the nurse continues to collect data and carries out the prescribed nursing activities or delegates the care to an appropriate person who validates the nursing care plan.

Evaluation: It is assessing the client's response to nursing interventions and then comparing the response to predetermined standards. These standards are often referred to as "outcome criteria". The nurse determines the extent to which the goals are predetermined and

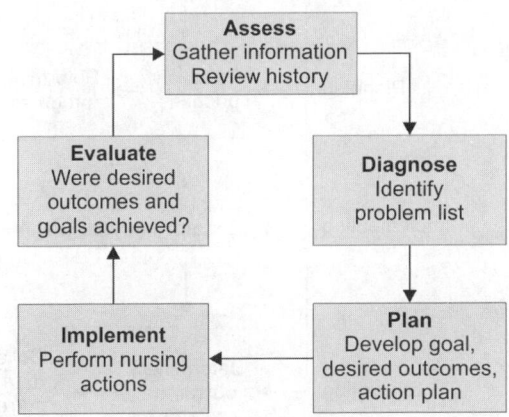

Fig. 16.5: Nursing process.
(Mnemonic: ADPIE)

the outcomes of care that have been achieved, partially achieved or not met.

BENEFITS OF NURSING PROCESS

Benefits for the Client

- **Quality clients care:** The nursing care is planned to meet the unique needs of the individual, family or community. Continuous evaluation and reassessment of the client's changing needs ensure an appropriate level of care.
- **Continuity of care:** The written care plan is accessible to all the persons involved in the client's care and it prevents the client from repeating information and preferences to each caretaker.
- **Participation by the client in their health care's:** The process can help the clients to develop skills related to their health care and to become more committed to the goals of care.

Benefits for the Nurse

- **Consistent and systematic nursing education:** The agency which accredits nursing education programs requires all graduates to be competent in using the nursing process.
- **Job satisfaction:** Well written care plans, has given the nurses to be confident about that nursing interventions which are based on correct identification of the clients problems, thus preventing the uncoordinated, trail and error nursing.
- **Professional growth:** By elevating the effectiveness of the nursing interventions, the nurse learns which interventions are most effective and which ones can be adapted to meet the needs of other clients.
- **Meet professional standards:** Learning and implementing the nursing process while providing client care is a basic requirement for professional nursing competence.

A Framework for Accountability

- Accountability is the condition of being answerable and responsible to someone for specific behaviors that are part of the nurse's professional role.
- The nursing process provides a framework for accountability and responsibility in nursing and maximizes accountability and responsibility for standards of care.
- Nurses are accountable to the client (public), to their professional statuary nursing body, to colleagues, to the employing agency and to themselves.
- The nursing process provides a framework for accountability in all areas. A professional nurse is accountable for activities in all five phases of the nursing process.

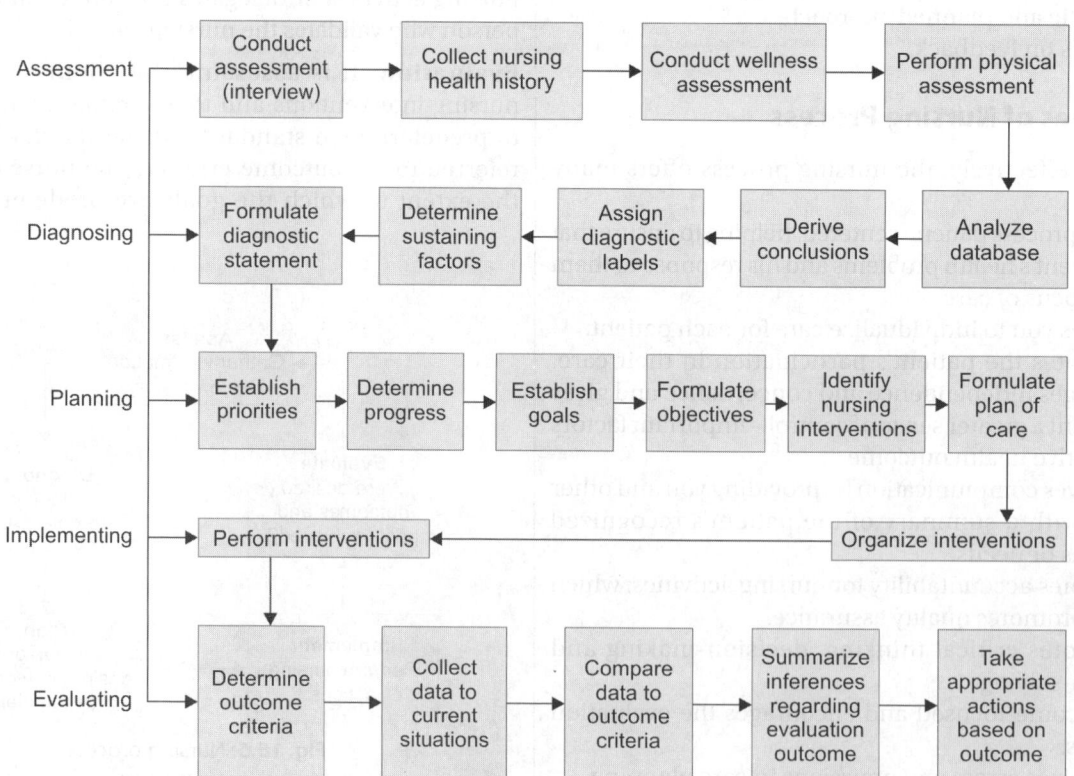

Fig. 16.6: Steps and application of nursing process model.

Domain	Nursing process	Education process
Assessment	Appraise physical and psychosocial needs	Determine learning needs, readiness to learn and learning styles
Planning	Develop care plan based on mutual goal sening to meet individuals needs	Develop teaching plan based on mutually pre-determined behavioral outcomes to meet individuals needs
Implementation	Perform nursing care interventions using standard procedures	Perform teaching using specific instructional methods and tools
Evaluation	Determine physical and psychosocial outcomes	Determine outcome changes (knowledge. attitudes and skills)

(Adopted from Bastable. (2006). Patient Education)

NURSING ASSESSMENT

The first step of nursing process is assessment. Assessment is the collection of data about the client from a variety of sources. Assessment is the continuous process carried out during all phases of the nursing process. It may be used during the diagnosis phase to validate a diagnosis.

Purposes of Nursing Assessment

- To gather information regarding clients health.
- To determine clients normal function.
- To organize the collected information.
- To confirm hypothesis growing out of the nurses interview.
- To enhance investigation of nursing problems.
- To frame nursing diagnosis.
- To increase greater managing skill of handling patients problems.
- To identify health problems.
- To identify clients strength.
- To identify need for health teaching.

Prerequisites to Assessment

- **Beliefs:** The nurse's belief encompasses a caring philosophy about the client's, responsibilities and health and illness and the role of nursing in health care. These philosophies do not blossom overnight but are molded during the course of nursing education by nurses, other students, instructors and clients.
- **Knowledge:** The knowledge base for nurses is extensive and nurses are required to use information from sciences such as nursing, anatomy, physiology, microbiology, pharmacology, chemistry and nutrition using all of these sciences is guidelines, the nurse can analyze data collected about the client.
- **Skill:** A variety of skills are required to perform a complete assessment of the client. They include psychomotor and interpersonal.

Psychomotor skills are the technical skills required in many phases and nursing process. During the assessment phase, the most common skills are those of physical assessment such as inspection, palpation and auscultation.

Interpersonal skills are important in all phases of nursing process but are a critical component of the assessment phase. The term therapeutic relationship is often used to describe the communication techniques that allow the client and family to share views and telling openly.

DATA COLLECTION

Data collected from a patient includes both objective and subjective data. Objective data are detectable by an observer. Examples of objective data are blood pressure recording, checking body temperature, detecting cyanosis in a patient. Subjective data are apparent only to the patient concerned. Examples of subjective data are feeling of pain, inching, etc.

Sources of Data

- **Client:** The chief source of data is usually the client unless the client is too ill, young or confused to

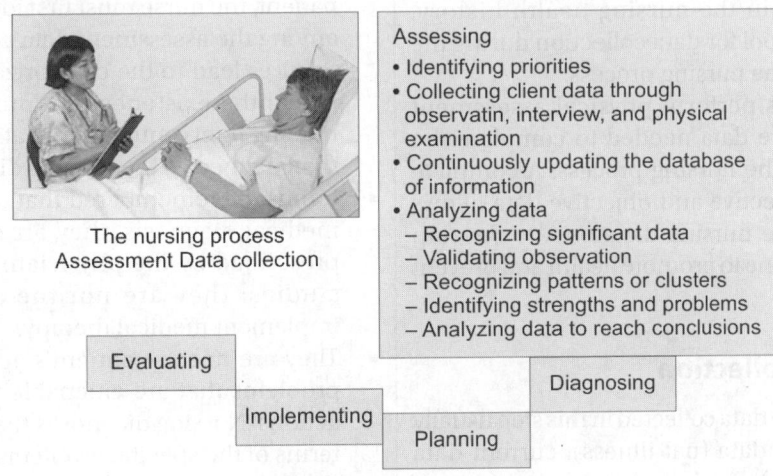

Fig. 16.7: Nursing assessment.

communicate clearly. The client can provide subjective data that no one else can offer.
- **Significant others:** Significant others are supporting person who knows the client well and often provide data. They might convey information about the stress the client was experiencing before the illness, family attitudes to illness and health and the client's home environment.
- **Health personnel:** Health personnel are often the sources of information about a client's health. Nurses, physicians, social workers and physiotherapist. Physician who knows the client's home setting may provide valuable data about the family and the environmental stress.
- **Medical records:** Medical records are often a source of a client's present and past health and illness patterns. This record can provide nurses with information about a client's coping behaviors, health practices, previous illness and allergies.
- **Other records and reports:** Other records and reports can also provide information pertinent to health, laboratory, tests are frequently ordered as part of the physician's initial examination to aid in a medical diagnosis.
- **Literature:** The review of nursing and related literature, such as professional journals and reference texts, can provide additional information for the database.

Methods of Data Collection

- **Observation:** The nurse observes mainly through sight, all of the senses are engaged during careful observations. Observation has two aspects: (1) noticing the stimuli and (2) selecting organizing and interpreting the data, i.e. perceiving them. Observation is a conscious, deliberate skill that is developed only through effort and with an organized approach.
- **Interviewing:** The nurse interviews the patient and his significant others obtain data by asking relevant questions. Interview is a planned communication or conversation with a purpose. Interviewing can be viewed as a process in the nursing health history, which is the primary tool for data collection during the assessment phase of the nursing process.
- **Examination:** Nurses perform physical assessment to obtain the objective data needed to complete the assessment phase of the nursing process. A complete database of both subjective and objective data allows the nurse to formulate nursing diagnosis, to develop client goals and intervene to promote health and prevent disease.

Guideline for Data Collection

- **The initial history:** The data collected in this step usually include the historical data (pat illness), current data (the current complaint) and demographic data (date of birth, address). It is helpful to address the client's chief complaint early in the interview process.
- **Symptom analysis:** When a client expresses a problem the nurse conducts a complete analysis of a symptom. This process begins with symptoms analysis which is the collection of subjective data about the problem. Symptoms analysis requires the client to identify the location of the symptoms, describe the symptoms, severity of the pain, and timing of the symptoms. (Including onset, duration and frequency). Aggravating and relieving symptoms and any associated symptoms. It is crucial that the nurse be able to perform a complete symptoms analysis. The data obtained can guide the nurse in detecting what the problem is and what degree of priority is should be given.
- **Approaches to history taking:** There are various approaches that can be used to provide a systematic guide to assessment. Gordon has devised functional health patterns and the North American Nursing Diagnosis Association (NANDA) has devised human response patterns-based on patterns of unitary persons.
- **Physical examination:** Physical examination of the client is the second portion of assessment. Examination allows the nurse to gain objective data through the use of inspection, percussion, palpation and auscultation. These data further define the client's response to the disorder, provide a baseline of data for further comparison, and elaborate on the subjective data provided in the client's history.

NURSING DIAGNOSIS

- Nursing diagnosis is actual or potential problems that are amenable to resolution by nursing actions are identified as nursing diagnosis.
- The five national conferences on the classification of nursing diagnosis held in 1970's and the early 1980's have provided an impetus for the identification and classification of nursing diagnosis according to symptomatology.
- When developing the nursing diagnosis for a particular patient, the nurse must first identify the commonalities among the assessment data collected. These common features lead to the categorization of related data that reveal the existence of a problem and the need for nursing intervention. The patient's nursing problem is then defined as the nursing diagnosis (**Fig. 16.8**).
- It must be remembered that nursing diagnosis are not medical diagnosis, they are not medical treatments prescribed by the physician; they are not diagnostic studies; they are not the equipment utilized to implement medical therapy.
- They are not the patient's actual or potential health problems that are amenable to resolution by nursing actions. Nursing diagnoses that are succinctly stated in terms of the specific problems of the patient will guide the nurse in the development of the nursing care plan.

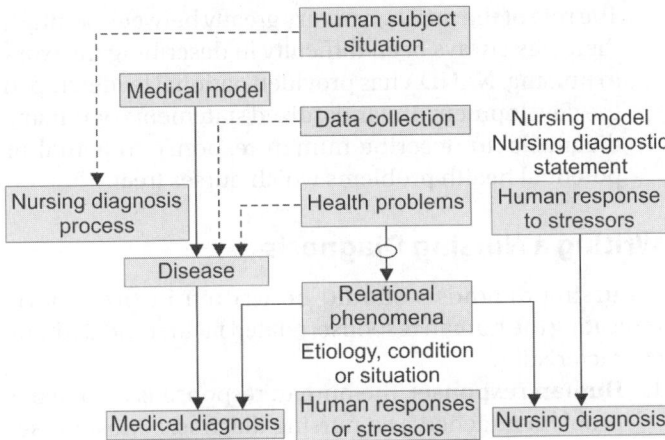

Fig. 16.8: Nursing and medical diagnosis.

Definition

- The nursing diagnosis is a conclusion drawn from the data collected about a client that serves as a means of describing a health need amenable to treatment by nurses. A uniform or standardized way of identifying, focusing on, and labeling specific phenomena allows the nurse to deal effectively with individual client responses.
- Nursing diagnosis is defined as "a clinical judgment about individual, family, or community experiences/responses to actual or potential health problems/life processes. A nursing diagnosis provides the basis for selection of nursing interventions to achieve outcomes for which the nurse has accountability."
- The process of assessing potential or actual health problems, including those pertaining to an individual patient, a family or community, that fall within the scope of nursing practice; a judgment or conclusion reached as a result of such assessment or derived from assessment data.
- A nursing diagnosis is a standardized statement about to the health of a client (individual, family, or community) for the purpose of providing nursing care. One organization for defining standard diagnoses is the North American Nursing Diagnosis Association now known as NANDA-International.

Purposes of Nursing Diagnosis

- To analyze collected data.
- To identify clients normal functional level statement.
- To identify the clients strength and weaknesses.
- To formulate a diagnostic weaknesses.

Characteristics of a Diagnostic Statement

- Clear and concise
- Specific and patient oriented
- Relates to the patient problem
- Accurate
- Based on reliable and relevant assessment data.

Nursing Diagnosis Classifications

The NANDA-I system of nursing diagnosis provides for four categories.

1. **Actual diagnosis:** "A clinical judgment about human experience/responses to health conditions/life processes that exist in an individual, family, or community". An example of an actual nursing diagnosis is: Sleep deprivation. An actual diagnosis is a statement about a health problem that the client has, and could benefit from nursing care. An example of an actual nursing diagnosis is: Ineffective airway clearance related to decreased energy and manifested by an ineffective cough.
2. **Risk diagnosis:** Describes human responses to health conditions/life processes that may develop in a vulnerable individual/family/community. It is supported by risk factors that contribute to increased vulnerability. An example of a risk diagnosis is: Risk for shock. A risk diagnosis is a statement about a health problem that the client doesn't have yet, but is at a higher than normal risk of developing in the near future. An example of a risk diagnosis is: Risk for injury related to altered mobility and disorientation.
3. **Health promotion diagnosis:** A clinical judgment about a person's, family's or community's motivation and desire to increase wellbeing and actualize human health potential as expressed in the readiness to enhance specific health behaviors, and can be used in any health state. An example of a health promotion diagnosis is: Readiness for enhanced nutrition.
4. **Syndrome diagnosis:** "A clinical judgment describing a specific cluster of nursing diagnoses that occur together, and are best addressed together and through similar interventions." An example of a syndrome diagnosis is: Rape-trauma syndrome related to anxiety about potential health problems and as manifested by anger, genitourinary discomfort, and sleep pattern disturbance.

Diagnostic Reasoning

- **Classification:** The initial step of data analysis is classification of the data. Data need to be organized in order to be clearly analyzed and the most logical means to organize data is to classify them. The body systems approach functional health pattern approaches are two convenient methods of classification. When these methods are used for taking a history and performing a physical examination, the data are already classified.
- **Validation:** The next step of data analysis is validation. In this step the nurse verifies the diagnosis by speaking to the client. The nurse can validate finding with the family, especially if the client is unable to communicate. For example, the nurse could ask about scars or wounds and therefore, expand the data base on the client. The

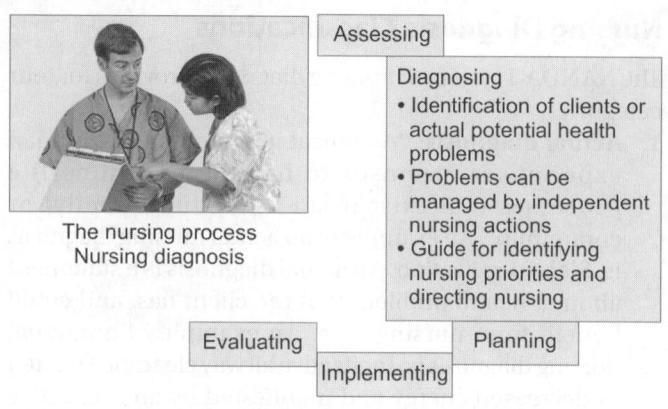

Fig. 16.9: Nursing diagnosis.

nurse can also validate the diagnosis by comparing it to textbook material or by talking to other nurses.
- **Inductive versus deductive reasoning:** The nurse may use inductive or deductive reasoning to interpret data. Inductive reasoning begins with a set of facts from which a conclusion is drawn. Inductive reasoning is the use of cues to draw a conclusion. Deductive reasoning begins with the facts that the client is on bed rest and taking narcotics and concludes (deduces) that the client is at an increased risk.

Errors in Diagnosis

- **Incomplete data:** Common cause of incomplete data occurs during the interview phase of assessment. Some clients withhold information intentionally because some they feel embarrassed or are unsure how the nurse would react to the information.
- **Inaccurate interpretation:** Data from the client can be misinterpreted in several ways. The problem can be diagnosed in several ways. The problem can be diagnosed before the data are completely collected. Sometimes the nurse can have a personal prejudice about the client.
- **Lack of knowledge or experience:** The clinical experience and knowledge may result in inaccurate data processing. Failure to recognize a problem is a common experience for most nurses. The inexperienced nurse may overlook important data or fail to realize the significance of the data.

Using a Nursing Diagnosis

- The diagnosis is anything abnormal or that concerns the client, or strengthens of the client. Diagnoses within the realm of nursing are the response of the client to a state of health or illness and include physical, psychological, spiritual and educational areas.
- These nursing diagnosis and their treatment are within the legal scope of nursing practice. The actual conditions that nurses are educated to handle and licensed to treat are called nursing diagnosis.
- The role of the nurses can vary greatly between settings; there has always been difficulty in describing the work in nursing. NANDA has provided national leadership in the development of standardized statements or nursing diagnosis, to describe human response to actual or potential health problems which nurses treat.

Writing a Nursing Diagnosis

A nursing diagnosis should be written in three parts indicating the human response, related factors and defining characteristics.
1. **Human response:** The human response is the client's problem attached as a nursing diagnosis. Most nurses use NANDA nursing diagnosis as the human response statement, but other form of problem statements are possible. The human response should always be stated as a response to care rather than as a need for care. Needs for care such as needs to be fed or needs to be turned every 2 hours, describe a nursing intervention rather than a client problem.
2. **The related factors:** The related factors are the possible causes or etiology of the problem. This section of the statement describes the factors associated with the problem. These factors may be environmental, psychological, physiological, sociocultural or spiritual. Because these factors direct nursing actions aimed at resolving, preventing or reducing the problem, the related factor should be directed at an aspect of the client response on which the nurse have an impact.
3. The defining characteristics are the data indicating the problem is present. When the client is at risk of developing a problem, the risk factors are identified rather than defining characteristics.

Ten Rules for Writing a Nursing Diagnosis

1. Write the diagnosis in terms of the client's response rather than nursing need.
2. Use "related to" rather than "due to" or "caused by" to connect the first two parts of the statement.
3. Write the diagnosis in legally advisable terms.
4. Write the diagnosis without value judgments.
5. Avoid reversing the parts of the statement.
6. Avoid using single cues as the first part of the statement.
7. The two parts of the statement should not mean the same thing.
8. Express the related factor in terms that can be changed.
9. Do not include the medical diagnosis in the nursing diagnosis.
10. State the diagnosis clearly and concisely.

Collaborative Problems

- As nurses have continued to work with nursing diagnosis, shortcomings of the system have been identified.

- Carpenito defines collaborative problems as the psychological complications that have resulted or may result from the pathophysiologic and treatment related conditions, and from other situations.
- Nurses monitor to detect the onset and status of complications and collaborate with physicians in treatment.

NURSING PLANNING

The next step in the nursing process is planning activities to promote healthy client responses or prevent, correct or reduce unhealthy client responses. Planning and setting expected outcomes begins by determining the priority of human response.

Definitions of Planning

- Planning is a deliberate systematic phase of the nursing process that involves decision making and problem solving- Cozier-1975.
- Planning is a category of nursing behavior in which client centered goals are established and interventions are designed to achieve the goals-potter and perry-2001.
- Planning is defined as the selecting and carrying out of series of action assigned to achieve stated goals-Kropt.
- Planning defined as the development of nursing strategies designed to alleviate client problems-Craven.

Purpose of Planning

- Give direction to client care activities.
- Enhance the continuity care.
- Permit the delegation of specific activities.

Types of Planning

There are three types of planning; they are initial planning, on-going planning and discharge planning.

1. **Initial planning:** The planning done immediately after the initial assessment is the initial planning. Planning must be started early because of the trend towards shorter hospital stay.
2. **On-going planning:** The on-going planning is done by all the nurses who give care to the client. They carry out daily planning by using on-going assessment.
3. **Discharge planning:** Discharge planning is the process of planning about the needs which will occur after discharge of client. It is a critical part of comprehensive health care and should be included in every clients nursing care plan.

Steps of Planning

- **Initial planning**
  – Done by the nurse who perform admission assessment in order to prioritize problems, identify goals and correlate nursing care to resolve the problems.
- **Ongoing planning**
  – Involves continuous updating of the client's plan. of care. Every nurse who cares for the client is involved in ongoing planning.
- **Discharge planning**
  – Involves anticipation and planning for the client's needs after discharge.

Phases of Planning

- The assessment of priorities to nursing diagnosis.
- The specification of short-term, intermediate and long-term goals of nursing action.
- The identification of specific nursing interventions appropriate for attaining the goals.
- The documentation of the nursing diagnosis, goals nursing interventions and expected outcomes in the nursing care plan.

Setting Priorities

- The assignment of priorities to the nursing diagnosis should be a joint effort by the nurse and the patient or his family members.
- Consideration must be given to the urgency of he problems. The most critical receiving the highest priorities.
- Maslow's hierarchy of needs provides a useful framework for the determination of priority problems. The use of this hierarchy requires that high priorities be given to physical needs.

Establishing Goals for Nursing Action

- After the priorities of the nursing diagnoses have been establish, the short-term goals and the nursing actions appropriate for attainment of the goals are identified.
- The patient and his family should be included in the establishment of the short-term intermediate and long-term goals of the nursing actions.
- Short-term goals are those that are of immediate concern and that can be reached in a short-period of time.
- The critical time periods provide a time for determining the effectiveness of the nursing interventions and the existence of a need for additional or altered nursing care.

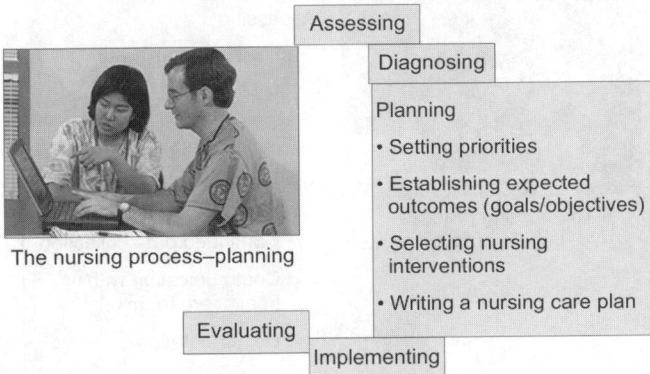

The nursing process–planning

Fig. 16.10: Nursing planning.

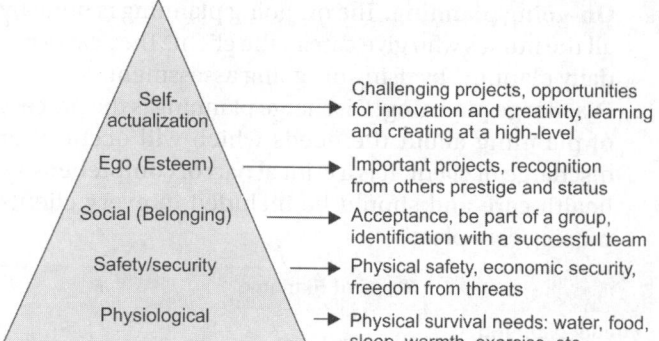

Fig. 16.11: Maslow's hierarchy of needs: The pyramid illustrates the five levels of human needs—the most basic are physiological and safety/security, shown at the base of the pyramid as one moves to higher-levels of the pyramid, the needs become more complex.

Team Planning

- Ideally the accomplishment of all aspects of the planning phase of the nursing process is a group effort.
- The nurse collaborates with other members of the nursing team, with the patient and his family and with appropriate resource persons from the health care agency and community agencies.
- It is also important to remember that the patient is part of a family. The family members have need that arises from the patient's illness.
- Another aspect of care planning takes into the account the fact that the patient comes from the community. Community agencies have an interest in the patient and are involved in planning.

Formulating the Nursing Care Plan

The nursing care plan serves to communicate the following information to all members of the nursing team:
- Nursing diagnosis and their priorities.
- The goals of the nursing interventions.
- The nursing interventions which are expressed in the form of nursing orders.
- The outcomes criteria, which identify the expected behavioral outcomes for the patient.
- The critical time period within which each outcome must be met.

NURSING IMPLEMENTATION

Nursing intervention is a nursing action. This action may be treatment, any diagnostic or therapeutic procedure or nursing activity. Nurse is performing an action to achieve outcome for a medical or nursing diagnosis to which nurse is accountable. Nursing interventions are the actual implementation of the care plan. Nursing interventions are designed to promote, maintain or restore the client's health.

Definition

- A nursing intervention is a single nursing action-treatment, procedure are activity-designed to achieve an outcome to a diagnosis—nursing or medical for which the nurse is accountable.
- Nursing intervention is any action taken by the nurse to help the client move from a present health state to the health state described in expected outcomes.

Purpose of Implementation

- To provide technical nursing care.
- To provide therapeutic nursing care.
- To help client to achieve optimum level of health.

Skills Required for Nurse in Implementation

In implementation phase of nurse process, nurse need to be competent in cognitive, interpersonal, technical and psychomotor skill.
- **Cognitive skills:** Cognitive skills involve application of nursing knowledge to anticipate and identify client's needs. Cognitive skills include problem solving, decision making and teaching. In order to enhance client's decision making ability, nurse gives him multiple choices to select choices to select which treatments are performed and in which sequence.
- **Interpersonal:** this is the ability to work with others to achieve a goal. As nurse is considered as backbone of the hospital, she must have knowledge and skill of developing and maintaining interpersonal and intrapersonal relations. Nurse uses communication skill to carry out planned nursing interventions.
- **Psychomotor skill:** It requires the integration of cognitive and motor activities. For giving intramuscular injection, nurse need to have knowledge of anatomy and physiology of body as well as preparing and administering injection such skill are important while doing dressing wounds, giving injection, suctioning and tracheotomy care.

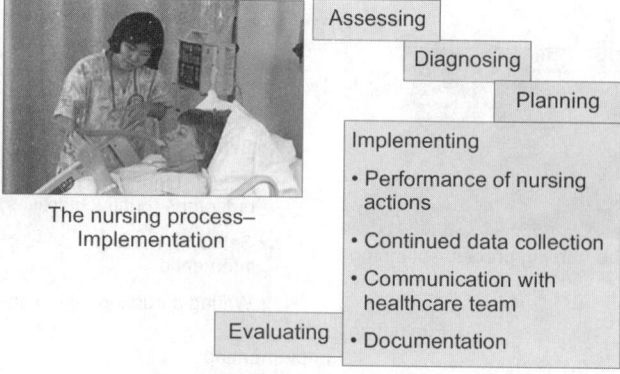

The nursing process—Implementation

Fig. 16.12: Nursing implementation.

- **Technical skills:** It is the skill needed to use equipment, machine, supplies in a particular specialty. Example: equipment such as ventilation, phototherapy machine, suctioning machine, infusion pump, etc.

Nursing Interventions have Following Seven Characteristics

1. Be congruent with the overall plan of care.
2. Be based on scientific principles.
3. Be individualized to the client.
4. Be designed to provide a safe and therapeutic environment.
5. Consider the need for teaching and learning.
6. Use resources appropriately.
7. Be clearly communicated.

Providing self-care: The nurse should identify what skills are required for providing the intervention. It is important to remember that when a skill is delegated to another health care team member, the registered nurse remains legally responsible for the client's outcome. Another aspect of providing self-care is continuous monitoring for complication. There are many complications that can allow surgery, medication administration and disease states. While the care is being given, the nurse continues to assess the client and evaluate his or her response to the care. The nurse also needs to consider which of the interventions could be modified, if the client shows no progress toward the desired outcome.

Nursing roles: Providing care teller into seven categories, according to Benner. Helper role, teaching coaching, diagnostic and patient monitoring, management of rapidly changing conditions, administering and monitoring therapeutic regimens, monitoring and ensuring quality of health care practices and organizational and work role competencies.

Rationale: At times, the scientific rationale for an intervention is required on a student care plan or listed within a standardized plan of care. It is important that the care given has its basis in scientific study, not in habit or old wives tales. The use of rationale assists in identifying the professional nurse from other providers of health care.

NURSING EVALUATION

The last step in the process is evaluation. Evaluation examines the degree of goal attainment and basically asks, "Did the client achieve the goal he or she was supposed to?" and if not why not? Evaluation begins with collecting data about the client's health status, closely reexamining the outcome criteria. The degree of outcome attainment is determined and a revised plan of care is established, if needed.

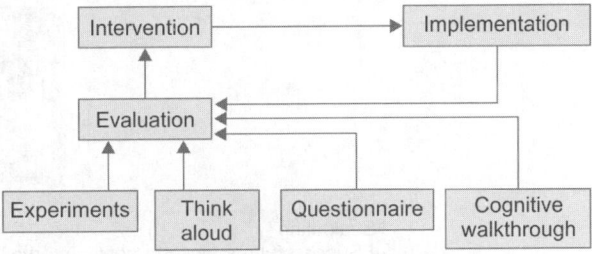

Fig. 16.13: Evaluation in nursing process.

Definition: Evaluation defined as the judgment of the effectiveness of nursing care to meet client goals, in this phase compares the client is behavioral responses with predetermined client goals and outcome criteria.

Evaluation will answer the following questions:
- Were the nursing diagnoses accurate?
- Did the patient meet the outcome criteria?
- Did the patient meet the criteria within the critical time periods?
- Have the patient's nursing problems been resolved?
- Have the patient's nursing needs been met?
- Should the nursing interventions be retained, altered or discontinued?
- Have new problems evolved for which nursing interventions have not been planned or implemented?
- What factors influenced the achievement or lack of achievement of the goals?
- Do priorities need to be reassigned?
- Should changes be made in the goals and outcome criteria?

Purpose of Evaluation

- Collect data for making judgments about nursing care delivered.
- Determine client's behavioral response to nursing interventions.
- Compare the client's response with predetermined outcome criteria.
- Apprise the extent to which clients goal were attained.
- Apprise/appreciate the involvement of client/family members in health care decisions.
- Assess the collaboration of client and health care team members.
- Identify the errors in the plan of care.
- Monitor the quality of nursing care.

Need of Evaluation in Nursing Process

- It determines the effectiveness of nursing plan of care.
- It evaluates whether the predetermined goal are achieved.
- It helps the nurse to discover/identify the errors in the previous steps of nursing process.

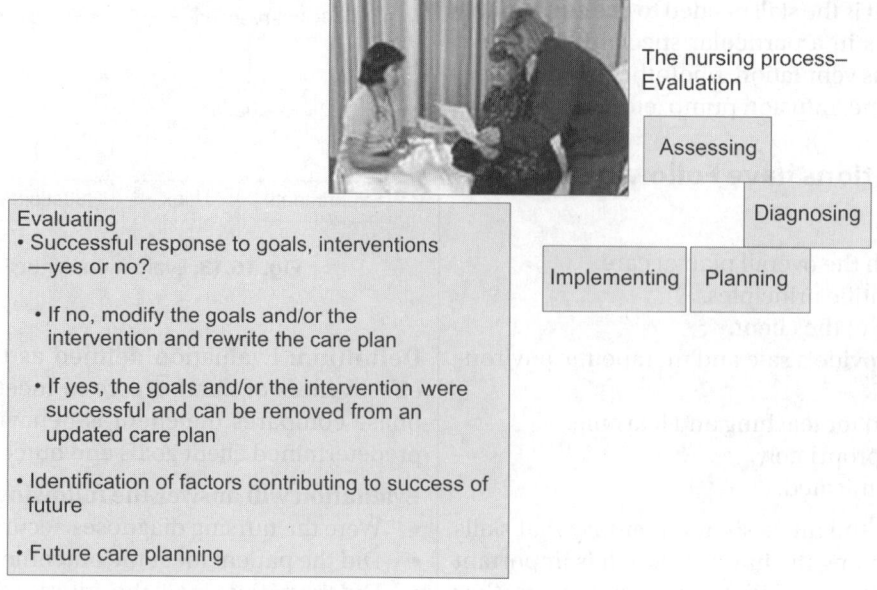

Fig. 16.14: Nursing evaluation.

- It helps the nurse to assess the clients behavioral responses to the planned course of action.

Activity in Evaluation Phase

Evaluation phase of nursing process involves following activities.
- **Review client goals and outcome criteria:** Nursing plan is very important to measure the goal attainment. Nurse will judge the attainment of goal by measuring the outcome criteria of planning phase.
- **Collect data:** Subjective and objective data is collected systematically to evaluate the goal attainment and outcome of care. Collection of data is also helpful to determine the effectiveness of nursing care provided. Sources for collecting the subjective data are client, family members, nursing personnel, other health care team members.
- **Goal:** Client will state that pain relived within 15 minutes after medication.
- **Measures of goal attainment:** After collecting the data, nurse forms a picture regarding clients behavioral response to the predetermined goals in planning phase.
- **Revision or modification of nursing care plan:**
  - Gather data to determine if new problem is arisen.
  - Look for all the factors resolved, need no intervention can be omitted.
  - Examine the list of nursing diagnosis and set new priorities.
  - Reassess the accuracy and appropriateness of the framed diagnosis.
  - Make goals realistic and accurate.
  - Examine the intervention that are identified, change or delete the inappropriate ones.
  - Incorporate factors leading to successful attainment of goal.
  - Do reevaluation again.

Evaluation Skills Required for Nurse

- Nurse must know the hospital policies, procedure and protocols of interventions and recording, etc.
- Nurse must have update knowledge and information of many subjects, such as psychology, pathophysiology, biochemistry, physiology, sociology, pharmacology. It helps her to understand client's response.
- Nurse must have intellectual and technical skills to monitor the effectiveness of nursing interventions.
- Nurse must have knowledge and skill of collecting subjective data and objective data.

Formal Evaluation Models

This type of evaluation can be viewed as informal. There is also a formal method of evaluation through a system called quality assurance.
- Quality assurance is the planned and systematic evaluation of care given to group of clients. The organization most actively involved in formal quality assurance is the joint commission for accreditation of health care organizations
- Quality assurance programs in nursing are viewed as evaluation system composed of three dimensions: Structure, process and outcome
- The structural dimension: Focuses on the organization within which nursing care is provided
- The process dimension: Focuses on patient welfare and end results of the care provided to the patient.

TABLE 16.2: Nursing care plan.

Assessment	Diagnosis	Inference	Planning	Intervention	Rationale	Evaluation
SUBJECTIVE: "Bakit kaya madalas ako mahilo?" (why do I always feel dizzy?) as verbalized by the patient. OBJECTIVE: • Request for information. • Agitated behavior • Inaccurate follow through of instructions. • Vital signs (V/S) taken as follows: T: 37.2 P: 84 R: 18 BP: 180/110	• Risk for prone bahavior related to lack of knowledge about the disease	• High blood pressure (HBP) or hypertension means high pressure (tension) in the arteries. Arteries are vessels that carry blood from the pumping heart to all the tissues and organs of the body. High blood pressure does not mean exessive emotional tension, although emotional tension and stress can temporary increase blood pressure. Normal blood pressure is below 120/80; blood pressure between 120/80 and 139/89 is called "prehypertension"	• After 8 hours of nursing interventions, the patient will verbalize understanding of the disease process and treatment regimen.	INDEPENDENT: • Define and state the limits of desired BP, Explain hypertension and its effect on the heart, blood vessels, kidney, and brain. • Assist the patient in identifying modifiable risk factors like diet high in sodium, saturated fats and cholesterol. • Reinforce the importance of adhering to treatment regimen and keeping follow up appointments. • Suggest frequent position changes, leg exercises when lying down	• Provides basis for understanding elevations of BP, and clarifies misconceptions and also understanding that high BP can exist without symptom or even when feeling well. • These risk factors have been shown to contribute to hypertension. • Lack of cooperation is common reason for failure of antihypertensive therapy. • Decreases peripheral venous pooling that may be potentiated by vasodilators	After 8 hours of nursing interventions, the patient was able to verbalize understanding of the disease process and treatment regimen.

Outcome criteria: Goals for accountability and quality assurance in nursing are being realized. The American Nurses Association has developed basic standards that provide a general model for nursing practice by which the quality of nursing practice may be evaluated. Record-Keeping has been revised to provide a problem-oriented approach to documentation of data. The use of outcome criteria as validations of the nursing process has become an accepted trend. The nursing audit has become an accepted method for comparing results of the actual nursing performance with the established criteria.

NURSING CARE PLAN

A nursing care plan (NCP) is a formal process that includes correctly identifying existing needs, as well as recognizing potential needs or risks. Care plans also provide a means of communication among nurses, their patients, and other healthcare providers to achieve health care outcomes. Without the nursing care planning process, quality and consistency in patient care would be lost.

Nursing care planning begins when the client is admitted to the agency and is continuously updated throughout in response to client's changes in condition and evaluation of goal achievement. Planning and delivering individualized or patient-centered care is the basis for excellence in nursing practice.

Types of Nursing Care Plans

Care plans can be informal or formal: Informal nursing care plan is a strategy of action that exists in the nurse's mind. A formal nursing care plan is a written or computerized guide that organizes information about the client's care. Formal care plans are further subdivided into standardized care plan, and individualized care plan: Standardized care plans specify the nursing care for groups of clients with everyday needs. Individualized care plans are tailored to meet the unique needs of a specific client or needs that are not addressed by the standardized care plan.

Objectives

The following are the goals and objectives of writing a nursing care plan:
• Promote evidence-based nursing care and to render pleasant and familiar conditions in hospitals or health centers.

- Support holistic care which involves the whole person including physical, psychological, social and spiritual in relation to management and prevention of the disease.
- Establish programs such as care pathways and care bundles. Care pathways involve a team effort in order to come to a consensus with regards to standards of care and expected outcomes while care bundles are related to best practice with regards to care given for a specific disease.
- Identify and distinguish goals and expected outcome.
- Review communication and documentation of the care plan.
- Measure nursing care.

Purposes of a Nursing Care Plan

The following are the purposes and importance of writing a nursing care plan:
- Defines nurse's role. It helps to identify the unique role of nurses in attending the overall health and well-being of clients without having to rely entirely on a physician's orders or interventions.
- Provides direction for individualized care of the client. It allows the nurse to think critically about each client and to develop interventions that are directly tailored to the individual.
- Continuity of care. Nurses from different shifts or different floors can use the data to render the same quality and type of interventions to care for clients, therefore allowing clients to receive the most benefit from treatment.
- Documentation. It should accurately outline which observations to make, what nursing actions to carry out, and what instructions the client or family members require. If nursing care is not documented correctly in the care plan, there is no evidence the care was provided.
- Serves as guide for assigning a specific staff to a specific client. There are instances when client's care needs to be assigned to a staff with particular and precise skills.
- Serves as guide for reimbursement. The medical record is used by the insurance companies to determine what they will pay in relation to the hospital care received by the client.
- Defines client's goals. It does not only benefit nurses but also the clients by involving them in their own treatment and care.

Components

A NCP usually includes nursing diagnoses, client problems, expected outcomes, and nursing interventions and rationales. These components are elaborated below:
- Client health assessment, medical results, and diagnostic reports. This is the first measure in order to be able to design a care plan. In particular, client assessment is related to the following areas and abilities—physical, emotional, sexual, psychosocial, cultural, spiritual/transpersonal, cognitive, functional, age-related, economic and environmental. Information in this area can be subjective and objective.
- Expected client outcomes are outlined. These may be long-and short-term.
- Nursing interventions are documented in the care plan.
- Rationale for interventions in order to be evidence-based care.
- Evaluation. This documents the outcome of nursing interventions.

Care Plan Formats

Nursing care plan formats are usually categorized or organized into four columns: (1) nursing diagnoses, (2) desired outcomes and goals, (3) nursing interventions, and (4) evaluation. Some agencies use a three-column plan wherein goals and evaluation are in the same column. Other agencies have a five-column plan that includes a column for assessment cues.

Step 1: Data collection or assessment: The first step in writing a nursing care plan is to create a client database using assessment techniques and data collection methods (physical assessment, health history, interview, medical records review, and diagnostic studies). A client database includes all the health information gathered. In this step, the nurse can identify the related or risk factors and defining characteristics that can be used to formulate a nursing diagnosis. Some agencies or nursing schools have their own assessment formats you can use.

Step 2: Data analysis and organization: Now that you have information about the client's health, analyze, cluster, and organize the data to formulate your nursing diagnosis, priorities, and desired outcomes.

Step 3: Formulating your nursing diagnoses: NANDA nursing diagnoses are a uniform way of identifying, focusing on, and dealing with specific client needs and responses to actual and high-risk problems. Actual or potential health problems that can be prevented or resolved by independent nursing intervention are termed nursing diagnoses.

Step 4: Setting priorities: Setting priorities is the process of establishing a preferential sequence for address nursing diagnoses and interventions. In this step, the nurse and the client begin planning which nursing diagnosis requires attention first. Diagnoses can be ranked and grouped as to having a high, medium, or low priority. Life-threatening problems should be given high priority.

Step 5: Establishing client goals and desired outcomes: After assigning priorities for your nursing diagnosis, the nurse and the client set goals for each determined priority. Goals or desired outcomes describe what the nurse hopes to achieve by implementing the nursing interventions and are derived from the client's nursing diagnoses. Goals provide direction for planning interventions, serve as criteria for evaluating client progress, enable the client and nurse to determine which problems have been resolved, and help motivate the client and nurse by providing a sense of achievement.

Short-term and long-term goals: Goals and expected outcomes must be **measurable** and **client-centered**. Goals are constructed by focusing on problem prevention, resolution, and/or rehabilitation. Goals can be **short-term** or **long-term**. In an acute care setting, most goals are short-term since much of the nurse's time is spent on the client's immediate needs. Long-term goals are often used for clients who have chronic health problems or who live at home, in nursing homes, or extended care facilities.

Short-term goal—a statement distinguishing a shift in behavior that can be completed immediately, usually within a few hours or days.

Long-term goal—indicates an objective to be completed over a longer period, usually over weeks or months.

Discharge plans—involves naming long-term goals, therefore promoting continued restorative care and problem resolution through home health, physical therapy, or various other referral sources.

Step 6: Selecting nursing interventions: Nursing interventions are activities or actions that a nurse performs to achieve client goals. Interventions chosen should focus on eliminating or reducing the etiology of the nursing diagnosis. As for risk nursing diagnoses, interventions should focus on reducing the client's risk factors. In this step, nursing interventions are identified and written during the planning step of the nursing process; however, they are actually performed during the implementation step.

Step 7: Providing rationale: Rationales, also known as scientific explanation, are the underlying reasons for which the nursing intervention was chosen for the NCP. Rationales do not appear in regular care plans; they are included to assist nursing students in associating the pathophysiological and psychological principles with the selected nursing intervention.

Step 8: Evaluation: Evaluating is a planned, ongoing, purposeful activity in which the client's progress towards the achievement of goals or desired outcomes, and the effectiveness of the NCP. Evaluation is an important aspect of the nursing process because conclusions drawn from this step determine whether the nursing intervention should be terminated, continued, or changed.

Step 9: Putting it on paper: The client's NCP is documented according to hospital policy and becomes part of the client's permanent medical record which may be reviewed by the oncoming nurse. Different nursing programs have different care plan formats, most are designed so that the student systematically proceeds through the interrelated steps of the nursing process, and many use a five-column format.

CONCLUSION

The nursing process is a process by which nurses deliver care to individuals, families, and/or communities and is supported by nursing theories. The nursing process was originally an adapted form of problem solving and is classified as a deductive theory. The nursing process is a cyclical and ongoing process that can end at any stage if the problem is solved. The nursing process exists for every problem that the individual/family/community has. The nursing process not only focuses on ways to improve physical needs, but also on social and emotional needs as well.

Nursing process is a deliberate activity utilized to organize nursing care within which the nurse (agent) assumes the role of provider of care, manager of care and member within the profession to empower the client toward self-care. The components include assessment, diagnosis, planning, implementation and evaluation. The entire process is recorded or documented in an agreed format in the record in order to inform all members of the interdisciplinary team about the contributions of nursing professionals to care, and to direct nurses in the performance, revision and evaluation of that care, as appropriate.

The nurse evaluates the progress toward the goals/outcomes identified in the previous phases. If progress towards the goal is slow, or if regression has occurred, the nurse must change the plan of care accordingly. Conversely, if the goal has been achieved then the care can cease. New problems may be identified at this stage, and thus the process will start all over again.

The nursing process is used by nurses every day to help patients improve their health and assist doctors in treating patients. Nursing requires the use of this process day in and day out. The process is based on theories and practices taught in nursing school. It is a form of problem solving. The nursing process is made up of a series of stages that are used to achieve the objective-The health improvement of the patient. The nursing process can stop at any stage as deemed necessary or can repeat as needed. This process is inclusive of physical health as well as the emotional aspects of patient health.

BIBLIOGRAPHY

1. Alfaro R. Applying Nursing Diagnosis and Nursing Process: A Step-by-step Guide, 2nd edition. Philadelphia: JB Lippincott, 1990.
2. American Nurses Association. Standard of Nursing Practice. Kansas City, Mo, 1973.
3. Becker BG, Fendler DJ. Vocational and Personal Adjustments in Practical Nursing, 7th edition. St. Louis: Mosby Year Book, Inc., 1994.

4. Carpenito LJ. Nursing Diagnosis: Application to Clinical Practice, 4th Ed. Philadelphia, 1992.
5. Carroll-Johnson RM (Ed). Classification of Nursing Diagnoses: Proceedings from the Ninth NANDA National Conference. Philadelphia: JB Lippincott, 1991.
6. Craven RF, Hirnle CJ. Fundamentals of Nursing: Human Health and Function. Philadelphia: JB Lippincott, 1992.
7. Gettrust KV, Brabec PD. Nursing Diagnosis in Clinical Practice: Guides for Care Planning, Albany, NY: Delmar Publishers, 1992.
8. Hickey PW, Nursing Process Handbook, St. Louis: Mosby Year Book, Inc., 1990.
9. Potter PA, Perry AG. Fundamentals of Nursing Concepts, Process and Practice, 3rd edition. St. Louis: Mosby Year Book, Inc., 1993.
10. Purtilo R. Health Professional and Patient Interaction, 4th edition. Philadelphia: WB Saunders, 1990.

REVIEW QUESTIONS

Long Essays

1. Define critical thinking; explain the components and importance of critical thinking in nursing.
2. Define nursing process; describe the steps of nursing process in detail.
3. Define nursing assessment; explain in detail about data collection in nursing process.

Short Essays

1. Skills required for critical thinking.
2. Critical thinking application in nursing practice.
3. Describe the levels of critical thinking in nursing.
4. Explain the benefits of nursing process for the patient and nurse.
5. Define nursing diagnosis; explain nursing diagnosis classifications.
6. Characteristic of nursing implementation.
7. Nursing care plan.
8. Define evaluation, explain the activity in evaluation phase.

Short Answers

1. Characteristics of nursing process.
2. Advantages of nursing process.
3. Accountability.
4. Methods of data collection.
5. Syndrome diagnosis.
6. Types of planning.
7. Setting priorities.
8. Time planning.
9. Formal evaluation models.

MULTIPLE CHOICE QUESTIONS

1. **The nurse in charge identifies a patient's responses to actual or potential health problems during which step of the nursing process?**
   a. Assessing
   b. Diagnosing
   c. Planning
   d. Evaluating

2. **A nurse is revising a client's care plan. During which step of the nursing process does such a revision take place?**
   a. Assessment
   b. Planning
   c. Implementation
   d. Evaluation

3. **Which intervention should the nurse in charge try first for a client that exhibits signs of sleep disturbance?**
   a. Administer sleeping medication before bedtime.
   b. Ask the client each morning to describe the quantity of sleep the night before.
   c. Teach the client relaxation techniques, such as guided imagery and progressive muscle relaxation.
   d. Provide the client normal sleep aids, such as pillows, back rubs, and snacks.

4. **Using Maslow's hierarchy of needs, a nurse assigns the highest priority to which client need?**
   a. Elimination
   b. Security
   c. Safety
   d. Belonging

5. **The nurse performs an assessment of a newly admitted patient. The nurse understands that this admission assessment is conducted primarily to:**
   a. Diagnose if the patient is at risk for falls
   b. Ensure that the patient's skin is intact
   c. Establish a therapeutic relationship
   d. Identify important data

ANSWERS

1. b   2. d   3. d   4. a   5. d

CHAPTER 17
Nutritional Needs

LEARNING OBJECTIVES
- Importance
- Factors affecting nutritional needs
- Assessment of nutritional status
- Review: Special diets—Solid, liquid, soft
- Review on therapeutic diets
- Care of patient with dysphagia, anorexia, nausea, vomiting
- Meeting nutritional needs: Principles, equipment, procedure, indications
  - Oral
  - Enteral: Nasogastric/Orogastric,
  - Introduction to other enteral feeds types, indications, gastrostomy, jejunostomy
  - Parenteral: TPN

TERMINOLOGY
- **Anorexia:** Loss of appetite.
- **Dyspepsia:** Indigestion, a feeling of fullness, discomfort, nausea and anorexia
- **Dysphasia:** Difficulty in swallowing
- **Nausea:** A sensation of sickness with inclination to vomit.
- **Nutrients:** Constituents of food, e.g. carbohydrate, protein, fat minerals, vitamins and water.
- **Regurgitation:** Back flow, e.g. back flow of partly digested food into the mouth from the stomach.
- **Vomiting:** Expulsion of stomach contents via the esophagus and the mouth.
- **Soft diet:** A diet that is soft in texture, low in residue, easily digested, and well tolerated. It provides the essential nutrients in the form of semisolid foods, such as eggs, cheese, custards and puddings, pureed vegetables, ground beef and lamb, fowl, fish; mashed, boiled or baked potatoes; soft-cooked cereals, and breads.
- **Therapeutic diet:** Normal diet which is modified to meet the altered requirements resulting from disease or injury; diet used in the treatment of a disease.
- **Low-oxalate diet:** A diet which excludes consumption of foods that are rich in oxalates such as beans, chocolate, cocoa, potatoes, spinach, tea and tomatoes (chemicals found in plant foods). This diet is prescribed for patients with urinary calculi composed of oxalate.
- **Obesity:** The generalized accumulation of excess adipose tissue in the body resulting in an increase of more than 20% of the desirable weight (ideal body weight). Obesity results when there is positive energy balance where the intake of calories (from food) is more than the expenditure of calories (physical activity).
- **Oliguric phase:** The early phase of acute renal failure when urine volume is reduced.
- **Parenteral nutrition:** The administration of nutrients by a route other than the alimentary canal, such as subcutaneously, intravenously, intramuscularly or intradermally. The parenteral fluids usually consist of physiologic saline solution with glucose, amino acids, electrolytes, vitamins, and medications.
- **Polydipsia:** Excessive thirst due to loss of body fluids, especially from the urine, as seen in diabetes mellitus.
- **Polyphagia:** 1. Swallowing abnormally large amounts of food at a meal. 2. Excessive appetite as in diabetes mellitus.
- **Polyuria:** Excessive secretion and discharge of urine as seen in diabetes mellitus.
- **Self-monitoring:** An important component of behavior modification in weight management. It includes maintaining a daily record of the place and time of food intake, as well as accompanying thoughts and feelings which stimulate food intake, It helps to identify physical and emotional settings in which eating occurs.
- **Food allergy:** Also referred to as food sensitivity. Any immunologically mediated adverse reaction related to the chemical composition of foods and their additives resulting from antigen-antibody combination.
- **Food exchanges:** Food exchanges are used to bring variety to the diet and to suit the family's economic capacity. Foods approximately containing the same calorie and protein values are grouped together, so that any item in that group can be chosen while formulating the daily menu. Food exchanges are specifically useful for patients with diabetes.
- **Food poisoning:** Any of a large group of toxic processes that result from the ingestion of a food contaminated by

toxic substances or by bacteria that contain toxins. Kinds of food poisoning include salmonella food poisoning, mushroom poisoning and shellfish poisoning.
- **Nutrition status:** It is defined as the extent to which a customary diet meets the body's requirement. In other words, it signifies the condition of body after the consumption of food The Condition of health of individuals as influenced by the utilization of nutrients. It can be assessed by dietary survey, anthropometry, clinical and laboratory investigations. A brief outline of the

Dietary information on the importance of various nutritional constituents that are present in foodstuffs is given in the following pages.

INTRODUCTION

Nutrition is the science of food values. It is relatively a new science, which was evolved from chemistry and physiology. The effect of food in our body is explained in nutrition. In other words, nutrition is defined as food at work in the body. In a broader sense nutrition is defined as "the science of foods, the nutrients and other substances their action, interaction, and balance in relationship to health and diseases, the process by which the organism ingests, digests, absorbs, transport and utilizes nutrients and dispose off their end products, in addition nutrition must be concerned with the social, economic, cultural and psychological implication of food and eating."

NUTRITION AND HEALTH

Definitions

- Nutrients are defined as the constituents of food, which perform important functions in our body. If these nutrients are not present in our food in sufficient amount, the result is ill health. Important nutrients include carbohydrates, proteins lipids, vitamins, minerals, and water.
- Food also contains many substances, which are non-nutrients e.g. coloring and flavoring substances in food.
- Dietetics: It is the branch of science that deals with the practical application of the principles of nutrition in health which is required to the human body.

Functions of Food

- **Physiological functions:**
  - Supplies nutrients for energy. Energy nutrients include carbohydrates, fats and proteins.
  - Supplies nutrients to build and maintain body tissues, nutrients needed in building and maintaining body are proteins, minerals and water.
  - Supplies nutrients needed for regulatory body processes. All the nutrients, except carbohydrates,

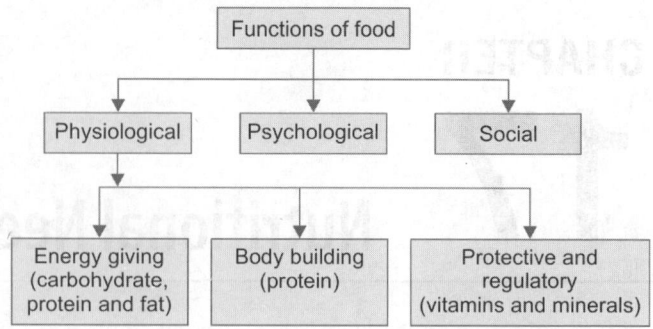

Flowchart 17.1: Different functions of food.

play an important role in the regulation of body process, such as circulation of food, maintenance of body temperature and digestion, etc.
- **Social function:** Food is served at many social events like teas, breakfasts, banquets, athletic award dinners, dances and meeting of all sorts. On all these occasions, food indirectly serves as an instrument to develop social support.
- **Psychological function:** Besides other functions, food satisfies certain emotional needs also. People often find it difficult to get adjusted to unfamiliar food, although it may be nutritionally sound. Traditional habits are characterized by certain foods, which are pleasing to persons of one culture and distasteful those of another.
- **Relationship of food to main functions:** Nutrition does the process or an activity by which the human body receives and uses all the food necessary for its growth, development and functions or activities.

Psychological function
- They give a sense of comfort, security, love and attention.
- Sharing of food among friend is a token of friendship and acceptance
- Friendly get together help in introducing us to new foods
- Foods are associated with emotions like sweets and chocolates for celebration
- Food is used for reward and punishment.

Physiological function
- Body building or growth
- Providing energy
- Regulation of body process (beating of the heart etc)
- Protective function (recovery from diseases)
- Maintenance and repairs

- Food supplies heat and energy for work and play.
- Food supplies materials for growth and repair of the body.
- Food supplies materials for regulation or control of body process and for protection of the body. All people are familiar with food but in order to understand now different foods are used in the body it is necessary to know what substances or materials are present in food. These substances are called nutrients. The nutrients

present in food these substances proteins, fats, minerals elements and vitamins.

Physiological Functions of Food

- **Energy yielding foods:** Foods rich in carbohydrates and fats are called energy yielding foods. They provide energy to sustain the involuntary processes essential for continuance of life, to carry out various professional, household and recreational activities and to convert food ingested into usable nutrients in the body. The energy needed is supplied by the oxidation of foods consumed. Cereals, roots and tubers, dried fruits, oils, butter and ghee are all good sources of energy.
- **Body building foods:** Foods rich in protein are called body building foods.
  Milk, meat, eggs and fish are rich in proteins of high quality. Pulses and nuts are good sources of protein but the protein is not of high quality. These foods help to maintain life and promote growth. They also supply energy.
- **Protective and Regulatory foods:** Foods rich in protein, minerals and vitamins are known as protective and regulatory foods. They are essential for health and regulate activities such as maintenance of body temperature, muscle contraction, control of water balance, clotting of blood, removal of waste products from the body and maintaining heartbeat. Milk, egg, liver, fruits and vegetables are protective foods.

> **Social function**
> - Food serves as a reason for get togethers.
> - Temples, gurudwaras serve same food to all
> - Birthdays, marriage and others celebrations become reasons to serve food
> - Males are given more and better food due to their higher status in the society
> - Refreshments served at get togethers bring more people together rather then dividing them
> - Food planned must be wholesome and enjoyable

- **Social functions of food:** Food has always been the central part of our community, social, cultural and religious life. It has been an expression of love, friendship and happiness at religious, social and family get-togethers.
- **Psychological functions of food:** In addition to satisfying physical and social needs, foods also satisfy certain emotional needs of human beings. These include a sense of security, love and acceptance. For example, preparation of delicious foods for family members is a token of love and affection.

Basic Food Groups

A well balanced diet contains food from the basic food groups:
- Milk and milk products.
- Meat, fish and poultry.

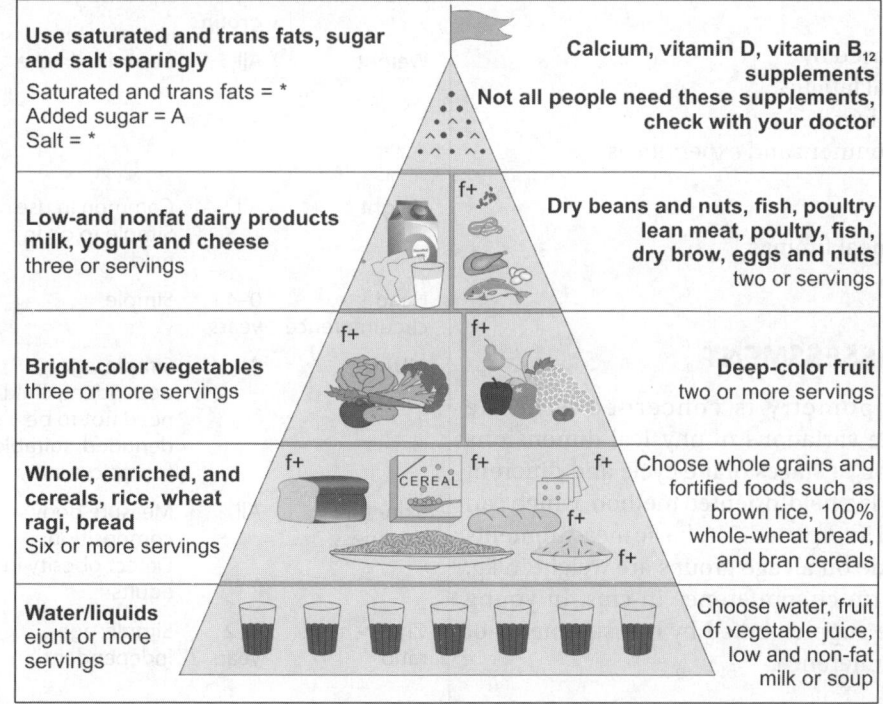

Fig. 17.1: Food guide pyramid.

(f+ = High fiber choices).

- Bread and cereals.
- Fruits and vegetables.

Purpose

- Food gives nourishment to body.
- It gives a feeling of security.
- It is used to promote a feeling of social acceptance.
- It is vitally important for our physical well being.
- Food is the fuel with which we run our bodies.

Essential Nutrients

- Carbohydrates: These are used as a source of energy. All cereals and root vegetable contain carbohydrates.
- Fats: They also are a source of energy. They are found in animals and plant seeds also in egg and milk.
- Proteins: The function of proteins in human body is the release of energy and building and repair of body tissues.

Factors Affecting Appetite

The appetite is increased by:
- Sight and smell of food (attractive serving)
- Food preference (likes and dislikes of the individual)
- Physical and mental relaxation (freedom from hurry, worry, pain, stress and fatigue)
- Regularity in eating (spacing of meals)
- Pleasant environment (attractive and cheerful atmosphere)
- Exercise

The appetite is decreased by:
- Physical and metal fatigue.
- Hurry, worry and fear.
- Unpleasant environment and experiences.
- Lac k of exercises.
- Irregular meals.
- Long spacing of meal timings.
- Hospitalization.

NUTRITIONAL ASSESSMENT

Nutritional anthropometry is concerned with the measurements of the variations of physical dimensions and body composition at stages of life cycle and different planes of nutrition. It is a field-oriented method, which can be easily adopted and interpreted. The basic measurements which should be made on all age groups are weight in kg, length/height and arm circumference in cms. In young children it should be supplemented by measurements of head and chest circumference.

Weight: Weight gain is an indicator of growth in children. It is measured with the help of the weighing scale. Body weight should be determined after the first void and before ingestion of food.

Anthropometric indices (weight for age): The Nutritional status can be interpreted using Gomez Classification as follows:

Weight: > 90% weight for age. Normal.
76–90% weight for age. Grade I malnutrition.
61 <75% weight for age. Grade II malnutrition.
<60% weight for age. Grade III malnutrition.

Linear measurements: Two types of linear measurements are commonly used.
- Height or length of the whole body
- Circumference of the head and the chest.

Height: The height of the individual is the sum of four components—leg, pelvis, spine and skull. For infants and children recumbent length (crown- heel length) is measured. The measurement is compared with the standards of the ICMR as given in Table 17.1 to assess nutritional status.

The desirable birth weight and length of an infant is 3 kg and 50 cm respectively. By the time the baby turns the first birth day, the birth weight is doubled and an increment of 25 cm in length is reached.

Head circumference: The measurement of head circumference is a standard procedure to detect pathological condition in children. Head circumference is related mainly to brain size. At birth the circumference of head is greater than that of the chest.

TABLE 17. 1: Anthropometry measurement.

Measurements	Age groups	Advantage	Disadvantage
Weight	All	Common in use	Difficult in field; Cannot tell body composition; Need accurate age; Need proper scale
Height	All	Common in use Simple to do in field	Differs by day time: Other factors play a role
Head circumference	0–4 years	Simple	Other factors play a role
MUAC	All	Simple, age dependent, child need not to be denuded, suitable for rapid survey	No limits for over nutrition and no standard for adults
Skin- fold thickness	All	Measure body composition: Detect obesity in adults	Need expensive callipers; difficult with the child and in the field
Chest - head ratio	1–2 years	Simple, age independent	For limited age— no classification method

Chest circumference: The circumference of the head and the chest are about the same at six months of age. After this the skull grows slowly and the chest more rapidly.

Therefore between the ages of six months and five years the chest/head circumference ratio of less than one may be due to failure to develop or due to wasting of muscle and fat of chest. In nutritional anthropometry the chest/head circumference ratio is of value in detecting under nutrition in early childhood.

Mid upper arm circumference (MUAC): Mid upper arm circumference at birth in a healthy child is between 10 and 11 cm. Over the first year the increment in MUAC is 3 to 4 cm as the muscles of the arms start to develop. In the preschool age the increase in MUAC is only one cm. Hence there is not much difference between the MUAC of a 3 year old from that of a 5 year old. So MUAC is an age independent index. The field workers in nutrition in our country have fixed the desirable value for MUAC as 12 cm for Indian preschool children.

The WHO has recommended 14 centimeter as a desirable value for MUAC for preschool children. Hence in screening malnourished children in a community this method is used with ease. When the value of MUAC is less than 12 cm among 1–5 year old children, they are designated as malnourished. In the field condition a bangle with a diameter of 4 centimeter can be used as a tool to detect malnutrition. When the bangle moves smoothly over the mid-upper arm of the child, it indicates malnutrition. The bangle test can be conducted with ease in field condition to screen malnourished children.

CARE OF PATIENT WITH DYSPHAGIA

Nutrition therapy is important for a patient who's having trouble swallowing, which affects the types and amounts of food he can eat. Because this patient is at risk for aspiration, a speech therapist should recommend the types and consistency of foods that would be safest for him.

Besides dietary recommendations, other interventions that can help ensure adequate nutrition include:
- Providing mouth care immediately before meals to help improve taste
- Encouraging the patient to rest before meals so he is not too tired to eat
- Offering him small, frequent meals
- Minimizing or eliminating distractions so he can focus his attention on eating and swallowing
- Placing him in high Fowler's position and having him tilt his head forward to help ease swallowing
- Using adaptive devices, such as mugs with spouts, as necessary. But avoid using straws, which can cause more liquid to flow into the mouth than the patient can handle, increasing the risk of aspiration.
- Encouraging him to take small bites and to chew thoroughly
- Offering praise and encouragement during mealtimes
- Providing foods that are cool or mildly warm to stimulate the swallowing reflex
- Adding flavor as necessary to stimulate salivation
- Helping the patient select nutritious foods.

Dysphagia types
- there are three types of swallowing disorder, divided on the basis of where the problem is occurring:
  - Oral dysphagia
  - Pharyngeal dysphagia
  - Esophageal dysphagia

Oral or pharyngeal dysphagia	Esophageal dysphagia
• Coughing or choking with swallowing	• Sensation of food sticking in the chest
• Difficulty initiating swallowing	• Oral or pharyngeal regurgitation
• Food sticking in the throat	• Food sticking in the throat
• Drooling	• Drooling
• Unexplained weight loss	• Unexplained weight loss
• Change in dietary habits	• Change in dietary habits
• Recurrent pneumonia	• Recurrent pneumonia
• Change in voice or speech	
• Nasal regurgitation	

Do
- Review the patient's medical record for risk factors for dysphagia and aspiration.
- If he is tired, your patient may have more difficulty swallowing. Wait 30 minutes, and then reassess his alertness before performing the test.
- Have suction equipment immediately available.
- Minimize environmental distractions and position him upright in a chair or elevate the head of the bed 60 to 90 degrees.
- Assess his mental status and make sure he can voluntarily cough, clear his throat, and swallow saliva before proceeding with the test. If he is managing his oral secretions, offer him small bites of ice chips or sips of water from a cup or a teaspoon. Observe him carefully before, during, and after each offering for cough, drooling, voice change (especially a wet or gurgling quality), and swallowing difficulty. Stop the test immediately if any of these occur and notify his health care provider.
- If he can swallow without his voice or breathing sounding wet, and without choking or coughing, proceed with a soft diet, then if tolerated to a regular diet as ordered.
- If he has difficulty tolerating water, try giving him thickened liquid (the consistency of honey) by spoon and try pureed semisolids. Observe him for choking or coughing. If tolerated, proceed with a pureed or thickened liquid diet as ordered until he's formally evaluated by a speech-language pathologist or place him on NPO. status based on your observations.
- Provide diligent oral care to all patients with dysphagia, including those who are NPO.
- Notify the patient's health care provider of the results of the swallow screen so she can order an appropriate diet and additional testing, as indicated. Document the test results and subsequent actions in the patient's medical record.

Don't

- Don't offer semisolids, liquids, or solids (including oral medications) to a patient who can't swallow saliva or voluntarily cough and clear his throat.
- Don't leave the patient unattended during the test.
- Don't administer sedatives and hypnotics, if possible, because they can impair the cough reflex and swallowing.

CARE OF PATIENT WITH ANOREXIA

Anorexia nervosa is a chronic and severe disorder with a high incidence of morbidity and mortality.

Individuals who have anorexia nervosa:
- Fear obesity;
- Have a disturbed perception of their own body image;
- Suffer significant weight loss;
- Refuse to maintain normal body weight.

The age of onset is usually adolescence but anorexia can affect individuals from pre-puberty to middle age. The condition primarily affects young women but there is an increase in the disorder among younger males and nurses need to be aware of this.

In some people anorexia may occur as an acute episode but it can become a chronic condition suffered over many years.

Signs and symptoms to look out for include:
- Weight loss;
- Refusal to eat;
- Appetite loss;
- Fear of becoming obese;
- Self-induced vomiting;
- Difficulty in swallowing;
- Use or abuse of laxatives;
- Constipation;
- Preoccupation with food, weight loss and/or body image.

Physical problems that stem from the condition—some of which can become life threatening—include electrolyte imbalance, bradycardia, hypotension, hypothermia, fatigue, edema and amenorrhoea.

Role of the Nurse

- Having knowledge and understanding will enable nurses to monitor food intake and observe for potential eating disorders. Treatment will depend on an individual's symptoms and relate specifically to the individual problem.
- It is essential to observe patients' nutritional status as eating disorders can be life threatening. It is also important to ensure they maintain adequate nutrition and electrolyte balance. If an eating disorder has been identified, the nurse must monitor weight on a regular basis.
- This can be achieved by encouraging the supervision of patients during and after mealtimes in order to prevent vomiting after eating. Setting time limits for each meal will help to set realistic expectations and encourage a relaxed atmosphere at mealtimes that will, in turn, help to reduce stress and anxiety.
- It is essential to monitor patients' elimination pattern as excessive use of diuretics and laxatives is common among patients with eating disorders. As a consequence, patients may require intervention to treat constipation.
- Monitoring skin condition for breakdown and poor healing is an important part of the nurse's role. A lack of protein, needed to aid tissue repair, makes the skin more likely to break down. In addition, it is vital that good oral hygiene is achieved as recurrent vomiting may cause dental problems.
- Finally, it is important to monitor patients' activity levels. With anorexia they may undertake excessive exercise that can be detrimental to their physiological state. Additionally, if they also have a physical illness, excessive exercise could slow their recovery.

CARE OF PATIENT WITH NAUSEA

Nausea defined as an unpleasant, wavelike sensation in the back of the throat, epigastrium, or throughout the abdomen that may or may not lead to vomiting.

Defining Characteristics

The nursing diagnosis is characterized by the following signs and symptoms:
- Allergy to food
- Excessive salivation

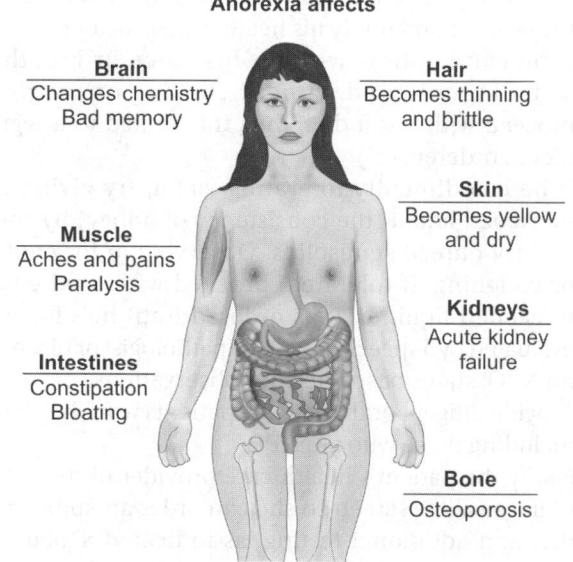

Fig. 17.2: Signs and symptoms of anorexia.

- Gagging sensation
- Increased swallowing
- Reports of nausea
- Sour taste in the mouth

Assess Nausea Characteristics

- History
- Duration
- Frequency
- Severity
- Precipitating factors
- Medications
- Measures used to alleviate the problem

Interventions

- Eat small, frequent meals. This may mean eating small amounts of food every 2-3 hours.
- Choose bland, non-spicy, non-fatty foods.
- Avoid foods that have caused nausea in the past.
- Remain sitting up or standing within one hour of eating. Do not lay down right after eating.
- Avoid foods with strong odors. Eat foods that are cool or can be eaten at room temperature as this will decrease the smell of these foods.
- Try dry foods such as crackers or toast. If you have nausea before getting out of bed, try having a cracker or two before getting up from bed.
- Avoid cooking methods that cause strong odors. Avoid using a crock-pot for cooking or cooking soups/stews as these will fill the house with cooking odors for a long period of time.
- Make sure to drink liquids to prevent dehydration. If possible, choose fluids with additional calories and protein.
- Avoid eating your favorite foods when you are extremely nauseated. This will allow you to still enjoy this food after your nausea has subsided.
- Try using ginger or ginger products such as ginger tea or ginger ale. You can also try ginger aromatherapy.
- Drink liquids in between meals/snacks.

CARE OF PATIENT WITH VOMITING

Vomiting is a complex reflex that is mediated by the vomiting center in the medulla oblongata of the brain.

Vomiting is spending gastric contents exclusively through the mouth with the help of contraction of the abdominal muscles. Necessary to distinguish between regurgitation, rumination, or gastroesophageal reflux.

Nursing diagnoses that may arise:
- Fluid volume deficit related to loss of active liquid.
- Imbalanced Nutrition: less than body requirements related to absorption disorders.
- Nausea related to gastric irritation.
- Ineffective tissue perfusion related to hypovolemia.

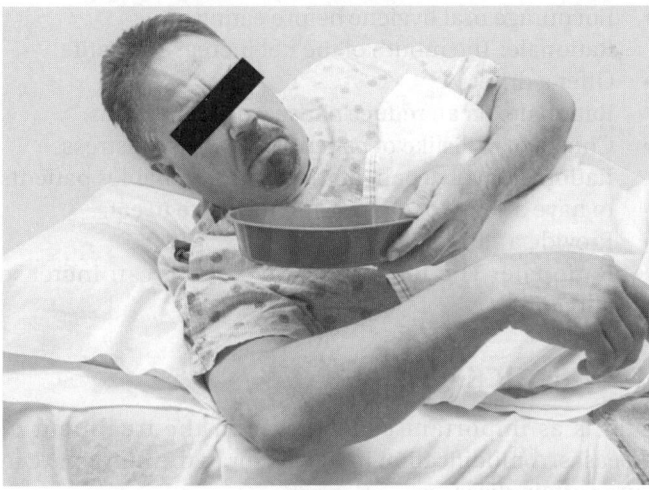

Fig. 17.3: Nursing care of patient vomiting.

- Risk for Impaired skin integrity related to disruption of metabolic status.
- Anxiety related to changes in health status.

Nursing Care Plan for Vomiting

Nursing diagnosis-1: Fluid volume deficit related to loss of active liquid.

Goal: Fluid and electrolyte deficit is resolved.

Expected outcomes: Signs of dehydration—none, mucosa of the mouth and lips moist, fluid balance.

Intervention:
- Observation of vital signs.
- Observation for signs of dehydration.
- Measure the input and output of fluid (fluid balance).
- Provide and encourage the family to drink a lot more than 2000 - 2500 cc per day.
- Collaboration with physicians in fluid therapy, laboratory tests electrolyte.
- Collaboration with a team of nutrition in low-sodium fluid administration.

Nursing diagnosis-2: Imbalanced nutrition—less than body requirements related to absorption disorders.

Goal: Nutrients are met.

Intervention:
- Assess the extent to which the inadequate nutrition clients.
  Rational: Analyze the causes implement interventions.
- Estimate/calculate the calorie intake, keep the comments about the appetite to a minimum.
  Rationale: Identifying deficiencies/nutritional needs to focus on the problem and create a negative atmosphere affects the input.
- Measure the weight as indicated.
  Rational: Overseeing the effectiveness in diet.
- Give eats little but often.
  Rational: Do not let boredom and nutrient intake can be increased.

- Encourage oral hygiene before eating.
  Rationale: The mouth of the net increase appetite.
- Offer a drink.
  Rationale: It can reduce nausea and relieve gas.
- Consul of a/dislike of patients who cause distress.
  Rational: Involve patients in planning, enables patients to have a sense of control and the drive to eat.
- Provide a varied diet.
  Rationale: The food was varied client can increase appetite.

DIET IN SICKNESS

Diet is as important as medicine in the treatment of diseases. A modification in the diet or in the nutrients can cure certain diseases.

Nutrition during illness should be adequate to prevent weight loss and weakness. An acutely ill or injured patient is in danger of malnutrition.

Purpose

- To meet the metabolic needs of human body..
- To prevent dehydration.
- To improve the appetite.
- To provide adequate nutrition.
- It is necessary for the growth and maintenance of bones and other tissues.

General Rules of Treatment

- The diet must be planned in relation to changes in metabolism occurring as a result of the disease.
- The diet must be planned to agree as nearly as possible with the patients food habits, his likes and dislikes and the amount of exercise he takes.
- Changes should be made gradually adequate explanation must be when given, it is necessary to make dietary changes gradually.
- There should be plenty or variety in the diet, hot food should be served hot and cold foods cold.

Problems during Sickness

- There will be disturbance of gastrointestinal function
- Anorexia (loss of appetite)
- Defective digestion and absorption
- Lack of exercise decreases need for energy
- The process of anabolism and catabolism are not normal in sickness.
- Vomiting and diarrhea are problems in which intravenous fluid administration is required.
- In some kinds of illness, protein requirements are more while in some others, both protein and carbohydrate are needed in large amounts.

Modifications of Nutrients in Therapeutic Diet

- Carbohydrates are usually well tolerated and are necessary to maintain the stores of liver glycogen. Adequate intake of carbohydrates can prevent ketosis.
- During sickness demand of protein is usually increased due to waste. So easily digestible protein should be given.
- The requirements of calcium and iron must be maintained during illness, sodium and potassium may sometimes need to be restricted especially if there is edema, ascites and hypertension.
- Fat soluble vitamin, e.g. vitamin A and D need to be added if the patient is on fat-restricted diet for a long time.
- Vitamin B complex may not be adequately absorbed in pathological conditions of the gastrointestinal tract.
- Requirement of vitamin C is greatly increased in fevers and is especially necessary for the healing of wounds after surgery.
- Fluids are very important to prevent dehydration especially in conditions like high fevers, diarrhea and vomiting, in such conditions the fluid intake within 24 hours should be 2,500 mL to 3,000 mL
- If adequate fluids cannot be given by mouth, they must be given intravenous maintain fluid balance by maintaining accurate intake output chart
- Infants require a higher amount of fluid compared to adult requirements they need 150 mL of fluid per kg of body weight.

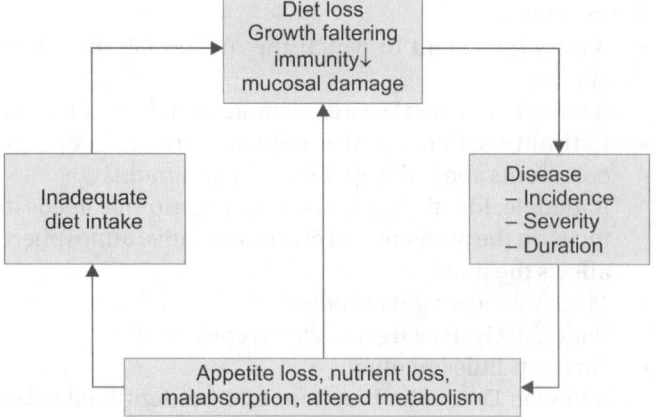

Fig. 17.4: Effects of diet on health.

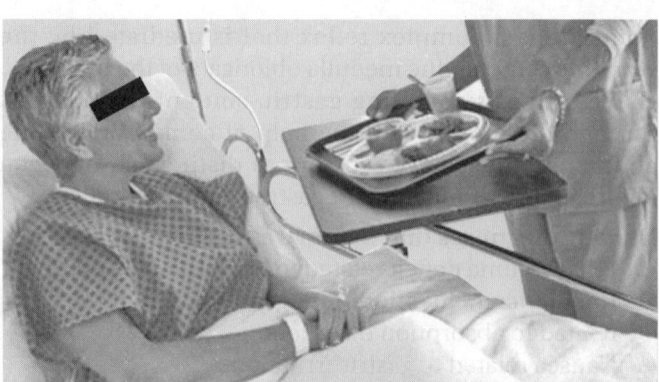

Fig. 17.5: Nurse providing normal hospital diet.

THERAPEUTIC DIET

Diet in disease must be planned as part of the complete care of the patient. Many modifications may have to be made according to the disease and the condition of the patient.

Objectives

- To improve the general health
- To meet the metabolic needs
- To promote healing
- To prevent dehydration
- To facilitate tissue repair and growth.

Principles Involved in Diet Therapy

- The diet must be planned in relation to changes in metabolism occurring as a result of disease.
- The diet must be planned according to the habits of the patient based on culture, religion, socioeconomic status, personal preferences, physiological and psychological conditions.
- As far as possible, changes in the diet should be brought gradually and adequate explanations are given with the changes made, if any.
- In short and acute illness, the food should not be forced because his appetite is very poor but he may soon recover the normal appetite.
- Whatever the diet prescribed, there should be variety of for selection.
- Small and frequent feeds are preferred to the usual three meals
- Hot foods should be served hot and cold foods should be served cold.

HOSPITAL DIET

- **Full diet:** It is a regular well balanced diet. It is vegetarian or non-vegetarian, this is for patients who do not need any special modification
- **Soft light diet:** It is given to provide light and easily digestible food with minimum residue. It contains food which requires little chewing and contains no fiber or no seasoning
- **Bland diet:** The foods are easily digestible, free from substances which might cause irritation of the gastrointestinal tract and generally or low roughage content, used mainly for patients with gastrointestinal conditions.

Liquid Diets

- **Liquid diets:** Must be used for patients who are unable to take or tolerate solid food this diet is given usually to patient having hyperpyrexia, postoperative patients and patients having gastrointestinal disturbances.
- **Clean fluids:** Used when there is a marked intolerance to food and roughage these include clear tea, weak black coffee, clear soups, whey water, strained fruit juices, clear fluid diet should be used only for a short time
- **Full liquid diet:** It is given as a total nutrition of the patient and has to be maintained by fluids for considerable time. This is necessary when the patient is unable to swallow solid food or if the patient is fed by intragastric or gastrostomy tubes.

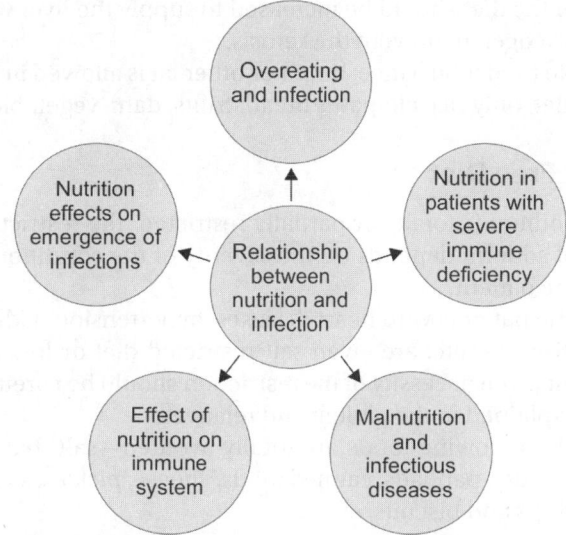

Fig. 17.6: Therapeutic diet functions.

Low Calorie Diet

- The total calorie intake is reduced to less than the body's requirements so that the remainder of the calories required can be derived from the stored fat.
- The aim of this diet is to slow steady loss of weight over a period of several weeks or even months. This diet is advised obese patients.
- The food stuffs like: Ghee, butter, sugar, sweets bread, rice, and potatoes are omitted from the diet. Use salads fruits and boiled vegetables. The patient must have plenty of bulk in the diet by using high fiber foods and low calorie beverages.

Low Protein Diet

- Low protein diet is advised in kidney diseases such as nephritis, uremia. In these disease the protein is avoided or given in low moderate type
- This type of diet is given to give the rest to kidneys because excessive protein intake acts as an additional load to the kidneys.
- The foodstuffs like: Milk; eggs and meat, etc. are omitted or restricted according to the prescribed protein intake.

Low Fat Diet

- Low fat diet is restricted from the diet patients with liver diseases and gallbladder diseases. Carbohydrates

in the diet should be increased to supply the liver with glycogen to prevent the ketosis.
- No fried food: Ghee, butter or other fat is allowed in the diet, only rice chapattis bread, fruits, dahi, vegetables.

Salt Free Diet

- Sodium is totally or partially restricted, the restriction of sodium depends on the severity of the condition of the patient.
- The patients with heart diseases, hypertension, kidney diseases, etc. are given salt restricted diet or low salt diet. The necessity of the restriction should be carefully explained to the patient and relatives.
- The following foods are totally avoided—salt, baking powder, pappads, canned foods, cheese, pickles, salted chips and biscuits, etc.

High Protein Diet

- High protein diet: The protein intake should be average from 75 to 100 gm per day for adult. In protein energy malnutrition cases easily digestible and high nutritive value protein, e.g. milk protein should be given.
- High protein diet is given to the patients such as operated cases, tuberculosis accident, burns, nephritic syndrome and emacided cases.
- The food stuffs contains rich protein are milk and milk proteins, eggs, fish meat, broth, dhals, dahi beans, soybean and ground nuts.

Diabetic Diet

- In diabetes mellitus the metabolism of carbohydrate, fat and protein are affected. Diabetes is a lifelong disease which can be treated but not cured. The dietary treatment depends upon the severity of the condition.
- The purpose of diabetic diet is to keep the patient in good health to keep the blood sugar level within normal level and to keep urine free from sugar.
- The diet should be balanced but there should be restriction of carbohydrates, e.g. rice, biscuits, sugar, jams, sweets, honey, carrots, and sweet potatoes. The patient should have egg, milk raw salads all types of green leafy vegetables.
- The total calories required 20 to 25 percent should be from protein 40 percent from carbohydrates and 40 percent from fat.

Diet in Anemia

- This type of patient requires the diet which is high in protein, high in iron and high in vitamins. The diet should provide necessary nutrients for the formation of new red blood cells or hemoglobin.
- The main purposes are to provide necessary nutrients for blood cell formation and to remove the cause of anemia.

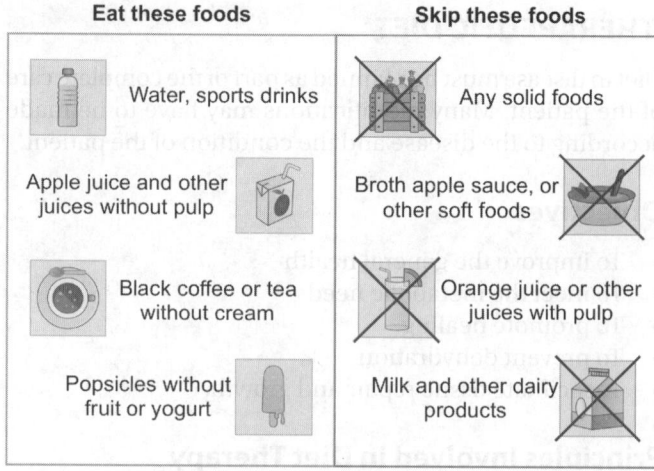

Fig. 17.7: Health food tips.

- The food stuffs recommended are liver, meat, eggs, spinach drumstick leaves, ragi, jaggery, etc.

Clear Fluid Diet

Whenever an acute illness or surgery produces a marked intolerance for food as may be evident by nausea. Vomiting, anorexia, distention and diarrhea, it is advisable to restrict the intake of food. In acute infection, in acute inflammatory conditions of the intestinal tract, following operations upon the colon or rectum when it is desirable to prevent evacuation from the bowel, clear fluid diet is suggested. This diet is also given to relieve thirst, to supply the tissues with water, to aid in the removal of gas.

The diet is made up of clear liquids that leave no residue, and it is non-gas forming action. This diet is entirely inadequate from a nutritional standpoint. Since it is deficient in protein, minerals, vitamins, and calories. It should not be continued for more than 24 to 48 hours. The amount of fluid is usually restricted to 30 to 60 ml per hour at first, with gradually increasing amounts being given as the patients tolerance improves. This diet can meet the requirement of fluids and some minerals and can be given in 1 to 2 hour intervals.

Conditions Necessitating the Use of Clear Liquid Diet

- Preoperative period e.g., as a preparation for bowel surgery.
- Prior to colonoscopic examination.
- Postoperative phase e.g., in the initial recovery phase after abdominal surgery or after a period of intravenous therapy.
- Acute illness and infections as in acute gastro intestinal disturbances such as acute gastroenteritis, when fluid and electrolyte replacement is desired to compensate for losses from diarrhea.
- As the first step in oral alimentation of a nutritionally debilitated person.
- In temporary food intolerance.

FULL FLUID DIET

This diet bridges the gap between the clear fluid and soft diet. It is used following operations in acute gastritis, acute infections and in diarrhea. This diet is also suggested when milk is permitted and for patients not requiring special diet but too ill to eat solid or semisolid foods. In this diet, foods which are liquid or which readily become liquid on reaching the stomach are given. This diet may be made entirely adequate and may be used over an extended time without fear of deficiencies developing, provided it is carefully planned. This diet is given at 2-4 hours interval.

Conditions Necessitating the Use of Full Fluid Diet

- Postoperative phase when progressing from clear liquids to solid foods.
- Acute gastritis and infections.
- Following oral surgery or plastic surgery of face or neck area.
- In chewing and swallowing dysfunction.
- In esophageal or stomach disorders causing intolerance to solid food intake.

SOFT DIET

It bridges the gap between acute illness and convalescence. It may be used in acute infections, following surgery, and for patients who are unable to chew. The soft diet is made up of simple, easily digestible food and contains no harsh fiber. Patients with dental problems are given mechanically soft diet. It is often modified further for certain pathologic conditions as bland and low residue diets. In this diet, three meals with intermediate feedings should be given.

Conditions Necessitating the Use of Soft Diet

- While progressing from full fluid diet to general diet.
- During postoperative phase when a patient is unable to tolerate normal diet.
- Gastrointestinal problems e.g. diarrhea.
- General debilitation and inadequate dentition.
- Convalescence.
- Transition from acute phase of illness to convalescence.
- Acute infections.

A soft diet can be modified as mechanical soft diet.

Mechanical soft diet: Many people require a soft diet simply because they have no teeth and such a diet is known as mechanical or a dental soft diet. It is not desirable to restrict the patient to the food selection of the customary soft diet and the following modifications to the normal diet may be made:

- Vegetables may be chopped or diced before cooking.
- Hard raw fruits and vegetables are to be avoided; tough skins and seeds to be removed.
- Nuts and dried fruits may be used in chopped or powdered forms.
- Meat to be finely minced or ground.

NORMAL DIET

It is used for ambulatory and bed patients whose conditions do not necessitate a special diet as one of the routine diets. Many special diets progress ultimately to a regular diet. The regular hospital diet is simple in character and preparation, easy of digestion and calculated to afford maximum nourishment with minimum effort to the body. The diet is well balanced, adequate in nutritional value and attractively served to stimulate a possible poor appetite.

A normal diet is defined as one which consists. of any and all foods eaten by a person in health. It is planned keeping the basic food groups in mind so that optimum amounts of all nutrients are provided. As there is no restriction of any kind of food, this diet is well balanced and nutritionally adequate.

Since the patient is hospitalized and/or is at bed rest, a reduction of 10% in energy intake should be made and too many fatty foods and fried foods be avoided as they are difficult to digest. The proteins are slightly increased (+10%) to counteract a negative nitrogen balance. All other nutrients are supplied in normal amounts.

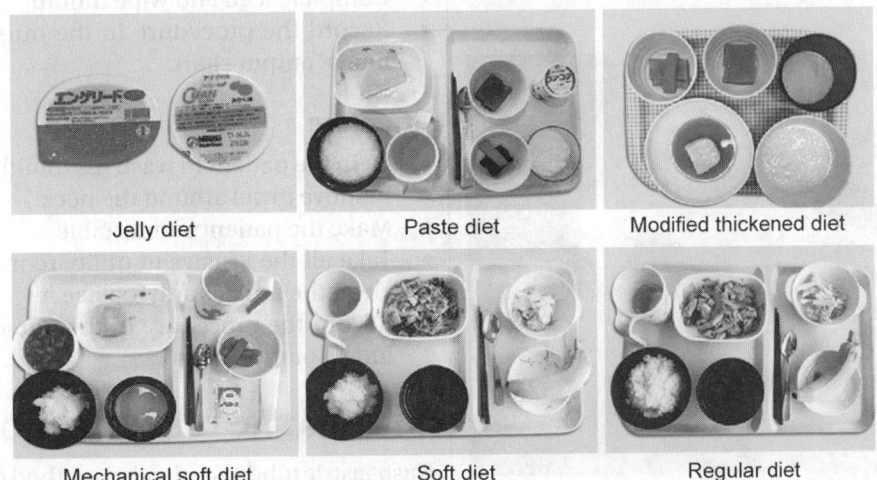

Fig. 17.8: Types of hospital diet.

FEEDING THE HELPLESS PATIENT

It is assisting a dependent patient to take food and fluids.

Purpose

- To assist the patient to eat meal.
- To meet the nutritional need.
- To promote health.
- To prevent dehydration.
- To improve appetite.

General Instructions

- The diet is prescribed by doctor planned by dietitian and sewed by nurse.
- Food should be sewed at correct time in a pleasant manner and in a pleasant atmosphere.
- Small and frequent meals are preferable for a sick person.
- Maintain a chart for intake of food and fluids for seriously ill patients.
- The patient should be free from pain and other discomfort during meal time.
- Food should be sewed in an attractive manner so that the sight and smell of should increase his appetite.
- Food should not be too hot or too cold.
- Meals should be sewed in clean and covered vessels.
- Give enough time for the patient to enjoy his food.
- Encourage the patient to develop a taste to his therapeutic regimen of diet.
- Be careful not to spill food. Wipe the patient's mouth and chin whenever necessary.
- Wash patient's hands and make him brush his teeth after meals.

Preliminary Assessment

Check

- Doctors order for any specific precautions.
- Patients likes and dislikes and socioeconomic status.
- Find out the food habits of the patient.
- General condition and the ability for self-care.
- Patients ability tom follows instructions.
- Ensure that the ordered diet is prepared properly and safety.
- The articles available in the patients unit.

Preparation of the Patient and the Environment

- Create a pleasant environment for the patient by well ventilated, free from noise, odor and unpleasant sight.
- Send the visitors away tactfully.
- Give bed pan or urinal to patient if required before meals.
- If patient can sit help him to have fowler's position with cardiac table or over bed table.
- Provide hand washing facilities to patient and if necessary help him, so that he will feel fresh.
- Place the towel over the chest and under the chin to protect clothing.

Equipment

A tray containing:

- A glass of water to give at the end of the meal
- Napkin to wipe the face in between
- Mackintosh and towel
- Feeding cup or spoon
- The required amount of feed in a mug at the right temperature
- Kidney tray.

Procedure

- Wash hands thoroughly.
- Make sure that patient is not starving for any procedure.
- Explain procedure to patient.
- Make sure that therapeutic restriction are considered.
- Cover patient below chin with face towel.
- Feed the patient either by using spoon or fingers.
- Offer water as required after meal, to rinse mouth and spit into K-basin.
- Complete feed and wipe mouth.
- Record the procedure in the nurse record sheet and intake output chart.

Aftercare

- Help the patient to wash his mouth and hands.
- Remove towel around the neck.
- Make the patient comfortable.
- Take all the articles to utility room, discard the waste, clean the articles and replace it.
- Record the procedure in the nurse's record sheet and intake output chart.

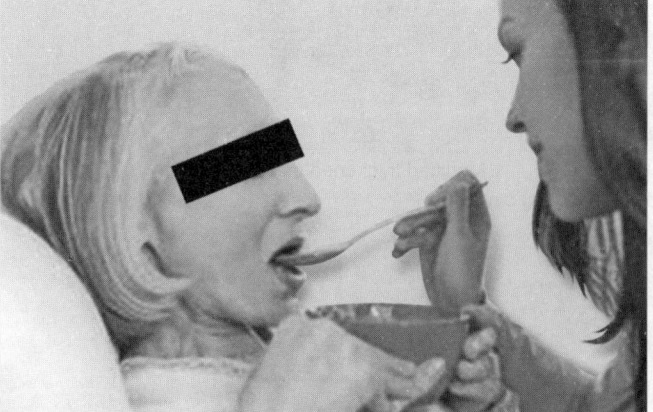

Fig. 17.9: Nurse feeding helpless patient.

NASOGASTIC TUBE INSERTION

Nasogastric tube insertion is a method of introducing a tube through nose into stomach.

Indications: By inserting a nasogastric tube, you are gaining access to the stomach and its contents. This enables you to drain gastric contents, decompress the stomach, obtain a specimen of the gastric contents, or introduce a passage into the GI tract. This will allow you to treat gastric immobility, and bowel obstruction. It will also allow for drainage and/or lavage in drug over dosage or poisoning. In trauma settings, NG tubes can be used to aid in the prevention of vomiting and aspiration, as well as for assessment of GI bleeding. NG tubes can also be used for enteral feeding initially.

Purpose

- To feed patient with fluids when oral intake is not possible.
- To dilute and remove consumed position.
- To instill ice cold solution to control gastric bleeding.
- To prevent stress on operated site by decompressing.
- To relieve vomiting and distention.
- To collect gastric juice for diagnostic purposes.

Equipment

A tray containing:
- Nasogastric tube of appropriate size.
- K-basin.
- Stethoscope.
- Bowl with water.
- Adhesive scissor.
- Syringe 20 cc or 10 cc.

Preliminary Assessment

Check

- Doctors order for any specific instruction.
- Patients ability to follow instructions.
- General condition of the patient.
- Articles available in the unit.

Preparation of the Patient and Unit

- Explain the sequence of procedure.
- Arrange the articles at the bedside.

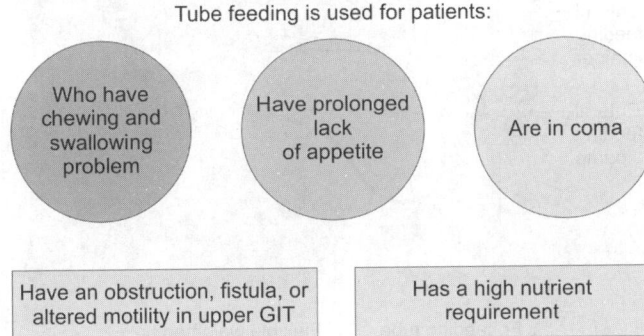

Fig. 17.10: Indications of tube feeding.

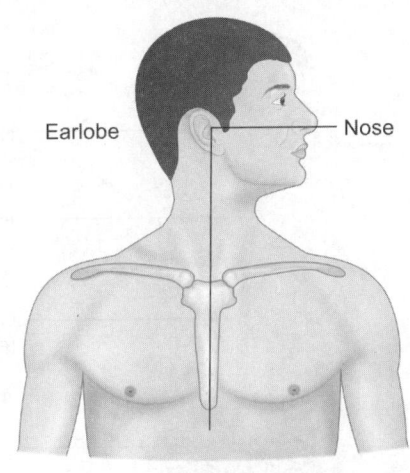

Fig. 17.11: Nasogastric tube measurement technique.

- Provide privacy.
- Provide comfortable position.
- Place the Mackintosh and towel across the chest.
- Remove the dentures, if any and place it in a bowel of clean water.
- Give mouthwash and help him to clean the teeth.
- Clean the nostrils, if there are secretions or crust formation, using swab stick dipped in saline.

Procedure

- Wash hands thoroughly.
- Measure distance of tube from tip of patient's ear lobe to nose to tip of xiphoid process.
- Mark the distance of the tube.
- Lubricate the tube for about 6 to 8 inches with the lubricant using a rag pieces or a paper square.
- Hold the tube coiled in the right hand and introduce the tip into the left nostril.
- Pass the tube gently but quickly backwards momentary resistance may occur as the tube is passed into the nasopharynx.
- When the tube reaches the pharynx the patient may gag. Allow him to rest for a movement.
- Have the patient take sips of water on command advance the tube 3 to 4 inches each time patient swallows.
- Make sure tube is in stomach.
- Once location of NG tube insured close other end of tube with spigot, secure tube on nose using adhesive in 'T' or butterfly.

Methods to Confirm NG Tube in the Stomach

- **Aspirate:** Attach the syringe to the end of NG tube and aspirate small amount of gastric contents.
- **Immerse distal end of tube:** Into bowel of water and check for air bubbles. If the tube is in the trachea, air bubbles will coincide with the expiration of each breath.
- **Auscultate:** Attach syringe to free end of NG tube, place diaphragm of stethoscope over left hypochondrium.

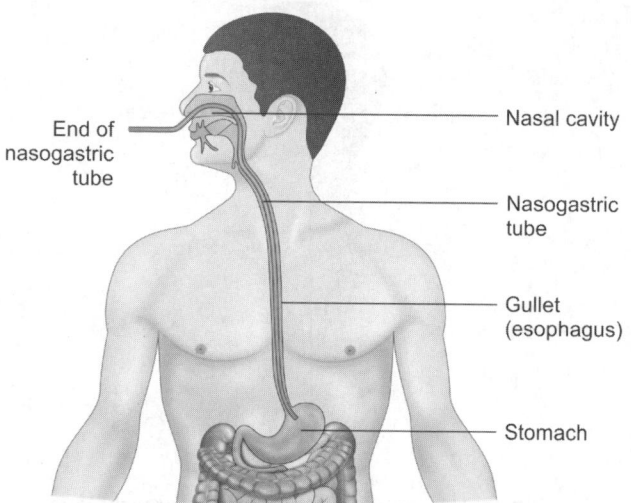

Fig. 17.12: Nasogastric tube insertion.

Inject 10 mL of air and auscultate abdomen for gushing sound.

Aftercare

- Offer a mouthwash. Clean the face and hands and dry them.
- Remove the Mackintosh and towel.
- Make the patient comfortable in bed.
- Take all the articles to the utility room discard the waste, clean it and replace it in a proper place.
- Wash hands.
- Record the procedure in the nurse's record sheet.

Contraindications: Nasogastric tubes are contraindicated in the presence of severe facial trauma (cribriform plate disruption), due to the possibility of inserting the tube intracranially. In this instance, an orogastric tube may be inserted.

Complications: The main complications of NG tube insertion include aspiration and tissue trauma. Placement of the catheter can induce gagging or vomiting, therefore suction should always be ready to use in the case of this happening.

GASTRIC GAVAGE

Gastric gavage or nasogastric tube feeding is given through tube which is inserted through patient's nose into stomach, when patient is unable to take food orally.

It is the administration of fluid food by means of tube passed into the stomach it is also called gastric gavage.

Purpose

- To provide adequate nutrition.
- To give large amounts of fluids for therapeutic purpose.
- To assess tolerance of feeds in postoperative patients.
- To introduce food into stomach when the patient is not able to take food in the usual manner.
- When the condition of mouth or esophagus makes swallowing difficult.

Indication for Tube Feeding

- Unconscious patient or semiconscious.
- After certain surgeries of the mouth and throat.
- Patients unable to swallow.
- Premature babies.
- When the patient is unable to retain the food, e.g. anorexia nervosa and vomiting.

General Instructions

- Give mouthwash frequently to avoid complications of a neglected mouth.
- Maintain accurate intake and output chart.
- Measure and drain the feed (fluid) to avoid blockage in the tube.
- Avoid introducing air into the stomach during each feed. Pinch the tube before the fluid run into to the stomach completely.
- Feeding may be given at intervals of 2,3, or 4 hours and the amount is not exceeding 150 to 300 mL per feed.
- Observe for complications such as nausea, vomiting, distension, diarrhea, aspiration pneumonia, asphyxia, fever, and water and electrolyte imbalance.

Advantages of Tube Feeding

- An adequate amount of all types of nutrients including distasteful foods and medication can be supplied.
- Large amount of fluids can be given safely.
- The danger of pererial feeding are avoided, e.g. venous thrombosis.
- Tube feeding may be continued for weeks without any danger to the patient.
- The stomach may be aspirated at any time is desired.
- Overloading of the stomach can be prevented by a drip method.

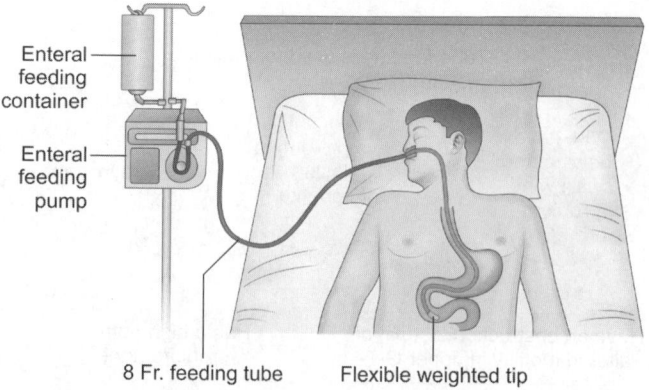

Fig. 17.13: Nasogastric tube feeding by feeding pump.

Principles Involved in Gastric Gavages

- A thorough knowledge of the anatomy and physiology of the digestive tract and respiratory tract, ensures safe induction of the tube (avoid misplacement of the tube).
- Tube feed is a process of giving liquid nutrients or medications through a tube into the stomach when the oral intake is inadequate or impossible.
- Microorganism enters the body through food and drink.
- Introduction of the tube into the mouth or nostrils is a frightening situation and the preparation of the patient facilitates introduction of the tube.
- Systematic ways of working adds to the comfort and safety of the patient and help in the economy of material, time and energy.

Preliminary Assessment

- Identify the correct patient.
- Check the doctor's order for any specific precautions.
- Check the level of consciousness of the patient.
- Check whether the feed is ready at hand.
- Articles available in the unit.

Preparation of the Patient and Environment

- Explain the sequence of the procedure
- Provide adequate privacy.
- Position the patient in sitting or semi fowlers
- Place the Mackintosh and towel around the neck.
- Arrange the articles at the bedside locker.
- Clean the mouth by providing mouthwash.

Equipment

A tray containing:
- Mackintosh and towel
- 20 cc syringe
- Stethoscope
- Bowl with water
- Adhesive with scissors
- Feeds and water
- Ounce glass.

Procedure

Syringe Method

- Wash hands thoroughly.
- Place towel around neck in such a way that patients clothing and bed linen are protected.
- Make sure the tube is in stomach before giving feeds.
- Remove spigot. Pinch tube to prevent air entry. Remove plunger from syringe and connect to tube.
- Keep syringe about 12 inches above patients head. Start feed with small measured amount of water and allow feed to follow slowly and steadily through tube in such a way, that air does not enter tube.
- Do not force fluid, allow to flow by gravity.
- At the end of feed flush tube by pouring small measured amount of water. Remove syringe and replace spigot.

Syphon Method

- Place towel around neck in such a way that patients clothing and bed linen are protected.
- Make sure that tube is in stomach before giving feeds.
- Immerse tip of tube in prepared feed immediately by avoiding air entry into tube.
- Raise fluid container about 12 inches above patients head and observe flow of fluid.
- When feed is over flash tube with small quantity of water.
- Pinch tube and close with spigot.

Aftercare

- Remove the Mackintosh and towel.
- Place the patient in comfortable position
- Replace the articles to utility room, clean it and replace it.
- Record the procedure in nurse's record sheet and intake and output chart.

GASTROJEJUNOSTOMY FEEDING

Gastrojejunostomy feeding is defined as enteral nutrition is the of a liquid food preparation directly into the stomach or small intestine via a tube. It is a ideal method of providing nutrition for the person who as unable to swallow food and drink normally but has intact gastrointestinal function. It is the introduction of liquid food through a tube or catheter which the surgeon has already introduced into the stomach through the abdominal wall.

Indications

- Tumors or operations on the upper gastrointestinal tract.
- Cancer of the esophagus.
- Stricture of the esophagus caused by poisoning in case of fistula.

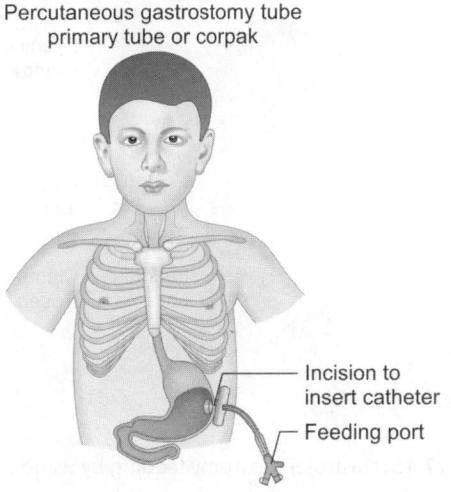

Fig. 17.14: Gastrojejunostomy feeding.

General Instructions

- It is essential that the area of the skin around the tube be kept clean and dry.
- A water proof ointment such as zinc oxide may be applied around the tube to protect the skin from the irritation of the hydrochloric acid.
- Foods given through the gastostomy tube are some as those given by nasogastric tube and the same amounts are given at the same intervals.

Methods of Administration

- **Intermittent feeding:** Given four to six times a day continuously is delivered as a bolus through a longer lumen tube. Volume for formula usually 250 mL to 450 mL is placed in a large syringe and inserted into the proximal end of the tube.
- **Intermittent gravity drip:** Administration delivers a similar volume 250 to 450 mL of feeding over 20 to 30 ml a minute, four to six times a day.
- **Continuous administration:** Delivers fluid through a small lumen tube at a constant rate via orogastric and nasogastric routes. The rate of flow is carefully regulated. The nurse should calculate the amount of fluid to be infused during an hour and regulates the infusion pump accordingly.

Preliminary Assessment

Check

- The doctors order for any specific instruction.
- Level of consciousness of the patient.
- Self-care ability of the patient.
- Mental status to follow instructions.
- Articles available in the unit.

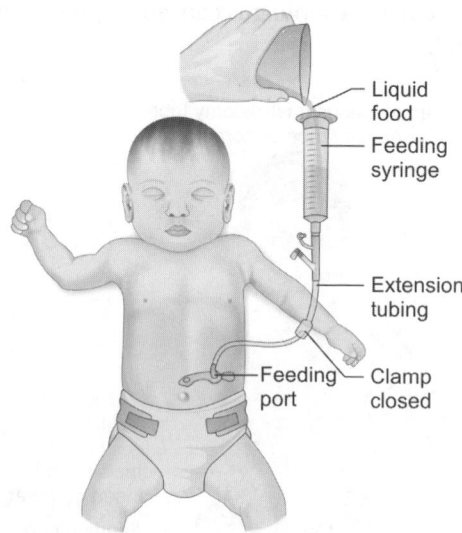

Fig. 17.15: Gastrojejunostomy feeding by using syringe.

Operation of the Patient and Environment

- Explain the sequence of the procedure.
- Provide privacy.
- Arrange the articles at the bedside.
- Place the patient in a comfortable position.
- Keep the environment clean and tidy.
- Keep ready with feed to be given.

Equipment

A clean tray containing:
- A funnel, rubber tubing, glass connection screw and a clamp.
- A glass of drinking water.
- Required amount of feed, temperature 100° F.
- Sterile lubricant to protect surrounding area.
- Sterile dressing and forceps in a dressing tray.
- Medicine as per order.
- Kidney tray.
- Many tailed binder if required.
- Mackintosh and towel.
- Stethoscope.
- Syringe.

Procedure

- Wash hands thoroughly.
- Place the mackintosh or towel; clean the surrounding area of the opening. Cover the wound with sterile piece of gauze.
- Unscrew the clamp from the gastrostomy tube and attach the funnel and rubber tubing; keep the tube pinched to prevent air from setting in.
- Aspirate the gastric contents by attaching a syringe.
- Pour some clean water into the funnel and lower a little to let our air.
- Then pour the feed before the funnel is empty.
- If any medicines are ordered, these are given after feed.
- Give water after giving medicines.
- Disconnect the tabbing and funnel.
- Clean and apply sterile instrument around the wound. Dress it with sterile dressing and apply the binder.

Aftercare

- Remove the mackintosh and towel.
- Position the patient comfortable.
- Secure the tube with plaster.
- Replace the articles to utility room.
- Hand wash
- Record the procedure in nurse record sheet.

Skin Care

It is very important to keep the skin site clean and dry so it does not get red and irritated. The skin around the GJ tube should be cleaned once a day with a bath or shower. To clean:

- Gently remove any tape and gauze. A small amount of clear or tan drainage is normal.
- Gently clean the skin around the GJ tube with soap and water. Rinse and pat dry.
- After the skin is dry, you may put a clean 2x2 gauze around the GJ tube, under the disc..
- Make sure the disc on the outside fits against the skin so that the tube does not move in or out easily.
- Cut four 3-inch pieces of tape.
- Tape the disc and gauze dressing to the skin.

BREASTFEEDING

Breastfeeding is the best food for the baby. It not only gives nourishment but also suffice the baby's emotional needs.

Advantages

- It is the best natural food for the baby.
- If fully meets the nutritional requirements of the infant and promotes optimal growth.
- It protects the baby from infections.
- It satisfies the sucking reflex of the child.
- It is always clean and sterile.
- It is available at the correct temperature and requires no preparation.
- Lactoferrin present in the breast milk inhibits the growth of bacteria.
- Gastrointestinal disturbances are less in breastfed children, due to presence of lactobacillus fibrous.
- It creates bonding between the mother and child
- It helps parents to space their children.
- It reduces infant mortality rate.
- It helps in involution of the uterus.
- It gives baby a sense of security.

Contraindication for Breastfeeding

Mother

- Breast diseases, e.g. mastitis, breast abscess.
- Cardiac diseases and active tuberculosis.
- Infectious diseases.
- Mental illness of mother.
- Unconscious mother.

Baby

- Babies with cleft lip and cleft palate.
- Premature and sick babies who have poor sucking reflex.
- Oral thrush.

General Instructions

- Mother should keep her body clean and wear clean cloths.
- Before each feed, clean the breasts and hands of the mother.
- Mother should be in comfortable position during feeding.
- Hold the nipple between index and middle finger.
- Feed the baby on demand; it helps the baby to gain weight.
- Feed the baby for minimum 10 minutes on each breast.
- Instruct the mother to feed the baby even when the child is ill.
- Burping should be done after each feed to expel the air from the air from the baby's stomach.
- When the baby is 4 to 6 months old start weaning, because, mother's milk is not sufficient to sustain growth after 6 months of age.
- If the baby's napkin is wet, dirty, change, the napkins and cloths before each feeding.
- Weigh the child every month and record it.
- Teach the mother to have adequate rest to avoid tension, fatigue and stress.

ARTIFICIAL FEEDING

Artificial feeding given to infants instead to the breast milk, Breast milk is often substituted by cow's milk. The cow's milk is substituted by dried milk, evaporated milk, etc.

Difference between Human Milk and Cow Milk

Points of difference	Human	Cow
Carbohydrate	7%	4%
Protein	1.5%	4%
Fat	3.5%	4%

Preparation of Formula

The milk formula should be planned to meet the nutritional requirement of the infant which is based on his age and weight.

- Caloric requirement: 110 calories per kg of baby weight.
- Fluid requirement: 165 mL per kg of baby weight.
- Milk requirement: 100 to 130 mL per kg of body weight.
- Number of feeds in 24 hours: 7 feeds.
- Time interval between each feed: 2 to 3 hours.

Preparation of Milk Formula for a Day

Take 460 mL of milk, 140 mL of water and add 9 teaspoonful of sugar and boil it and keep it in the refrigerator, for each feed, take 85 mL of milk, ward it and feed the baby.

Different Ways of Feeding an Infant

- By using the feeding bottle and teat.
- By nasal tubes.
- By belcroy feeder.
- By dropper.
- By using spoon.

General Instructions

- Plan the formula according to the nutritional requirement of the baby.
- The feeding bottle, teat and other articles used for the feeding should be sterile,
- The milk feed should be warm.
- The mother and the child should be in a comfortable position.
- Ensure a slow and steady flow of milk by making a hold in the teat neither too big nor too small.
- Change the napkin before the feed, if it is wet or soiled.
- The feeds should be given at regular intervals.
- The mother should wash her hands thoroughly before preparing the feed and feeding the child.
- Offer a small quantity of water at the end of each feed.
- Never pinch the baby's nose to make him to open his mouth instead press his cheeks.

Preliminary Assessment

Check

- The doctors order for any specific instructions.
- Plan the formula according to the nutritional needs of the infant.
- Time at which the last feed was given.
- General condition of the baby.
- Baby's ability for sucking.
- Articles available in the unit.

Preparation of the Infant and the Environment

- Arrange the articles at the bedside.
- Provide privacy.
- Change the napkin if it is wet.
- Bath the baby in necessary.
- Keep the feeding bottle ready.

Equipment

A tray containing:
- Mackintosh and towel.
- Baby dress and napkin.
- Feeding bottle and teat in a sterile container.
- Required amount of feed (sterile).
- Sterile water in a bottle.
- A piece of clean towel or flannel.
- Gown and mask for the nurse.

Procedure

- Wash hands thoroughly.
- Hold the baby in a position similar to one used for breastfeeding.
- Check the temperature of the feed by dropping few drops on the inner aspect of the wrist joint.
- Hold the bottle in an angle of 45 degree and bring the teat to the lips and then into the mouth of the baby.
- Take care to keep the teat filled with milk throughout the feeding.
- Break the wind (burping) in between the feeds.
- When the feed is finished, give sterile water to the baby.

Aftercare

- Keep the baby on the shoulders and pat over his back.
- Wipe the face.
- Remove the towel and lay the baby in the cradle.
- Replace the articles in the proper place after cleaning.
- Wash hands.
- Record the procedure in the nurse's record sheet.

TOTAL PARENTERAL NUTRITION

Parenteral nutrition, also known as intravenous feeding, is a method of getting nutrition into the body through the veins. While it is most commonly referred to as total parenteral nutrition (TPN), some patients need to get only certain types of nutrients intravenously. Parenteral nutrition is often used for patients with Crohn's disease, cancer, short bowel syndrome, and ischemic bowel disease.

Definition: Parenteral nutrition (PN) is sterile intravenous solution of protein, dextrose and fat in combination with electrolytes, vitamins, trace elements and water. PN is used to treat children who cannot be adequately fed by the oral or enteral route.

TPN bypasses the normal way the body digests food in the stomach. It supplies the fuels the body needs directly into the blood stream through a central IV line. The body needs three kinds of fuel-carbohydrates, protein and fat.

- Carbohydrates provide calories to the body. They supply most of the energy or fuel the body needs to run. The main energy source in TPN is dextrose (sugar).
- Protein is made up of amino acids, which are the "building blocks" of life. The body uses protein to build muscle, repair tissue, fight infections and carry nutrients through the body.
- Fat or lipids are another source of calories and energy. Fat also helps carry vitamins in the blood stream. Fat supports and protects some of your organs and insulates your body against heat loss. Fat is white in color.

TPN also contains other nutrients, such as vitamins and minerals, electrolytes and water.

- Vitamins added to the TPN provide the needed daily amounts of vitamins A, B, C, D, E and K. It is the vitamins that are added to the TPN mixture that turns it yellow. The body also needs minerals. These minerals are zinc, copper, chromium, manganese and selenium. The vitamins and minerals in the TPN are needed for the body's growth and good health.
- Electrolytes are important for bone, nerve, organ and muscle function. Electrolytes, such as calcium, potassium, phosphorus, magnesium, sodium, chloride and acetate, are also added to the TPN mixture.

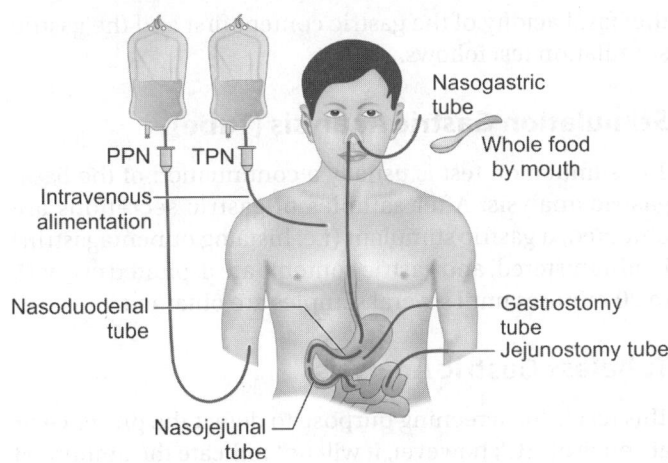

Fig. 17.16: Different types of feeding techniques.

- Water is a vital part of TPN. It prevents patients from becoming dehydrated (too little fluid). The amount of water in the TPN is based on your child's height and weight.

Roles of Professionals in TPN

- **Medical**: Assess patient, assess fluid balance, contact dietician to assess nutritional status, refer to nutrition support team to develop nutrition plan, complete ordering and prescribing of PN (ordering prior to 1200), ensure monitoring in place, reassess patient (ongoing).
- **Nursing**: Assess patient, fluid balance recording, daily weight of patient, check PN prescription, ensuring specific PN solution written (g/L protein and g/L glucose), check PN solution, line care and connection/running of intravenous PN infusions.
- **Dietetics**: Assess patient, provide energy and protein requirements, and assessment of enteral intake.
- **Pharmacy**: Check ordering PN, manufacturing, checking and dispensing PN.
- **Clinical nutrition team** (nurse coordinators, dietician, medical staff, pharmacy): Assess a) patient, b) fluid balance charts, c) dietician advice, d) PN ordering and prescribing and e) special circumstances and provide an overarching nutritional plan and consultation based advice.

Initial Preparation

- Document patient's weight and weight loss
- Complete consult form for Clinical Nutrition Program and page Nutrition Support Nurse Coordinator
- Organize dietician review of nutritional state and estimated nutritional requirements (energy, protein and specific nutrient) or use equations to calculate basal metabolic rate and adjustments.
- Consider access type (CVC or peripheral) and duration it will be needed. Only day 1 (10% dextrose) solutions can be run through a peripheral line. In general the smallest caliber single lumen central line is preferable.

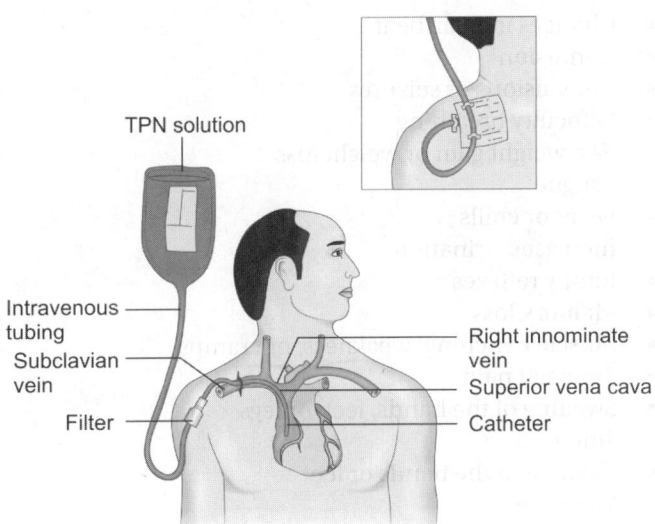

Fig. 17.17: Total parenteral nutrition method.

- Perform baseline bloods (creatinine, urea and electrolytes, calcium magnesium and phosphate, liver function tests, full blood count, triglycerides, blood sugar, venous blood gas) and correct electrolyte abnormalities before starting PN. See drug doses for potassium, phosphate, and magnesium corrections. Corrections can often be given by the enteral route (e.g. potassium, phosphate) if the child is receiving other medications by this route.

Fluid Calculations

- Calculate total fluid volume requirement (mL/hr and total volume over 24 hours)
- Consider losses (upper GIT, lower GIT, drains, urine)
- Consider other fluids being given to the patient over 24 hrs (antibiotics, other infusions, blood or albumin)
- Determine the volume available for PN (total fluid volume requirement minus the volume required for other infusions).
  Note: sometimes the volume available may not be enough to provide adequate nutrition, especially in patients who are fluid restricted - other infusion volumes should be minimal volume, liaise with clinical nutrition team to ensure the patient is receiving adequate nutrition
- Calculate mL/kg/day = volume available for PN/weight Lipid is not usually included in volume calculations
- Calculate mL/hr = volume available for PN/24. Note PN may be run over a shorter time in which case the denominator will change.
- In children with significant refeeding risk, PN may be started at lower volumes (giving a lower % of their EER and reducing the risk of refeeding)

Side effects of TPN: The most common side effects of parenteral nutrition are mouth sores, poor night vision, and skin changes. Patients should speak with their doctors if these conditions do not go away. Other, less common side effects include.

- Changes in heartbeat
- Confusion
- Convulsions or seizures
- Difficulty breathing
- Fast weight gain or weight loss
- Fatigue
- Fever or chills
- Increased urination
- Jumpy reflexes
- Memory loss
- Muscle twitching, weakness, or cramps
- Stomach pain
- Swelling of the hands, feet, or legs
- Thirst
- Tingling in the hands or feet
- Vomiting.

GASTRIC ANALYSIS

The gastric analysis test examines the acidity of the gastric secretions in the basal state (without stimulation) and the maximal secretory ability (with stimulation, i.e. with histamine phosphate, betazole hydrochloride (histalog) indicate a peptic ulcer (stomach or duodenal), and an absence of free HCl (achlorhydria) could indicate gastric atrophy (possibly caused by gastric malignancy) or pernicious anemia. In addition, gastric contents can be collected for cytological examinations. Gastric analysis by tube (basal and stimulation) and tube less gastric analysis (urine examination after a resin dye and stimulant are administered) are the methods used for evaluating gastric secretions.

Major Constituents of Gastric Secretions

Constituents	Source	Major functions
HCl (acid)	Parietal cells	Kills microbes, dissolves food particles, activates pepsinogen into pepsin and provides optimum pH for pepsin
Pepsinogens (pepsin)	Chief cells	Begins initial hydrolysis of proteins (optimum pH 2–4)
Rennin (only in infants)	Stomach	Causes milk clotting and promote its digestion by preventing rapid passage from the stomach.
Gastric lipase	Chief and mucous cells	An acid stable lipase that digest short chain fatty acid
Gastrin	G cells	Stimulates acid secretion by stomach
Mucus	Mucous cells	Protects stomach, moistens food

Basal Gastric Analysis (Tube)

Gastric secretions are aspirated through a nasogastric tube after a period of fasting. Specimens are obtained to evaluate the basal acidity of the gastric content first and the gastric stimulation test follows.

Stimulation Gastric Analysis (Tube)

The stimulation test is usually a continuation of the basal gastric analysis. After samples of gastric secretions are obtained, a gastric stimulant (i.e. histalog or pentagastrin) is administered, and gastric contents are aspirated every 15 to 20 minutes until several samples are obtained.

Tubeless Gastric Analysis

This test is for screening purpose to detect the presence or absence of HCl; however, it will not indicate the amount of the free acid in the stomach. A gastric stimulant (caffeine, histalog) is given, and an hour later a resin dye (azuresin, diagnex blue) is taken orally by the client. The free HCl releases the dye from the resin base; the dye is absorbed by the gastrointestinal tract and is excreted in the urine. Absence of the dye in the urine 2 hours later is indicative of gastric achlorhydria. This test method saves the client the discomfort of being intubated with nasogastric tub; however, it does lack accuracy.

Normal Findings

Fasting: 1.0 to 5.0 mEq/L/h

Stimulation: 10 to 25 mEq /L/h

Tubeless: Detectable dyes in the urine.

Purposes

- To evaluate gastric secretions.
- To detect an increase or decrease of free HCl.

Clinical Problems

Decreased Level

- Pernicious anemia.
- Gastric malignancy (atrophy).
- Atrophic gastritis.

Elevated Level

- Peptic ulcer (duodenal).
- Zolliner-Ellison syndrome.

Client Preparation

- Explain the purpose and procedure of the tube or tubeless gastric analysis test to the client. Check with the health care providers before you give your explanation to find out whether he or she will perform both basal and stimulation gastric analysis. List the steps of the test on paper for the client, if needed.
- Tell the client how the nasogastric tube is inserted (i.e. the tube is lubricated and passes through the nose or

mouth) and that he or she will be asked to swallow or will be given sips of water as the tube is passed into the stomach. The end of the tube may be attached to low intermittent suction.
- Notify the health care provider, if the client is receiving the following categories of drugs: antacids, antispasmodics, anticholnergics, adrenergic blocker, cholinergics and steroids. Drugs from the above groups and a few others should be withheld for 24 to 48 hours before the gastric analysis. Drugs that cannot be withheld should be listed on the request slip.
- Monitor vital signs. Observe for possible side-effects for use of stimulants (i.e. dizziness, flushing, tachycardia, headache and a lower systolic blood pressure).
- Label the specimens (gastric or urine) with the client's name, the date, the time and the specimen's number.
- Be supportive of the client. Encourage the client to express his or her concerns or fear. Answer questions or her refer them to appropriate health professions.

Procedure

- The client should be NPO for 8 hours to 12 hours prior to the test. Smoking should be restricted for hours.
- Certain groups (i.e. anticholinergics, cholinergics, adrenergic blockers, antacid, and steroids) and alcohol and coffee should be restricted for at least 24 hours before the test. It should be noted on the request slip, if the drugs cannot be withheld.
- Baseline vital signs should be recorded.
- Loose dentures should be removed.
- A lubricated nasogastric tube is inserted through the nose or mouth.
- A residual gastric specimen and four additional specimens taken 15 minutes apart should be aspirated and labeled with the client's name, the time, and a specimen number. The nastrogastric tube may be attached to low intermittent suction.

Stimulation test: A continuation of the basal gastric analysis.
- A gastric stimulant is administered (i.e. betazole hydrochloride (histalog) or histamine phosphate intramuscularly, pentagastrin subcutaneously).
- Several gastric specimens are obtained over a period of 1 to 2 hours (histamine four 15 minute specimens in 1 hour and histalog eight 15-minute specimens in 2 hours). Specimens should be labeled with the client's name, the date, the time, and specimen numbers.
- Vital signs should be monitored. Emergency drugs such as epinephrine (adrenalin) should be available.
- The test usually takes 2 and half hours for both parts (basal and stimulation).

Tubeless Gastric Analysis

- The client should be NPO for 8 to 12 hours before the test.
- The morning urine specimen is discarded.
- Certain drugs are withheld for 48 hours before the test (i.e. antacids, quinine, iron, vitamin B complex), with the health care providers permission.
- Give the client caffeine sodium benzoate 500 mg in a glass of water.
- Collected a urine specimen 1 hour later. This is control urine specimen.
- Give the client the resin dye agent (azuresin or diagnex blue) in a glass of water.
- Collect a urine specimen 2 hours later. The urine may be colored blue or blue green for several days. Absence of color in the urine usually absence of HCl in the stomach.

Factors Affecting Diagnostic Results

- Incorrect labeling of specimens could affect test results.
- Drugs antacids, anticholinergics, and histamine blockers (cimetidine, ranitidine) could decrease HCl levels; antacids, electrolyte and iron preparations, vitamin B complex, and quinidine could fastly elevate the diagnex blue level.
- Stress, smoking and sensory stimulation could increase HCl secretions.

CONCLUSION

Nutrition is defined as the science of food and its relationship to health. Nutrition is food at work in the body. It includes everything that happens to food. It is the study of nutrients and processes by which they are used by the body. It is concerned with the part played by nutrients in the body-growth, development and maintenance. Proper nutrition is important for staying healthy and is particularly vital for the elderly. The nutritional state of a patient often affects patient outcomes during illness and recovery. The nurse is the logical person to provide nutritional information because nurses are the primary interface between the patient and the healthcare system. Nursing plays a key role in nutrition education because nutrition is a part of patient outcomes. The healing of the body can take place only when the nutrients that provide the building blocks for repair are present. The nurse as a nutrition educator is a vital role in the overall healthcare system. Prehospital nursing has the opportunity to provide nutrition education that can help to preserve the health of all populations and particularly of older adults.

BIBLIOGRAPHY

1. Bartali B, Frongillo E, Bandinelli S, et al. Low nutrient intake is an essential component of frailty in older persons. J Gerontol A Biol Sci Med Sci. 2006;(61A):589-93.
2. Fried LP, Tangen CM, Walston J, et al. Frailty in older adults: evidence for a phenotype. J Gerontol A Biol Sci Med Sci. 2001;(56):M146-M156.
3. Fulgoni VL 3rd, Miller GD. Dietary reference intakes for food labeling. Am J Clin Nutr. 2006;(83):1215S-1216S.

REVIEW QUESTIONS

Long Essays

1. Explain the functions of food; discuss in detail about physiological functions of food.
2. Explain diet in sick; enumerate the modifications of nutrients in therapeutic diet.
3. Discuss in detail about nasogastric tube insertion procedure.

Short Essays

1. Enumerate nutritional assessment.
2. Care of patient with dysphagia.
3. Care of patient anorexia.
4. Care of patient with nausea.
5. Care of patient with vomiting.
6. Therapeutic diet.
7. Feeding helpless patient.
8. Gastric gavages.
9. Gastrojejunostomy feeding.
10. Total parenteral nutrition.
11. Gastric analysis.

Short Answers

1. Basic food groups.
2. Factors affecting appetite.
3. Linear measurements.
4. Hospital diet.
5. Diabetic diet.
6. Soft diet.
7. Methods to confirm NG tube in the stomach.
8. Advantages of tube feeding.
9. Breastfeeding.
10. Artificial feeding.
11. Difference between human milk and cow milk.

MULTIPLE CHOICE QUESTIONS

1. **What is the daily calorie requirement of an adult with average body weight?**
   a. 1500 calories
   b. 2000 calories
   c. 3000 calories
   d. 2500 calories

2. **Which of the following food item believed to be complete meal or balanced diet?**
   a. Vegetables
   b. Fruits
   c. Milk
   d. Honey

3. **Which one of the following is known as "Poor man's meat"?**
   a. Cow milk
   b. Soya bean
   c. Apple
   d. Chicken

4. **How much BMI or body mass index scores for obesity?**
   a. 20 to 25
   b. More than 15
   c. More than 30
   d. Less than 18

5. **Which disease is caused is caused by the deficiency of protein?**
   a. Pellagra
   b. Marasmus
   c. Beri-Beri
   d. Rickets

ANSWERS

1. d   2. c   3. b   4. c   5. b

CHAPTER 18
Elimination Needs

LEARNING OBJECTIVES

Urinary Elimination
- Review of physiology of urine elimination, composition and characteristics of urine
- Factors influencing urination
- Alteration in urinary elimination
- Facilitating urine elimination: Assessment, types, equipment, procedures and special considerations
- Providing urinal/bed pan
- Care of patients with condom drainage, intermittent catheterization, indwelling urinary catheter and urinary drainage, urinary diversions, bladder irrigation

Bowel Elimination
- Review of physiology of bowel elimination, composition and characteristics of feces
- Factors affecting bowel elimination
- Alteration in bowel elimination
- Facilitating bowel elimination: Assessment, equipment, procedures, enemas, suppository bowel wash, digital evacuation of impacted feces, care of patients with ostomies (bowel diversion procedures)

TERMINOLOGY

- **Anuria:** Technically, no urine is voided or 24-hour urine output is less than 100 mL.
- **Dysuria:** Difficulty in voiding, may or may not be associated with pain, a feeling of warm local irritation occurring during voiding is called 'burning'.
- **Enuresis:** Most often used to refer to the child who involuntarily urinates during night, i.e. bedwetting.
- **Frequency increased incidence of voiding:** Glycosuria—presence of sugar in the urine. It may be due to an unusually large intake of sugar or to marked emotional disturbance. It is temporary.
- **Hematuria:** Presence of blood in the urine. Hesitancy delay or difficulty in initiating voiding.
- **Incontinence:** Inability to voluntarily control the discharge of urine.
- **Nocturia:** Frequency of urination during the nights.
- **Oliguria:** Scanty or greatly diminished amount of urine voided in a given time (24 hours urine output is 100–400 mL).
- **Orthostatic albuminuria:** Presence of albumin in urine that is voided after periods of standing, walking or running. It is a phenomenon of circulatory systems.
- **Pneumaturia:** Passage of urine containing gas.
- **Polyuria:** Excessive output of urine (diuresis).
- **Proteinuria:** Presence of protein, usually albumin in the urine.
- **Pyuri:** Pus in the urine. Urine appears cloudy.

URINARY ELIMINATION

Urinary elimination, a natural process in which the body excretes waste products and materials those exceeded bodily needs, usually is taken for granted. When the urinary system fails to function properly, virtually organ systems can be affected. Persons with alterations in urinary elimination may also suffer emotionally from body image changes. The proper functioning of the urinary system is vital to the body's physical well-being to life itself and a person's general sense of well-being. Nursing therapies promote or minimize factors that influence urinary elimination. Each client has a different pattern of elimination. The nurse must assess this pattern and design therapies to promote normal urinary elimination when necessary. The nurse uses devices such as a condom or an indwelling catheter to assist the client with urinary elimination. The nurse assisting a client with urination or intervening to resolve health problems related to urinary needs may have specialized abilities.

DEFINITION

- Urinary elimination is defined as expulsion of waste products from the body through the urinary system
- Elimination from the urinary tract helps to remove the waste products from body. It is essential to the body's physical well being.

PHYSIOLOGY OF URINE ELIMINATION

Urinary elimination depends on the function of the kidneys, ureters, bladder, and urethra. Kidneys remove waste from the blood to form urine. Ureters transport urine from the kidneys to the bladder. The bladder holds urine until the urge. It influences urination. Usually, infants or children with 6 to 8 kg excrete 400 to 500 mL per day and child cannot withhold urination. The adult normally voids 1500 to 1600 mL per day, has a normal urine color and; also has control over urination. Aging impairs urination, e.g. elder adults. Food and fluid foods, high in water content, increase urine production. Certain foods affect the color and odor of urine. Certain fluid needed to urinate develops. Urine leaves the body through the urethra.

All organs of the urinary system must be intact and functional for successful removal of urinary wastes. The process of emptying the bladder is known as micturition or voiding or urination. The bladder normally holds as much as 600 mL of urine. However, the desire to urinate can be sensed when the bladder contains only a small amount of urine (150 to 200 mL in adults and 50 to 200 mL in a child). As the volume increases, the bladder walls stretch, sending sensory impulses to micturition center in the sacral spinal cord. Parasympathetic impulses from the center stimulate the detrusor muscle to contract rhythmically. The internal sphincter also relaxes so that urine may enter the urethra, although voiding does not yet occur. As the bladder contracts, nerve impulses travel up the spinal cord to the midbrain and cerebral cortex. A person is thus conscious of the need to urinate. If the person chooses not to void, the external urinary sphincter remains contracted, and the micturition reflex is inhibited. However, when a person is ready to void, the external sphincter relaxes, the micturition reflex stimulates the detrusor muscle to contract and urination occurs. The act of micturition normally is painless.

CHARACTERISTICS OF URINE

Table 18.1 shows characteristics of urine.

DIAGNOSTIC EXAMINATION

Diagnostic examination of the urinary system can also influence micturition, for example, IVP.

Conditions which alter urinary elimination: The most common conditions which alter urine elimination encountered by the nurse, involve disturbance in the act of micturition. These disturbances result from impaired bladder function, obstruction to urine outflow, or inability of voluntary control of micturition. The common renal conditions causing alteration in urinary elimination are as follows:

I. Prerenal conditions
   - Decreased intravascular volume, dehydration, hemorrhage, burns shock
   - Altered peripheral vascular resistance, sepsis, anaphylactic shock and reactions

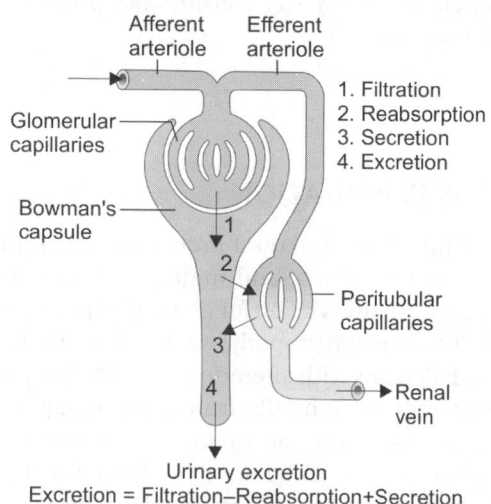

Fig. 18.1: Physiology of urine elimination.

TABLE 18.1: Characteristics of urine.

Sl. No.	Characteristics	Normal	Abnormal	Nursing action
1.	24 hours urine in adult	1200–1500 mL	Below 1200 mL, a large amount over intake	Check for total intake and output if it is less than 30 mL/hr indicates decreased blood flow to the kidneys and it should be reported immediately
2.	Color, clarity	Straw, amber transparent	Dark amber, Cloudy, Dark orange, Red or dark brown, Mucus plug, viscid and thick	Check for Concentrated urine is darker in color, diluted urine will be clear, pale yellow, hematuria indicate red blood cells in urine evident as pink, bright red or rusty brown urine, menstrual bleeding can color urine, WBC bacteria, pus, bright red or rusty urine, contaminants like prostate fluid, sperm, vaginal drainage may cause cloudy urine
3.	Odor	Faint aromatic	Offensive	Check for and infected urine. It has fetid odor, with high glucose. It has sweet odor, and some foods e.g. asparagus cause musty odor
4.	Sterility	No microorganisms present	Microorganisms present	Collecting a sterile specimen is important to interpret correct results, urine in the bladder is sterile but it may be contaminated from perineum
5.	pH	4.5–8	Over 8, under 4.5	Check whether the urine is acidic or alkaline, normally urine is acidic

- Cardiac pump failure, congestive heart failure, myocardial infarction, hypertensive heart disease, valvular disease, pericardial tamponade.

II. **Renal conditions**
   - Use of nephrotoxic agents (e.g. gentamicin)
   - Transfusion reactions
   - Diseases of the glomeruli (e.g. nephritis)
   - Neoplasms
   - Systemic diseases (e.g. diabetes)
   - Hereditary diseases (e.g. polycystic kidney)
   - Infections.

III. **Postrenal conditions**
   - Ureteral, bladder or urethral obstructions, due to calculi, blood clot, tumors, strictures
   - Prostatic hypertrophy
   - Neurogenic bladder
   - Pelvic tumor
   - Retroperitoneal fibrosis.

TABLE 18.2: General characteristics of normal urine.

Characteristic	Normal range
pH	4.5–8 f(average 6.0)
Specific gravity	1.003–1.030
Osmotic concentration (osmolarity)	855–1335 mOsm/L
Water content	93–97%
Volume	700–2000 mL/day
Color	Clear yellow
Odor	Varies with composition
Bacterial content	None (sterile)

FACTORS AFFECTING URINARY ELIMINATION

There are numerous factors which affect the amount and quality of urine produced by the body and manner which it is excreted. These are as follows: When person is dehydrated to maintain fluids and electrolyte balance. According to lifestyle, some sociocultural variables influence a person's normal voiding habits.

Developmental considerations are concerned; Infants are born without voluntary control of urination and with little ability to concentrate urine. Older children and adults have general control of urination voluntarily. Physiological may affect urination.

Lifestyle: Many individuals' families and sociocultural variables influence a person's normal voiding habits. For some individuals voiding is a very personal and private act.

Fluid and food intake: The healthy body maintains a sensitive balance between the amount of fluid ingested and the amount of fluid eliminated. When fluid intake increases, the output also increases.

Environment: During summer, due to excessive perspiration urine output is less. During winter, due to lack of perspiration, urine output is more.

Factors affecting urinary elimination

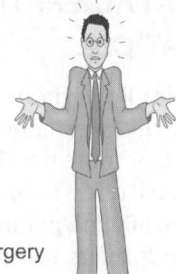

- Fluid
- Diet
- Response to urge
- Stress
- Psychosocial factors
- Activity
- Pathological conditions
- Medications
- Developmental level
- Medical diagnosis or surgery

Psychological factors: Stress can also interfere with the ability to relax external urethral sphincter as a result, emptying the bladder completely becomes difficult or impossible.

Muscle tone and activity: People who exercise regularly will have good muscle tone increased body metabolism and good urine production.

Pathological conditions: Endocrine disorders such as diabetes insipidus increase urine formation. Diseases of the kidney themselves can reduce kidney function and perhaps eventually result in renal failure.

Surgical and diagnostic procedure: Surgery on structures adjacent to the urinary tract can also affect voiding because of swelling in the lower abdomen and often necessitates the use of retention catheter for a short time.

Privacy and adequate time to urinate are usually important for most people; they think voiding is private act. The nurse approach in or to a client's elimination must consider cultural and social habits. Psychologic variables like anxiety and stress do not change the characteristics of urine but may cause a sense of urgency and increase frequency of urination.

Activity and muscle tone: Due to regular exercise increases the metabolism and helps in optimal urine production and elimination. Weak abdominal and pelvic floor muscles impair bladder contraction and control of external urethral sphincter. In pathologic condition, several diseases can affect the ability to micturate. Any lesion of peripheral nerves leading to the bladder causes loss of bladder tone, reduced sensation of bladder-fullness and difficulty in controlling urination (e.g. diabetis mellitus).

Medications: These have numerous effects on urine production and elimination. Diuretics prevent reabsorption of water and certain electrolytes to increase urine output. Urinary retention may be caused by use of anticholenergics, antihistamines, antihypertensive and beta-adrenergic blockers. Certain drugs also change the color of urine. For example, diuretics lead to pale yellow, B complex preparations lead to green or blue-green. Iron tablets lead to brown or black color urine.

COMMON ALTERATIONS IN URINARY ELIMINATION

- **Polyuria:** Polyuria or diuresis refers to production of abnormally large amounts of urine by the kidneys, about 2500 mL or more per day.
- **Oliguria:** It refers to voiding scanty amount of urine such as 100 to 500 mL per day.
- **Anuria:** It refers to voiding less than 100 mL per day. The terms complete kidney shutdown, renal failure and urinary suppression have the same meaning.

Altered in urinary elimination

- **Frequeny:** Void at frequent intervals due to cystitic stress pressure on bladder are some of the causes listed.
- **Nocturia/nycturia:** Incresed frequency at night. Don't give diuretics at night. Take by 5 pm.
- **Urgency:** Urgent need to void
- **Dysuria:** Painful voiding, injury, infection, sturctural problems.
- **Enuresis:** Involuntary passage of urination after age 4–5 years (primary and secondary)
- **Urinary incontinenece:** Urine overflows or dribbles Types: Total, stress, urge, functional and reflex incontinence

---

- **Nocturia:** It is an increased frequency at night. That is not the result of an increase in fluid intake. It is expressed in terms of the number of times the person gets out of bed to void.
- **Dysuria:** It means voiding that is either painful or difficult. It can be caused by stricture of the urethra, urinary infection and injury to the bladder of urethra.
- **Enuresis:** It is defined as repeated involuntary urination in children beyond 4 to 5 years of age, when voluntary bladder control is normally acquired. Enuresis can be nocturnal (night time) and diurnal (day time) or both.
- **Heritancy:** It is defined as delay or difficulty in initiating voiding. It may be due to urethral structure, prostatic enlargement post catheterization and urethritis.
- **Urinary incontinence:** It is the ability to control passage of urine to continence may be caused by stress, neurological impairment and injury to urethral sphincter.
- **Urinary retention:** It is the accumulation of urine in the bladder associated with inability of the bladder to empty itself.

Renal Condition Causing Alteration in Urine Elimination

- **Prerenal conditions:** Dehydration hemorrhage, burns, shock, sepsis, anaphylactic, reactions, congestive heart failure, myocardial infarction and hypertensive heart disease.
- **Renal condition:** Use of nephrotoxic agents, glomerulo-nephritis, neoplasms and infections.
- **Postrenal condition:** Urinary tract obstruction, calculi, prostatic, hypertrophy, neurogenic bladder and pelvic tumor.

URINARY RETENTION

Urinary retention is the inability to empty the bladder. Urinary retention can be acute or chronic. Acute urinary retention is a medical emergency. Urinary retention is most common in men in their 50s and 60s because of prostate enlargement. A woman may experience urinary retention if her bladder sags or moves out of the normal position (cystocele) or pulled out of position by a sagging of the lower part of the colon (rectocele).

Causes: Causes of urinary retention include an obstruction in the urinary tract such as an enlarged prostate or bladder stones, infections that cause swelling or irritation, nerve problems that interfere with signals between the brain and the bladder, medications, constipation, urethral stricture, or a weak bladder muscle.

Symptoms: Symptoms of acute urinary retention are severe discomfort and pain, an urgent need to urinate but you simply can't, and bloated lower belly. Chronic urinary retention symptoms are mild but constant discomfort, difficulty starting a stream of urine, weak flow of urine, needing to go frequently, or feeling you still need to go after you've finished.

Diagnosis: Tests to diagnose urinary retention include taking a urine sample, bladder scan, cystoscopy, X-ray and CT scan, blood test for prostate-specific antigen (PSA), prostate fluid sample test, and urodynamic tests to measure the bladder's ability to empty steadily and completely.

Treatment: Treatment for urinary retention includes catheterization, treating prostate enlargement, and surgery.

Surgical management:
- Bladder neck repair: Urethroplasty
- Suprapubic cystotomy

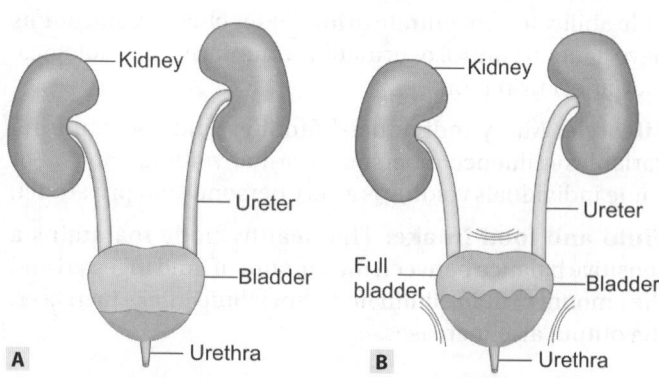

Figs. 18.2A and B: (A) Healthy bladder; (B) Bladder in retention.

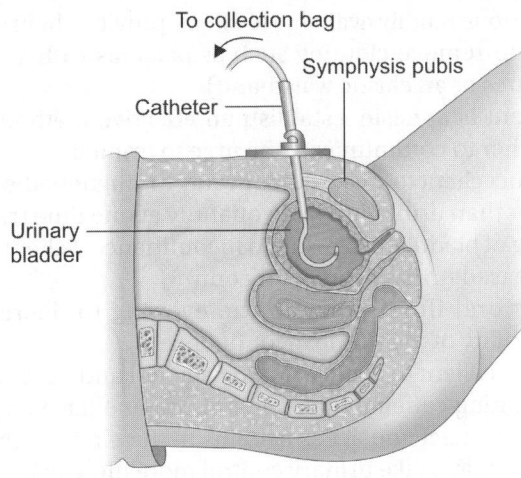

Fig. 18.3: Suprapubic catheterization.

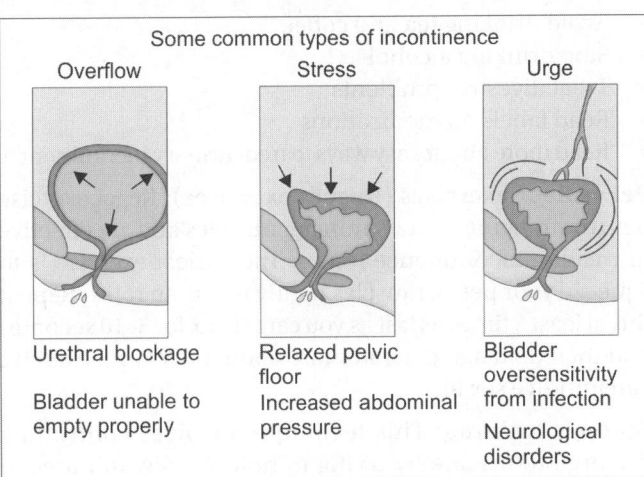

Fig. 18.4: Types of urinary incontinence.

Nursing management:
- Assess the urine output pattern.
- Observe for oliguria and anuria.
- Percussion over the bladder produces a dull sound.
- Clients experience increased discomfort and need to urinate.
- Implement measures to stimulate independent voiding.
- Provide privacy.
- Place the patient in a comfortable position (squatting position).
- Warm bath on the perineum for muscle relaxation.
- A running hydrogen or flushing toilet within ear short of the client may encourage voiding.
- Apply ice or gently stroke in the inner thigh.
- Relaxation therapy.
- Catheterization of client.
- Prevent infection by hand wand washing techniques.
- Maintain a closed drainage system.
- Avoid back flow of urine.
- Prevent colonization of bacteria.
- Maintain patency of catheter.
- Encourage increased fluid intake.
- Prophylactic antibiotics.

URINARY INCONTINENCE

Urinary incontinence is unintentional or uncontrolled urine leakage that occurs due poor functioning of muscles called urinary sphincter which enable to hold urine in the urinary bladder. It is more common in women than in men.

Types of incontinence: There are four different types of urinary incontinence:

1. **Stress incontinence,** which occurs when urine leaks from the bladder when you cough, laugh, sneeze or do any other activity that places stress on the abdomen.
2. **Urge incontinence:** The leakage of urine associated with a great urgency or desire to urinate, which cannot be suppressed. For example, it kicks in when (even if you've been fine up until that moment) you get close to a toilet and suddenly find you can't make it all the way.
3. **Overflow incontinence** happens when someone has difficulty passing urine, which causes the bladder to be permanently full. As the kidneys continue to produce urine, the excess spills out through the urethra—almost like a dam that's overflowing.
4. **Total incontinence** is the continuous leakage of all the urine. It is most often caused by an abnormal communication between the bladder and the vagina (called vesicovaginal fistula).

Causes: Incontinence mainly occurs when the pressure due to a completely filled bladder exceeds a certain threshold. Here are some factors that can increase this pressure and cause incontinence.
- Over-active bladder
- Blockage in the urinary system
- Mental health problems
- Poor muscle control
- Medications
- Prostate problems
- Excess urine production
- Secondary causes due to underlying medical condition.

Treatment: Most cases of urinary incontinence can be treated with lifestyle changes and bladder training exercise but medication and other coping strategies like use of diapers (that can soak the excess urine) are also used if the problem is due to urgency or mixed incontinence.

Severity	Definition
Stress urinary incontinence grade 0	No urine loss found
Stress urinary incontinence grade I	Urine loss in droplets while standing
Stress urinary incontinence grade II	Urine loss in a stream while standing
Stress urinary incontinence grade III	Urine loss in a stream while lying down

Lifestyle changes: There are a few effective ways to put an end to your battle with leakage problems such as:
- Drink fluids in moderation
- Empty the bladder completely
- Lose weight

- Avoid drinking tea and coffee
- Stop drinking alcohol
- Treat digestive problems
- Read labels on medications
- Read more about easy ways to treat urinary incontinence.

Pelvic floor exercises (Kegel's exercises): Kegel exercise help to strengthen your sphincter muscles and are effective in treating incontinence issues. The easiest exercise is to squeeze your pelvic muscles tightly and then relax. Repeat this at least 5 times as fast as you can. Relax for 5–10 seconds, and then do it again. Read more about how kegel exercise can improve sex life.

Bladder training: This technique involves controlling the urge to urinate by trying to hold for few minutes to delay urination. It is recommended till you urinate every few hours. In some cases, double voiding (emptying your bladder completely) is also found to provide better results.

Medications: The common medications that provide great relief for patients suffering from urinary incontinence are anticholinergics and alpha blockers.

Percutaneous tibial nerve stimulation: It is a technique where the nerve at the ankle is stimulated using an electrode. This impulse in turn stimulates the spinal nerve responsible for bladder stimulation.

Botox treatment: In this, Botox is injected into the muscles of the bladder to reduce sensitivity of the bladder offering better control.

Assessment: Assess client's pattern of fluid intake and urination (e.g. times and amounts of fluid intake, types of fluids consumed, times and amounts of voluntary and involuntary voiding, reports of sensation of need to void, activities preceding incontinence).

Nursing diagnosis:
- Increased reflex activity of the bladder and loss of voluntary control of urinary elimination associated with upper motor neuron involvement if it has occurred;
- Decreased ability to control urination associated with decreased level of consciousness or inability to recognize sensation of bladder fullness;
- Inability to get to bedside commode or bathroom in a timely manner associated with:
  - Delay in obtaining assistance resulting from inability to communicate the urge to urinate
  - impaired physical mobility.

Implement measures to reduce the risk of urinary incontinence:
- Offer bedpan or urinal or assist client to bedside commode or bathroom every 2-4 hours if indicated
- Allow client to assume a normal position for voiding unless contraindicated in order to promote complete bladder emptying
- Perform actions to reduce delays in toileting (e.g. have call signal within client's reach and respond promptly to requests for assistance; have bedpan, urinal, or bedside commode readily available to client; provide client with easy-to-remove clothing such as pajamas with Velcro closures or an elastic waistband)
- If client is aphasic, establish an effective method for him/her to communicate the urge to urinate
- Instruct client to space fluids evenly throughout the day rather than drinking a large quantity at one time (rapid filling of bladder can result in incontinence if client has decreased urinary sphincter control)
- Limit oral fluid intake in the evening to decrease possibility of nighttime incontinence
- Instruct client to avoid drinking alcohol and beverages containing caffeine (alcohol and caffeine have a mild diuretic effect and act as irritants to the bladder; these factors may make urinary control more difficult).

If urinary incontinence persists, consult physician about intermittent catheterization, insertion of indwelling catheter, or use of external catheter.

MONITORING URINARY OUTPUT

Normal urinary output is approximately 1.5 liters in 24 hours and the usual frequency of micturition is between 5 and 10 times in that period. However, this can be influenced significantly by the amount of fluid a person drinks and how much fluid they are losing through sweating, mental state and lifestyle.

Urine normally consists of: 96% water, 2% urea, 2% uric acid, creatinine, sodium, potassium, chlorides, phosphates, sulphates, oxalates. These are all waste products of the body's utilization of food and fluid.

The intensity of color of normal urine depends on the concentration, and usually ranges from yellow to amber. Fresh urine does not have a strong odor and it should be clear when voided.

When monitoring a client's urine, important clues can be gained simply by careful observation. For example, greenish or yellow-brown urine could contain bile pigments and may indicate problems with liver function, whilst blood

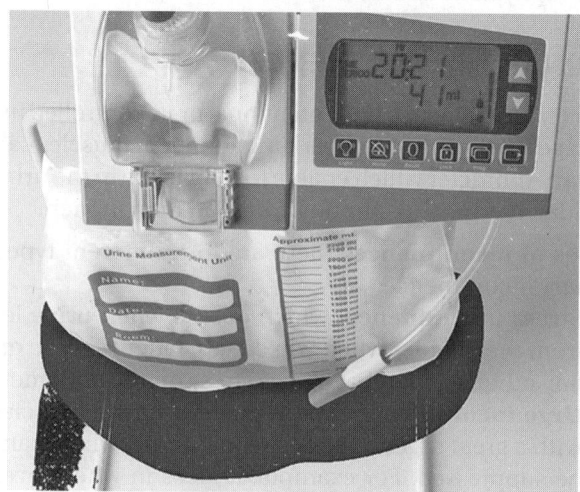

Fig. 18.5: Monitoring urinary output.

and hemoglobin will give a red-brown color if present in quite large quantities. Some drugs, foods and dyes may also change the color of urine. If any abnormalities are found they should be documented, reported and further investigations undertaken in consultation with the medical staff. If you suspect that blood is present in the urine, and if the client is female, check whether or not they are menstruating before reporting, as menstrual blood can give a false positive result.

USE OF URINAL

Urinal is used for male patients to void the urine, the nurse should assist the bedridden to void into a urinal (a plastic or metal receptacle for urine) in bed.

In case of female patients nurse should provide bedpan for bedridden to collect the urine.

Purposes

- To promote comfort.
- To assist to void.
- To prevent bed wetting.
- To maintain the urinary output record.
- To minimize the physical strain.

Factors Influences

- Normal urinary elimination habits.
- Nature of disease condition.
- Environment (privacy).
- The amount of intake (food and fluids).
- Availability of equipment and personal.

Preliminary Assessment Check

- Doctors order for specific precautions such as movements and position.
- Level of consciousness.
- Self care ability of the patient.
- Frequency of urination.
- Articles available in the unit.

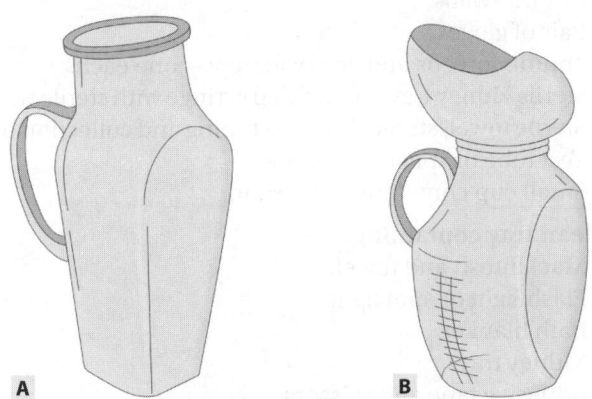

Figs. 18.6A and B: Types of urinals.

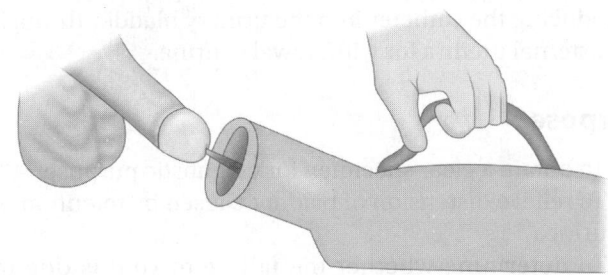

Fig. 18.7: Providing urinals for male patients.

Preparation of the Patient and Environment

- Provide adequate privacy.
- Arrange the article (urinal) ready at bed side.
- Place the Mackintosh and draw sheet.
- Place the patient in proper body alignment.

Equipment

- Clean urinal.
- Disposable gloves.
- Clean linen if required.
- Hand washing basin, mug and water.
- Soap with soap dish.
- Measuring jar.

Procedure

- Wash hands thoroughly.
- If the patient is conscious, allow him to place or else position penis into urinal.
- Prevent soiling of urine on bed or patients body.
- Remain with helpless patient; get assistance from relatives if needed.
- Remove urinal after patient has voided.
- Measure and empty the urine in sluice room.

Aftercare

- Assist the patient to wash perineal area and hands.
- Place the patient in a proper body alignment.
- Change the bed linen, if required.
- Replace the articles used after cleaning.
- Wash hands.
- Record the procedure in nurse's record sheet and the amount in intake output chart.

CATHETERIZATION OF THE URINARY BLADDER

Urinary catheterization is the introduction of a tube (a catheter) through the urethra into the urinary bladder to drain the bladder.

Urinary catheterization is an aseptic method of introducing the catheter into the urinary bladder through the external urethra for withdrawal of urine.

Purpose

- To obtain a clear specimen for diagnostic purpose.
- To relieve distension of bladder caused by retention of urine.
- To determine whether the failure to void is due to retention or suppression.
- To determine the amount of residual urine present in the bladder.
- To empty the bladder prior to surgery, bladder, irrigation or before instillation of a drug.
- To avoid soiling and infection of the wound following operations on the genital region.
- To manage incontinency, when all other measures to prevent skin breakdown have failed.
- To provide for intermittent or continuous bladder drainage and irrigation.
- To prevent urine from passing over a wound, e.g. after repair of the perineum.

Principles Involved

- Pathogenic organisms are transmitted from the source to a new host directly on by contaminated articles.
- Urinary bladder is a sterile cavity and the urinary meatus acts as a portal of entry for pathogenic organisms.
- Cleaning an area minimize the spread of organisms.
- A break in the integrity of the skin and mucus membrane provides ready entrance for microorganism.
- Lubrication reduces friction.
- Through knowledge of anatomy and physiology of the genitourinary system facilitates catheterization of the urinary bladder.
- Systematic ways of doing saves time, energy and material.
- Unfamiliar situation produce anxiety.

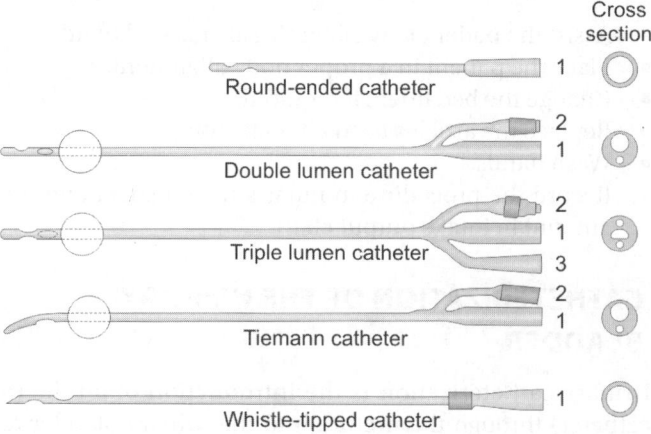

Fig. 18.8: Types of urinary catheters.

General Instruction

- Apply all the nursing measures to induce urination before the catheterization of the bladder.
- Observe strict aseptic techniques to prevent the urinary tract infection.
- Catheterization should be done slowly and never use force.
- Always catheterize in a good light.
- Clean the perineum from the pubis downwards to the anal region.
- Use one cotton ball for one swabbing.
- Do not touch the portion of the catheter that is going into the urinary tract.
- Lubricate the catheter well before introducing into the urinary tract.
- Keep the patient relaxed by providing privacy and adequate explanations.

Preliminary Assessment Check

- Doctors order for any specific precautions.
- Identify the purpose of catheterization.
- Level of consciousness.
- Any contraindications.
- General condition of the patient.
- Mental status to follow instructions.
- Articles available in the unit.

Preparation of Patient and Environment

- Explain the sequence of the procedure.
- Arrange the articles at the bed side locker.
- Provide privacy.
- Position the patient in dorsal recumbent.
- Place the mackintosh and towel under the buttocks.
- Provide adequate light by placing extra spotlight.

Equipment

A sterile tray containing:
- Catheter of correct size.
- Small bowl containing an antiseptic.
- Cotton swabs.
- Pair of gloves.
- Thumb forceps and artery forceps—one each.
- Sterile kidney tray—1 prefilled syringe with sterile water.
- Sterile towel, sterile drainage tubing and collection bag.
- Test tube or specimen bottle.
- Small cup containing lubricant.

A clean tray containing:
- Mackintosh and towel.
- Flash light or spot light.
- Bath blanket.
- Kidney tray.
- Adhesive tape and scissors.
- Bed-pan to empty the urine from the kidney tray

Elimination Needs

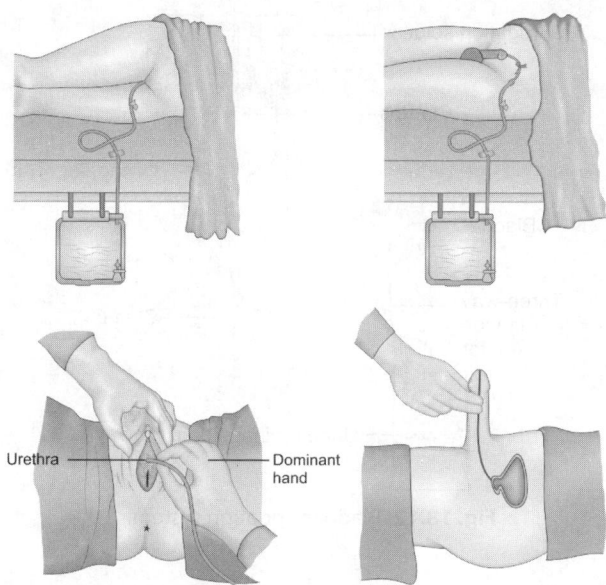

Fig. 18.9: Catheterization procedure.

- Measuring jar.
- Urobag or collection bag.

Procedure

- Scrub hands for a surgical procedure.
- Lift the draping sheet back towards abdomen.
- Open the sterile tray with aseptic techniques.
- Place the sterile towel and the slit in position.
- Place the sterile kidney tray on the sterile towel in front of the patient.
- Lubricate the catheter and place it in the sterile tray ready for insertion.
- Clean the perineum with the cotton balls dipped in the antiseptic lotion using the forceps.
- Discard the swab in the paper bag and discard the forceps in an unutterable kidney tray.

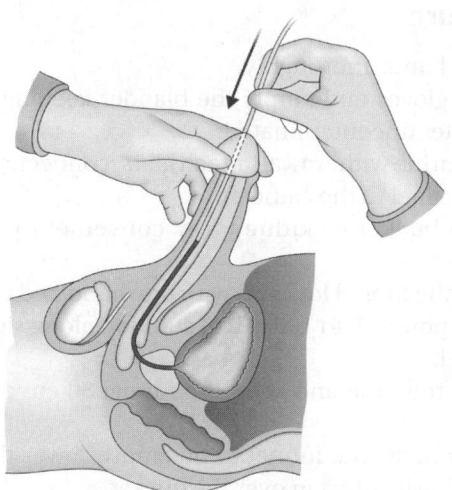

Fig. 18.10: Urinary catheter insertion technique.

- Pick up the catheter with the gloved hand, holding it about 7.5 cm from the tip and place the distal end in the sterile kidney tray.
- Gently insert the catheter about 5 to 7.5 cm (female) the urine will flow into the kidney tray.
- Collect the urine specimen if required. Attach the drainage tubing if an indwelling catheter is put in.

Cleaning the Perineum in Female Patients

- Clean only in one direction.
- Use one swab for one swabbing.
- Clean labia majora on both sides.
- Clean the inside of the labia majora on both sides.
- Clean the labia minora on the both sides.
- Clean the vulva.

Cleaning the Perineum for Male Patients

- Retract the foreskin during the cleaning process.
- Draw the penis upward and forward at 90 degree angle to the patients leg in order to straighten the urethra before the catheter is introduced.
- Foreskin is replaced as quickly as possible after the insertion of the catheter.

Aftercare

- Wash and dry the perineum.
- Remove the drapes, replace the garments and bed covers.
- Place the patient comfortably.
- Take all the articles to the utility room, clean it and replace it.
- Send specimen to the lab immediately.
- Wash Hands.
- Record the procedure in the nurse's record sheet.

Types of Catheterization

- Intermittent catheterization.
- Short term indwelling catheterization.
- Long term indwelling catheterization.

BLADDER IRRIGATION

Bladder irrigation or wash is defined as washing of the urinary bladder directly by a stream of solution into the bladder through the urinary meatus by means of a catheter tubing and funnel.

Purpose

- To cleanse the bladder from decomposed urine bacteria, excess mucus and pus.
- To medicate the lining of the bladder of antiseptic irrigation.
- To prepare the bladder for surgery as a preoperative measure.

- To promote healing.
- To relieve congestion and pain in case of inflammatory conditions of cystitis.
- To arrest bleeding and prevent clothing of blood.

Solution Used

- Normal saline 0.9 percent
- Boric acid solution 2 percent
- Sterile water
- Acetic acid 1:4000 to treat pseudomonas infection
- Sodium nitrate 1:8000 to prevent clot formation
- Potassium permanganate 1:5000–1:10,000
- Acriflavin 1:10,000
- Silver nitrate 1:5,000
- Mercury compounds in low concentration.

General Instructions

- The temperature of the solution needed for cleaning purpose body temperature in enough.
- The temperature of the solution needed for therapeutic purposes ranging from 100 to 110° F.
- The maximum amount of solution used for cleaning is 2 pints and also depends on the patient's condition.

Methods of Administration

- Funnel and tubing method (open method).
- Irrigation can, rubber tubing and Y connection.
- Asepto syringe (open method).

Preliminary Assessment Check

- Doctors order for specific precautions and instructions.
- General condition of the patient.
- Diagnosis of the patient.
- Self-care ability of the patient.
- Mental status to follow instructions
- Articles available in the unit.

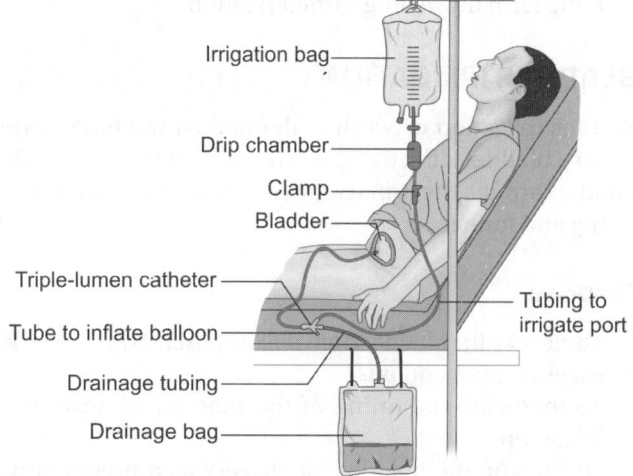

Fig. 18.11: Bladder irrigation.

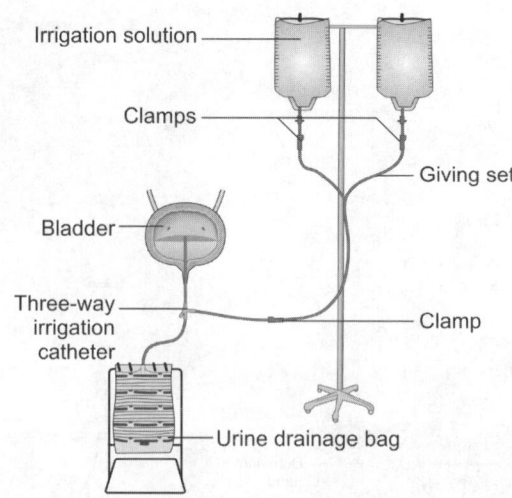

Fig. 18.12: Bladder irrigation system.

Preparation of the Patient and Environment

- Explain the sequence of the procedure.
- Arrange the articles at the bedside.
- Provide privacy.
- Place the patient in comfortable position
- Place the Mackintosh under the buttocks.

Equipment

Sterile catheterization pack.

A sterile tray containing:

- Funnel, tubing 3 feet long which fits the connection screw clip and glass connection.
- A small mug or pint measures to pour solution.
- A sterile pint jug with required solution.
- Solution thermometer kept in antiseptic solution in a bottle if available.
- Medication if ordered.
- Bucket for emptying the return flow.
- Litmus paper.

Procedure

- Wash hands thoroughly.
- Wear gloves and empty the bladder keeping outlet of catheter uncontaminated.
- After urine withdrawal, attach glass, connection, tubing and funnel to the catheter.
- Place bucket or kidney tray conveniently near the meatus.
- Hold the funnel lowered with one hand and with other hand pours 75 to 100 mL of solution along sides of the funnel.
- Raise the tube and keep the funnel 30 cm above bed level.
- Never allow the funnel to be empty, lower the funnel and slowly invert in over the bucket.
- Repeat procedure until the return flow is clear.

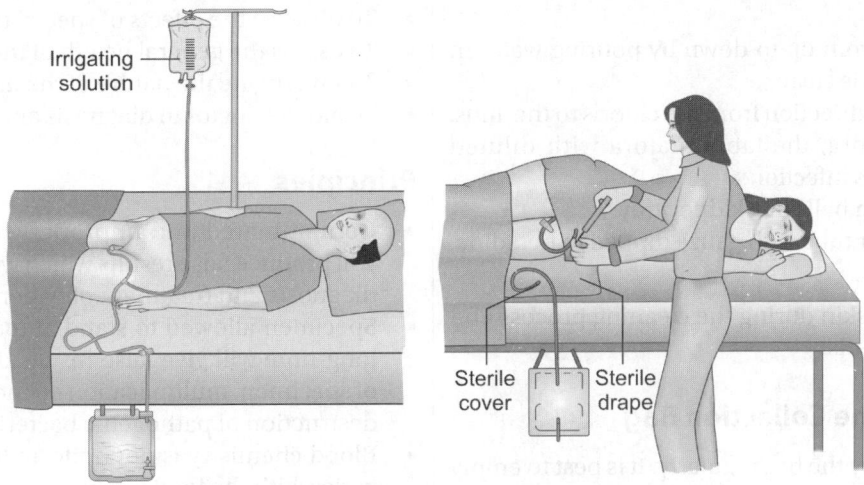

Fig. 18.13: Nurse assisting in bladder irrigation.

- At the end of the procedure, clamp tubing disconnects glass connection, tubing and funnel, gently remove catheter and complete.
- In case of self-retaining catheter, connect it to the drainage bag.

Aftercare

- Provide catheter care.
- Remove the Mackintosh and position the patient comfortably.
- Cover the patient with bed sheets.
- Replace the articles after cleaning.
- Wash hand thoroughly.
- Record the procedure and observations in the nurse's record sheet.

CATHETER CARE

Always wash hands before and after handling a catheter. Follow all of the instructions the doctor has given. Also:
- Make sure that urine is flowing out of the catheter into the urine collection bag. Make sure that the catheter tubing does not get twisted or kinked.
- Keep the urine collection bag below the level of the bladder.
- Make sure that the urine collection bag does not drag and pull on the catheter.
- It is okay to shower with a catheter and urine collection bag in place, unless the doctor says not to.
- Check for inflammation or signs of infection in the area around the catheter. Signs of infection include pus or irritated, swollen, red, or tender skin.
- Clean the area around the catheter twice a day with soap and water. Dry with a clean towel afterward.
- Do not apply powder or lotion to the skin around the catheter.
- Do not tug or pull on the catheter.
- Talk with your doctor about your options for sexual intercourse while wearing a catheter.
- At night it may be helpful to hang the urine collection bag on the side of the bed.

Articles Used

- A dressing tray containing: Artery forceps, thumb forceps, cotton balls, gauze pieces
- Bed pan.
- Soap, water in a basin, betadine, mackintosh, kidney tray.

Procedure

- Wash hands.
- Lift the draping sheet back towards the abdomen with the elbow to expose only the perineum.
- Place the mackintosh and slide the bed pan under the buttocks.
- Take the artery forceps with wet big cotton balls, and clean the perineum with water and soap including groins.

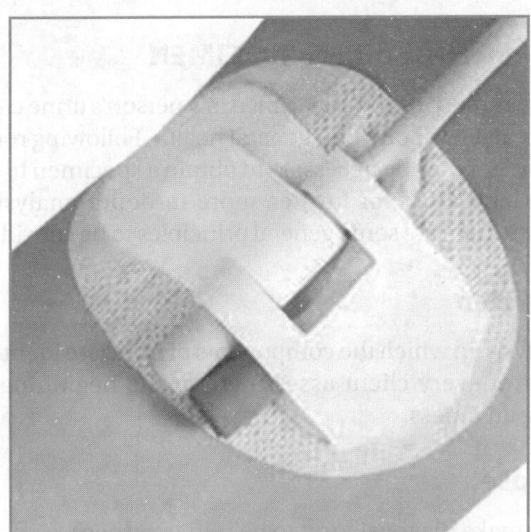

Fig. 18.14: Care of urinary catheter.

In female patients:
- Clean the vulva from up to down by pouring water in the left hand till it is clean.
- Clean only in one direction from the clitoris to the anus.
- Clean labia minora, the labia majora with diluted betadine if there is infection.
- Discard the cotton balls in a kidney tray.
- Clean the catheter tube with gauze dipped in betadine.

In male patients:
- Retreact the fore-skin during the cleaning process and clean the glans penis.

To Empty the Urine Collection Bag

You will need to empty the bag regularly. It is best to empty the bag when it's about half full or at bedtime. If the doctor has asked you to measure the amount of urine, do that before you empty the urine into the toilet.
- Wash your hands with soap and water. If you are emptying another person's collection bag, you may choose to wear disposable gloves.
- Remove the drain spout from its sleeve at the bottom of the collection bag. Open the valve on the spout.
- Let the urine flow out of the bag and into the toilet or a container. Do not let the tubing or drain spout touch anything.
- After you empty the bag, close the valve and put the drain spout back into its sleeve at the bottom of the collection bag.
- Wash your hands with soap and water.

Aftercare

- Remove the drapes.
- Position the patient for correct body alignment.
- Take all articles to the utility room and clean them.
- Wash hands.
- Record the procedure on the nurse's record with date and time.

COLLECTING URINE SPECIMEN

Observing and testing a specimen of a person's urine can tell us a great deal about their general health. Following routine urinalysis it may be necessary to obtain a specimen to send to the laboratory for further, more in-depth analysis. In doing so there are some general principles to be considered:

Definition

Urinalysis, in which the components of urine are identified, is part of every client assessment at the beginning and during an illness.

Purpose

- To make diagnosis and to help in treatment.
- To note progress or recess of a disease.
- To observe the effects of special treatment and drugs.
- To assess the general health of the patient.
- To investigate the nature of the diseases.
- To aid the doctor in diagnosis and treating the diseases.

Principles

- Contaminated and improperly collected specimens will produce false results which will adversely affect the diagnosis and treatment of patient.
- Specimen allowed to stand at room temperature for a long-time will give false results due to decomposition of specimen, multiplication of undesirable bacteria and destruction of pathogenic bacteria.
- Blood chemistry is not uniform throughout the day. It varies with the food intake.
- The accuracy and reliability of findings depend upon the correct method collection. Transportation of the specimens to the laboratory and recording of reports.
- Inaccurate results may lead the physician in wrong diagnosis and treatment of patients.
- Specimens serve as a media for transmission of disease producing organisms to the personnel who handle them carelessly.

General Instructions

- Provide adequate explanations regarding collection of specimens.
- Ask the patient to wash the external genital area with soap and water then rinse with water alone before collecting urine specimens.
- Equipment used for the collection of specimen should be clean and dry.
- No antiseptic should be present in the specimen bottle.
- As far as possible morning specimens should be collected.
- Specimens should be always be fresh for the laboratory examination.
- Bacteria multiply in the room temperature so, the specimens which are not tested immediately should be kept in the refrigerator, because cold temperature inhibits the growth of bacteria.
- Insist the patient and the personnel to wash hands thoroughly after handling the specimen bottles.
- Container should have a wide mouth to prevent spilling of the spilling of the specimens, on the outer side of the bottle.
- Containers of the proper size are used according to the nature of specimen.

Procedure

- Instruct patient to wash perineum.
- Instruct to avoid directly into clean, dry container or into bedpan and then transfer.
- Instruct not be contaminate outside of container.
- Instruct to collect 3/4th of container.
- Wear gloves while handling urine.

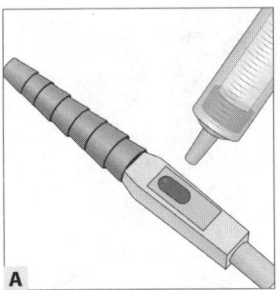
A
A sampling port can be found on the tubing of the catheter drainage bag–urine should only be obtained from this point

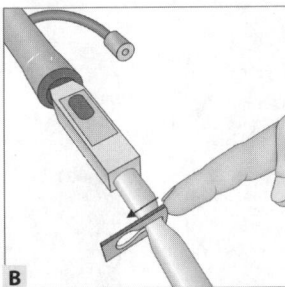
B
Clamp the catheter below the port so that urine can collect above it in the tubing. Some catheter bags have an integral clamp.

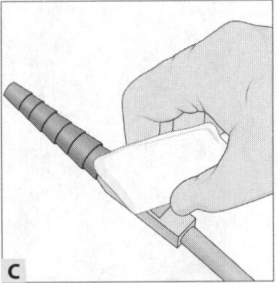
C
Swab the sampling port with an alcohol-impregnated swab following local policy to reduce the risk of cross infection and contamination of the specimen.

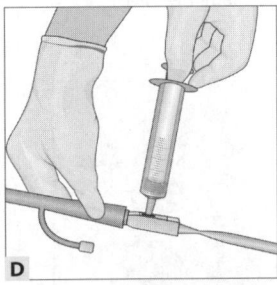
D
Insert the syringe tip into the sampling port and withdraw the urine following manufacturer's instruction

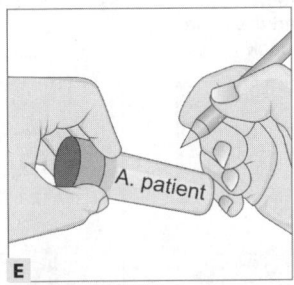
E
Place sample in the specimen pot, avoiding contact with the syringe. Secure top to prevent leakage and contamination, then label, place in a specimen bag and seal.

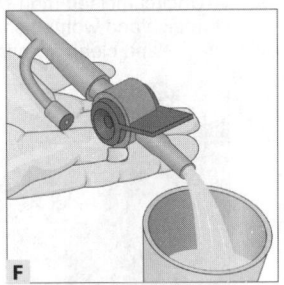
F
If the sample is taken from a catheter valve, the valve must be cleaned with an alcohol-impregnated swab first to reduce the risk of cross infection

Figs. 18.15A to F: Urinary sample (culture) collection from urinary catheter.

Nursing Alert

- Label specimen containers or bottles before the client voids (Rationale: Reduce handling after the container or bottle is contaminated).
- Note on the specimen label if the female client is menstruating at that time (Rationale: One of the tests routinely performed is a test for blood in the urine. If the female client is menstruating at the time a urine specimen is taken, a false-positive reading for blood will be obtained).
- To avoid contamination and necessity of collecting another specimen, soap and water cleansing of the genitals immediately preceding the collection of the specimen is supported (Rationale: Bacteria are normally present on the labia or penis and the perineum and in the anal area).
- Maintain body substances precautions when collecting all types of urine specimen (Rationale: To maintain safety).
- Wake a client in the morning to obtain a routine specimen (Rationale: If all specimen are collected at the same time, the laboratory can establish a baseline. And also this voided specimen usually represents that was collecting in the bladder all night).
- Be sure to document the procedure in the designated place and mark it off on the Kardex (Rationale: To avoid duplication).

COLLECTING A SINGLE VOIDED SPECIMEN

Urine specimens should be tested as soon after collection as possible. Consequently if specimens cannot be transported to the laboratory and examined within two hours of collection they must be stored in an appropriate refrigeration unit at 40°C. However, they should not be stored for longer than 24 hours otherwise any findings will be inaccurate.

Assessment of the client's physical and mental capacity prior to collecting a specimen of urine is essential in order to ensure that they can comply with the needs of the procedure, particularly if a mid-stream specimen (MSU) or a 24-hr collection is required. For an MSU, the client must urinate in the toilet or other receptacle, stop, pass urine into the specimen container or sterile receptacle, stop and then finish urinating as normal. If you wish to collect all the urine that the client passes in a 24-hr period (24-hr urine collection), special bottles containing preservatives and other chemicals are usually obtainable from the laboratory.

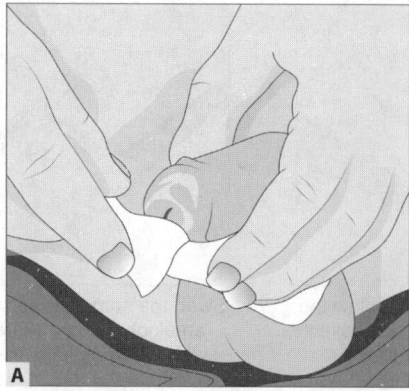

A
Ask the patient to clean around the urethra meatus to reduce the risk of contamination. Uncircumcised men should retract the foreskin and women should part the labia and clean from front to back

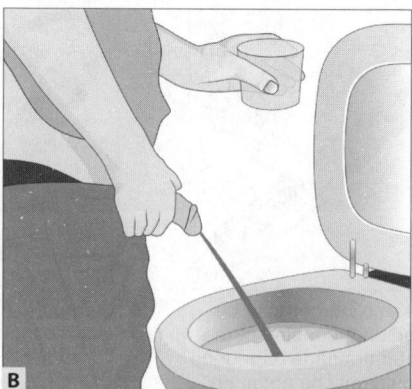

B
Ask the patient to pass 15–30mL of urine into the toilet to wash away any bacteria colonising the distal urethra

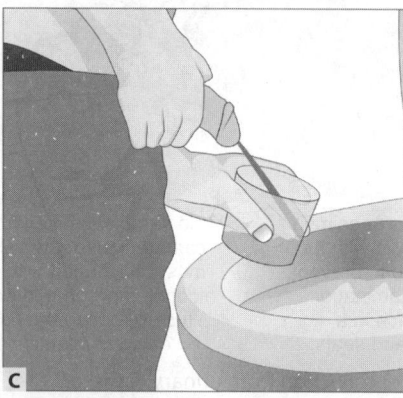

C
Ask the patient to collect the middle part of the stream in a wide-neck sterile container and void the remaining urine in the toilet

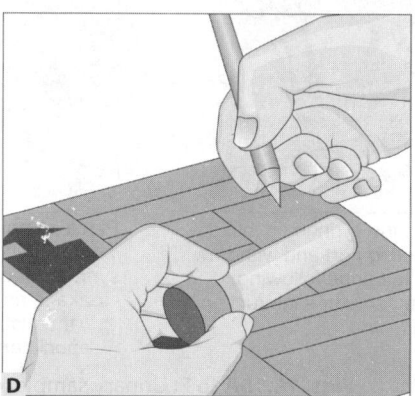

D
Complete the specimen request form and on the specimen pot, and document in the patient's notes that the sample was taken

Figs. 18.16A to D: Mid-stream urine sample collection.

Equipment Required

- Laboratory form
- Clean container with lid or cover (1): wide-mouthed container is recommended
- Bedpan or urinal (1): as required
- Disposable gloves (1): if available
- Toilet paper as required

Procedure

- Explain the procedure
- Assemble equipment and check the specimen form with client's name, date and content of urinalysis
- Label the bottle or container with the date, client's name, department identification, and Dr's name.
- Perform hand hygiene and put on gloves
- Instruct the client to void in a clean receptacle.
- Remove the specimen immediately after the client has voided
- Pour about 10–20 mL of urine into the labeled specimen bottle or container and cover the bottle or container
- Dispose of used equipment or clean them. Remove gloves and perform hand hygiene.
- Send the specimen bottle or container to the laboratory immediately with the specimen form.
- Document the procedure in the designated place and mark it off on the Kardex.

24 HOURS URINE COLLECTION

Collection of 24 hours urine specimen means the collection of all the urine voided in 24 hours, without any spillage of wastage.

Purpose

- To detect kidney and cardiac conditions.
- To measure total urine protein and creatinine.
- To measure total urine electrolytes, 17 ketogenic steroid, oxylate, porphyrins, drugs and vitamins.

Normal Characteristics of Urine

- Volume: 1000 to 2000 mL excreted in 24 hours.
- Appearance: Clear
- Odor: Aromatic odor, if kept for some time, ammonia smell.

- Color: Straw or amber in color
- Reaction: Acidic
- Specific gravity: 1.010 to 1.020
- Constituents of urine: 96 percent water, 2 percent urea and 2 percent uric acid. Urates, creatin chlorides, phosphates, sulphates and oxalates also may be present in minute's quantities.

Preliminary Assessment Check

- Doctor order for any specific instructions.
- General condition and diagnosis of the patient.
- Self ability of the patient.
- Mental status to follow directions.
- Articles available in the unit.

Preparation of the Patient and Environment

- Explain the sequence of the procedure.
- Provide privacy.
- Keep the articles at the bedside.
- Obtain lab request and container.

> **First morning/24 hour urine specimens**
> - **First morning specimen:** This is the specimen of choice for urinalysis and microscopic analysis, since the urine is generally more concentrated (due to the length of time the urine is allowed to remain in the bladder)
> - **Urine for 24 hours**
> - **Purpose:** This procedure checks the function of your kidneys or measures certain products in your urine
> - A special container is used to collect the urine
> - A preservative is in the container
> - Refrigerate the container during collection, the urine must be kept cold

Equipment

- Bed pan or urinal.
- Dry container (24 hours collection bottle).
- Clean pouring (measuring) jar.
- Funnel.

Procedure

- Before beginning 24 hours urine collection, patient is asked to void.
- Discard the sample and note the time.
- Document the starting time of urine collection in the nurses record.
- Advise not to spill urine.
- All urine passed over next 24 hours is collected in large container.
- Exactly 24 hours after, patient is instructed to void and specimen is included.

Aftercare

- Send the sample immediately to the laboratory with lab request.
- Replace the articles after cleaning.
- Record the procedure in the nurse's record sheet.

General Instructions

- The entire collected urine should be stored in a covered container in a cool place.
- Add preservatives to the urine to prevent decomposition and multiplication of bacteria, e.g. boric acid, formalin, chloroform, etc.
- The urine should be thoroughly mixed and all or part sent to the laboratory in a clean bottle.
- Requisition form must be duly filled and signed.

URINE CULTURE

Collection of midstream specimen of urine without contaminating container and urine specimen.

Purpose

- To collect uncontaminated urine specimen for culture and sensitivity test.
- To detect the micro-organism causing urinary tract infection (UTI).
- To diagnose and treat with specific antibiotic.

General Instructions

- Urine should be collected in sterile containers.
- Urine specimens for culture should be collected in the morning.
- After washing the perineal area and drying collect a midstream specimen of urine in a sterile bottle.
- For bed-ridden patients cauterized specimen of urine is taken.

Preliminary Assessment Check

- The doctors order for any specific instruction.
- General condition and diagnoses of the patient.
- Self-care ability of the patient.
- Mental status to follow instructions.
- Articles available in the unit.

Preparation of the Patient and Environment

- Explain the procedure to the patient.
- Provide privacy.
- Arrange the articles at the bedside.
- Collect and arrange the culture bottle- from the laboratory.
- Keep the lab request ready.

Equipment

- Basin and soap
- Towel and sterile gloves
- Gauze pads 2 to 3 (if patient on strict bed rest)

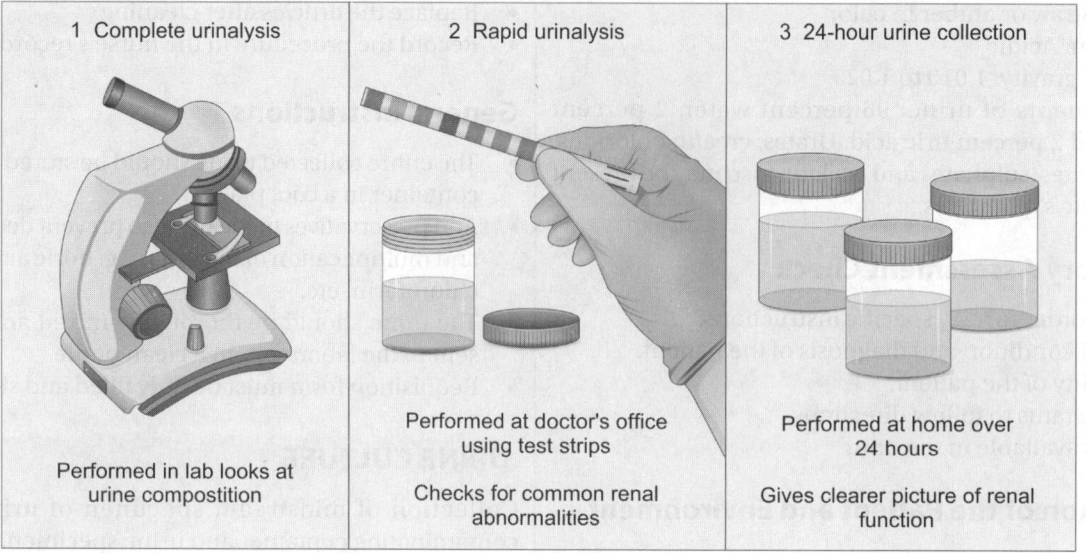

Fig. 18.17: Different methods of urine test.

- Sterile culture bottle.
- Lab request form.
- Sterile K-basin (if needed).

Procedure

- Instruct patient to clean perineum with soap and water.
- Open container and leave cover facing inside up.
- Instruct patient to void into sterile K-basin. If patient is unable to get out of bed.
- Instruct patient to void directly into sterile container.
- Collect 30 to 50 mL (1/2 to 3/4 of container) at midstream point of voiding.
- Emphasize first and last portions of voiding to be discarded.
- Cap container securely without touching inside of liquid.

Aftercare

- Label container with patient's name, hospital number and date.
- Send container to lab immediately with lab request.
- Record the procedure in nurse record sheet and register in microbiology lab note book.

URINE TESTING

Urine analysis methods comprise testing reaction, specific gravity, albumen sugar bile, acetone, pus, blood and yeasts microscopically.

Purpose

- To detect reaction, in cystitis the reaction is alkaline.
- To detect sugar, it is present in diabetes mellitus.
- To detect protein, it is present in kidney damage, pre-eclampsia and is called proteinuria.
- To detect acetone, it is present due to incomplete metabolism of fat.
- To detect bile, it is seen in cases of obstructive jaundice or hemolytic diseases.
- To detect pus cells, it is present due to urinary tract infection.
- To detect blood, it is seen in snake bite, fracture pelvis, etc.

Characteristics of Normal Urine

- Volume: 1,000 to 2,000 mL in 24 hours.
- Appearance: Clear
- Odor: Aromatic odor
- Color: Amber or pale straw in color.
- Reaction: Normal urine is slightly acidic,
- Specific gravity: 1.010 to 1.025
- Constituents of the normal urine: Water 96 percent, urea 2 percent and uric acid, urates, creatinine, chlorides, phosphates, sulphates, oxlates-2 percent.

Characteristics of Abnormal Urine

Volume

- Polyuria: Increased in volume.
- Oliguria: Decreased in volume.
- Anuria: Total absence or marked decrease of urine.
- Suppression: Failure of the kidney to secrete urine.

Color

- Green or brownish-yellow: Bile salts and bile pigments.
- Reddish brown: Urobilinogen.
- Bright red: A large amount of fresh blood.

- Smokey brown: Blood pigment.
- Milk white: Chyluria due to filariasis.

Appearance
- Mucus: Appears as a flocculent cloud.
- Pus: Settles at the bottom as a heavy cloud.
- Stones: As fine sand.
- Uric acid: As grains of pepper.

Odor
- Sweetish or fruity odor: Seen in diabetes.

Reaction
- Alkaline: Cystitis
- Specific gravity
- Diabetes mellitus: Increased specific gravity
- Renal disease: Low specific gravity
- Constituents of urine
- Kidney damage: Albumin.

Types of Examination of the Urine
- **Physical examination:** Color appearance, volume, reaction, specific gravity and odor.
- **Chemical examination:** Routine tests such as for albumin and sugar. Special tests such as tests for acetone, bile pigments and bile salts. Microscopic examination-Crystals, casts, RBC, pus cells, epithelial and bacteria.

Preliminary Assessment
- The doctor order for any instructions.
- Articles available in the unit.
- General condition and diagnosis of the patient.
- Self-care ability of the patient.

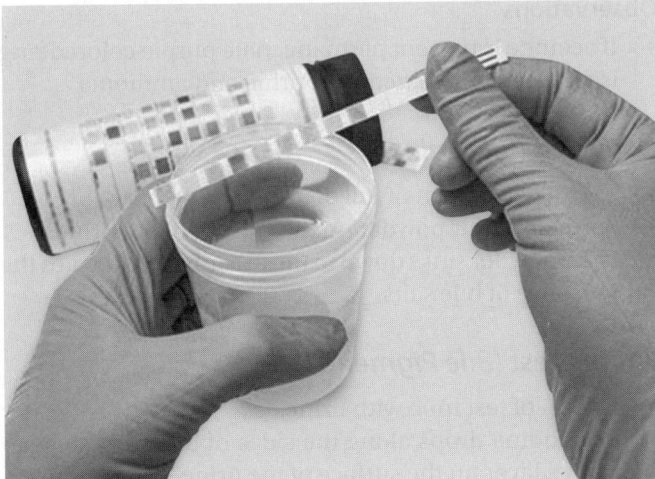

Fig. 18.18: Dip stick method of urine testing.

Preparation of the Patient and Environment
- Explain the procedure to the patient.
- Keep the urine sample ready.
- Arrange the articles ready in the treatment.
- Provide labeled container for collecting urine.

Equipment
- Test tubes 4 to 6 on a test tube.
- Test tube holder—1.
- Spirit lamp—1.
- Match box—1.
- Kidney tray with lining to discard the wastes.
- Duster or rag piece: To wipe the outside of the test tube before heating.
- Acetic acid: To test urine for albumin.
- Nitric acid or sulphosalic acid: To test urine for albumin.
- Red and blue litmus paper: To tests the reaction of the urine.
- Urinometer: To measure the specific gravity of the urine.
- Benedict's solution: To test urine for sugar.
- Ammonium sulphate crystals, sodium nitroprusside crystals and liquor ammonia to test urine for acetone.
- Weak solution of Tr. Iodine to test for bile pigments.
- Sulphur power: To test for bile salts.
- Glass jar: To measure the amount of the urine.
- Pipettes—2: To measure drops of urine and reagents.
- A small bottle brush: To clean the test tubes.

Procedure

Sugar Test
- Take test tube and fix in holder.
- Pour 5 mL of Benedict's solution into test tube.
- Light spirit lamp and heat Benedict solution till it boils.
- Holding test tube mouth facing away from nurse.
- Add 8 drops of urine using dropper and allow to boil for few seconds.
- Put off flame and cool test tube under running water.

Observations
- Blue: Nil (Negative)
- Green: + (25%)
- Yellow: ++ (50%)
- Orange: +++ (75%)
- Brick red: ++++ (100%)

Albumin Test

A. Hot Test
- Fill 2/3 of test tub with urine, secure test tube holder at very top.
- Heat the upper third of test tube over flame.
- If there is precipitation, it denotes the presence of wither protein or phosphate.
- Add 2–4 drops of 2 percent acetic acid.

Benedict's qualitative test-
Principle: Alkali and heat
Cupric ions (blue)+ suger→ cuprous oxide(red color) +cuprous hydroxide (yellow).
Method: Take 5 mL of Benedict's reagent in a test tube, and 0.5 mL of urine and mix well. boil over flame for 2 min.
Allow to cool.
Note chane in color.

Sensitivity-200 me/dl of reducine agent in urine

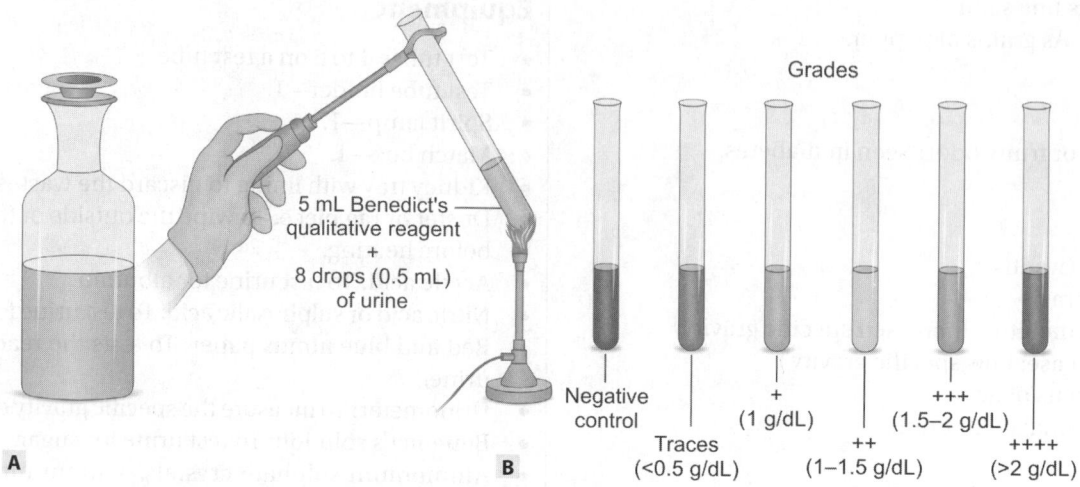

Figs. 18.19A and B: (A) Benedict's test; (B)Semiquantitative interpretation.

- If precipitate dissolves it is due to phosphates present in normal urine.
- If precipitate does not dissolve it denotes presence of albumin.

Observation
- Trace: +
- Cloudy: ++ (100 mg /dL)
- Thick cloudiness: +++ (500 gm /dL)

B. Cold Test
- Pour a small quantity of nitric acid or sulphosalic acid 3 percent in to a clean test tube.
- Allow equal quantity of urine to trickle down the sides of the test tube.
- If albumin present, a white precipitate will be seen where two fluids meet.

Urine pH
- Collect and keep ready with urine sample
- Dip litmus strip in urine and keep for one minute.
- Note color change.
- Discard strip into container for infected waste.

Urine Specific Gravity
- Fill 3/4 of jar with urine.
- Gently place urinometer into jar.
- When urometer stops bobbing read specific gravity directly from scale marked on calibrated stem of urinometer.
- Make sure that instrument floats freely and does not touch sides of jar.
- Read scale at lowest point of meniscus to ensure an accurate reading at eye level.

Rothera's Test (Acetone)
- Take 2 cm depth of ammonium sulphate crystals in a small test tube.
- Add equal volume of urine and one crystal of sodium nitroprusside.
- Close the test tube with a cork and shake the test tube.
- Take liquor ammonia and add to it the urine, trickling through the sides.
- Read the results immediately.

Observations
- If acetone is present permanganate purple colored ring is formed at the junction of urine and ammonia.

Hays Test (Bile Salts)
- Take a test tube, half full of urine.
- Sprinkle sulfur powder on the surface of the urine.
- If the powder sinks down to the test tube, it indicates the presence of bile salts.

Smiths Test (Bile Pigments)
- Fill 3/4 of test tube with urine.
- Add iodine drops along the sides of the tube, so as to form a layer on the surface of the urine.
- A green color at the junction of the two liquids indicates the presence of bile pigments.

Aftercare

- Discard the urine in the sluice room.
- Wash the test tube with soap and water.
- Dry the tube, holder and urinometer with jar.
- Replace the article after cleaning.
- Wash hands thoroughly.
- Record the procedure in the nurses' record sheet and diabetics chart.

ROLE OF NURSE IN URINARY ELIMINATION

The nursing role in relation to the assessment and management of urinary retention, urinary incontinence and catheterization are considered using recent literature and best practice statements. Retention of urine and incontinence has a major detrimental impact on a person's life and nurses have an important role to play in supporting patients. Catheterization is often necessary for acute retention of urine but is the last resort for incontinence. However, when catheter use is appropriate, asepsis technique during insertion and continuing management can help to minimize associated problems. Urinary elimination problems are embarrassing and distressing and nurses need to deal with them with sensitivity and empathy.

The role and responsibilities of nurse, when managing the urinary elimination in his her clients include the following:

- Taking nursing history pertaining to client with partial emphasis on urinary elimination
- Conducting or assessing physical assessment of kidneys, bladder, urethral orifice, skin integrity and hydration and urine
- In addition, carrying out the following assessment measures like measuring urine output, collecting urine specimens, determining the presence of abnormal constituents, assisting with diagnostic procedure.

BOWEL ELIMINATION

Defecation is the expulsion of feces from the anus and the rectum. It is also called a bowel movement.

The peristaltic waves move the feces into the sigmoid colon and the rectum, the sensory nerves in the rectum are stimulated and the individual becomes aware of the need to defecate.

Defecation reflex: There are two centers governing the reflex to defecate. One is situated in the medulla and subsidiary one is in the spinal cord. When parasympathetic stimulation occurs, the internal anal sphincter relaxes and the colon contracts. The defecation reflex is stimulated chiefly by the fecal mass in the rectum. When the rectum is distended the intrarectal pressure rises, the defecation reflex is stimulated by the muscle stretch, and the desire to eliminate results.

FACTORS AFFECTING BOWEL ELIMINATION

- **Age and development:** There is a marked difference between the stools of an infant and an older person. The very young are unable to control elimination until the neuromuscular system is developed, usually between the ages of 2 to 3 years.
- **Daily patterns:** Most people have regular patterns of bowel elimination which include frequency, timing considerations, position and place changes in any of these may upset a person routine and actually lead to constipation.
- **Lifestyles:** Many individual's family and sociocultural variables influences a person's usual elimination habits. The long-term effect of bowel training, the availability of toilet facilities, embarrassment about a odors and need to privacy, also affect the fecal elimination patterns.
- **Fluids:** Both the type and amount of fluid ingested affect elimination. Healthy fecal elimination is facilitated by a daily intake of 2000 to 3000 mL.
- **Activity and muscle tone:** Regular exercise improves gastrointestinal motility and muscle tone while inactivity decreases both. Adequate tone in the abdominal muscles, the diaphragm and the perineal muscles is essential to case in defecation.
- **Psychological factors:** Emotional stress affects the body in many ways. Persons with anxiety causes increased intestinal motility and persons with depression causes slower intestinal motility resulting in constipation.
- **Pathological conditions:** Spinal cord and head injuries decrease sensory stimulation for defecation. Impaired

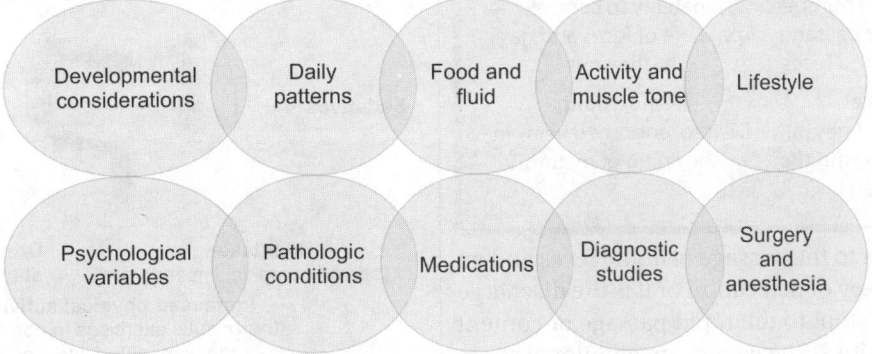

Fig. 18.20: Factors affecting bowel elimination.

mobility limits the patient's ability to respond to the urge to defecate. Ribbon like stools in appearance due to tumor in the colon.
- **Medications:** Narcotic analgesics cause constipation by decreased gastrointestinal mobility. Many medications have diarrhea as undesirable side effect.
- **Diagnostic procedure:** Barium salts used in radiologic examinations. It Hardens, if allowed to remain in the colon, producing constipation and sometimes an impaction.
- **Surgery and anesthesia:** Direct manipulation of the bowel during abdominal surgery inhibits peristalsis causing a condition termed as paralytic lieu's. General anesthetic agents that are inhaled also inhibit peristalsis by blocking the parasympathetic impulses to the intestinal muscle.
- **Irritants:** Spicy, foods, bacterial toxins and poisons can irritate the intestinal tract and produce diarrhea and often large amounts of flatus.
- **Pain:** Patients who are experience discomfort when defecating, e.g. following hemorrhoid surgery will often suppress the urge to defecate to avoid the pain.

COMMON PROBLEMS IN BOWEL ELIMINATION

- **Constipation:** It refers to the passage of small, dry hard stool or the passage of no stool for a period of time. The causes are irregular defecation habits, inappropriate diet, insufficient fluid, insufficient exercises and increased psychological stress.
- **Fecal impaction:** It is a mass or collection of hardened feces in the folds of the rectum. The causes are prolonged retentions and accumulation of fecal material, poor defecation habits and constipation and medication.

Common bowel elimination problems	
Constipation A symptom, not a disease infrequent stool and/or hard, dry, small stools that are difficult to eliminate	**Impaction** Results from unrelieved constipation; a collection of hardened feces wedged in the rectum that a person cannot expel
Diarrhea An increase in the number of stools and the passage of liquid, unformed feces	**Incontinence** Inability to control passage of feces and gas to the anus
Flatulence Accumulation of gas in the intestines causing the walls to stretch	**Hemorrhoids** Dilated, engorged veins in the lining of rectum

- **Diarrhea:** It refers to the passage of liquid feces and an increased frequency of defecation or it is the discharge of frequent loose stool to the rapid passage of content through the intestines. The causes are emotional stress and infection.
- **Fecal incontinence:** It refers to loss of voluntary ability to control fecal and gaseous discharge through the anal sphincter or inability to control the expulsion of feces. The causes are spinal cord trauma and tumors of the external sphincter muscles.
- **Flatulence:** It is the presence of excess in the intestine and leads to stretching and inflation of the intestines (intestinal distension) air or gas in the gastrointestinal tract is called flatus.

CONSTIPATION

Constipation means hard stools, difficulty passing stools (straining), or a sense of incomplete emptying after a bowel movement. The cause of each of these symptoms of constipation varies, so the approach to each should be tailored to each specific person. The number of bowel movements generally decreases with age. Most adults have bowel movements between three and 21 times per week, and this would be considered normal. The most common pattern is one bowel movement a day, but this pattern is seen in less than half the people. Moreover, most people are irregular and do not have bowel movements every day or the same number of bowel movements each day.

Signs and Symptoms of Constipation

- Infrequent bowel movements
- Straining to have bowel movements
- Hard and/or small stools
- Sense of incomplete evacuation after bowel movements
- Lower abdominal discomfort
- Abdominal bloating, occasionally distension
- Anal bleeding or fissures from the trauma caused by hard stools
- Occasionally diarrhea due to obstruction of the colon by hard stool

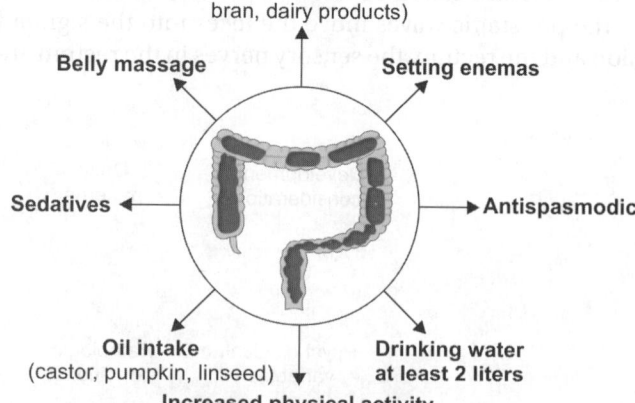

Fig. 18.21: Constipation treatment.

- Rarely colonic perforation
- Psychological distress and/or obsession with having bowel movements
- Possible aggravation of diverticular disease, hemorrhoids and rectal prolapse.

Management for Constipation

Initial treatment measures for constipation include manual disimpaction and transrectal enemas. A well-lubricated gloved finger might be required in patients with lower anorectal impactions. These initial measures are then followed by elective evaluation of the causes of the constipation.

Medical care should focus on dietary change and exercise rather than laxatives, enemas, and suppositories, none of which really address the underlying problem. The key to treating most patients with constipation is correction of dietary deficiencies, which generally involves increasing intake of fiber and fluid and decreasing the use of constipating agents (e.g., milk products, coffee, tea, and alcohol).

Medications to treat constipation include the following:
- **Bulk-forming agents (fibers; e.g., psyllium):** Arguably the best and least expensive medication for long-term treatment.
- **Emollient stool softeners (e.g., docusate):** Best used for short-term prophylaxis (e.g., postoperative).
- **Rapidly acting lubricants (e.g., mineral oil):** Used for acute or sub acute management of constipation
- **Prokinetics (e.g., tegaserod):** Proposed for use with severe constipation-predominant symptoms.
- **Stimulant laxatives (e.g., senna):** Over-the-counter agents commonly but inappropriately used for long-term treatment of constipation.

DIARRHEA

Diarrhea is loose, watery stools. Having diarrhea means passing loose stools three or more times a day. Acute diarrhea is a common problem that usually lasts 1 or 2 days and goes away on its own. Diarrhea lasting more than 2 days may be a sign of a more serious problem. Chronic diarrhea (diarrhea that lasts at least 4 weeks) may be a symptom of a chronic disease. Chronic diarrhea symptoms may be continual or they may come and go. Diarrhea of any duration may cause dehydration, which means the body lacks enough fluid and electrolytes (chemicals in salts, including sodium, potassium, and chloride) to function properly. Loose stools contain more fluid and electrolytes and weigh more than solid stools.

Causes of Diarrhea

Acute diarrhea is usually caused by a bacterial, viral, or parasitic infection. Chronic diarrhea is usually related to a functional disorder such as irritable bowel syndrome or an intestinal disease such as Crohn's disease. The most common causes of diarrhea include the following:

- **Bacterial infections.** Several types of bacteria consumed through contaminated food or water can cause diarrhea. Common culprits include *Campylobacter, Salmonella, Shigella,* and *Escherichia coli (E. coli).*
- **Viral infections.** Many viruses cause diarrhea, including rotavirus, norovirus, cytomegalovirus, herpes simplex virus, and viral hepatitis. Infection with the rotavirus is the most common cause of acute diarrhea in children. Rotavirus diarrhea usually resolves in 3 to 7 days but can cause problems digesting lactose for up to a month or longer.
- **Parasites.** Parasites can enter the body through food or water and settle in the digestive system. Parasites that cause diarrhea include *Giardia lamblia, Entamoeba histolytica,* and *Cryptosporidium.*
- **Functional bowel disorders.** Diarrhea can be a symptom of irritable bowel syndrome.
- **Intestinal diseases.** Inflammatory bowel disease, ulcerative colitis, Crohn's disease, and celiac disease often lead to diarrhea.
- **Food intolerances and sensitivities.** Some people have difficulty digesting certain ingredients, such as lactose, the sugar found in milk and milk products. Some people may have diarrhea if they eat certain types of sugar substitutes in excessive quantities.
- **Reaction to medicines.** Antibiotics, cancer drugs, and antacids containing magnesium can all cause diarrhea.

Signs and Symptoms of Diarrhea

Diarrhea may be accompanied by cramping, abdominal pain, nausea, an urgent need to use the bathroom, or loss of bowel control. Some infections that cause diarrhea can also cause a fever and chills or bloody stools.

Dehydration: Diarrhea can cause dehydration. Loss of electrolytes through dehydration affects the amount of water in the body, muscle activity, and other important functions. Dehydration is particularly dangerous in children, older adults, and people with weakened immune systems. Dehydration must be treated promptly to avoid

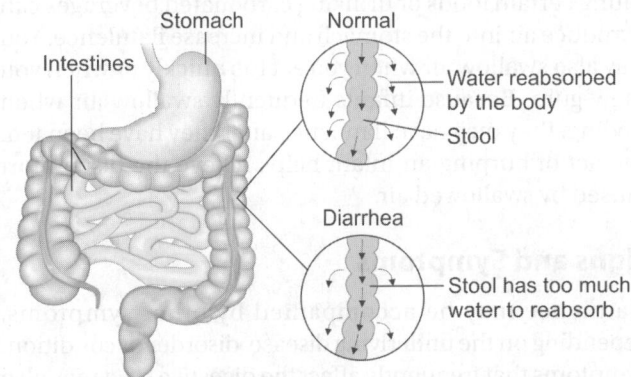

Fig. 18.22: Changes occurring in colon due to diarrhea.

serious health problems, such as organ damage, shock, or coma-a sleeplike state in which a person is not conscious.

Treatment and Medications

Most cases of diarrhea resolve spontaneously within a few days and all that is needed is preventing dehydration by replacing lost fluids, according to the NIH. In the meantime, various over-the-counter medications may help firm the stool and decrease the urgency for bowel movements. These include loperamide hydrochloride (commonly known as the brand name Imodium AD), bismuth subsalicylate (brand name Pepto-Bismol) and attapulgite (brand name Kaopectate.

These medications however are not recommended for diarrhea caused by bacterial infection or parasites, according to the NIH, since organisms will be trapped in the intestines if the diarrhea ceases before they are completely excreted. The Cleveland Clinic recommends drinking two to three quarts or liters of liquids daily while recovering from diarrhea. While water is fine, it does not replace lost salt or nutrients, so better choices are broth, tea with honey, sports drinks and pulp-free juices. Avoid milk products, caffeine, alcohol, and apple and pear juices since they may worsen diarrhea. Soft, bland foods are recommended as well, including bananas, plain rice, toast, crackers, boiled potatoes, smooth peanut butter, cottage cheese, noodles and applesauce. Because yogurt, cheese and miso contain probiotics, which contain strains of bacteria similar to those in a healthy intestine, they are also good choices. Avoid fatty, high-fiber or heavily seasoned foods for several days.

FLATULENCE

Flatulence is defined in the medical literature as "flatus expelled through the anus" or the "quality or state of being flatulent" which is defined in turn as "marked by or affected with gases generated in the intestine or stomach; likely to cause digestive flatulence" The root of these words is from the Latin *flatus* – "a blowing, a breaking wind". Flatus is also the medical word for gas generated in the stomach or bowels.

Flatulence is the expulsion of gas from the gastrointestinal tract through the rectum. Daily, the average person produces one to four pints of gas and expels it up to 14 times. Eating certain foods or drinking carbonated beverages can introduce air into the stomach and increase flatulence. You may also swallow air when you eat too quickly or when you chew gum. Because infants frequently swallow air when feeding, they may have flatulence after they have been fed. The act of burping an infant helps relieve the discomfort caused by swallowed air.

Signs and Symptoms

Flatulence may be accompanied by other symptoms, depending on the underlying disease, disorder or condition. Symptoms that frequently affect the digestive tract may also involve other body systems.

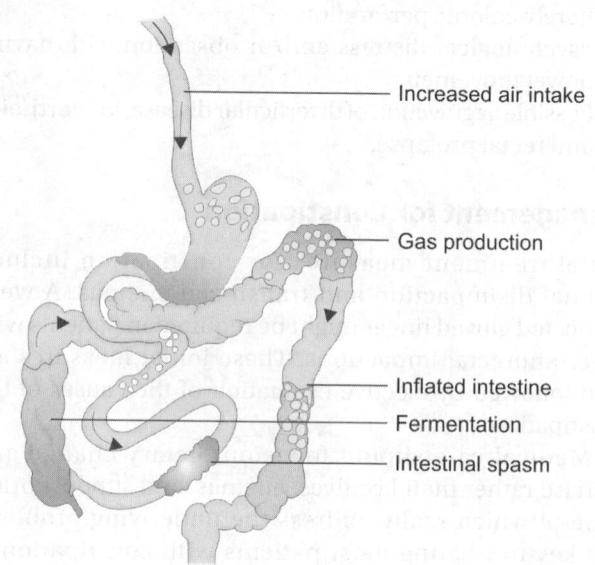

Fig. 18.23: Causes of flatulence.

Flatulence may accompany other symptoms affecting the digestive tract including:
- Abdominal swelling, distension or bloating
- Bad breath
- Belching
- Change in bowel habits
- Constipation
- Diarrhea
- Heartburn
- Nausea with or without vomiting

INSERTION OF A FLATUS TUBE

Flatus tube or a rectal tube inserted into the rectum to relieve flatulence and gaseous distension of the abdomen.

Passing of flatus tube is defined as an introduction of a tube into the rectum for expulsion of gas.

Purpose

- To remove flatulence from the lower bowel.
- To relieve abdominal distension.
- Used before giving a retention enema.

General Instructions

- Introduce the rectal tube into 4 to 6 inches.
- Rectal tube should not leave more than 30 minutes.
- Longer periods of insertion can lead to permanent sphincter damage.
- The tube can be reinserted every 3 to 4 hours if necessary.

Preliminary Assessment Check

- The doctors order for any specific precautions.
- Patients general condition.
- Diagnosis of the patient.

- Self-care ability of the patient.
- Mental status to follow instructions.
- Articles available in the unit.

Preparation of the Patient and Environment

- Explain the sequence of the procedure.
- Provide privacy.
- Provide left lateral position.
- Arrange the articles at the bedside.
- Place the mackintosh under the buttocks of the patient.

Flatus tube: It is reusable rubber tube used for the removal of flatus. It is also used for the treatment of sigmoid volvulus and intussusception. It is used also for barium enema.

Equipment

A clean tray containing:
- Flatus tube in a kidney tray with water
- Vaseline
- Wet swabs in a bowl
- Paper or Mackintosh or towel
- Paper bag
- Long artery forceps
- Screen.

Procedure

- Wash hand thoroughly.
- Place the patient in left lateral position.
- Lubricate the flatus tube and insert 4 to 6 inches into the anal canal.
- The free end of the tube is kept in water in a kidney tray.
- Keep the tube in a place for 20 minutes.
- Presence of air bubbles in the water indicates that flatus is being expelled.
- Remove the tube and place it in the K-basin.

Aftercare

- Clean and area with wet cotton swabs.
- Position the patient comfortably.
- Replace the article after cleaning.
- Wash hand thoroughly.
- Record the procedures and findings in the nurses record sheet.

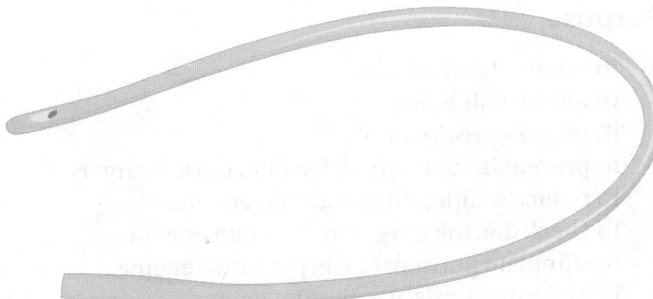

Fig. 18.24: Flatus tube.

USE OF BEDPAN

Bedpan is made from steel or plastic device to meet elimination need of patient confined to bed.

Bedpan may be used by a person who is unable to get out of bed. Bedpans used by females for elimination of urine and faces of by males for elimination of feces.

Purpose

- To provide comfort.
- To facilitate bowel and bladder elimination.
- To collect specimen for diagnostic purposes.
- To promote continence during bowel and bladder training.
- To give perineal wash.

Indications

- Patient with spinal injury.
- Postoperative patients.
- Patients with fracture and traction.
- Chronic bedridden patients.
- Patients those who are strict bedrest.

Types of Bedpan

- **Regular bedpan:** Made of metal or hard plastic has a curved, smooth upper end and a tapered lower end. The pan is approximately 5 cm deep.
- **Fracture pan:** Designed for patients with body or leg casts, the shallow upper end approximately 13 cm deep that slips easily under the patient.
- **Offering bedpan:** A bedpan for patients confined to bed provides a means to collect stool Female bedpan to pass urine and feces, For male bedpans only for defecation Sitting on a bedpan can be extremely uncomfortable. The caregiver should help the patient assume a position similar to the natural squatting position.

Preliminary Assessment Check

- The doctors order for specific precautions such as movements and positions.
- General condition of the patient.

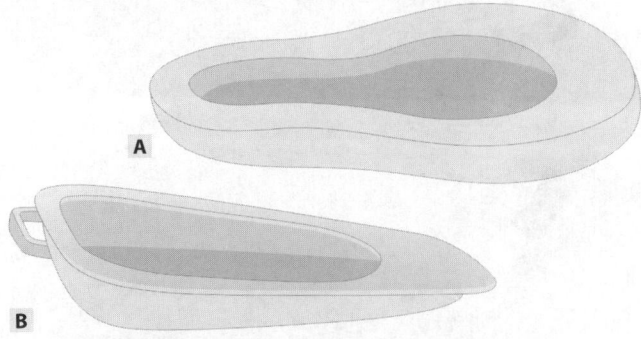

Figs. 18.25A and B: Types of bedpan used for patient bowel elimination.

- Level of consciousness.
- Mental healthy to follow instructions.
- Self-care ability.
- Articles available in he unit.

Preparation of Patient and Environment

- Explain to assist (hip to lift).
- Arrange the article at the bedside.
- Provide privacy.
- Position the patient for easy lifting.
- Place mackintosh under the buttocks to prevent soiling.

Equipment

- Bedpan with lid
- Clean gloves
- Draw mackintosh if needed
- Water and mug
- Tissue paper
- Soap with soap dish K-basin and towel.

Procedure

- Assess patient's condition for level of consciousness and limitation in movements.
- Explain the procedure to the patient and relatives.
- Provide privacy.
- Encourage patient to assume normal position for defecation if possible.
- Elevate the head end of bed if patient is alert.
- Roll draw sheet towards one side of the bed.
- Place the mackintosh under the patients buttocks.
- Place dry bed pan under patients buttocks by following any of the methods **(Figs. 18.26 A and B)**.
- Flex patient's knees and bring heels towards buttocks. Assist patient to lift buttocks. Instruct patient to raise the hip and buttocks, fold back the gown and slide the bedpan under the buttocks. Make sure that wider and flat surface of bedpan is placed under the buttocks.
- Turn the patient to side line position and place the bedpan firmly close to the buttocks. Roll the patient on the bedpan. Once patient is on the bedpan give enough time to pass stool/urine.

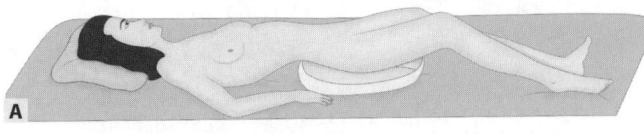

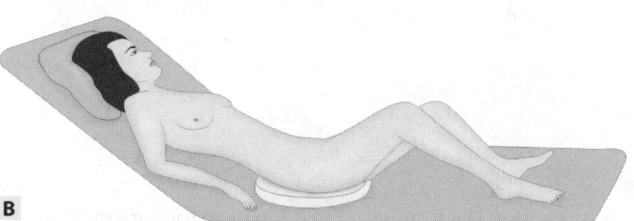

Figs. 18.26A and B: Bed pan provided for bed-reddened patient.

- Keep the patient covered well to avoid embarrassment.
- Once patient has finished, permit patient to self clean by assisting in pouring of water.
- Use measured quantity of water if output is to be maintained.
- If patient is unable to clean, pour water and clean with long artery forceps and cotton swabs.
- Remove the bedpan by lifting the patient carefully.
- Cover it with a newspaper/card board immediately. Dry the mackintosh if it is wet.
- Secure draw sheet and position the patient comfortably.
- Provide water and soap to wash hands. Note the color, amount and consistency of bowel contents.
- Empty the contents into toilet and flush properly.
- Wash the bedpan in following manner.
- Rinse the bedpan.
- Clean outside with liquid soap.
- Using separate brush, clean inside of the bedpan and disinfect with any antiseptic solution hypochlorite solution for half hour.
- Rinse off the soap/vim under place it to dry.
- Replace all articles in respective areas.
- Record frequently of bowl movements and any abnormalities noticed.

Aftercare

- Cover bedpan immediately and dry mackintosh of wet.
- Secure draw sheet and position the patient comfortably.
- Provide water and soap to wash hands.
- Empty the articles in to stop—hopper in sluice room.
- Replace the articles after cleaning.
- Wash hands thoroughly.
- Record the procedure in the nurse's sheet.

ENEMA

Enema (Clysis) is defined as a introduction of the fluid into the rectum.

An enema is an introduction of fluid into the bowel through the rectum for the purpose of cleansing or to introduce nourishment.

An enema is an introduction of fluid into the lower bowel through the rectum for the purpose cleaning, medicinal, diagnostic or such other purpose.

Purpose

- To remove fecal matter.
- To relieve flatulence.
- To relieve constipation.
- To prevent involuntary defecation during surgery.
- To reduce temperature, e.g. cold enema.
- To check diarrhea, e.g. starch opium enema.
- To stimulate peristalsis, e.g. purgative enema.
- To make diagnosis, e.g. barium enema.
- To cleanse the bowel before X-ray studies.

- To induce anesthesia, e.g. anesthetic enema.
- To administer medications.
- To destroy intestinal parasites, e.g. anthelminitic enema.
- To administer fluids and nutrients.
- To relieve inflammation.
- To establish regular bowel functions during bowel training program.

Contraindications

- Acute myocardial infarction and cardiac problems.
- Acute renal failure.
- Appendicitis.
- Obstetrical and gynecological contraindications.

Classification of Enema

Soap water enema: It is otherwise called saline enema. In this normal saline (sodium chloride 1 teaspoon) to half-liter of water. The amount of solution used for adult 500 to 1000 mL children 250 to 500 mL and infants 250 mL or less. The temperature of the solution in adult 105 to 110°F and children 100°F.

Oil enema: It is given to soften fecal matter in cases of serve constipation. The enema must be retained ½ or 1 hour to soften the feces.

The solutions used are olive oil gingelly oil, castor oil and olive oil 1:2 the amount of solution used is 115 to 175 mL the temperature of the solution is 100° F (37.7° C).

Carminative enema: It is also called antispasmodic enema. It is given to relieve gaseous distension of abdomen by increasing peristalsis and expulsion of flatus. The solution used is 8 to 16 mL of turpentine mixed thoroughly with 600 to 1200 mL of soap solution. Milk and molasses 90 to 230 mL well mixed with equal quantity of warm milk.

Antihelmentic enema: It is given to destroy and expel worms from the intestine cleansing enema must be given prior to antihelmentic enema so that the drug comes in direct contact with worms and the lining of intestine.

The solution used is infusion of quassia 15 gm of chips to 600 mL of water or hypertonic saline solution sodium chloride 60 mL with 600 mL of water. The amount of solution given is 250 mL.

Cold enema: Cold enema or ice-water enema is given to reduce body temperature in hyperpyrexia and heat stroke. it is given in the form of colonic irrigations. The temperature of the solution is 80 to 90° F (27 to 32° C).

Glycerin enema: Glycerin enema is given to children to fever patients and postoperative patient. Pure glycerin and water 1:2 are used.

Astringent enema: Astringent enema contracts the tissues and blood vessels checks bleeding and inflammation lessens the amount of mucus discharge and gives a temporary relief in the inflamed area. It is usually given in colitis and dysentery. The solution used are tannic acid 25 gm to 600 mL water, alum 30 gm to 600 mL of water and silver nitrate 2 percent (silver nitrate is dissolved in the distilled water).

Sedative enema: Sedative enema contains an anesthetic drug to produce anesthesia in the patient. The commonly used drugs are paraldehyde and over tin. Dose is given as per doctor's order.

Stimulant enema: Stimulant enema is given in the treatment of shock and collapse. Coffee enema is given in

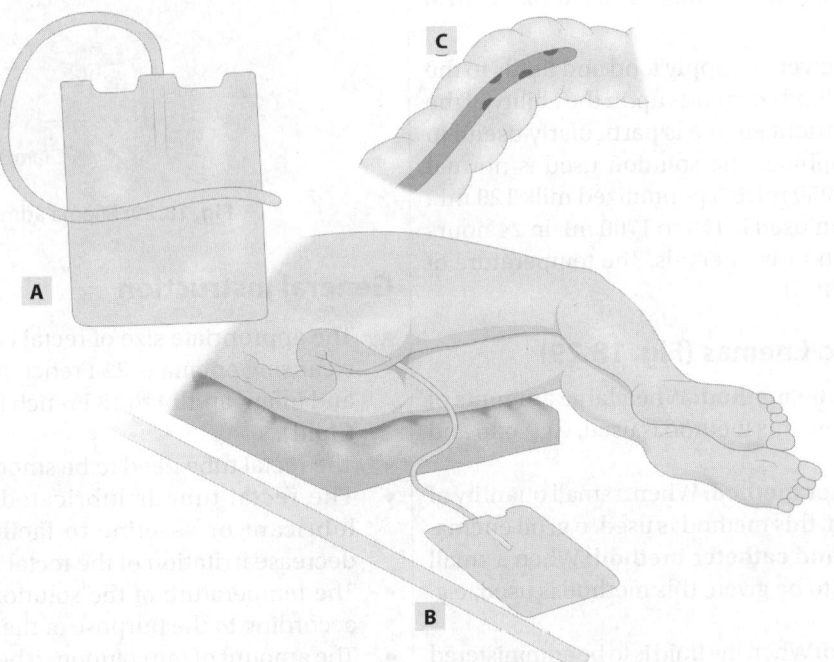

Figs. 18.27A to C: Left lateral position used for enema.

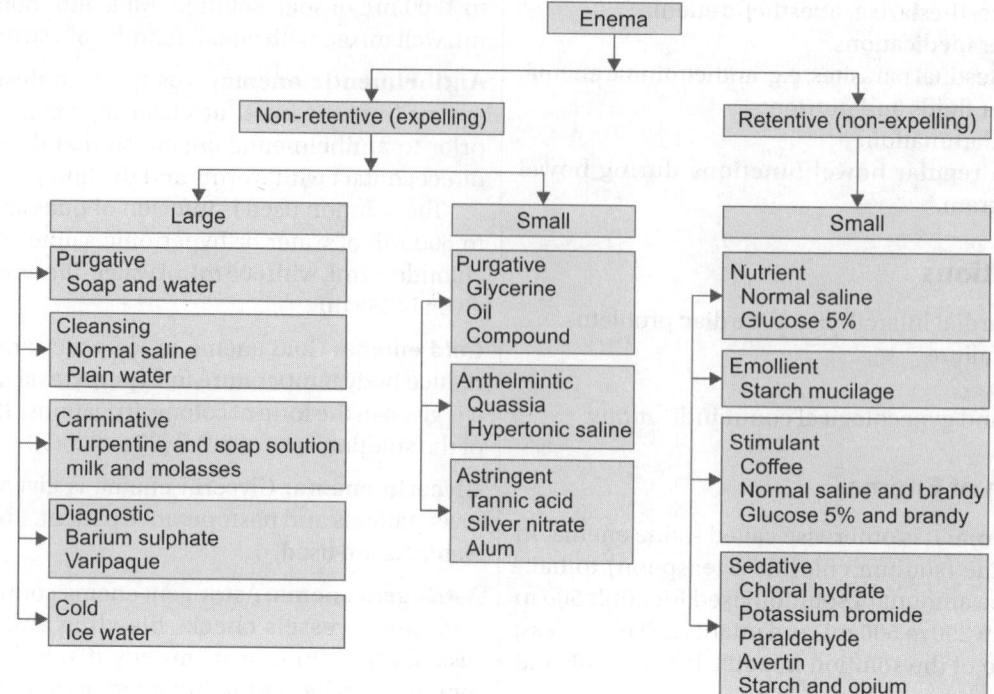

Fig. 18.28: Types of enema.

case of opium poisoning. Solution used are black coffee-1 tables spoon coffee powder to 300 mL of water and l5 mL of brandy added to 120 to 180 mL of glucose saline. The amount of solution used is 180 to 240 mL and the temperature of solution is 108 to 110° F (42 to 43° C).

Emollient enema: Emollient enema or starch enema is given in case of diarrhea to relieve irritation in an inflamed mucous membrane. The solution used is starch and opium. 1 to 2 mL added to 120 to 180 mL of starch mucilage or rice water. The temperature of the solution is 100 to 105° F (37.8 to 40.5° C).

Nutrient enema: It is given to supply food and fluids to the body. Selection of the fluids depends upon the ability of the colon to absorb it. Nutrient enema is particularly useful in conditions like hemophilia. The solution used is normal saline; glucose saline 250 mL 5% peptonized milk 120 mL. The amount of solution used is 110 to 1700 mL in 24 hours or 180 to 270 mL at 4 hourly intervals. The temperature of solution is 100° F (37.8° C).

Methods of Giving Enemas (Fig. 18.29)

- **Enema can and tube method:** When large amounts of fluids are to be given, this method is used, e.g. soap and water enema.
- **Funnel and catheter method:** When a small quantity of fluids is to be given, this method is used, e.g. oil enema.
- **Glycerin syringe and catheter method:** When a small quantity of fluid is to be given, this method is used, e.g. purgative enema.
- **Rectal drip method:** When the fluid is to be administered very slowly in order to aid in its absorption, e.g. nutrient enema.

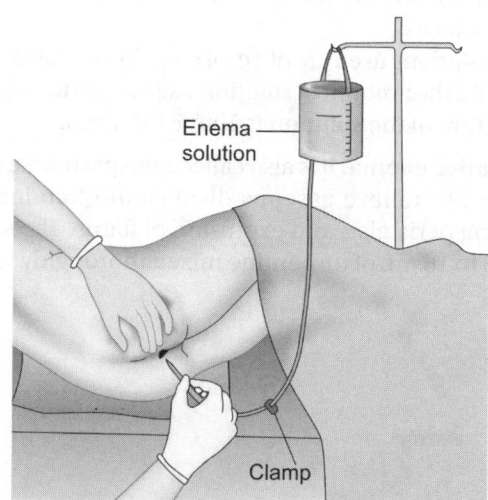

Fig. 18.29: Enema administration.

General Instruction

- The appropriate size of rectal catheter or rectal tube of cleansing enema is 22 French for adults, 12 French for and infant and 14 to 18 French for children (School age Child).
- The rectal tube need to be smooth and flexible.
- The rectal tube is lubricated with a water soluble lubricant or vaseline to facilitate insertion and to decrease irritation of the rectal mucosa.
- The temperature of the solution needs to be adjusted according to the purpose of the enema.
- The amount of the solution to be administered depends up on the type of enema and the age and size of the person.

- The patient usually placed in left lateral position, when an enema is administered. In this position sigmoid colon is below the rectum, thus facilitating instillation of the fluid.
- The distance to which the tube is inserted depends upon the age and the size of the patient. For an adult it is normally inserted 7.5 to 10 cm (3 to 4 inches), for children it is 2.5 to 3.75 cm (into 1 ½ inches).
- The height of the enema can should not be above 18 inches (20 cm) from the anus.
- The length of time that the enema solution is retained will depend up on the purpose of enema oil retention enema are usually retained for 2 to 3 hours. Other cleansing enemas are normally retained 5 to 10 minutes.
- Prepacked enema will have their own instruction which need to be followed.
- Prevent air from entering into rectum, by expelling air from the tube.
- If the rectum is impacted, attempt to remove the fecal matter with a gloved finger.
- Make sure the whole apparatus use for the administration of enemas is in a good working condition.
- Regulate the flow of fluid according to the type of enema.
- Listen to the complaints of the patient and should not ignore any discomfort however small they are.

Preliminary Assessment

- Doctors order for any specific precautions.
- Diagnosis of the patient.
- Abilities and limitations concerning movements.
- Level of consciousness to follow directions.
- Availability of the articles.
- Extra help needed.
- Lesions on the rectal and perineal area.
- Nature of enema ordered.

Preparation of the Patient and Environment

- Explain the sequence of the procedure.
- Arrange the articles at the bedside.
- Provide privacy.
- Cover the patient with bed sheet.
- Place the mackintosh and towel under the patient's buttocks.
- Place the patient in the left lateral position.
- Keep the bedpan under the bed over a stool.
- Adjust the IV pole to hold the enema can at the required height.

Equipment

A clean tray containing:
- Enema cans, rubber tubing, glass connection, screw clamp.
- Mackintosh and towel.
- Rectal tube (adjusts) or rectal catheter placed in a kidney tray.
- Vaseline.
- Pint measure.
- Soap jelly in a bottle.
- IV Stand.
- Toilet tray.
- Bedpan-2.
- Clean linen if needed.
- Bath thermometer.
- Rag pieces and K-basin.

Procedure

- Wash hands thoroughly.
- Attach tubing to enema can and clamp tube.
- Prepare solution at required temperature and check temperature with bath thermometer.
- Attach rectal tube to tubing, expel air and clamp tube. Air entry into rectum may cause discomfort.
- Hang enema can with solution on IV stand and adjust height to 18 inches from bed.
- Lubricate tip of rectal tube.
- Use rag pieces to separate patients buttocks and visualize anus clearly. Insert rectal tube gently to a distance of 2 to 4 inches.
- Encourage patient to take a deep breath while inserting tube. Note level of fluid and make sure there is free flow.
- Encourage patient to take deep breaths during administration of fluid.
- Clamp or pinch the rectal tube if the fluid is about to get over.
- Use rag pieces to remove the rectal tube.

Aftercare

- Instruct patient to hold solution for 10 to 15 minutes.
- Discard rag pieces in K-basin, detach rectal tube and place in same K-basin.
- Position the patient in supine and assist to toilet or provide a bedpan.
- Assist patient to wash perineal area if not able to do so.
- Remove the articles to utility room, clean and replace it.
- Keep the patient dry and comfortable.
- Wash hands.
- Record the procedure in the nurse's record.

BOWEL WASH

Bowel wash or colonic lavage or enteroclysis is defined as washing out colon with large quantities of solution.

Bowel irrigation or enteroclysis is defined as washing out of the colon after the feces has been expelled by using large quantities of prescribed solution.

Purpose

- To prepare for diagnostic examination or before certain surgery.
- To relieve inflammation.
- To stimulate peristalsis.

- To supply fluid and electrolyte those are absorbed from intestine.
- To dilute and remove toxic agents.
- To reduce temperature in hyperpyrexia.
- To relieve fecal incontinence.
- To supply medications locally.
- To clean the colon of feces, gas and barium.
- To treat infection and other pathological condition of colon.

Contraindications

- Rectal infection.
- Fistula in anus.
- Painful and bleeding hemorrhoids.
- Painful skin lesions around the anus.
- Massive carcinoma or tumors of the rectum.
- Loose sphincter.
- Polypus and diverticula of the intestine.

General Instructions

- A cleaning enema should be given one hour before the colon irrigation.
- The bladder should be emptied before colonic irrigations.
- The temperature of the solution is kept constant throughout the procedure.
- Allow only 200 to 300 mL of fluid to run into the rectum at a time.
- Make sure that the return flow is not blocked.
- Use a smooth and flexible rectal tube and lubricate it well.
- Prevent air entry into the intestines.
- Stop the procedure temporarily the patient complaints of pain.
- Listen to the complaints of the patient and should not ignore any discomfort however small they may be.

Methods Used for Bowel Irrigation

- Funnel and catheter.
- Y-connection and a rectal tube.
- Two tube method.

Solution Used

- Tap water
- Cold water
- Normal saline
- Sodium bicarbonate 1 to 2 percent
- Antiseptic solution $AgNO_3$
- $KMNO_4$ 1:5000
- Boric solution 1 to 2 percent
- Tannic acid 1:100
- Alum 1:100.

Temperature of the Solution

- Cleaning purpose 104° F (40° C)
- Thermal effect 110 to 115° F (43.3 to 46° C)

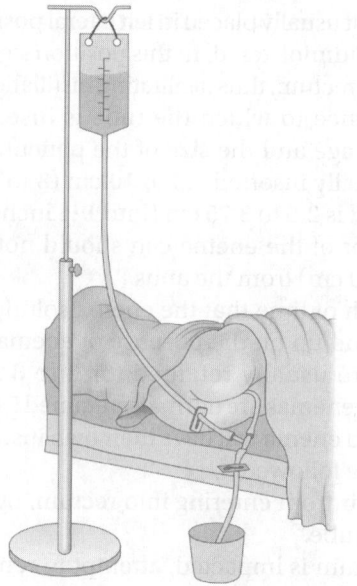

Fig. 18.30: Bowel washes procedure.

- Reducing temperature 80 to 90° F (27 to 32° C), amount of solution used for bowl, irrigation is 2 to 3 liters or till the return flow is clear.

Preliminary Assessment Check

- Doctors order for any specific precautions.
- Diagnosis of the patient.
- General condition of the patient.
- Self-care ability of the patient.
- Mental status to follow instructions.
- Any contraindication.
- Need for any extra help.
- Articles available in the unit.

Preparation of the Patient and Environment

- Explain the sequence of the procedure.
- Arrange the articles at the bedside.
- Provide privacy.
- Place the Mackintosh and towel under the patient.
- Place the patient in left lateral position.
- Keep the bucket on a low stool to receive the out flow of fluid.
- Remove the back rest and extra pillows.

Equipment

A clean tray containing:
- Funnel and tubing with glass connection.
- Mackintosh and towel.
- Rectal tube placed in a kidney tray.
- Vaseline.
- Rag pieces in a container.
- Hot and cold water in jugs.
- Prescribed solution in jug.
- Paper bag.
- Bucket.

- Toilet tray if needed.
- Clean linen if needed.
- Bath thermometer.

Procedure

- Wash hands thoroughly.
- Prepare the solution at the required temperature.
- Attach the tubing and the rectal tube with the funnel, pour solution in it and check for any leakage.
- Lubricate the tip of the rectal tube about 4 inches.
- Separate patient's buttocks to visualize anus clearly and insert tip of tube about 4 to 5 inches, while patient takes deep breath.
- Lower funnel below level of rectum and empty return flow into bucket.
- Fill funnel again. Pour 200 to 300 mL of fluid each time. Raise funnel and allow fluid to run continuously. When 200 to 300 mL of fluid has gone in pinch tube before tunnel is completely. Lower and invert tunnel over bucket and siphon fluid, noting characteristics of return flow.
- Repeat this process, till return flow is clear.
- Remove the rectal tube by using rag pieces.

Aftercare

- Remove rectal tube by using rag pieces.
- Discard rag piece in to K-basin.
- Place patient comfortably.
- Provide bedpan if needed.
- Change linen if soiled.
- Replace equipment after cleaning.
- Hand wash.
- Record the procedure in nurse's record sheet.

STOOL: ROUTINE AND CULTURE

Collection of stool specimen for specific or routine tests (stool culture to detect abnormal characteristics).

Purpose

- To identify specific pathogens.
- To determine presence of blood, ova and parasites.
- To determine presence of fat.
- To do gross examination of stool characteristics such as colour, consistency and odor.

Normal Characteristics of Feces

- **Color:** Light to dark down
- **Odor:** Pungent smell
- **Frequency:** 1 to 2 times per day
- **Quantity:** 4 to 5 ounces per day
- **Composition:** 30 percent water, shed epithelium from the intestine, a considerable quantity of bacteria and a small quantity of nitrogenous matter.
- **Stool of infants:** At birth the stool of infants is dark green and it is called "meconium".

Abnormal Characteristics of Feces

Color

- **Tarry black stools:** Bleeding in the upper gastro-intestinal tract.
- **Black color stool:** Melena, administration of iron or charcoal.
- **Clay colored stool:** Obstruction to the flow of bile.
- **White colored stool:** Presence of barium salts after barium tests.

Odor

Melena and dysentery: Foul smell.

Frequency

- Diarrhea: Increased frequency
- Constipation: Decreased frequency and low residue diet.

Consistency and Form

- Watery stools: Diarrhea
- Rice water stools: Cholera
- Pea soup stools: Typical of typhoid fever.

Appearance

- Fresh blood in large amounts: Bleeding piles.
- Blood and mucus stool: Amebic or bacillary dysentery.
- Worm or segments or worms in stool: Parasitic cysts, ova or larvae.

General Instructions

- Fecal specimens are collected for chemical bacteriological or parasitological analysis.
- Fecal specimens should be collected in the early stages of disease preferably before antibiotic treatment is given.
- Stool specimens should be collected in a sterile container (making use of the scoop provided in the container) with a tight-fitting leak proof-lid.
- After collection, the lid should be immediately replaced tightly.
- After proper labeling, the collected stool should be handed over to the laboratory without delay.

Preliminary Assessment Check

- The doctors order for any specific instructions.
- General condition and diagnosis of the patient.
- Assessment of the self-care ability.
- Mental status to follow instructions.
- Articles available in the unit.

Preparation of the Patient and Environment

- Explain the procedure to the patient.
- Provide privacy.

- Arrange the articles at bedside.
- Obtain lab request and container.

Equipment

- Appropriate specimen container.
- Spatula (clean for routine, sterile for culture).
- Bedpan or portable commode.
- Gloves.
- Waste paper.

Procedure

- Instruct patient to defecate into clean dry bedpan or commode.
- Instruct not to contaminate specimen with urine.
- Nurse to wear gloves while collecting specimen.
- Collect stool specimen with clean spatula for routine stool test and with sterile spatula into culture container.
- Cover the container tightly.

Aftercare

- Remove the gloves.
- Wrap spatula in waste paper and discard appropriately.
- Label specimen container with name, hospital number and date.
- Send to laboratory immediately (fresh specimen provides more accurate results).
- Replace equipment and after cleaning.
- Record the procedure in nurse's record sheet.

COLOSTOMY IRRIGATION

Colostomy irrigation, similar to an enema, in a form of stoma management used only for clients who have sigmoid colostomy or descending colostomy.

Colostomy is an operations in which artificial opening is made into the colons on the anterior abdominal wall to permit the escape of feces and flatus.

Purpose

- To establish regularity of evacuation.
- To cleanse the intestinal tract of gas, mucus and feces.
- To prevent excoriations of the skins around stoma.
- To remove any irritant foods ingested by the patient.
- To teach patient and his relatives the care of colostomy.

Types of Colostomy

- Temporary and permanent colostomy.
- Double barreled colostomy and end colostomy.
- Wet colostomy and dry colostomy.

Solutions Used for Colostomy Irrigation

- Normal saline.
- Plain water.
- Soapy solutions.

Preliminary Assessment

- Which the name, bed number and other identification of the patient.
- Check the diagnosis and purpose of irrigation.
- Check the type of colostomy done. Make sure of the proximal and distal loop of the colors.
- Check the patient's ability for self-care.
- Check the doctor's order for specific instructions and the precautions, if any, regarding the colostomy irrigations, movement of the patient, etc.
- Check the understanding of the patient to follow instructions.
- Check the articles available in patient's unit.

Preparation of the Patient and the Environment

- Explain the procedure to the patient.
- Make the patient sit on a chair in the bathrooms. A rubber sheet placed on the lap of the patient can be

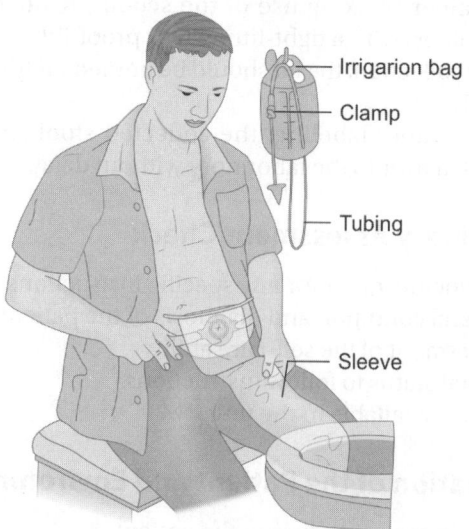

Fig. 18.31: Patient preparing for self-colostomy irrigation.

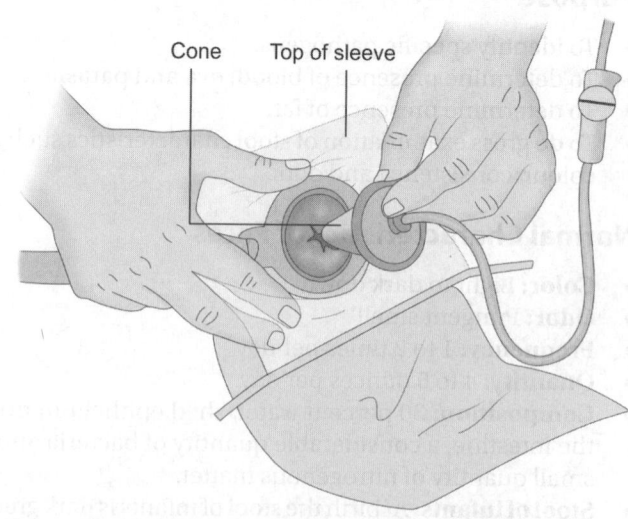

Fig. 18.32: Colostomy irrigation technique.

used as a through leading into the toilet to receive returns flow.
- Provide privacy. Remove undergarments.
- Clean the skin around the stoma with clears cotton swabs or rag pieces.

Preparation of the Article

- Irrigating can with tubing, clamp and catheter.
- IV stand.
- A jug with solution at the temperature of 100 to 105°C.
- Water soluble jelly.
- Clean cotton swabs.
- Kidney tray.
- Dressing, protective ointments.
- Mackintosh.
- Clean linen.
- Bucket.

Procedure

- Wash hands.
- Fill the irrigating can with the solutions and hang it at a required height.

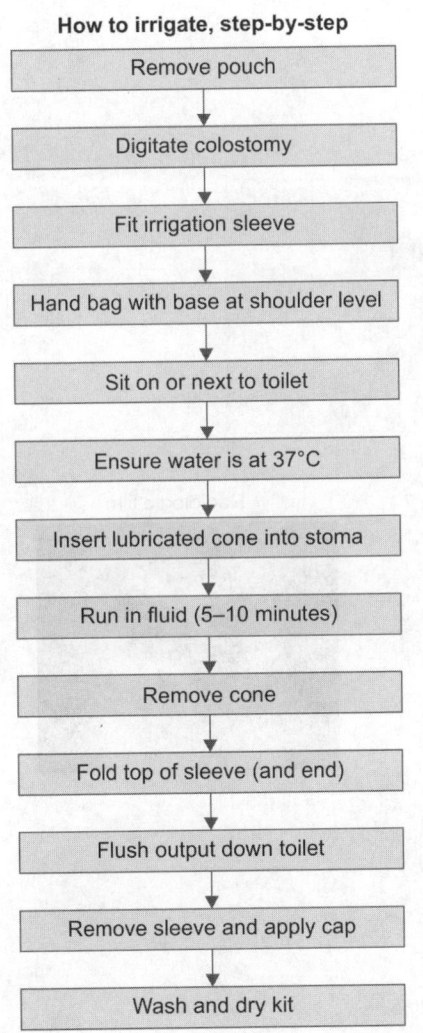

Fig. 18.33: Step by step process of colostomy irrigation.

- Expel the air from the tubing and clamp it remove the froth if any.
- Unite colostomy bag and remove the dressing.
- Introduce the catheter through the teat and the tip of the catheter is lubricated with water and jelly.
- Pour some solutions over stoma.
- Introduce catheter into stoma about 4 inches. Do not use any force.
- Allow the solutions to pass slowly, involving about 20 minutes.
- Clamp the tube before the entry of entire fluid.
- Remove the catheter from stoma. Disconnect it from the tubing and place it is the kidney tray.
- Wait for the return flow. Divert the attention of the patient.

Postprocedure Care

- When return flow is complete, remove the mackintosh clean the skin around the colostomy opening of and dry use skin thoroughly.
- Apply a clean dressing or a clear colostomy bed over the stoma.
- Change the dressing of incision aspects technique.
- Take all the articles in utility room. Clean the equipment immediately.
- Patients are instructed for the care and deamy of colostomy bags to prolong its life and keep it fete from odor.
- Chart the procedure in the patient's record.

BARIUM ENEMA

When barium is instilled rectally to visualize the lower GI tract, the procedure is called a barium enema.

Purpose

- To detect the presence of polyps, tumors and other lesions of the large intestine.
- To demonstrate any abnormal anatomy or malfunction of the bowel.
- To detect diverticula's, stenoses, obstructions, inflammations and ulcerative colithis.
- For the radiographic examination of the large intestine.

Types

- Barium sulfate (single-contrast technique) or barium sulfate.
- Air (double-contrast technique).

Principles

- Clear liquid diet for two days before the test.
- Procedure takes about 15 to 30 minutes during which time X-ray images are taken.
- If bowel is clear, clear images are obtained.

Preliminary Assessment

- See the doctor's order or prescription.
- See the patient's condition.
- See whether any allergic reaction is there for patient.
- See whether the patient can follow the orders.
- Check for all articles in the patients unit.

Preparation of the Patient

- Explain the procedure to the patient.
- Do colonic irrigation.
- Take the ultrasonography and colonoscopy.
- Check all the prescriptions of the patient.

Equipment

- Barium sulphate.
- Sterile water.
- Enema and tubing's.
- Syringe with needle.
- A water soluble iodinated contrast agent.
- Laxatives.
- Fluoroscopy screen.
- X-ray instruments.
- Warm water, air pump, pint measuring jar.

Procedure

- Prepare the patient, equipment and seat the patient to the X-ray section.
- Barium is mixed with equal amount of water to the suspension used for barium meal.
- The enema is set and is allowed to sum slowly through the rectal tube while the radiologist examines the patient under the fluoroscopic screen.
- The mixture should be at body temperate and stirred continuously during administration.
- It should not be further given without instruction.

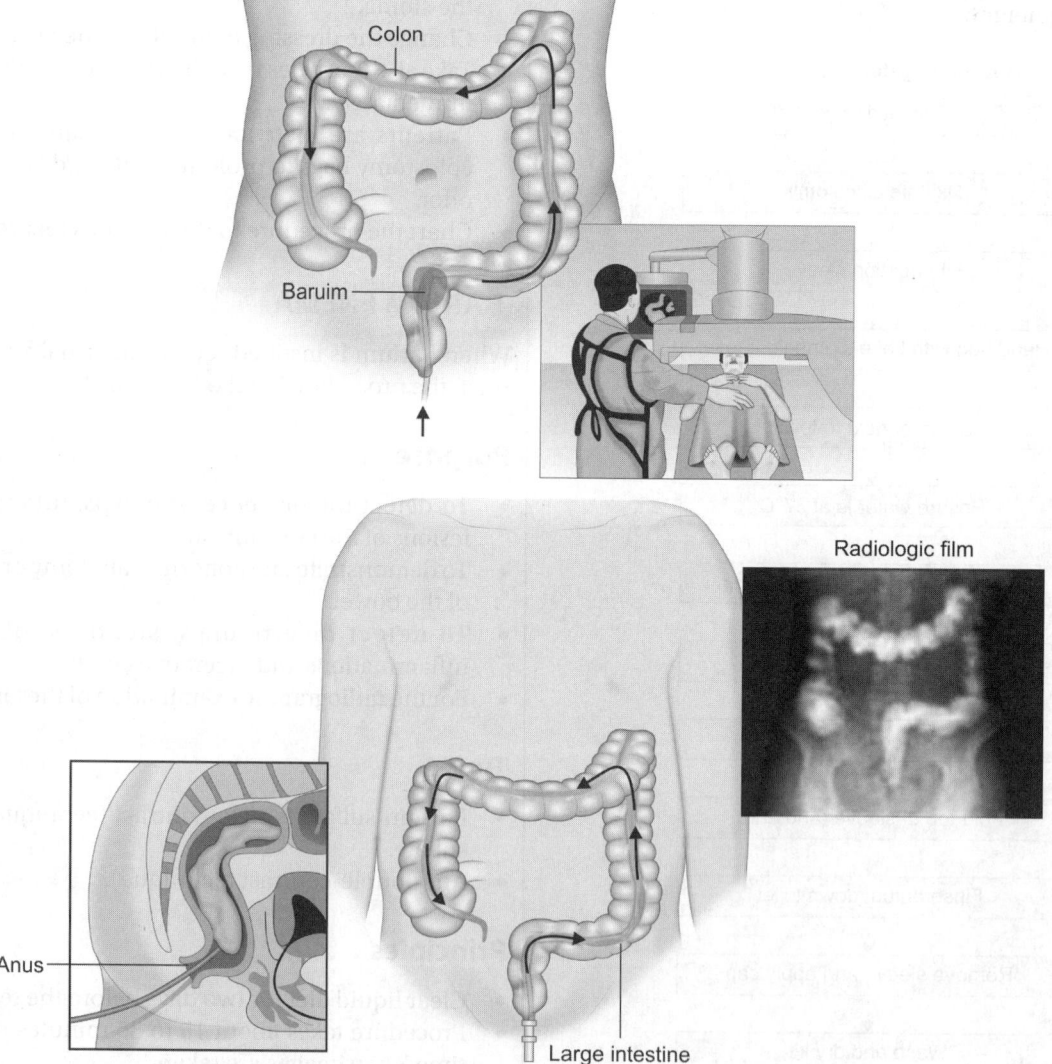

Fig. 18.34: Barium enema procedure.

- Various X-rays are taken to diagnose the problem.
- Then it is removed by cleansing enema or by a laxative.

Aftercare

- A laxative or cleansing enema is often given after the test to empty the large bowel.
- Stools are white for 24 to 72 hours after the examination.
- Encourage the client to increase the liquid intake to prevent fecal impaction.
- Instruct the client to report any pain, bloating, absence of stool or bleeding.

Complications

- Fecal impaction, if the bowel is not cleaned immediately.
- Pain bleeding, etc. can occur.

ROLE OF NURSE IN BOWEL ELIMINATION

The aims of effective bowel management are to "achieve regular, predictable emptying, at a socially acceptable time and place, avoiding constipation and unplanned evacuations." Bowel problems include: Constipation—dry, hard stool that is difficult to expel because it is stuck in the lower intestine. The stool can appear like small round pellets or balls. Causes include lack of stool softeners, not using suppositories, lack of adequate fluid intake, lack of exercise and certain foods such as rice, potatoes, pasta, cheese, bananas. *Diarrhea:* Loose water stools, and can be caused by flu, illness, medications and foods, and can be a sign of impaction. Causes include high anxiety, occasionally antibiotics or other medications, constipation and certain foods such as papayas, mangoes, excessive alcohol intake, beans. Hemorrhoids: condition in which the veins in and around the anus or lower rectum become inflamed and swollen. They can begin to itch, bleed and cause pain. They can be internal or external. The best way to prevent hemorrhoids is to keep stools soft so they can pass easily. Many creams are available to decrease the symptoms however, in some cases they may have to be surgically removed. A colostomy my be performed in extreme cases. A colostomy is a cut in the large intestine to create an artificial opening to the exterior of the abdomen. It serves as an artificial anus in which bowel movements fall into a collection pouch that is anchored to the abdominal skin.

BIBLIOGRAPHY

1. Craven R, Himle C. Fundamentals of Nursing, 2nd edition. Philadelphia: Lippincott. 1996.
2. Craven RF, Hirnle CJ. Fundamentals of Nursing: Human Health and Function. Philadelphia: JB. Lippincott, 1992.
3. Dean M, Harris JD, Regnard C, Hockley J. Constipation. Symptom Relief in Palliative Care. Oxford, United Kingdom. Radcliffe Publishing, 2006:75-9.
4. Goodman ML, Low J, Wilkinson S. Constipation Management in Palliative Care: A Survey of Practices in the United Kingdom. Journal of Pain and Symptom Management. March, 2005.
5. Gould CV, Umscheid CA, Agarwal RK, Kuntz G, Pegues DA. Guideline for prevention of catheter associated urinary tract infections 2009. Infect Control Hosp Epidemiol. 2010; 31(4).
6. Harkness-Hood G, Dincher JR. Total Patient Care: Foundations and Practice of Adult Health Nursing, 8th edition. St. Louis: Mosby-Year Book, Inc. 1992.
7. Jarman H. Consultant nurses as clinical leaders. Nursing Management. 2007; 14(3):22-6.
8. Jepson RG, Craig JC. Cranberries for preventing urinary tract infections. Cochrane Database Syst Rev, 2008.
9. Lindberg JB, et al. Introduction to Nursing Concepts, Issues and Opportunities. Philadelphia: JB. Lippincott Co, 1990.
10. Potter PA, Perry AG. Fundamentals of Nursing Concepts, Process and Practice 3rd edition. St. Louis: Mosby-Year Book, Inc. 1993.
11. Wiesel P, Bell S. Bowel dysfunction: assessment and management in the neurological patient. In: Norton C, Chelvanayagam S (Eds). Bowel Continence Nursing. Beaconsfield: Beaconsfield Publishers, 2004.

REVIEW QUESTIONS

Long Essays

1. Define urinary elimination; explain the physiology of urine elimination.
2. Define bowel elimination; explain the factors affecting bowel elimination.

Short Essays

1. Factors affecting urinary elimination.
2. Care of patient with urinary retention.
3. Care of patient with urinary incontinence.
4. Catheterization of the urinary bladder.
5. Bladder irrigation.
6. Catheter care.
7. Explain urine testing procedure.
8. Role of nurse in urinary elimination.
9. Nursing care of constipation and diarrhea.
10. Insertion of a flatus tube.
11. Define enema; enumerate the classification of enema.
12. Define bowel wash; explain the bowel wash procedure.
13. Colostomy irrigation.
14. Role of nurse in bowel elimination.

Short Answers

1. Characteristic of urine.
2. Common alterations in urinary elimination.
3. Monitoring urinary output.
4. Collecting urine specimen.
5. 24 hours urine collection.
6. Urine culture.
7. Rothera's test.
8. Hays test.
9. Smiths test.
10. Common problems in bowel elimination.
11. Causes of diarrhea.

12. Flatulence.
13. Carminative enema.
14. Use of bedpan.
15. Barium enema.

MULTIPLE CHOICE QUESTIONS

1. The normal specific gravity of urine is:
   a. 1.002–1.020
   b. 1.003–1.030
   c. 1.004–1.040
   d. 1.005–1.050
2. Common bowel elimination problems is:
   a. Constipation
   b. Impaction
   c. Diarrhea
   d. All of the above
3. The nurse would expect the least formed stool to be present in which portion of the digestive tract?
   a. Ascending
   b. Descending
   c. Transverse
   d. Sigmoid
4. Which of the following is not a function of the large intestine?
   a. Absorbing nutrients
   b. Absorbing water
   c. Secreting bicarbonate
   d. Eliminating waste
5. Methods of emptying the colon of feces is:
   a. Enemas
   b. Rectal suppositories
   c. Digital removal of stool
   d. All of the above

ANSWERS

1. d   2. d   3. a   4. a   5. d

CHAPTER 19
Diagnostic Testing

LEARNING OBJECTIVES

Phases of diagnostic testing (pre-test, intra-test and post-test) in common investigations and clinical implications:
- Complete blood count
- Serum electrolytes
- LFT
- Lipid/lipoprotein profile
- Serum glucose: AC, PC, HbA1c
- Monitoring capillary blood glucose (glucometer random blood sugar—GRBS)
- Stool routine examination
- Urine testing-Albumin, acetone, pH, specific gravity
- Urine culture, routine, timed urine specimen
- Sputum culture
- Overview of radiologic and endoscopic procedures

TERMINOLOGY

- **Endoscopy:** It is a direct visual examination of the internal body parts by means of an endoscope passed along the interior of hallows organs or cavities. Endoscopy is a term used to for the visualization of more than one organ with the same endoscope.
- **Larynogoscopy:** Larynx is visualized internally by direct or an indirect laryngoscope.
- **Bronchosopy:** It refers to the examination of tracheo-bronchial tree and bronchopulmonary segments. It may be done under local or general anesthesia. A bronchoscopic examination is performed by passing a fibro-optic bronchoscope into the trachea and bronchi through the trans-oral route.
- **Esophagogastroduodenoscopy:** It is a procedure done to visualize the inner surface of esophagus, stomach and even the duodenum. Fibro-optic gastroscopy allows greater flexibility and permits visualization of all the areas of the esophagus to duodenum.
- **Endoscopic retrograde cholangiopancreatography:** This is an investigation which permits radiographic imaging of bile ducts and pancreatic ducts using long, flexible and side viewing fibro optic endoscope.
- **Colonoscopy:** This investigation permits direct viewing of the large intestine (colon) by means of a long, flexible, fibro-optic instrument called colonoscopy.
- **Protoscopy:** It is the examination of the anus and rectum using a protoscope.
- **Sigmoidoscopy:** This is the visualization of the anus, rectum and sigmoid colon. This sigmoidoscope is a long and narrow tubular instrument which can be passed into the sigmoid colon through the anus.
- **Laparoscopy:** It is a procedure through which the abdominal and pelvic organs are visualized by means of a laparoscope. Laparoscopies are rigid telescope varying in diameters incorporating an optical system with a system of illumination.
- **Cystoscope:** It is the direct visualization of the urinary tract with cystoscope introduced into the bladder via urethra.
- **Fundoscopy:** The fundus of the eyes is visualized by means of an ophthalmoscope. The blood vessels of an interior eyes as well as other structure can be visualized and magnified. The fundus of the eye is the only area in the body where the blood vessels can be directly observed.
- **Biopsy:** A biopsy is the removal and examination of tissue for diagnostic purposes. It may be performed by a surgical excision at the time of exploratory surgery (open biopsy) or through a special needle or bore (needle biopsy) which does not necessitate a surgical incision or by means of an endoscope (endoscope surgery).
- **Bone marrow biopsy:** This is one of the diagnostic procedures performed in blood dyscrasisas in which a specimen of bone morrow is taken from the stream, iliac crest, posterior superior iliac spine, spine of the vertebra or tibia (in children) by mean of a hollow thick needle.
- **Thoracentesis:** It refers to the puncture by needle through the chest wall into the pleural space for the purpose of removing pleural fluid (blood, serous fluid, pus etc). This is done for diagnostic purpose.
- **Pericardial aspiration:** It is the removal of fluid from the pericardial sac. It is usually carried out either to relieve pressure or to obtain a specimen for diagnostic purpose.
- **Abdominal pracentesis:** It is the removal of fluid from the peritoneal cavity.
- **Lumbar puncture:** A lumbar puncture (LP, spinal tap, spinal puncture) is the insertion of a needle into the

lumbar region of the spine, in such a manner that the needle enters the lumbar arachnoid space of the spinal cannal below the level of the spinal cord.
- **Cisternal puncture:** It is the puncture of the cistern magna, a small reservoir of the CSF between the cerebellum and the medulla oblongata by introducing a short bevel lied needle below the occipital bone and between the first cervical lamina and the rim of the foramen magnum.
- **Liver biopsy:** Liver biopsy may be an open or closed procedure. In an open biopsy, a wedge of the liver is removed for study and the remaining edges are sutured together.
- **Liver aspiration:** It is an introduction of a needle into the liver substance to drain an abscess.
- **Renal biopsy:** Renal tissue may be obtained for examination either by an open or a closed biopsy technique. An open biopsy requires the surgical procedure-involving an incision through the flank.
- **Cervical biopsy:** It is the removal of a small piece of tissue from the cervix for the histopathological examination. It can be done as punch biopsy or cervical conization.
- **Endometrial biopsy:** It is done by spacing the lining of the uterine cavity with a curctte. It can be done as an outpatient procedure using novak curette.
- **X-ray examination:** X-ray examination is a form of electromagnetic energy of very short wave length, because of their short wavelength, they have the ability to penetrate into matter and it is this characteristic that makes them useful in the study of tissues.
- **Bronchography:** It is a radiological examination of the tracheobroncheal tree and the lungs after an installation of an opaque medium (radio-opaque oil or water soluble dye) into the bronchi.
- **Angiography:** It is the roentgenography visualization of the blood vessels anywhere in the body following the injection of a contrast medium. It is useful in evaluating the disorders of the brain, heart, lungs and other body parts.
- **Angiocardiography:** It is the study of the chambers of the heart and the large thoracic blood vessels done in conjunction with the cardiac catheterization.
- **Pulmonary angiography:** It is the roentgenography visualization of the blood vessels of the lungs. It is helpful in diagnosing such conditions are pulmonary embolism, lung tumors, aneurisms, vascular changes associated with emphysema, congenital defects, space occupying lesions within the thorax.
- **Cerebral angiography:** Cerebral angiography allows X-ray visualization of the brains vascular system. The dye may be injected directly into the common carotid artery.
- **Venography:** It is designed to identify and locate deep vein thrombosis and other structural abnormalities of the veins. A radio-opaque dye is injected into the various systems of the affected limbs under fluoroscopy and X-ray films are taken.
- **Cardiac catheterization:** It is a complex procedure involves the insertion of a catheter into the heart and surrounding vessels to obtain detailed information about the structure and functions of the heart, its valves and circulatory system.
- **Barium X-ray:** The plain X-ray abdomen shows the shadows of the relative densities of the structure photographed, but the inside of the gastrointestinal tract can be visualized unless a contrast medium is ingested or instilled into it.
- **Barium swallow:** It may be performed as a part of the barium meal. The filling and emptying of the esophagus is studied by barium swallow. The client drinks the barium sulphate solution.
- **Barium meal:** It is useful in diagnosing obstructions, ulcerations and growths within the esophagus, stomach and duodenum and to find out the structural and functioning abnormalities of the small intestine.
- **Barium enema:** A large colon is studied with barium given per rectum. About 2 to 3 pints of barium sulphate is given to distend the bowel and the X-rays are taken, it will show any abnormalities in the structure of the colon or a space occupying tumors in the abdominal cavity.
- **Cholecystography:** It is the radiographic examination of the gallbladder after administration of opaque medium for detection of gallstones and to estimate its ability to fill, concentrate its contents, contract and empty in normal states.
- **Retrograde pyelograpgy:** It is a procedure in which radio-opaque agents similar to those used in the IVP are introduced directly into the urinary tract following cystoscopy and catheterization of the ureter.
- **Hysteron-salphingography:** This is an X-ray study of the uterus and fallopian tubes using a contrast medium, in order to evaluate the uterine abnormalities and tubal patency in sterility problems.
- **Myelography:** It is the radiographic examination of the spinal cord and its canal after the injection of a radio-opaque substance into the subarachnoid space of the spinal canal through a lumbar puncture needle.
- **Peumoecephalography:** It is the radiographic examination of the ventricles of the brain and the sub-arachnoid spaces. It involves withdrawal of some CSF and the injection of air or oxygen into the subarachnoid space through a spinal/cisternal punctures.
- **Electrocardiogram:** It is a graphic record of the electrical impulses that are generated by depolarization and repolarization of the myocardium. These impulses are conducted to the external surface of the body where they are detected by electrodes and measured by galvanometer.
- **Electroencephalogram:** The electroencephalogram may be compared with electrocardiogram, in that

electrodes are placed over the skull in many areas and the electric activity of the various segments of the brain is recorded.
- **Electromyelography:** It is the recording of the electrical activity associated with enervation of skeletal muscles. Electrical currents are produced by skeletal muscles called muscle action potential.
- **Scanning:** Scanning is a process by image obtained for the examination of organs or regions of the body by gathering information with a sensing device. Examples of scanning procedures are bone scan, computerized axial tomography (CAT) scan, spiral CAT scan, nuchal fold scan, and thyroid scan.
- **Aspirin:** Once the Bayer trademark for acetylsalicylic acid, now the common name for this anti-inflammatory pain reliever.
- **Biopsy:** The removal of a sample of tissue for examination under a microscope to check for cancer cells or other abnormalities
- **Enteroscopy:** The use of a flexible instrument (a "scope") to examine the small intestine, a very long hollow tube located between the stomach and colon (large intestine) and made up of the duodenum, jejunum, and ileum
- **Sigmoidoscopy:** A procedure in which a physician inserts a viewing tube (sigmoidoscope) into the rectum for the purpose of inspecting the lower colon and rectum. If an abnormal area is detected, a biopsy can be performed.

INTRODUCTION

A diagnostic test is any approach used to gather clinical information for the purpose of making a clinical decision (i.e., diagnosis). Some examples of diagnostic tests include X-rays, biopsies, pregnancy tests, medical histories, and results from physical examinations

SALIENT FEATURES OF DIAGNOSTIC TESTING

The following are the salient features of diagnostic testing:
- The diagnostic test takes up where the formative test leaves off.
- A diagnostic test is a means by which an individual profile is examined and compared against certain norms or criteria.
- Diagnostic test focuses on individual's educational weakness or learning deficiency and identify the gaps in pupils.
- Diagnostic test is more intensive and act as a tool for analysis of learning difficulties.
- Diagnostic test is more often limited to low ability students.
- Diagnostic test is corrective in nature.
- Diagnostic test pinpoint the specific types of error each pupil is making and searches for underlying causes of the problem.
- Diagnostic test is much more comprehensive.

COMPLETE BLOOD COUNT

A complete blood count (CBC) is a blood test used to evaluate your overall health and detect a wide range of disorders, including anemia, infection and leukemia. A complete blood count test measures several components and features of your blood, including: Red blood cells, which carry oxygen

A complete blood count test measures several components and features of your blood, including:
- Red blood cells, which carry oxygen
- White blood cells, which fight infection
- Hemoglobin, the oxygen-carrying protein in red blood cells
- Hematocrit, the proportion of red blood cells to the fluid component, or plasma, in your blood
- Platelets, which help with blood clotting.

A CBC Test Usually Includes

- **White blood cell (WBC, leukocyte) count:** White blood cells protect the body against infection. If an infection develops, white blood cells attack and destroy the bacteria, virus, or other organism causing it. White blood cells are bigger than red blood cells but fewer in number. When a person has a bacterial infection, the number of white cells rises very quickly. The number of white blood cells is sometimes used to find an infection or to see how the body is dealing with cancer treatment.
- **White blood cell types (WBC differential):** The major types of white blood cells are neutrophils,

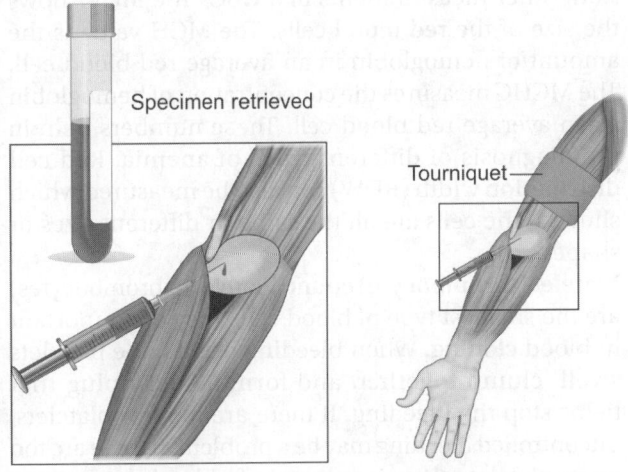

Fig. 19.1: Phlebotomy procedure.

lymphocytes, monocytes, eosinophils, and basophils. Immature neutrophils, called band neutrophils, are also part of this test. Each type of cell plays a different role in protecting the body. The numbers of each one of these types of white blood cells give important information about the immune system. Too many or too few of the different types of white blood cells can help find an infection, an allergic or toxic reaction to medicines or chemicals, and many conditions, such as leukemia.

- **Red blood cell (RBC) count:** Red blood cells carry oxygen from the lungs to the rest of the body. They also carry carbon dioxide back to the lungs so it can be exhaled. If the RBC count is low (anemia), the body may not be getting the oxygen it needs. If the count is too high (a condition called polycythemia), there is a chance that the red blood cells will clump together and block tiny blood vessels (capillaries). This also makes it hard for your red blood cells to carry oxygen.
- **Hematocrit (HCT, packed cell volume, PCV):** This test measures the amount of space (volume) red blood cells take up in the blood. The value is given as a percentage of red blood cells in a volume of blood. For example, a hematocrit of 38 means that 38% of the blood's volume is made of red blood cells. Hematocrit and hemoglobin values are the two major tests that show if anemia or polycythemia is present.
- **Hemoglobin (Hgb):** The hemoglobin molecule fills up the red blood cells. It carries oxygen and gives the blood cell its red color. The hemoglobin test measures the amount of hemoglobin in blood and is a good measure of the blood's ability to carry oxygen throughout the body.
- **Red blood cell indices:** There are three red blood cell indices: mean corpuscular volume (MCV), mean corpuscular hemoglobin (MCH), and mean corpuscular hemoglobin concentration (MCHC). They are measured by a machine, and their values come from other measurements in a CBC. The MCV shows the size of the red blood cells. The MCH value is the amount of hemoglobin in an average red blood cell. The MCHC measures the concentration of hemoglobin in an average red blood cell. These numbers help in the diagnosis of different types of anemia. Red cell distribution width (RDW) can also be measured which shows if the cells are all the same or different sizes or shapes.
- **Platelet (thrombocyte) count:** Platelets (thrombocytes) are the smallest type of blood cell. They are important in blood clotting. When bleeding occurs, the platelets swell, clump together, and form a sticky plug that helps stop the bleeding. If there are too few platelets, uncontrolled bleeding may be a problem. If there are too many platelets, there is a chance of a blood clot forming in a blood vessel. Also, platelets may be involved in hardening of the arteries (atherosclerosis).

Complete Blood Count with Differential (CBC with diff)

Test	Conventional	SI Units
Red blood cell (RBC)	Male: 4.6–6.2 × 10⁶ cell/μL	4.6–6.2 × 10^{12} cells/L
	Female: 4.2–5.9 × 10⁶ cell/μL	4.2–5.9 × 10^{12} cells/L
Hemoglobin (Hgb)	Male: 13–18 g/dL	Male: 130–180 g/L
	Female: 12–16 g/dL	Female: 120–160 g/L
Hematocrit (Hct)	Male: 45–52%	Male: 0.45–0.52
	Male: 37–48%	Female: 0.37–0.48
MCV	80 to 100 μm³	80 to 100 μm³
MCH	27 to 31 pg/cell	27 to 31 pg/cell
MCHC	32 to 36 g/dL	32 to 36 g/dL
White blood cells (WBC)	4,300–10,800 cells/mm³	4.3–10.3 × 10^9/L
WBC differential		
• Neutrophils, bands	0–5%	0.03–0.08
• Neutrophils, segmented	54–65%	0.54–0.65
• Lymphocytes	25–40%	0.25–0.40
• Monocytes	2–8%	0.02–0.08
• Eosinophils	1–4%	0.01–0.04
• Basophils	0–1%	0–0.01
Platelets	150,00–450.000/mm³	150–450 × 10^9/L

- **Mean platelet volume (MPV):** Mean platelet volume measures the average amount (volume) of platelets. Mean platelet volume is used along with platelet count to diagnose some diseases. If the platelet count is normal, the mean platelet volume can still be too high or too low.

Procedure

During a CBC, a lab technician will draw blood from a vein, typically from the inside of your elbow or from the back of your hand. The test will take only a few minutes. The technician:
- Cleans your skin with an antiseptic wipe
- Places an elastic band, or tourniquet, around your upper arm to help the vein swell with blood
- Inserts a needle in the your and collects a blood sample in one or more vials
- Removes the elastic band
- Covers the area with a bandage to stop any bleeding
- Label your sample and send it to a lab for analysis

A blood test can be slightly uncomfortable. When the needle punctures your skin, you might feel a prick or pinching sensation. Some people also feel faint or light-headed when they see blood. Afterwards, you may have minor bruising, but it will clear up within a few days.

Most CBC results are available within a few hours to a day after testing.

SERUM ELECTROLYTES

An electrolyte test can help determine whether there's an electrolyte imbalance in the body. Electrolytes are salts and minerals, such as sodium, potassium, chloride and bicarbonate, which are found in the blood. They can conduct electrical impulses in the body. The test is sometimes carried out during a routine physical examination, or it may be used as part of a more comprehensive set of tests.

Normal Values and Mass Conversion Factors

Electrolytes	Normal plasma values	Mass conversion
Sodium(Na^+)	135–145 mEq/L	23 mg = 1 mEq
Potassium (K^+)	3.5–5.0 mEq/L	39 mg = 1 mEq
Chloride (Cl^-)	98–107 mEq/L	35 mg = 1 mEq
Bicarbonate (HCO_3^-)	22–26 mEq/L	61 mg = 1 mEq
Calcium (Ca^{2+})	8.5–10.5 mg/dL	40 mg = 1 mmol
Phosphorus	2.5–4.5 mg/dL	31 mg = 1 mmol
Magnesium (Mg^{2+})	1.8–3.0 mg/dL	24 mg = 1 mmol
Osmolality	285–295 mOsm/kg	-

Definition: Electrolytes are positively and negatively charged molecules called ions that are found within the body's cells and extracellular fluids including blood plasma. A test for electrolytes includes the measurement of sodium, potassium, chloride, and bicarbonate. These ions are measured to assess renal (kidney), endocrine (glandular), and acid-base function, and are components of both renal function and comprehensive metabolic biochemistry profiles. Other important electrolytes routinely measured in serum or plasma include calcium and phosphorus. These are measured together because they are both affected by bone and parathyroid diseases, and often move in opposing directions. Magnesium is another electrolyte that is routinely measured. Like calcium, it will cause tetany (uncontrolled muscle contractions) when levels are too low in the extracellular fluids.

Purpose: Tests that measure the concentration of electrolytes are needed for both the diagnosis and management of renal, endocrine, acid-base, water balance, and many other conditions. Their importance lies in part with the serious consequences that follow from the relatively small changes that diseases or abnormal conditions may cause. For example, the reference range for potassium is 3.6-5.0 mmol/l. Potassium is often a STAT (needed immediately) test because values below 3.0 mmol/l are associated with arrhythmia (irregular heartbeat), tachycardia (rapid heartbeat), and cardiac arrest, and values above 6.0 mmol/L are associated with bradycardia (slow heartbeat) and heart failure. Abnormal potassium cannot be treated without reference to bicarbonate, which is a measure of the buffering capacity of the plasma. Sodium bicarbonate and dissolved carbon dioxide act together to resist changes in blood pH.

Measurement of electrolytes: Electrolytes are measured by a process known as potentiometry. This method measures the voltage that develops between the inner and outer surfaces of an ion selective electrode. The electrode (membrane) is made of a material that is selectively permeable to the ion being measured. This potential is measured by comparing it to the potential of a reference electrode. Since the potential of the reference electrode is held constant, the difference in voltage between the two electrodes is attributed to the concentration of ion in the sample.

Precautions: Electrolyte tests are performed on whole blood, plasma, or serum, usually collected from a vein or capillary. Special procedures are followed when collecting a sweat sample for electrolyte analysis. This procedure, called pilocarpine iontophoresis, uses electric current applied to the arm of the patient (usually an infant) in order to convey the pilocarpine to the sweat glands where it will stimulate sweating. Care must be taken to ensure that the collection device (macroduct tubing or gauze) does not become contaminated and that the patient's parent or guardian understands the need for the electrical equipment employed.

Preparation: Usually no special preparation is necessary by the patient. Samples for calcium and phosphorus and for magnesium should be collected following an eight-hour fast.

Aftercare: Discomfort or bruising may occur at the puncture site, or the person may feel dizzy or faint. Pressure to the puncture site until the bleeding stops reduces bruising. Applying warm packs to the puncture site relieves discomfort.

Risks: Minor temporary discomfort may occur with any blood test, but there are no complications specific to electrolyte testing.

Normal Results

Electrolyte concentrations are similar whether measured in serum or plasma. Values are expressed as mmol/L for sodium, potassium, chloride, and bicarbonate. Magnesium results are often reported as milliequivalents per liter (mEq/L) or in mg/dL. Total calcium is usually reported in mg/dL and ionized calcium in mmol/L. Since severe electrolyte disturbances can be associated with life-threatening consequences such as heart failure, shock, coma, or tetany, alert values are used to warn physicians of impending crisis. Typical reference ranges and alert values are cited below:

- Serum or plasma sodium: 135–145 mmol/L; alert levels: less than 120 mmol/L and greater than 160 mmol/L
- Serum potassium: 3.6–5.4 mmol/L (plasma, 3.6–5.0 mmol/L); alert levels: less than 3.0 mmol/L and greater than 6.0 mmol/l
- Serum or plasma chloride: 98–108 mmol/L
- Sweat chloride: 4–60 mmol/L
- Serum or plasma bicarbonate: 18–24 mmol/L (as total carbon dioxide, 22–26 mmol/L); alert levels: Less than 10 mmol/L and greater than 40 mmol/L
- Serum calcium: 8.5–10.5 mg/dL (2.0–2.5 mmol/L); alert levels: less than 6.0 mg/dL and greater than 13.0 mg/dL
- ionized calcium: 1.0–1.3 mmol/L
- Serum inorganic phosphorus: 2.3–4.7 mg/dL (children, 4.0–7.0 mg/dL); alert level—less than 1.0 mg/dL
- Serum magnesium: 1.8–3.0 mg/dL (1.2–2.0 mEq/L or 0.5–1.0 mmol/L)
- ionized magnesium: 0.53–0.67 mmol/L
- Osmolality (calculated): 280–300 mOsm/kg.

LIVER FUNCTION TEST

Liver function tests are blood tests used to help diagnose and monitor liver disease or damage. The tests measure the levels of certain enzymes and proteins in your blood. Some of these tests measure how well the liver is performing its normal functions of producing protein and clearing bilirubin, a blood waste product. Other liver function tests measure enzymes that liver cells release in response to damage or disease.

Liver function tests can be used to:
- Screen for liver infections, such as hepatitis
- Monitor the progression of a disease, such as viral or alcoholic hepatitis, and determine how well a treatment is working
- Measure the severity of a disease, particularly scarring of the liver (cirrhosis)
- Monitor possible side effects of medications

Liver function tests check the levels of certain enzymes and proteins in your blood. Levels that are higher or lower than normal can indicate liver problems. **Some common liver function tests include:**
- Alanine transaminase (ALT): ALT is an enzyme found in the liver that helps convert proteins into energy for the liver cells. When the liver is damaged, ALT is released into the bloodstream and levels increase.
- Aspartate transaminase (AST): AST is an enzyme that helps metabolize amino acids. Like ALT, AST is normally present in blood at low levels. An increase in AST levels may indicate liver damage, disease or muscle damage.
- Alkaline phosphatase (ALP): ALP is an enzyme found in the liver and bone and is important for breaking down proteins. Higher-than-normal levels of ALP may indicate liver damage or disease, such as a blocked bile duct, or certain bone diseases.

Test	Normal range
Bilirubin total	0–1 mg/dL
Conjugated (direct bilirubin)	0–0.35 mg/dL
Unconjugated (direct bilirubin)	0.2–0.65 mg/dL
SGOT	10–40 IU/L
SGPT	10–40 IU/L
Alkaline phosphatase	40–112 U/L
Total protein	6–8.5 gm/dL
Albumin	3.5–5 gm/dL
Globulin	2–3.5 gm/dL

(SGOT: serum glutamic oxaloacetic transaminase; SGPT: serum glutamic pyruvic transaminase)

- Albumin and total protein: Albumin is one of several proteins made in the liver. Your body needs these proteins to fight infections and to perform other functions. Lower-than-normal levels of albumin and total protein may indicate liver damage or disease.
- Bilirubin: Bilirubin is a substance produced during the normal breakdown of red blood cells. Bilirubin passes through the liver and is excreted in stool. Elevated levels of bilirubin (jaundice) might indicate liver damage or disease or certain types of anemia.
- Gamma-glutamyltransferase (GGT): GGT is an enzyme in the blood. Higher-than-normal levels may indicate liver or bile duct damage.
- L-lactate dehydrogenase (LD): LD is an enzyme found in the liver. Elevated levels may indicate liver damage but can be elevated in many other disorders.
- Prothrombin time (PT): PT is the time it takes your blood to clot. Increased PT may indicate liver damage but can also be elevated if you're taking certain blood-thinning drugs, such as warfarin.

Risks

The blood sample for liver function tests is usually taken from a vein in your arm. The main risk associated with blood tests is soreness or bruising at the site of the blood draw. Most people don't have serious reactions to having blood drawn.

Preparation: Certain foods and medications can affect the results of your liver function tests. Your doctor will probably ask you to avoid eating food and taking some medications before your blood is drawn.

During the test: The blood sample for liver function tests is usually drawn through a small needle inserted into a vein in the bend of your arm. The needle is attached to a small tube, to collect your blood. You may feel a quick pain as the needle is inserted into your arm and experience some short-term discomfort at the site after the needle is removed.

After the test: The blood will be sent to a laboratory for analysis. If the lab analysis is done on-site, you could have your test results within hours. If your doctor sends your blood to an off-site laboratory, you may receive the results within several days.

Results: Normal blood test results for typical liver function tests include:
- ALT: 7 to 55 units per liter (U/L)
- AST: 8 to 48 U/L
- ALP: 40 to 129 U/L
- Albumin: 3.5 to 5.0 grams per deciliter (g/dL)
- Total protein: 6.3 to 7.9 g/dL
- Bilirubin: 0.1 to 1.2 milligrams per deciliter (mg/dL)
- GGT: 8 to 61 U/L
- LD: 122 to 222 U/L
- PT: 9.4 to 12.5 seconds

These results are typical for adult men. Normal results vary from laboratory to laboratory and might be slightly different for women and children.

LIPID/LIPOPROTEIN PROFILE

Lipid tests are routinely performed on plasma, which is the liquid part of blood without the blood cells. Lipids themselves are a group of organic compounds that are greasy and cannot be dissolved in water, although they can be dissolved in alcohol. Lipid tests include measurements of total cholesterol, triglycerides, high-density lipoprotein (HDL) cholesterol, and low-density lipoprotein (LDL) cholesterol.

LIPID PROFILE

	Desirable	Borderline	High risk
Cholesterol	<200 mg/dL	200–239 mg/dL	240 mg/dL
Triglycerides	<150 mg/dL	150–199 mg/dL	200–499 mg/dL
HDL cholesterol	60 mg/dL	25–45 mg/dL	<35 mg/dL
LDL cholesterol	60–130 mg/dL	130–159 mg/dL	160–189 mg/dL
Cholesterol/HDL ratio	4.0	5.0	6.0

Lipid tests may also be performed on amniotic fluid, which is the fluid that surrounds the fetus during pregnancy. Prenatal lipid tests include tests for lecithin and other pulmonary (lung) surfactants that cover the air spaces in the lungs with a thin film.

Purpose: The purpose of blood lipid testing is to determine whether abnormally high or low concentrations of a specific lipid are present. Low levels of cholesterol are associated with liver failure and inherited disorders of cholesterol production. Cholesterol is a primary component of the plaques that form in atherosclerosis and is therefore the major risk factor for the rapid progression of coronary artery disease (CAD). High blood cholesterol may be inherited or result from such other conditions as biliary obstruction, diabetes mellitus, hypothyroidism, and nephrotic syndrome. In addition, cholesterol levels may be increased in persons who eat foods that are rich in saturated fats and cholesterol, and who lead a sedentary lifestyle.

Description: Cholesterol screening can be performed with or without fasting, but it should include tests of total and HDL cholesterol levels. The frequency of cholesterol testing depends on the patient's risk of developing CAD. Adults over 20 with total cholesterol levels below 200 mg/dL should be tested once every five years. People with higher levels should be tested for LDL cholesterol levels, and tested at least once per year thereafter if their LDL cholesterol is 130 mg/dL or higher. The National Cholesterol Education Program (NCEP) suggests further evaluation when the patient has any of the symptoms of CAD, or if she or he has two or more of the following risk factors for CAD:
- High blood pressure
- History of cigarette smoking
- Diabetes
- Low HDL levels
- Family history of CAD
- Age over 45 years (men) or 55 years (women)

Measurements of cholesterol and triglyceride levels are routinely performed in all patients.

Preparation: Patients who are scheduled for a lipid profile test should fast (except for water) for 12 to 14 hours before the blood sample is drawn. If the patient's LDL cholesterol is to be measured, he or she should also avoid alcohol for 24 hours before the test. When possible, patients should also stop taking any medications that may affect the accuracy of the test results. These drugs include corticosteroids; estrogen or androgens; oral contraceptives; some diuretics; antipsychotic medications, including haloperidol; some antibiotics; and niacin. Antilipemics are drugs that lower the concentration of fatty substances in the blood. When these medications are taken by the patient, blood testing may be done frequently to evaluate liver function as well as lipid levels.

Aftercare: Aftercare following blood lipid tests includes routine care of the skin around the needle puncture. Most patients have no aftereffects, but some may have a small bruise or swelling. A washcloth soaked in warm water usually relieves any discomfort. In addition, the patient can resume taking any prescription medications that were discontinued before the test.

Risks

The primary risk to the patient from blood tests of lipid levels is a mild stinging or burning sensation during the venipuncture, with minor swelling or bruising afterward.

Although amniocentesis is much safer in the third trimester, and is less risky when it is performed with the guidance of ultrasound technology, does present a risk of miscarriage and fetal injury. The mother should be monitored for any signs of bleeding, infection, or impending labor.

Results: The normal values for serum lipids depend on the patient's age, sex, and race. Normal values for people in Western countries are usually given as 140–220 mg/dL for total cholesterol in adults, although as many as 5% of the population have a total cholesterol higher than 300 mg/dL. Among Asians, the figures are about 20% lower. As a rule, both total and LDL cholesterol levels rise as people get older. Normal values for HDL cholesterol are also age- and sex-dependent. The range for males between 20 and 29 years is approximately 30–63 mg/dL; for females of the same age group it is 33–83 mg/dL. Normal values for fasting triglycerides are also age- and sex-dependent. The reference range for adult males 20 to 29 years is 45–200 mg/dL; for females of the same age group it is 37–144 mg/dL. As with cholesterol, the normal range rises with age.

Since a person's diet and lifestyle affect normal values, which are determined by the interval between the 5th and 95th percentile of the group, it is more helpful to evaluate cholesterol and triglycerides from the perspective of desirable plasma levels. The desirable values defined by the Nation Cholesterol Education Program (NCEP) in 2001 are as follows:

- Total cholesterol: Less than 200 mg/dL; 200–239 mg/dL is considered borderline high and greater than 240 mg/dL is high.
- HDL cholesterol: Less than 40mg/dL is low.
- LDL cholesterol: Less than 100 mg/dL is optimal; near-optimal is 100–129 mg/dL; borderline high is 130-159 mg/dL; high is 160–189 mg/dL; and very high is any value over 190 mg/dL.
- Total cholesterol: HDL ratio: Under 4.0 in males; 3.8 in females.

SERUM GLUCOSE: AC (FASTING PLASMA GLUCOSE), PC (POSTPRANDIAL PLASMA GLUCOSE), HBA1C (GLYCATED HEMOGLOBIN A1C)

Many types of glucose tests exist and they can be used to estimate blood sugar levels at a given time or, over a longer period of time, to obtain average levels or to see how fast body is able to normalize changed glucose levels. Eating food for example leads to elevated blood sugar levels. In healthy people these levels quickly return to normal via increased cellular glucose uptake which is primarily mediated by increase in blood insulin levels.

Random blood glucose level: A sample of blood taken at any time can be a useful test if diabetes is suspected. A level of 11.1 mmol/L or more in the blood sample indicates that you have diabetes. A fasting blood glucose test may be done to confirm the diagnosis.

Fasting blood glucose level: A glucose level below 11.1 mmol/L on a random blood sample does not rule out diabetes. A blood test taken in the morning before you eat anything is a more accurate test. Do not eat or drink anything except water for 8-10 hours before a fasting blood glucose test. A level of 7.0 mmol/L or more indicates that you have diabetes.

If you have no symptoms of diabetes but the blood test shows a glucose level of 7.0 mmol/L or more, the blood test must be repeated to confirm you have diabetes. If you do have symptoms and the blood test shows a glucose level of 7.0 mmol/L or more, the test does not need to be repeated.

Oral glucose tolerance test: This test is not now usually used to diagnose diabetes. However, the test may be done if it is thought your body doesn't control glucose levels normally but not badly enough to be called diabetes. This is referred to as pre-diabetes (impaired glucose tolerance). The test may also be used to see whether a woman has developed diabetes associated with pregnancy.

For this test, you fast overnight. In the morning you are given a drink which contains 75 g of glucose. A blood sample is taken two hours later. Normally, your body should be able to deal with the glucose and your blood level should not go too high. A glucose level of 11.1 mmol/L or more in the blood sample taken after two hours indicates that you have diabetes.

The HbA1c blood test: If you have diabetes, your HbA1c level may be done every 2-6 months by your doctor or nurse. This test measures your recent average blood sugar (glucose) level. Because it is an average measurement you do not need to fast on the day of the test. The test measures a part of the red blood cells. Glucose in the blood attaches to part of the red blood cells. This part can be measured and gives a good indication of your average blood glucose over the previous 2-3 months.

Comparing DCCT-HbA1c and IFCC-HbA1c results

DCCT-HbA1c (%)	IFCC-HbA1c (mmol/mol)
6.0	42
6.5	48
7.0	53
7.5	59
8.0	64
9.0	75

(DCCT: Diabetes Control and Complications Trial; IFCC: International Federation of Clinical Chemistry)

For people with diabetes, treatment aims to lower the HbA1c level to below a target level which is usually agreed between you and your doctor. Ideally, the aim is to maintain your HbA1c to less than 48 mmol/mol (6.5%). However, this may not always be possible to achieve and the target level of HbA1c should be agreed on an individual basis between you and your doctor. (For example, by increasing the dose of medication, improving your diet, etc.).

MONITORING CAPILLARY BLOOD GLUCOSE (GLUCOMETER RANDOM BLOOD SUGAR)

A blood sugar test is done to measure the amount of glucose content in your blood. You can check your sugar level at a doctor's office or even at your home! The main source

Diagnostic Testing

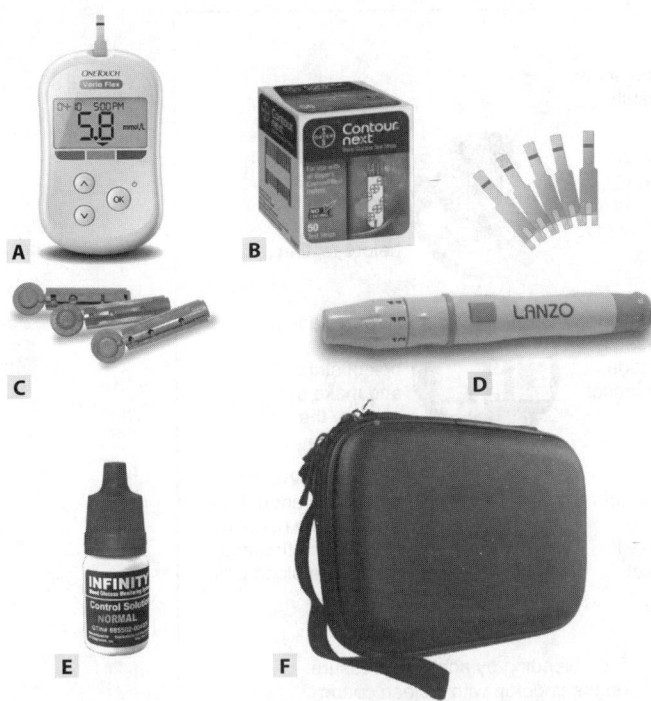

Figs. 19.2A to F: Included with your kit: (A) Meter (battery include); (B) Test strips; (C) Lancing device; (D) Sterile lancet; (E) Control solution; (F) Carrying case.

of glucose in your blood is caused due to the breakdown of carbohydrates. Insulin, a hormone produced by the pancreas, is responsible for the breakdown of sugar in our body. When it malfunctions, the sugar level in the blood may increase or decrease. Although glucose is the main source of energy for our body, extremely high or low levels of it is harmful for our very existence.

Procedure

The steps are similar for many meters, and generally look like this:
- Wash and dry your hands—using warm water may help the blood flow.
- Turn on the meter and prepare a test strip as outlined in your owner's booklet. Many Accu-Chek meters turn on automatically when a strip is inserted.
- Choose your spot—don't check from the same finger all the time. Using the side of the fingertip may be less painful than the pads.
- Prepare the lancing device according to the user guide provided, then lance your fingertip or other approved site to get a drop of blood.
- Touch and hold the test strip opening to the drop until it has absorbed enough blood to begin the test.
- View your test result and take the proper steps if your blood sugar is high or low, based on your healthcare professionals' recommendations.
- Discard the used lancet properly.
- Record the results in a logbook, hold them in the meter's memory or download to an app or computer so you can review and analyze them later.

SPECIMEN COLLECTION

Specimen collection is defined as collection of a required amount of tissue of fluid for laboratory examination.

Specimen may be defined as small quantity of a substance, which shows the kind and quality of the whole.

Purpose

- To make diagnosis and to help in treatment.
- To note progress or recess of a disease.
- To observe the effects of special treatment and drugs.
- To assess the general health of the patient.
- To investigate the nature of the diseases.
- To aid the doctor in diagnosis and treating the diseases.

Principles

- Contaminated and improperly collected specimens will produce false results which will adversely affect the diagnosis and treatment of patient.
- Specimen allowed to stand at room temperature for a long-time will give false results due to decomposition of specimen, multiplication of undesirable bacteria and destruction of pathogenic bacteria.
- Blood chemistry is not uniform throughout the day. It varies with the food intake.
- The accuracy and reliability of findings depend upon the correct method collection. Transportation of the specimens to the laboratory and recording of reports.
- Inaccurate results may lead the physician in wrong diagnosis and treatment of patients.
- Specimens serve as a media for transmission of disease producing organisms to the personnel who handle them carelessly.

General Instructions

- Provide adequate explanations regarding collection of specimens.
- Ask the patient to wash the external genital area with soap and water then rinse with water alone before collecting urine specimens.
- Equipment used for the collection of specimen should be clean and dry.
- No antiseptic should be present in the specimen bottle.
- As far as possible morning specimens should be collected.
- Specimens should be always be fresh for the laboratory examination.
- Bacteria multiply in the room temperature so, the specimens which are not tested immediately should be kept in the refrigerator, because cold temperature inhibits the growth of bacteria.

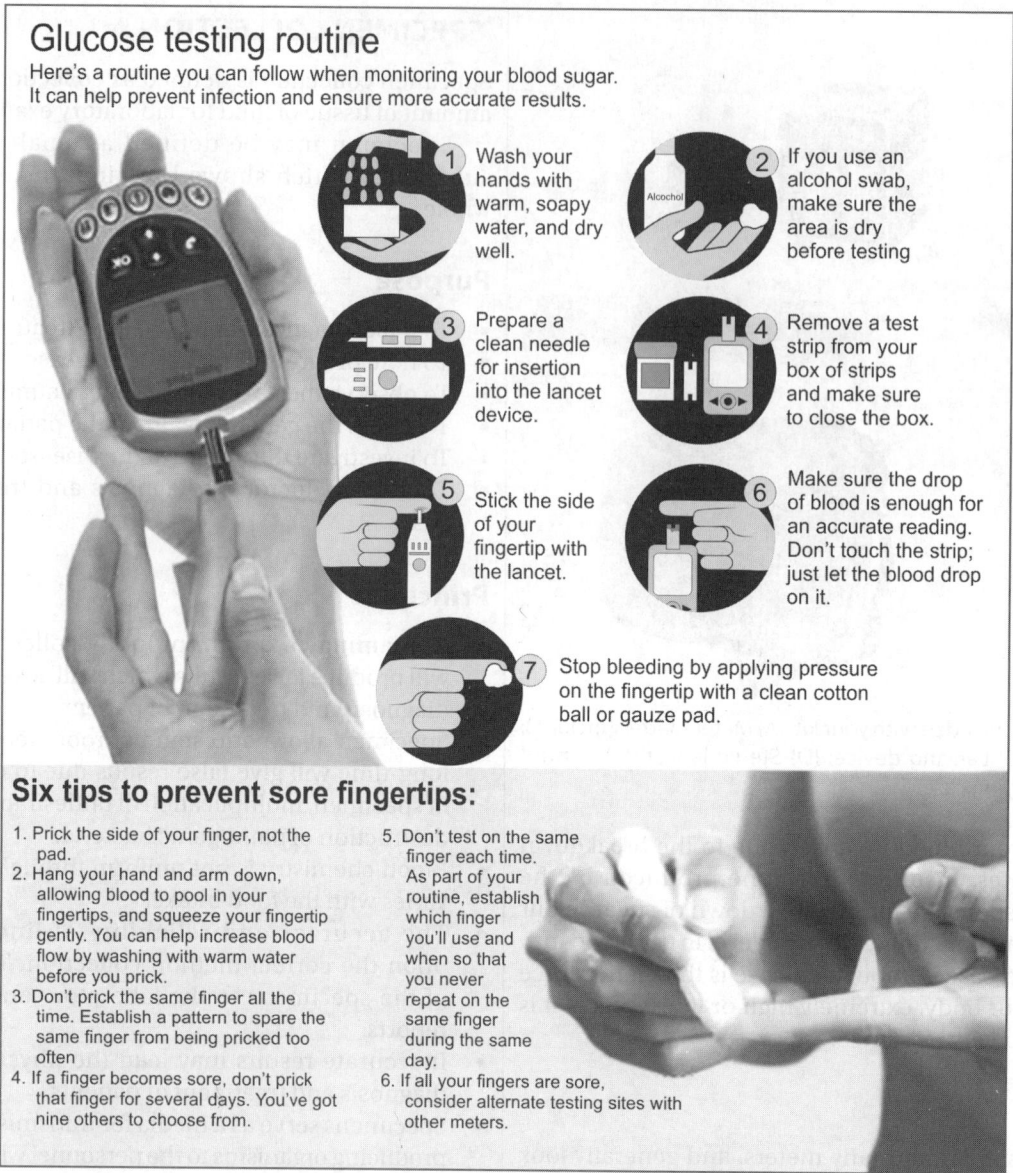

Fig. 19.3: Blood sugar measurement procedure.

- Insist the patient and the personnel to wash hands thoroughly after handling the specimen bottles.
- Container should have a wide mouth to prevent spilling of the spilling of the specimens, on the outer side of the bottle.
- Containers of the proper size are used according to the nature of specimen.

Equipment

- Dry container
- Bed
- Sterile gauze
- Artery forceps
- K-Basin.

Procedure

- Instruct patient to wash perineum.
- Instruct to avoid directly into clean, dry container or into bedpan and then transfer.
- Instruct not be contaminate outside of container.
- Instruct to collect 3/4th of container.
- Wear gloves while handling urine.

URINE COLLECTIONS FROM CATHETER

- Clamp tubing for about 15 to 30 minutes before obtaining sample.
- Wash hands thoroughly.
- Disconnect bladder drainage tubing.

- Cover distal end of drainage tube with sterile gauze till procedure is over.
- Clean tip of urinary catheter with antiseptic.
- Release clamp and collect urine in container.
- Remove gauze and discard in K—basin.
- Reconnect tubing.
- Wear glove while handling urine.

Aftercare

- Clean the outer part of the container.
- Label the container.
- Send immediately to laboratory with lab request.
- Wash hands thoroughly.
- Record the procedure in nurse's record sheet.

The 24-Hour Urine Collection

Collection of 24 hours urine specimen means the collection of all the urine voided in 24 hours, without any spillage of wastage.

Purpose

- To detect kidney and cardiac conditions.
- To measure total urine protein and creatinine.
- To measure total urine electrolytes, 17 ketogenic steroid, oxylate, porphyrins, drugs and vitamins.

Normal Characteristics of Urine

- Volume: 1000 to 2000 mL excreted in 24 hours.
- Appearance: Clear
- Odor: Aromatic odor, if kept for some time, ammonia smell.
- Color: Straw or amber in color
- Reaction: Acidic
- Specific gravity: 1.010 to 1.020
- Constituents of urine: 96 percent water, 2 percent urea and 2 percent uric acid. Urates, creatin chlorides, phosphates, sulphates and oxalates also may be present in minute's quantities.

Preliminary Assessment Check

- Doctor order for any specific instructions.
- General condition and diagnosis of the patient.
- Self ability of the patient.
- Mental status to follow directions.
- Articles available in the unit.

Preparation of the Patient and Environment

- Explain the sequence of the procedure.
- Provide privacy.
- Keep the articles at the bedside.
- Obtain lab request and container.

Equipment

- Bed pan or urinal.
- Dry container (24 hours collection bottle).
- Clean pouring (measuring) jar.
- Funnel.

Procedure

- Before beginning 24 hours urine collection, patient is asked to void.
- Discard the sample and note the time.
- Document the starting time of urine collection in the nurses record.
- Advise not to spill urine.
- All urine passed over next 24 hours is collected in large container.
- Exactly 24 hours after, patient is instructed to void and specimen is included.

Aftercare

- Send the sample immediately to the laboratory with lab request.
- Replace the articles after cleaning.
- Record the procedure in the nurse's record sheet.

General Instructions

- The entire collected urine should be stored in a covered container in a cool place.
- Add preservatives to the urine to prevent decomposition and multiplication of bacteria, e.g. boric acid, formalin, chloroform, etc.
- The urine should be thoroughly mixed and all or part sent to the laboratory in a clean bottle.
- Requisition form must be duly filled and signed.

URINE CULTURE

Collection of midstream specimen of urine without contaminating container and urine specimen.

Purpose

- To collect uncontaminated urine specimen for culture and sensitivity test.
- To detect the micro-organism causeing urinary tract infection (UTI).
- To diagnose and treat with specific antibiotic.

General Instructions

- Urine should be collected in sterile containers.
- Urine specimens for culture should be collected in the morning.
- After washing the perineal area and drying collect a midstream specimen of urine in a sterile bottle.
- For bed-ridden patients cauterized specimen of urine is taken.

Preliminary Assessment Check

- The doctors order for any specific instruction.
- General condition and diagnoses of the patient.

- Self-care ability of the patient.
- Mental status to follow instructions.
- Articles available in the unit.

Preparation of the Patient and Environment

- Explain the procedure to the patient.
- Provide privacy.
- Arrange the articles at the bedside.
- Collect and arrange the culture bottle-from the laboratory.
- Keep the lab request ready.

Equipment

- Basin and soap
- Towel and sterile gloves
- Gauze pads 2 to 3 (if patient on strict bed rest)
- Sterile culture bottle.
- Lab request form
- Sterile K-basin (if needed).

Procedure

- Instruct patient to clean perineum with soap and water.
- Open container and leave cover facing inside up.
- Instruct patient to void into sterile K-basin. If patient is unable to get out of bed,
- Instruct patient to void directly into sterile container.
- Collect 30 to 50 mL (1/2 to 3/4 of container) at midstream point of voiding.
- Emphasize first and last portions of voiding to be discarded.
- Cap container securely without touching inside of liquid.

Aftercare

- Label container with patient's name, hospital number and date.
- Send container to lab immediately with lab request.
- Record the procedure in nurse record sheet and register in microbiology lab note book.

STOOL: ROUTINE AND CULTURE

Collection of stool specimen for specific or routine tests (stool culture to detect abnormal characteristics).

Purpose

- To identify specific pathogens.
- To determine presence of blood, ova and parasites.
- To determine presence of fat.
- To do gross examination of stool characteristics such as color, consistency and odor.

Normal Characteristics of Feces

- Color: Light to dark down
- Odor: Pungent smell
- Frequency: 1 to 2 times per day
- Quantity: 4 to 5 ounces per day
- Composition: 30 percent water, shed epithelium from the intestine, a considerable quantity of bacteria and a small quantity of nitrogenous matter.
- Stool of infants: At birth the stool of infants is dark green and it is called "meconium".

Abnormal Characteristics of Feces

Color

- Tarry black stools: Bleeding in the upper gastro—intestinal tract.
- Black color stool: Melena, administration of iron or charcoal.
- Clay colored stool: Obstruction to the flow of bile.
- White colored stool: Presence of barium salts after barium tests.

Odor

- Melena and dysentery: Foul smell.

Frequency

- Diarrhea: Increased frequency
- Constipation: Decreased frequency and low residue diet.

Consistency and Form

- Watery stools: Diarrhea
- Rice water stools: Cholera
- Pea soup stools: Typical of typhoid fever.

Appearance

- Fresh blood in large amounts: Bleeding piles.
- Blood and mucus stool: Amebic or bacillary dysentery.
- Worm or segments or worms in stool: Parasitic cysts, ova or larvae.

General Instructions

- Fecal specimens are collected for chemical bacteriological or parasitological analysis.
- Fecal specimens should be collected in the early stages of disease preferably before antibiotic treatment is given.
- Stool specimens should be collected in a sterile container (making use of the scoop provided in the container) with a tight-fitting leak proof-lid.
- After collection, the lid should be immediately replaced tightly.
- After proper labeling, the collected stool should be handed over to the laboratory without delay.

Preliminary Assessment Check

- The doctors order for any specific instructions.
- General condition and diagnosis of the patient.
- Assessment of the self-care ability.

- Mental status to follow instructions.
- Articles available in the unit.

Preparation of the Patient and Environment
- Explain the procedure to the patient.
- Provide privacy.
- Arrange the articles at bedside.
- Obtain lab request and container.

Equipment
- Appropriate specimen container.
- Spatula (clean for routine, sterile for culture).
- Bedpan or portable commode.
- Gloves.
- Waste paper.

Procedure
- Instruct patient to defecate into clean dry bedpan or commode.
- Instruct not to contaminate specimen with urine.
- Nurse to wear gloves while collecting specimen.
- Collect stool specimen with clean spatula for routine stool test and with sterile spatula into culture container.
- Cover the container tightly.

Aftercare
- Remove the gloves.
- Wrap spatula in waste paper and discard appropriately.
- Label specimen container with name, hospital number and date.
- Send to laboratory immediately (fresh specimen provides more accurate results).
- Replace equipments and after cleaning.
- Record the procedure in nurse's record sheet.

SPUTUM CULTURE

Collection of coughed out sputum for culture studies to identity respiratory pathogens.

Purpose
- To detect abnormalities.
- To diagnose disease condition.
- To detect the microorganism causes respiratory tract infections.
- To treat with specific antibiotics.

Characteristics of Sputum
- Quantity: Normally no sputum is expectorated. The amount of sputum coughed up in 24 hours varies with the diseases.
- Consistency: The sputum may be classified into various types according to its consistency and appearance, e.g. serous, frothy, mucoid, purulent, seropurulent and hemorrhagic.
- Odor: Normally the sputum is odorless in case of lung abscess; carcinoma and bronchiectasis the sputum will bad foul smelling
- Color: Sputum consisting of mucus may be:
  - Colorless and translucent
  - Yellowish color: Presence of pus
  - Blackish sputum: Excessive smoking
  - Blood: Hemoptysis
  - Red and frothy sputum: Freshly bleeding from lungs.
  - Rusty color: Altered hemoglobin as seen in pneumonia.
  - Greenish color: Bronchiectasis
  - Brown color: Gangrenous condition of the lungs.
- If sputum is examined microscopically, a few WBC and epithelial cells may be seen. Eosinophils are found in such conditions as asthma. RBC is found only when there is hemoptysis. The main organism that is looked for in stained sputum is tubercle bacilli (AFB).

General Instructions
- Give water proof disposal sputum mug on the previous evening and instruct to raise the material from the lungs by coughing and not the saliva.
- Collect the sputum in the morning.
- Ask the patient to rinse the mouth with plain water. Do not use any antiseptic mouth washes.
- If sterile specimens are required sterile bottle with cover is given to the patient.

Preliminary Assessment Check
- The doctors order for specific instructions.
- General condition and diagnosis of the patient.
- Self-care ability.
- Mental status to follow instructions.
- Articles available in the unit.

Preparation of the Patient and Environment
- Explain the procedure to the patient.
- Arrange the articles at the bedside.
- Provide privacy if needed.

Equipment
- Sterile sputum container.
- Sputum mug or cup.
- Tissue paper.
- K-basin.

Procedure
- Instruct to collect specimen early morning before brushing teeth, to obtain overnight accumulated secretions.
- Instruct to remove and place lid facing upward.
- Instruct not to contaminate inside of lid and container, as well as outside of container.

- Instruct to cough deeply and expectorate directly into specimen container.
- Collect at least 10 mL of sputum.
- Close the container immediately after sputum is collected.

Aftercare

- Label the container with patient's name, date and hospital number.
- Send specimen to laboratory immediately along with request.
- Replace the equipment after cleaning.
- Wash hands thoroughly.
- Record the procedure in nurse's sheets.

BLOOD SMEAR

It is a process of taking two to three drops of blood by pricking the finger tip by using a lancet. Thereby smearing the expressed drop of blood on the slide.

Purpose

- To diagnose blood borne disease such filarial and malaria.
- To detect carcinogenic cells.
- To detect abnormal blood cell counts.

General Instructions

- The lancet (needle) used for communicable disease, e.g. HIV. Patients discard it after use.
- The slides should be clean and fresh.
- The procedure should do in an aseptic manner.
- The person doing blood smear should wear clean gloves.

Preliminary Assessment Check

- Doctors order for specific instructions.
- General condition and diagnosis.
- Mental status to follow instructions.
- Articles available in the unit.

Preparation of the Patient and Equipment

- Explain the procedure to the patient.
- Provide privacy if needed.
- Arrange articles at bedside.
- Obtain request from the doctor.
- Obtain slide from the laboratory or arrange technician from the laboratory.
- Make the patient to sit or lie in the bed comfortable.

Equipment

A clean tray containing:
- Clean slides—2.
- Sterile needle in a container (lancet).
- Methylated spirit in a bottle.
- Paper bag.
- Cotton swab.

Procedure

- Wear clean gloves.
- Clean the patient's finger tip with spirit opposite side away from you.
- Press the finger tip and give a prick with the sterile needle.
- Allow a drop of blood to fall on each slide.
- Make the smear by taking one slide on your left hand and another with the right hand.
- Make the smear with the edge of the slide by spreading the blood. Make 2 or 3 slides.
- Provide spirit swab to apply gentle pressure.

Aftercare

- Dry and send the slide to the laboratory for examination.
- Replace the articles after cleaning.
- Remove the gloves.
- Wash hands thoroughly.
- Record the procedure in the nurse's record sheet.

BLOOD CULTURE

Collection of blood for blood culture is a sterile procedure. Surgical (Scrub) preparation and techniques are used in collection, storage, transport of blood sample.

Purpose

- To detect the micro-organism.
- To treat the disease condition with correct antibiotics.
- To detect the right antibiotic to kill the particular micro-organisms.
- When the patient has chills or a temperature hike, blood culture is done.

General Instructions

- Special type of culture bottles are used for blood culture sample collection.
- All blood culture bottles should be carefully examined for clarity of media, any medium showing turbidity should not be used.
- Only disposable syringes and needles should be used for collection of blood.
- The top of the bottle must be carefully disinfected (with 70% alcohol) just before the bottle is inoculated.
- Blood should never be taken from an IV line or above the IV line.
- If blood culture bottles are available, blood should be immediately added to the culture medium (broth).
- If blood culture bottles are not available, blood may be transported in a sterile tube containing a sterile anticoagulant solution.

- The amount of blood collected is 10 mL for adult, 2 to 5 mL for children and 1-2 mL for infants and to neonates.
- Blood for culture should be taken before antibiotics are administered.

Preliminary Assessment Check

- The do ctors order for specific instructions.
- General condition and diagnosis of the patient.
- Mental status to follow instruction.
- Self-care ability of the patient.
- Articles available in the unit such as culture bottles, etc.

Preparation of the Patient and Environment

- Explain the procedure to the patient.
- Arrange the articles at the bedside.
- Obtain lab request and culture bottles.
- Arrange extra help (if needed any).
- Label and number the container in order wise.

Equipment

- Mackintosh and towel.
- Surgical gloves.
- Surgical dressing packs to clean the skin over the vein.
- Surgical spirit and betadine solution.
- Disposable syringe 10 mL with needles.
- Culture bottles—3.
- Cotton swabs.
- Paper bag and K-basin.
- Tourniquet.

Procedure

- Choose the vein to be drawn by touching the skin before it has been disinfected.
- Cleanse the skin over the venipuncture site in a circle approximately 5 cm in diameter with 70 percent alcohol, rubbing vigorously.
- Starting in the centre of the circle, apply 2 percent iodine (or povidone iodine).
- Allow the iodine to remain on the skin for at least 1 mts.
- Insert the needle into the vein and withdraw blood.
- After the needle has been removed, the site should be cleaned with 70 percent alcohol again.
- Apply gentle pressure with cotton ball over the punctured site.
- Transfer the blood in the syringe in to the culture bottles.

Aftercare

- Clean the culture bottle led with spirit swab.
- Insert the needle and pour blood into culture bottle.
- Mix the solution and blood gently by moving sideways.
- Label the culture bottles and send immediately to the laboratories.
- Replace the articles after cleaning.
- Remove the gloves and wash hands thoroughly.
- Record the procedure in the nurse's record sheet.

THROAT SWAB

The specimen is collected from the patients with upper respiratory tract infection. The upper respiratory tract can be the site of several types of infection.

Purpose

- To detect the causative microorganism.
- To diagnose the disease condition.
- To detect the correct antibiotics for effective treatment.

Indications

- Pharyngitis sometimes involving tonsillitis and giving rise to a "sore throat".
- Nasopharyngitis.
- Otitis media.
- Sinusitis.
- Epiglottitis.

General Instructions

- Pharyngitis is by far the most frequent one. Most cases of pharyngitis have a viral etiology and follow a self-limiting course.
- Approximately 20 percent are caused by bacteria and usually require treatment with appropriate antibiotics.
- Specimen should be collect by a physician or other trained personnel.
- Swab can be collected after asking the patient to gargle with sterile saline.

Preliminary Assessment Check

- The doctors order for any specific instructions.
- General condition and diagnosis.
- Mental status to follow instructions.
- Self-care ability of the patient.
- Articles available in the unit.

Preparation of the Patient and Environment

- Explain the procedure to the patient.
- Arrange the articles at the bedside.
- Provide privacy if needed.
- Obtain lab request and specimen container.
- Place the patient comfortably in sitting or semi-sitting position.

Equipment

- Sterile or clean gloves.
- Specimen container.
- Gauze pieces.

- Paper bag and K-basin.
- Torch light (if needed).
- Tongue depressor.

Procedure

- The patient should sit in from of a light source.
- Tongue should be kept down with a tongue depressor and a cotton wool swab is rubbed vigorously over each tonsil, over the back wall of the pharynx and over any other inflamed area.
- Care should be taken not to touch the tongue or buccal surfaces.
- It is preferable to take 2 swabs from the same area.
- One can be used to prepare a smear, while the other is placed into glass or plastic sterile container.

Aftercare

- Label and send the container immediately to the laboratory.
- Discard the disposable items used.
- Replace the articles after cleaning.
- Wash hands thoroughly.
- Record the procedure in the nurse's record sheet.

VAGINAL SWAB/SMEAR

Vaginal specimen (swab) collected for cervical cytology to detect the abnormalities.

Purpose

- To detect the abnormalities.
- To do routine examination.
- To diagnose and treat the infection.
- To identify carcinogenic cells.
- To do cytohormonal study, to know the progesterone status.

Indications

- Cervical: Suspected cervix to exclude premalignant or malignant lesion.
- Vaginal: Vaginitis—to know the specific pathogen and cytohormonal status.

General Instructions

- Smear means to make a fine film of vaginal discharge on a slide and send it for examination of the vaginal discharge.
- Minimum two slides with smear should be sent to the laboratory.
- When trichomones vaginitis is to be tested the vaginal discharge is collected in a test tube or a hanging drop made on a slides.

Preliminary Assessment Check

- The doctors order for any specific instruction.
- General condition and diagnosis of the patient.
- Self-care ability of the patient.
- Mental status to follow instructions.
- Articles available in the unit.

Preparation of the Patient and Environment

- Explain the procedure to the patient.
- Arrange the equipment at the bedside.
- Provide privacy.
- Obtain lab request and specimen container and slides.
- Position the patient comfortably.
- Instruct the patient to empty bladder.

Equipment

- Draw mackintosh and sheet.
- Sterile swab container or slides.
- Sterile gloves or clean gloves.
- Paper bag and K-basin.
- Torch light or spotlight.
- Sterile speculum and water soluble jelly.

Procedure

- Give dorsal positions.
- Wear clean gloves.
- Take the vaginal discharge with sterile swab stick.
- Smear it on one side of the slide and make thin film over the sides.
- Dry in the slides, then wrap in paper and send to the laboratory.

Aftercare

- Place the position comfortably.
- Label and send the specimen to the laboratory.
- Replace the articles after cleaning.
- Wash the hands thoroughly.
- Record the procedure in the nurse's record sheet.

URINE TESTING

Urine analysis methods comprise testing reaction, specific gravity, albumen sugar bile, acetone, pus, blood and yeasts microscopically.

Purpose

- To detect reaction, in cystitis the reaction is alkaline.
- To detect sugar, it is present in diabetes mellitus.
- To detect protein, it is present in kidney damage, pre-eclampsia and is called proteinuria.
- To detect acetone, it is present due to incomplete metabolism of fat.

- To detect bile, it is seen in cases of obstructive jaundice or hemolytic diseases.
- To detect pus cells, it is present due to urinary tract infection.
- To detect blood, it is seen in snake bite, fracture pelvis, etc.

Characteristics of Normal Urine

- Volume: 1,000 to 2,000 mL in 24 hours.
- Appearance: Clear
- Odor: Aromatic odor
- Color: Amber or pale straw in color.
- Reaction: Normal urine is slightly acidic,
- Specific gravity: 1.010 to 1.025
- Constituents of the normal urine: Water 96 percent, urea 2 percent and uric acid, urates, creatinine, chlorides, phosphates, sulphates, oxalates—2 percent.

Characteristics of Abnormal Urine

Volume

- Polyuria-Increased in volume
- Oliguria-Decreased in volume
- Anuria-Total absence or marked decrease of urine
- Suppression-Failure of the kidney to secrete urine.

Color

- Green or brownish-yellow: Bile salts and bile pigments.
- Reddish brown: Urobilinogen.
- Bright red: A large amount of fresh blood.
- Smokey brown: Blood pigment
- Milk white: Chyluria due to filariasis.

Appearance

- Mucus: Appears as a flocculent cloud.
- Pus: Settles at the bottom as a heavy cloud.
- Stones: As fine sand.
- Uric acid: As grains of pepper.

Odor

- Sweetish or fruity odor: Seen in diabetes.

Reaction

- Alkaline: Cystitis
- Specific gravity
- Diabetes mellitus: Increased specific gravity
- Renal disease: Low specific gravity
- Constituents of urine
- Kidney damage: Albumin.

Types of Examination of the Urine

- Physical examination: Color appearance, volume, reaction, specific gravity and odor.
- Chemical examination: Routine tests such as for albumin and sugar. Special tests such as tests for acetone, bile pigments and bile salts. Microscopic examination-Crystals, casts, RBC, pus cells, epithelial and bacteria.

Preliminary Assessment

- The doctor order for any instructions.
- Articles available in the unit.
- General condition and diagnosis of the patient.
- Self-care ability of the patient.

Preparation of the Patient and Environment

- Explain the procedure to the patient.
- Keep the urine sample ready.
- Arrange the articles ready in the treatment.
- Provide labeled container for collecting urine.

Equipment

- Test tubes 4 to 6 on a test tube.
- Test tube holder—1.
- Spirit lamp—1.
- Match box—1.
- Kidney tray with lining to discard the wastes.
- Duster or rag piece: To wipe the outside of the test tube before heating.
- Acetic acid: To test urine for albumin.
- Nitric acid or sulphosalic acid: To test urine for albumin.
- Red and blue litmus paper: To test the reaction of the urine.
- Urinometer: To measure the specific gravity of the urine.
- Benedict's solution: To test urine for sugar.
- Ammonium sulphate crystals, sodium nitro prusside crystals and liquor ammonia to test urine for acetone.
- Weak solution of Tr. Iodine to test for bile pigments.
- Sulphur power: To test for bile salts.
- Glass jar: To measure the amount of the urine.
- Pipettes—2: To measure drops of urine and reagents.
- A small bottle brush-To clean the test tubes.

Procedure

Sugar Test

- Take test tube and fix in holder.
- Pour 5 mL of Benedict's solution into test tube.
- Light spirit lamp and heat Benedict solution till it boils.
- Holding test tube mouth facing away from nurse.
- Add 8 drops of urine using dropper and allow to boil for few seconds.
- Put off flame and cool test tube under running water.

Observations

- Blue: Nil
- Green: +
- Yellow: ++

- Orange: +++
- Brick red: ++++

Albumin Test

Hot Test

- Fill 2/3 of test tub with urine, secure test tube holder at very top.
- Heat the upper third of test tube over flame.
- If there is precipitation, it denotes the presence of wither protein or phosphate.
- Add 2–4 drops of 2 percent acetic acid.
- If precipitate dissolves it is due to phosphates present in normal urine.
- If precipitate does not dissolve it denotes presence of albumin.

Observation

- Trace: +
- Cloudy: ++ (100 mg/dL)
- Thick cloudiness: +++ (500 g/dL)

Cold Test

- Pour a small quantity of nitric acid or sulphosalic acid 3 percent in to a clean test tube.
- Allow equal quantity of urine to trickle down the sides of the test tube.
- If albumin present, a white precipitate will be seen where two fluids meet.

Urine pH

- Collect and keep ready with urine sample
- Dip litmus strip in urine and keep for one minute.
- Note color change.
- Discard strip into container for infected waste.

Urine Specific Gravity

- Fill 3/4 of jar with urine.
- Gently place urinometer into jar.
- When urometer stops bobbing read specific gravity directly from scale marked on calibrated stem of urinometer.
- Make sure that instrument floats freely and does not touch sides of jar.
- Read scale at lowest point of meniscus to ensure an accurate reading at eye level.

Rothera's Test (Acetone)

- Take 2 cm depth of ammonium sulphate crystals in a small test tube.
- Add equal volume of urine and one crystal of sodium nitroprusside.
- Close the test tube with a cork and shake the test tube.
- Take liquor ammonia and add to it the urine, trickling through the sides.
- Read the results immediately.

Observations

- If acetone is present permanganate purple colored ring is formed at the junction of urine and ammonia.

Hays Test (Bile Salts)

- Take a test tube, half full of urine.
- Sprinkle sulfur powder on the surface of the urine.
- If the powder sinks down to the test tube, it indicates the presence of bile salts.

Smiths Test (Bile Pigments)

- Fill 3/4 of test tube with urine.
- Add iodine drops along the sides of the tube, so as to form a layer on the surface of the urine.
- A green color at the junction of the two liquids indicates the presence of bile pigments.

Aftercare

- Discard the urine in the sluice room.
- Wash the test tube with soap and water.
- Dry the tube, holder and urinometer with jar.
- Replace the article after cleaning.
- Wash hands thoroughly.
- Record the procedure in the nurses' record sheet and diabetics chart.

ENDOSCOPIES

Endoscopy means looking inside and typically refers to looking inside the body for medical reasons using an endoscope, an instrument used to examine the interior of a hollow organ or cavity of the body. Unlike most other medical imaging devices, endoscopes are inserted directly into the organ.

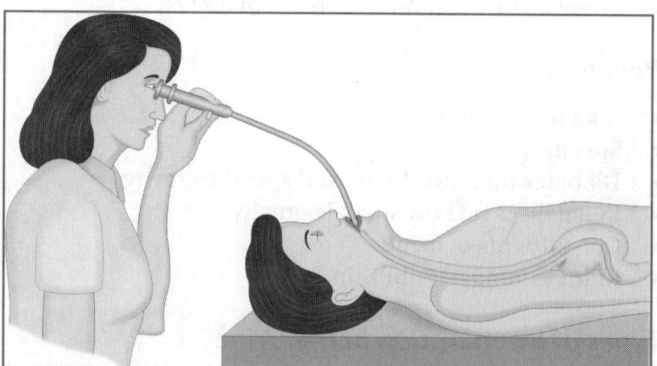

Fig. 19.4: Endoscopy procedure.

Laryngoscopy

Laryngoscopy is a visual examination below the back of the throat, where the voice box (larynx) containing the vocal cords is located. It is an effective procedure for discovering the causes of voice and breathing problems, pain in the throat or ear, difficulty in swallowing, narrowing of the throat (strictures or stenosis), and blockages in the airway.

Purpose of Laryngoscope

Laryngoscopy is performed to:
- Diagnose a persistent cough, throat pain, bleeding, hoarseness, or bad breath
- Check for inflammation
- Discover a possible narrowing or blockage of the throat
- Remove foreign objects
- Visualize or biopsy a mass or tumor in the throat or on the vocal cords
- Diagnose difficulty swallowing
- Evaluate causes of persistent earache
- Diagnose voice problems, such as weak voice, hoarse voice, breathy voice, or no voice

Types of Laryngoscope

The procedure is relatively painless, but the idea of having a scope inserted into the throat can be a little scary, so it helps to understand how a laryngoscopy is done. The following basics will help you understand what is happening and help put your child at ease.

Indirect laryngoscopy: The indirect procedure can be performed in the doctor's office using a small hand mirror, which is held at the back of the throat. The doctor will aim a light at the back of the throat, usually by wearing headgear that has a bright light attached. This technique will help the doctor examine the larynx, vocal cords, and hypopharynx, which is a part of the passageway to the lungs and stomach. Indirect laryngoscopy is not typically used with children, as it tends to cause gagging and can be hard for kids to tolerate.

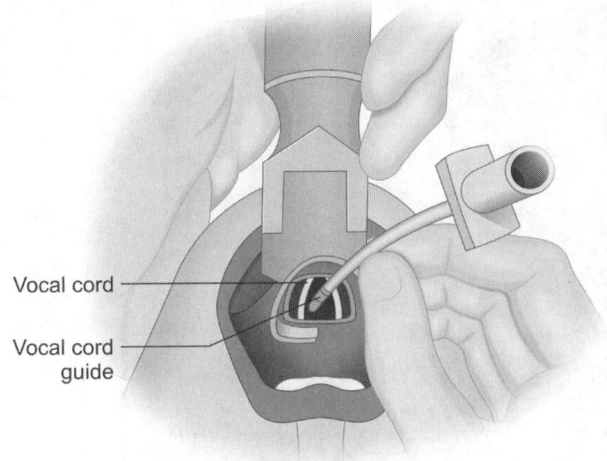

Fig. 19.6: Laryngoscope used for examination of larynx.

Fiber-optic (flexible) laryngoscopy / Direct laryngoscopy: Fiber-optic or direct laryngoscopy examinations allow doctors to see deeper into the throat by using either a flexible or rigid telescope. Rigid telescopes are more often used as part of a surgical procedure in evaluating children with **stridor** (a noisy, harsh breathing) and removing foreign objects in the throat and lower airway. They are also used in collecting tissue samples (a**biopsy**), laser treatments, and in locating cancer of the larynx.

During the Procedure: Indirect laryngoscopy and fiber-optic laryngoscopies often are performed in the doctor's office, usually using local anesthetic. These procedures usually take only 5 to 10 minutes.

Indirect laryngoscopy: the patient will be asked to sit up straight in a high-backed chair with a headrest. The chair will allow your child's head and jaw to move forward. The patient will open his or her mouth wide, and the doctor will spray the throat with an anesthetic or numbing medication. The patient will gargle and then spit out. The doctor will then cover the tongue with gauze and hold it down. The doctor will hold up a warm mirror to the back of the throat.

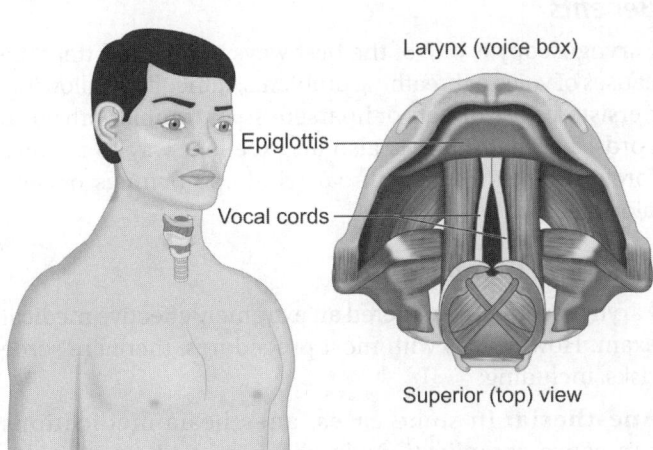

Fig. 19.5: Anatomical structure of larynx.

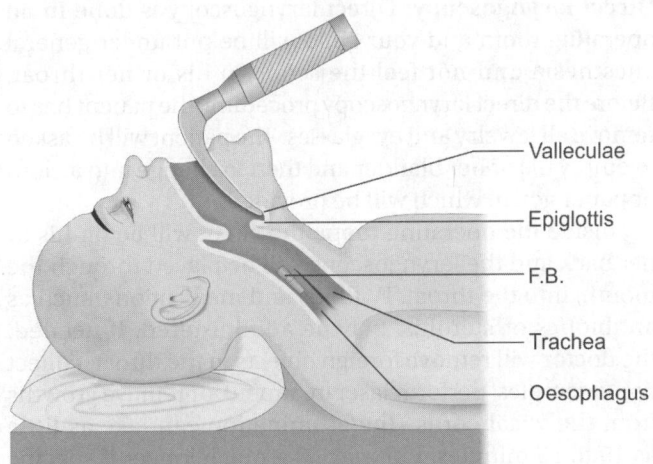

Fig. 19.7: Laryngoscope application technique.

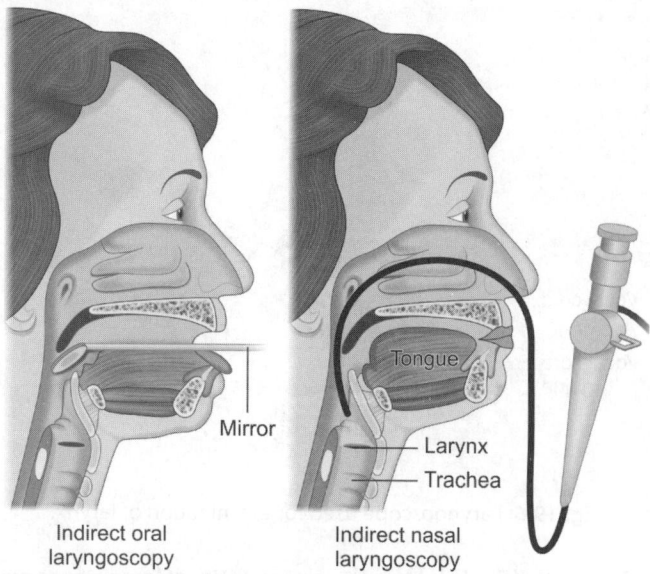

Fig. 19.8: Fiber-optic laryngoscope used for diagnostic purposes.

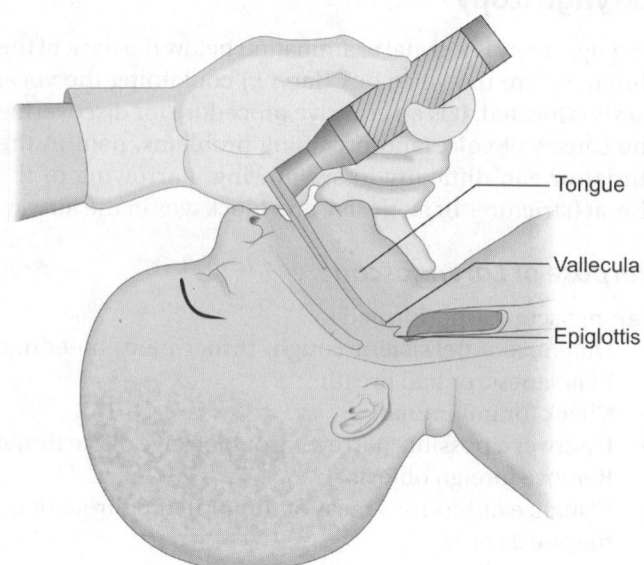

Fig. 19.9: Pediatric blade used for children.

With a light that is usually attached to headgear the doctor is wearing, the doctor will tilt the mirror to view various areas of the throat. The patient may be asked to make high-pitched or low-pitched sounds so that the doctor can view the larynx and see the vocal cords move.

Fiber-optic laryngoscopy: In a fiber-optic laryngoscopy the doctor will use a fiber-optic laryngoscope, which is a thin, flexible instrument that lights and magnifies images, providing a better view of the larynx and vocal cords. The doctor will determine if this procedure is to be done in the operating room under general anesthesia or in the office. The procedure typically does not require a hospital stay. Sometimes numbing medication is sprayed or swabbed in the nose or throat before the procedure. The flexible scope will be inserted through the nostril or the mouth. The doctor will examine the throat area through the scope's eyepiece. Sometimes the images are displayed on a monitor so that family members can see what the doctor is seeing.

Direct laryngoscopy: Direct laryngoscopy is done in an operating room and your child will be put under general anesthesia and not feel the scope in his or her throat. Before the direct laryngoscopy procedure, the patient has to remove all jewelry and eyeglasses. The patient will be asked to empty his or her bladder and then to change into a cloth or paper gown, which will be provided.

Inside the operating room, the client will lie on his or her back and the laryngoscope will be placed through the mouth, into the throat. IV fluids and medications, such as antibiotics or steroids, may be administered. If needed, the doctor will remove foreign objects in the throat, collect tissue samples, perform laser treatment, or remove growths from the vocal cords. The examination can take as little as 15 to 30 minutes, but may take much longer if specific treatments are required.

After the Procedure

If a local anesthetic or topical numbing spray was used during the examination, it will wear off in about 30 minutes. The client should not eat or drink anything for about 2 hours, until the spray has worn off and the throat is no longer numb.

Direct laryngoscopy: After a direct laryngoscopy, your child will be watched by a nurse until fully awake and able to swallow. This usually takes about 2 hours. In some cases, an overnight hospital stay may be required. The client may have some nausea, general muscle aches, and feel tired for a day or two. Gargling and sucking on throat lozenges will help with the soreness, and pain medication will be given, if needed. The client may sound hoarse or have noisy breathing for a few days after the procedure. This is normal. If the hoarseness persists, or your child is having difficulty breathing, check with doctor.

Benefits

Laryngoscopy is one of the best ways to find and treat the causes of voice or breathing problems, difficulty swallowing, persistent sore throats or hoarseness, or trouble with vocal cords. Laryngoscopy is also an excellent way to retrieve foreign objects from the throat, windpipe, or lungs, or clear blockages in the airway.

Risks and Complications

Laryngoscopy is considered an extremely effective medical exam. However, as with most procedures, there are some risks, including:

Anesthesia: In some cases, anesthesia medications can cause complications in children, such as irregular heartbeats and breathing problems. These complications are not common. Allergic reactions also are not common. If they do occur, they typically develop within a few minutes after the anesthesia is given. The doctors can provide immediate medical attention if that happens.

Blocked airway: Inserting a laryngoscope down the throat has the potential to cause swelling of the airways and breathing difficulties. Sometimes the airway is already blocked by the foreign body or condition that caused the problem in the first place. In very rare cases, doctors may need to perform a tracheotomy (a small incision made in the neck and windpipe, or trachea) to allow air into the lungs.

Bleeding or infection: If a biopsy was taken, there's the rare possibility of bleeding or infection at the site.

Bronchoscopy

Bronchoscopy is a medical procedure involving the direct examination of one's air passages (the larynx, trachea, and bronchi) via the use of a flexible, lighted tube called a bronchoscope.

Definition

- Bronchoscope is an endoscope diagnostic procedure involving the inspection and observation of the trachea, larynx and bronchi.
- Bronchoscope is the examination of the interior of the tracheo-bronchial tree through a bronchoscope.

Purpose

Diagnostic Purpose
- To visualize
- Tumors
- Obstructions
- Secretion
- Bleeding sites and foreign objects in the tracheobronchial system.

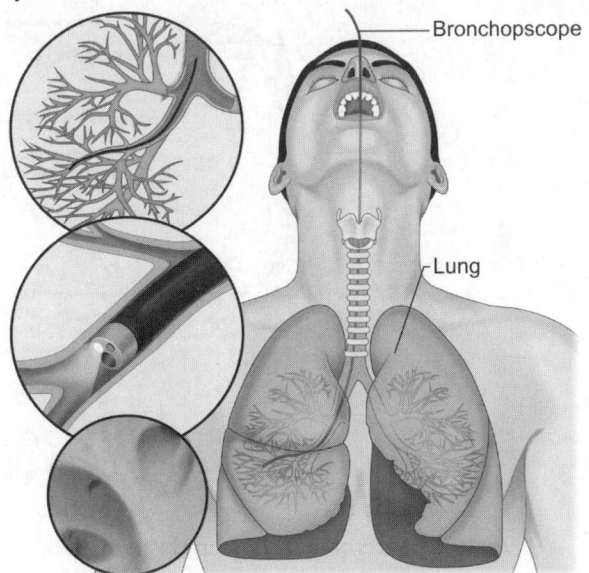

Fig. 19.10: Examination of lung segments.

Relationship between bronchi and order
Primary bronchus — 0th order
Intermediate bronchus — 0th to 1st order
Lobar bronchi (superior lobe, middle lobe, inferior lobe) — 1st order
Superior segmental bronchus, lingular bronchus, basal bronchus — 1st to 2nd order
Segmental bronchi — 2nd order — B^1
Sub-segmental bronchi — 3rd order — $B^1a \cdot B^1b$
Sub-segmental bronchi — 4th order — $B^1ai \cdot B^1aii$
5th order — $B^1ai\alpha \cdot B^1ai\beta$

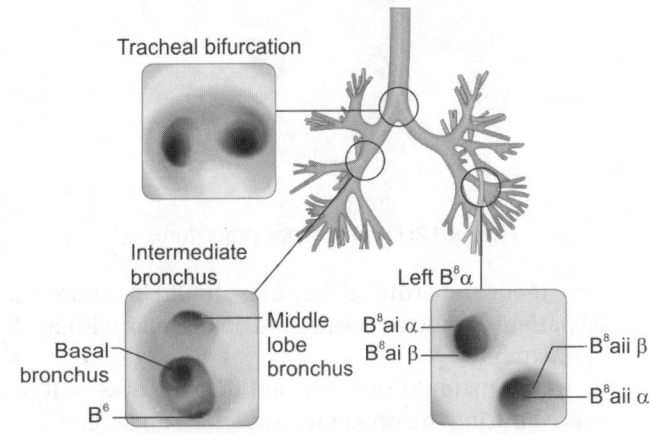

Fig. 19.11: Examining various segments of the lungs.

- Collection of secretions for cytological and bacteriologic study.
- Assessing tumors for potential resection.
- Tissue for lung biopsy may be obtained.

Therapeutic Purpose
- To remover secretions that obstructing the air passages.
- To fulgurate (electro desiccate) and excise lesions.

Principle
- The knowledge of the anatomy and physiology of the body is essential for the safe administration of the injection.
- Micro-organism are present everywhere so strict aseptic technic should be practiced.
- Any unfamiliar situation produces anxiety.
- Organization and planning results in the economy of fenie, material and effort.

General Instruction
- Proper explanation about the procedure should be given to the patient.
- Sedation should be given 30–60 minutes before the procedure.
- Procedure is done in a darkened room.
- Instruction should be given to the patient to keep his mouth clean.
- Nothing should be given to the patient 6–8 hours before the procedure.

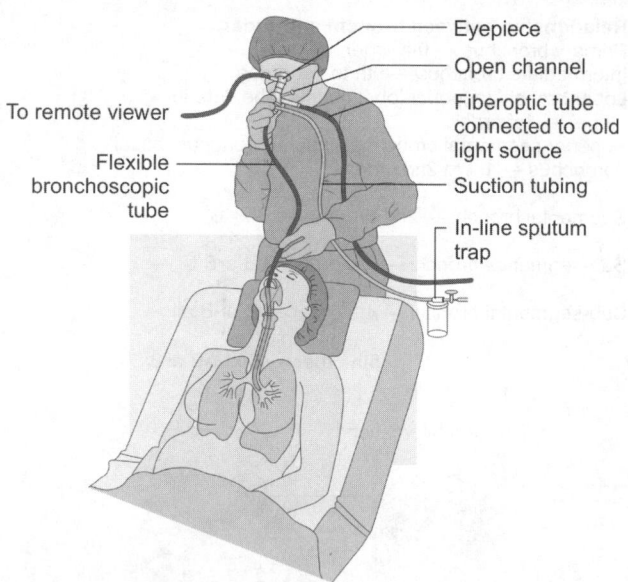

Fig. 19.12: Bronchoscopy procedure.

- Loose teeth and artificial dentures should be removed.
- The patient should be positioned on his back with neck hyperextended.
- The patient should be informed that his eyes will be covered during the procedure to reduce anxiety.
- The patient should be told that the doctor and his assistants will be masked and gloved.

Preliminary Assessment

- Identify the patient with name, bed no: Qp. no: etc.,
- Check the physician's order.
- Check the general condition of the patient.
- Assess the abilities and limitations of the patient.
- Check the article available in the patient's unit.

Preparation of the Patient Unit

- Ensure that a signed consent form has been obtained.
- Obtain a medication history to determine whether the patient is receiving anticoagulation therapy or aspirin preparations.
- Explain the purpose and procedure of the test. Warn the patient that the local anesthetic may taste bitter.
- Record baseline vital signs.
- Check for articles available in the unit.

Equipment: The bronchoscope is a piece of equipment that can be directed and moved around the bends in the larynx, trachea, and bronchi. These images are transmitted through the bronchoscope either to the eyepiece or a video screen. An open channel in the scope allows other instruments to be passed through it to take tissue samples (biopsies) or to remove fluid.

Articles needed: Bronchoscope (flexible fiber optic bronchoscope).

A sterile tray containing:
- Gown
- Gloves
- Mask.

An unsterile tray containing: Normal saline.

Procedure

- A rigid or flexible fiber optic bronchoscope may be used.
- The bronchoscope is inserted through the nose (most common) or through the mouth.
- The tube is inserted as the physician observes the condition of the upper airways through the eyepiece and guides the tube to the area of the lung to be evaluated.

Parts of Flexible Fiberoptic Bronchoscope

- Eyepiece.
- Open channel.
- Fiber optic tube connected to cold light source.
- Section tubing.
- In-line sputum trap.

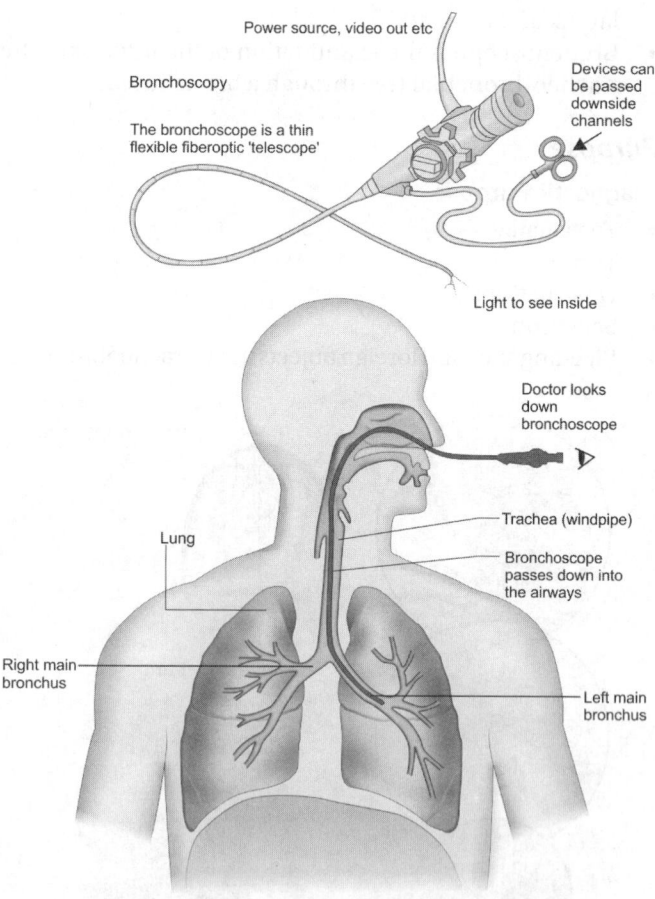

Fig. 19.13: Parts of bronchoscopy instrument.

Post-procedural Care

- Vital signs are monitored as per hospital protocol
- The client is observed for signs of respiratory distress including dyspnea, changes in respiratory rate, use of accessory muscles and changes in or absent lung sounds.
- Expectorated secretions are inspected for evidence of any hemoptysis.
- Nothing is given by mouth until the cough and swallow reflexes have returned, which is usually in 1 to 2 hours.
- Once the client can swallow, feeding may begin with ice chips and small sips of water.
- Lung sounds are monitored for 24 hours. Development of adventitious sound should be reported to the physician.

Aftercare

- If bronchoscope is done under general anesthesia, position the patient in a head low position, flat with head turned to one side.
- If not under general anesthesia semi Fowler's position.
- Save all the sputum for lab studies.
- Observe the patient for impaired respiration laryngeal spasm and laryngeal edema.
- Laryngeal strider, dyspnea and shortness of breath should be noticified to the doctor.
- Provide emergency resuscitation as necessary.
- Give treatment as prescribed.
- Give nothing by mouth until his gay reflex returns.
- Give warm, soothing, soft fluids.
- Observe the patient for toxicity of anesthetic drugs.
- Treat the sore throat.
- An ice collar may; be used to minimize edema and soreness.
- Lozenges and smooth garyles are given to the patient.
- Instruct the patient not to clear his throat, cough or talk.

Findings

- A telectasis
- Bleeding
- Bronchial adenomas
- Foreign objects
- Infection
- Lung cancer
- Sarcoidosis
- Seuetions
- Tuberculosis
- Tumors.

Complications

- Bleeding
- Drug reactions
- Hypotension
- Laryugospasm
- Bronchospasm
- Hypoxia
- Dyssrhythymia
- Cardiopulmonary arrest.

Side Effects and Risks

Bronchoscopy is a safe test that carries little risk. Complications are rare, but if they occur, they may include collapsed lung, bleeding from the sample site, and an allergic reaction to medicines, hoarseness, and slight fever. Only rarely do patients experience other more serious complications. Due to sedation, the patient should not drive or operate machinery for the remainder of the day following the exam.

Colonoscopy

Colonoscopy is a procedure that enables an examiner (usually a gastroenterologist) to evaluate the inside of the colon (large intestine or large bowel). The colonoscope is a four foot long, flexible tube about the thickness of a finger with a camera and a source of light at its tip. The tip of the colonoscope is inserted into the anus and then is advanced slowly, under visual control, into the rectum and through the colon usually as far as the cecum, which is the first part of the colon.

Definition: It is diagnostic procedure which provides visualization of the lining of the large intestine. Through a flexible endoscope.

Purpose

Diagnostic Purposes
- To detect colon cancer or polyps
- To detect inflammation & disease of bowel.

Therapeutic Purpose
- To remove the polyps
- Detection & prevention of colorectal cancer

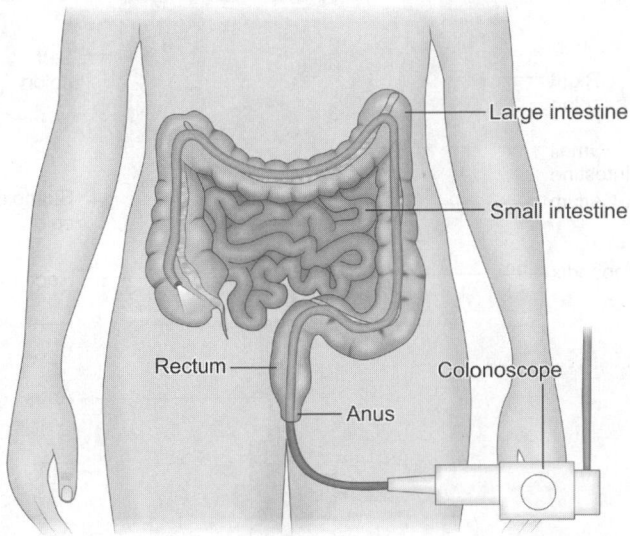

Fig. 19.14: Examination of colon.

- To treat bleeding or stricture.

Indication
- Unexplained constipation/Diarrhea
- Rectal bleeding, lower abdominal pain.

Principles
- A thorough knowledge about the anatomy & physiology of the GI tract.
- Mental & physical preparation of the patient facilitates introduction of the tulee.
- Systematic way of doing saves, time, energy & Material
- Any unfamiliar situation procedure fear & Anxiety.

General Instruction
- Explain the procedure to the client to uein his confidence & co-operation.
- Limit the intake of fluids for 24-72 has before the examination.
- Fleet or saline enema should be given until the return is clear.
- Lavage solutions are used for effective cleansing of bowel.
- Instruct the pt not to take routine medication when lavage solution is ingested.
- Achieve the diabetic pt to consult his/her physician about medication adjustment.
- Instructing all the pts especially elderly to maintain adequate fluid, electrolyte & caloric intake.
- NSAIDs must be discontinued before the test & for 2 weeks after the procedure.
- The patients having cardio vascular disease requires careful cardiac monitoring during the procedure.
- Colono scopy cannot be performed if there is a suspected colon perforation, Acute severe duvertucytutus.
- The patients taking heparin must consult physician for specific instruction.

Preliminary Assessment
- Identify the patient name, age, sex, diagnosis, uracel and bed no.
- Check the doctor's order for specific precaution.
- Check the general condition of the pt.
- Check for any lesion on the rectal area.
- Check the consciousness and ability to follow the Instructions.
- Check the articles available in the unit.
- Check the purpose of the procedure.
- Check the medical order for the collection of specimen.

Preparation of the Article
- Colonoscope
- Draping sheet.
- Lubricant
- Cotton suvales
- Gloves
- Emesis basin.
- Toilet tissue.
- Kidney teay & paper bag.
- Biopsy forceps

Preparation of the Patient
- Explain the procedure to the patient.
- Provide privacy with curtains.

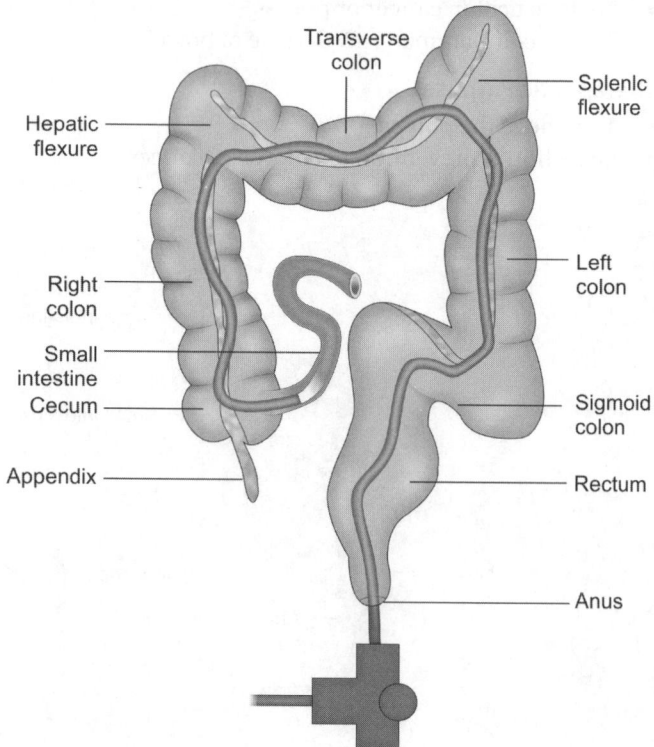

Fig. 19.15: Colonoscopy introduced through rectum.

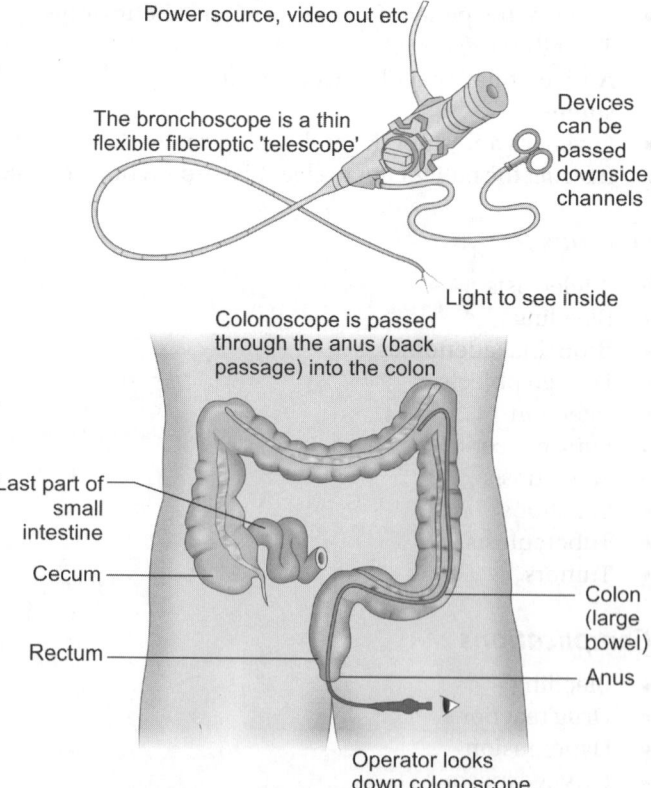

Fig. 19.16: Parts of colonoscope and application procedure.

- Cover the patient with sheet or bath blanket.
- The patient receiver NPO after midnight before the test.
- Place the patient in a left lateral position.
- Keep the entire article on the bed side & check the articles for good working condition.
- Remove the bottom gaements or raise it up above the waist level.
- Get the written consent from the client.

Procedure: The patient assumes left lateral position ask him to relax as much as possible. The client is usually given [IV] sedation with valium, Demerol vessel. The lubricated colonoscope is inserted into the Anus. A small amount of ai is instilled to help the physician visualize the bowel lumen. When the4 colonoscope reaches the sigmoid junction, the client may move to the supine position making it easier to advance the colonoscope past the splence flexuce. During the test encourage the client to relax. Monitor the vital signs throughout the procedure watching for a vasovagal response teaching to hypotension & bradycardia.

Aftercare
- Place the pt in a comfortable position.
- Monitor the vital signs
- Assess for the signs of perforation
- Administer the IV fluids with sedation.
- Client may develop nausea which may ticated with IV Antiemetic Recording & Reporting (Time, Date, Pt response, Complication).

Complication
- Bleeding.
- Intestinal perforation.

Sigmoidoscopy

The sigmoid colon is the final portion of the bowel that is joined to the rectum. A sigmoidoscope is a small tube with an attached light source about the thickness of your finger. A doctor or nurse inserts the sigmoidoscope into the anus and pushes it slowly into the rectum and sigmoid colon. This allows the doctor or nurse to see the lining of the rectum and sigmoid colon. The procedure is not usually painful but it may be a little uncomfortable.

Definition: Sigmoidoscopy is defined as an examination of the distal sigmoid colon, rectum and anal canal.

Purpose
- To diagnose malignant and benign neoplasm.
- To detect hemorrhoids, polyps, fissures and fistula.
- To detect abscesses within the anal canal and rectum.
- before the rectal surgery.
- To evaluate rectal bleeding, acute or chronic diarrhea.

Principles
- Microorganism are found everywhere; nurse takes care to prevent the transference of microorganism.

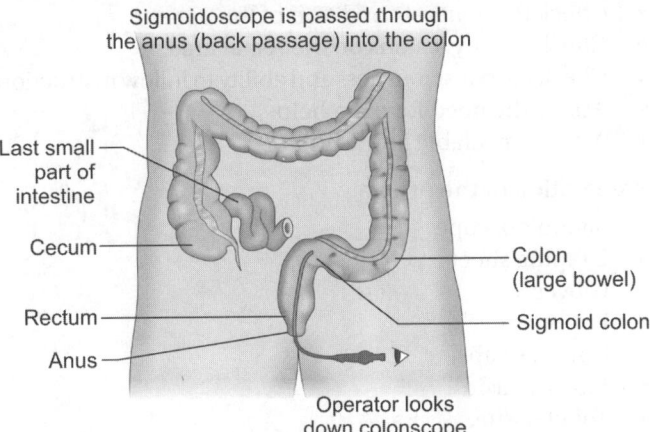

Fig. 19.17: Sigmoidoscopy procedure.

- A thorough knowledge about the anatomy and physiology of the GI tract.
- Mental and physical preparation of the patient facilitates introduction of the tube.
- Systematic may be doing sacs time, energy and material
- Any unfamiliar situation produces fear and anxiety.

Types of Sigmoidoscopy

There are two types of sigmoidoscope that can be used. The most commonly used is the flexible sigmoidoscope. This instrument allows your doctor to see around bends in the colon. A flexible sigmoidoscope gives doctors a better view of the lower colon and usually makes the examination more comfortable. The rigid sigmoidoscope has generally been replaced by the flexible version and is now used less often. It allows your doctor to look into the rectum and the bottom part of the colon but it does not reach as far into the colon as the flexible sigmoidoscope.

General Instruction
- Explain the procedure to the client and urine his confidence and co-operation.
- The Client assumes a knee-chest position.
- The client is instructed to eat a light evening meal prior to the examination.
- Catharactice are seldom used in preparation for this examination.
- Enema should be given until the return is clear before the examination.
- The nurse should remain with client. Watch his general condition and monitor the vital signs skin color.
- Both doctor and nurse should follow strict aseptic technique.
- Lubricate the instrument before introducing into the rectum.
- Do not expose the patient unnecessarily.

Preliminary Assessment
- Identify the patient name, age, ward, bed no, sex and diagnosis.
- Check doctors order for specific precautions.

- Check the general condition of the patient
- Check for any lesions on the rectal area.
- Check the consciousness and ability to follow instruction
- Assess the need for extra help.
- Articles available in the unit.

Preparation of the Article
- Sigmoidoscope
- Draping sheet
- Gloves
- Lubricant
- Cotton swabs.
- Emesis basin
- Toilet tissue.
- Biopsy forceps
- Suction machine
- Paper bag.

Preparation of the Patient
- Explain the procedure to the client.
- Provide privacy with curtains and adequate draping.
- Cover the patient with sheet or bath blanket.
- Remove the backrest and extra pillows.
- Place the Mackintosh and towel under the patient.
- Place the patient in a knee-chest position.
- Keep all the article arranged on the bedside locker and check the article for good working condition.
- Remove the bottom garments or raise it up above the waist level.
- Fold back a small portion of the sheet or bath blanked to expose only the anal region.

Procedure: The client assumes a knee chest position and encouraged him to relax, as much as possible and to take deep breathing. The physician usually first examines the rectum with gloved fingers. After that 25-30 on sigmoid scope is inserted into the anus to visualize the distal sigmoid colon and rectum. A flexible sigmoid scope also makes it possible to visualize the descending colon and rectum. The examines may obtain specimen from suspicious looking access of anus.

Aftercare
- The client is observed for signs of perforation such as bleeding, fever.
- Label and send the specimen to the laboratory.
- Allow the pt to take rest.
- Size may be ordered for rectal discomfort.
- Replace all the articles
- Recording and reporting (time, data, patient responses to the procedure, complication if any).

Complication
- Bleeding
- Intestinal perforate.

Laparoscopy

Laparoscopy is a procedure through which the abdominal and pelvic organs are visualized by means of a laparoscope.

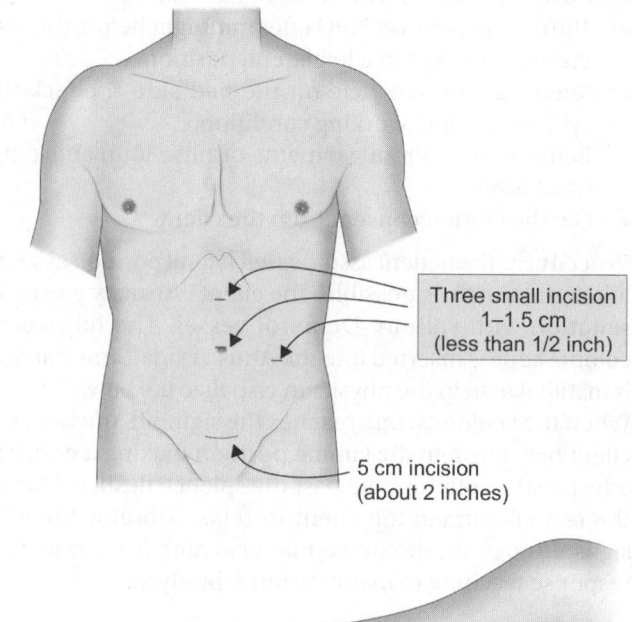
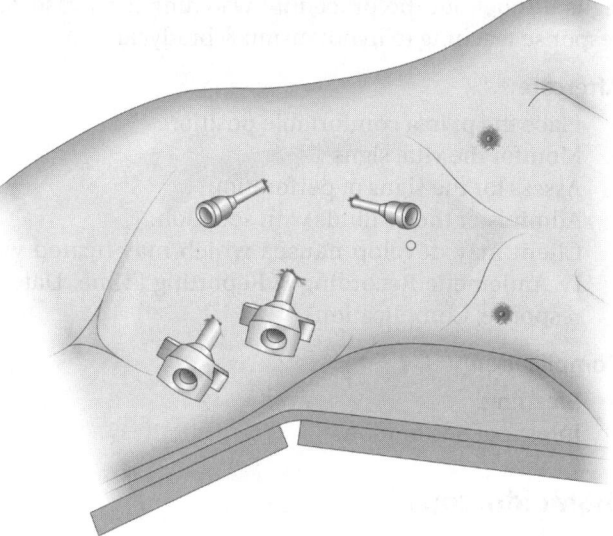

Fig. 19.18: Area of inserting laparoscopy tubes.

Laparoscopes are rigid telescope varying in diameter incorporating an optical system with a system of illumination. A variety of ancillary instruments such as punch biopsy forceps, hook scissors, coagulation points, diathermy points, knives, probes, traumatic forceps etc. are used with the laparoscopes. These instruments are used for measurements, aspirations, biopsies, dividing adhesions, coagulations, tubal ligations and operations.

Definition: Laparoscopy is a minimally invasive procedure used as a diagnostic tool and surgical procedure that is performed to examine the abdominal and pelvic organs, or the thorax, head, or neck. Tissue samples can also be collected for biopsy using laparoscopy and malignancies treated when it is combined with other therapies. Laparoscopy can also be used for some cardiac and vascular procedures.

Indication: Laparoscopy may be performed to diagnose variety of conditions. A laparoscopy is safe and convenient procedure with the added benefits of being usable for outpatients having a short postoperative period and minimal incision scarring. It may be used for the following:

- To diagnose ectopic pregnancy, follicular activity in the ovaries in case of sterility, pelvic masses, pelvic conditions such as endometriosis, adhesions, tubal occlusions etc.
- To diagnose conditions that is affecting the uterus, bladder and cul-de-sac.
- To find out the etiology of abdominal and pelvic pains, endocrinopathies and/or amenorrhea.
- To take a biopsy from any part of the abdominal area.
- To do tubal sterilization by electrocoagulation.

Types of Laparoscope

There are two types of laparoscope: (1) a telescopic rod lens system, that is usually connected to a video camera (single chip or three chip), or (2) a digital laparoscope where a miniature digital video camera is placed at the end of the laparoscope, eliminating the rod lens system.

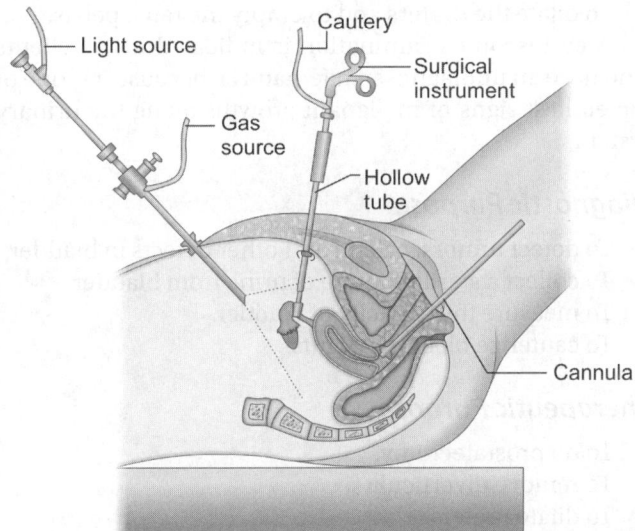

Fig. 19.19: Types of laparoscopic instrument.

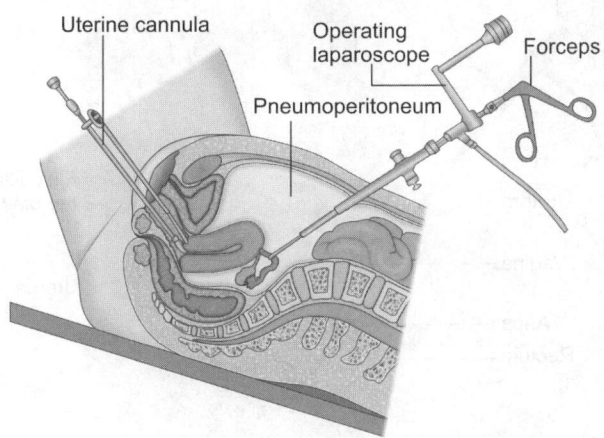

Fig. 19.20: Method of handling laparoscopic instruments.

The mechanism mentioned in the second type is mainly used to improve the image quality of flexible endoscopes replacing traditional fiberscopes. Nevertheless, laparoscopes are rigid endoscopes. The rigidness is required in clinical practice. The rod lens based laparoscopes are highly dominant in practice, due to their fine optical resolution (typically, dependant on the aperture size used in the objective lens), and the image quality can be better than the digital cameras if necessary. The second type is very rare in the laparoscope market and hospitals.

Procedure

Laparoscopy is typically performed in the hospital under general anesthesia, although some laparoscopic procedures can be performed using local anesthetic agents. Once under anesthesia, a urinary catheter is inserted into the patient's bladder for urine collection. To begin the procedure, a small incision is made just below the navel and a cannula or trocar is inserted into the incision to accommodate the insertion of the laparoscope. Other incisions may be made in the abdomen to allow the insertion of additional laparoscopic instrumentation. A laparoscopic insufflation device is used to inflate the abdomen with carbon dioxide gas to create a space in which the laparoscopic surgeon can maneuver the instruments. After the laparoscopic diagnosis and treatment are completed, the laparoscope, cannula, and other instrumentation are removed, and the incision is sutured and bandaged.

Laparoscopes have integral cameras for transmitting images during the procedure, and are available in various sizes depending upon the type of procedure performed. The images from the laparoscope are transmitted to a viewing monitor that the surgeon uses to visualize the internal anatomy and guide any surgical procedure. Video and photographic equipment are also used to document the surgery, and may be used postoperatively to explain the results of the procedure to the patient.

Robotic systems are available to assist with laparoscopy. A robotic arm, attached to the operating table may be used to hold and position the laparoscope. This serves to reduce unintentional camera movement that is common when a surgical assistant holds the laparoscope. The surgeon controls the robotic arm movement by foot pedal with voice-activated command, or with a handheld control panel. Microlaparoscopy has become more common over the past few years.

The procedure involves the use of smaller laparoscopes (that is, 2 mm compared to 5-10 mm for hospital laparoscopy), with the patient undergoing local anesthesia with conscious sedation (during which the patient remains awake but very relaxed) in a physician's office. Video and photographic equipment, previously explained, may be used.

Laparoscopy has been explored in combination with other therapies for the treatment of certain types of malignancies, including pelvic and aortic lymph

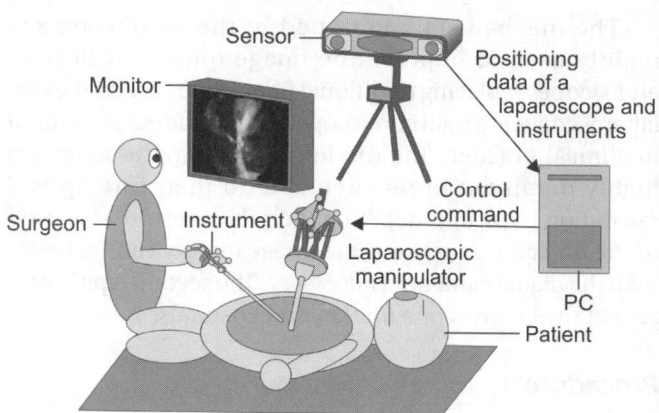

Fig. 19.21: Video-assisted method of laparoscopic procedure.

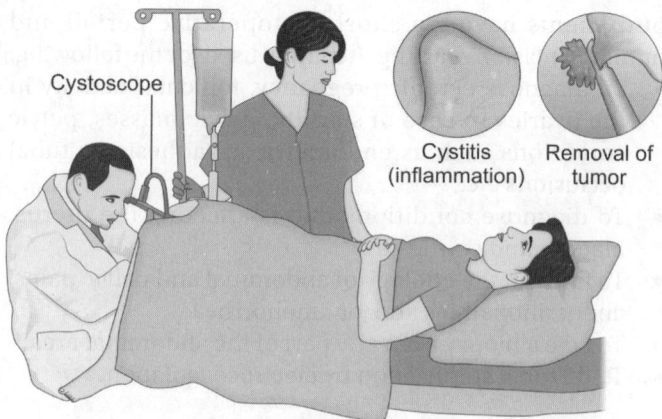

Fig. 19.22: Visual examination of bladder and urethra with cystoscope.

node dissection, ovarian cancer, and early cervical cancer. Laparoscopic radiofrequency ablation is a technique whereby laparoscopy assists in the delivery of radiofrequency probes that distribute pulses to a tumor site. The pulses generate heat in malignant tumor cells and destroy them. The introduction of items such as temperature-controlled instruments, **surgical instruments** with greater rotation and articulation, improved imaging systems, and multiple robotic devices will expand the utility of laparoscopic techniques in the future. The skills of surgeons will be enhanced as well with further development of training simulators and computer technology.

Complications

- Injury to the blood vessels, perforation of the viscera and bladder due to careless passage of an instrument.
- Gas embolism and overdistension of the abdomen with gas.
- Cardio-respiratory failure.
- Dangers associated with electro-coagulation. Burns may take place on the bowels or other viscera and on other parts of the body where any metal part of the table which is in contact with the client creates a passage to the earth.
- Bleeding at the site of biopsy.

Cystoscopy

Cystoscopy is the visualization of bladder and urethra with the help of a cystoscope.
- Visualizations of the urinary bladder: - Cystoscopy
- Visualization of the urethra: - Cystourethroscopy.

Purpose of Cystoscopy

Cystoscopy is useful for both diagnostic and therapeutic purposes. The purpose for which cystoscopy may be done is:
- To diagnose tumor, ulcers, calculi and other defects in the urinary bladder.
- To collect urine directly from the kidney pelvis and from each kidney separately in order to assess the bladder functions.
- To visualize the kidney pelvis and ureters through the retrograde pyelography.
- To measure the capacity of the bladder (cystometry).
- Resection of tumors (enlarged prostate) or diverticula.
- Removal of stones or foreign bodies.
- To locate a point of hemorrhage and to cauterize the bleeding point.
- To implant radium seeds.
- To dilate the ureters and to empty the renal pelvis.

A cystoscopic examination is indicated for all clients who have an undiagnosed haematuria, because it is one of the earliest signs of malignant growths along the urinary system.

Diagnostic Purpose

- To detect tumors, calculi and other defects in bladder.
- To collect a sterile sample of urine from bladder.
- To measure the capacity of bladder.
- To cauterize bleeding points.

Therapeutic Purpose

- To do prostatectomy.
- To remove diverticula's.
- To dilate ureters.

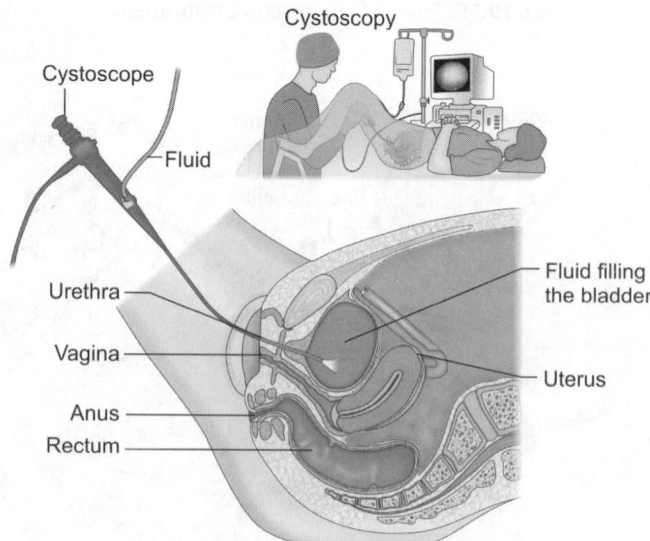

Fig. 19.23: Cystoscopy procedure.

Principles
- Through knowledge of anatomy and physiology of urinary treat.
- Microorganisms are found everywhere. So strict aseptic techniques should be followed.
- An unfamiliar situation produces fear and anxiety.
- Systematic way of doing saves time energy, and material.

General Instructions
- Explain the procedure to the patient to win his confidence, and co-operation and to allay his anxiety.
- If cystoscopy is done under general anesthesia, prepare him for general anesthesia.
- An enema is given to empty bowels.
- Shaving and cleaning of perineum.
- Change his dress and make him put on hospital dress.
- Give a sedative one hour before the procedure.
- Antibiotics are started prior to the procedure to prevent infection.
- Place the patient in the lithotomy position, safe for cystoscopy.
- Stay with the patient throughout the procedure.
- Give rest to the patient after cystoscopy.
- Observe his vital signs.
- Observe for pain and report immediately.
- Observe the urinary output, heamaturia, fullness of bladder and burning micturition.
- Give him plenty of fluids us he is out of anesthesia.
- Provide not drinks and extra warmth to prevent chills.
- Record the procedure in the nurse's record.
- Sterile catheters are present; tape them individually to both the thighs, marking right and left, to collect specimens f4rom renal pelvis.

Preliminary Assessment
- Check the doctor's order for the procedure.
- Check the doctor's order for specific precautions.
- Check the general condition of the patient.
- Check the abilities and limitations of the patient.
- Check for articles available in the unit.
- Obtain written consent from the patient.

Preparation of the Patient Unit
- Explain the procedure to the patient.
- Provide privacy.
- Position the patient kept ready for the procedure.
- Administer anesthesia before 20–30 minutes.
- Empty the bladder and bowels.
- Perineal shave and perineal car.

Articles Needed
Unsterile Tray
- Solutions—betadine
- Mackintosh and towel
- Kidney tray and paper-bag
- Lubricting agent.

Sterile Tray
- Sterile dressing towel
- Small bowls
- Cotton balls, gauge piece
- Gown, mask and gloves.

Procedure
- With the patient under local anesthesia, the cystoscope is inserted through the urethra into the urinary bladder.

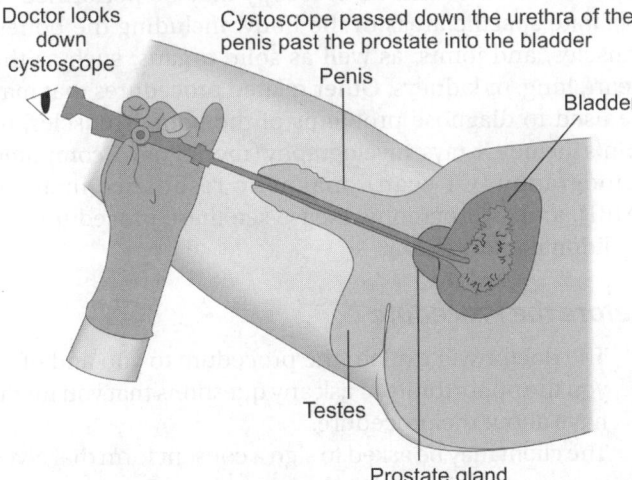

Fig. 19.24: Parts of cystoscopy instrument.

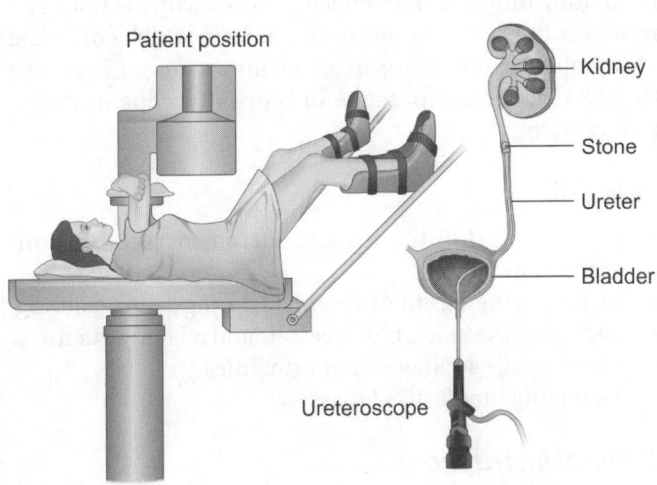

Fig. 19.25: Patient position for cystoscopy procedure.

- Once the bladder is filled with saline for irrigation, all aspects of the bladder walls are examined.
- Biopsy samples for tissue examination and cell washings for cytologic analysis may be carried out.
- Urine samples may be collected from the bladder or from each ureter.
- The procedure takes 30–45 minutes.

Aftercare

- Check vital signs and record the results.
- Assess for pain or bladder spasms and medicate us needed.
- Encourage extra-oral fluids to promote adequate hydration.
- Instruct the patient to void within 8 hours after the rest.
- Instruct the patient to take the prescribed antibiotics.
- Record the procedure and findings.

Findings

- Cancer of the bladder.
- Polyps.
- Diverticulum's of the bladder.
- Bladder fistula.
- Bladder stones.
- Bladder neck stricture.
- Congenital anomaly.
- Benign prostatic hypertrophy.
- Cancer of the prostate gland.

Complication

- Persistent bleeding.
- Infection.
- Urinary obstruction.

Fluoroscopy

Fluoroscopy uses X-ray to observe deep structure in motion. Instead of producing a signal, still image, a fluoroscopy screen registers a constant image of the chest (or other part body) being examined. This makes if possible for the chest and intrathoracic structures to be observed while they function dynamically. Fluoroscopy is not used routinely but rather in those situations in which continual observation of the thorax in an advantage (e.g., to observe the transbronchial passage of biopsy forceps during a bronchoscopy).

Indications

- Observing the diaphragm during inspiration and expiration.
- Detecting mediastinal movement during deep breathing.
- Assessing the heart, blood vessels and related structures.
- Identifying esophageal abnormalities
- Detecting mediastinal masses.

General Instructions

- In a darkened room, a client is positioned between a fluorescent screen and an X-ray source (X-ray tube), and

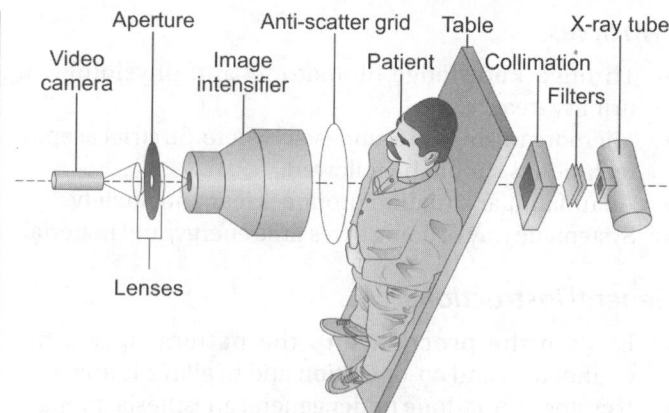

Fig. 19.26: Fluoroscopy procedure.

images of the moving internal structures are projected on a screen.
- Sometimes a radiopaque medium is administered to help distinguish the structures being assessed.
- Imges projected by fluoroscopy are not as clear and definitive as those produced by a standard by a standard chest film. However, if abnormalities are discovered, still photographs and cinefluorography may be done for a permanent record.
- Cineflurorographys are motion pictures that allow more leisurely study and re-study of the area photographed, without exposure of either radiology personnel other client to unnecessary radiation.

Procedure

Fluoroscopy is a study of moving body structures--similar to an X-ray "movie." A continuous X-ray beam is passed through the body part being examined. The beam is transmitted to a TV-like monitor so that the body part and its motion can be seen in detail. Fluoroscopy, as an imaging tool, enables physicians to look at many body systems, including the skeletal, digestive, urinary, respiratory, and reproductive systems. Fluoroscopy may be performed to evaluate specific areas of the body, including the bones, muscles, and joints, as well as solid organs, such as the heart, lung, or kidneys. Other related procedures that may be used to diagnose problems of the bones, muscles, or joints include X-rays, myelography (myelogram), computed tomography (CT scan), magnetic resonance imaging (MRI), and arthrography. Please see these procedures for additional information.

Before the Procedure

- The doctor will explain the procedure to you and offer you the opportunity to ask any questions that you might have about the procedure.
- The client may be asked to sign a consent form that gives your permission to do the procedure. Read the form carefully and ask questions if something is not clear.
- The specific type of procedure or examination being done will determine whether any preparation prior to

the procedure is required. Your doctor will notify you of any preprocedure instructions.
- Notify your doctor if you have ever had a reaction to any contrast dye, or if you are allergic to iodine.
- If the client is pregnant or suspect that should notify your doctor

After the procedure: The type of care required after the procedure will depend on the type of fluoroscopy that is performed. Certain procedures, such as cardiac catheterization, will likely require a recovery period of several hours with immobilization of the leg or arm where the cardiac catheter was inserted. Other procedures may require less time for recovery. If you notice any pain, redness, and/or swelling at the IV site after you return home following your procedure, you should notify your doctor as this could indicate an infection or other type of reaction.

Funduscopy

The retina is the only portion of the central nervous system visible from the exterior. Likewise the fundus is the only location where vasculature can be visualized. So much of what we see in internal medicine is vascular related and so viewing the fundus is a great way to get a sense for the patient's overall vasculature. But the fundoscopic exam can discover pathological process otherwise invisible, examples are plentiful, and include recognizing endocarditis, disseminated candidemia, CMV in an HIV infected patient, and being able to stage both diabetes and hypertension.

Large/medium/small light source: Ophthalmoscopes usually have 2 or 3 sizes of light to use depending on the level of pupil dilation. The small light is used when the pupil is very constricted (i.e. well lit room, no pupil dilators used). The large light is best if using mydriatic eye drops to dilate. Most commonly in a dark, non-dilated pupil, the medium sized light is used.

Half light: If, for example, the pupil is partially obstructed by a lens with cataracts, the half circle can be used to pass light through only the clear portion of the pupil to avoid light reflecting back

Red free: Used to visualize the vessels and hemorrhages in better detail by improving contrast. This setting will make the retina look black and white.

Slit beam: Used to examine contour abnormalities of the cornea, lens and retina.

Blue light: Some ophthalmoscopes have this feature that can be used to observe corneal abrasions and ulcers after fluorescein staining.

Grid: Used to make rough approximations of relative distance between retinal lesions.

Types of Funduscope

Each type of ophthalmoscopy has a special type of ophthalmoscope:

The direct ophthalmoscope is an instrument about the size of a small flashlight (torch) with several lenses that can magnify up to about 15 times. This type of ophthalmoscope is most commonly used during a routine physical examination.

An indirect ophthalmoscope, on the other hand, constitutes a light attached to a headband, in addition to a small handheld lens. It provides a wider view of the inside of the eye. Furthermore, it allows a better view of the fundus of the eyes; even if the lens is clouded by cataracts. An indirect ophthalmoscope can be either monocular or binocular. It is used for peripheral viewing of the retina.

Technique

Traditional Direct Ophthalmoscope
- Darken room, ask patient to look at the same point as far as possible in the room (this will help to dilate the pupil).
- Wedge scope against your cheek with hand and then head/hand/scope should move as one unit.

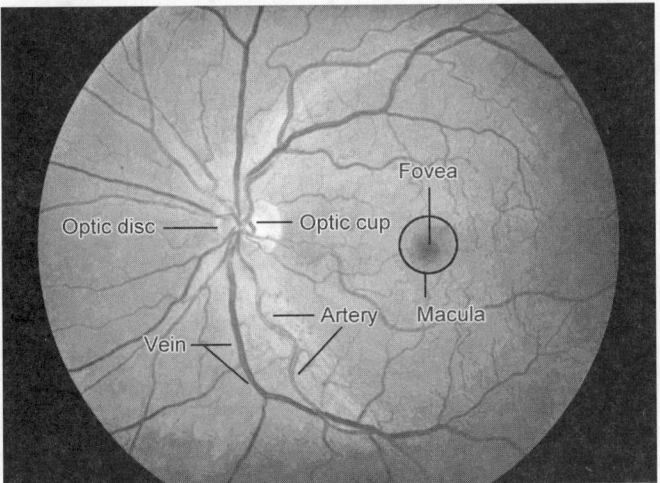

Fig. 19.27: Retinal image obtained by funduscopy.

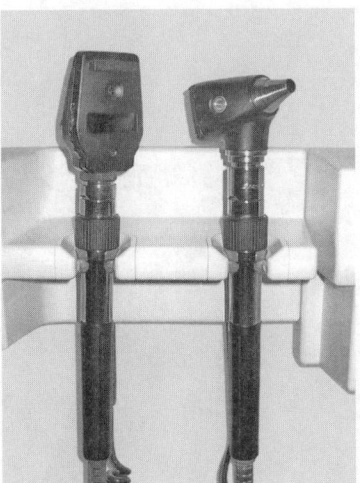

Fig. 19.28: Ophthalmoscope used for examination of fundus of eye.

- Use your right hand & your right eye to look at the patient's right eye.
- Look through the ophthalmoscope, if you are nearsighted and have taken off your glasses, you may need to adjust the focusing wheel towards the negative/red until what you see at a distance is in focus.
- **Finding the retina:** Direct the ophthalmoscope 15 degrees from center and look for the **red reflex** (see video). Simply follow the red reflex in until you see the retina. If you lose the red reflex, come back until you find it again and repeat.
- To look around the retina using a traditional direct ophthalmoscope, you should "pivot" the ophthalmoscope, angling up, down, left and right.

PanOptic Ophthalmoscope: Although the PanOptic is very similar to the traditional ophthalmoscope, there are a number of differences. Additionally, the view of the PanOptic is 4-5x wider.

- Use the scope to view an object approximately 15 feet away and adjust the focus until clear (unless you're wearing glasses and are taking them off, you'll likely be in perfect focus at a setting of zero). (You will NOT need to use your right eye, patient's right eye and your right hand as usually instructed with the traditional ophthalmoscope. You can hold the Panoptic however you are most comfortable.)
- Darken room, ask patient to look at the same point as far as possible in the room (this will help to dilate the pupil).
- **Finding the retina:** Stand back! Direct the ophthalmoscope 15 degrees from center and look for the **red reflex** (see video). Simply follow the red reflex in until you see the retina. If you lose the red reflex, come back until you find it again and repeat.
- To see other regions around the retina, rather than angling the ophthalmoscope, you simply ask the patient to look up to see the upper retina, down to see the lower retina, medial to see the medial retina, lateral to see the lateral retina and to look towards the light to see the macula.

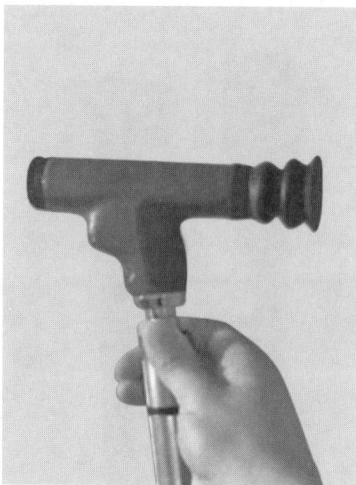

Fig. 19.29: PanOptic ophthalmoscopic instrument used for eye examination.

Esophagogastroduodenoscopy

Esophagogastroscopy includes gastroscopy and esophagoscopy. If duodenoscopy is included with the endoscopic examination, the term is esophagogastroduodenoscopy. A flexible fiberoptic endoscope is used for direct visualization of the internal structures of the esophagus, stomach, and duodenum. Biopsy forceps or a cytology brush can also be inserted through a channel of the endoscope. Suction can be applied for the removal of secretions and foreign bodies.

This test is performed under local anesthesia or IV sedation (benzodiazepine or narcotics), in a gastroscopy room of a hospital or clinic, usually by a gastroenterologist. This procedure can be done on an emergency basis for removal of foreign objects (a bone, a pin, etc.) and for diagnostic purposes. The major complications that can occur from esophagogastroduodenoscopy are perforation and hemorrhage.

Purposes

- To visualize the internal esophagus, stomach, and duodenum.
- To obtain a cytological specimen.
- To confirm the presence of gastrointestinal pathology.

Clinical Problems

S.N.	Areas	Description
1.	Esophageal	Esophgitis, hiatal hernia, esophageal stenosis, achalasia, esophageal neoplasm (benign or malignant tumors), esophageal varices, Mallory-Weiss tear.
2.	Gastric	Gastritis, gastric neoplasm (benign or malignant), gastric ulcer (acute or chronic), gastric varices.
3.	Duodenal (small intestinal)	Duodenitis, diverticula, duodenal ulcers, neoplasm (benign or malignant)

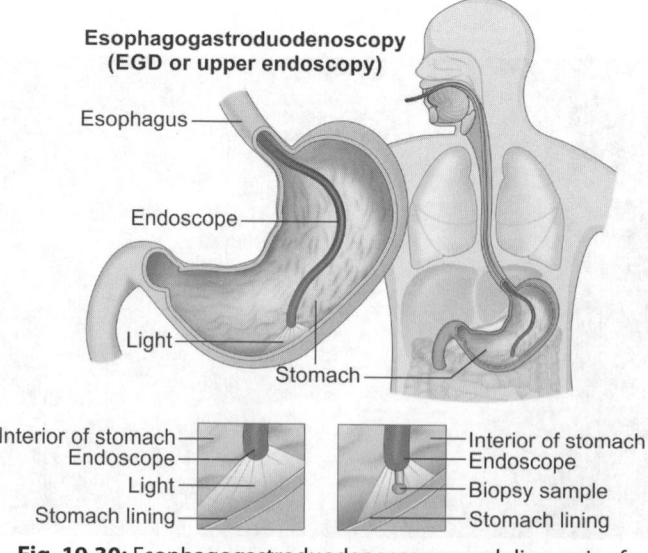

Fig. 19.30: Esophagogastroduodenoscopy used diagnosis of stomach and duodenal problems.

Client Preparation

- Recognize that a gastroscopy test for visualizing the esophageal, gastric and duodenal mucosa is actually an esophagogastroduodenscopy. These names are frequently used interchangeably.
- Explain the procedure to the client. Inform the client that instrument is flexible; the procedure will be done under local anesthesia (the throat will be sprayed) premeditations will be given before the test and usually IV sedation is given with the test; dentures are jewelry should be removed; and food and fluids will be restricted for 8 to 12 hours before the test.
- Cheek the client dentures, eyeglasses and jewellary are removed. Give the client a hospital gown.
- Have the client void. Take vital signs.
- Check the consent form has been signed before giving the client premeditations. Once the sedative and the narcotic analgesic are given, the client should remain in bed with side up. Tell him or her that these medications will cause drowsiness.
- Explain to the client that he or she may feel some pressure with the insertion of the endoscope and may feel some fullness in the stomach and intestine areas.
- Be a good listener. Allow the client time to ask questions and to express concerns or fear.

Procedure

- A consent should be signed
- The client should be NPO for 8 to 12 hours before the test. When this procedure is used during an emergency and NPO cannot be enforced, the client's stomach is lavaged (suctioned) to prevent aspiration.
- The client may take prescribed medications at 6 AM on the day of the test. Check with laboratory or health care provider for any changes.
- A sedative / tranqualizer, a narcotic analgesic, and atropine may be given an hour before the test, or they can be titrated intravenously immediately prior to the procedure and during the procedure as needed.
- A local anesthetic may be used.
- Dentures, jewelry and clothing should be removed from the neck to the wrist.
- Record baseline vital signs. The client should void before the procedure.
- Specimen containers should be labeled with the client's name, the date and the type of tissues.
- Emergency drugs and equipment should be available for hypersensitivity to medications (premeditations and anesthetic) and for severe laryngospasms.
- The test takes approximately 1 hour or less.
- The client should not drive self home following the test because of possible aftereffects of sedation.

Post-procedural Care

- Check the gag reflexes before offering food and fluids by asking the client to swallow or by touching the posterior pharynx with a cotton swab or tongue blade if the throat was sprayed with an anesthetic.
- Monitor vital signs (blood pressure, pulse, respirations) as ordered.
- Give the client throat lozenges or analgesics for throat discomfort. Inform the client that he or she may have flatus or burp-up gas, which is normal. This is caused by instillation of air during the procedure for visualization purposes.
- Observe the client for possible complications
- Be supportive of the client and family.

Complications: Perforation in the gastrointestinal tract from the endoscope. Symptoms could include pain (epigastric, abdominal and back pain), dyspnea, fever, tachycardia and subcutaneous emphysema in the neck.

Factor affecting diagnostic results: Barium from a recent gastrointestinal images series can decrease visualization of the mucosa. This test should not be performed within 2 days after such tests. An X-ray film of the abdomen can be taken to see if barium is in the stomach or duodenum.

RADIOLOGICAL STUDIES

Chest X-ray

Chest X-ray studies provide information about the chest that may not be available through other assessment means. Also, they often graphically illustrate the cause of respiratory dysfunction. Chest films may reveal abnormalities when there are no physical signs or symptoms of pulmonary disease.

Purposes

- It is done as part of routine screening procedures.
- To identify the pulmonary disease conditions
- To monitor the status of respiratory disorders and abnormalities (pleural effusion, atelectasis and tuberculous cavity lesions).

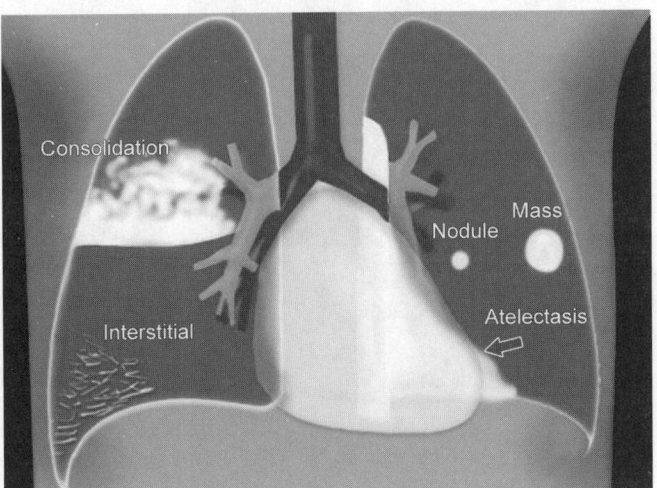

Fig. 19.31: Chest X-ray studies.

- To confirm endotracheal or tracheotomy tube placement.
- To conform the traumatic chest injury.
- The radiographic information helps the management of the respiratory problem

Indication

- Chest films show the bony structures (ribs, sternum, clavicles, scapulae, and upper portions of the humerus).
- The vertebral column is visible vertically through the middle of the thorax.
- It provides information about two diaphragms. It normally appear rounded, smooth, and sharply defined, with the right hemi diaphragm slightly elevated above the left.
- To get the information about the junction of the rib cage and the diaphragm. The junction of rib cage otherwise called the costophrenic angle, it is normally clearly visible and angled.
- To get information about heart and lung tissue. The heart tissue is dense and appears white but less intensely white than bony structures. The lung tissue appears black on X-ray.
- It provides information about heart shadow, the heart shadow is normally clearly outlined and extends primarily onto the lift side of the thorax and occupies no more than one third of the chest width.

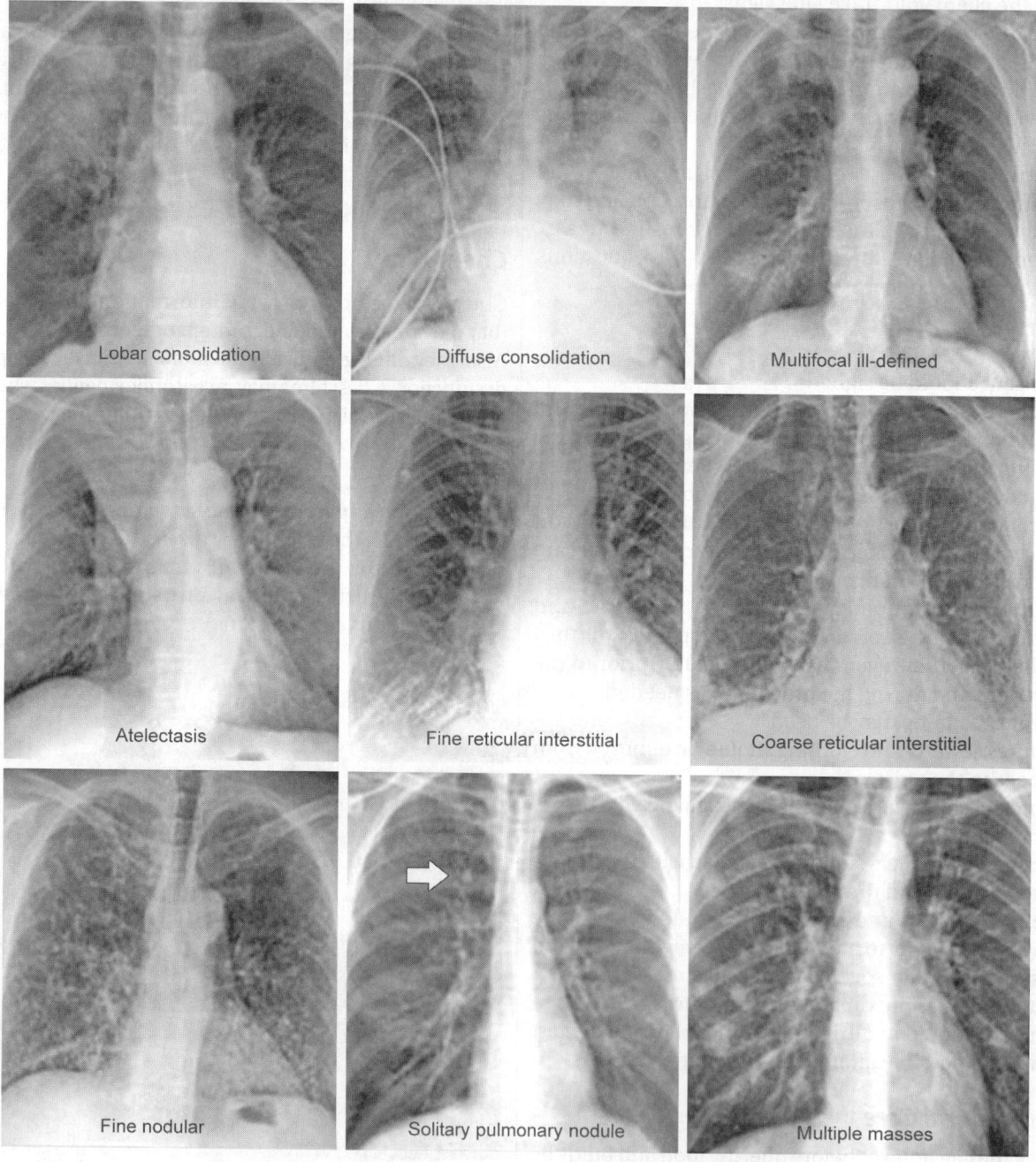

Fig. 19.32: Radiological images (chest X-ray) of various lung diseases.

- Close observation shows the trachea in the upper middle chest almost superimposed over the cervical and thoracic vertebrae. The trachea bifurcates bronchi.
- The pulmonary blood vessels, bronchi and lymph nodes of the midthorax. The vascular lung tissues are visible as white, thin, wispy strings fanning out from the hilum.

Standard Radiographical Positions

- Routine adult chest X-ray studies are taken with the client standing or sitting facing the X-ray film, with the chest and shoulders in direct contact with the film cassette.
- The shoulders are rotated forward to pull the scapulae away from the lung field.
- The X-ray cathode penetrates from the posterior. This position is called the posteroanterior (PA) position.
- The radiographs taken on expiration are sometimes requested for demonstrating the degree of diaphragm movement or for assisting in the assessment and diagnosis of pneumothorax.

For Immobilized Clients

- For clients unable to be transported to the radiology department, portable chest radiography may be taken.
- Portable radiographs are usually with the film placed behind the client, and the X-ray beam penetrates from the front of the chest-the anterioposterior (AP) position. Because the X-ray beam enters from the anterior chest, the heart will appear larger than it really is and larger than on a PA view.

Lateral View

- Lateral view, which usually accompanies a standard PA view. It is taken from either the right or left side of the chest.
- The arms are raised above the head, and the side of he chest is placed against the film.
- The lateral view allows better visualization of the heart and the diaphragm dome.
- When used in conjunction with a PA film, a lateral position gives a three-dimensional view, allowing more specific identification of an abnormality's location.

Lateral Decubitus Position

- Lateral decubitus position, which may be used when it is necessary to determine whether opaque areas on the pleura are due to solid or liquid media.
- This view is taken with the client lying on either the right or left side, depending on which side of the chest is being assessed.
- In a left lateral decubitus position, the client is lying on the left side. The term decubitus refers to a lying-down position.

Oblique Position

- Oblique position, which is used to see behind and around underlying structures.
- The shoulders are rotated either to the right or left of the film. By turning the client, the angle at which the X-ray beam passes through the chest is shifted.
- In a right oblique position, the right side is closest to the film. The view may be taken from either an anterior or posterior position.

Lordotic Position

- Lordotic positions, which are useful if clearer visualization of the upper lung fields is needed.
- The angle of the X-ray cathode is lowered and the bam directed at an upward angle. This angle removes the clavicles and first and second ribs from the field of vision.

Bronchography

Bronchography is a radiological technique, which involves X-raying the respiratory tree after coating the airways with contrast Bronchography is rarely performed, as it has been made obsolete with improvements in computerized tomography and bronchoscope.

A bronchography is a radiographic (x-ray) examination of the interior passageways of the lower respiratory tract. The structures of the lower respiratory tract, which include the larynx (voice box), trachea (windpipe), and bronchi (larger branching airways to the lungs), become visible on x-ray film after contrast dye is instilled through either a catheter or bronchoscope (narrow, flexible, lighted tube) into these areas. Contrast dye is a substance that causes a particular organ, tissue, or structure to be more visible on x-ray or other diagnostic images.

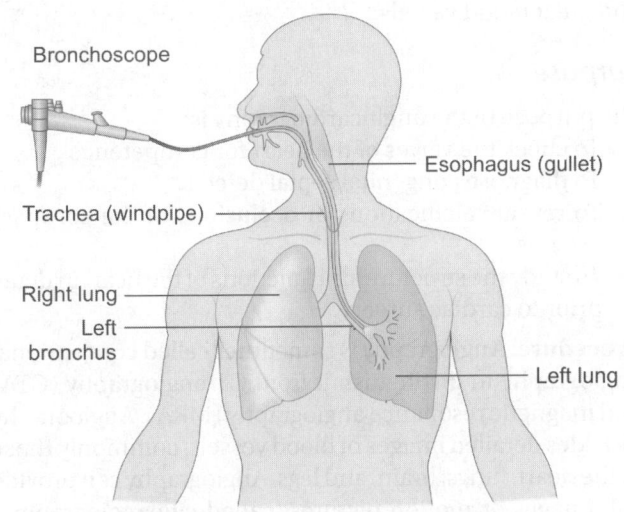

Fig. 19.33: Bronchoscopy procedure.

The contrast dye is released as the catheter or bronchoscope is inserted through the nose or mouth and advanced down the throat into the trachea and bronchi. The contrast dye forms a coating on the lining of the interior walls of these structures, thus outlining their anatomy on x-ray. In addition, abnormalities such as tumors, cavities, cysts, and obstructions may be revealed. As a result of improved computerized tomography (CT scan) and bronchoscopy technology, as well as increased availability of these procedures, bronchography is performed on an infrequent basis.

Reasons for the procedure: A bronchography may be performed to diagnose structural or functional abnormalities of the larynx, trachea, and/or bronchi. Abnormalities may include, but are not limited to, the following:
- Bronchiectasis—an irreversible enlargement of the bronchi as a result of deterioration of the muscle and elastic tissue of the bronchial walls. Generally, this is the result of chronic inflammation from various causes.
- Hemoptysis—coughing up blood
- Tracheoesophageal fistula—abnormal tract between trachea (windpipe) and esophagus (hollow tube used for swallowing)
- Tumors (abnormal growths)
- Chronic pneumonia or bronchitis

Angiography

Angiography is the roentgenographic visualization of the blood vessels anywhere in the body following the injection of a contrast medium. It is useful in evaluating the disorders of the brain, heart, lungs and other body segments.

Meaning

It is the study of the chambers of the heart and the large thoracic blood vessels done in conjunction with the cardiac catheterization. Immediately after the dye is injected, a series of x-ray films are taken which will reveal the course of the dye as it circulates through the client's heart, lungs and great blood vessels.

Purpose

The purpose of the angiocardiography is:
- To check the valves of the heart for competence.
- To diagnose congenital septal defects.
- To reveal calcifications or occlusions of the coronary arteries.
- To study the structure and functions of the heart in detail prior to cardiac surgery.

Procedure: Angiography is sometimes called conventional angiography to distinguish it from CT angiography (CTA) and magnetic resonance angiography (MRA). Angiography provides detailed images of blood vessels, commonly those in the heart, lungs, brain, and legs. Angiography can provide still images or motion pictures (called cineangiography). IV contrast is injected through a catheter inserted into a blood vessel that connects with the vessel to be imaged. A local anesthetic or a sedative may be used. If the catheter is inserted into an artery, the insertion site must be steadily compressed for 10 to 20 min after all instruments are removed to reduce the risk of bleeding at the puncture site. Patients may also need to lie flat for several hours or be hospitalized to reduce this risk.

Types of Angiography

- **Pulmonary angiography:** Pulmonary angiography is the roentgenographic visualization of the blood vessels of the lungs. It is helpful in diagnosing such conditions as pulmonary embolism, lung tumors, aneurisms, vascular changes associated with emphysema, congenital defects, space occupying lesions within the thorax. Like anglo-cardiography, the pulmonary angiography also involves the cardiac catheterization.
- **Cerebral angiography:** A cerebral angiography allows x-ray visualization of the brain's vascular system. The dye may be injected directly into the common carotid artery (percutaneous carotid arteriogram) or with the insertion of a catheter into the brachial artery or femoral artery to the descending aorta and from there into the desired vessels of the heart. Once the appropriate vessel has been reached, the contrast material is injected and a series of films are rapidly taken.

Common uses of conventional angiography include the following:
- **Coronary angiography** is usually done before percutaneous or surgical interventions involving the coronary arteries or heart valves. It is usually done with cardiac catheterization.
- **Cerebral angiography** may be indicated after stroke or transient ischemic attack (TIA) e.g. if stenting or carotid endarterectomy is being considered.
- **Iliac and femoral angiography** may be indicated before interventions to treat peripheral arterial disease.
- **Aortography** is sometimes done to diagnose and provide anatomic detail about aortic aneurysms, aortic dissection, and aortic regurgitation.
- **Angiography of the eye arteries** can be done using fluorescein dye.
- **Conventional pulmonary angiography** used to be the gold standard for diagnosis of pulmonary embolism; now, it has largely been replaced by CT pulmonary angiography [CTPA], which is less invasive.

Conventional angiography is usually done before therapeutic angiographic procedures such as angioplasty, vascular stenting, and embolization of tumors and vascular malformations.

Disadvantages

The injection site may bleed if the injected blood vessel ruptures; a painful hematoma can form. Rarely, the site becomes infected; it becomes red and swollen and exudes a purulent discharge within a few days after the injection.

Rarely, an artery is injured by the catheter, or an atherosclerotic plaque dislodges, causing an embolism distally. Very rarely, shock, seizures, renal failure, and cardiac arrest occur.

Risk of complications is higher in the elderly, although it is still low. The radiation dose used in angiography can vary and be significant (eg, coronary angiography is associated with an effective radiation dose of 4.6 to 15.8 mSv). Angiography must be done by highly skilled physicians, usually specially trained interventional radiologists or cardiologists.

Pulmonary Angiography

Pulmonary angiography is a procedure that uses a special dye (contrast material) and x-rays to see how blood flows through the lungs. Angiography is an imaging test that uses x-rays and a special dye to see inside the arteries. Arteries are blood vessels that carry blood away from the heart.

This test is done in a special unit of a hospital. You will be asked to lie on an x-ray table.

- Before the test starts, you will be given a mild sedative to help you relax.
- An area of your body, usually the arm or groin, is cleaned and numbed with a local numbing medicine (anesthetic).
- The radiologist inserts a needle or makes a small cut in a vein in the area that has been cleaned, and inserts a thin hollow tube called a catheter.
- The catheter is placed through the vein and carefully moved up into and through the right-sided heart chambers and into the pulmonary artery, which leads to the lungs. The doctor can see live x-ray images of the area on a TV-like monitor, and use them as a guide.
- Once the catheter is in place, dye is injected into the catheter. X-ray images are taken to see how the dye moves through the lungs' arteries. The dye helps detect any blockages to blood flow.

- Your pulse, blood pressure, and breathing are monitored during the procedure. Electrocardiogram (ECG) leads are taped to your arms and legs to monitor your heart.
- After the x-rays are taken, the needle and catheter are removed.
- Pressure is immediately applied to the puncture site for 20-45 minutes to stop the bleeding. After that time the area is checked and a tight bandage is applied. The leg should be kept straight for 6 hours after the procedure.
- Rarely, this test can be used to deliver medications to the lungs when a blood clot has been found.

Cerebral Angiography

Cerebral angiography is an X-ray study of the cerebral circulation following injection of contrast material into a selected artery. Cerebral angiography is the primary investigative tool for intracranial aneurysm, arteriovenous malformation, cerebral vascular occultation disease and study of collateral blood flow.

Definition: Cerebral angiography is the X-ray study by injecting radiopaque contrast medium into an artery visualization of intracranial and extracranial blood vessels.

Purposes

- To diagnose intra cranial lesions.
- To detect abnormalities of blood vessels such as stenosis, aneurysms and arteriovenous malformation
- To detect any displacement of cerebral vessels due to cysts, tumors or abscess.
- To visualize the cerebral arteries and veins to determine the size and nature of pathological process.
- It is done as a preparatory investigation to neurovascular interventional therapy.
- It also has value in localizing mass lesion and may aid in preparative diagnosis.
- It is frequent done prior to craniotomy.

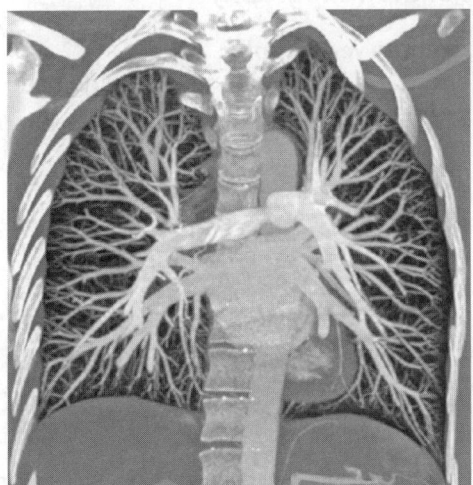

Fig. 19.34: Pulmonary angiography images.

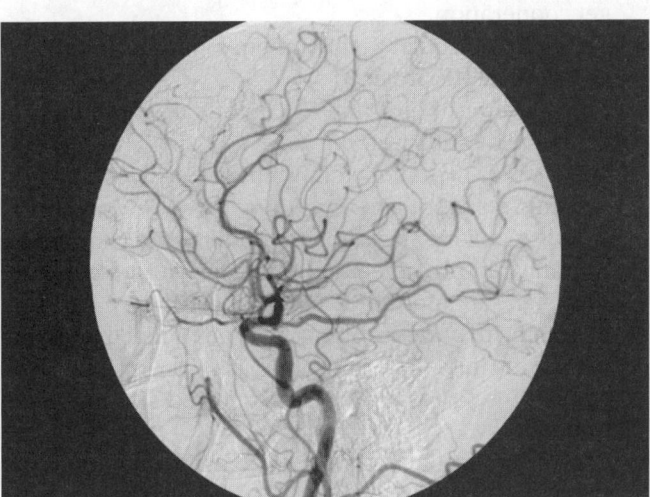

Fig. 19.35: Cerebral angiography images.

General Instructions

- The client needs to prepare physiologically and psychologically.
- The majority of cerebral angiograms are done by the transfemoral route, but the procedure may be accomplished by direct puncture of the carotid / vertebral artery or by retrograde injection of contrast medium into the brachial artery.
- The skin to be shaved at puncture site, for direct puncture. In male client, beard and neck to be shaved. For transfemoral approach shaving to be done for both male and females from umbilicus to mid thigh on both sides.
- The client should be informed that the lie still during the procedure and he will feel a burning sensation during the injection for 4-6 seconds.
- Indwelling catheter for female and condom connected to urosac placed for male clients.
- Keep the client nothing per oral for 6-8 hours, those posted under general anesthesia.
- Mark the appropriate peripheral pulses with a felt tipped pen on the skin.

Client Preparation

- Explain the procedure to the client that X-ray films will be taken from different angles during procedure.
- Obtain informed consent from the client.
- Remove any metal objects and jewellery from the client.
- Assess the client for allergic reactions to dye.
- Maintain nothing per oral before six hours to the procedure.
- Perform skin preparation and remove the hair from the sites of catheter insertion.
- Monitor the baseline neurological signs
- Explain the client the local anesthesia is administered before insertion of catheter.

Procedure

- The nurse in the angiogram room will receive the client.
- The nurse explain the entire procedure thoroughly to get cooperation
- The client placed in the treatment table comfortably
- Legs and hands are fixed
- Blood pressure cuff and ECG leads are applied and connected to the monitor.
- The client is hydrated with IV fluids
- Xylocain test dose given
- Painting and draping is done for femoral artery puncture
- Administration of injection heparin given after puncture
- Vital signs are monitored continuously
- At the end of puncture, heparin is neutralized by giving protamine injection
- Apply direct pressure over punctured site for 15-20 minutes
- Pressure crape bandage is applied in the punctured site
- Check the peripheral pulse after conformation shift the client to the ward.

Aftercare

- Maintain strict bed rest for 12-24 hours.
- Observe for bleeding, swelling, redness and changes in the temperature.
- After bleeding stops, apply a pressure dressing and place sand bag over the dressing.
- If the punctured site is femoral artery, the leg is immobilized for 24 hours to prevent bleeding.
- Monitor vital signs and neurological signs.
- Ice bags may also be used to provide pressure and relieve tenderness.

Complications

- Cerebral embolus caused by the catheter dislodging a segment of atherosclerotic plaque in the vessel.
- Hemorrhage or clot formations at the insertion site.
- Vasospasm of a vessel caused by the irritation of catheter placement
- Thrombosis of the extremity distal to the injection site.
- Allergic reaction to the contrast medium.

Venography

Lower extremity venography is a test used to see the veins in the leg. X-ray are a form of electromagnetic radiation like light, but of higher energy, so they can go through the body to form an image on film. Structures that are dense (such as bone) will appear white, air will be black, and other structures will be shades of gray. Veins are not normally seen in an x-ray, so a special dye (called contrast) is used to highlight them.

Leg venography, also called lower extremity venography or phlebography, offers a way for doctors to see the veins in your legs. Veins do not normally show up on X-rays. In a venogram, a doctor injects a special kind of dye into your veins. This dye, called **contrast material**, is visible on X-rays, and enables your doctor to take images of the veins in your leg.

Purpose of the Venography

Lower extremity venography:

- To identify and locate blood clots in the deep veins of the legs (deep vein thrombosis)

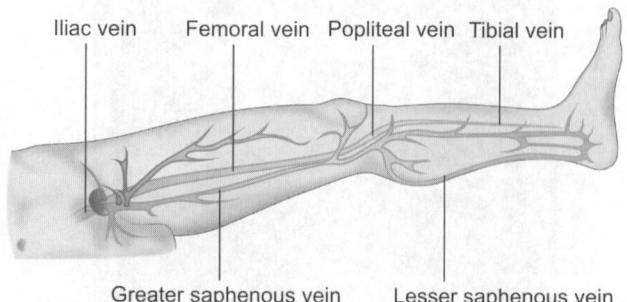

Fig. 19.36: Lower extremity venography procedure.

- To distinguish between a blood clot and an obstruction caused by a large pelvic tumor encroaching on the venous system
- To assess congenital venous malformations
- To evaluate the competence of valves in the leg veins (which can aid in identifying the causes of leg swelling)

Renal venography:
- To detect and evaluate blood clots, tumors, or abnormalities in the renal veins of the kidney
- To collect blood samples from the renal vein to evaluate renovascular hypertension (increased blood pressure due to narrowing of the artery that leads to the kidney).

Adrenal venography: To obtain blood samples from the adrenal gland veins to aid in the detection of diseases such as Cushing's syndrome (marked by increased secretion of the hormone cortisol) and pheochromocytoma (a tumor marked by increased secretion of the hormones epinephrine or norepinephrine).

Portal Venography

- To diagnose and assess portal hypertension (high pressure in the portal vein, which empties into the liver)
- To detect and locate a suspected blood clot in the portal or splenic vein
- To assess the progression of cirrhosis of the liver
- To assess the patency of shunts that were constructed to treat portal hypertension (portal-systemic shunts)

Special Concerns about Venography

- Pregnant women should not undergo this test because exposure to ionizing radiation may harm the fetus.
- People with allergies to iodine or shellfish may experience an allergic reaction to iodine-based contrast dyes.
- In people with kidney disorders or chronic dehydration, the contrast dye can worsen kidney function and may cause renal failure. To determine whether the dye can be administered safely, your doctor may perform a blood test to assess your kidney function before the test.
- This procedure may not be safe for people who have bleeding disorders. Coagulation studies may be performed prior to the test to ensure that your blood will clot normally.
- The presence of feces, gas, or residual barium in the abdomen from recent contrast x-rays may make it difficult to obtain clear pictures of abdominal veins.

Before the Venography

- You may be asked to observe certain dietary restrictions for variable periods before the test, depending on the specific procedure.
- Report to your doctor any medications, herbs, or supplements you are taking. You may be advised to discontinue certain of these agents before the test.
- Inform your doctor if you have a known shellfish or iodine allergy or have ever had an adverse reaction to x-ray contrast dyes. You may be given preventive medication to reduce the risk of an allergic reaction, or a noniodinated dye may be used.
- Tell your doctor if you are pregnant or may be pregnant.
- An intravenous (IV) line is inserted into a vein in your arm so that any necessary medications can be administered during the procedure.
- Empty your bladder before the procedure.
- You will be given a sedative to help you relax during the examination.

During Procedure

Lower extremity venography (ascending):
- You are positioned lying down on a tilting x-ray table. The table is inclined so that your feet are elevated.
- The skin on the top of your foot is cleansed with an antiseptic, and a local anesthetic is injected. A tourniquet may be tied around the ankle to make the foot veins fill with blood.
- A catheter is inserted into a selected foot vein, and contrast dye is infused into the vein.
- The movement of the dye up the leg is followed using continuous x-ray imaging, or fluoroscopy. Spot x-ray films are also obtained as the dye circulates through different regions of the leg.
- The catheter is withdrawn, and a bandage is applied to the insertion site.
- The procedure may take 30 to 45 minutes.

Lower extremity venography (descending):
- You are positioned lying down on a tilting x-ray table.
- The skin over a vein in your arm or neck is cleansed with an antiseptic solution, and a local anesthetic is injected.
- A catheter is inserted into the selected vein. Under the guidance of fluoroscopic imaging, it is carefully guided to a selected pelvic or leg vein.
- Contrast dye is injected through the catheter and the table is inclined so that your feet are lowered.
- The movement of the dye down the leg is followed using continuous x-ray imaging, or fluoroscopy. Spot x-ray films are also obtained to document any "leaking" valves in the veins of the legs.
- The catheter is withdrawn, and a bandage is applied to the insertion site.
- The procedure may take 30 to 45 minutes.

Renal and adrenal venography:
- You will lie on your back on an x-ray table.
- The skin over the catheter insertion site—usually the femoral vein in the groin—is cleansed with an antiseptic solution and (if necessary) shaved. A local anesthetic is injected to numb the area.
- A catheter is inserted into the femoral vein. Under the guidance of fluoroscopic imaging, it is carefully guided to either the renal or adrenal veins in the abdomen.

- A contrast dye is injected through the catheter. This may cause a transient burning or flushing sensation.
- As the contrast agent flows through the selected veins, a series of x-ray films is obtained.
- If applicable, blood samples are then obtained and sent to a laboratory for analysis.
- The catheter is withdrawn, and a bandage is applied to the insertion site.
- The procedure takes about 1 hour.

Portal Venography

- You will lie on your back on an x-ray table.
- The skin over the catheter insertion site—usually the femoral artery in the groin—is cleansed with an antiseptic solution and (if necessary) shaved. A local anesthetic is injected to numb the area.
- A catheter is inserted into the femoral artery. Under the guidance of fluoroscopic imaging, it is carefully guided to a selected abdominal artery.
- A contrast dye is injected through the catheter. This may cause a transient burning or flushing sensation.
- Fluoroscopy is used to follow the flow of the dye from the selected artery into draining veins and then into the portal vein near the liver.
- The catheter is withdrawn, and a bandage is applied to the insertion site.
- The procedure takes about 1 hour.

Risks and Complications of Venography

- Possible risks include blood clot formation, bleeding, blood vessel damage, or infection at the site of catheter insertion.
- Some people may experience an allergic reaction to the iodine-based contrast dye, which can cause symptoms such as nausea, sneezing, vomiting, hives, and occasionally a life-threatening response called anaphylactic shock. Emergency medications and equipment are kept readily available.
- Venogram causes deep vein thrombosis in rare cases.
- Renal failure may occur as a result of exposure to the contrast dye, especially in elderly patients with chronic dehydration or mild renal impairment.
- Cellulitis, inflammation of connective tissue, and pain may occur if the contrast dye infiltrates into the tissues under the skin.

After the Venography

- Your vital signs will be monitored until they are stable. Depending on the procedure, you may be advised to rest in bed for a certain period of time.
- Cold compresses can help to relieve any swelling or discomfort at the puncture site.
- You are encouraged to drink clear fluids to avoid dehydration and to help flush the contrast dye out of your system.
- You may resume your normal diet and any medications discontinued before the test, according to your doctor's instructions.
- If bleeding or any other complications develop, call your doctor or emergency medical service immediately.

Results of Venography

- A physician will examine the recorded images and other test data for evidence of venous abnormalities.
- This test usually establishes a definitive diagnosis. Based on the findings, your doctor will recommend an appropriate course of medical or surgical treatment.

Cardiac Catheterization

Cardiac catheterization is an invasive procedure that permits the assessment of anatomic abnormalities of the heart. It may be right sudden catheterization, a left side catheterization, or both. Cardiac catheterization is complex procedure involves the insertion of a catheter into the heart, valves and circulatory system.

Definition: Cardiac catheterization is an invasive diagnostic procedure, in which one or more catheters are introduced into heart and selected blood vessels, to measure pressures and to determine oxygen saturation in the various heart chambers.

Purposes

- To assess potency of coronary arteries.
- To decide on appropriate treatment such as Percutaneous transluminal coronary angioplasty/Coronary artery bypass grafting (PTCA/CABG) if atherosclerosis is present.
- To measure pressure in various chambers of the heart.
- To obtain blood samples for measurement of hematocrite and oxygen saturation.
- To conform diagnosis of heart disease and to determine the extend to which the disease has affected structure and function of heart.
- To obtain clear picture of cardiac anatomy prior to heart surgery.
- To determine cardiac output.
- To obtain endocardial biopsies1to the occluded coronary artery to restore coronary blood flow.
- To allow infusion of fibrinolytic agents directly in the occulted coronary artery to restore coronary blood flow.
- To detect shunts.
- To determine congenital abnormalities.
- To obtain a clear picture of cardiac anatomy prior to heart surgery.

Types/Classification

- **Right-side catheterization:** Passing a radio-opaque catheter from antecubital or femoral vein into the right atrium, right ventricle and pulmonary vasculature.

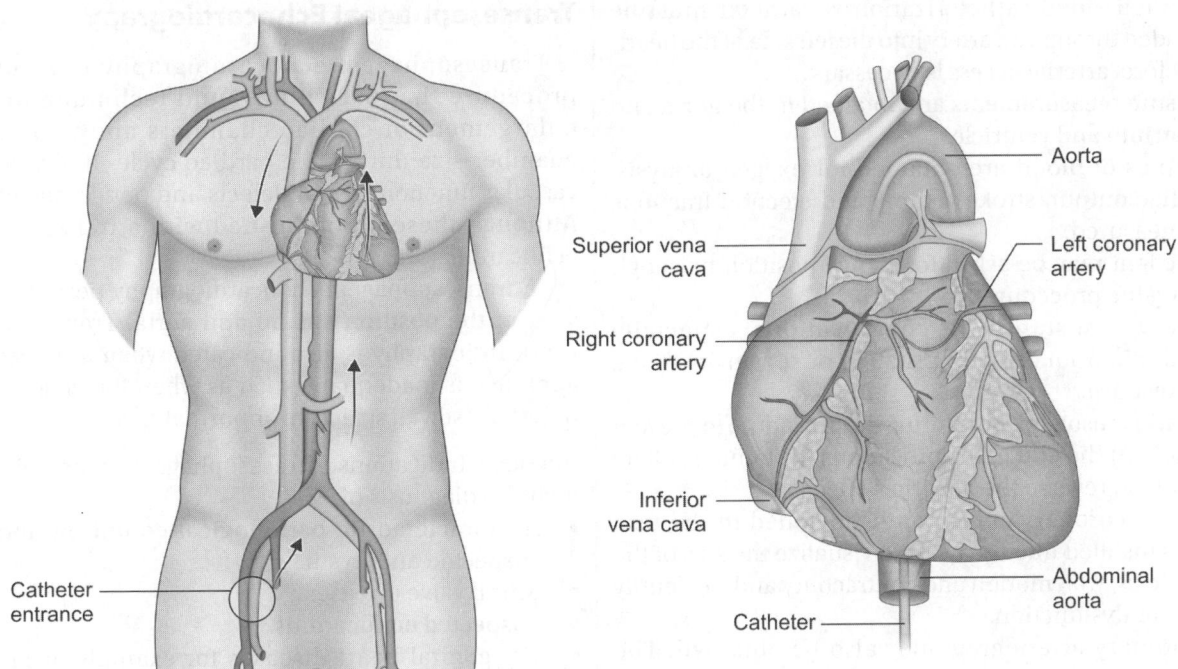

Fig. 19.37: Cardiac catheterization procedure.

- **Left-side catheterization**: Insertion of catheter into right brachial artery or femoral artery, ascending aorta and into left ventricle. It can also be performed transseptally from right atrium into left atrium and then left ventricle.

Client Preparation

- Instruct the client about the purpose and procedure.
- Inform the client that the table rotates and that the physician may ask the client to change positions or cough
- Explain the client that when the dye is given, a feeling of warmth or flushing or a metallic taste may be sensed.
- Assist the precatheterization evaluation—blood test, including a prothrombin time test and a partial thromboplastin time test; an electrocardiogram; and chest X-ray.
- Obtain client's height and weight.
- Assess the client's fear and anxiety. Correct any misconceptions and reassure the client that the nurse, physician and technicians to assist during the procedure will be continuously present.
- If contrast dye is going to be used, cheek for allergies
- Keep the client nothing per oral after midnight, except if the catheterization is planned for late in the afternoon. In that case, a clear liquid breakfast may be given.
- Withhold the cardiac drugs as per the physicians order
- Prepare catheter site according to laboratory protocols. The femoral artery is commonly used for the percutneous of the catheter. Usually both sides of the groin are prepared.
- Premedication is given as ordered to reduce the client's anxiety. In some catheterization laboratories, the client is premeditated to decrease the risk of allergic reaction to the contrast dye.
- Instruct the client to void before going to the catheterization laboratory.

Equipment

- Cardiac monitor
- Pressure monitoring device
- Fluoroscope
- Sterile radiopaque cardiac catheters
- Radiopaque dye
- Sterile linen for draping
- Cleaning solutions
- Sterile gloves
- Cardiac catheterization pack
- cut down set
- Scalpel blade
- Emergency articles
- Sterile gown
- Local anesthetic agent
- Sterile syringes and needles.

Procedure

- Provide emotional support and reinforce with adequate explanations
- Continuous cardiac monitoring is maintained throughout the procedure.
- Help the physician to administer local anesthic agent
- Left-sided catheterization is performed in a cardiac catheterization laboratory.
- This laboratory is designed with fluoroscopy, electrocardiography equipment and emergency equipment and drugs.

- For a left-sided catheterization, a catheter must be threaded through an artery into the left side of the heart; therefore, arterial access is necessary.
- Pressure measurements are obtained in the aorta and left atrium and ventricle.
- Samples of blood are obtained for oxygen analysis. Cardiac output, stroke volume and ejection fractions are measured.
- The client may be asked to change position or cough during the procedure
- Observe constantly for complications, especially dysrthmia from catheter irritation or sensitivity to the contrast dye.
- Heparin is usually given during the procedure to prevent emboli. At the end of the procedure, protamine sulfate is given to reverse the heparin's effect.
- When a coronary angiogram is included in the test, dye is instilled into the heart to visualize the size of the ventricles, wall motion and contractility and to identify valvular dysfunction.
- A coronary arteriogram may also be obtained. The catheter is withdrawn from the left ventricle and positioned at the coronary ostia, where small boluses of dye are injected into the coronary arteries while a series of X-ray films are taken.

Aftercare

- Observe the insertion site of bleeding. Palpate around the punctured site to detect bleeding into tissue.
- If bleeding is present, exert pressure just proximal to the puncture site with a gloved hand for a minimum of 15 minutes.
- Monitor vital signs and cardiac monitor according to hospital protocol.
- Cheek the distal pulse for artery patency.
- Report immediately if any significant changes in vital signs, rhythm and circulation or occurrence of chest pain
- Assess post-procedure laboratory values such as blood count, prothrombin time, electrolytes and creatine.
- Instruct the client about strict bed rest for 12–24 hours and to keep affected extremity straight for 12 hours.
- Encourage plenty of oral fluids.
- Record type of cardiac catheterization done and client's tolerance of the procedure.

Contraindications

- Pregnancy because of radioactive iodine crossing the blood placental barrier.
- Cardiomyopathy.
- Severe dysrhythias.
- Uncontrolled congestive heart failure.
- Patient allergic to local anesthesia, iodine or radiopaque contrast material.
- Bleeding disorders.
- Drug toxicity.
- Renal insufficiency.

Transesophageal Echocardiograpy

A Transesophageal echocardiography is an invasive procedure that uses ultrasound technique to detect enlargement of cardiac chambers and variations in chamber size during the cardiac cycle. It also assesses vascular function, septal defects and pericardial effusion. Although these accomplished with a transesophageal echocardiogram.

A transesophageal echocardiography permits a better view of the position atrium and aorta. Transesophageal echocardiography is also indicated when a transthoracic approach is inadequate, such as when the client is obese or has chest wall structure abnormalities.

Purpose: Indications of trasesophageal echocardiography includes diagnosis of:
- A thoracic aortic pathological condition, including suspected aneurysm.
- Mitral valve disease.
- Suspected endocarditis.
- Congenital heart diseases for example atrial septal defect.
- Left atrial intracranial thrombi.
- Cardiac tumors.
- It also used to assess cardiac function during minimally invasive cardiac surgery (MICS) and to assess prosthetic valves.

Interfering factors: Transesophageal echocardiography should not be performed if the client has a history of irradiation of the mediastinum, esophageal, dysphagia or structural abnormalities.

Client Preparation

- Ensure that a signed informed consent form has been obtained
- Ask the client about any disorder of the esophagus, stomach, throat or vocal cord.
- Inquire if the client has dentures, bridges or plates.
- Report to the physician any history of arthritis of the neck, respiratory problems or anticoagulation therapy.
- Maintain the client on a nothing by mouth starts for 6 to 8 hours.
- Describe the procedure to the client, especially the need for a mouth guard, positioning and the need to swallow when asked.
- If the client has prosthetic heart valves, prophylactic antibiotics may be prescribed.
- Report any indications in the mouth or throat.
- Administer antianxiety medication as prescribed.

Procedure

- The procedure may also be used intraoperatively where conventional echocardiography is ineffective.
- The client needs to be in bed or an table with ECG leads attached. ECG and BP are monitored.

- The throat is anesthetized and sedation is given.
- Instruct the client to gargle with various lidocaine and then to swallow.
- Warn the client that it will make the tongue and throat fell swollen.
- A mouthy guard is placed to prevent the client from biting down on the endoscope.
- The client is positioned on the left side in the chin-chest position. The head may be supported with a small pillow.
- The probe is lubricated with lidicaine jelly and slowly inserted as the client swallows.
- Monitor the client for a vasovagal response from the medication given to dry up secretions.
- Check the client for gagging and observe the oximeter for oxygen saturation is reading.

Aftercare

- Assess the client for return of the gag reflex before resuming oral intake.
- Instruct the client to avoid hot liquids or foods for 2 hours.
- If an outpatient, the client should be accompanied home by another person.
- Give lozenges for relief of throat discomfort.

Advantages

- Transesophageal echocardiography (TEE) gives a higher quality picture of the heart than does a regular echocardiogram.
- It is especially useful in clients who have thickened lung tissue or thick chest walls or are obese.
- TEE allows clear visibility of the heart and its structures it is most useful in diagnosis of cardiac masses, prosthetic valve function and aneurysm.

Complication: TEE has several complications that are related to the placement of the probe in the esophagus including esophageal perforation, transient hypoxia, dysrthythmias and vasovagal response.

Vectorcardiogram

A vectorcardiogram is a graphic recording of electric forces of the heart. It is a non-invasive procedure that graphically records the direction and magnitude of the heart's electric forces by means of a continuous series of vector loops. Three planes of the heart are recorded (frontal, sagittal and horizontal).

Purpose: A ventor cardiogram is used to assess ischemia, conduction defects and chamber enlargement (hypertrophy or dilation).

Client Preparation

- Explain to the client the purpose and procedure for vector cardiogram, no risk is involved.
- No present restrictions are required.
- Because electrode is applied to the four extremities and the chest, clothing should permit easy access.
- If the male client's chest is excessively hairy, the sites may need to be shaved.

Procedure

- Establish a relaxed environment.
- Place the client in a supine position.
- Conduction jelly is placed on the electrodes and the electrodes are applied and recording is made.

Aftercare

- Remove the conduction jelly
- Help the client to a comfortable position.

Findings

- Axis deviation
- Conduction disturbances
- Dysrthmias
- Hypertrophy of the ventricles
- Therapeutic drug effects or toxicity.

Roentgenogram

- A cardiac roentgenogram is a routine screening procedure in clients suspected or known cardiac disorders. It provides information regarding the size of the heart, its shape and location of the cardiac structure and great vessels.
- The X- ray may also be used to evaluate pulmonary vasculature and determine the placement of evasive catheter and pacemaker wires.

Purpose

- Various views of the chest are usually obtained in a cardiac X –ray series. The four views commonly obtained are anteroposterior, lateral, right anterior oblique.
- During acute cardiac status, only portable chest X-ray studies are available to evaluate the client's progress. Because the plate is positioned under the client, an anterioposterior view is obtained.
- This film is obtained routinely for hospitalized and preoperative clients to screen for tuberculosis and other serious pulmonary or cardiac diseases.
- It also provides a preoperative comparison film for the post operative clients whom a pulmonary or cardiac complication develops, and it is a basic radiological procedure for the clients with a suspected pulmonary disorder.

Indications

- The chest X-ray provides data about the heart including its size and shape.
- In congenital and acquired cardiac disease, the enlargement of the heart and its atria or ventricles

provides information about the improper function of the cardiac valves, pulmonary or aortic arterial hypertension and venous pulmonary conduction that affect heart size.

Findings
- Pneumothorax
- Atelectasis
- Pleural effusion
- Pleurisy
- Cystic Fibrosis
- Pulmonary fibrosis
- Tumor or cyst
- Silicosis.

Interfering Factors
- Excessive movement
- Failure to remove jewellery or other metal from the X-ray field
- Improper positioning.

Client Preparation
- Instruct the client to remove all clothes and put on a hospital gown.
- Instruct the client to remove all jewellery and metal objects from the area that is to be imaged.
- Provide reassurance to the client. Young children often fear the equipment, strange room, isolation and separation from the parents.

Procedure
- Ensure the client's safety at all times, particularly when there is a risk of the client's falling.
- The radiography table has no side rails. A Velcro waist restraint may be used, but sometimes the restraint interferes with the positioning and imaging needed.
- Position the client for the specific views needed.
- Instruct the client to remain motionless during the imaging.
- Sometimes the client is instructed to inhale deeply and hold the breath until the image is taken.
- The client must often wait in the imaging area as the decision is made concerning whether to take additional X-ray films.
- Provide a blanket or extra gown for the client who is chilled in the cool room.

Aftercare
- Assist the client in dismounting from the radiography table and getting dressed, as needed.
- Record the entire procedure in the nurses record.

Cholecystography

Cholecystography, X-ray of the gall bladder and biliary channels, following the administration of a radiopaque dye, one of the techniques of diagnostic imaging. In oral cholecystography, the dye is ingested, absorbed by the intestine, and concentrated by the gallbladder, which normally appears well opacified in the X ray. Abnormalities (*e.g.*, gallstones) may be demonstrated by radiolucent areas. Oral cholecystography is usually indicated in cases of suspected gallbladder disease.

Newer dyes that permit visualization of the bile channels without concentration by the gallbladder are administered intravenously to determine or rule out the presence of intermittent obstruction of the bile ducts or recurrent biliary disease after biliary surgery.

Definition: A cholecystogram is an x-ray procedure used to help evaluate the gallbladder. For the procedure, a special diet is consumed prior to the test and contrast tablets are also swallowed to help visualize the gallbladder on x-ray. The test is used to help in diagnosing disorders of the liver and gallbladder, including gallstones and tumors.

Oral cholecystography is a procedure used to visualize the gallbladder by administering, by mouth, a radiopaque contrast agent that is excreted by the liver. This excreted material will collect in the gallbladder, where reabsorption of water concentrates the excreted contrast. Since only 10% of gallstones are radiopaque, the remaining 90% will appear as translucent on an opaque background in an abdominal X-ray. Current medical practice prefers ultrasound and CT over oral cholecystography. If needed, IV cholecystography and cholangiography may be done.

Purpose
- To detect gallstones.
- To test the contractibility of the gallbladder.
- To find out filling ability of the gallbladder.
- To find out its ability to concentrate, its contents, and its condition when it is empty in normal states.

Preparation of the Patient
- Explain the procedure to the patient to relieve tension and worries.

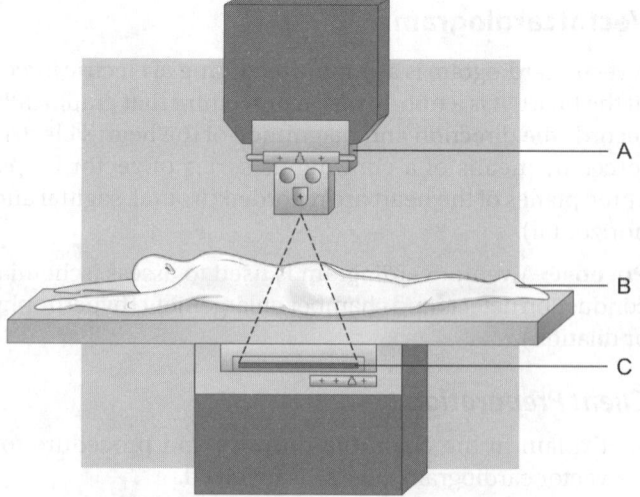

Fig. 19.38: Cholecystography procedure.

- Stop medications which contain iodine compounds and bismuth three days prior to the test.
- Check whether the patient is allergic to iodine or sea food before giving the dye.
- Record the patient's weight to calculate the dose of the dye.
- The patient is given a low-fat evening meal to avoid gallbladder contraction. Thereafter, no food and water should be given to the patient until the X-ray examinations are complete.
- The bowel is cleansed with saline enema.
- The emergency drugs and resuscitation equipment should be kept ready to resuscitate the patient.

Procedure

- The patient is given a light diet at 7 pm without fat.
- A laxative like dulcolax is given to clear the bowels.
- At 10 pm the patient is given 6 telepaque tablets to swallow.
- This dye is opaque to X-rays and is absorbed from the intestines, and is excreted by the liver.
- When the gallbladder is normal, this dye gets concentrated in the gallbladder, which becomes visible by X-ray.
- X-ray pictures are taken on the following day approximately 14, 18 and 19 hours after the drug has been administered, i.e. at 12 noon, 4 pm and 5 pm.
- No food is given during this period.
- Then, to test the contractibility of the gallbladder, the patient is fed with a fatty meal, one hour before the last X-rays taken at 12 noon and 4 pm, but it empties itself after the fatty meal taken at 4 pm and is, therefore, not visible in the X-ray taken at 5 pm.
- An abnormal gallbladder may not get filled properly or may fail to empty itself.

Aftercare

- Observe the patient for allergic reactions. Check the vital signs of the patient.
- Accompany the patient throughout the procedure.
- Make the patient comfortable.

Complications

Severe reactions to dye may lead to:
- Respiratory difficulty.
- Urticaria.
- Shock.
- Collapse.

Endoscopic Retrograde Cholangiopancreatography

Endoscopic retrograde cholangiopancreatography (ERCP) is an imaging technique in which the biliary pancreatic ducts are examined endoscopically after contrast medium is injected into the duodenal papilla. The purpose for this procedure is to identify the cause of a biliary obstruction, which could be stricture, cyst, stones, or tumor, jaundice is usually present. ERCP is performed following abdominal ultrasound, computed tomography, liver scanning and/or biliary tract X-ray studies to confirm or diagnose hepatobiliary or pancreatic disorders.

Purposes

- To detect biliary stones, strictures, cyst or tumor
- To identify biliary obstruction, such as stones or strictures
- To conform a biliary or pancreatic disorders.

Indications

- biliary stones
- Biliary strictures, cyst or tumor,
- Primary cholangitis
- Cirrhosis
- Pancreatic stones
- Stricture, cysts or pseudocyst or tumor
- Chronic pancreatitis
- Pancreatic fibrosis or duodenal papilla tumors.

Client Preparation

- Obtain a client history of allergies to seafood, iodine and contrast dye. Report allergic findings.
- Determine whether the anxiety level may interfere with the client's ability to absorb information concerning the procedure.
- Cheek that the concern forms has been signed prior to premeditations.
- Explain to the client that when the contrast medium is injected, there usually is a transient flushing sensation.
- Be supportive of the client prior to and during the test procedure.
- Monitor the vital signs during the test and compare them to baseline vital signs. An increase in the pulse rate could be due to atropine. Rupture within the gastrointestinal tract caused by endoscope perforation could cause shock.
- Inform the client that the endoscope will not obstruct breathing.
- Inform the client that atropine will make the mouth dry and the tongue feels large or swollen.
- Inform the client that the test takes approximately 1 hour and that lying still on the x-ray table is important.

Procedure

- Food and fluids are restricted for at least 8 hours before the test.
- The consent form should be signed prior to premeditations.
- Obtain baseline vital signs. Have the client void.
- Premedicate with mild narcotic or sedative. Atropine may be given prior to or after insertion of the endoscope.

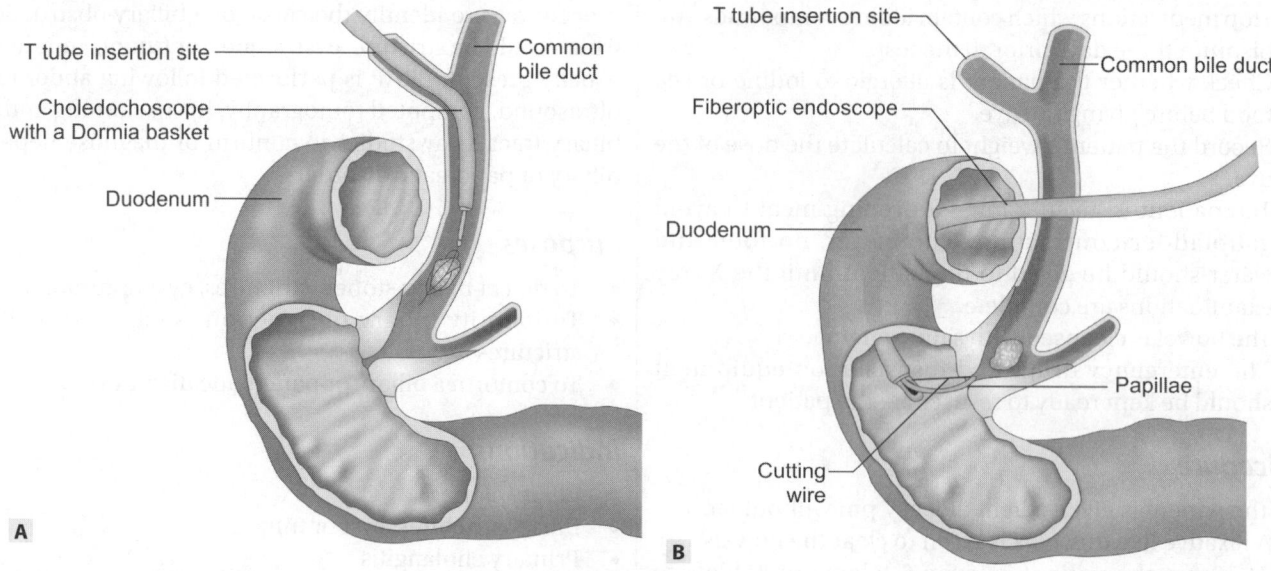

Figs. 19.39A and B: Choledochoscopic removal of gallstones: (A) Approach through T-tube insertion site; (B) Approach through duodenum.

Atropine relaxes gastrointestinal motility and will cause dryness of mouth.
- Local anesthetic is sprayed in back of throat (pharynx) to decrease the gag reflex prior to the insertion of the fiberoptic endoscope.
- Secretion may be given intravenously to paralyze the duodenum. Contrast medium is injected after the endoscope is at the duodenal papilla and the catheter is in the pancreatic duct.

Post-procedural Care

- Monitor vital signs. A rise in temperature might indicate (bacteremia or septicemia). Cheek respirations for respiratory distress resulting from anesthetic spray and/or the endoscope.
- Cheek the skin color. Increased or decreased jaundice is an indicator of a disease process or the result of therapy.
- Check the gag reflex before offering food or drink.
- Check signs and symptoms of urinary retention caused by atropine.

Factor affecting diagnostic results: Inability to cannulate biliary and / or pancreatic duct.

Client Teaching

- Suggest warm saline gargle and / or lozenges to decrease throat discomfort
- Explain to the client that he or she has a sore throat foe a few days after the test. This is due to the endoscope.

Myelography

A myelogram is an X-ray of the spinal subarachnoid space taken after an opaque medium or air is injected into the spinal subarachnoid space through a spinal puncture. It is also a diagnostic procedure used to visualize the lumbar, thoracic or cervical areas or whole spinal axes for diagnosis of a spinal tumor, a herniated intervertebral disc or a ruptured disc.

Definition: Myelography is an X-ray examination of the spinal subarachnoid space taken after an opaque medium or air is injected into the spinal subarachnoid space through a spinal puncture. It shows any distortion of the spinal cord or spinal dural sac caused by tumors, cysts, herniated intervertebral discs or other lesions.

Purposes

- To identify space-occupying lesions of the spinal cord.
- To help diagnosis a herniated nucleus pulposus.
- To diagnose intramedullary tumors.
- To identify the traumatic lesion and cysts of the vertebrae or the spinal cord.

Indications

- Spinal cord tumors
- Traumatic lesions of the spinal cord
- Herniated intervertebral disc.

General Instructions

- The client should be prepared physiologically and psychologically.
- Strict aseptic technique should be followed throughout the procedure.
- The client should be informed that the X-ray table may be tilted in varying positions during the study.
- The commonly used dyes are mertrizamide (amipaque) and iophendylate (pantoopaque) so the sensitivity should be checked.

Diagnostic Testing

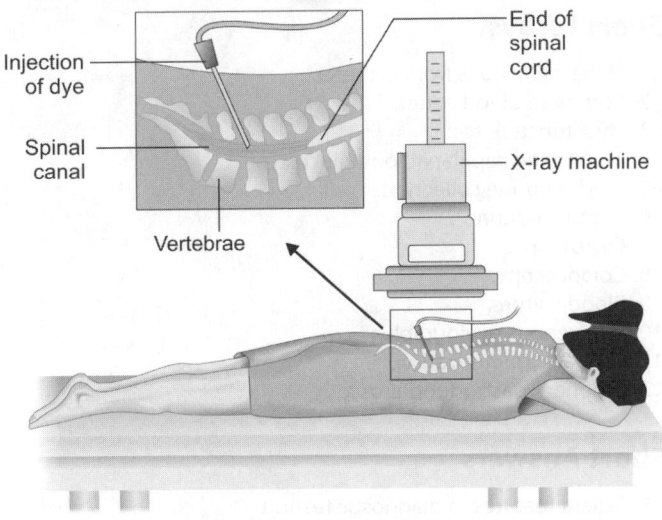

Fig. 19.40: Myelography procedure.

- Instruct the client to remain supine for 12 to 24 hours after the procedure.
- Inform the client that the procedure is done in X-ray department.

Client Preparation
- Explain the procedure to the patient and relatives
- Obtain informed consent
- The meal that would normally be eaten prior to the procedure is omitted.
- The client may be given a light sedative to help cooperate.
- Sensitivity test for the dye must be checked.

Procedure
- Place the client on the X-ray table
- Position the client for lumbar puncture.
- LP needle is inserted L4-L5.
- Approximately 10 mL of CSF is removed.
- Water soluble nonionic contrast medium is then injected.
- The table is tilted to allow the column of the dye to move up and down within the subarachnoid space.
- By minimal changes in position of the table and patient, various regions of the spine are screened and films taken at appropriate levels.

Aftercare
- Keep the client strict bed rest
- Position the client's head elevated 30 degrees
- Check the neurological and vital signs
- Encourage more oral fluids
- Provide light soft diet if no nausea and vomiting
- Mild analgesics may be given if headache persists.
- Check the client's ability to void
- Observe for fever, stiff neck, photophobia or the signs of chemical or bacterial meningitis.

Intravenous Pyelography

An intravenous pyelogram also called an excretory urogram, is an X-ray exam of your urinary tract. An intravenous pyelogram lets your doctor view your kidneys, your bladder and the tubes that carry urine from your kidneys to your bladder (ureters). An intravenous pyelogram may be used to diagnose disorders that affect the urinary tract, such as kidney stones, bladder stones, enlarged prostate, kidney cysts or urinary tract tumors. During an intravenous pyelogram, you'll have an X-ray dye (iodine contrast solution) injected into a vein in your arm. The dye flows into your kidneys, ureters and bladder, outlining each of these structures. X-ray pictures are taken at specific times during the exam, so your doctor can clearly see your urinary tract and assess how well it's working.

Indications: An intravenous pyelogram may be used to help diagnose conditions that affect the urinary tract, such as:
- Kidney stones
- Bladder stones
- Enlarged prostate
- Kidney cysts
- Urinary tract tumors
- Structural kidney disorders, such as medullary sponge kidney—a birth defect of the tiny tubes inside the kidneys.

In the past, intravenous pyelogram was the most frequently used imaging test for evaluating possible urinary tract disorders. Since the development of kidney (renal) ultrasound and CT scans-which take less time and don't require X-ray dye- use of intravenous pyelograms has become less common. However, an intravenous pyelogram still can be a helpful diagnostic tool, particularly for:
- Identifying certain structural urinary tract disorders
- Detecting kidney stones
- Providing information about urinary tract obstruction.

Risk factors: In some people, the injection of X-ray dye can cause side effects such as:
- A feeling of warmth or flushing
- A metallic taste in the mouth
- Lightheadedness
- Nausea
- Itching
- Hives.

Rarely, severe reactions to the dye occur, including:
- Extremely low blood pressure
- A sudden, full-body allergic reaction that can cause breathing difficulties and other life-threatening symptoms (anaphylactic shock)
- Cardiac arrest.

CONCLUSION

Proper sample collection and handling is an integral part of obtaining a valid and timely laboratory test result. Specimens must be obtained using proper phlebotomy techniques, collected in the proper container, correctly labeled (in the presence of the patient) and promptly transported to the laboratory. It is the policy of the laboratory to reject samples when there is failure to follow these guidelines. All specimens should be handled with universal precautions, as if they are hazardous and infectious. Careful attention to routine procedures can eliminate most of the errors outlined in this section. Materials provided by the laboratory for specimen collection can maintain the quality of the specimen only when they are used in strict accordance with the instructions provided. All laboratory specimens shall be placed in leak proof containers (i.e. culturettes, vacuum tubes), then bagged in single, biohazard specimen bags. Place the requisition slip in the outside pocket of the biohazard specimen bag.

BIBLIOGRAPHY

1. Alice L Price. The Art, Science and Spirit of Nursing, Philadelphia, WB Saunders Company, 3rd edition, 1968.
2. Clinical Microbiology Procedures Handbook; 1992; Isenberg; American Society for Microbiology.
3. Henry, J. B. Clinical Diagnosis and Management of Laboratory Methods, 20th edition. Philadelphia: W. B. Saunders Company, 2001.
4. Kozier Barbara B, Du Gas Beverly Witter. Fundamentals of Patient Care: A Comprehensive Approach to Nursing; WB Saunders Company; 1967.
5. McClosky, JC, Grace HK. Current Issues in Nursing, 4th edition. St. Louis: Mosby Year Book, Inc, 1994.
6. Mitchell PR, Grippando GM. Nursing Perspectives and Issues, 5th edition Albany, New York: Delmar Publishers, Inc., 1993.
7. Potter P Perry A. Fundamentals of Nursing: Concepts, Process and Practice 3rd edition. Mosby Year Book; 1993.
8. Shafer Kathleen, et al. Medical-Surgical Nursing 6th edition. Saint Louis; CV Mosby Co; 1975.
9. Shakuntala Sharma 'Birpuri', Principles and Practice of Nursing. Jaypee Brothers Medical Publishers (P) Ltd, New Delhi, 1997.
10. Sr. Nancy. Principles and Practice of Nursing; Vol. 1, 3rd edition. NR Brothers, Indore, 1992.
11. Taylor C, Lillis C, LeMone P. Fundamentals of Nursing: The Art and Science of Nursing Care. Philadelphia: JB Lippincott, 1993.
12. Thresvamma CP. Fundamentals of Nursing, Procedure Manual for General Nursing Course, PC Mathew, Kottayam, Kerala, January, 1992.
13. Tierney, Lawrence M, Stephen J. McPhee, Maxine A Papadakis. Current Medical Diagnosis and Treatment 2001, 40th edition. New York: Lange Medical Books/McGraw-Hill, 2001.
14. Virginia Henderson. Principles and Practice of Nursing, New York, MacMillan Publishing Co. 1970.
15. Wallach, Jacques. Interpretation of Diagnostic Tests, 7th edition Philadelphia: Lippincott Williams & Wilkins, 2000.

REVIEW QUESTIONS

Long Essays

1. Define specimen collection, explain the purpose, principles.
2. Define endoscopies, explain bronchoscopy procedure.
3. Define radiological studies, explain in brief about X-ray procedure.

Short Essays

1. Urine collections from catheter.
2. Complete blood count.
3. Liver function test.
4. Monitoring capillary blood glucose.
5. 24-Hour urine collection.
6. Sputum culture.
7. Cystoscopy.
8. Colonoscopy.
9. Blood culture.
10. Intravenous pyelography.
11. Cardiac catheterization.
12. Esophagogastroduodenoscopy.

Short Answers

1. Salient features of diagnostic testing.
2. Red blood cell (RBC) count.
3. Serum electrolytes.
4. Lipid/lipoprotein profile.
5. Types of sigmoidoscopy.
6. Throat swab.
7. Blood smear.
8. Vaginal swab/smear.
9. Fluoroscopy.
10. Types of angiography.
11. Venography.
12. Roentgenogram.
13. Endoscopic retrograde cholangio-pancreatography.

MULTIPLE CHOICE QUESTIONS

1. **Which of the method or test is used for hemoglobin estimation?**
   a. Snellen's chart
   b. Rothera test
   c. Nitric acid test
   d. Sahli's method
2. **Normal fasting blood sugar value:**
   a. 80–140 mg/dL
   b. 70–110 mg/dL
   c. Less than 60 mg/dL
   d. Less than 140 mg/dL
3. **Specimen used for occult blood:**
   a. Blood
   b. Sputum
   c. Stool
   d. Surgical drain
4. **Which of the following is to be evaluated in order to assess risk for cardiovascular disease?**
   a. VLDL and hematocrit
   b. LDL and HDL
   c. LDL and Hb
   d. VLDL and Hb
5. **Which of the following abnormal blood value would not be improved by dialysis?**
   a. Hypernatremia
   b. Hyperkalemia
   c. Elevated serum creatinine level
   d. Decreased hemoglobin level

ANSWERS

1. d   2. b   3. c   4. b   5. d

CHAPTER 20
Oxygenation Needs

LEARNING OBJECTIVES

- Review of cardiovascular and respiratory physiology
- Factors affecting respiratory functioning
- Alterations in respiratory functioning
- Conditions affecting:
  - Airway
  - Movement of air
  - Diffusion
  - Oxygen transport
- Alterations in oxygenation
- Nursing interventions to promote oxygenation—assessment, types, equipment used and procedure
  - Maintenance of patent airway
  - Oxygen administration
- Suctioning—oral, tracheal
- Chest physiotherapy—percussion, vibration and postural drainage
- Care of chest drainage—principles and purposes
- Pulse oximetry—factors affecting measurement of oxygen saturation using pulse oximeter, interpretation
- Restorative and continuing care:
  - Hydration
  - Humidification
  - Coughing techniques
  - Breathing exercises
  - Incentive spirometry

TERMINOLOGY

- **Aerobic:** With oxygen.
- **Anaerobic:** Without oxygen.
- **Anoxia:** No oxygen reaching the brain.
- **Apnea:** Absence of breathing.
- **Apneustic breathing:** Prolonged gasping inspiration and short inefficient expiration.
- **Asthmatic breathing:** Difficulty on expiration with an audible expiratory wheeze. Caused by spasm of the respiratory passages and partial blockage by increased mucus secretion.
- **Biot's respirations:** Periods of hyperpnea occurring in normal respiration. Sometimes seen in clients with meningitis.
- **Bradypnea:** Slow but regular breathing. Normal in sleep but may be a sign of opiate use, alcohol indulgence or brain tumor.
- **Cheyne-Stokes respirations:** Gradual cycle of increased rate and depth followed by gradual decrease with the pattern repeating every 45 seconds to three minutes. Also associated with periods of apnea, particularly in the dying.
- **Cyanosis:** A bluish appearance of the skin and mucous membranes caused by inadequate oxygenation.
- **Dyspnea:** Difficulty breathing.
- **Expiration:** The act of breathing out.
- **Hemoptysis:** Blood in the sputum.
- **Homeostasis:** The automatic self-regulation of man to maintain the normal state of the body under a variety of environmental conditions.
- **Hypercapnia:** High partial pressure of carbon dioxide.
- **Hyperpnea:** Deep breathing with marked use of abdominal muscles.
- **Hyperventilation:** Increased rate and depth of breathing.
- **Hypoventilation:** Irregular, slow, shallow breathing.
- **Hypoxia:** A lack of oxygen concentration.
- **Hypoxemia:** A lack of oxygen in the blood.
- **Inspiration:** The act of breathing in.
- **Kussmaul's respirations:** Increased respiratory rate (above 20 rpm), increased depth, panting labored breathing. Causes include diabetic ketoacidosis and renal failure.
- **Orthopnea:** The ability to breathe easily only when in an upright position.
- **Perfusion:** The flow of oxygenated blood to the tissues.
- **Stridor:** A harsh, vibrating, shrill sound produced during respiration. Usually indicates an obstruction.
- **Tachypnea:** Increased rate of breathing.
- **Tracheostomy:** Making of an opening into the trachea or windpipe.
- **Ventilation:** The movement of air in and out of the lungs.

INTRODUCTION

Oxygen is vital for metabolic processes in cells and therefore the function of tissues within the body. The atmospheric content of oxygen within room air is only 21%. Although this amount is adequate for healthy individuals, those with certain diseases can benefit from an increased oxygen fraction in the gas they breathe, which will increase the oxygen content of their blood. Oxygen therapy refers to the administration of supplemental oxygen as part of managing illness. In healthy individuals, oxygen is absorbed from the air in adequate amounts, but certain diseases and conditions can prevent some people from absorbing enough oxygen. It may be administered as a medical intervention to manage short-term (acute) or emergency situations or as a part of long-term patient care. Oxygen therapy may therefore be a key tool in the hospital setting to manage a medical emergency or in the home setting to manage long-standing illness.

REVIEW OF CARDIOVASCULAR PHYSIOLOGY

The human heart is a hollow organ that lies between the left and right lungs, slightly on the left side and quite close to the center of the chest. It is protected within the body by the ribs. The heart is an involuntary muscle that contracts and relaxes so that it is able to send and pump blood throughout the entire body. This pumping action is enabled by the electrical impulses that it conducts from and to the areas of the heart itself.

The heart cycle consists of two phases which are systole and diastole. Systole is the contraction of the heart and diastole is the rest phase of the heart. Each beat of the heart consists of both systole and diastole. The "lub dub" of the heart is systole and diastole, respectively.

Under normal circumstances, the heart beats from 60 to 100 times per minute or from 3,600 beats to 6,000 per hour. A pulse rate of less than 60 per minute is called bradycardia or a slower than normal heart rate and a pulse rate of more than 100 per minute is referred to as tachycardia or a more rapid than normal heart rate.

The right side of the heart has the pulmonary circulation pathway which moves blood to the lungs for reoxygenation and the left side of the heart has the systemic circulation which moves oxygenated blood to the rest of the body.

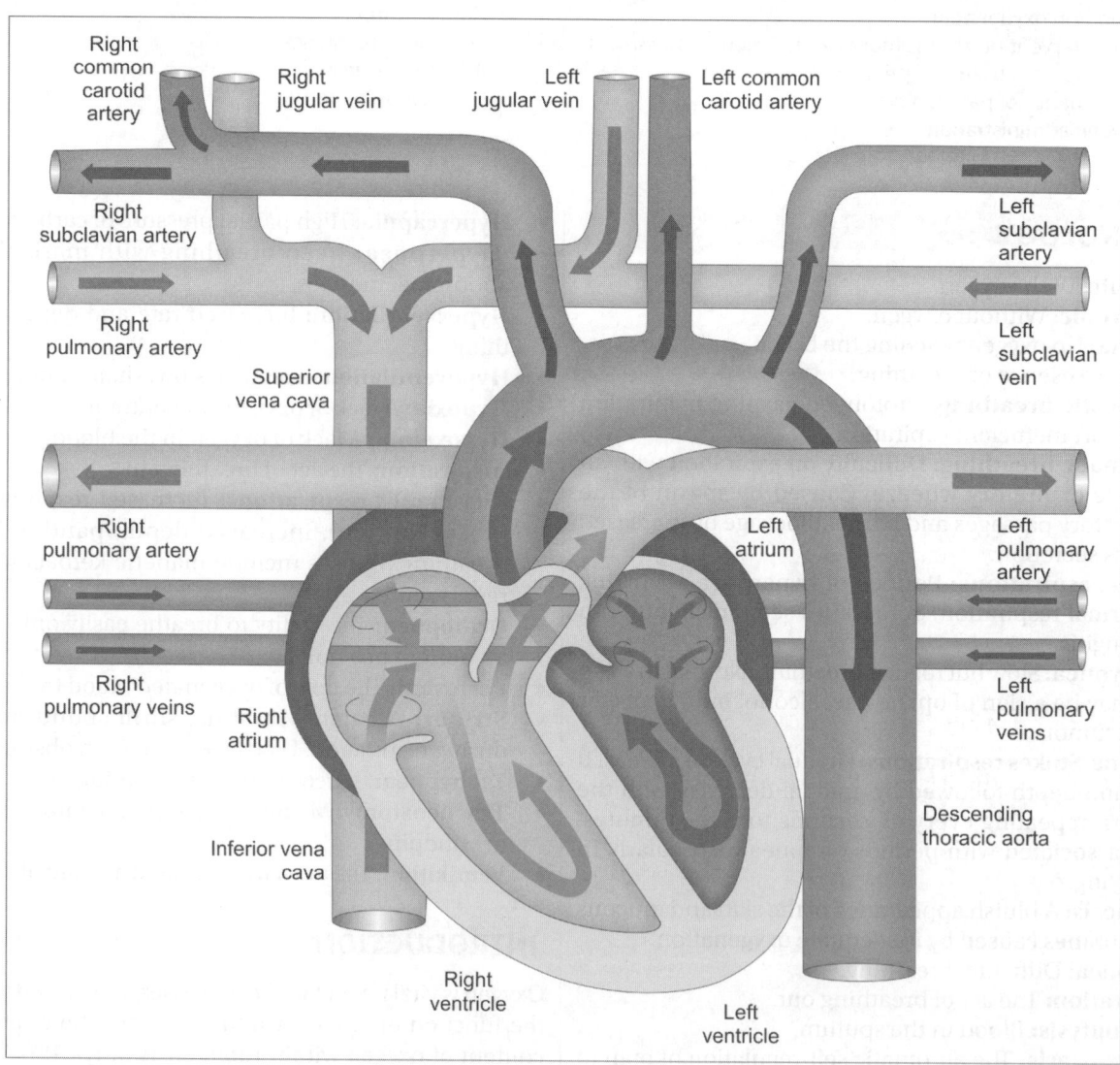

Fig. 20.1: Blood circulation in the heart.

The pulmonary circulation pathway, in the correct sequential order, consists of:
- Deoxygenated blood is sent into the right atrium from the superior and inferior vena cava which are the major veins of the body.
- Deoxygenated blood from the right atrium goes through the right atrioventricular valve into the right ventricle.
- The right ventricle contracts.
- The deoxygenated blood from the right ventricle goes through the pulmonary valve into the pulmonary artery.
- The pulmonary artery carries the deoxygenated blood into the lungs for reoxygenation.

The systemic circulation pathway begins after the last phase of the pulmonary circulation pathway. The systemic circulation pathway begins after the pulmonary artery carries the deoxygenated blood into the lungs for reoxygenation.

The systemic circulation pathway, in the correct sequential order, consists of:
- The newly oxygenated blood goes through the pulmonary veins from the lungs into the left atrium of the heart.
- The blood from the left atrium of the heart flows into the left ventricle after it passes through the left atrioventricular valve.
- The left ventricle contracts.
- The blood from the left ventricle of the heart flows into the aorta and then to the rest of the body after it passes through the aortic valve.

REVIEW OF RESPIRATORY PHYSIOLOGY

The organs of the respiratory system include the nose, pharynx, larynx, trachea, bronchi, and their smaller branches, and the lungs, which contain the alveoli.

The functions of the respiratory system are:
- Oxygen supplier: The job of the respiratory system is to keep the body constantly supplied with oxygen.
- Elimination: Elimination of carbon dioxide.
- Gas exchange: The respiratory system organs oversee the gas exchanges that occur between the blood and the external environment.
- Passageway: Passageways that allow air to reach the lungs.
- Humidifier: Purify, humidify, and warm incoming air.

Physiology of the Respiratory System

The major function of the respiratory system is to supply the body with oxygen and to dispose of carbon dioxide. To do this, at least four distinct events, collectively called respiration, must occur.

Respiration

- Pulmonary ventilation: Air must move into and out of the lungs so that gases in the air sacs are continuously refreshed, and this process is commonly called breathing.
- External respiration: Gas exchange between the pulmonary blood and alveoli must take place.
- Respiratory gas transport: Oxygen and carbon dioxide must be transported to and from the lungs and tissue cells of the body via the bloodstream.
- Internal respiration: At systemic capillaries, gas exchanges must be made between the blood and tissue cells.

Mechanics of Breathing

- Rule: Volume changes lead to pressure changes, which lead to the flow of gasses to equalize pressure.
- Inspiration: Air is flowing into the lungs; chest is expanded laterally, the rib cage is elevated, and the diaphragm is depressed and flattened; lungs are stretched to the larger thoracic volume, causing the intrapulmonary pressure to fall and air to flow into the lungs.
- Expiration: Air is leaving the lungs; the chest is depressed and the lateral dimension is reduced, the rib cage is descended, and the diaphragm is elevated and dome-shaped; lungs recoil to a smaller volume, intrapulmonary pressure rises, and air flows out of the lung.
- Intrapulmonary volume: Intrapulmonary volume is the volume within the lungs.
- Intrapleural pressure: The normal pressure within the pleural space, the intrapleural pressure, is always negative, and this is the major factor preventing the collapse of the lungs.
- Nonrespiratory air movements: Nonrespiratory movements are a result of reflex activity, but some may be produced voluntarily such as cough, sneeze, crying, laughing, hiccups, and yawn.

FACTORS AFFECTING RESPIRATORY FUNCTIONING

Lung function reference values are traditionally based on anthropometric factors, such as weight, height, sex, and age. Forced vital capicity (FVC) and forced expiratory volume in 1 second (FEV_1) decline with age, while volumes and capacities, such as residual volume (RV) and functional residual capacity (FRC), increase. Total lung capacity (TLC), vital capacity (VC), RV, FVC and FEV_1 are affected by height, since they are proportional to body size.

Men have longer airways than women, causing greater specific resistance in the respiratory tract. The increased work of breathing to increase ventilation among women means that their consumption of oxygen is higher than men under similar conditions of physical intensity. Lung volumes are higher when the subject is standing than in other positions.

Factors Influence Respiration

- Sex: Female has slightly rapid respiration than the male.
- Exercise: Exertion of any type increase the metabolic rate and stimulate respiration
- Rest and sleep: During rest and sleep metabolize decreased so respiration rate is normal or decreased.

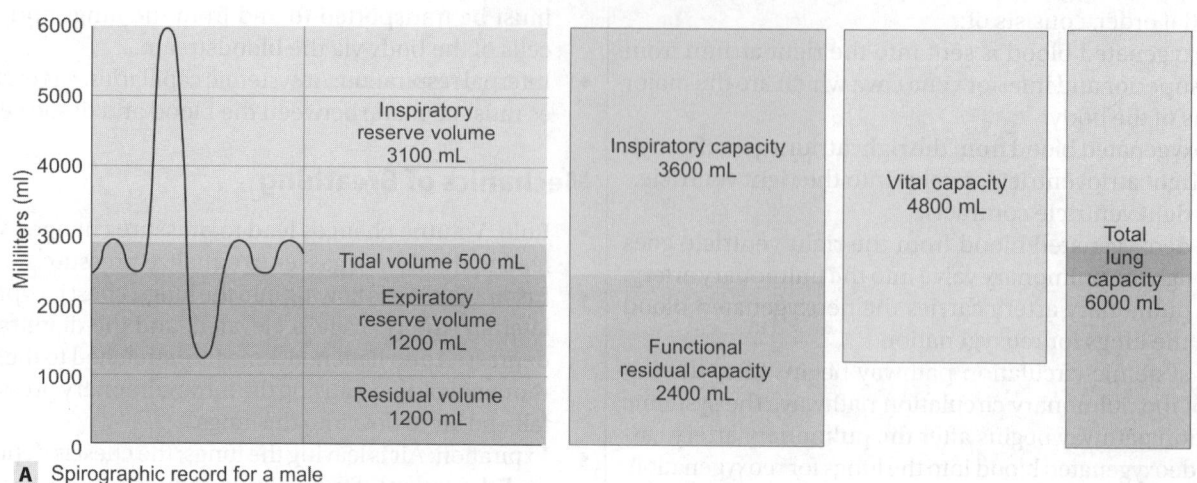

Figs. 20.2A and B: Respiratory volumes and capacities: (A) Spirographic record for a male; (B) Summary of respiratory volumes and capacities for males and females.

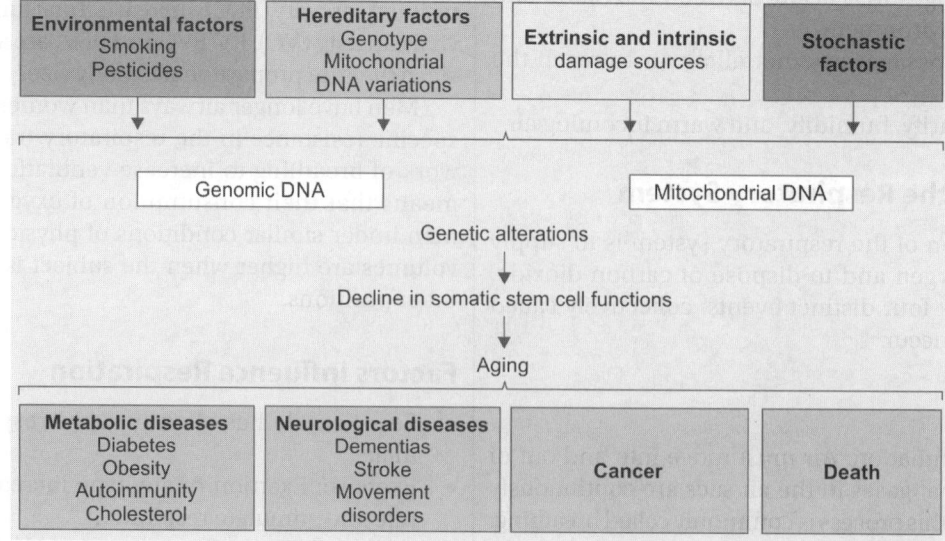

Fig. 20.3: Factors affecting oxygen status.

- **Emotions:** Sudden stressful condition such as fear and anxiety influences the respiratory rate.
- **Changes in atmospheric pressure:** In high altitudes the content of oxygen in the atmosphere is very low. So rate of respiration is increased and the increased demand of oxygen is fulfilled.

RESPIRATION: TYPES, ASSESSMENT, MANAGEMENT

Respiration is the act of breathing. It includes the intake of oxygen and the output of carbon dioxide, i.e. respiration consist of inspiration and expiration.

Types of Respiration

- **External respiration:** The exchange of gases between the blood and the air in the lungs is called as external or pulmonary respiration.
- **Internal respiration:** The exchange of gases between the blood and the tissue cells is called as internal or tissue respiration.
- **Regulation of respiration:** It is a rhythmical movement's respirations, which are regulated by respiratory centre in the brain called medulla oblongata, nerve fibers of the autonomic nervous system and the chemical composition of the blood.

Normal Rates

- At birth—30 to 40 breaths/minute
- One year—26 to 30 breaths/minute
- 2 to 5 years—20 to 26 breaths/minute
- Adolescence—20 breaths/minute
- Adults—16 to 20 breaths/minute
- Old age—10 to 24 breaths/minute.

Characteristics of Respiration

- Normal breathing is effortless.
- It is painless, quiet and automatic.
- Normal respiration consists of rhythmical rising and falling of the chest wall.
- Respiratory rate in resting adult is 16 to 18 breaths/minute.
- Eupnea: It is regular, even and produces no noise.

Abnormalities in Respiration

- **Apnea:** Respiration ceases for several seconds.
- **Dyspnea:** Difficult respiration. Increased effort has to be made in inspiration and expiration.
- **Bradypnea:** Rate of breathing is less than 10/minute of regular respiration.
- **Tachypnea:** Rate of breathing is more than 20/minute of regular respiration.
- **Hyperpnea:** Respiration is increased in depth and rate.
- **Orthopnea:** It is a respiratory condition in which a person must sit or stand to breathe comfortably.
- **Cheyne-Stokes respiration:** Respiratory rhythm is irregular, characterized by alternating periods of apnea and hyperventilation.
- **Kussumaul's respiration:** Respiration is abnormally deep but regular. Rate is increased. It is seen in diabetic ketoacidosis.
- **Biot's respiration:** It is shallow breathing interrupted by irregular periods of apnea, seen in central nervous system disorders.

TABLE 20.1: Types of normal and abnormal breathing patterns.

Breathing patterns		
Pattern	Condition	Description
～～～	Eupnea	Normal breathing rate and pattern
∧∧∧∧∧∧	Tachypnea	Increased respiratory rate
⌒⌒	Bradypnea	Decreased respiratory rate
———	Apnea	Absence of breathing
∧∧∧∧	Hyperpnea	Increased depth and rate of breathing
∧_∧∧∧_∧	Cheyne-Stokes	Gradual increases and decreases in respirations with periods of apnea
∧_∧∧_∧	Biot's	Abnormal breathing pattern with groups/clusters of rapid respiration of equal depth and regular apnea periods
∧∧∧∧∧∧	Kussmaul's breathing	Tachypnea and Hyperpnea
⊓⊓⊓⊓	Apneustic	Prolonged inspiratory phase with a prolonged expiratory phase

- **Sighing:** It expands the small air ways. It is a protective mechanism.
- **Noisy respiration:** Stertorous, grunting, expiration is forced; stridor-inspiration is forced; yawning inspiration is forced due to air hunger.
- **Hiccough:** It is due to spasms of diaphragm and glottis.

CARE OF PATIENT WITH DYSPNEA

Dyspnea is a clinical sign of hypoxia and manifests as breathlessness. It is the subjective sensation of difficult or uncomfortable breathing.

Dyspnea is shortness of breath associated with exercise a excitement but in some clients dyspnea may be present without any relation, to activity or exercise.

Dyspnea is associated with many conditions such as pulmonary diseases cardiovascular diseases, neuromuscular conditions and anemia. In addition dyspnea may occur in the pregnant women in the final months of pregnancy. Last environmental factors such as pollution cold air and smoking may also cause worsen dyspnea.

Causes

- Obstructions in air passages, e.g. mucus, vomit, blood or other fluid inhaled or foreign body such as teeth may occur during operation or tooth extraction.
- Pressure from outside, e.g. growth in the chest or neck or abdominal distension.
- Respiratory diseases such as asthma, pneumonia, tuberculosis.
- Heart failure anemia.

Types

- Dyspnea exertion
- Orthopnea.

These are commonly accompanying congestive heart failure and paroxysmal nocturnal dyspnea is an early sign of left ventricular failure.

Clinical Manifestations

- Exaggerated respiratory effort.
- Use of accessory muscles of respiration.
- Nasal flaring.
- Marked increases in the rate and depth of respirations.
- Cough.
- Wheezing.

Alterations in respiratory functioning	
Hypoventilation	**Hyperventilation**
Alveolar ventilation inadequate to meet the body's oxygen demand or to eliminate sufficient carbon dioxide	Ventilation in excess of that required to eliminate carbon dioxide produced by cellular metabolism
Hypoxia	**Cyanosis**
Inadequate tissue oxygenation at the cellular level	Blue discoloration of the skin and mucous membranes

Pathophysiology: Although dyspnea is a relatively common problem, the pathophysiology of the uncomfortable sensation of breathing is poorly understood. Unlike those for other types of noxious stimuli, there are no specialized dyspnea receptors (although recent MRI studies have identified a few specific areas in the midbrain that may mediate perception of dyspnea). The experience of dyspnea likely results from a complex interaction between chemoreceptor stimulation, mechanical abnormalities in breathing, and the perception of those abnormalities by the CNS. Some authors have described the imbalance between neurologic stimulation and mechanical changes in the lungs and chest wall as neuromechanical uncoupling.

Dyspnea Management

The underlying process that cause or worsen dyspnea must be treated and stabilized initially and then four additional therapies should be administered.

- **Medication (pharmacological) management**, e.g. bronchodilators, steroids, mucolytics, low dose antianxiety medications.
- **Oxygen therapy** as indicated: Oxygen therapy can reduce dyspnea associated with exercise.
- **Physical techniques**, e.g. cardiopulmonary reconditioning through exercises, breathing technique and enough control can reduce dyspnea.
- **Psychosocial technique,** e.g. relaxation technique biofeed back and meditations are physiological measure that can lessen the sensations of dysphone
  - Airway maintenance.
  - Mobilization of pulmonary secretions.
  - Humidification.
  - Nebulization.
  - Chest physiotherapy.
- **Postural drainage:** Postural drainage is the use of positioning technique that draw secretions from specific segments of the lungs and bronchi into the trachea.
- **Coughing or suctioning** usually removes secretions from the trachea.

Nursing care of dyspnea: Dyspnea is "a subjective experience of breathing discomfort that consists of qualitatively distinct sensations that vary in intensity". The causes of dyspnea are multiple, encompassing physiologic, psychological, social, and environmental etiologies that may lead to secondary physiologic and behavioral responses.

Nursing diagnosis: Ineffective breathing pattern related to hypoxia as evidence by shortness of breath with activity, use of accessory muscles, O_2 saturation of 85%, and abnormal ABGS.

Subjective data: Patient states she has been extremely short of breath for the past 12 hours, patient states her normal oxygen setting is 2 L but since she has became short of breath she increased it to 4 liters but says it hasn't helped and that is why she come to the ER.

Objective data: The patient breathing is fast and irregular (especially on activity and exertion). You hook the patient up to cardiac monitor and find her oxygen saturation to be 85%, HR 112, BP 150/86, and RR 36. Lungs sounds are diminished and hard to hear. Chest X-ray shows hyper-inflated lungs with flatten diaphragm correlating with. Chronic obstructive pulmonary disease (COPD). Arterial blood gases (ABGs) show PCO_2 60, pH 7.25, PO_2 50, O_2 Sat 85%.

Nursing outcomes:
- Patient oxygen saturation will be 90-100% throughout hospitalization.
- Patient respiratory rate will be 12-20 breaths per minute throughout hospitalization.
- Patient will demonstrate two breathing techniques to use during dyspneic episodes within 12 hours.
- Patient will verbalize two ways on how to prevent COPD exacerbation.

Nursing intervention:
- The nurse will place the patient on bilevel positive airway pressure (BiPAP) per minute order and assess patient's oxygen saturation every 30 minutes.
- The nurse will assess pt respiratory rate every 30 minutes within the first 8 hours and then every 4 hours when the patient's respiratory rate is 12-20 breaths per minute during hospitalization.
- The nurse will verbalized and demonstrate to the patient 4 breathing techniques to use during dyspnea episodes within 6 hours of the hospitalization.
- The nurse will verbalize four ways on how to prevent COPD exacerbation to the patient within 12 hours of hospitalization.

NEED OF OXYGEN THERAPY

Some acute and long-term (chronic) illnesses can reduce the amount of oxygen that is transferred from the alveoli in the lungs to the blood. Examples of these conditions include chronic obstructive pulmonary disease (COPD) and pneumonia. In people with these conditions, oxygen therapy can help them function better and become more active. A doctor performs tests such as the pulse oximetry test or arterial blood gas test to decide whether or not a person has a low oxygen level and requires oxygen therapy For most of the diseases that affect oxygen absorption, increasing the oxygen fraction to around 30 % to 35% is enough to make a significant improvement. This can be done using a nasal cannula, which is made up of two plastic tubes that are fitted into the nostrils. When 100% oxygen is needed, a tight-fitting face mask can be used and for infants, a 100% oxygen can be delivered to an incubator.

ACUTE DISEASES AFFECT BLOOD OXYGEN LEVEL

Oxygen therapy may be administered in hospital if someone suddenly develops an illness that prevents proper oxygen absorption. This therapy is stopped once the person has recovered from the condition. Some examples of illnesses where this short-term oxygen therapy is administered include the following:
- **Pneumonia:** This is a lung infection that can cause extreme inflammation of the alveoli and prevent oxygen moving from these air sacs into the bloodstream.
- **Bronchopulmonary dysplasia or respiratory distress syndrome in premature babies:** These are both serious lung conditions that can develop in premature babies. Such babies may be administered supplemental oxygen using a ventilator, a tube placed in the nostril or a nasal continuous positive airway pressure machine.
- **Asthma attack:** A severe asthma attack can inflame and narrow the airways, therefore requiring oxygen therapy if the attack cannot be managed using the medication a patient has been prescribed.
- **Chronic diseases that affect the blood oxygen level:** People with certain chronic diseases may require long-term oxygen therapy at home. Examples of these conditions include the following:
  - **Cystic fibrosis:** Cystic fibrosis is a genetic condition that affects the secretory glands that produce mucus and sweat. Patients with this condition develop a buildup of viscous, sticky mucus in their airways. This provides an environment that promotes bacterial growth and people with cystic fibrosis experience recurrent and severe lung infections that eventually cause serious lung damage.
  - **Chronic obstructive pulmonary disease:** Here, permanent damage to the alveoli prevents oxygen from moving out of the alveoli and into the blood. As the condition is progressive, COPD only worsens over time.
  - **Late-stage heart failure:** Here, the heart fails to pump enough blood around the body to provide it with an adequate level of oxygen.
  - **Sleep apnea:** This is a sleep disorder characterized by shallow or infrequent breathing that can lead to a low blood oxygen level while a patient is asleep.

FACTORS AFFECTING OXYGENATION

Sl. No.	Factors	Description
1.	Anemia	• Hemoglobin transports 99% of oxygen to tissues • Decreased Hb production, increased RBC destruction, blood loss
2.	Toxic inhalation	• Decreased binding sites • Carbon monoxide
3.	Increased metabolic rate	• Increased rate increased oxygen demand • Oxygenation decreased if unable to meet demand • Exercise, pregnancy, fever • Prolonged or high fever • Protein breakdown and muscle wasting • RR and depth to rid waste products (CO_2)
4.	Aging	Structural changes • Chest wall compliance, elastic recoil, functioning alveoli • Defense mechanisms • Cilia function, cough force, immunity • Respiratory control • Response to hypoxemia, hypercapnia

Contd...

Contd...

Sl. No.	Factors	Description
5.	Deceased inspired O_2 concentration	• Upper or lower airway obstruction • Decreased environmental oxygen • Incorrect setting on oxygen delivery equipment
6.	Hyperventilation	• in excess of cellular need for oxygen • Enhances alveolar ventilation and flushes out CO_2 • Decreased pCO_2 producing alkalosis • Usually self limiting • Increases Hb affinity for O_2, O_2 held onto the RBC
7.	Respiratory risk factors	Increased age • Nutrition • Cigarette smoking • Substance abuse • Exercise • Environmental pollution • Stress/anxiety

ALTERATIONS IN OXYGENATION: HYPOXIA

Hypoxia is lack of oxygen at the tissue level while hypoxaemia implies a low arterial oxygen tension below the normal expected value (85–100 mm Hg).

Definition: Hypoxia is an insufficient supply of oxygen to meet the demands of the body.

Types: There are four basic types of hypoxia.
- **Hypoxic hypoxia** occurs when there is a deficiency in oxygen exchange in the lungs. Some causes include:
  - Decreased partial pressure of oxygen available at altitude.
  - Conditions that block the exchange at the alveolar capillary level (e.g. pneumonia, pulmonary edema, asthma, drowning).
- **Anemic (hypemic) hypoxia** occurs when the body cannot transport the available oxygen to the target tissues.
  Causes include:
  - Anemia from acute or chronic blood loss.
  - Carbon monoxide poisoning.
  - Medications: such as aspirin, sulfonamides and nitrites.
  - Methemoglobinemia.
  - Sickle cell disease.
- **Stagnant hypoxia** occurs when there is insufficient blood flow. Causes include:
  - Heart failure.
  - Decreased circulating blood volume.
  - Vasodilatation.
  - Venous pooling due to G-forces.
  - Continuous positive pressure ventilation.
  - G-forces.
- **Histotoxic (histologic) hypoxia** occurs when the body's tissues are not able to use the oxygen that has been delivered to them. This is not a "true hypoxia" because the tissue oxygenation levels may be at or above normal. Causes include:
  - Cyanide poisoning.
  - Alcohol consumption.
  - Narcotics.

Susceptibility to Hypoxia

Factors: Everyone becomes hypoxic to some degree when exposed to decreased partial pressures of oxygen at altitude. Some factors beyond atmospheric pressure can cause some people to react as they would at altitude even when they are at sea level. These are what create a person's physiologic altitude. The following factors affect physiologic altitude.
- Smoking (due to high baseline levels of carboxyhemoglobin)-3 quick cigarettes or 1–1.5 pk/day = 2,000 foot physiological altitude.
- Alcohol consumption (due to histotoxic hypoxia)—one ounce of alcohol = 2,000 foot physiological altitude.
- Coffee (secondary to the stimulant effects of caffeine)—5 cups = 2,500 foot physiological altitude.
- Anemia (due to anemic hypoxia).

The following factors also can affect the body's response to changes in altitude:
- Medications, such as aspirin, nitrites and sulfa.
- Chronic obstructive pulmonary disease (COPD).
- Diet.
- Level of physical fitness.
- Emotional state.
- Baseline metabolic rate.
- Fever or low body temperature (higher temperature tends to lower hemoglobin (Hgb) O_2 saturation).
- High or low pH:
  - Low pH makes it harder for the hemoglobin to bind to oxygen (requiring a higher partial pressure to achieve the same oxygen saturation), but it makes it easier for the hemoglobin to release bound oxygen.
  - High pH makes it easier for the hemoglobin to pick up oxygen but harder for it to release it to the tissues.
  - Duration of exposure to altitude-the longer the exposure, the more profound the affect.
  - Change in altitude-the greater the change in altitude, the greater the affect.

The sum of a person's actual altitude, his or her physiological altitude, along with the duration of exposure and the degree of change in altitude help determine how each person will react during air medical transport flights.

Stages of Hypoxia

There are four stages of hypoxia. The amount of time spent in any one of these four stages may vary, and each patient and provider is likely to respond differently to the same conditions. The air medical escort needs to be alert to the signs and symptoms of hypoxia. There are four stages of hypoxia:

- **Asymptomatic or indifferent:** People are not generally aware of the effects of hypoxia at this stage. The primary symptoms are a loss of night vision and a loss of color vision. These changes can occur at relatively modest altitudes (as low as 4,000 feet) and are probably most significant to pilots operating at night. Arterial oxygen saturations are typically between 90 and 95 percent.
- **Compensatory:** In healthy people, this stage may occur at altitudes between 10,000 and 15,000 feet. The body generally has the ability to stave off further effects of hypoxia by increasing the rate and depth of ventilation and cardiac output. Arterial oxygen saturations during this phase are typically between 80 and 90 percent.
- **Deterioration or disturbance:** In this state, people are unable to compensate for the lack of oxygen. Unfortunately, not everyone recognizes or experiences the signs and symptoms associated with this stage. If they do not, they cannot take steps to correct the problem. Arterial oxygen saturations during this phase typically are between 70 and 80 percent.
- **Critical:** This is the terminal stage leading up to death. People are almost completely incapacitated physically and mentally. People in this stage will lose consciousness, have convulsions, stop breathing and finally die. Arterial oxygen saturations are less than 70 percent.

Monitoring oxygen levels: Pulse oximeters are the most common device for monitoring patients' oxygen status. While a useful tool, pulse oximeters are not a replacement for an arterial blood gas or for looking at the patient. They simply measure the saturation of the hemoglobin present in the blood, not the actual amount of oxygen in the blood. Pulse oximeters cannot differentiate which gas is bound to the hemoglobin, so readings are falsely elevated in carbon monoxide poisoning. Low flow states (shock), cold, and bright light can also make the readings unreliable.

CARE OF OXYGEN CYLINDERS

Nurses frequently have to administer oxygen but it should be remembered that oxygen could have harmful effects as well as beneficial ones; it is often forgotten that oxygen is a drug that has to be prescribed. Prior to administering any drug the nurse is expected to have a sound knowledge of what is being administered, along with contraindications and its side-effects. The aim of this article is to update nurses on the properties of oxygen, how it should be prescribed, different ways of administering and what the indications are for administering the oxygen in the first place. For the purpose. **Oxygen therapy** is the administration of oxygen as a medical intervention, which can be for a variety of purposes in both chronic and acute patient care. Oxygen is essential for cell metabolism, and in turn, tissue oxygenation is essential for all normal physiological functions. Room air only contains 21% oxygen, and increasing the fraction of oxygen in the breathing gas increases the amount of oxygen in the blood. It is often only required to raise the fraction of oxygen delivered to 30 to 35% and this is done by use of a nasal cannula. When 100% oxygen is needed, it may be delivered via a tight-fitting face mask, or by supplying 100% oxygen to an incubator in the case of infants.

- Handle the cylinder with care.
- Oxygen stand should be used to prevent falling and causing injury to someone or to the equipment.
- It should be always placed at the head of the bed.
- Oxygen does not cause fire but it supports combustion. So avoid any source of fire from the cylinder for fear of fire.
- Visitors and other patients may need to be reminded. Hang "No smoking" board to the oxygen cylinder.
- Oxygen cylinders should be stored in a cool temperature, because high temperature can cause expansion of the gas with consequent loss of gas through the safety valve.
- Do not use electric appliances close to oxygen.
- Oil or grease should not be used on the regulator, because in the presence of high oxygen concentration, oil is likely to catch the fire and the cylinder may explore.
- Mark empty cylinder, replace protection cap, and set aside from full cylinders.
- Inspect the apparatus at frequent intervals and make sure that it is in working condition. The nurse should learn the working of cylinders, its regulators etc. before handling the apparatus.

Precautions:
- Giving oxygen is an emergency procedure, so it should be ready for 24 hours.
- The nurse should see that the cylinders are full and all the apparatus is in working condition, the key is attached with the cylinder in a bag.

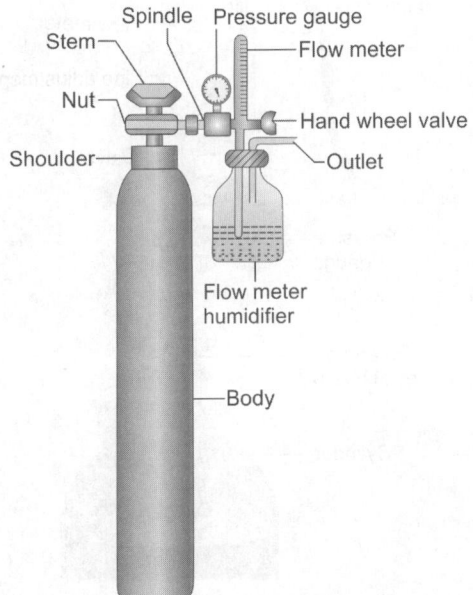

Fig. 20.4: Oxygen delivery system.

- There should not be any leakage in rubber tubing.
- There should be written order for O_2 inhalation and specific does must be prescribed to avoid oxygen toxicity.
- Use regular to reduce the pressure of the oxygen in the cylinder to a safer level.
- Measure the flow in litres per minute. Adjust the flow of oxygen 2 to 4 litres per minute for adults when the nasal catheter is used.
- Use sterile or disposable nasal catheters to avoid infection.
- The catheter should be changed at least every 8 hourly to avoid blockage of catheter.
- The catheter may be taped to the forehead for the comfort of the patient and to keep it in place.
- Patient's nostrils should be lubricated with petroleum jelly, if there is any sign of irritation.
- Oxygen administration must never be stopped until the cause of hypoxia is reversed.
- If nurse is leaving the patient for short period, leave a call bell near the patient.
- The premature babies should be given oxygen inhalation only for a short time and at a very low concentration to avoid retrolental fibroplasia.
- Observe the patient, receiving oxygen inhalation continuously to detect early signs of oxygen toxicity.
- Since oxygen helps in combustion, fire precautions are to be taken when the oxygen is on flow.

Dangers of oxygen therapy: There are three types of risks associated with oxygen use.

- **Physical risks:** Oxygen being combustible, fire hazard and tank explosion is always there. This is more with high concentration of oxygen, use of pressure chambers, and in smokers. Catheters and masks can cause injury to the nose and mouth. Dry and non-humidified gas can cause dryness and crusting.
- **Functional risks:** Patients who have lost sensitivity to CO_2 and are upon the hypoxic drive are in danger of ventilator depression as seen in patients of COPD. Hypoventilation can lead to hypercapnia and CO_2 narcosis although the risk is small with low flow oxygen therapy. Arterial pH may be a better guide than $PaCO_2$ for monitoring oxygen therapy. As long as pH does not suggest acidosis, long term oxygen therapy can benefit the patients with CO_2 retention.
- **Cytotoxic damage:** COPD patients on long term oxygen therapy, on autopsy, show proliferative and fibrotic changes in their lungs. In acute conditions, most of the structural damage occurs from high FiO_2 as the oxygen can lead to the release of various reactive species which attack the DNA, lipids, and SH containing proteins.

OXYGEN ADMINISTRATION

Oxygen administration treats the effects of oxygen deficiency (anoxemia) but it does not correct the underlying causes.

Oxygen therapy is important to keep a healthy level of tissue oxygenation.

Purpose:
- To supply O_2 in conditions when there is interference with normal oxygenation of blood.
- To reduce the effects of anoxemia.
- To maintain healthy level in tissue oxygenation.

Classification: Oxygen is administered by either low flow or high flow systems. Low flow administration devices include nasal cannula, oxygen mask, oxygen tent, etc. High flow administration devices include venturi mask, some devices can be used for both low and high flow administration, e.g. oxygen hood incubator, etc.

NASAL CANNULA

It is the most important low flow device used to administer oxygen of a rubber or plastic tube that extends around the face with 6-1. Curved prongs that fit into the nostrits. One side of the tube connects to oxygen tubing and oxygen

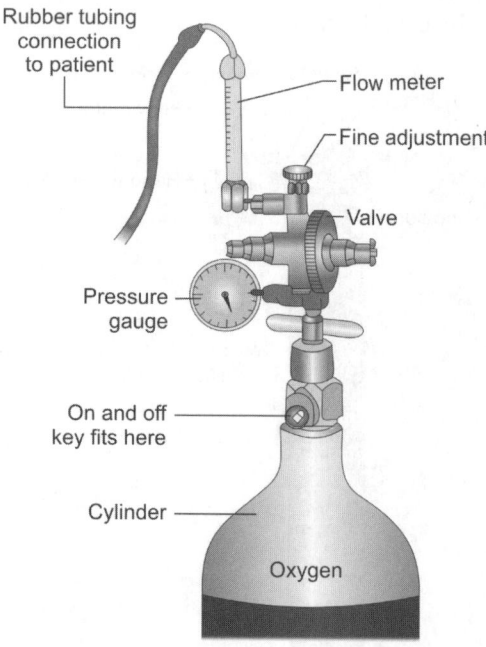

Fig. 20.5: Oxygen cylinder and connections.

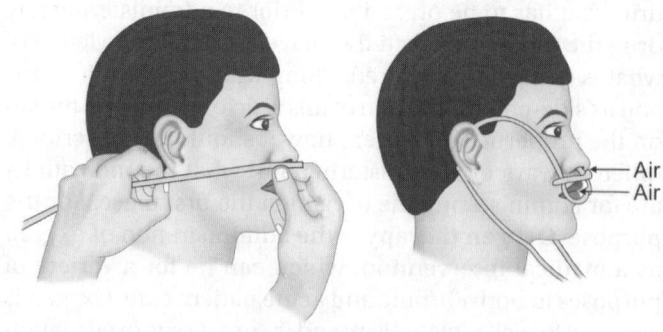

Fig. 20.6: Oxygen administration by nasal cannula.

supply. The cannula is often held in place by an elastic band that fits around the clients head or under the chin.

The nasal cannula is easy to apply and does not interfere with client's ability to eat or talk. It is very comfortable and permits some freedom of movement. Oxygen is delivered via the cannula with a flow rate of up to 4 L/min. Higher flow rates dry air mucous and do not further increases inspired oxygen concentrations.

Equipment

- Oxygen supply with a flow meter.
- Humidifier with sterile distilled water.
- Nasal cannula and tubing.
- Tape if needed to secure the cannula in place.
- Gauze to pad the tubing over the cheek.

Procedure

- Determine the need for oxygen therapy and the physicians order.
- Assist the client to a semi-Fowler's position as possible. It permits easier chest expansion easier breathing.
- Explain about the procedure and inform the client and support persons about safety precautions connected with oxygen use.
- Set-up the oxygen equipment and humidified.
- Turn on the oxygen at the prescribed rate and ensure proper functioning.
- Put the cannula over the client's face.
- If the cannula will not stay in place tape if at sides of face.
- Slip gauze pads under the tubing over the cheek bones to prevent skin irritation as necessary.
- Assess the client regularly.
- Assess the vital signs, color, breathing pattern and chest movement.
- Check the equipment are working regularly.
- Make sure that safety precautions are being followed.
- Record initiation of therapy and all nursing assessments.

NASAL CATHETER

Nasal catheters are used infrequently but they are not absolute. The procedure involves inserting an oxygen catheter into the nose to the nasopharynx. Because securing the catheter must be changed at least every 8 hours and inserted into the other nostril, for this reason, the nasal catheter is a less described method because the client may have pain when the catheter is passed into nasopharynx and because trauma can occur to the nasal mucosa. The nasal catheter permits free movements for the patient and nursing care may be given with much more ease (Figs. 20.7A and B).

OXYGEN MASK

An oxygen mask is a device used to administer oxygen, humidity it is shaped to fit tightly over the mouth and nose

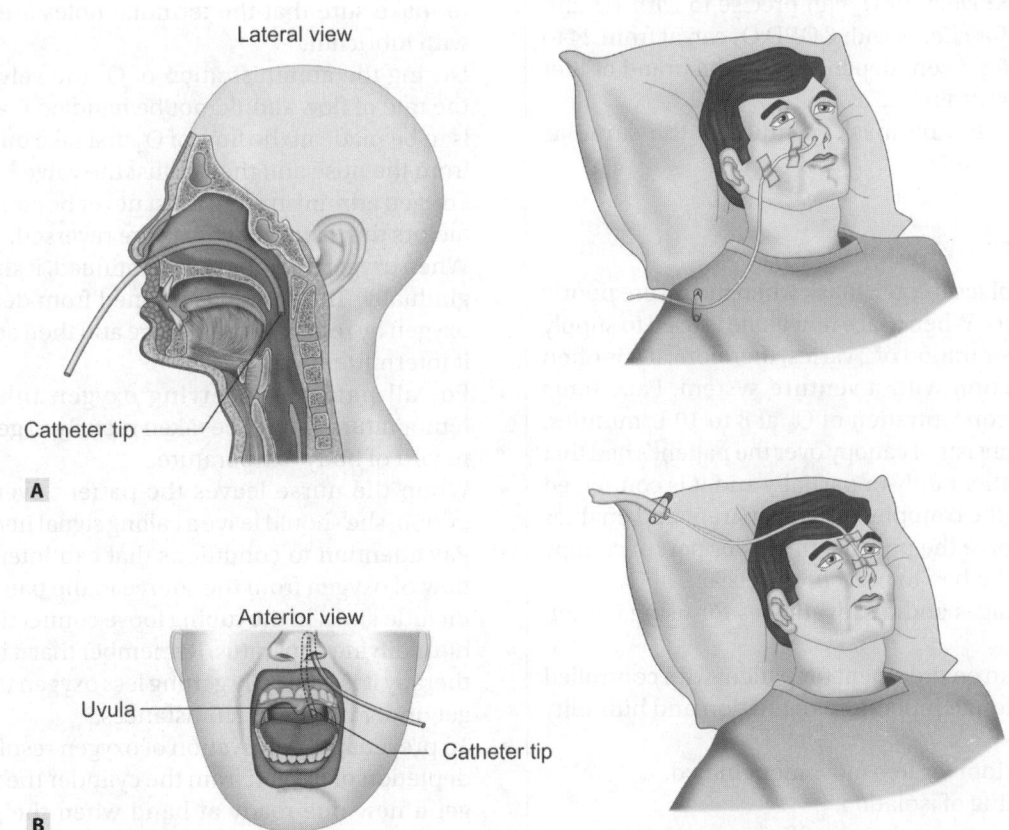

Figs. 20.7A and B: Oxygen administration by nasal catheter: (A) Lateral view; (B) Anterior view.

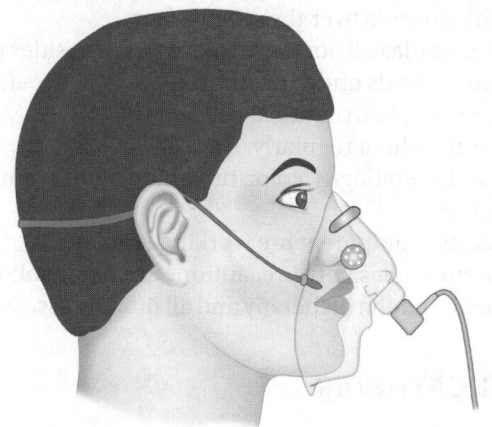

Fig. 20.8: Oxygen administration by simple face mask.

and is secured in place with a strap. There are four types of oxygen masks:

i. **Simple face masks:** Used for short-term oxygen therapy. If delivers O_2 concentration from 40 to 60 percent at liter flows of 5 to 8 liters per minute.
ii. **The partial rebreather mask:** Delivers O_2 concentrated of 60 to 90 percent liter flows of 6 to 10 L per minute (Fig. 20.8).
iii. **The nonrebreather mask:** Delivers the highest O_2 can possible by means other than inhibition or mechanical ventilation that is 95 to 100 percent at liter flows of 6 to 15 L/minutes.
iv. **Venturi mask:** Delivers O_2 can precise to with 1.1 and is often used for clients with COPD O_2 can at from 24 to 40 percent/50 percent depending on the brand at liter flows of 4 to 8 L/minute.

Initiating oxygen by mask in mucous the same as initiating O_2 by cannula.

OXYGEN TENT

Fact tents can replace oxygen mask when masks are poorly tolerated by clients. When a face tent alone is used to supply oxygen, the concentration of 2 varies, therefore, if it is often used in conjunction with a venture system. Face tents provide varying concentration of O_2 at 8 to 10 L/minutes. An oxygen tent consists of canopy over the patient's bed that may cover the patient fully or partially and it is connected to a supply of O_2 the canopies are transparent and enables the nurse to observe the patient. The lower part of canopy is tucked under the bed to prevent the escape of O_2. There are some advantages and disadvantages for using oxygen tent these are:

- If it provides an environment for patient with controlled 2 concentration, temperature regulation and humidity control.
- It allows freedom for free movement in bed.
- It creates feeling of isolation.
- There is an increased chance of fire.
- It requires much time and effort to clean and maintain a tent.
- Loss of desired concentration occurs each time, the tent is opened to provide care for patient.
- Since it requires high volume of oxygen, it cannot be made available ordinarily.

General Instructions

- Since oxygen acts as a drug. It must be prescribed and administered in specific dose in order to avoid oxygen toxicity. The dosage of O_2 is started in terms of concentration and rate of flow.
- When using oxygen cylinder, use a regulator and humidifiers. The purpose of the regulator is to reduce the pressure of the O_2 in the cylinder to a safer level. The humidifier helps to saturate the oxygen with water vapour to prevent the drying of the mucus membranes of respiratory tract.
- The glass tube should be summered under the water so that oxygen is bubbled through the water.
- Every drop of water of the apparatus should be clean to prevent infection.
- Use disposable nasal catheters or sterilized rubbed catheters
- Change the nasal catheters at least every 8 hours or more often.
- Lubricate the nasal catheter sparingly while the O_2 is flowing. Then hold tip of the catheter in a glass of H_2O to make sure that the terminal holes are not plugged with lubricant.
- During the administration of O_2 the valve controlling the rate of flow should not be handled if any alteration is to be made in the flow of O_2 first take out the catheter from the nose and then adjust the valve.
- Oxygen administration must never be stopped until the factors that caused hypoxia are reversed.
- When oxygen therapy is discontinued, it should be done gradually. The patient is weaned from dependence on oxygen by reducing the dosage and then administrating it intermittently.
- For all patients receiving oxygen inhalation, the temperature should be taken rectally to get an accurate record of body temperature.
- When the nurse leaves the patient even for a short period, she should leave a calling signal near the patient.
- Pay attention to conditions that can interfere with the flow of oxygen from the source to the patient. This may include kinks in the tubing loose connection and faulty humidifying apparatus. Remember that it is not unusual therapy it is generally getting less oxygen than he would get under normal circumstances.
- To prevent the deprivation of oxygen resulting from the depletion of oxygen from the cylinder the nurse should get a new one ready at hand when the gauge shows about 1/4 level in the pressure.

- For fear of retrolental fibroplaisa the premature babies are given oxygen inhalation only for a short period at a very low concentration.
- Watch the patients receiving oxygen therapy continuously to detect the early signs of oxygen toxicity.
- When oxygen is administrated through the nasal catheters, the catheter is not directed distension of abdomen.
- Since oxygen supports combustion, fire precautions are to be taken when the oxygen is a flow.

Preparation of Patient and Environment

- Explain the procedure to the patient to win his confidence and cooperation. Answer his questions and allay the anxiety. Explain the sequence of the procedure and tell him how he can cooperate in the procedure. Explain the purpose of the procedure to the relatives also.
- Instruct the patient the family members and the visitors, if any about the safety precautions required during the oxygen therapy.
- Put up the instructions regarding fire precautions in the unit.
- Remove the cigars matches, electric appliances and other inflammable articles from patient's unit.
- Assemble the equipment and arrange them conveniently in the unit.
- Place the patient in a comfortable position (Fowler's position) to help in the expansion of the lungs.
- Clears the nostrils, if there is crust formation.
- Protect the bed and garments by spreading the Mackintosh and towel.

Equipments

- Oxygen cylinder with its stand and accessories.
- Nasal catheter.
- Water soluble lubricating jelly.
- Adhesive tapes.
- Bowl of water.
- Flash light and tongue depressor.
- Normal saline in a container.
- Kidney tray.
- Paper bag.
- Mackintosh.
- Towel.
- Rag pieces in a container.

Procedure

- Explain the procedures to the patient and relatives to get the cooperation and win the confidence.
  What you are going to do and reassure him. Explain the purpose of procedure.
- Put the instructions regarding the fire precautions in the ward or unit. Instruct the relatives or visitors regarding safety measures required during the oxygen inhalation.
- Observe vital signs and breathing pattern.
- Collect the necessary articles at the bedside.
- Give comfortable position to the patient.
- Screen the bed of the patient.
- Wash hands to prevent cross-infection.
- Measure catheter from the tip of the nose to ear label for distance to enter, mark the length with ink.
- Check the apparatus for working condition. Open the main valve in an anti-clockwise direction.
  Observe for pressure reading on the gauge. Open the wheel valve on the regulator and see the reading on the meter adjust the flow of O_2 2 to 4 L for adults or as desired. When the wheel valve is opened the oxygen will start bubbling through the water in the Wolf's bottle. Attach the catheter to the connecting tube, oxygen will start bubbling through the water in the Wolf's bottle. Attach the catheter to the connecting tube and check the flow of O_2 through the catheter to prevent by dipping it under the water in the bowl.
- Lubricate the tip of catheter with water soluble jelly inserts it through nortred into pharynx.
- Bring catheter across check and scope securely with adhesive tape.

Aftercare of the Patient

- Be with the patient fill he is at case.
- Keep the patient warm and comfortable.
- Observe the patient's progress by assessing vital signs and color.
- Observe patient's progress at specified intervals to make sure that the state of anoxemia is treated.
- When the O_2 is discontinued. Unscrew regulator he the leter flow disconnect the catheter and put it in kidney tray.
- Clean the catheter, first with cold water, then with warm soapy water and finally with clean water bill it for, 3 to 5 minutes, dry it and store in a cool dry place.
- All other articles must be cleaned with soap and clean water dried and then replaced to their usual places.
- Wash hands.

Patient Education

- Educate the client and visitors about the hazard of smoking with oxygen in use.
- Request other clients in the room and visitors to smoke in areas provided elsewhere in the hospitals.
- Educate the patients about the short-circuit spark of electrical equipment.
- Educate the patient, about safety precautions.

Complications

- The use of contaminated equipment can spread infection in the patient.
- Fire is a potential hazard when oxygen is administered.
- If there is no sufficient humidity, there is a chance of drying and irritation of mucous membrane.

- Prolonged exposure to a high concentration causes damage to the lung tissue and atelectasis.
- If there are increased oxygen concentrations in inspired air, there is a chance of collapse of alveoli.
- The oxygen therapy may affect eyes.
- Ulceration, edema and visual impairment, etc. result from the toxic effects of O_2 on the cornea and lens of adult.

HOME OXYGEN THERAPY

Home oxygen therapy is available to clients who require continuous oxygen therapy at home. It is usually delivered by nasal cannula.

Purpose

To provide continuous oxygen therapy for patients.

Preparation

- Explain the procedure step by step to the patients and their relatives to confidence.
- Explain about the safety precautions.

Classification

In this therapy 3 types of oxygen is used:
- Compressed oxygen.
- Liquid oxygen.
- Oxygen concentrations.

Equipment

- Nasal cannula equipment.
- Primary and portable liquid oxygen source for ambulation.

Procedure

- Explain the procedure to client and family.
- Wash hands.
- Demonstrate steps for preparation and completion of oxygen therapy.
- Prepare primary and portable oxygen.
- Place primary oxygen source in clutter free environment.
- Check oxygen levels of both sources by reading gauge on top.
- Check oxygen gauge to determine fullness of portable source.
- Select prescribed rate.
- Connect nasal cannula and O_2 tubing to oxygen.
- Have client and family perform each step with guidance from the nurse.

Patient Education

- Explain or teach about the home oxygen therapy.
- The nurse coordinates the efforts of the client and family, home call nurse, home respiratory therapist and home oxygen equipment vendor.
- The nurse must assist the client and family in learning about home oxygen and ensure their ability to maintain the oxygen delivery system.

Complications

Bulky, possibly unsightly, frequent refilling necessary with continuous use.

AIRWAY MANAGEMENT

Airway management is a set of medical procedures performed in order to prevent airway obstruction and thus ensuring an open pathway between a patient's lungs and the outside world. This is accomplished by clearing or preventing obstructions of airways, often referred to as choking, caused by the tongue, the airways themselves, foreign bodies or materials from the body itself, such as blood or stomach content, the latter resulting in aspiration.

Airway management can be divided into two categories: basic and advanced airway management. Basic techniques are simple to perform even by non-health care professionals and do not require use of medical equipment, whereas advanced techniques require special training and medical equipment. Advanced airway management is further categorized in increasing order of invasiveness into supraglottic devices, such as oropharyngeal or nasopharyngeal airways, followed by infraglottic techniques, such as tracheal intubation, and finally surgical methods.

OROPHARYNGEAL AIRWAY

An oropharyngeal airway (also known as an oral airway, OPA or Guedel pattern airway) is a medical device called an airway adjunct used to maintain or open a patient's airway. It does this by preventing the tongue from covering the epiglottis, which could prevent the person from breathing. When a person becomes unconscious, the muscles in their jaw relax and allow the tongue to obstruct the airway

Oropharyngeal airways are indicated only in unconscious people, because of the likelihood that the device would stimulate a gag reflex in conscious or semi-conscious persons. This could result in vomit and potentially

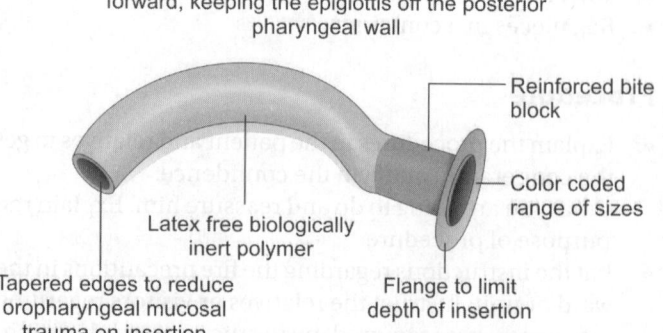

Fig. 20.9: Parts of oropharyngeal airway.

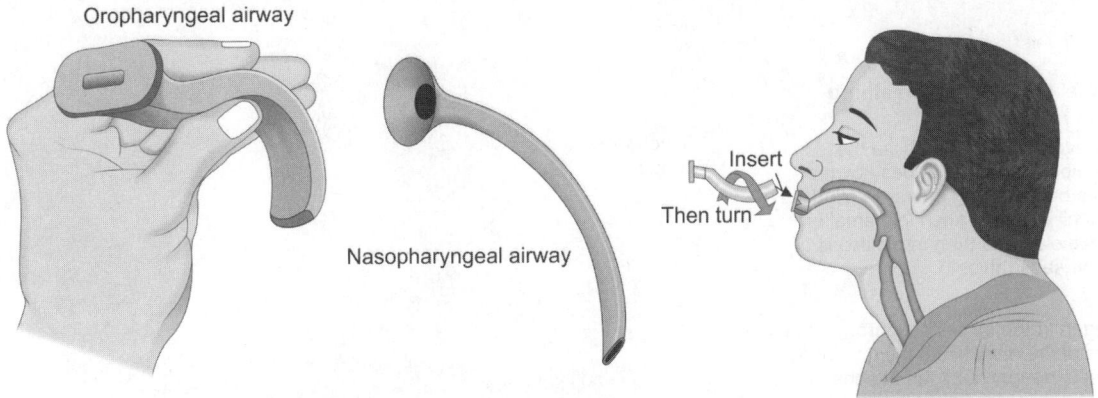

Fig. 20.10: Types of oropharyngeal airway.

lead to an obstructed airway. Nasopharyneal airways are mostly used instead as they do not stimulate a gag reflex. In general oropharyngeal airways need to be sized and inserted correctly to maximize effectiveness and minimize possible complications such as oral trauma.

Procedure: Oral airways are inserted upside down from the side or top of the mouth then twisted 180 degrees around so the distal tip is positioned in the inferior oropharynx. Care should be taken during insertion that the tongue is not inadvertently pushed down into the throat. A tongue depressor can aid insertion. To determine proper airway size, place the airway along the cheek and measure the distance from the corner of the mouth to the tragus of the ear (the cartilaginous point near the opening). Tubes too long can put pressure on the epiglottis and may obstruct the airway. A tube too short can push the tongue back and decrease ventilation. If the flange sticks out more than a few millimeters, select a smaller airway. Oropharyngeal airways are to be used only with the unconscious patient as they may cause vomiting and laryngospasm in the alert or semiconscious patient.

Problems associated with orotracheal Tubes:
- They are poorly tolerated in conscious and semiconscious patients.
- They are difficulty to stabilize and may be easily dislodged.
- Inadvertent extubation is common.
- A bite block may be necessary to prevent biting of tube
- Vagal stimulation may cause bradycardia and hypotension.

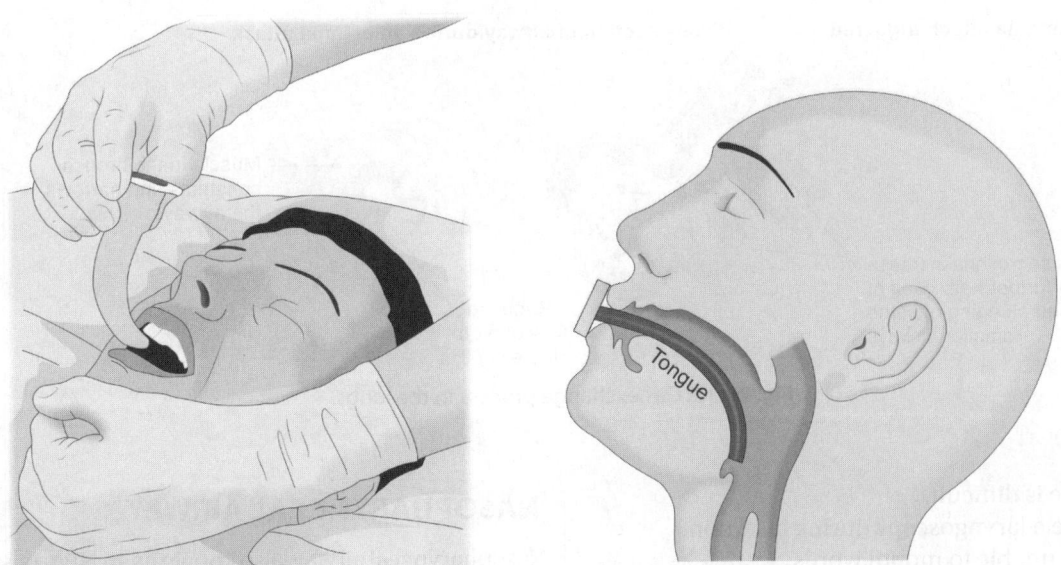

Fig. 20.11: Oropharyngeal airway application procedure.

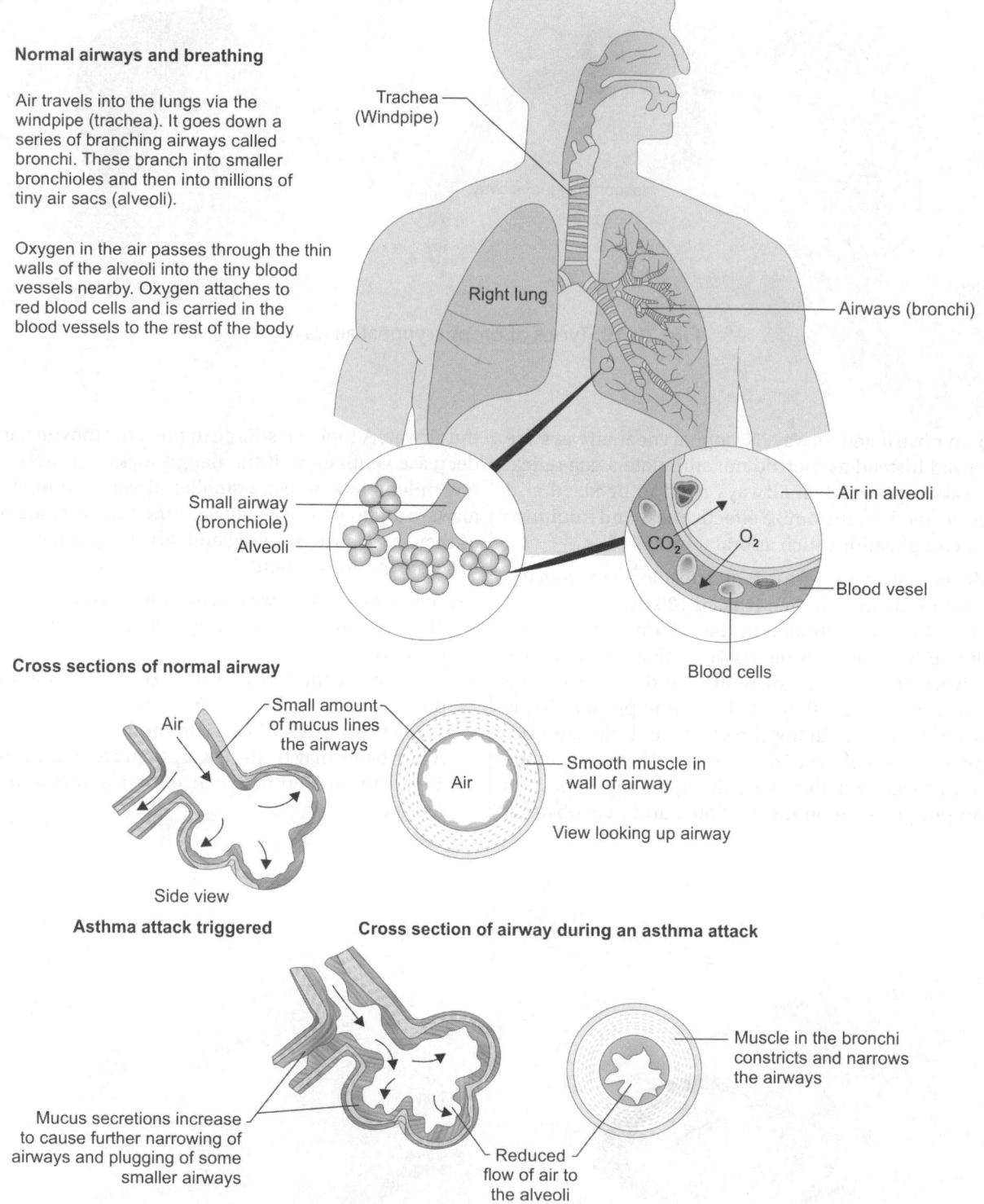

Fig. 20.12: Gas exchange process in the lungs.

- Oral hygiene is difficult.
- They require a laryngoscopy during insertion.
- Patients are unable to mouth words.
- Lips may be lacerated.

NASOPHARYNGEAL AIRWAY

Nasopharyngeal airway, also known as an NPA, nasal trumpet (because of its flared end), or nose hose, a type of airway

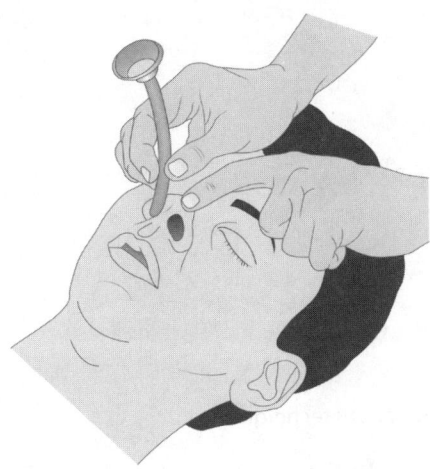

Fig. 20.13: Nasopharyngeal airway insertion technique.

adjunct, is a tube that is designed to be inserted into the nasal passageway to secure an open airway. When a patient becomes unconscious, the muscles in the jaw commonly relax and can allow the tongue to slide back and obstruct the airway. The purpose of the flared end is to prevent the device from becoming lost inside the patient's nose.

Size: As with other catheters, NPAs are measured using the French catheter scale, but sizes are usually also quoted in millimeters. Typical sizes include: 6.5 mm/28FR, 7.0 mm/30FR, 7.5 mm/32FR, 8.0 mm/34FR, and 8.5 mm/36FR.

Indications and contraindications: These devices are used by emergency care professionals such as emergency medical technicians (EMTs) and paramedics in situations where an artificial form of airway maintenance is necessary, but tracheal intubation is impossible, inadvisable, or outside the practitioner's scope of practice. An NPA is often used in conscious patients where an oropharyngeal would trigger the gag reflex.

Insertion of an NPA is absolutely contraindicated in patients with severe head or facial injuries, or has evidence of a basilar skull fracture-battle's sign, raccoon eyes, cerebrospinal fluid/blood from ears, etc.) due to the possibility of direct intrusion into brain tissue. Nasopharyngeal airways are also used, though very rarely, by people who have severe sleep apnea, inserted by the patient themselves at home.

Insertion techniques: The correct size airway is chosen by measuring the device on the patient—the device should reach from the patient's nostril to the earlobe or the angle of the jaw. The outside of the tube is lubricated with a water-based lubricant so that it enters the nose more easily. The device is inserted until the flared end rests against the nostril. Some tubes contain a safety pin to prevent inserting the tube too deeply. Care must be taken to ensure the pin does not stick into the nostril. In the event that a pin is not available, you may also stop insertion just short of the natural gag reflex and tape the remaining exposed portion of the NPA to the surrounding facial tissue.

Advantages of nasotracheal tubes:
- Easier to stabilize
- May be better tolerated by some patients
- May be inserted blindly (laryngoscopy is unnecessary in most cases)
- Oral hygiene is easily accomplished
- The patient is able to mouth words
- Attachment of equipment is easier and safer; there is less torque on the trachea.

Problems associated with nasotracheal tubes:
- The tip of the tube moves when the patient's head position changes
- Pressure necrosis in area of the alaenasi may occur
- Sinus drainage may be obstructed, and acute sinusitis may result
- Eustachian tube drainage may be obstructed, and otitis media may result
- The incidence of vocal cord damage after 3 to 7 days (also seen with oral ETT's) increases
- Vagal stimulation is possible, but it occurs less frequently than with the oral ETT
- Skilled personnel are necessary for placement
- The nasal passage limits the tube size; a tube at least 0.5 mm ID smaller than the oral route is required.

ENDOTRACHEAL TUBES

An endotracheal tube (ETT) is indicated when a patient's airway requires airway protection, tracheal suctioning or when ventilation is necessary. Endotracheal tubes can be inserted nasally or orally. Oral endotracheal tubes have a preformed curve at a 450 angle. Nasal endotracheal tubes have a preformed curve curved at a 600 angle. Once the selected tube is in place, the distal tip rests in the trachea just above the carina. Most have an opening (Murphy's eye) in the wall near the distal tip. Should the tip be occluded, ventilation may still be possible through this opening.

There also is an inflatable cuff attached near the distal end of adult tubes. Cuff inflation seals the airway so all ventilation must occur through the endotracheal tube. The cuff is inflated via a pilot balloon valve and line attached to the endotracheal tube. Infant tubes have no cuff. Endotracheal tubes less than sizes 5.0 are generally uncuffed. Some 5.0 tubes are manufactured with and without cuffs.

TRACHEOSTOMY TUBES

Tracheostomy tubes also are inserted in the trachea, but insertion is through a tracheal stoma. They are similar to an endotracheal tube but much shorter and more rigid. Most tracheostomy tubes have an inner and outer cannula, obturator, and inflatable cuff. Some have no inner cannula or cuff. The obturator provides a smooth surface to ease insertion and prevent tissue and blood debre from entering the tube during insertion. The obturator is removed when

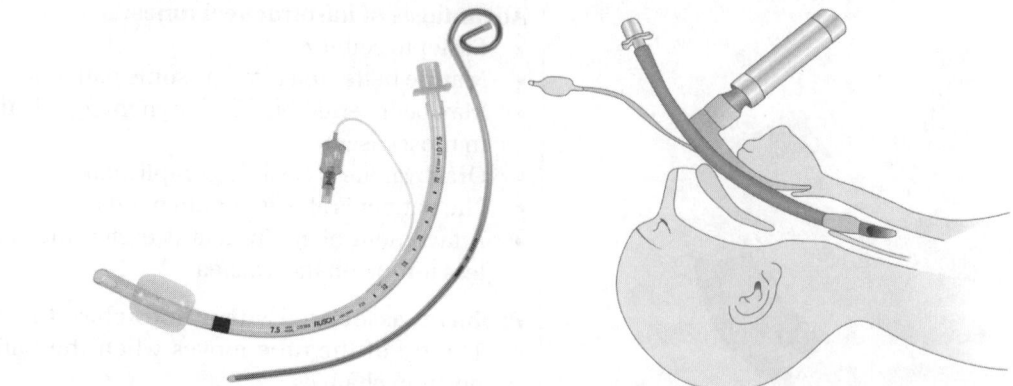

Fig. 20.14: Endotracheal tube and inserting (intubation) technique.

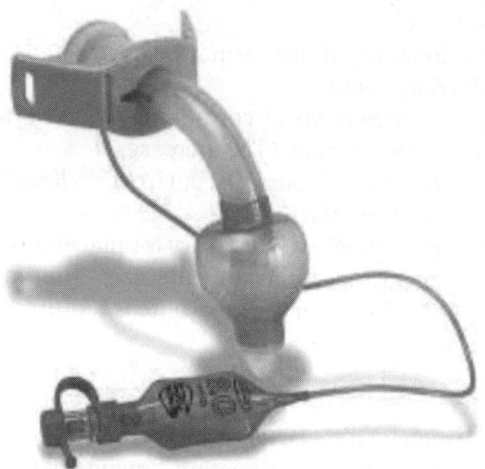

Fig. 20.15: Tracheostomy tube.

the airway is in place. Inner cannulas can be removed and cleaned periodically. Some inner cannulas are disposable. Most tubes also come with a decannulation plug.

The variation in tracheostomy tubes is endless. Sizes, materials, style and specific applications differ. The practitioner must learn the basic theory of operation of tracheostomy tubes and the wide array that exists. Basically, each tracheotomy tube consists of a neck flange, tube body and cuff.

Inner cannula: This device can be removed to clean secretions and blood from the interior surface without removing the entire tube. Shiley manufactures tracheostomy tubes with disposable inner cannulas.

Obturator: The obturator prevents blood or mucus from entering the tube as it is being inserted and provides a smoothly tapered surface to facilitate introduction of the tube into the airway and is removed when the tube is in the proper position.

15mm connector: This is the standard connector, which allows connection to resuscitation bags and other respiratory equipment.

Neck plate or flange: This enables the tube to be secured around the patients' neck with ties or collar. Some surgeons initially suture the flange to the patients' neck. These sutures are removed in approximately 3–5 days by the surgeon or respiratory therapist. They are replaced with the standard tracheostomy ties or alternative commercially available ties.

Cuffs: Cuffs seal the airway to allow positive pressure ventilation and minimize the risk of aspiration of stomach contents into the lungs. They do not eliminate aspiration; even the best cuffs have microscopic air leakage. Aspiration of pharyngeal secretions commonly occurs with cuffed artificial airways. Tubes that remain connected to continuous suction can suction above the cuff and lower the risk of aspirated secretions, but these systems have not gained wide use since their introduction and cost may be a factor. Knowing these facts, we cannot emphasize enough the importance of oral care, oral suction and proper procedures prior to and during deflation of cuffs.

Pilot balloon: The cuff is inflated (not foam cuffs) using a syringe. A spring-loaded one-way valve on the pilot balloon maintains cuff inflation when the syringe is removed. The pilot balloon functions to show an inflated, or not inflated, condition of the cuff. It is impossible to judge the pressure within the cuff by squeezing the pilot balloon. The best practice is to use minimal leak technique (MLT) minimal occlusion technique (MOT) to determine the lowest amount of air aspirated in to seal the cuff.

ARTIFICIAL AIRWAY MANAGEMENT

An artificial airway is a tube that is inserted at the mouth or nose or level of the second or third tracheal ring to permit mechanical ventilation and facilitate secretion removal. The distal end of the tube is located in the trachea below the vocal cords.

Indications

- Acute respiratory failure, CNS depression, neuro-muscular disease, pulmonary disease, chest wall injury.
- Upper airway obstruction.
- Anticipated upper airway obstruction from edema or soft tissue swelling due to head and neck trauma some postoperative head and neck procedures involving

the airway facial or airway burns, decreased level of consciousness.
- Aspiration prophylaxis.
- Fractured cervical vertebrae with spinal cord injury requiring ventilatory assistance.

Route of Insertion

Endotracheal: May be inserted through nose or mouth. A cuff is always located at the distal end of the tube.
- **Orotracheal:** Insertion of an oral tube is technically easier, since it is done under direct visualization. Disadvantages are increased oral secretions, decreased patient comfort, difficulty with stabilization, and inability of patient to use lip movement as a communication means.
- **Nasotracheal:** It may be more comfortable to the patient and is easier to stabilize. Disadvantages are that blind insertion is required, possible development of pressure necrosis of the nasal airway, sinusitis and otitis media.

Tube Types

- Vary according to length and inner diameter in millimeters. Usual sizes for adults are 6.0, 7.0, 8.0, 9.0 mm.
- Vary according to cuff most are high volume low pressure with self-sealing inflation valves or the cuff may be foam rubber (foam cuff).
- Vary according to composition and cuff type synthetic teflon, nylon, polyvinyl chloride, polyethylene or silastic. May or may not have inner cannula. Usually are cuffed.
- Tubes with high volume, low pressure cuff self-sealing inflation valves. With or without inner cannula.
    - Pressure limiting cuffs.
    - Polyurethane foam filled cuffs.
    - Speaking tracheotomy tube.
    - Fenestrated.
- Usual sizes for adult are 6.0, 7.0, 8.0, and 9.0 mm.

General Instructions

Physical Management

- Ensure adequate ventilation and oxygenation through the use of mechanical ventilation, continuous positive airway pressure device, Briggs T-piece adapter.
- Provide adequate humidity, since the natural humidifying pathway of the oropharynx is bypassed. Clear airway of secretions as needed with suctioning.
- Use aseptic technique when entering the artificial airway. The artificial airway is sterile below the level of the vocal cords.
- Frequently assess the patient's need for ventilatory assistance.
- Elevate the patient to a semi-Fowler's or sitting position, when possible, since these positions resulting improved lung compliance. The patient's position, however, should be changed at least every 2 hours to ensure ventilation of all lung segments and prevention of secretion stagnation. Position changes are also necessary to avoid skin breakdown.
- Nutrition:
Endotube: Recognizes that the tube holds open the epiglottis. Therefore only the inflated cuff prevents the aspiration of oropharyngeal contents into the lungs. The patient must not receive oral feeding. Nutrition must take the form of enternal tube feedings.
- Be aware of the complications and damage that inflated cuffs may have on the tracheal mucosa. Endotracheal tune cuffs should be inflated continuously and deflated only during intubations, extubation, and tube repositioning. The internal cuff pressure should be checked every 2 hours.
- External tube site care:
Endotube—Patients with endotracheal tubes have mouth care every shift, or a frequently as needed. Oral secretions tend to stagnate and risk oral infection is increased. An oral endotracheal tube may also stimulate as increase in the production of oral secretions. The tube must be secured at all times and the ventilator, CPAP or T piece tubing supported so that traction is not applied to the tube.
- Have available at al times at the patient's bedside a resuscitation bag, oxygen bag source and mask to ventilate the patient in the event of accidental removal anticipate your course of action in such an event.
Endotracheal tube—Know the location and assembly of reintubation equipment. Know the method of contact personnel capable of reintubation.

Psychological Care of the Patient

- Recognize that the patient is usually apprehensive particularly about choking inability to communicate verbally, being unable to remove secretions, difficulty in breathing, or mechanical failure.
- Explain the function of the equipment carefully.
- Inform the patient and his family that he will not be able to speak while the tube is in place being a tracheotomy tube.

Equipment

- Laryngoscope with curved or straight blade and working light source.
- Endotracheal tube with low pressure cuff and adapter to connect tube to ventilator or resuscitation bag.
- Stylet to guide the endotracheal tube.
- Oral airway or bite block to keep the patient from biting into and occluding the endotracheal tube.
- Adhesive tape or tube fixation system.
- Sterile anesthetic lubricant jelly.
- Syringe.
- Suction source.

- Suction catheter and tonsil suction
- Resuscitation bag and mask connected to oxygen source.
- Anesthetic spray.

Preparation of the Patient and the Environment

- Monitor the patient's heart rate, level of consciousness and respiratory status.
- Remove the patient's dental bridgework and plates.
- Remove headboard of bed.

Procedure

- Suction endotracheal tube.
- Suction oropharyngeal airway above the endotracheal cuff as thoroughly as possible.
- Loosen tape or endotracheal tube securing device.
- Extubate the patient.
  - Ask the patient to take as deep as a breath as possible.
  - At peak inspiration deflate the cuff completely and pull the tube out in the direction of the curve.
- Once the tube is fully removed, ask the patient to cough or exhale forcefully to remove secretions. Then suction the back of the patient's airway with the tonsil suction.
- Evaluate immediately for any signs of airway obstruction, stridor or difficult breathing. If the patient develops any of the above problems, attempt to ventilate the patient with the resuscitation bag and mask and prepare for reintubation.
- Administer oxygen as directed.

Aftercare

- Observe patient closely post extubation for any signs and symptoms of airway obstruction or respiratory insufficiency.
- Observe character of voice.

Complications

Mechanical:
- Cuff leaks
- Cuff herniation
- Tube obstruction
- Tube displacement.
- Inadvertent extubation.
- Right main stem intubation.

Laryngeal and tracheal:
- Sore throat
- Hoarse voice
- Glottic edema
- Ulceration of tracheal mucosa
- Vocal cord ulceration, granuloma, or polyps
- Vocal cord paralysis
- Laryngotracheal web: Formation of a web fibrin and cellular debris initiated by neuro tissue at the glottic or subglottic level.
- Post extubation tracheal stenosis.
- Formation of tracheoesophageal fistula.
- Formation of tracheoarterial fistula.
- Innominate artery erosion.
- See additional complications under specific procedures dealing with artificial airways.

NURSING PROCESS IN AIRWAY MANAGEMENT

Maintaining a patent airway is vital to life. Coughing is the main mechanism for clearing the airway. However the cough may be ineffective in both normal and disease states secondary to factors such as pain from surgical incisions/trauma, respiratory muscle fatigue, or neuromuscular weakness. Other mechanisms that exist in the lower bronchioles and alveoli to maintain the airway include the mucociliary system, macrophages, and the lymphatics. Factors such as anesthesia and dehydration can affect function of the mucociliary system. Likewise, conditions that cause increased production of secretions (pneumonia, bronchitis, chemical irritants) can overtax these mechanisms. Ineffective airway clearance can be an acute (e.g., postoperative recovery) or chronic (e.g., from cerebrovascular accident [CVA] or spinal cord injury) problem. The elderly who have an increased incidence of emphysema and a higher prevalence of chronic cough or sputum production are at high risk.

Related factors:
- Decreased energy and fatigue
- Ineffective cough
- Tracheobronchial infection
- Tracheobronchial obstruction (including foreign body aspiration)
- Copious tracheobronchial secretions
- Perceptual/cognitive impairment
- Impaired respiratory muscle function
- Trauma.

Defining characteristics:
- Abnormal breath sounds (crackles, rhonchi, wheezes)
- Changes in respiratory rate or depth
- Cough
- Hypoxemia/cyanosis
- Dyspnea
- Chest wheezing
- Fever
- Tachycardia.

Expected outcome:
Patient's secretions are mobilized and airway is maintained free of secretions, as evidenced by clear lung sounds, eupnea, and ability to effectively cough up secretions after treatments and deep breaths.

Airway assessment:
- **Assess airway for patency.** *Maintaining the airway is always the first priority, especially in cases of trauma, acute neurological decompensation, or cardiac arrest.*

- **Auscultate lungs for presence of normal or adventitious breath sounds, as in the following:** Decreased or absent breath sounds: *May indicate presence of mucus plug or other major airway obstruction.*
  Wheezing: *May indicate increasing airway resistance.*
  Coarse sounds: *May indicate presence of fluid along larger airways.*
- **Assess respirations; note quality, rate, pattern, depth, flaring of nostrils, dyspnea on exertion, evidence of splinting, use of accessory muscles, position for breathing:** *Abnormality indicates respiratory compromise.*
- **Assess changes in mental status:** *Increasing lethargy, confusion, restlessness, and/or irritability can be early signs of cerebral hypoxia.*
- **Assess changes in vital signs and temperature:** *Tachycardia and hypertension may be related to increased work of breathing. Fever may develop in response to retained secretions/atelectasis.*
- **Assess cough for effectiveness and productivity:** *Consider possible causes for ineffective cough—respiratory muscle fatigue, severe bronchospasm, thick tenacious secretions, and others.*
- **Note presence of sputum; assess quality, color, amount, odor, and consistency:** *May be a result of infection, bronchitis, chronic smoking, and others. A sign of infection is discolored sputum (no longer clear or white); an odor may be present.*
- **Send a sputum specimen for culture and sensitivity as appropriate:** *Respiratory infections increase the work of breathing; antibiotic treatment is indicated.*
- **Monitor arterial blood gases (ABGs):** *Increasing $PaCO_2$ and decreasing PaO_2 are signs of respiratory failure.*
- **Assess for pain:** *Postoperative pain can result in shallow breathing and an ineffective cough.*
- **If patient is on mechanical ventilation, monitor for peak airway pressures and airway resistance:** *Increases in these parameters signal accumulation of secretions/fluid and possibility for ineffective ventilation.*
- **Assess patient's knowledge of disease process:** *Patient education will vary depending on the acute or chronic disease state as well as the patient's cognitive level.*

Nursing intervention for airway management:
- Maintenance of a patent airway is critical when providing care to a client, and suctioning and tracheostomy care are procedures that nurses must be knowledgeable about to ensure a patent airway.
- Whenever possible, the client should be encouraged to cough. Coughing is more effective than artificial suctioning at moving secretions into the upper trachea or laryngopharynx.
- Airway suctioning involves the use of a suction machine and catheter to remove secretions from the airway.
- A tracheotomy is a sterile surgical incision into the trachea for the purpose of establishing an airway. A tracheostomy is the stoma/opening that results from a tracheotomy and the insertion and maintenance of a cannula.

COUGHING TECHNIQUES

Coughing is one of the most important lung defense mechanisms, and unfortunately it is significantly impaired in COPD. While the nasal passages provide a mechanism to warm and humidify the incoming air, and trap dirt particles and germs, inevitably some undesirable foreign material penetrates down into the lungs. Coughing is needed to clear undesirable material from the bronchial tubes. This module will teach you a more efficient way to do a COPD cough, called "**Huff Coughing.**" To understand Huff Coughing you first need to have some understanding of normal coughing. Coughing is effective in maintaining a patient airway; it permits the client to remove secretions from both the upper and lower airways.

The various coughing techniques are given below:

Sl. No.	Types	Description
1.	Cascade cough	In this technique, the client is asked to take slow deep breath and hold it for two seconds. While contracting expiratory muscles, tell the client to open the mouth and perform a series of coughs throughout exhalation, thereby coughing at lowered lung volumes.
2.	Huff cough	In this the client on exhalation opens the glottis by say the word huff. The huff cough stimulates a natural cough reflex. This method is useful for clearing central airway.
3.	Quad cough	This is used for clients without abdominal muscle control e.g., clients with spinal cord injuries. The client or nurse pushes inward and outward on the abdominal muscles to the diaphragm while the client breaths with maximal expiratory efforts, causing the cough.
4.	Controlled coughing	Ask the client to take two slow, deep breaths, inhaling through nose and exhaling through mouth. Inhale deeply third time and hold breath to count of 3. Cough fully for two or three consecutive coughs without inhaling between cough. Tell the client to push all air out of lungs.

SUCTIONING PROCEDURE

Suctioning into the nose and mouth to remove mucus (thickened nose and throat secretions) will make it easier for him or her to breathe and eat.

Suctioning is the process of sucking. The removal of gas or fluid from a cavity or rather container by means of reduced pressure. When a patient is unable to clear respiratory tract secretion with coughing, the nurse must use suctioning to clear the airways.

Oral/nasal suctioning: Oral/nasal suctioning is suctioning of the upper airway passages of the nose, mouth, and pharynx. This procedure is used to assist the patient in eliminating secretions before he has regained full consciousness and cannot spit out secretions. The catheter used should be soft and pliable. When you employ suctioning, you must make every effort to prevent the introduction of pathogens (disease causing microorganisms) into the lower airways.

Oropharyngeal and nasopharyngeal: The orophaynx extends behind the mouth from the soft palate above the level of the hyoid bone and contains the tensil the nasopharyx is located behind the nose and extends to the level of soft palate. This suctioning is used when the patient is able to cough effectively but is unable to clears secretions by expectorating or swallowing.

Orotrachial and nasotrachial: It is necessary when the client with pulmonary secretion is unable to cough and does not have an artificial airway present.

Tracheal suctioning: Tracheal suctioning is accomplished through an artificial airway such an endotracheal tube or tracheotomy tube.

Equipment

- Laryngoscope with curved on straight blade and working light sources.
- Endotracheal tube with low pressure cuff and adapter to connect tube to ventilator style to guide the endotracheal tube.
- Oral airway.
- 10 mL syringe.
- Suction sources.
- Suction catheter.
- Sterile towel.
- Gloves.
- Face should.
- End trial CO_2 detector.
- Resuscitation buy and mask connected to 02 source.

Procedure

Preparation Phase

- Assess the patient's heart rate, level of consciousness and respiratory status.

Performance Phase

- Remove the patient dental bridgework and plates
- Remove headboard of bed
- Prepare equipment
- Aspirate stomach consents if nasogastric tube is in place.

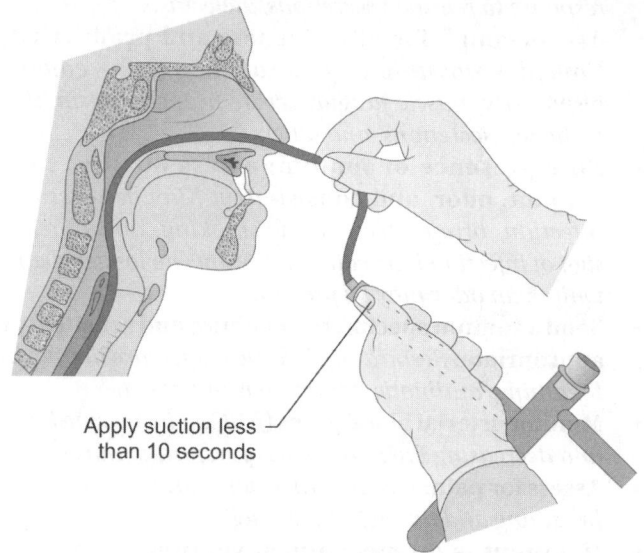

Fig. 20.17: Nasopharyngeal suctioning procedures.

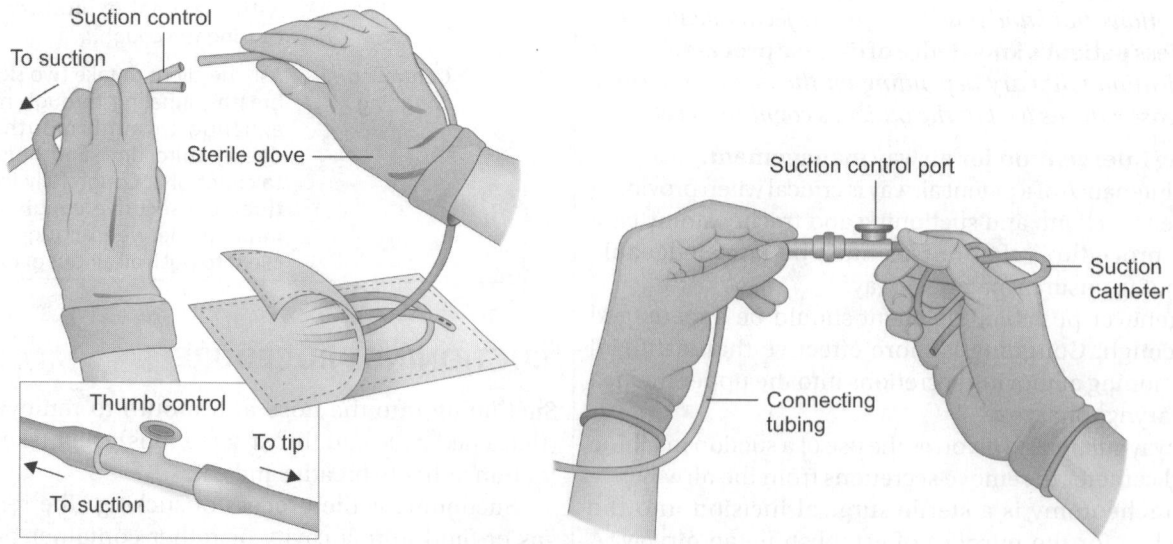

Fig. 20.16: Method of connecting suction catheters.

- If time allows inform the patient of impending inability to talk and discuss alternative means of communication.
- If the patient is confused it may be necessary to apply soft wrist restraints.
- Put on gloves and face shield.
- During oral intubations if cervical spine is not injured place patients head an a "sniffing" position anesthetic sprat if time is a valuable.
- Spray the back of the patients throat with anesthesia spray if time is available.
- Ventilate and oxygenate the patient with the resuscitation bug and mask before intubations.
- Hold the handle of the laryngoscope in the left hand and hold the patient's mouth open with the right hand by placing crossed hungers on the teeth.
- Insert the curve blade of the laryngoscope along the right side of the tongue, push the tongue to the left and use right thumb and index finger to pull patient lower lip away from lower teeth.
- Lift the laryngoscopes forward to expose the epiglottis.
- Lift the laryngoscopes forward at 45 degree angle to expose glottis and visualize vocal cards.
- As the epiglottis is left forwards the vertical opening of the larynx between the vocal cords will come into vein.
- Once the vocal cord are visualized insert the tube into the right corner of the mouth and pass the tube while keeping vocal cords in continent view.
- Gently push the tube through the triangular space formed by the vocal cards and buck wall of trachea.
- Stop insertion just after the tube cuff has disappeared from vein beyond the cards.
- Withdraw laryngoscope while holding endotracheal tube, attach bug to ET tube, and ventilate the patient.
- Inflate cuff with the minimal amount of air required to include the teacher.
- Insert bite black if necessary
- Ascertain expansion of both side of the chest by observation and auscultation of breath sound.
- Record distance from proximal end of tube to the point where the tube reaches the teeth.
- Secure tube to the patients face with adhesive tape of applies a commercially available endotracheal tube stabilization device.
- Obtain chest X-ray to verify tube position.

TRACHEOSTOMY SUCTIONING

Tracheostomy is an artificial airway which requires being maintained secretion free, thereby insuring adequate ventilation for the patient.

Purpose
- To clear secretions from the artificial airway or tracheobronchial tree.
- To maintain the patency of the tracheostomy tube.
- To ensure maximum ventilation of the patient.
- To reduce the risk of respiratory infection.

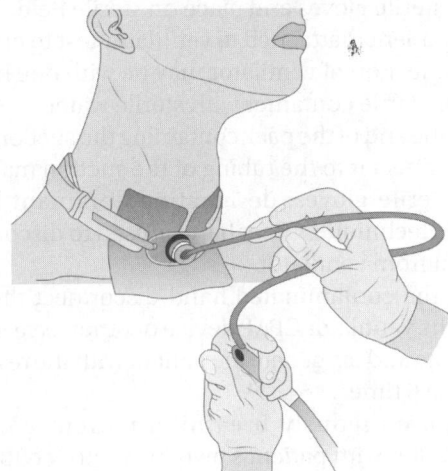

Fig. 20.18: Tracheostomy suctioning procedure.

Equipment
- A clean tray.
- Sterile suction catheters size 14, 16 adult 10, 12 pediatric with thumb control.
- Sterile gloves.
- Sterile towel.
- Sterile container and water or normal saline for flushing the catheter and tubing.
- Normal saline for installation.
- Sterile syringe 2 mL, 5 mL.
- Resuscitation bag with reservoir connected to 100 percent oxygen source. Add positive end-expiratory pressure valve to exhalation valve on resuscitation bag in an amount equal to that on the ventilator or positive airway pressure (PAP), continuous positive airway pressure (CPAP) device.
- Receptacle for disposables.
- Suction apparatus, e.g. portable machine or wall suction set at 80 to 120 mm Hg.

Preliminary Assessment
- Check physician's order, progress notes and nursing care plan.
- Explain the procedure to the patient. Include instructions on how to splint the surgical incision as coughing will be induced during the procedure.
- Ensure the patient's privacy.
- Position the patient in suitable position.
- Monitor heart rate, respiration rate and type and arterial blood pressure. If blood gases are ordered, know baseline values.
- Collect and assemble equipment. Check function of suction and resuscitation bag connected to 100 percent oxygen source.
- Wash and dry hands.

Procedure
- Open sterile towel and place in bib like fashion on patient's chest.

- Open sterile gloves and place on sterile field.
- If the patient is attached to ventilator test to ensure that disconnection of ventilator may be with one hand.
- Fill the sterile container with sterile water.
- Open the end of the pack containing the suction catheter and connect it to the tubing of the suction machine.
- Don sterile gloves, designating dominant hand for aseptic technique. Other hand is used to disconnect the patient from ventilator.
- Using the contaminated hand disconnect the patient from the ventilator CPAP device or other oxygen source.
- Ventilate and oxygenate the patient with the resuscitator bag 5 to 6 times.

In the spontaneously breathing patient coordinate ventilation with patient's own inspiratory effort.

- Slide the cover off the catheter and rinse it through with sterile water/saline to lubricate it.
- Insert the catheter into the tracheotomy as for as possible without applying suction.
- Apply suction and quickly rotate the catheter while it is being withdrawn.
- Limit suction time 10 to 15 seconds. Discontinue if heart rate decreases by 20 beats per minute or if cardiac ectopy is observed.
- Ventilate the patient between suction with 4–5 manual ventilation.
- Sterile normal saline 2 to 3 mL may be instilled into the airway followed by manual ventilation then suction.
- Rinse catheter between suctioning. Procedure with sterile water/saline.
- Continue procedure as necessary to a maximum of 4 suction passes.
- Give the patient 6 to 8 'sigh' breaths with the bag.
- Return the patient to the ventilator or apply CPAP or other oxygen delivery device.
- Suck oral secretions from the oropharynx above the artificial cuff.
- Deliver tracheotomy care as required.
- If patient is not an respiratory assistance apply filter or humidifier as indicated.
- Check vital signs.
- Leave the patient as comfortable as possible.
- Clear and clean equipment.
- Wash and dry hands.
- Document the procedure including patient's response in appropriate nursing notes.

STEAM INHALATION

Inhalation is defined as the drawing of air or other vapors into lungs through mouth or nose.

Steam inhalation is defined as utilization of moist heat to loosen lung congestion and help liquefy secretions.

Purpose

- To relieve inflammation of the mucus membrane in acute colds and in sinusitis.
- To relieve irritation in bronchitis and whooping cough by moistening.
- To provide antiseptic action on the respiratory tract.
- To provide warm and moist air following operation, e.g. tracheotomy.
- To soften thick, tenacious mucus and relieve coughing.

Types of Inhalations

Dry-inhalation: Ether, chloroform, nitrous, oxide, menthol, eucalyptus and spirit ammonia.

Water moist inhalation: Plain steam, tincture benzoic, menthol in alcohol and oil of eucalyptus solution.

Indication of Tr. Benzoin Inhalation

- Purulent bronchitis.
- Bronchiectasis.
- Lung abscess.
- Common cold and sore throat.

General Instructions

- The temperature of the water should be remaining between 120 and 160°F or 54.4 and 76.7° C.
- Water in the inhaler should remain just below the spout to avoid scalding.
- The spout of the inhaler must be placed in such a way that the patient cannot touch it or put his face too near.
- Keep the patient warm and prevent drought before, during and after the inhalation.
- When volatile groups like menthols are used to keep his eyes closed to prevent the drug irritating the conjunctiva.
- Observe the patient closely throughout the procedure.

Preliminary Assessment Check

- The doctors order for any specific instructions.
- General condition and diagnosis of the patient.
- Self-care ability to follow instructions.
- Type, duration and medication of inhalation.
- Articles available in the unit.

Preparation of the Patient and Environment

- Explain the procedure to the patient.
- Allow the patient to empty to the bladder and towels if necessary. Given bedpan or urinal to a bedridden patient.
- Provide Fowler's position with back rest, cardiac table and extra pillows.
- Close windows, doors and put off fan to prevent drought.
- Provide sputum cup within the reach of the patient.
- Provide a face towel to remove sweat from face during inhalation.
- Mouth piece should be boiled and cooled before serving the patient.
- Arrange the articles at the bedside.

Equipment

A tray containing:
- Nelson's inhaler in a large bowl.
- Face towel and patient towel—1.
- Bath blanket.
- Tr. Beazoine.
- Teaspoon, drooper.
- Kettle with boiling water.
- Gauze pieces.
- Cotton swabs.
- Swab sticks.
- Kidney tray and paper bag.

Procedure

- Wash hands.
- Open sterile inhaler mouthpiece and cover with sterile gauze and attach to clean inhaler.
- Close spout of inhaler with cotton ball. Pour boiling water up to spout. Add medicine (tincture benzoine) if needed. Close inhaler with mouth piece and take to bedside.
- Face spout away from patient and remove cotton ball.
- Instruct to take in deep breath through mouth and breathe out through nose.
- Continue procedure for 15 to 20 minutes, keep patient warm throughout to prevent chilling.
- Give chest physiotherapy and encourage patient to bring out sputum.

Aftercare

- Remove the inhaler from the patient.
- Use face towel to wipe of perspiration from his face.
- Remove the accessories and make the patient comfortable.
- Replace the articles after cleaning.
- Wash hands.
- Record the procedure in nurse's record sheet.

POSTURAL DRAINAGE

Drainage of secretion from lung segments by gravity utilizing specific positioning techniques.

Purpose

- To drain lung secretion before and after surgery.
- To aid for easy breathing in bronchial or lobar pneumonia, lung abscess.

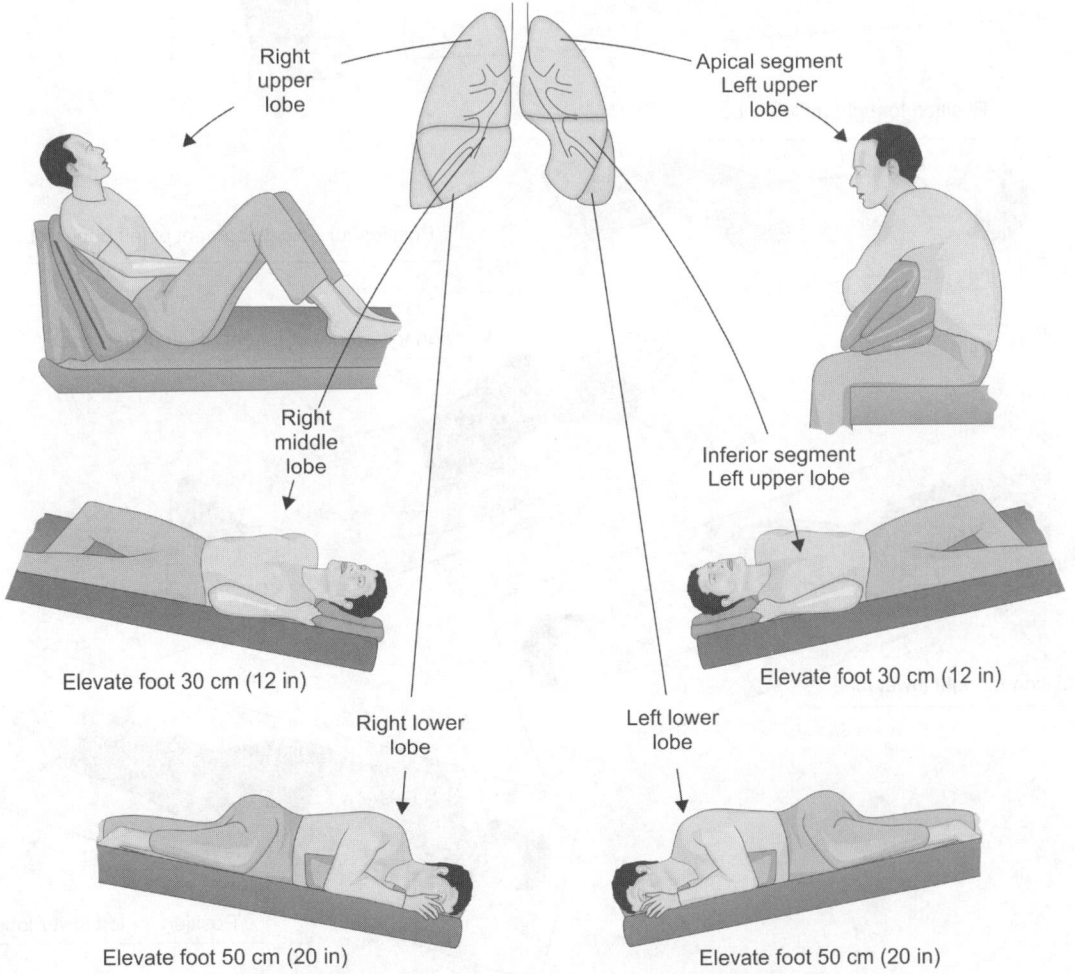

Fig. 20.19: Postural drainage on affected lobes of the lung.

- To treat patient with, e.g. bronchiectasis, chronic bronchitis and cystic fibrosis.
- To assist patient who are unable to cough and bring out sputum, viz. unconscious, debilitated, quadriplegic patient.

Equipment

- Pillows—3-4
- Sputum cup
- Tissue paper
- Sputum measuring glass.

General Instructions

- Perform postural drainage for patient on empty stomach before meals.
- Avoid postural drainage for patient with hemoptysis.

Procedure

- Explain purpose an procedure to patient.
- Locate affected lung with help of X-rays, auscultation and percussion.
- Administer bronchodilators before procedure.

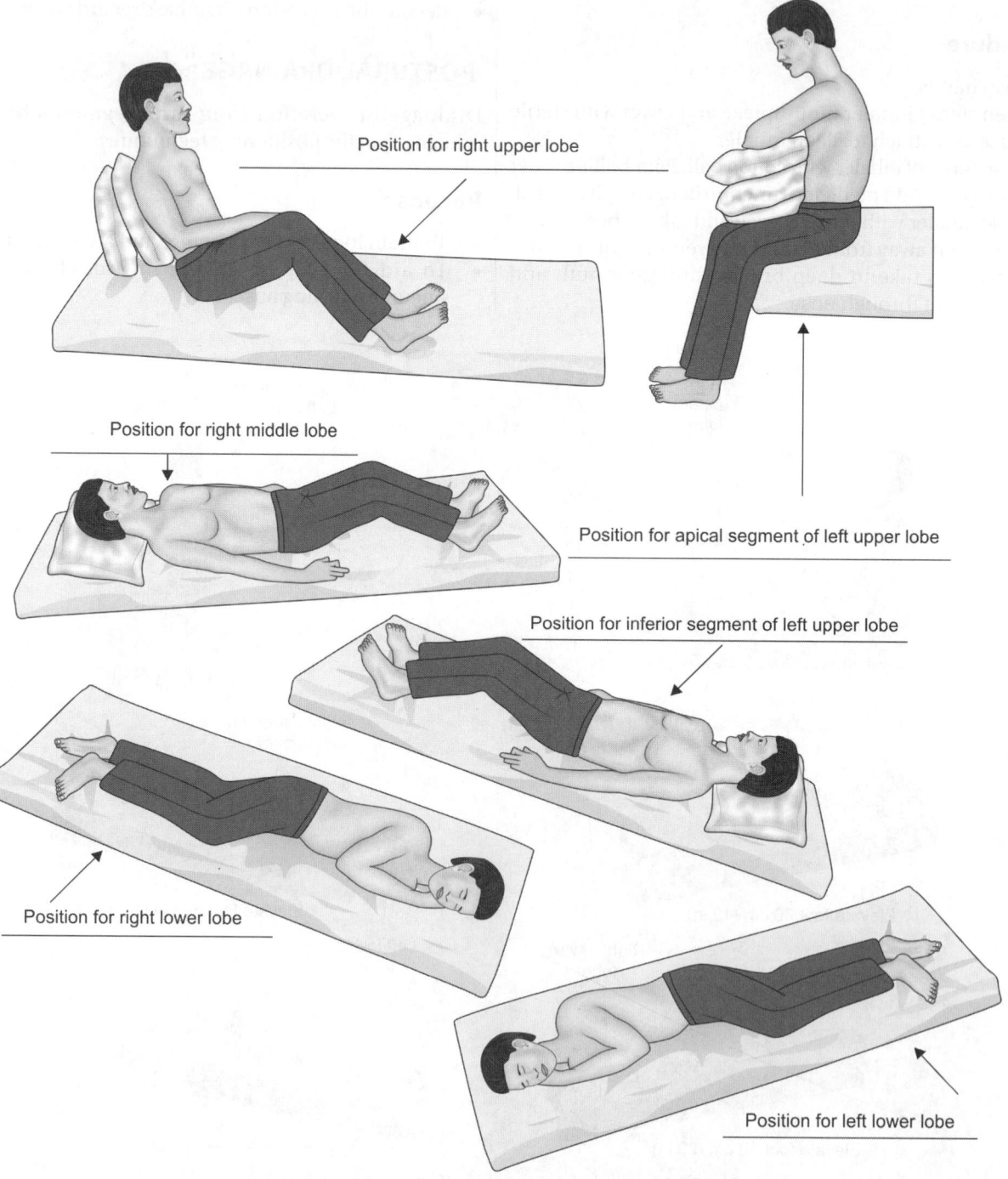

Fig. 20.20: Different positions used for postural drainage.

- Give steam inhalation to patient after obtaining doctor's written order.
- Position patient according to lung segment to be drained.

  Postural drainage techniques:
  - **Upper lobes**
    - Upper segments: Place patient in high Fowler's position in chair or bed.
    - Anterior segments: Place patient in semi-fowler's position in chair or bed.
    - Posterior segments: Place patient in Fowler's position in chair or bed, provide a cardiac table.
    - Lateral segments: Place patient in lateral position elevated to about 45 degree, first to one side and then to other side. When out of bed ask patient to lean on arm, resting on chair or table for support.
  - **Right middle lobes**
    - Anterior segment (right side): Place patient flat on left side with a pillow under chest. Right shoulder and body are kept forward.
    - Posterior segment: Place patient in prone with chest and abdomen elevated.
  - **Lower lobes**
    - Anterior segments: Place patient in supine, Trendlenberg with hips elevated with pillows, so that hips are higher than shoulders.
    - Posterior segments: Place patient prone, Trendlenberg or hips elevated with pillows so that hips are higher than shoulders.
    - Lateral segments: Place patient in right side lying Trendlenberg for left lung and left side lying Trendlenberg for right lung or hips elevated with pillows to keep hips higher than shoulders.
- Perform chest percussions and vibrations on areas to be drained.
- Encourage patient to cough out secretions and collect in sputum container.
- Do suctioning if coughing is not possible.
- Make patient comfortable and ask to rest flat for ten to fifteen minutes before allowing sitting or getting out of bed.
- Dispose sputum container in infectious waste container. Replace articles.
- Document, time, amount and color of sputum drained, response of patient to therapy.

Percussion technique:

- Perform postural drainage for patient on empty stomach before meals.
- Avoid postural drainage for patient with hemoptysis.

Procedure

- Explain purpose and procedure to patient.
- Locate affected lung with help of X-rays, auscultation and percussion.
- Administer bronchodilators before procedure.
- Give steam inhalation to patient after obtaining doctor's written order.
- Position patient according to lung segment to be drained.
  - **Upper lobes**
    - Upper segments: Place patient in high Fowler's position iii chair or bed.
    - Anterior segments: Place patient in semi-fowler's position in chair or bed.
    - Posterior segments: Place patient in Fowler's position in chair or bed, provide a cardiac table
    - Lateral segments: Place patient in lateral position elevated to about 45 degree, first to one side and then to other side. When out of bed ask patient to lean on arm, resting on chair or table for support.
  - **Right middle lobes**
    - Anterior segment (right side): Place patient flat on left side with a pillow under chest. Right shoulder and body are kept forward.
    - Posterior segment: Place patient in prone with chest and abdomen elevated.
  - **Lower lobes**
    - Anterior segments: Place patient in supine, Freedenberg with hips elevated with pillows, so that hips are higher than shoulders.

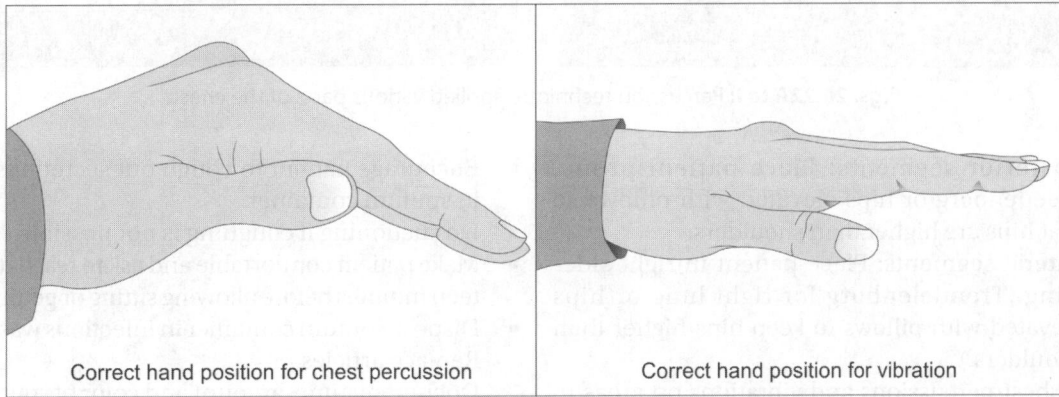

Fig. 20.21: Position of hand for percussion technique.

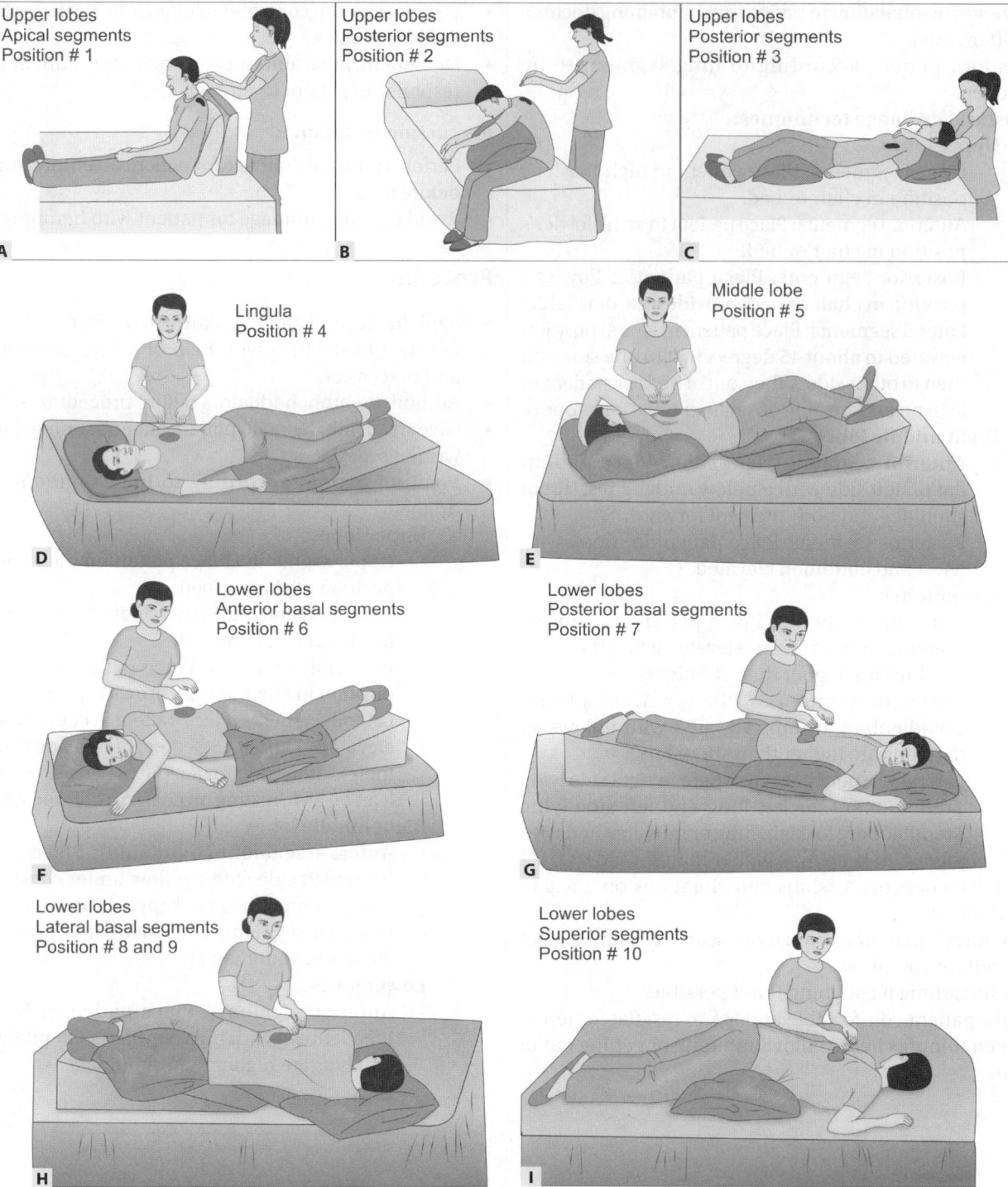

Figs. 20.22A to I: Percussion technique applied various parts of the chest.

- Posterior segments: Place patient prone, Freedenberg or hips elevated with pillows so that hips are higher than shoulders.
- Lateral segments: Place patient in right side-lying. Trendelenburg for right lung or hips elevated with pillows to keep hips higher than shoulders.
• Perform chest percussions and vibrations on areas to be drained.
• Encourage patient to cough out secretions and collect in sputum container.
• Do suctioning if coughing is not possible.
• Make patient comfortable and ask to rest flat for ten to fifteen minutes before allowing sitting or getting out of bed.
• Dispose sputum container in infectious waste container. Replace articles.

Document, time, amount and color of sputum drained, response of patient to therapy.

PULSE OXIMETRY

Pulse oximetry offers a reliable, noninvasive, painless alternative to frequent needle sticks usually required for arterial oxygen monitoring. The pulse oximeter continuously tracks arterial oxygen saturation levels using noninvasive light. A transducer (sensor) shines red and infrared light through tissues when attached to the client's body (e.g., a finger or toe). A photo detector records the relative amount of each color absorbed by arterial blood and transmits the data to a monitor, which displays the information with each heart beat. Alarms sound if the oxygen saturation level or pulse rate exceeds or drops below limits set by the user.

The oximeter eliminates delays associated with laboratory analysis of blood samples and instantly alters you to changes in the client's oxygen saturation levels so the nurse can take immediate action. It also monitors pulse rate and amplitude and can detect changes in the client's oxygenation status within 6 seconds.

Types of oxygen transducers: The type oxygen transducer used depends on the client's age, size and clinical condition.
- Neonatal foot transducer
- Infant toe transducer
- Pediatric finger transducer
- Adult finger transducer for clients engaging in limited activity
- Adult nasal transducer for inactive clients (typically used during surgery)
- Ear transducer
- Forehead reflectance transducer.

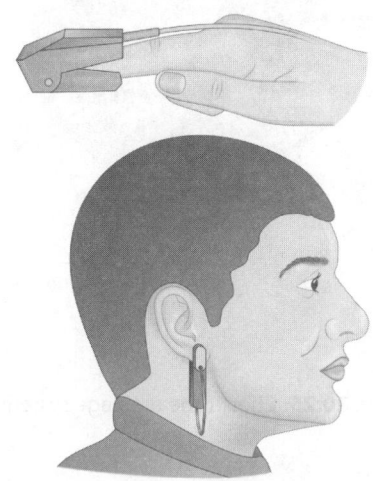

Fig. 20.23: Placement of pulse oximetry probe.

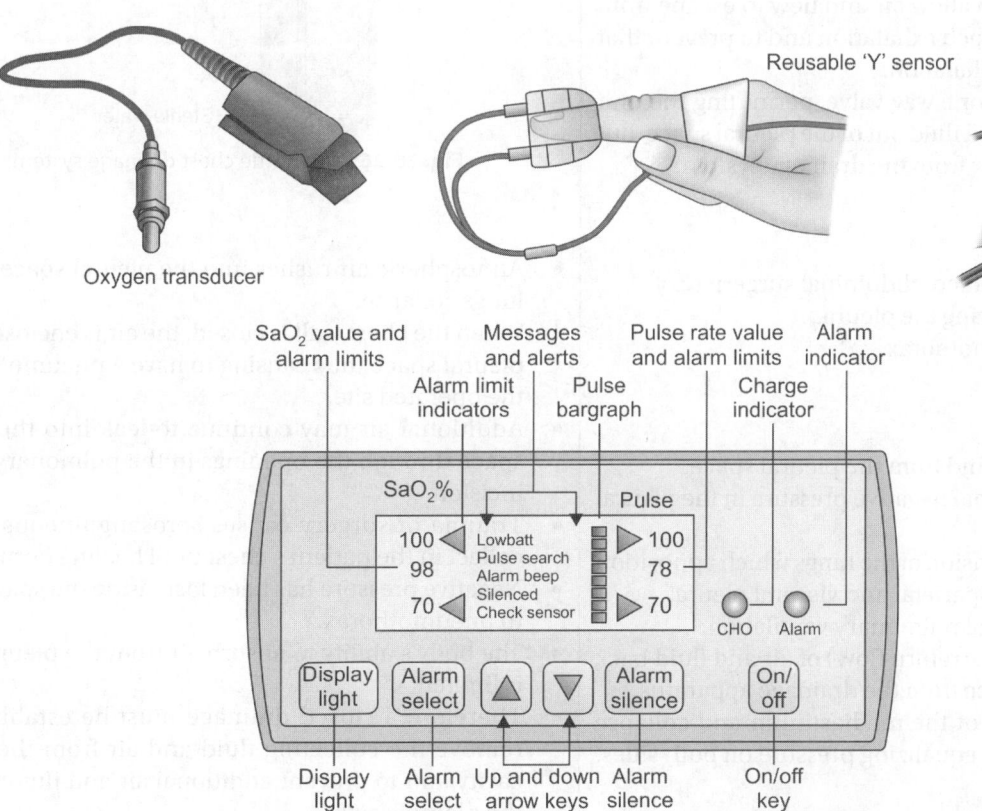

Fig. 20.24: Digital display screen of pulse oxymetry and settings.

Nursing Consideration

- The site selected for transducer requires no special preparation. For best results with the ear transducer, attach it to the fleshy parts of the earlobe, not on the cartilage.
- Attach a finger transducer to the client's index finger and keep the finger at heart level.
- Don't attach any transducer to an extremity that has a blood pressure cuff or an arterial catheter in place; the reduced blood flow will yield erroneous data.
- Protect the transducer from exposure to strong light.
- Cheek the transducer site frequently to make sure the device is in place and examines the skin for abrasion and circulatory impairment.
- Rotate the transducer at least every 4 hours to avoid skin irritation.
- If oxymetery has been performed properly, the oxygen saturation readings are usually within 2% of arterial blood gas values when saturations range between 84% and 98%.

WATER SEAL CHEST DRAINAGE

Water seal chest drainage means that a column of water in a bottle seals off the atmospheric air preventing from entering the chest drainage tube and thereby in the pleural space.

Water seal drainage system or so called "closed chest drainage" is indented to allow air and flew to escape from the pleural space with each exhalation and to prevent that return flow with each inhalation.

Water seal acts as a one way valve, permitting the unit directional flow of air and fluid out of the pleural space, but permitting none to enter from the drainage system.

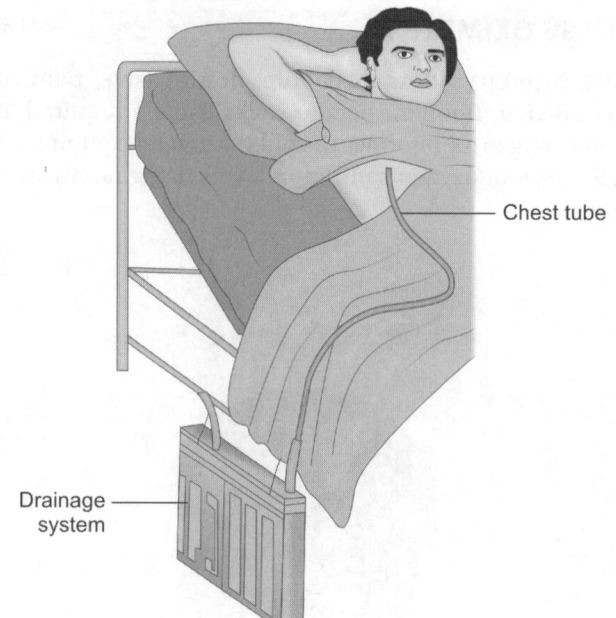

Fig. 20.25: Chest tube drainage system.

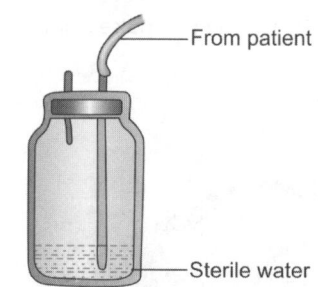

Fig. 20.26: One bottle chest drainage system.

Indications

- After thoracic or thoraco-abdominal surgeries.
- Chest injuries involving the pleura.
- Spontaneous pneumothorax.

Objectives

- To remove air and fluid from the pleural space.
- To re-establish normal negative pressure in the pleural space.
- To promote re-expansion of the lungs which apposition and cohesion of the parietal and visceral pleura.
- To restore the normal pulmonary ventilation.
- To prevent the reflex (return flow) of air and fluid back into the pleural space from the drainage apparatus.
- To prevent shifting of the mediastinum and collapse of the lung tissue by equalizing pressure on both sides.

Mechanism

- In a thoracic surgery the parietal pleura is incised and pleural space is opened.
- Atmospheric air rushes into the pleural space and the lungs collapse.
- When the chest wall is closed, the air is enclosed in the pleural space thus causing to have a pneumothorax in the operated site.
- Additional air may continue to leak into the pleural space through the openings in the pulmonary pleural incision.
- Trauma of surgery causes serosanguineous fluid to collect in the patient's chest until healing occurs.
- Negative pressure has been lost inside the space owing to pneumothorax.
- The body's ability to absorb air from the pleural cavity is limited.
- Therefore a closed drainage must be established to remove the collecting fluid and air from the pleural cavity and to prevent additional air and fluid entering the pleural cavity.
- A closed drainage system is used postoperatively to remove air and sero-sanguineous fluid form the pleural cavity.

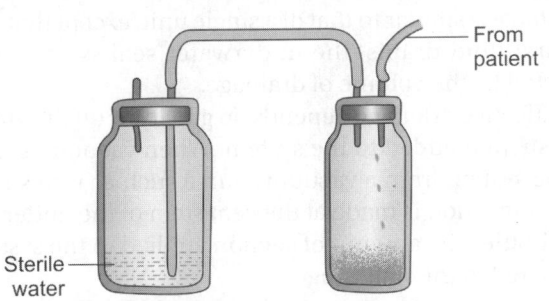

Fig. 20.27: Two bottle chest drainage system.

Factors Affecting the Chest Drainage

- **Proper placement of chest catheters:** Usually two catheters are placed in the chest, one of them is placed anteriorly through the second intercostal space to permit the escape of air rising in the pleural space. The lower catheter is placed posteriorly through the eighth or ninth intercostals space in the maxillary line to drain off serosanguineous fluid accumulating in the lower portion of the pleural space.
- **Proper placement of drainage apparatus:** The drainage apparatus for closed chest drainage must always located at a level lower than the patient's chest. Thus this helps drainage by gravity. At the same time it prevents backflow of air and fluid in pleural space.
- **Length of the drainage tubing:** Drainage tubing which connect the chest catheters to the drainage apparatus should be neither too long nor too short. It should fall in a straight line to the drainage apparatus with no dependent ioops. Dependent loops of the tubing, that contain fluids obstruct the flow of air and water into the drainage bottle and create back pressure thus impairing the drainage of air or fluid.
- **Maintaining the patency of the drainage tubing:** Patency of the drainage tubing and the chest catheter are checked frequently. Kinks and pressure on the tubing will cause obstruction in the flow of drainage. Observe the amount of drainage per hour to make sure that the tube is not internally plugged with pus or blood clots. Milking the tube helps to dislodge any clot that is formed in the drainage tubes.
- **Maintenance of an air tight drainage system:** Closed drainage system must be maintained air-tight. The bottles are sealed with tight stoppers and all connection of the tubes is taped to ensure its air tightness.
- **Position of the patient:** The patient is placed in a Fowler's position. This position helps to locate the fluid in the lower portion of the pleural space and drainage thorough the chest tubes, which are placed in the lower chest.
- **Activity of the patient:** The movement of the patient in bed helps to drain the chest. Coughing and deep breathing exercises help the patient to promote lung expansion and expulsion of air and fluid from the pleural space by increasing the intrapulmonic and intrapleural pressure.

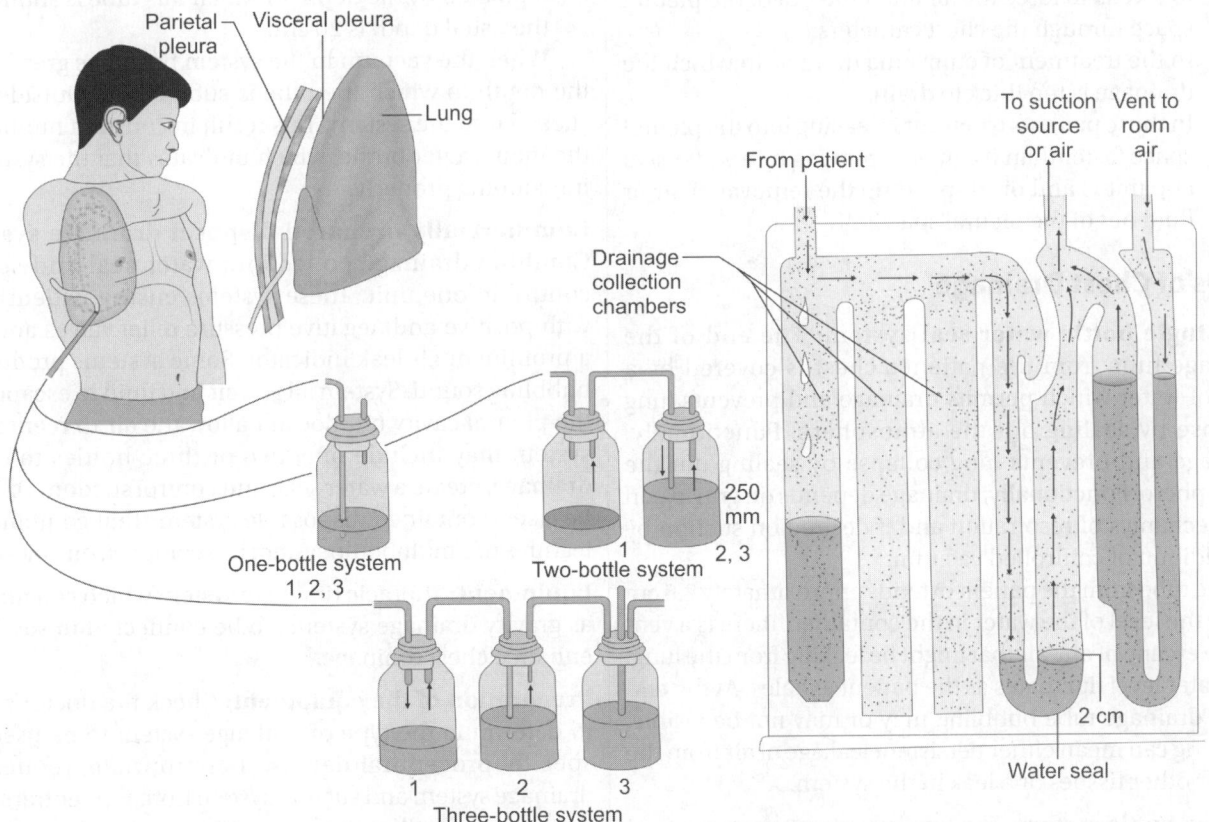

Fig. 20.28: Different types of chest drainage system.

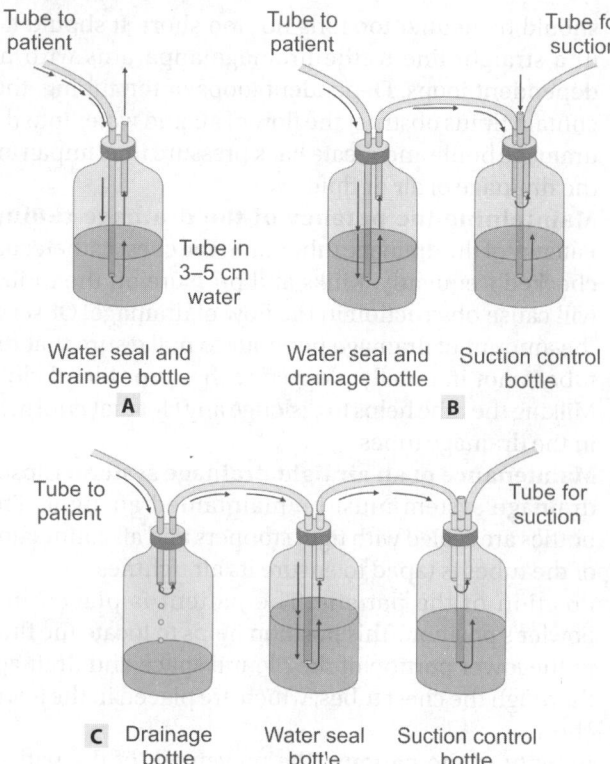

Figs. 20.29A to C: Tubing connections between the bottles in chest drainage.

- **Application of mechanical suction on the water seal drainage system.**
    - Continuous and gentle cough and respirations are too weak to force the air and fluid out of the pleural space through the chest catheters.
    - In the treatment of empyema thoracic in which the drainage is too thick to drain.
    - In those patients where air is leaking into the pleural space faster than it can be removing by a water seal apparatus and or to speed up the removal of air or fluid out of the pleural space.

Types of Chest Drainage

The single bottle water seal system: The end of the drainage tube from the patient's chest is covered by a layer of water which permits drainage and prevents lung collapse by sealing out the atmosphere. Functionally, drainage and prevents lung collapse by sealing out the atmosphere. Functionally, drainage depends on gravity, on the mechanics of respiration and if desired on suction by the addition of controlled vacuum.

The tube from the patient extends approximately 2.5 cm below the level of the water in the container. There is a vent for the escape of any air that might be leaking from the lung. The water level fluctuates as the patient exhales. At the end of the drainage tube bubbling may or may not be visible. Bubbling can mean either persistent leakage of air from the lung or other tissues or a leak in the system.

The two bottle system: The two bottle system consists of the same water seal chamber plus a fluid collection bottle. Drainage is similar to that of a single unit, except that when pleural fluid drains, the underwater seal system in not affected by the volume of drainage.

Effective drainage depends on gravity or on the amount of a suction added to the system. When vacuum is added to the system from a vacuum source such as wall suction, the connection is made at the vent stem of the underwater seal bottle. The amount of suction applied to the system is regulated to the wall gauge.

The three bottle system: This system is similar in all respect to the two bottle system, except for the addition of a third bottle to control the amount of suction applied. The amount of suction is determined by the depth to which the tip of the venting glass tube is submerged. In the three bottles system drainage depends on gravity or the amount of suction applied. The amount of suction in the system is controlled by the manometer bottle. The mechanical suction motor or wall suction creates and maintains a negative pressure throughout the entire closed drainage system.

The manometer bottle regulates the amount of the vacuum in the system. This bottle contains three tubes:
i. A short tube above the water level comes from the water seal bottle.
ii. Another short tube leads to the vacuum or suction motor or wall suction.
iii. The third tube is a long tube which extends below the water level in the bottle and which is open to the atmosphere outside the bottle. This is in the tube that regulates the amount of vacuum in the system. This is regulated by the depth to which this tube is submerged the usual depth is 20 cm.

When the vacuum in the system becomes greater than the depth to which the tube is submerged, Outside air is sucked into the system. This result in constant bubbling in the manometer bottle, which indicates that the systems is functioning properly.

Commercially prepared disposal drainage systems: Combine drainage collection, water seal and suction control in one unit. These systems ensure patient safety with positive and negative pressure relief valves and have a prominent air leak indicator. Some systems produce no bubbling sound. System allows air and fluid to escape from the pleural cavity but doesn't allow the air to reenter. The system may include one, two or three bottles to collect drainage, create a water seal, and control suction. Or it may be a self-contained disposable system. That combines the features of a multibottle system in a compact, one piece unit.

Equipment: Thoracic drainage system which can function as gravity drainage systems to be connected to suction to enhance chest drainage.

Preparation of the equipment: Check the doctor's order to determine the type of drainage system to be used and specific procedural details, if appropriate, request the drainage system and suction system from the central supply department. Collect the appropriate equipment and take it to the patient's bedside.

Oxygenation Needs 457

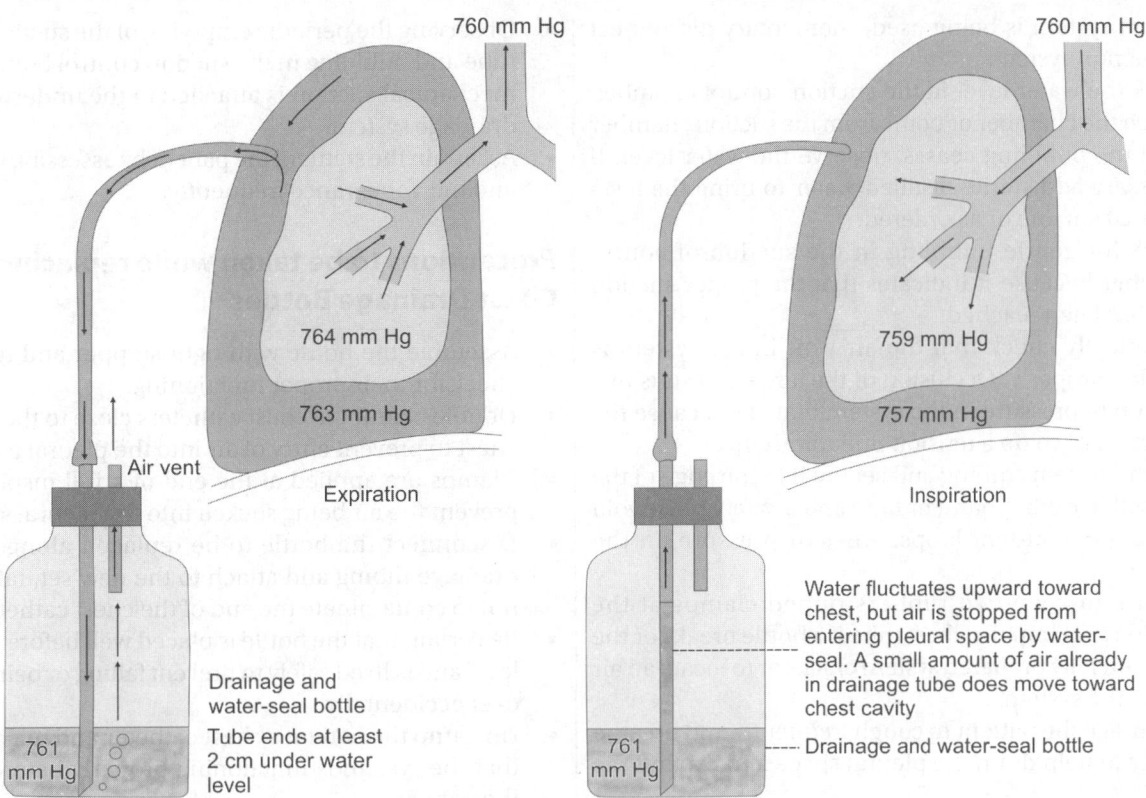

Fig. 20.30: Expiration and inspiration with pneumothorax and a chest tube using one-bottle gravity drainage system.

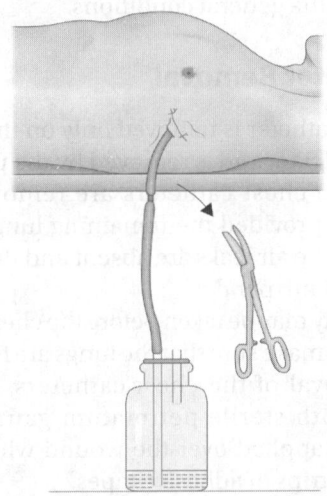

Fig. 20.31: Method of closing/clamping the drainage tube with artery forceps.

Implementation

- Explain the procedure to the patient and wash your hands.
- Maintain sterile technique throughout the entire procedure and whenever you make changes in the system or alter any of the connections to avoid introducing pathogens into the pleural space.

Setting Up a Commercially Prepared Disposable System

- Open the packaged system and place it on the floor in the rack supplied by the manufacture to avoid accidental knocking it over or dislodging the components. After the system is prepared, it may be hung from the side of the patient's bed.
- Remove the plastic connector from the short tube that is attached to the water seal chamber. Using a 50 mL catheter tip syringe instill sterile distilled water into the water seal chamber.
- If suction is ordered remove the cap on the suction control chamber to open the vent. Next instill sterile distilled water until it reaches the 0 cm mark or the ordered level and recap the suction control chamber.
- Using the long tube connect the patient's tube to the closed drainage system to the suction source, and turn on the suction. Gentle bubbling should begin in the suction chamber, indicating that the correct suction level has been reached.

Managing Closed Chest Underwater Seal Drainage

- Repeatedly note the character, consistency and amount of drainage collection chamber.
- Mark the drainage level in the drainage collection chamber by noting the time and date at the drainage level on the chamber every 8 hours.
- Check the water level in the water seal chamber every 8 hours, if necessary; carefully add sterile distilled water until level reaches the 2 cm mark indicated on the water seal chamber of the commercial system.
- Check for fluctuation in the water seal chamber as the patient breathes. To check for fluctuation when a

- suction system is being used, momentary disconnect the suction system.
- Check the water level in the suction control chamber. Detach the chamber or bottle from the suction chamber when the bubbling ceases, observe the water level. If necessary add sterile distilled water to bring the level to the 20 cm line or as ordered.
- Check for gentle bubbling in the suction of contra chamber because it indicates that the proper suction level has been reached.
- Periodically check that the air vent in the system is working properly. Occlusion of the air vent results in a buildup of pressure in the system that could cause the patient to develop a tension pneumothorax.
- Coil the systems tubing and secure it to the edge of the bed with a rubber band or tape and a safety pin. Avoid creating dependent loops, kinks or pressure on the tubing.
- Be sure to keep two rubbers tipped clamps at the bedside to clamp the chest tube if a bottle breaks or the commercially prepared system cracks or to locate an air leak in the system.
- Encourage the patient to cough frequently and breathe deeply to help drain the pleural space and expand the lungs.
- Check the rate and quality of the patient's respirations and auscultate his lungs periodically to assess air exchange in the affected lung.
- Tell the patient to report any breathing difficulty immediately. Notify the doctor immediately if the patient develops cyanosis rapid or shallow breathing, subcutaneous emphysema chest pain or excessive bleeding.
- When clots are visible you may be able to strip the tubing depending on your facility policy. This is a controversial procedure because it creates high negative pressure that could suck viable lung tissue into the drainage.
- Check the chest tube dressing at least every 8 hours. Palpate the area surrounding that dressing for crepitus or subcutaneous emphysema, which indicates that air is leaking into the subcutaneous tissue surrounding the insertion site.
- Encourage active or passive range of motion (ROM) exercises for the patient's arm or the affected side if he has been splint his arm to decrease his discomfort.
- Remind the ambulatory patient to keep the drainage system below chest level and to be careful not to disconnect the tubing to maintain the water seal.

Assessment of Proper Functioning

- Observing the oscillating movements of the fluid up and down in the water sealed tube.
- Observing the intermittent bubbling in the water seal bottle.
- Observing the collection of drainage in the water seal or drainage bottles.
- Observing the periodic emptying of the suction control tube and bubbling in the suction control bottle when a mechanical suction is attached to the underwater seal drainage system.
- Ascertain the status of the patient by assessing vital signs and the appearance frequently.

Precautions to be taken while replacing the Chest Drainage Bottles

- Assemble the bottle with tight stopper and tubes and check for their proper functioning.
- Double clamp the chest catheters close to the patient's chest to prevent entry of air into the pleural cavity.
- Clamps are applied at the end of a full inspiration to prevent the air being sucked into the pleural space.
- Disconnect the bottle to be replaced along with the drainage tubing and attach to the new set, taking care not to contaminate the end of the chest catheters.
- Be certain that the bottle is placed well before the chest level and is fixed safely to prevent falling or being kicked over accidentally.
- Unclamp the patient's chest catheter and make certain that the system is functioning properly before leaving the patient.
- Watch the patient's vital signs for few minutes to see any changes in the general conditions.

Chest Catheter Removal

- The chest catheter is removed only on the return order of the physician, and is removed by the physician.
- Usually the chest catheters are removed in two or three days, provided the remaining lung tissue is well expanded, the air leaks are absent and fluid drainage is less than 75 mL per day.
- A chest X-ray may be taken before the chest catheters are removed to make sure that the lungs are fully expanded.
- After removal of the chest catheters, the wound is covered with sterile petrolatum gauze and a firm dressing is applied over the wound which is secured with wide strips of adhesive tapes.
- After removal of the catheters the patient is observed closely for the development of respiratory distress.

Discharge Teaching

The following advice is given to these patients on discharge from the hospital.
- To have deep breathing and coughing exercise.
- To maintain good nutrition.
- to maintain good hygiene especially oral hygiene.
- To avoid activities or environment that can cause irritation of trachea bronchial tree.
- They are advised not to smoke, to avoid dusty place and to avoid exposure to the persons having respiratory infections.

- To consult the physician if symptoms of upper reparatory infections or other ailments develop.
- To obtain a fitness certificate before they join their duty.

Common Problems and Suggested Actions

Lack of Drainage

Causes: Kinking, looping or pressure on the tubing may cause reflux of fluid into the intrapleural space or may impede drainage, causing blocking of the intrapleural drain.

Nursing action: Check the system and straighten tubing as required. Secure the tubing to prevent a recurrence of the problem.

No Fluctuation of Fluid in Tubing from the Underwater Seal

Causes
- Re-expansion of the lung.
- Tubing is obstructed by blood clots fibrin.
- Failure of the suction apparatus.

Nursing action: Ask medical staff if the drain may be removed following chest X-ray. The purpose of the drain has been fulfilled. Keeping the drain in any longer than necessary may lead to hazards from infection or air re-entry. "Milk" the tubing towards the drainage bottle to try to dislodge the obstruction and re-establish potency. Straighten tubing as required. Secure the tubing to prevent a recurrence. Disconnect the suction apparatus and ensure drain is patent.

Constant Bubbling of Fluid in the Drainage

Causes: An air leak in the system.

Nursing action: Clamp the intrapleural drain momentarily close to the chest wall and establish whether there is a leak in the rest of the system. Clamping the tubing shows whether the leak is below the level of the clamp.

Patient Shows Signs of Rapid Shallow Breathing, Cyanosis, Pressure in the Chest, Subcutaneous Emphysema or Hemorrhage

Causes: Tension pneumothorax, mediastinal shift, postoperative hemorrhage, severe incision pain, pulmonary embolus or cardiac tamponade.

Nursing actions: Observe record and report any of these signs to a doctor immediately.

Incision Pain

Nursing actions: Provide analgesia as prescribed to reduce the patient's discomfort and to enable deep breathing exercises to be performed and mobilization to ensure adequate drainage and to avoid complications.

Accidental Disconnection of the Drainage Tubing from the Intrapleural Drain

Nursing action: Apply an artery clamp to the drain immediately in order to avoid air entering the pleural space. Reestablish the connection as soon as possible in order to reestablish drain age. If necessary use cleans sterile drainage tube tubing may have been contaminated when it became disconnected.

Patient needs to be moved to Another Area

Nursing action: Place the drainage bottle below the level of the intrapleural drain as close to the floor as possible in order to prevent reflux of fluid into the pleural space. Do not clamp the drain unless the doctor has ordered it.

Intrapleural Brain Falls Out

Nursing Action: Pull the purse string suture immediately to close the wound. Cover the wound with an occlusive sterile dressing. Inform a doctor. The objective is to minimize the amount of air entering the pleural space. The drain will probably need reinserting. Reassure the patient with appropriate explanations.

CARDIOPULMONARY RESUSCITATION

Cardiopulmonary resuscitation (CPR) is a life saving technique useful in many emergencies, including heart attack or near drowning, in which someone's breathing or heartbeat has stopped. The air we breathe in travels to our lungs where oxygen is picked up by our blood and then pumped by the heart to our tissue and organs. When a person experiences cardiac arrest—whether due to heart failure in adults and the elderly or an injury such as near drowning, electrocution or severe trauma in a child—the heart goes from a normal beat to an arrhythmic pattern called ventricular fibrillation, and eventually ceases to beat altogether. This prevents oxygen from circulating throughout the body, rapidly killing cells and tissue. In essence, cardio (heart) pulmonary (lung), resuscitation

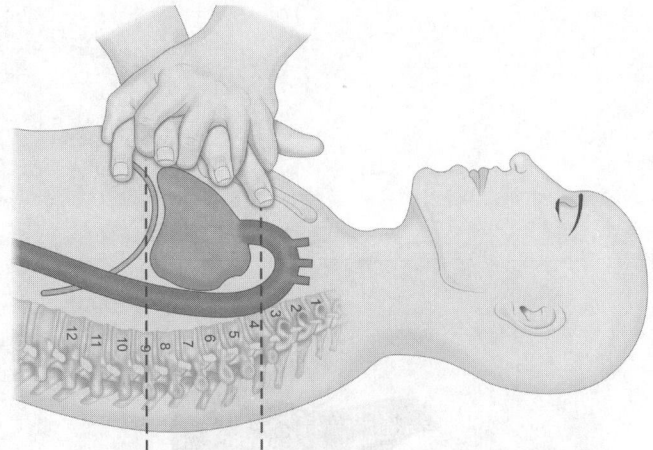

Fig. 20.32: Placement of hands during cardiopulmonary resuscitation.

(revive, revitalize) serves as an artificial heartbeat and an artificial respirator.

Cardiopulmonary resuscitation or CPR is an emergency life-support procedure. It includes artificial respiration and manual cardiac massage. Both these procedures are applied to prevent irreversible brain damage or death in the case of cardiac arrest. They should be performed only by someone trained in the technique after making sure that the victim's heart has stopped or respiration has ceased. The first step is to check if a victim's pulse has stopped and then to check the pulse rate in the neck or groin. If no pulse can be felt the rescuer can assume that the victim's heart has stopped and start CPR at once, if he is properly trained. If untrained in CPR one should seek emergency medical help as soon as possible. Those who are performing the CPR may shout out to someone nearby to call for medical help.

Definition

Artificial ventilation accompanied by cardiac massage to facilitate normal breathing and heart action in the event of cardiac arrest.

Purpose

To reestablish effective ventilation and circulation.

Equipment

- Cardiac board.
- Suction apparatus.
- Oxygen supply.
- Box containing Ambu bag (Fig. 20.33).
- Sterile endotracheal tube (2.5 to 5.5 mm).
- Extra batteries.
- Laryngoscope with 0, 1, 2 size tongue blades and stillet, Magill forceps, adhesive scissors, Airway syringes 1, 2, 5, 10 cc.
- Intracardiac needle 20 G, 22 G, 6 to 8 cm length.
- Needles 23 and 20 G.
- Elastoplasts bandage.

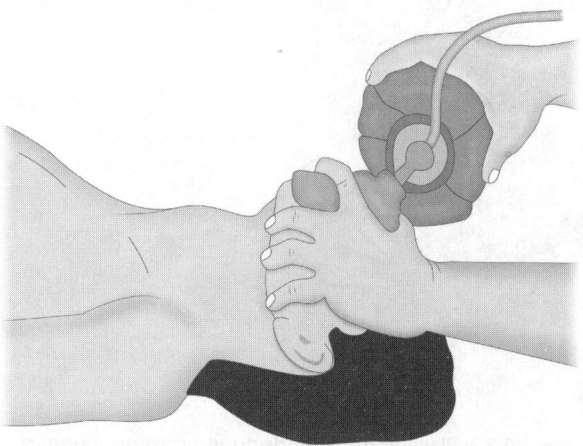

Fig. 20.33: Ventilation given with Ambu bag.

General Instructions

- Identify "Red Flag" signs of critically ill child- changes in level of consciousness, flaccid posturing, cyanosis severe chest retractions, grunting respiration, increased respiratory rate, shallow respiration, see saw respiration, i.e. abdominal protrusion with inhalation, irregular respirations with periodic deep sighs, apneas, absent pulse, absent heart rate, absent carotid pulse, dilated pupils, unrecordable blood pressure, cold clammy skin.
- Act quickly! As child can go into cerebral hypoxia within 3 to 4 minutes which will lead to permanent brain damage.
- Assess child (look, listen, feel) and if not breathing call for help.
- Immediately start cardiopulmonary resuscitation (CPR).
- Equipment for CPR to be always accessible and in functioning condition.
- All CPR equipment to be checked at beginning of each shift.
- All staff to be skillful at CPR.

Procedure

A. **Airway:** Establish patent airway by suctioning oropharynx with catheter, and deflate stomach by aspirating stomach contents.

B. **Breathing:** Establish breathing by artificial ventilation. Place Ambu bag on mouth and nose, and connect to 100 percent oxygen (Fig. 20.35). Select ET tube using the formula:

$$\frac{\text{Age in years} + 4}{4}$$

Calculate size of ET tube approximately as diameter of child's little finger. The ET tube is inserted.

C. **Circulation:** Initiate cardiac compression to a distance calculated using the formula (ET size × 3 cm).
   Method: Serial rhythmic compressions of chest that help to circulate oxygen containing blood to vital organs.
   - **Infant**
     - Site: Sternum compression—below level of infant's nipples.
     - Width one finger breadth.
     - Depth ½ inch to 1 inch.
     - Rate 100 times per minute.
   - **Child**
     - Site: Lower margin of child's rib cage to notch where ribs and sternum meet.
     - Avoid compression over notch.
     - Place heel of nurse's hand over lower half of sternum (between nipple line and notch).
     - Depth: 1 to 1½ inches.
     - Rate: 100 times per minute.

Ratio of Cardiac Compression to Ventilation

2 persons—30:1.
1 person—30:2.

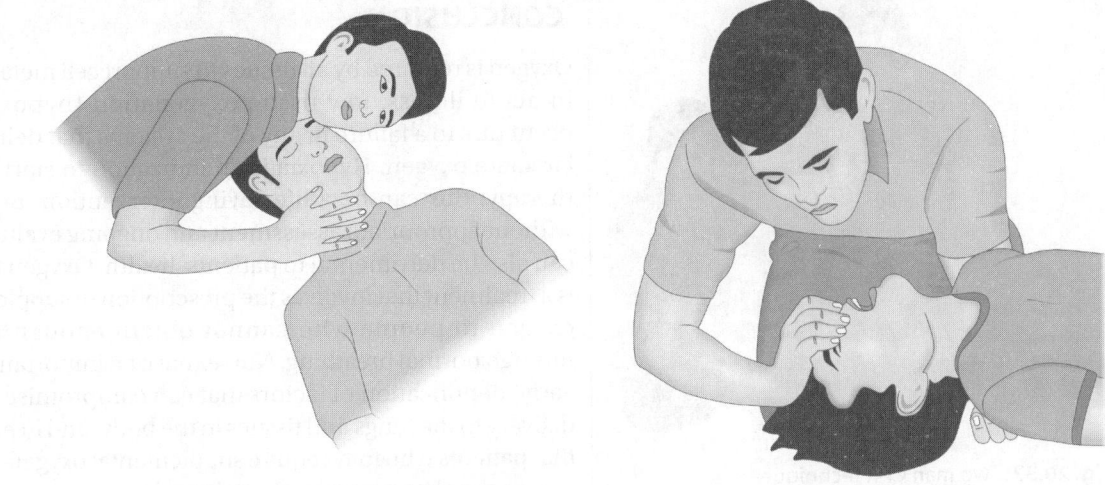

Fig. 20.34: Assessment of circulation and breathing.

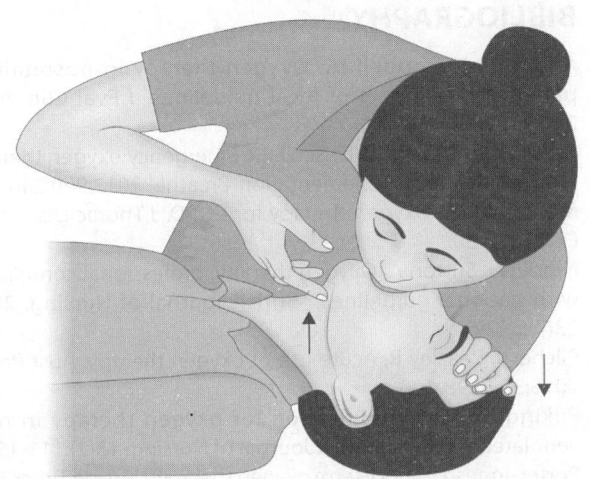

Fig. 20.35: Ventilation by mouth to mouth.

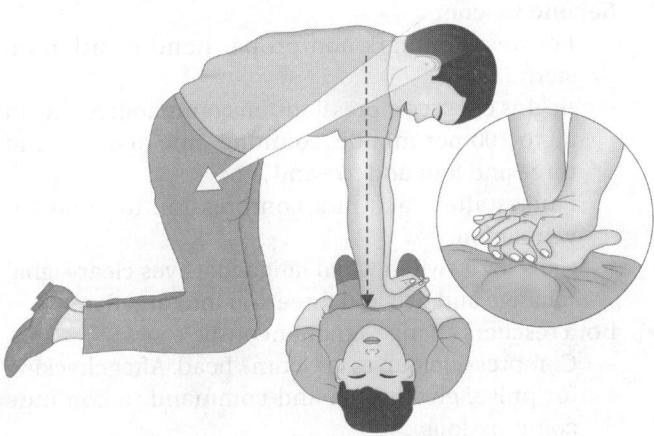

Fig. 20.36: External cardiac massage.

One Rescuer CPR

Shake shoulders and ask "Are you OK? ", shout for help.

Open the airway: The most important action for successful resuscitation is immediate opening of the airway. Tilt the head by applying firm backward pressure on the victim's forehead with palm of one hand. Place two or three fingers of the other hand under the bony part of the lower jaw near the chin and lift the chin.

Check for breathing: Place check close to victim's mouth and nose. Look at chest to see if it rises and falls. Listen and feel for exhaled air (for at least 5 seconds)

Breathe: Maintain an open airway. Pinch nose, seal lips around victims mouth and deliver two full breathe watching for chest to rise and fall with each breath.

Check for Circulation

Feel for a carotid pulse. Again shout for help/activate emergency medical services (EMS) system. If pulse is present, continue to give artificial ventilation at the rate of 1 breath or 12 mm.

Circulate: If pulse is absent, run fingers along the lower rib to notch in center of the heart where ribs meet sternum. With middle finger in notch, place index finger on lower end of sternum. Place heel of other hand on lower ½ of sternum next to index finger. Put the heel of 1st hand on top. With shoulders directly over sternum and elbows locked, compress straight up and down 15 times, at the rate of 80 to 100 times a minute, using the count "one and two and three and", etc. Return quickly to victims head to deliver two breaths. Compression depth should be 1½ to 2 inches (Fig. 20.36).

Two Rescuers CPR

Two medical professional arriving at same time—no.

CPR in Progress

- **First rescuer**
  - Determine unresponsiveness
  - Opens the airway
  - Checks for breathing

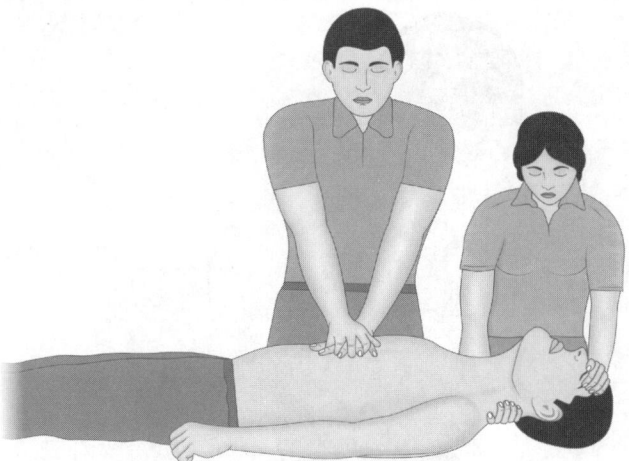

Fig. 20.37: Two man CPR technique.

– Ventilates twice, watching chest movement.
– Checks for carotid pulse: Gives command to begin compressions if pulse is absent.
- **Second rescuer**
  – Locates landmark and proper hand position on sternum.
  – Begins chest compressions on command: At rate of 80 to 100 per minute, counting "one and two and three and four and five and", etc.
  – Pauses after each fifth compression to allow for ventilation.
  – Calls for a switch when fatigued. Gives clear signal "change and two and three and four and five".
- Both rescuers change simultaneously
  – Compression moves to victim's head. After checking for pulse, give breath and command to continue compressions.
  – Ventilator moves to chest: Finds landmark and properly positions hands, begins compressions on command pausing after each 5th compression for breath.

If CPR is in progress by lay person, rescue team enters after completion of cycle of 15 compressions and 2 ventilations and start with a reassessment.

If CPR is in progress by a professional rescuer, the 2nd professional rescuer takes over compressions at the end of a cycle and after 1st rescuer reassesses pulse and gives another breath.

Complications

- Damage to the cervical spine due to hyperextension of the neck.
- Fracture of the rib and xiphoid process.
- Hemopericardium.
- Pneumothorax.
- Intra abdominal hemorrhage.
- Gastric distention of air.
- Aspiration of the vomitus into the lungs.

CONCLUSION

Oxygen is required by all tissues to support cell metabolism; in acute illness, low tissue oxygenation (hypoxia) can occur due to a failure in any of the systems that deliver and circulate oxygen. Hypoxia is an indication to start oxygen therapy; this can be a life-saving intervention, but given without appropriate assessment and ongoing evaluation, it can also be detrimental to patients' health. Oxygen therapy is a treatment that involves the prescription of supplemental oxygen to people who cannot obtain enough oxygen through normal breathing. Nurses have an important role in early identification of factors that can compromise oxygen delivery to the lungs and tissues in the body, and in ensuring that patients who may require supplemental oxygen therapy are assessed and managed safely and competently.

BIBLIOGRAPHY

1. Akbar FA, Campbell IA. Oxygen therapy in hospitalized patients: the impact of local guidelines. J Eval Clin Pract. 2006;12(1):31-36.
2. Kane B, Decalmer S, O'Driscoll BR. Emergency oxygen therapy: From guideline to implementation. Breathe. 2013;9(4):246-253.
3. McDonald CF. Oxygen therapy for COPD. J Thorac Dis. 2014;6 (11):1632-39.
4. Nippers I, Sutton A. Oxygen therapy: professional compliance with national guidelines. British Journal of Nursing. 2014; 23(7):382-6.
5. Pilcher J, Beasley R. Acute use of oxygen therapy. Aust Prescr. 2015;38(3):98-100.
6. Pilkington F. Humidification for oxygen therapy in non-ventilated patients. British Journal of Nursing. 13(2):111-15.
7. Porter-Jones, G. Short-term oxygen therapy. Nursing Times Plus. 2004;98(40):53-6.
8. Pruitt WC, Jacobs M. Breathing lessons: basics of oxygen therapy. Nursing Times Plus. 33(10): 43-45;2003.
9. Ramsey K. Oxygen therapy and oxygen delivery principles (respiratory therapy). Mosby's Skills. St. Louis, 2012.
10. Ridler N, et al. Oxygen therapy in critical illness. Friend or foe? A review of oxygen therapy in selected acute illnesses. Journal of Intensive Care Society. 2014;15:3,190-8.
11. Sheppard M, Davis S. Oxygen therapy–1. Nursing Times. 2000;96(29):43-4.
12. Vines DL, Shelledy DC, Peters J. Current respiratory care. Pt 1: Oxygen therapy, oximetry, bronchial hygiene. Journal of Critical Illness. 2000;15:507–10, 513-15.

REVIEW QUESTIONS

Long Essays

1. Discuss respiration. Explain the types, assessment and management.
2. Define dyspnea. Explain care of patient with dyspnea.
3. Define oxygen therapy. Explain the factors affecting oxygenation.
4. Nursing process in airway management
5. Tracheostomy suctioning.

Short Essays

1. Factors affecting respiratory functioning.
2. Alterations in oxygenation.
3. Care of oxygen cylinders
4. Nasal cannula.
5. Artificial airway management.
6. Coughing techniques.
7. Suctioning procedure.
8. Postural drainage.
9. Pulse oximetry.
10. Water seal chest drainage.
11. Cardiopulmonary resuscitation.

Short Answers

1. Types of respiration.
2. Characteristics of respiration.
3. Abnormalities in respiration.
4. Stages of hypoxia.
5. Nasal catheter.
6. Oropharyngeal airway.
7. Endotracheal tubes.
8. Tracheostomy tubes.
9. Types of inhalations.
10. Steam inhalation.
11. Factors affecting the chest drainage.
12. Types of chest drainage.

MULTIPLE CHOICE QUESTIONS

1. **Gas exchange takes place in the:**
   a. Pharynx
   b. Larynx
   c. Alveoli
   d. Trachea
2. **Findings in a patient with pneumothorax include:**
   a. A dull percussion note
   b. Decreased to absent breath sounds
   c. Increased tactile fremitus
   d. Late inspiratory crackles
3. **Involuntary breathing is controlled by:**
   a. The pulmonary arterioles
   b. The bronchioles
   c. The alveolar capillary network
   d. Neurons located in the medulla and pons
4. **Soft and low-pitched breath sounds normally heard over most of both lungs are:**
   a. Bronchovascular
   b. Bronchial
   c. Tracheal
   d. Vesicular
5. **The purpose of oxygen therapy is:**
   a. To supply O_2 in conditions when there is interference with normal oxygenation of blood
   b. To reduce the effects of anoxemia
   c. To maintain healthy level in tissue oxygenation
   d. All of the above

ANSWERS

1. c   2. b   3. d   4. d   5. d

CHAPTER 21
Fluid, Electrolyte and Acid-Base Balances

LEARNING OBJECTIVES

- Review of physiological regulation of fluid, electrolyte, and acid-base balances
- Factors affecting fluid, electrolyte, and acid-base balances
- Disturbances in fluid volume:
  - Deficit—hypovolemia dehydration
  - Excess—fluid overload edema
- Electrolyte imbalances (hypo and hyper)
  - Acid-base imbalances
    - Metabolic—acidosis and alkalosis
    - Respiratory—acidosis and alkalosis

- Intravenous therapy
- Peripheral venipuncture sites
- Types of IV fluids calculation for making IV fluid plan
- Complications of IV fluid therapy measuring fluid intake and output
- Administering blood and blood components
- Restricting fluid intake
- Enhancing fluid intake

TERMINOLOGY

- **Total body water (TBW):** Percentage of body composition consisting of water, approximately 60% of body weight, less in obesity and more in infants.
- **Intracellular fluid (ICF) volume:** That part of the TBW contained within the cells, approximately 40% of body weight and two-thirds of TBW. Muscle cells contain 75% water and fat cells have <5% water.
- **Extracellular fluid (ECF) volume:** That portion of the TBW outside the cells, approximately 20% of body weight and one-third of TBW, sustained osmotically mainly by sodium.
- **Interstitial fluid volume:** That portion of the ECF outside the circulation and surrounding the cells.
- **Anabolism:** The synthesis of large molecules from small ones, e.g. protein from amino acids or glycogen from glucose.
- **Catabolism:** The breakdown of large molecules into small ones, e.g. protein to amino acids or glycogen to glucose.
- **Solution:** Fluid consisting of a solvent, e.g. water, in which a soluble substance or solute, e.g. sugar or salt, is dissolved.
- **Crystalloid:** A term used commonly to describe all clear glucose and/or salt containing fluids for IV use (e.g. 0.9% saline, Hartmann's solution, 5% dextrose, etc.).
- **Colloid:** A fluid consisting of microscopic particles (e.g. starch or protein) suspended in a crystalloid and used for intravascular volume expansion (e.g. 6% hydroxyethyl starch, 4% succinylated gelatin, 20% albumin, etc.).
- **Balanced crystalloid:** A crystalloid containing electrolytes in a concentration as close to plasma as possible (e.g. Ringer's lactate, Hartmann's solution, Plasmalyte, Sterofundin, etc.).
- **Osmosis:** This describes the process by which water moves across a semi-permeable membrane (permeable to water but not to the substances in solution) from a weaker to a stronger solution until the concentration of solutes are equal on the two sides.
- **Maintenance:** Provide daily physiological fluid and electrolyte requirements.
- **Replacement:** Provide maintenance requirements and add like for like replacement for ongoing fluid and electrolyte losses (e.g. intestinal fistulae).
- **Resuscitation:** Administration of fluid and electrolytes to restore intravascular volume

REVIEW OF PHYSIOLOGICAL REGULATION OF FLUID, ELECTROLYTE, AND ACID-BASE BALANCES

Body fluids are contained in three compartments. Most of the fluids of the body are inside the cells called the intracellular compartment. The fluid outside the cell is called extracellular fluid. The extracellular fluid is divided into two parts. The fluid that is within the vessel is called intravascular fluid. The fluid between the cells is called interstitial fluid. The kidneys excrete the largest quantity of body fluid, but fluid leaves the body also via gastrointestinal tract, lungs, and skin. Two sources of body fluid are through ingestion and digestion of fat, carbohydrate, and protein. About 10 mL of water is released in the metabolism of 100 calories of fat, carbohydrate, or protein.

Electrolytes description: Electrolytes are ionized molecules found throughout the blood, tissues, and cells of the body. These molecules, which are either positive (cations) or negative (anions), conduct an electric current and help to balance pH and acid-base levels in the body. Electrolytes also facilitate the passage of fluid between and within cells through a process known as osmosis and play a part in regulating the function of the neuromuscular, endocrine, and excretory systems.

The serum electrolytes include:
- **Sodium (Na):** A positively charged electrolyte that helps to balance fluid levels in the body and facilitates neuromuscular functioning.
- **Potassium (K):** A main component of cellular fluid, this positive electrolyte helps to regulate neuromuscular function and osmotic pressure.
- **Calcium (Ca):** A cation or positive electrolyte, that affects neuromuscular performance and contributes to skeletal growth and blood coagulation.
- **Magnesium (Mg):** Influences muscle contractions and intracellular activity.
- **Chloride (Cl):** An anion or negative electrolyte, that regulates blood pressure.
- **Phosphate (HPO_4):** Negative electrolyte that impacts metabolism and regulates acid-base balance and calcium levels.
- **Bicarbonate (HCO_3):** A negatively charged electrolyte that assists in the regulation of blood pH levels. Bicarbonate insufficiencies and elevations cause acid-base disorders (i.e., acidosis, alkalosis).

Medications, chronic diseases, and trauma (e.g. burns or fractures, etc.) may cause the concentration of certain electrolytes in the body to become too high (hyper-) or too low (hypo-).

Acid-base balance: An important property of blood is its degree of acidity or alkalinity. Body acidity increases when the level of acidic compounds in the body rises (through increased intake or production, or decreased elimination) or when the level of basic (alkaline) compounds in the body falls (through decreased intake or production, or increased elimination). Body alkalinity increases with the reverse of these processes. The body's balance between acidity and alkalinity is referred to as acid-base balance.

One mechanism the body uses to control blood pH involves the release of carbon dioxide from the lungs. Carbon dioxide, which is mildly acidic, is a waste product of the metabolism of oxygen (which all cells need) and, as such, is constantly produced by cells. As with all waste products, carbon dioxide gets excreted into the blood. The blood carries carbon dioxide to the lungs, where it is exhaled. As carbon dioxide accumulates in the blood, the pH of the blood decreases. The brain regulates the amount of carbon dioxide that is exhaled by controlling the speed and depth of breathing. The amount of carbon dioxide exhaled, and consequently the pH of the blood, increases as breathing becomes faster and deeper. By adjusting the speed and depth of breathing, the brain and lungs are able to regulate the blood pH minute by minute.

FLUID INTAKE

Under normal circumstances most of our fluid intake is oral, but remember that all food contains some water and electrolytes and also that water and CO_2 are end products of the oxidation of foodstuffs to produce energy. This metabolic water is a small but significant contribution to net intake. Our drinking behavior is governed by the sensation of thirst, which is triggered whenever our water balance is negative through insufficient intake or increased loss. It may also be triggered by a high salt intake, which necessitates the intake and retention of extra water in order to maintain the ECF sodium concentration and osmolality in the normal range.

Although, in the elderly, the thirst mechanism becomes blunted, it ensures, on the whole, that our intake matches the needs of bodily functions, maintaining a zero balance in which intake and output are equal and physiological osmolality (280-290 mOsm/kg) is maintained. More than a century ago, Claude Bernard coined the term 'volume obligatoire' to describe the minimum volume of urine needed to excrete waste products, e.g. urea, in order to prevent them accumulating in the blood. This concept implies that, if sufficient fluid has been drunk or administered to balance insensible or other losses and to meet the kidney's needs, there is no advantage in giving additional or excessive volumes. Indeed, excessive intakes of fluid and electrolytes may be hazardous under certain circumstances (see below) and overwhelm the kidney's capacity to excrete the excess and maintain normal balance. Salt and water retention becomes clinically apparent in the form of edema when the ECF has been expanded by at least 2-3 liters.

SOURCES OF WATER INTAKE

Water is taken in from 3 major sources:
1. Water in food: 0.7 liters
2. Metabolic water (which is produced in the body during biochemical reactions): 0.3 liters
3. Drinking: 1.5 additional liters.

Water is the preferred drink to hydrate the body. Water is an essential nutrient for healthy hydration without bringing any other elements into the body. An over-consumption of sugar sweetened beverages can lead to excessive calorie intake; substitution of sugary beverages by water is one of the healthy habits which help to fight against overweight/obesity risk..

Water Requirements

Requirements of water vary with climate, dietary constituents, activities and surface area of the body. As a rule, a person should take enough water to excrete about 1200–1500 mL of urine per day. In tropics because of greater water loss through perspiration increased water intake is required to maintain urine volume. Normal intake of water ranges between 8–10 glasses per day.

Daily Water Input

In tropical countries like India, the daily water input amounts to 2400–3000 mL of water through food, as fluid drinks and as metabolic water.
- As fluid drinks—water, tea, coffee, milk soups 1500–1750 mL
- Water intake through solid food—600–900 mL
- Oxidation of carbohydrate, fat—300–350 mL proteins (metabolic water)

Total 2400–3000 mL

Daily Output of Water

- Urine 1200–1500 mL (kidney)
- Perspiration 700–900 mL (skin)
- Respiration 400 mL (lung)
- Feces 100–200 mL (intestine)

Total 2400–3000 mL

Therefore the water intake and output is fairly kept constant. This is called water balance. The average adult metabolizes 2.5–3 liters of water and a constant balance is maintained between intake and output. Inadequate water intake disturbs water equilibrium resulting in decreased urinary output, thereby causing changes in extracellular fluid (ECF) and intracellular fluid (ICF). The water equilibrium is maintained by kidneys, lungs, intestine and pituitary gland. The water balance coordinates with both electrolyte and acid-base balance.

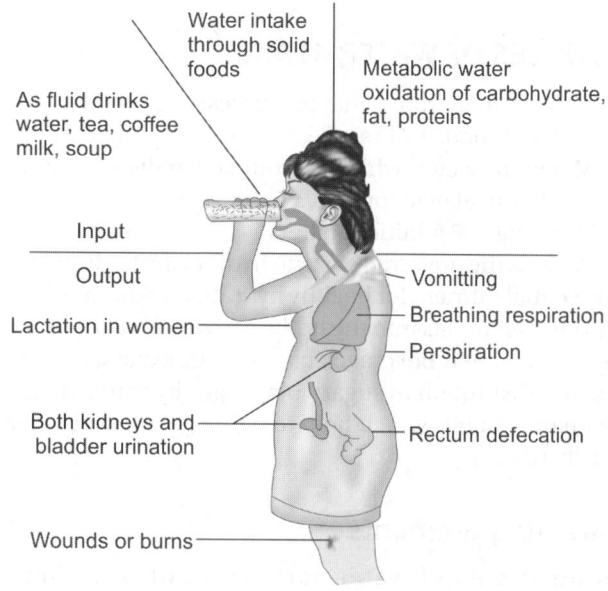

Fig. 21.1: Water intake and output.

> **Factors affecting fluid balance**
>
> Lifestyle factors
> - Nutrition
> - Exercise
> - Stress
>
> Developmental factors
> - Infants and children
> - Adolescents and middle-aged adults
> - Older adults
>
> Physiological factors
> - Cardiovascular
> - Respiratory
> - Gastrointestinal
> - Renal
> - Integumentary
> - Trauma
>
> Clinical factors
> - Surgery
> - Chemotherapy
> - Medications
> - Gastrointestinal intubation
> - Intravenous therapy

PHYSIOLOGY OF BODY FLUIDS

The primary body fluid, i.e. water is the most important nutrient of life. Whereas life can be sustained for many days without food but it can be sustained for only a few days without water. The primary functions of water in the body are as follows:
- Provides a medium for transporting nutrients to cells and wastes from cells and transporting substances such as hormones, enzyme, blood platelets, and red and white blood cells
- Facilitates cellular metabolism and proper cellular chemical functioning
- Acts as a solvent for electrolytes and nonelectrolytes
- Helps to maintain normal body temperature
- Facilitates digestion and promotes elimination
- Acts as a tissue lubricant.

Regulation of Body Fluids: As water moves through all parts of the body it is constantly being lost. Fluid leaves the body through the kidneys, lungs, skin, and GI tract. To maintain homeostasis, the normal daily loss must be met by the normal daily intake. Homeostasis is a relatively constancy in the internal environments of the body, naturally maintained by adaptive responses and that promote healthy survival. An approximate daily water intake and output of an adult eating 2500 calories per day.

> **Movement of fluid and electrolytes**
>
> **A. Passive transport (no energy required):**
> - **Osmosis:** *Fluid* move from higher concentration to lower concentration
> - **Diffusion:** *Molecules* move from higher concentration to lower (concentration gradient)
> - **Filtration:** *Fluid and diffusible substances* move together across a membrane; moving from ↑ pressure to ↓ pressure
> - **Hydrostatic pressure:** Fluids moves from an area of higher pressure to area of lower pressure
>
> **B. Active transport (energy required):** Sodium-potassium pump

FACTORS AFFECTING FLUID MOVEMENT

- **Diffusion:** Molecules move from a solution of higher concentration to solution of lower concentration. Increase in the temperature increases the rate of diffusion.
- **Osmosis:** The diffusion water molecules through a permeable membrane from an area of lesser solute concentration.
- **Hydrostatic pressure:** It is the pressure exerted by a fluid within a closed system. Counterbalancing the osmotic pressure of the plasma, which attract fluid into the vascular system.
- **Dialysis:** The diffusion of molecules of soluble constituents through a permeable membrane is known as dialysis.
- **Filtration:** It may be defined as the passage of fluids and dissolved substances across membranes because of differences in mechanical pressure on two sides of the membrane.
- **Selective permeability of membranes:** In body the capillary and the cell membranes are described as selective permeable.

MECHANISMS CONTROLLING FLUID AND ELECTROLYTE MOVEMENT

There are many different processes which control the movement of fluid and electrolytes between the ICF and ECF spaces. These processes include simple diffusion, facilitated diffusion, active transport, osmosis, fluid presence (hydrostatic pressure and oncotic pressure).

Simple diffusion: It is defined as the natural tendency of a substance or solutes to move from an area of higher concentration to that of lower concentration. It occurs through the random movement of ions and molecules. It occurs in liquids, gases, and solids. For example, exchange of oxygen and carbon dioxide between pulmonary capillaries and alveoli. Net movement of the molecules stops when the concentrations are equal in both areas. The membrane separating the two areas must be permeable to the diffusing substance for the process to occur. These molecules move without external energy. Diffusion is an efficient mechanism for the movement of molecules in and out of cells. Diffusion does not require energy.

Facilitated diffusion: Some molecules diffuse slowly into the cell because of the composition of cellular membrane. However, when they are combined with a specific carrier molecule, the rate of diffusion accelerates. Like simple diffusion, facilitated diffusion moves molecules from an area of high concentration to one of low concentration. Glucose transport into the cell is an example of facilitated diffusion. The hormone insulin increases the rate of facilitated diffusion of glucose in most tissues.

Active transport: It is a process in which molecules move in the absence of a favorable diffusion gradient. In which, the physiologic pump that moves fluid from an area of lower concentration to one of higher concentration. External energy is required for this process because molecules are being moved against a concentration gradient. Active transport requires adenosine triphosphate (ATP) for energy. The energy production depends on oxygen and glucose availability.

The concentration of sodium and potassium differs greatly, intracellularly and extracellularly. By active transport, sodium moves out of the cell and potassium moves into the cell. The energy source for the sodium-potassium pump is ATP which is produced in the mitochondria. By definition, active transport implies that energy expenditure must take place for the movement to occur against a concentration of gradient.

Osmosis: Osmosis, a special type of diffusion, is the flow of water between too compartments separated by a membrane permeable to water but not to solute. Here the movement of fluid across a semipermeable membrane from an area of low solute concentration to an area of high solute concentration. This process stops when the solute concentrations are equal on both sides of the membrane. In this, water moves from the compartments that is more dilute (has more water) to the side that is more concentrated (has less water). The semipermeable membrane prevents movement of solute particles. Osmosis requires no outside energy sources and stops when concentration differences disappear. In addition to diffusion, osmosis is very important for maintaining the chemical stability of body cells.

Osmotic pressure for force: Osmotic pressure is a term used to describe the movement of water by the process of osmosis. It can be described as a pulling of water. Osmotic pressure is an important factor in the movement of water between fluid compartments. 'Osmolarity' and 'osmolality' both are measurements of osmotic pressure.

- **Osmolality:** It measures the osmotic force of solute per unit of weight of solvent. It reflects the concentration of fluid that affects the movement of water between fluid compartments by osmosis. It measures the solute concentration per kilogram in blood and urine. It is measured in milliosmole per kg of water (mosm/kg). The normal osmolality of body fluids is between 275 and 295 mmol/kg or mosm/kg. The major determinants of osmolality are sodium, glucose, and urea with sodium. Increase in the concentration of these substances in the plasma causes fluid movement into plasma because of its increased osmotic pressure.
- **Osmolarity:** It measures the total milliosmole of solutes per unit of a total volume of solution. The number of osmoles, the standard unit of osmotic pressure per liter of solution. It is expressed as milliosmole per liter (mosm/L) used to describe the concentration of solutes

or dissolved particles. In clinical practice, osmolality is used most frequently. Serum osmolality may be measured directly through laboratory tests or estimated at the bedside by doubling the serum sodium level or by utilizing the following formula:

In osmotic movement of fluid, cells are affected by the osmolality of the fluid that surrounds them. Where fluids are added to the body those that have same osmolality as cell interior are "isotonic". Solutions that contain more water than the cell are "hypotonic" (hypo-osmolar), those with less water than the cell are hypertonic (hyperosmolar).

Fluid pressure: As a result of pressure, body fluids shift between the interstitial space and the vascular space within the capillary. The pressure in the body fluids are either hydrostatic or oncotic.

- **Hydrostatic pressure:** It is the force exerted by a fluid against the walls of its container. The heart is a main component in generating pressure in blood vessels. Hydrostatic pressure in the vascular system gradually decreases as the blood moves through the arteries until it is about 40 mm Hg at the arterial end of a capillary. Because of the size of the capillary bed and fluid movement into the interstitial, the pressure decreases to about 10 mm Hg at the venous end of the vessel. Hydrostatic pressure in the capillaries tends to filter fluid out of the vascular compartment into the interstitial fluid.
- **Oncotic pressure (colloidal osmotic pressure):** Oncotic pressure is an osmotic pressure exerted by colloidal, in solution. In plasma, proteins and molecules attract water and contribute to the total osmotic pressure in the vascular system. Unlike electrolytes, the large molecular size prevents proteins from leaving the vascular space through pores in capillary walls. Plasma oncotic pressure is approximately 25 mm Hg. Some patients are found in the interstitial space, and they exert an oncotic pressure of approximately 1 mm Hg.

Filtration: The movement of the fluid through a capillary via the above stated two pressures (hydrostatic and oncotic) is called 'filtration'. An example of filtration is the passage of water and electrolytes from the arterial capillary bed to the interstitial fluid. In this instance, the hydrostatic pressure is furnished by the pumping action of the heart. Through filtration, absorption or reabsorption, and resorption will take place.

- **Absorption:** It usually refers to the initial movement of substances such as end products of digestion or medications from organ such as GI tract or tissues such as the muscle, subcutaneous or dermal tissue, buccal or pharyngeal tissues, into the vascular system.
- **Reabsorption:** It refers to movement of water, electrolytes, vitamins, amino acids, glucose, lactate or other essential substances from one compartment, such as the interstitial or renal tubules, back into vascular capillaries.
- **Resorption:** It refers to the process of calcium salts leaving the bone and moving to the blood in a form.

REGULATION OF FLUIDS AND ELECTROLYTES OR HOMEOSTATIC MECHANISM

The body is equipped with remarkable homeostatic mechanisms to keep the composition and volume of body fluid within narrow limits of normal. Organs involved in the homeostatic mechanism or regulation of fluid and electrolytes include hypothalamus, pituitary gland, adrenal gland, kidney, GI tract, parathyroid gland, heart and blood vessels, lungs, etc.

Hypothalamus: Water ingestion in the conscious client is regulated by the thirst receptors located in the hypothalamus. The thirst mechanism is stimulated by the hypotension and increased serum osmolality. In addition thirst may result from polyuria, fluid volume depletion as small as 0.5 percent, excess sodium intake, hypertonic feedings and hypertonic IV fluids. Although thirst can be reported and is an important clinical manifestation of fluid imbalances, it is not a true indicator of fluid balance in all persons. The thirst mechanism is depressed in the elderly. The desire to consume fluids is also affected by social and psychological factors not related to fluid balance. A dry mouth will cause the person to drink, even when there is no measurable body water deficit. Water ingestion will equal water excretion in the individual who has free access to water, a normal thirst and ADH mechanism and normally functioning kidneys.

Pituitary gland: The hypothalamus manufactures a substance known as antidiuretic hormone (ADH) which is stored in vesicle in the posterior pituitary gland and released as needed. ADH regulates water retention by kidneys. The distal tubules and collecting ducts in the kidneys respond to the ADH by becoming more permeable in water so that water is absorbed into the blood and not excreted. When there is a normal plasma osmolality and normal circulating plasma volume, continued ADH secretion is called "syndrome inappropriate to antidiuretic hormone (SIADH)". ADH is released in response to many conditions.

An increase in plasma osmolality, ECF volume depletion, pain, stress, and use of certain medications such as narcotics, barbiturates, and anesthetics—stress may be physiologic or psychologic. The factors which suppressing ADH include hypo-osmolality of the ECF, increased blood volume, exposure to cold, acute alcohol ingestion, carbon dioxide inhalation, administration of some diuretics, lithium and some antipsychotic medications. ADH prevents urine production and promotes water reabsorption from the renal tubules. Stimulation of the thirst mechanism and ADH release usually occur concurrently in response to a body fluid deficit.

Adrenal gland: Adrenal gland fluid volume is maintained by combinations of hormonal influences. ADH helps only water reabsorption. Hormones released by the adrenal cortex helps to regulate both water and electrolytes. Two

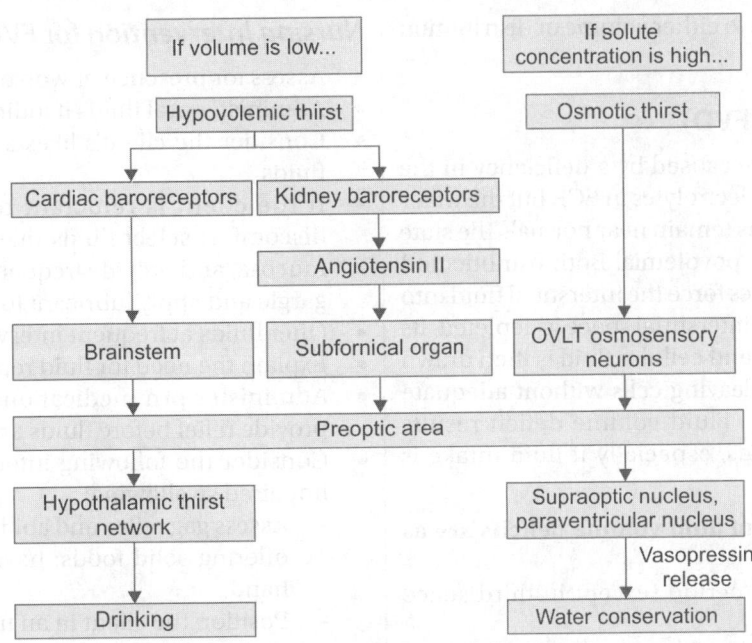

Fig. 21.2: Water regulatory mechanism.

groups of hormones secreted by the adrenal cortex include glucocorticoids and mineralocorticoids.

Extra cellularcoids primarily have an anti-inflammatory effect and increase serum glucose; whereas mineral affects corticoids (e.g. aldosterone) enhances sodium retention and potassium excretion. When sodium is reabsorbed, water follows as a result of osmotic charges. "Cortisol" is most common hormone which has both gluco and mineralocorticoids properties. Adrenocorticotrophic hormone (ACTH) from the anterior pituitary is necessary for aldosterone secretions. Hypovolemia is a common clinical condition in which aldosterone is secreted to maintain homeostasis.

Kidneys: The kidneys maintain fluid volume and concentration of urine by filtering the ECF through the glomeruli. Reabsorption and excretion of ECF occur in the renal tubules in response to ADH, aldosterone and ANP (atrial natriuretic peptides). ANP released from the atria in response to atrial distention, vasoconstriction, or direct cardiac failure. These factors increase the excretion of sodium and water and results in vasodilatation. The major functions of kidneys in maintaining normal fluid balance include the following:
- Regulation of ECF volume and osmolality by selective retention and excretion of body fluids. Regulation of electrolytes level in the ECF by selective retention of needed substances and excretion of unneeded substances
- Regulation of pH of ECF by retention of hydrogen ions
- Excretion of metabolic wastes and toxic substances.

Parathyroid gland: The parathyroid glands embedded in the corners of thyroid gland; regulate calcium and phosphate balance by means of parathyroid hormone (PTH). PTH influences bone resorption, calcium absorption from the intestine and renal tubules.

Gastrointestinal tract: Daily water intake and output are between 2000 mL and 3000 mL. The gastrointestinal tract accounts for the most of the water intake. Water intake includes fluids, water from foods metabolism and water present in solid goods. Lean meal has approximately 70 percent water whereas the water content of many fruits and vegetables approaches 100 percent. Most of the body water is excreted by kidneys. A small amount of water eliminated by GI tract through feces.

Lungs: The lungs are also vital in maintaining homeostasis. Insensible water loss, which is unavoidable vaporization from the lungs and skin assists in regulating body temperature. Normally, about 900 mL of water per day is lost. The amount of water loss is increased by accelerated body metabolism, which occurs with increased body temperature and exercise. Through exhalation, the lungs remove approximately 300 mL of water daily in the normal adult.

Heart and blood vessels: The pumping action of the heart circulates blood through the kidneys under sufficient pressure for urine to form. Failure of the pumping action interferes with renal perfusion and thus with water and electrolytic regulation.

Neural mechanism: In addition, neural mechanisms also contribute to the balance of water and sodium. Mechanoreceptors and baroreceptors are nerve receptors involved in neural mechanism.

FLUID IMBALANCES

Fluid imbalances occur when the body's compensating mechanisms are unable to maintain homeostatic state.

Fluid imbalance may relate to either volume or distribution of water or electrolytes.

Fluid Volume Deficit (FVD)

Fluid volume deficit can be caused by a deficiency in the amount of both water and electrolytes in ECF, but the water and electrolytes proportions remain near normal. The state is commonly known as 'hypovolemia'. Both osmotic and hydrostatic pressure changes force the interstitial fluid into intravascular space. As the interstitial space is depleted, its fluid becomes hypertonic, and cellular fluid is then drawn into the interstitial space, leaving cells without adequate fluid of function properly. Fluid volume deficit results from the loss of body fluids, especially if fluid intake is simultaneously decreased.

The main characteristics of fluid volume deficits are as follows:

- Weight loss over short period (except in third space losses)
- Decreased skin and tongue turgor
- Dry mucous membranes
- Urine output less than 30 mL per hour in adult
- Postural hypotension (systolic pressure drops by more than 15 mm Hg when client moves from lying to standing or sitting position)
- Weak, rapid pulse
- Slow-filling peripheral veins
- Decreased body temperature, such as 95 to 98°F (38 to 36.7°C) unless infection is present
- Central venous pressure (CVP) less than 4 cm H_2O
- Blood urea nitrogen (BUN) elevated out of proportion to serum creatinine
- Specific gravity (urine) high
- Hematocrit elevated
- Flat neck veins in supine position
- Marked oliguria, late
- Altered sensorium

Lab Values for Fluid and Electrolyte Status

Test	Usual Reference Range	SI Units
Serum sodium	135–145 mEq/L	135–145 mmol/L
Serum potassium	3.5–5.3 mEq/L	3.5–5.3 mmol/L
Total serum calcium	8.6–10 mg/dL (approx 50% in ionized form)	2.15–2.5 mmol/L
Serum magnesium	1.3–2.5 mEq/L	0.65–1.25 mmol/L
Serum phosphorus	2.5–4.5 mg/dL	0.87–1.45 mmol/L
Serum chloride	97–107 mEq/L	97–107 mmol/L
Carbon dioxide content	22–30 mEq/L	22–30 mmol/L
Serum osmolality	280–300 mOsm/kg H_2O	280–300 mmol/kg H_2O
Blood urea nitrogen (BUN)	5–20 mg/dL	1.8–7.1 mmol/L
Serum creatinine	Females: 0.5–1.1 mg/dL	44–97 mmol/L
	Males: 0.6–1.2 mg/dL	53–105 mmol/L

Nursing Intervention for FVD

- Assess for presence or worsening of FVD
- Administer oral fluids if indicated
- Consider the client's likes and dislikes when offering fluids
- If the client is reluctant to drink because of oral discomfort select fluids that are non-irritating to the mucosa, and provide frequent mouth care (offer saline gargle and apply lubricant to lips)
- Offer fluids at frequent intervals
- Explain the need for fluid replacement to the client
- Administer prn medications if nausea is present, to provide relief before fluids are offered.
- Consider the following interventions for clients with impaired swallowing:
  - Assess gag reflex and ability to swallow water before offering solid foods; have a suction apparatus on hand
  - Position the client in an upright position with head and neck flexed slightly forward during feeding (tilting the head backward during swallowing predisposes to aspiration because this position opens the airway)
  - Provide thick fluids or semisolid foods (such as pudding or gelatine). These are more easily swallowed because of their consistency and weight than are thin liquids.
  - If the client is unable to eat and drink, discuss possibility of tube feeding or TPN with the physician.
  - Monitor response to fluid intake, either orally or parenterally.
  - Monitor clients with tendency for abnormal fluid retention (such as renal or cardiac problems) for signs of overload during aggressive fluid replacement.
  - Turn client frequently, apply moisturizing agents on the skin.

Sometimes dehydration is used as synonym for hypovolemia; technically it is wrong. Dehydration refers only to a decreased volume of water; but water is not decreased without electrolyte charges also. Hydration is the union of a substance with water and is often used to indicate that there is normal water volume in the body.

Signs and Symptoms of Fluid Volume Deficit (Hypovolemia) and Fluid Volume Excess (Hypervolemia)

Fluid Volume Deficit (Hypovolemia)	Fluid Volume Excess (Hypervolemia)

Mild fluid loss
• Orthostatic hypotension, increased heart rate
• Restlessness, anxiety
• Weight loss
Moderate fluid loss
• Confusion, dizziness, irritability
• Extreme thirst
• Nausea—cool, clammy skin
• Rapid pulse
	• Tachypnea, dyspnea, crackles
	• Rapid or bounding pulse
	• Hypertension (unless in heart failure)
	• Distended neck and hand veins
	• Acute weight gain
	• Edema
	• Pulmonary edema
	  – Dyspnea
	  – Crackles

Contd...

Contd...

Fluid Volume Deficit (Hypovolemia)	Fluid Volume Excess (Hypervolemia)
• Decreased urine output (10–30 mL/hr) **Severe fluid loss** • Decreased cardiac output • Unconsciousness • Hypotension • Weak or absent peripheral pulses	– Orthopenea (difficult in breathing when supine)

Fluid Volume Excess (FVE)

Excessive retention of water and sodium in ECF in near-normal proportions results in a condition termed as fluid volume excess. It is also called "hypervolemia". Over hydration refers only to above-normal amounts of water in extracellular spaces. Malfunction of the kidneys causing an inability to excrete, the success and failure of the heart to function as a pump resulting in accumulation of fluid in the lungs and dependant parts of the body, are common causes.

Due to increased extracellular osmotic pressure from the retained sodium, fluid is pulled from the cells to equalize the tonicity. By the time intracellular and extracellular spaces are isotonic to each other, an excess of both water and sodium are in ECF, while the cells are nearly depleted. The excessive ECF may accumulate in tissue spaces, and is known as edema. Edema can be observed around eyes, fingers, ankles and sacral space and also accumulate in or around body organs. It may result in a weight gain in excess of 5 percent. When the excess fluid remains in the intravascular space, the concentration of solids in the blood is decreased.

Interstitial to plasma shift is the movement of fluid from the space surrounding the cells to the blood. The shift, also called hypervolemia is a compensatory response to volume or osmotic pressure changes of the intravascular fluid. Although the body attempts to maintain normal balance in all fluid spaces, the intravascular fluid is usually protected at the expense of interstitial fluid and ICF:

The common related factors which lead to fluid volume excess are as follows:
Compromised regulatory mechanisms such as
- Renal failure
- Congestive heart failure
- Cirrhosis of liver
- Cushing's syndrome
- Overzealous administration of sodium containing IV fluids
- Excessive ingestion of sodium containing substances in diet or sodium containing medication.

The characteristics of fluid volume excess include the following:
- Weight gain over short period
- Peripheral edema (excess of fluid in interstitial space)
- Distended neck veins
- Distended peripheral veins
- Slow-emptying peripheral veins
- CVP over 11 cm H_2O
- Crackles and wheezes in lungs
- Polyuria (if renal function normal)
- Ascitis, pleural effusion (when FVE is severe, fluid transudates into body cavities)
- Decreased BUN (due to plasma dilution)
- Decreased hematocrit (due to plasma dilution)
- Bounding, full pulse
- Pulmonary edema, if severe.

Common Laboratory Tests to Evaluate Body Fluid Disturbances

Hypovolemia	Hypervolemia
• Serum electrolytes • Serum urea nitrogen (SUN)/creatinine • Hematocrit • Urine electrolytes and specific gravity serum albumin • 24-hour urine for creatinine clearance	• Serum electrolytes • Urine-specific gravity • 24-hour urine for creatinine clearance • Total protein • Cholesterol • Liver enzymes bilirubin

Nursing Intervention for FVE

- Assess the presence or worsening of FVE
- Encourage adherence to sodium restricted diet, if prescribed
- Teach client requiring sodium restrictions to avoid over-the-counter drugs without first checking with the healthcare adviser/nurse
- When fluid retention persists despite adherence to dietary sodium intake, consider hidden sources of sodium, such as water supply or use of water softener
- When indicated, encourage rest period, lying down favors diuresis of edema fluid
- Monitor the client's response to diuretics. Discuss significant findings with physician
- Monitor the rate of parenteral fluids and the client response. Discuss significant finding with physician
- Teach self-monitoring of eight and intake and output measurements to clients with chronic fluid retention (such as those of ECF, renal failure, cirrhosis of liver)
- If dyspnea or orthopnea are present, position the client in semi-Fowler's position to facilitate lung expansion
- Turn and position the client frequently, beware that edematous tissue is more prone to skin breakdown than in normal tissue.

ELECTROLYTES

Electrolytes are substances whose molecules dissociate or split into ions when placed in water. These substances are found in ECF and ICF that dissociate into electrically charged particles known as 'ions'. 'Cations' are positively charged ions. For example, sodium (Na), potassium (K), calcium (Ca_2) and magnesium (Mg), hydrogen (pH) ions. 'Anions' are negative charged ions. For example, bicarbonates (HCO_3), chloride (Cl) and phosphate (PC43) ions and proteins. The ionic charge is termed 'valence'. Cations and anions combine according to their valency.

The concentration of electrolytes can be expressed in mol per deciliter (mol/dL), millimol per liter (mmol/L) or milliequivalent per liter (mEq/L). See the normal level of electrolytes in appendix. The role of electrolytes in cellular functions includes the following:
- Regulation of water distribution and osmolality
- Regulation of acid-base balance
- Transmission of nerve impulses, i.e. neuromuscular activity
- Contraction of muscles
- Clotting of blood
- Enzyme reaction.

IMPORTANCE OF ELECTROLYTES

Electrolytes play a vital role in maintaining homeostasis within the body. They help to regulate heart and neurological function, fluid balance, oxygen delivery, acid-base balance and much more. Electrolyte imbalances can develop by the following mechanisms—excessive ingestion; diminished elimination of an electrolyte; diminished ingestion or excessive elimination of an electrolyte. The most common cause of electrolyte disturbances is kidney failure.

Ion	Symbol	Function
Calcium	Ca^{2+}	Necessary for clotting blood, digestion, formation of bones and teeth, action of muscle (heart)
Iron	Fe^{2+}	Necessary for formation of hemoglobin and cytochromes
Sodium	Na^+	Extracellular positive ion
Potassium	K^+	Intracellular positive ion
Chloride	Cl^-	Negative ion
Bicarbonate	HCO_3^-	Extracellular negative ion and blood buffer
Iodide	I^-	Present in hormones
Ammonium	NH_4^+	Maintaining acid-base balance
Phosphate	PO_4^{3-}	Necessary for formation of bones and teeth
Magnesium	Mg^{2+}	Activator for many enzyme systems

Electrolytes are important because they are what cells (especially nerve, heart and muscle cells) use to maintain voltages across their cell membranes and to carry electrical impulses (nerve impulses, muscle contractions) across themselves and to other cells. Kidneys work to keep the electrolyte concentrations in blood constant despite changes in the body. For example, during heavy exercise, electrolytes are lost in sweat, particularly in form of sodium and potassium. These electrolytes must be replaced to keep the electrolyte concentrations of the body fluids constant.

Regulation or Electrolytes: Electrolytes regulate water distribution, regulate acid-base balance and maintain a balanced degree of neuromuscular excitability. There are many different kinds of electrolytes in the body. These include sodium (Na^+), potassium (K), calcium (Ca), magnesium (Mg_2), chloride (Cl), bicarbonate (HCO_3), phosphate (PO_4), etc.

Sodium

Sodium is the chief electrolyte of ECF. It moves easily between intravascular and interstitial spaces and moves across cell membrane by active transport. Many chemical reactions in the body are influenced by sodium, particularly in nervous tissue cells and muscle tissue cells.

The functions of sodium are as follows:
- It controls and regulates the volume of body fluids
- It maintains water balance throughout the body
- It is the primary regulator of ECF volume
- It influences ICF volume
- It participates in the generation and transmission of nerve impulses
- It is an essential electrolyte in the sodium-potassium pump.

Sources and Losses of Sodium
- An average daily intake is not known, but the average adult intake is eliminated to be between 6 and 15 mg and the RDA for sodium for adults is approximately 500 mg for 0.5 gm
- Sodium is found in many foods, particularly bacon, ham, sausage, catsup, mustard, relish, processed cheese, canned vegetables, bread, cereal, and salted snack food. It is found in table salt (NaCl) which has about 46 percent sodium
- Sodium excess are eliminated primarily by the kidneys, small amounts are lost in feces and perspiration.

Regulation of Sodium
- Sodium normally is maintained in the body within a relatively narrow range, and deviations quickly result in a serious health problem
- Salt intake regulates sodium concentrations
- Sodium is conserved through reabsorption in the kidneys, a process of stimulation by aldosterone
- The normal extracellular concentrations of sodium is 135 to 145 mEq/L (mmol/L).

Potassium

Potassium is the major cation of ICF. Potassium and sodium work reciprocally. For example, an excessive intake of sodium results in an excretion of potassium and vice versa.

The functions of potassium are as follows:
- It is the chief regulator of cellular enzyme activity and cellular water content
- It plays a vital role in such process as the transmission of electric impulses, particularly in nerve, heart, skeletal, intestinal, and lung tissue; protein and carbohydrate metabolism and cellular building
- It assists in regulation of acid-base balance by cellular exchange with H.

Sources and Losses of Potassium

- An average daily requirement of K is not known; but an intake of 50 to 100 mEq daily maintains potassium balance
- A well-balanced diet contains adequate quantities of potassium. Major sources include bananas, peaches, kiwi, figs, dates, apricots, oranges, prunes, melons, raising, broccoli, and potatoes. Meat and dairy products also provide adequate amounts of potassium
- Potassium excreted primarily by the kidneys. The kidneys have no effective method of conserving potassium. Therefore, deficits develop readily if excreted in excess amount without being replaced simultaneously
- Gastrointestinal secretions contain potassium in large quantities. Some is also found in perspiration and saliva.

Regulation of Potassium

- Cellular potassium is conserved by the sodium pump when sodium is excluded
- The kidneys conserve potassium when cellular K is decreased
- Aldosterone secretions trigger potassium excretion in urine
- The normal range for serum potassium is 3.5 to 5 mEq/L.

Calcium

Calcium is the most abundant electrolyte in the body. Upto 99 percent of the total amount of calcium in the body is found in bones and teeth in ionized form. There is close link between concentration of calcium and phosphorus. The functions of calcium are as follows:

- It is necessary for nerve impulse transmission and blood clotting
- It is catalyst for muscle contraction. Strength of contractions (especially cardiac muscle contraction) is directly related to the serum concentration of calcium ions
- It is needed for vitamin B12 absorption and for its use by body cells
- It acts as a catalyst for many cell chemical activities
- It is necessary for strong bones and teeth
- It establishes thickness and strength of cell membrane.

Sources and Losses of Calcium

- The average daily requirements for calcium is about 1 gm for adults. Higher amounts are required according to body weight; for children, for pregnant and lactating women, and postmenopausal women
- Calcium is found in milk, cheese and dried beans. Some calcium is present in meats and vegetables
- Use of calcium is stimulated by vitamin D. The most active form of vitamin D (calciferol) promotes calcium absorption and limits calcium excretion when levels are inadequate
- It leaves bones and teeth to maintain normal blood calcium levels, if necessary
- It is excreted in urine, feces, bile, digestive secretion and perspiration.

Regulation of Calcium

- When ECF calcium levels decrease, the parathyroid glands increase the secretions of PTH, which acts on bones to increase the release of calcium into the blood and acts on the kidney, tubules and the intestinal mucosa to increase the absorption of calcium from the kidneys and the intestine chloride
- A high serum phosphate concentration increases serum calcium; a low serum phosphate concentration decreases serum calcium
- Calcitonin, a hormone secreted by the thyroid gland has an opposite effect on calcium than PTH. Increase in calcitonin reduces the serum calcium concentration primarily by opposing osteoclast bone resorption.

Magnesium

Most of the cation magnesium is found within body cells. It is present in heart, bone, nerve, and muscle tissues. Magnesium is the second most important cation of ICF. The functions of magnesium are as follows:

- It is important for the metabolism of carbohydrates and proteins
- It is important for many vital reactions related to the body's enzymes
- It is necessary for protein and DNA synthesis, DNA and RNA transcription, and translation of RNA
- It maintains normal intracellular levels of potassium
- It serves to help or maintain electric activity in nervous membranes and muscle membranes.

Sources and Losses of Magnesium

The average daily adult requirement for magnesium is about 18 to 30 mEq. Children are required larger amount. Magnesium is found in most foods but especially in vegetables, nuts, fish, whole grains, peas and beans.

Regulation of Magnesium

- Magnesium is absorbed by the intestines and secreted by the kidneys
- Plasma concentration of magnesium range from 1.3 to 2.1 mEq/L with about one-third of that amount bound to plasma proteins.

Chloride

Chloride the chief extracellular anion is found in blood, intestinal fluid, and lymph and in minute amounts in intracellular fluid.

The functions of chlorides are as follows:

- It acts with sodium to maintain the osmotic pressure of the blood
- It plays a role in the body's acid-base balance
- It is important in buffering action when O_2 and CO_2 exchange in RBCs
- It is essential for the production of HCL in gastric juices

- The average daily requirement of chlorides is unknown. It is found in foods rich in sodium, in dairy products and meat.

Regulation of Chloride

- It is normally paired with sodium and excreted and conserved with sodium by the kidneys
- Chloride deficit leads to potassium deficit and vice-versa.
- Normal serum chloride levels range from 95 to 105 mEq/L.

Bicarbonate

The bicarbonate molecule is an anion. It is the major chemical base buffer within the body and is found in both ECF and ICF. It is essential for acid-base balance. Bicarbonate and carbonic acid constitute the body's primary buffer systems.

Phosphate

The phosphate ion is the major anion in body cells. It is a buffer anion in both ICF and ECF.

The functions of phosphate are as follows:
- It helps maintain acid-base balance
- It is involved in important chemical reactions in the body. For example, it is necessary for many vitamins to be effective; helps promote nerve and muscle action, and plays role in carbohydrate metabolism.
- It is important for cell division and for the transmission of heredity or hereditary traits. An average daily requirement for phosphorus is similar to those for calcium. It is found in most foods by especially in beef, pork, and dried peas and beans. It is metabolized in the same manner as calcium.
- Phosphate is regulated by PTH and by activated vitamin D. Calcium and phosphates are inversely proportional and increase fn one results in a decrease in the other. The normal range of phosphate is 2.5 to 4.5 mEq/L (mmol/L).

ELECTROLYTE IMBALANCES

Human body contains quite a large volume of water as ICF and ECF and the fluid contains several inorganic ions such as sodium, potassium, chloride, bicarbonate, sulfate, phosphate, calcium and magnesium. The complex mechanism of human life maintains the concentration and volume of the body fluids at a constant level and in general, it is not influenced by dietary intake and metabolism, while kidneys play a vital role in maintaining the balance. When clients presents with deficit or excesses of sodium, potassium, calcium, magnesium or phosphate, special nursing care is required. A brief description of the common electrolyte imbalances are as follows:

Hypernatremia
"Yoo Are Fried"
F-Fever (low), flushed skin
R-Restless (irritable)
I-Increased fluid retation and increased BP
E-Edema (peripheral and pitting)
D-Decreased urinary output, dry mouth

Can also use this one
SALT
S-Skin flushed
A-Agitation
L-Low grade fever
T-Thirst

Hypocalcemia
"CATS"
C-Convelsions
A-Arrhythmias
T-Tetany
S-Spasms and stridor

Cancer Assessment
CAUTION
C-Change in bowel/bladder habits
A-A sore that doesn't heal
U-Unusual bleeding or discharge
T-Thickening or lump
I-Indigestion or difficulty swallowing
O-Obvious changes in a wart or mole
N-Nagging cough or hoarseness

Hyperkalemia
Signs and symptoms increased
Serum K+
MURDER
M-Muscle weakness
U-Urine, oliguria, anuria
R-Respiratory distress
D-Decreased cardiac contractiltry
E-ECG changes
R-Reflexes, hyperreflexia or areflexia (flaccid)

Sx's minor bleeding
Beep
B-Bleeding gums
E-Ecchymosis (bruise)
E-Epistaxis (nosebleed)
P-Petechiae (tiny purplish spots)

ABG's
ROME
Respiratory Opposite Metabolic Equal

Hyperkalemia causes
Increase serum K+
Machine
M-Medication—ACE inhibitors, NSAIDS
A-Acidosis—Metabolic and respiratory
C-Cellular destruction—Bursa, traumatic injury
H-Hypoaldosteronism/hemolysis
I-Intake—Excessive
N-Nephrons, renal failure
E-Excretion—Impaired

"Hook" for serum sickness
Each letter stands for a key sign or symptoms of serum sickness.
F-Fever
A-Arthralgias
R-Rash
M-Malaise

Respiratory depression inducing drugs
"STOP breathing"
S-Sedatives and hypnotics
T-Trimethoprim
O-Opiates
P-Polymyxins

Hyponatremia

Hyponatremia refers to a sodium deficit in ECF caused by loss of sodium or gain of water. It is a condition on lowered level of plasma volume. In this condition, osmotic pressure changes result in ECF, moving into the cells. When this occurs, an examiner's fingerprints tend to remain on the client's skin over the sternum where pressure is applied with the fingers.

The related factors leading to hyponatremia are as follows:

- Loss of sodium as in; loss of CI fluids, use of diuretics; adrenal insufficiency
- Gains of water as in—excessive administration of D5W, diseases associated with SIADH; pharmacological agents that impair renal water excretion
- Hyponatremia or sodium depletion occurs from loss of body fluids through sweating, vomiting, diarrhea, intestinal fistula, dialysis and from aspiration of gastric contents
- Chronic pyelonephritis, chronic uremia, diuretic phase of acute renal failure, diabetic ketoacidosis, cystic diseases of the kidney, and excessive or prolonged use of diuretics result in excessive loss of sodium through urine
- Endocrine diseases show as myxoedema, Addison's disease, hyperaldosteronism, and uncontrolled diabetes mellitus also lead to sodium depletion
- Excessive loss of sodium can also occur through the skin as in extensive burns, generalized dermatitis, etc. in children with cystic fibrosis.

Sodium is mainly an extracellular ion, and its depletion causes migration of water in the intracellular compartments, making the extracellular fluid hypotonic. Consequently, plasma becomes hypo-osmolar and plasma volume falls.

Main Characteristics

- Anorexia
- Fingerprint over sternum
- Nausea and vomiting
- Muscular twitching
- Lethargy
- Seizures
- Confusion
- Coma
- Muscle cramps
- Serum sodium below 135 mEq/L.

This condition presents with tiredness, lethargy, muscular weakness, mental confusion, and in severe cases, convulsions and coma. The skin appears cold, pale and inelastic. Tongue is dry. Reduction in plasma volume causes reduction in cardiac output and results is tachycardia, fall of blood pressure and raised pulse rate. The eyeballs become soft due to reduced intraocular pressure, urine output is reduced and soon oliguria supervenes and finally leads to uremia. When the plasma serum concentration falls exaggeratedly to 120 mmol/L of blood or less, muscle cramps occur. It can produce acidosis and circulatory failure as complication.

Treatment

Mild cases are treated with frequent drink of water with added sodium chloride or with isotonic (0.9%) saline solution by IV injection. In other cases, 2 to 4 liters of isotonic saline solution is given IV infusion for over 6 to 12 hours. More severe cases are treated with 2 to 3 liters of IV isotonic solution in first 2 to 3 hours, followed by further 2 to 5 liters within 24 to 48 hours. If there is associated water intoxication, water intake is restricted to 500 to 1000 mL in 24 hours. In addition, the client is given treatment for the underlying condition.

Nursing Intervention

- Identify clients at risk for hyponatremia
- Monitor fluid losses and gains. Look for loss of sodium containing fluids, particularly in conjunction with low sodium intake
- Monitor presence of gastrointestinal symptoms, such as anorexia, nausea, vomiting, and abdominal cramping
- Monitor laboratory date for serum sodium levels less than normal
- Check specific gravity of urine
- With clients able to consume a general diet, encourage foods and fluids with high sodium content
- Be familiar with the sodium content of commonly used parenteral fluids. Monitor client with cardiovascular disease receiving sodium-containing fluids closely for sign of circulatory overload, such as moist rales in the lungs
- Use extreme caution when administering hypertonic saline solution (3 to 5% NaC1). Beware that these fluids can be lethal if infused carelessly
- Avoid giving large water supplements to clients receiving isotonic tube feedings, particularly if routes of abnormal sodium loss are present or water is being retained abnormally.

Hypernatremia

Hypernatremia or sodium excess refers to surplus of sodium in ECF that can result from excess water loss or overall excess of sodium. Because of the increased extracellular osmotic pressure, fluids move from the cells, leaving them without sufficient fluid. It is a condition which excess of sodium occurs in the ECF, giving rise to cellular dehydration.

The related factors which lead to hyponatrema are as follows:

- Deprivation of water, most common in those unable to perceive or respond to thirst
- Hypertonic tube feeding with inadequate water supplements
- Increased insensible water loss (as in hyperventilation)
- Ingestion of salt in unusual amounts
- Excessive parenteral administration of sodium-containing solution
- Hypertonic saline (3 or 5% NaCl)

- 7.5 percent sodium bicarbonate
- Isotonic saline
- Profuse sweating
- Diabetes insipidus
- Heat stroke
- Drowning in sea water
- Hypernatremia also occurs when water losses of the body exceed sodium loss as is seen in diabetes insipidus, marked glycosuria, hypercalcemia, hypokalemia, chronic renal failure, and recovery phase of acute renal failure
- Sodium excess may occur along with water excess when due to inadequate clearance of the kidneys both sodium and water accumulate in the extracellular space, leading to edema, for example, nephritic syndrome, cardiac failure, nutritional or thiamine deficiency, cirrhosis of liver, and in cases of usage of drugs such as corticosteroids, androgens, phenylbutazone, oral contraceptive and carbenoxelone. It causes retention of sodium, increased volume of ECF and edema in the interstitial compartment.

	Cause	
↓Na+ (135–145)	H2O↑, fluid loss, renal disease, adernal↓, SIADH, head trauma, hyperglycemia, heart failure **MEDS:** Diuretics, oxytocin	Anorexia, lethargy, dizzy, confusion, muscle cramp/weak/twitch, seizures, papilledema, dry skin, ↑pulse, ↓BP, weight gain, edema
↑Na+ (135–145)	H₂O↓, *diabetes insipidius*, heatstroke, hypertonic IVs, sea water, burns, hyperventilation, watery diarrhea **MEDS:** Corticosteroid, Na+ bicarbonate/chloride	Thirst, ↑ temp, lethargy, ↑BP, ↑pulse, restless, weak, swollen tongue
↓K+ (3.5–5)	Diarrhea, vomiting, gastric suction, hyperaldosteronism, bulimia, osmotic diuresis, alkalosis, starve **MEDS:** Corticosteroid, carbenicillin, amphotericin b, diuretics, digoxin toxicity	Fatigue, anorexia, polyuria, ↓ bowel motility, ventricular asystole or fibrillation, paresthesias, leg cramps, ↓ BP, ileus, ABD distention, ↓ reflexes **ECG:** Flat T waves, prominent U waves, ST ↓, prolonged PR
↑K+ (3.5–5)	Pseudohyperkalemia, oliguric renal failure, metabolic acidosis, Addison's disease, crush injury, burns, blood transfusions **MEDS:** ACE inhibitors, NSAIDs, cyclosporine, K+sparing diuretics	Muscle weak, dysrhythmias, flaccid paralysis, paresthesias, intestinal colic, cramps, abdominal distention, irritability anxiety **ECG:** Tall tented T waves, prologed PR interval and QRS duration, absent P waves, ST↓

Contd...

	Cause	
↓Ca+ (8.6–10.2)	Hypoparathyroidism (surgery), malabsorption, pancreatitis, alkalosis, ↑vitamin D, SC infection, peritonitis, citrated blood transfusion, chronic diarrhea, diuretic phase of renal failure, ↑PO₄, fistulas, burns, alcoholism	Numb, tingling, ↓BP, anxiety, Trousseau and Chvostek's sign, seizures, carpopedal spasms, ↑DTRs, irritability, bronchospasm, ↓clotting time, ↓prothrombin, diarrhea **ECG:** Prolonged QT interval
↑Ca+ (8.6–10.2)	Hyperparathyroidism, malignant neoplastic disease, prolonged immobilization, oliguric renal failure, acidosis, ↑parathyroid hormone **MEDS:** Thiazide diuretic, Ca+ corticosteroid, digoxin toxicity, vitamin-D	Constipation, anorexia, polyuria, polydipsia, dehydration, ↓ lethargy, bone pain, HTN, fractures, flank pain, Ca+ stones **ECG:** Shortened ST segment and QT interval, bradycardia, heart blocks

Main Characteristics

- Thirst
- Elevated body temperature
- Tongue dry and swollen, sticky mucous membranes
- In severe hypernatremia:
  - Disorientation
  - Hallucinations
- Lethargy when disturbed
- Irritable and hyper-reactive when stimulated
- Focal or grandmal seizures, coma, low blood pressure, tachycardia

It may produce hyponatremia, hyperglycemia and shock as complication.

Treatment

Management of the condition for an immediate attention and treatment instituted within 24–48 hours can avoid occurrence of cerebral edema.

Mild cases are given IV infusion 5 percent dextrose solution. Other cases need restriction of water and salt by mouth. Management of the condition depends upon the underlying condition. Diuretics and other measures are taken on the advice of the physician according to condition of patient.

Nursing Intervention

- Identify clients at risk of hypernatremia
- Monitor fluid losses and gains. Look for abnormal losses of water or low water intake; and for large gains of sodium as might occur with ingestion of proprietory drugs with high sodium content. And also consider

that prescription drugs may have high sodium content. Of course one should look for excessive intake of high sodium foods
- Monitor changes in behavior—such as restlessness, disorientation and lethargy
- Look for excessive thirst, and elevated body temperature. If present, evaluate in relation to other signs.

Prevent hyponatremia in debilitated clients who are unable to perceive or respond to thirst by offering them fluids at regular intervals. If fluids intake remains inadequate, consult the physician in order to plan an alternate route for intake, either by tube feedings or by the parenteral route. If tube feedings are used, give sufficient water to keep the serum sodium and the BUN level within normal limits. Higher the osmolity of the feeding, the greater the need for water supplements.

Hypokalemia

Hypokalemia refers to a potassium deficit in ECF. When the extracellular potassium level falls, potassium moves from the cell, creating an intracellular potassium deficiency. Sodium and hydrogen ions are then retained by the cells to maintain isotonic fluids. These electrolyte shifts influence normal cellular functioning, the pH of ECF, and function of most of the body systems. Skeletal muscles are generally the first to demonstrate a potassium deficiency. It is a condition associated with depletion of potassium characterized by muscular weakness, leg cramps, apathy, mental confusion and paralysis.

The related factors leading to hypokalemia are as follows:
It develops from excessive loss of potassium in the urine and stool and from severe water depletion Potassium-losing diuretics, i.e. frusemide, thiazide, etc.

Main Characteristics

- Fatigue
- Anorexia, nausea and vomiting
- Muscle weakness
- Decreased bowel motility (intestinal ileus)—paralytic ileus
- Cardiac arrhythmia
- Increased, sensitivity to digitalis
- Polyuria, nocturia, dilute urine (if hypokalemia prolonged)
- Mild hyperglycemia below 3.5 mEq/L
- Paresthesis or tender muscles
- ECG changes—flattened T waves, ST segment depressions
- Respiratory hyperventilation.

Treatment

Management of the condition requires adequate management of the underlying conditions.

Nursing Intervention

- Beware of clients at risk for hypokalemia and monitor for its occurrence
- Assess digitalized clients at risk for hypokalemia especially closely for symptoms of digitalis toxicity
- Take measures to prevent hypokalemia when possible
- Prevention may take the form of encouraging extra potassium intake for at-risk patient (when the diet allows)
- In case of hypokalemia due to abuse of laxatives or diuretics education of the client may help alleviate the problems
- Administer oral potassium supplement when prescribed
- Beware that clients may not need potassium supplements if they are using salt substitutes because these substances usually contain amounts of potassium
- Be thoroughly familiar with the critical facts related to administering potassium intravenously.

Hyperkalemia

Hyperkalemia refers to a condition with excess of potassium in ECG, characterized by conduction defect in the heart and myoneural junction of the muscle.

The related factors which lead to hyperkalemia are as follows:
Decreased potassium excretions as in:
- Oliguric renal failure
- Potassium-conserving diuretic usage
- Hypoaldosteronism
- High potassium intake, especially in presence of renal insufficiency
- Improper use of oral potassium supplements
- Rapid excessive administration of IV potassium
- High-dose potassium penicillin
- Foods high in potassium (such as dried apricots).
- Shift of potassium out of cells due to acidosis, tissue trauma, and malignant cell lysis
- Potassium excess also occurs in acute renal failure, severe crush injuries and burns and severe hemorrhages and adrenal insufficiency
- It is also seen in diabetic ketoacidosis.

Main Characteristics

- Vague muscular weakness is usually first sign
- Cardiac arrhythmias, bradycardia and heart block can occur
- Paresthesias of face, tongue, feet and hands
- Flaccid muscle paralysis (spreads from legs to trunk and arms, respiratory muscle may be affected)
- Gastrointestinal symptoms such as nausea, intermittent intestinal colic, or diarrhea may occur
- ECG changes falls, peaked T waves, absent P waves widened QRS complex

- Serum K, above 5.0 mEq/L (mmol/L) can produce cardiac arrest, metabolic acidosis and respiratory acidosis as complications.

Treatment

Management of the condition is done by replacements of water loss and correction of electrolyte imbalance. The client is given diet with restricted protein but with as much as fat and carbohydrate and also managing the underlying condition.

Nursing Intervention

- Beware of clients at risk for hyperkalemia and monitor for its occurrence. Hyperkalemia is life-threatening; it is imperative to detect it easily
- Take measures to prevent hyperkalemia when possible by following guidelines for administering potassium safely both intravenously or orally
- Follow rules for safe administration of potassium
- Avoid administration of potassium-conserving diuretics, potassium supplements or salt substitutes to client with renal insufficiency
- Caution client to use salt substitute sparingly if they are taking other supplementary form of potassium or taking potassium-conserving diuretics (e.g. spironolactone, triamaterine, and amiloride)

Caution hyperkalemic clients to avoid foods high in potassium content. Some of these are coffee, cocoa, tea, dried fruits, dried beans, whole grain breads.

Hypocalcemia

Hypocalcemia refers to a calcium deficit in ECF. If the condition is prolonged calcium is taken from bones. This results in osteomalacia, which is characterized by soft and pliable bones. Common signs and symptoms for hypocalcemia include numbness and tingling of fingers, muscle cramps and tetany.

The related factors leading to hypocalcemia are as follows:

- Surgical hypoparathyroidism (may follow thyroid surgery or radical neck surgery for cancer)
- Malabsorption
- Vitamin D deficiency
- Acute pancreatitis
- Excessive administration of citrated blood
- Primary hypothyroidism
- Alkalotic states (decreased ionized calcium)
- Hyperphosphatemia
- Medullary carcinoma of thyroid
- Hypoalbuminemia (as in cirrhosis, nephrotic syndrome and starvation)
- Hypomagnesemia
- Increased/decreased ultraviolet exposure.

Main Characteristics

- Numbness, tingling fingers, circumoral region and toes
- Cramps in the muscle of extremities
- Hyperactive deep tendon reflexes (such as patellar and triceps)
- Trousseau's sign
- Chvostek's sign
- Mental changes such as confusion and alteration in mood and memory
- Convulsions, usually generalized but may be focal
- Spasm of laryngeal muscles
- ECG shows prolonged QT interval
- Spasms of muscles in abdomen
- Total calcium level below 8.5 mg/dL or ionized level below normal (below 50%)
- Hypocalcemic state occurs when calcium loss occurs causing a fall in serum calcium level. This may eventually cause tetany and teeth.
- It is usually asymptomatic and the neurological manifestation develop slowly

BOX 1: Selected clinical features of hypocalcemia.

- Laryngospasm
- Tetany
- Infant feeding problems
- Muscle cramps (especially with exercise)
- Seizure
- Paresthesia
- Numbness
- Chvostek's sign
- Trousseau's sign
- Lengthened QTc interval (> 450 milliseconds)

- It then gives rise to diffused encephalopathy, depression and psychosis
- In severe cases there may be laryngospasm and general convulsion
- It may also give rise to papilledema and cataract.

Treatment

Most cases respond well to adequate or supplement calcium and phosphorus. The patient may be given calcium carbonate, 2.52 to 3.78 gm daily orally or calcium gluconate 0.5 to 1.5 gm along with calciferol 15.45 mg daily orally. Otherwise, 10 mL of 10 percent calcium gluconate is given by slow IV. Adequate management and control of predisposing causes can prevent the occurrence of the condition.

Nursing Interventions

- Beware of at risk for hypocalcemia and monitor its occurrence
- Be prepared to take seizures precautions
- Monitor condition of airway closely because laryngeal stridor can occur

- Take safety precautions if confusion is present
- Beware of factors related to the safe administration of calcium replacement salts
- Educate people in high-risk groups for osteoporosis (especially postmenopausal women not on estrogen therapy). If adequate amounts are not consumed in the diet (as is often the case), calcium supplements should be considered
- Educate people at risk for osteoporosis about the value of regular physical exercise in decreasing bone loss
- To prevent osteoporosis in later years, educate young women about the need for a normal diet to ensure adequate calcium intake. Also discuss the calcium-losing aspects of alcohol and nicotine use.

Hypercalcemia

Hypercalcemia refers to an excess of calcium in ECF. It presents an emergency situation because this condition often leads to cardiac arrest. It is a condition of excess of calcium and is characterized by polyuria, polydipsia, skeletal muscle weakness and hypertension.

The related factors that lead to hypercalcemia are as follows:
- Hyperparathyroidism
- Malignant neoplastic disease
- Prolonged immobilization
- Large doses of vitamin D
- Overuse of calcium containing antacids or calcium supplements thiazide diuretics
- Milk-alkali syndrome
- Sarcoidosis
- It is also seen in person with Paget's disease, myxoedema, Addison's disease and osteoporosis in aged persons.

Main Characteristics

- Muscle weakness
- Tiredness, restlessness, lethargy
- Constipation
- Anorexia, nausea, and vomiting
- Decreased memory span, decreased attention span, and confusion
- Polyuria and polydipsia
- Renal stones
- Neurobic behavior progressing to frank psychosis may occur (reversible with correction of hypercalcemia)
- Cardiac arrest may occur in hypercalcemic crisis
- ECG shows shortened QT interval
- Serum calcium over 10.5 mg/dL
- It may produce renal failure, shock and death in complication.

Treatment

In mild cases, adequate rehydration is often effective. Management of the condition also includes management of the underlying conditions. In other cases, intravenous infusion of isotonic saline is given to promote calciuria. Calcium is also eliminated or maintained in the lower level by giving sodium phosphate 1 to 2 gm orally daily, and client is encouraged to take more fluids.

Nursing Intervention

- Beware of clients at risk for hypercalcemia and monitor its occurrence
- Increase client mobilization when feasible
- Encourage the oral intake of sufficient fluids to keep the client well hydrated
- Discourage excessive consumption of milk products and other high calcium foods
- Encourage adequate bulk in the diet to offset the tendency for constipation
- Take safety precautions if confusion or other mental symptoms by hypercalcemia are present
- Beware that cardiac arrest can occur in clients with severe hypercalcemia be prepared to deal with this emergency
- Beware that bones may fracture more easily in clients with chronic hypercalcemia because bone resorption has been excessive, weakening the bony structure.
- Educate home-bound oncology clients with a predisposition for hypercalcemia and their families, to be alert for symptoms that occur with this condition and to report them to the healthcare providers before they become severe
- Be alert for signs of digitalis toxicity when hypercalcemia occurs in digitalized clients help prevent formation of calcium renal stones in clients with longstanding hypercalcemia or immobilization by:
  - Forcing fluids to maintain dilute urine, thus avoiding super saturation of precipitates
  - Encouraging fluids that yield an acid ash (prune or cranberry milk) because a urinary pH less than 6.5 favors calcium deposits
  - Preventing urinary stasis by turning the immobilized client, elevating head of the bed and having the client sit up if this can be tolerated.

Hypomagnesemia

Magnesium is an important and plentiful cation, and is essential for many enzymatic system associated with protein, carbohydrate and lipid metabolism.

Hypomagnesemia refers to magnesium deficit. It is condition of low plasma concentration of magnesium, characterized by neuromuscular and CNS hyperirritability.

The related factors which lead to hypomagnesemia are as follows:
- Chronic alcoholism
- Intestinal malabsorption syndrome
- Diarrhea
- Nasogastric suction-prolonged
- Aggressive refeeding after starvation (as in TPN).

Drugs: Prolonged use of diuretics, aminoglycoside, antibiotics (e.g. gentamycin), and cisplatin. Excessive dose of vitamin-D or calcium supplements citrate preservative in blood products, pancreatitis, thyrotoxicosis, hyperparathyroidism, severe osteofibrosis, PEM.

Main Characteristics

- It presents with multiple metabolic and nutritional deficiency
- It gives rise to anorexia, lethargy, vomiting, weakness, and tetany.

Neuromuscular Irritability

- Increased reflex
- Course tremors
- Positive Chvostek's and Trousseau's signs
- Convulsions.

Cardiac manifestations will include:

- Tachyarrhythmias
- Increased susceptibility to digitalis toxicity
  ECG changes in severe cases, PR and QT interval prolongation, widened QRS complex, ST segment depression and T-wave inversion
- Mental changes
- Disorientation in memory
- Mood changes
- Intense confusion
- Hallucination
- Serum magnesium level below 1.3 mEq/L.

Treatment

Treatment for repletion of the cases is done through magnesium sulfate and chloride. It is customary to give double the amount required because half of magnesium given is excreted by the kidneys. The repletion is done gradually and is given orally or intravenously; in severe cases by IV only.

Nursing Intervention

- Be prepared to take seizure precautions for client at risk for hypomagnesemia, especially watch closely for symptoms of digitalis toxicity because a deficit of magnesium predisposes to toxicity
- Monitor condition of airway, because laryngeal stridor can occur
- Take safety precautions if confusion presents. Be familiar with magnesium replacement salts and factors related to this safe administration
- Beware that magnesium-depleted clients may experience difficulty in swallowing
- When magnesium deficit is due to abuse of diuretics in laxatives, educating the client may help alleviate problem
- Beware that most commonly used IV fluids have either no magnesium or relatively small amount.
- When indicated, discuss the need for magnesium replacement with physicians
- For clients experiencing abnormal losses, but able to consume a general diet, encourage intake of magnesium-rich foods (such as green-leafy vegetables, nuts, legumes and fruits such as bananas, oranges and grape fruits).

Hypermagnesemia

Hypermagnesemia refers to a magnesium excess. It can occur especially in end stage renal failure when kidneys fail to excrete magnesium and excessive amounts are administered therapeutically. It is a condition associated with excess of magnesium and is characterized by muscular weakness and ECG changes.

The related factors which lead to hypermagnesemia are as follows:

- Renal failure (particularly when magnesium containing medications are administered)
- Adrenal insufficiency
- Excessive magnesium administration during treatment of eclampsia
- Hemodialysis with excessively hard water or with dialysate inadvertantly high in magnesium content
- Magnesium has a direct action on the myoneural junction. Its excess produces blockage causing impairment of neuromuscular transmission and that results diminished excitability of the muscle cells.

Main Characteristics

- Early signs (serum level of mg of 3 to 5 mEq/L)
- Flushing and a sense of skin warmth (due to peripheral vasodilation)
- Hypotension (due to blockage of sympathetic ganglia)
- Depressed respiration
- Drowsiness, hypoactive reflexes and muscular weakness
- Cardiac abnormalities—cardiac arrest may develop
- Weak or absent cry in newborn
- ECG shows prolonged PR interval, widened QRS complex and elevated T-wave amplitude
- Elevated serum magnesium level.

Treatment

In severe cases and also in other cases cardiac and respiratory support is given by IV injection of 10 to 20 mL of 10 percent calcium gluconate. Maintenance of adequate hydration is essential. The client is also given frusemide by IV injection to promote excretion of magnesium. In more severe cases, hemodialysis is done.

Nursing Intervention

Beware of client at risk for hypermagnesemia and assess for its presence. When it is suspected, assess the following parameters:

- *Vital signs:* Look for low blood pressure and shallow respirations with periods of apnea
- *Level of consciousness:* Look for drowsiness, lethargy and coma
- Do not give magnesium containing medication to clients with renal failure or compromised renal function
- Be particularly careful in following 'standing order' for bowel preparation for X-ray because some of these include the use of magnesium citrate
- Caution clients with renal disease to check with their healthcare providers before taking over the counter medication
- Beware of factors related to safe parenteral administration of magnesium salts.

Hypophosphatemia

Hypophosphatemia refers to a below normal serum concentration of inorganic phosphorus. It is a clinical manifestation of phosphate depletion, characterized by progressive encephalopathy and osteomalacia.

The related factors which lead to hypophosphatemia are as follows:
- Inadequate intake or absorption of phosphorus—malabsorption
- It is associated with vomiting and diarrhea
- Prolonged injection of alluminium hydroxide or bicarbonate.

It is also seen in:
- Prolonged use of glucose insulin, fructose, administrations
- Refeeding after starvation
- Hyperalimentation
- Alcohol withdrawal
- Diabetic ketoacidosis
- Respiratory alkalosis
- Phosphate-binding antacids use
- Recovery phase after severe burns
- Use of anabolic steroids
- Chronic hemodialysis.

Main Characteristics
- Progressive encephalopathy
- Paresthesias
- Muscle weakness
- Muscle pain and tenderness
- Mental changes, such as apprehension, confusion, delirium coma
- Cardiomyopathy
- Acute respiratory failure
- Seizures
- Decreased tissue oxygenation
- Joint stiffness
- Serum phosphate below 2.5 mg/dL
- Phosphate compounds are present in all normal foods and are essential for metabolism of carbohydrate, protein and fat. They are also responsible for changes, transfer or depletion occurring from prolonged negative phosphate balance and chronic malnutrition.

Treatment
Management of the condition includes treatment of the underlying cause, repletion of phosphate, and maintenance of body fluids.

Nursing Intervention
- Identify clients at risk for hypophosphatemia
- Severely malnourished clients
- Alcoholic clients
- Clients with diabetic ketoacidosis
- Monitor clients at risk for the presence of hypophosphatemia
- Beware that severely hypophosphatemic clients are thought to be at greater risk for infection because of changes in WBCs
- Administer IV phosphate products cautiously
- Beware that in adults the usual maintenance dose of phosphorus is 10 to 15 mmol/L of TPN solution
- Beware of the need to introduce hyperalimentation gradually in clients who are malnourished
- Because it is possible to give too much phosphorus when administering phosphate solutions, monitor for signs of hyperphosphatemia and of the salt in which it is administered
- Monitor for diarrhea in clients taking oral phosphorus supplements; consult physician if it persists or is severe
- Powdered oral phosphorus supplements with chilled or ice water to make them more palatable.

Hyperphosphatemia

Hyperphosphatemia refers to above normal serum concentrations of inorganic phosphorus. It is a condition associated with increased level of phosphate and is characterized by hypocalcemia.

The related factors which lead to hyperphosphatemia are as follows:
- Excessive intake of phosphate
- Hypervitaminosis D—large vitamin D intake indicates acute renal failure
- Chronic renal insufficiency
- Chemotherapy, particularly for acute lymphoblastic leukemia and lymphoma
- Large intake of milk
- Use of cow's milk in infants
- Excessive intake of phosphate containing laxatives
- Overzealous administration of phosphorus supplements (oral or IV)
- Excessive use of fleet's phospho soda as enema solution particularly in children and people with slow bowel elimination

- Hypoparathyroidism
- Hyperthyroidism.

Main Characteristics

This condition by itself does not give rise to any symptoms but manifested with that of hypocalcemia.

This includes:
- Short-term consequences—symptoms of tetany, such as tingling of fingertips and around mouth, numbness and muscle spasms
- Long-term consequences—precipitation of calcium phosphate in nonosseous sites; such as kidney, joints, arteries, skin of cornea
- Serum phosphate above 4.5 mg/dL.

Treatment

Management of the condition requires correction of underlying condition.

Nursing Intervention

- Identify clients at risk for hyperphosphatemia
- Monitor signs of tetanus and other features of hypocalcemia
- Beware that soft-tissue calcification can be long-term complication of a chemically elevated serum phosphate level. Calcification may occur in site such as kidney, arteries, joints, etc.
- Administer prescribed oral or IV phosphate supplements cautiously and monitor serum phosphorus levels periodically during their use
- When appropriate, instruct clients that use of phosphate, containing laxatives may result in acute phosphate poisoning
- Beware that phosphate containing enema can result in hyperphosphatemia if used injudiciously, particularly in children and those with slow bowel emptying, instruct clients accordingly
- When low-phosphorus diet is prescribed, instruct clients to avoid foods high in phosphorus content. Such foods include hard cheese or cream, nuts and nut products; whole grain cereals (e.g. bran and oatmeal), dried fruits, dried vegetables; special meats such as kidneys, sardines, sweet breads and desserts made with milk.

ACID-BASE BALANCES

An important property of blood is its degree of acidity or alkalinity. Blood acidity increases when the level of acidic compounds in the body rises (through increased intake or production, or decreased elimination) or when the level of basic (alkaline) compounds in the body falls (through decreased intake or production, or increased elimination). Blood alkalinity increases with the reverse processes. The body's balance between acidity and alkalinity is referred to as acid-base balance. The acidity or alkalinity of any solution, including blood, is indicated on the pH scale. The blood's acid-base balance is precisely controlled because even a minor deviation from the normal range can severely affect many organs. The body uses different mechanisms to control the blood's acid-base balance.

Role of Lungs: One mechanism the body uses to control blood pH involves the release of carbon dioxide from the lungs. Carbon dioxide, which is mildly acidic, is a waste product of the metabolism of oxygen (which all cells need) and, as such, is constantly produced by cells. As with all waste products, carbon dioxide gets excreted into the blood. The blood carries carbon dioxide to the lungs, where it is exhaled. As carbon dioxide accumulates in the blood, the pH of the blood decreases (acidity increases). The brain regulates the amount of carbon dioxide that is exhaled by controlling the speed and depth of breathing. The amount of carbon dioxide exhaled, and consequently the pH of the blood, increases as breathing becomes faster and deeper. By adjusting the speed and depth of breathing, the brain and lungs are able to regulate the blood pH minute by minute.

Role of Kidneys: The kidneys are able to affect blood pH by excreting excess acids or bases. The kidneys have some ability to alter the amount of acid or base that is excreted, but because the kidneys make these adjustments more slowly than the lungs do, this compensation generally takes several days.

Buffer Systems: Another mechanism for controlling blood pH involves the use of buffer systems, which guard against sudden shifts in acidity and alkalinity. The pH buffer systems are combinations of the body's own naturally occurring weak acids and weak bases. These weak acids and bases exist in pairs that are in balance under normal pH conditions. The pH buffer systems work chemically to minimize changes in the pH of a solution by adjusting the proportion of acid and base. The most important pH buffer system in the blood involves carbonic acid (a weak acid formed from the carbon dioxide dissolved in blood) and bicarbonate ions (the corresponding weak base).

ACID-BASE IMBALANCES

Acidosis and alkalosis are not diseases but rather are the result of a wide variety of disorders. The presence of acidosis or alkalosis provides an important clue to doctors that a serious problem exists. Acidosis and alkalosis are categorized as metabolic or respiratory, depending on their primary cause. Metabolic acidosis and metabolic alkalosis are caused by an imbalance in the production of acids or bases and their excretion by the kidneys. Respiratory acidosis and respiratory alkalosis are caused primarily by changes in carbon dioxide exhalation due to lung or breathing disorders.

Acid-base disorders				
Disorder	pH	[H⁺]	Primary disturbance	Secondary response
Metabolic acidosis	↓	↑	↓ [HCO₃⁻]	↓ pCO₂
Metabolic alkalosis	↑	↓	↑ [HCO₃⁻]	↑ pCO₂
Respiratory acidosis	↓	↑	↑ pCO₂	↑ [HCO₃⁻]
Respiratory alkalosis	↑	↓	↓ pCO₂	↓ [HCO₃⁻]

Acidosis and Alkalosis: There are two abnormalities of acid-base balance.
1. **Acidosis:** The blood has too much acid (or too little base), resulting in a decrease in blood pH.
2. **Alkalosis:** The blood has too much base (or too little acid), resulting in an increase in blood pH.

Sl. No.	Types	Description
1.	Respiratory acidosis	It is marked by an increased arterial carbon dioxide concentration, excess carbonic acid and increased hydrogen-ion concentration. Respiratory acidosis is caused by hypoventilation or any condition that depresses ventilation in respiratory acidosis, the cerebrospinal fluid becomes acidic. Hypoxemia occurs because of respiratory depression.
2.	Respiratory alkalosis	It is marked by decreased carbon dioxide concentration and decreased hydrogen ion concentration. Respiratory alkalosis results from excessive exhalation of carbon dioxide or hyperventilation. The signs and symptoms of respiratory alkalosis are headache, irritability, dizziness, dysarythmias, tachypnea, and tingling sensation of extremities.
3.	Metabolic acidosis	It results from a rise in hydrogen ion concentration in the extracellular fluid, caused by increased in hydrogen ion levels or a decrease in bicarbonate levels. Its causes are starvation, diabetic ketoacidosis, renal failure, shock, and diarrhea. It is manifested by headache, lethargy, confusion, tachypnea, deep respiration, abnormal cramps and flushed skin.
4.	Metabolic alkalosis	It is marked by heavy loss of acid from the body or by increased level of bicarbonate. The most common cause is vomiting. Other causes are hypokalemia, prolonged gastric suctioning, and cushing syndrome, use of certain drugs such as steroids, bicarbonate and diuretics. The signs and symptoms are headache, irritability, lethargy, dysrhythmias, abnormal cramps, numbness, tingling, muscle cramps and tetany.

INTRAVENOUS CATHETER INSERTION

Intravenous injection is the introduction of a small quantity of drug into the vein by venous puncture. Introduction of drug directly into the blood stream is called intravenous injection.

Purpose

- To have a fast action of the medicine as in emergency.
- To give medicines those are irritating or ineffective when given by other routes.
- To have the action of medicines on the blood stream or the blood vessels.

Common Sites of IV Injection (Fig. 21.3)

- Ventral aspect of elbow or forearm median cubical, basilica or cephalic veins.
- Doral aspect of hand—brachial, cephalic or metacarpal veins.
- In the infants, the scalp vein is used.

General Instructions

Expel the air from the syringe before giving the injection by holding it in upright position and gently pressing the piston until a drop of solution comes out to the tip of the needle.

- Always dissolve the drug in correct amount of fluid to minimize the risk of adverse effect of the medicine.
- Observe the patient closely for the signs of adverse reaction of the medicine and have emergency drugs and the antidote in hand while injecting the medicine.
- Do not give the medicine if the injection site shows any edema or intravenous solution is not following properly to avoid accidental administration of medicine in to the surrounding tissues.
- While giving iron preparation always confirms that the patient is not sensitive to it by giving a test dose.

Types of IV Administration

- Adding the medicine in intravenous solution bottle (intravenous infusion).
- Existing intravenous line for continuous infusion.
- Bolus—direct intravenous push for immediate or fast action.

Selection of Syringe and Needle

- The size of syringe used for intravenous infusion depends upon the amount of fluids to be injected.
- Size of the needle used 18 to 21 gauge or 1 to 2 inches.

Preliminary Assessment Check

- The diagnosis and age of the patient.
- The purpose of injection.
- The doctors order for the type, dosage, time and route of administration.
- The patient's name and bed number.
- The nurses record to find out the time at which the last dose was given.
- The symptoms of overdose or allergic reaction.

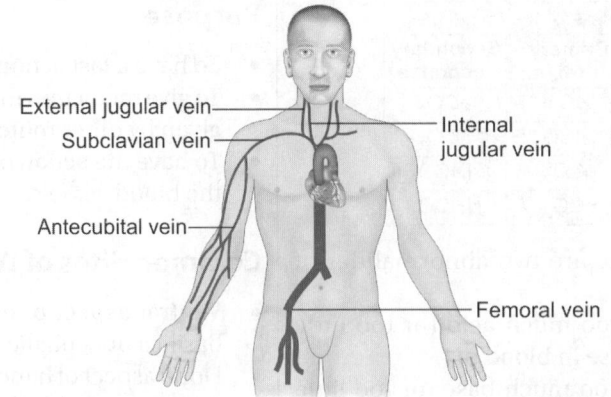

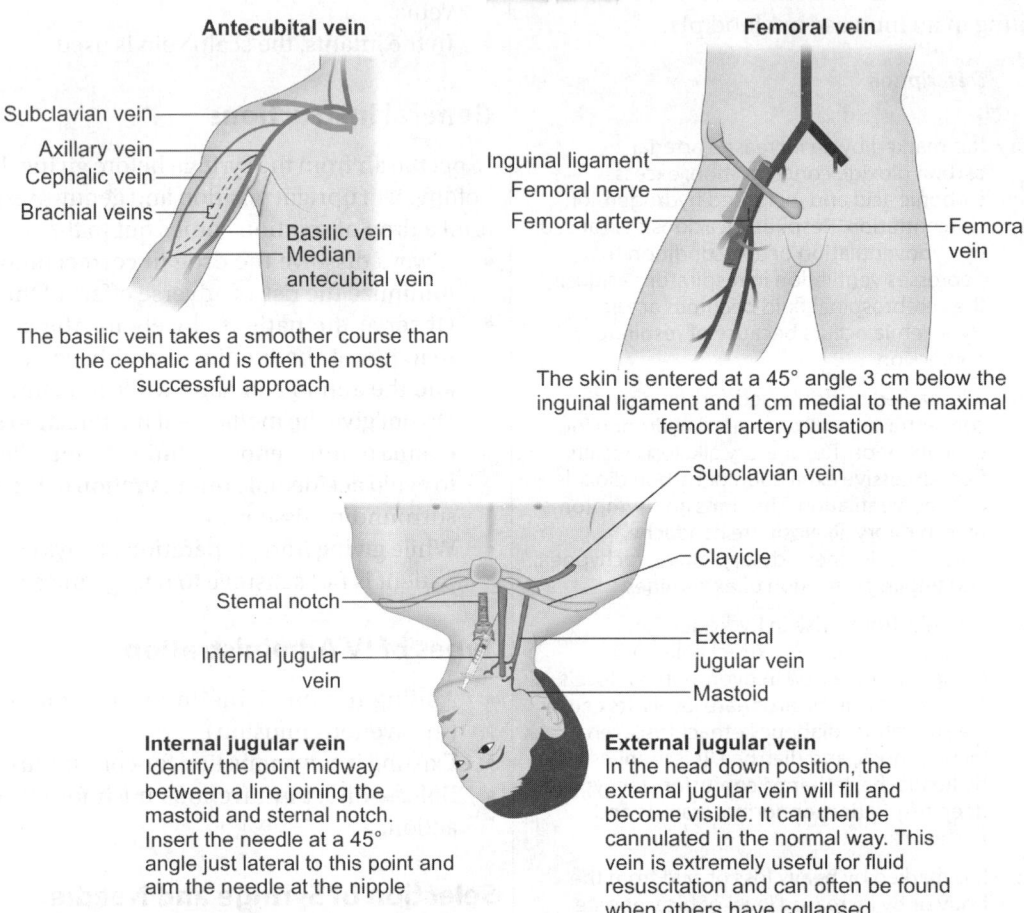

Fig. 21.3: Intravenous catheter sites.

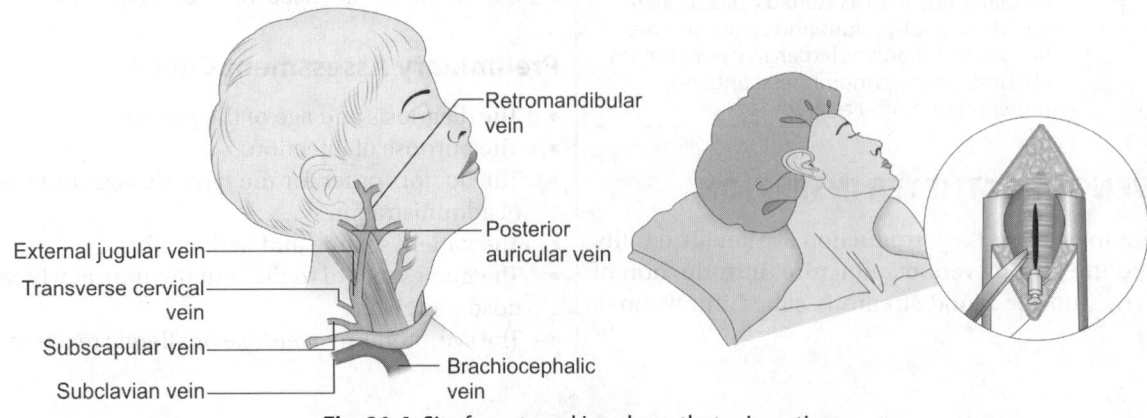

Fig. 21.4: Site for external jugular catheter insertion.

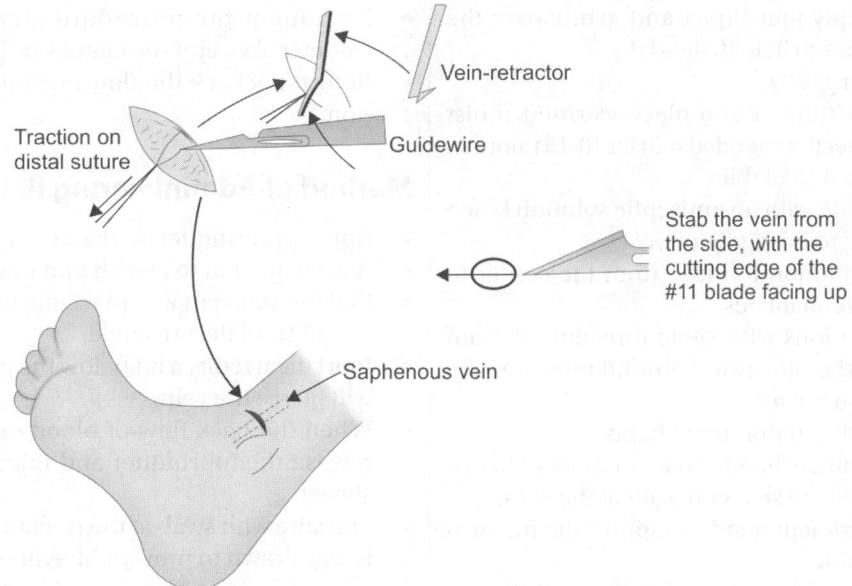

Fig. 21.5: Saphenous vein for intravenous catheter insertion.

- The necessity for giving test dose.
- The form of the medicine available and correct method of administration.
- The level of consciousness of the patient.
- The site and previous experience of the patient.

Equipment

A tray containing:
- Syringe and needles of various sizes according to the need in a covered tray (sterile).
- Transfer forceps in a jar containing antiseptic solution.
- Sterile cotton swabs and gauze pieces in sterile containers.
- Methylated spirit in a container.
- Bowl with water.
- Tourniquet.
- Water for injection.
- Drug order sheet.
- File to cut open the ampoules.
- Small covered tray (sterile).

Preparation of Tile Patient and Environment

- Identify the patient correctly.
- Explain the procedure to the patient.
- Provide privacy.
- Place the patient in comfortable and relaxed position suitable of intravenous injection.
- Select a site suitable for the route of administration, quantity of medication to be given and characteristics of medication.

Procedure

- Assemble all equipment and bring to bedside
- Check IV solution and medication.
- Explain procedure to the client
- Prepare IV solution and tubing:
  - Maintain aseptic technique when opening sterile packages and IV solution
  - Clamp tubing, uncap spike, and insert into entry site on bag as manufacturer directs
  - Squeeze drip chamber and allow it to fill at least one-third to halfway
  - Remove cap at end of tubing, release clamp, allow fluid to move through tubing. Allow fluid to flow until all air bubbles have disappeared
  - Close clamp and recap end of tubing, maintaining sterility of set up
  - If an electric device is to be used, follow manufacturer's instructions for inserting tubing and setting infusion rate
  - Apply label if medication was added to container
  - Place time-tape (or adhesive tape) on container as necessary and hang on IV stand
- Preparation the position:
  - Have the client in supine position or comfortable position in bed.
  - Place protective pad under the client's arm.
- Selection the site for venipuncture:
  - Select an appropriate site and palpate accessible veins
  - Apply a tourniquet 5-6 inches above the venipuncture site to obstruct venous blood flow and distend the vein.
  - Direct the ends of the tourniquet away from the site of injection.
  - Check to be sure that the radial pulse is still present.
- Palpation the vein
  - Ask the client to open and close his/her fist.
  - Observe and palpate for a suitable vein
  - If a vein cannot be felt and seen, do the following:
    - Release the tourniquet and have the client lower his/her arm below the level of the heart to fill the

veins. Reapply tourniquet and gently over the intended vein to help distend it
- Tap the vein gently
- Remove tourniquet and place warmed-moist compress over the intended vein for 10-15 minutes.
- Put on clean gloves if available
- Cleanse the entry site with an antiseptic solution (such as spirit) according to hospital policy.
    - Use a circular motion to move from the center to outward for several inches
    - Use several motions with same direction as from the upward to the downward around injection site approximate 5-6 inches
- Holding the arm with undominant hand
    - Place an undominant hand about 1 or 2 inches below entry site to hold the skin taut against the vein.
    - Place an undominant hand to support the forearm from the back side
    - *Nursing Alert:* Avoid touching the prepared site.
- Puncturing the vein and withdrawing blood:
    - Enter the skin gently with the catheter held by the hub in the dominant hand, bevel side up, at a 15-30 degree angle.
    - The catheter may be inserted from directly over the vein or the side of the vein.
    - While following the course of the vein, advance the needle or catheter into the vein.
    - A sensation can be felt when the needle enters the vein.
    - When the blood returns through the lumen of the needle or the flashback hamber of the catheter, advance either device 1/8 to 1/4 inch farther into the vein.
    - A catheter needs to be advanced until hub is at the venipuncture site
- Connecting to the tube and stabilizing the catheter on the skin:
    - Release the tourniquet.
    - Quickly remove protective cap from the IV tubing
    - Attach the tubing to the catheter or needle
    - Stabilize the catheter or needle with nondominant hand
- Starting flow
    - Release the clamp on the tubing
    - Start flow of solution promptly
    - Examine the drip of solution and the issue around the entry site for sign of infiltration
- Fasten the catheter and applying the dressing:
    - Secure the catheter with narrow non-allergenic tape
    - Place strictly sided-up under the hub and crossed over the top of the hub
    - Loop the tubing near the site of entry
- Bring back all equipment and dispose in proper manner
- Remove gloves and perform hand hygiene
- If necessary, anchor arm to an arm board for support
- Adjust the rate of IV solution flow according to doctors order
- Document the procedure including the time, site catheter size, and the client's response
- Return to check the flow rate and observe for infiltration.

Method of Administering IV Infection

- Apply a tourniquet on the upper arm.
- Ask the patient to clench and unclench the hand.
- Pull the skin taut and place the needle in line with vein at a 15 to 45 degree angle.
- Inert the needle, a bit below the point where the needle will pierce the vein.
- When the back flow of blood occurs into the syringe release the tourniquet and injects the medicine very slowly.
- Pressure with swab at the puncture site after the needle is withdrawn to prevent bleeding.

After Care

- Observe the area for bleeding if bleeding occurs, apply pressure but do not massage.
- Give comfortable position to the patient.
- Ask the patient to take rest at least 15 to 30 minutes so that you can observe him for any reaction.
- Observe the patient for any allergic reaction.
- Replace the equipment used for injection.
- Clean all other articles and replace them in their proper place.
- Wash hands.
- Record the procedure on the nurse recordsheet and medication sheet.

Complications

- Allergic reactions.
- Pain.
- Injection abscess.
- Injury of nerves.
- Air embolism.

MAINTENANCE OF IV SYSTEM

Definition: Maintenance of IV system is defined as routine care to keep well condition of IV therapy.

Purpose

- To protect injection site from infection
- To provide safe IV therapy
- To make the client comfort with IV therapy
- To distinguish any complications as soon as possible

Equipment Required

- Steel tray (1)
- Spirit swab

- Dry gauze or cotton
- Adhesive tape
- IV infusion set if required
- Kardex, client's record
- Kidney tray (1)

Procedure

Maintenance of IV system: General caring for the client with an IV

- Make at least hourly checks of the rate, tubing connections, and amount and type of solution present. If using an electronic infusion device (pump or controller), check that all settings are correct.
- Watch for adverse reactions. One such problem is infiltration, in which the IV solution infuses into tissues instead of the vein. Check the insertion site for redness, swelling, or tenderness hourly. Document that you have checked the site.
- Report any difficulty at once. The doctor may order the IV line to be discontinued or to be irrigated.
- Safeguard the site and be aware of tubing and pump during transfers, ambulation, or other activities.
- Change the IV dressing every 72 hours and if it becomes wet or contaminated with drainage.
- Wear gloves when changing dressings or tubing.
- Be sure to double-check all clamps when changing tubing, adding medications, or removing IV tubing (from a pump or controller).
- If the rate of flow is not regulated properly, it could result in the client receiving a bolus of medication.
- Always check to make sure medications, solutions, or additives are compatible before adding the into existing solutions.
- Protect the IV site from getting wet or soiled.
- If the client will be away from the nursing unit for tests or procedures, be sure there is adequate solution to be infused while he/she is gone.

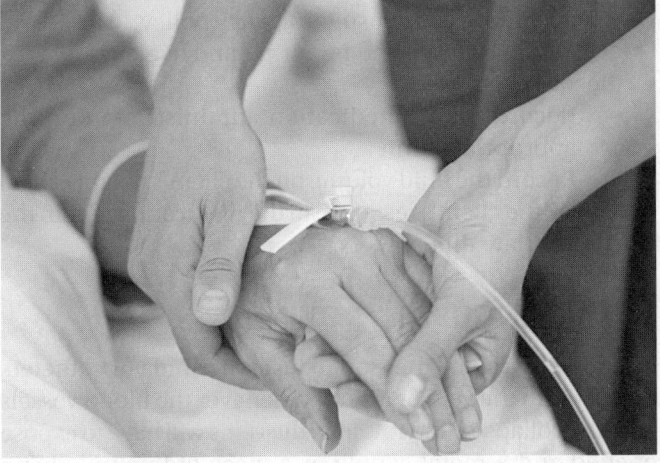

Fig. 21.6: Care of intravenous cannulation.

Maintenance of IV system: Changing of IV System

- Check IV solution.
- Determine the compatibility of all IV fluids and additives by consulting appropriate literature.
- Determine client's understanding of need for continued IV therapy.
- Assess patency of current IV access site.
- Have next solution prepared and accessible (at least 1 hour) before needed. Check that solution is correct and properly labeled. Check solution expiration date and for presence of precipitate and discoloration.
- Prepare to change solution when less than 50 mL of fluid remains in bottle or bag or when a new type of solution is ordered.
- Prepare client and family be explaining the procedure, its purpose, and what is expected of client.
- Be sure drip chamber is at least half full.
- Perform hand hygiene.
- Prepare new solution for changing. If using plastic bag, remove protective cover from IV tubing port. If using glass bottle, remove metal cap.
- Move roller clam to stop flow rate.
- Remove old IV fluid container from IV stand.
- Quickly remove spike fro mold solution bag or bottle and, without touching tip, insert spike into new bag or bottle.
- Hang new bag or bottle of solution on IV stand.
- Check for air in tubing. If bubbles form, they can be removed by closing the roller clamp, stretching the tubing downward, and tapping the tubing with the finger.
- Make sure drip chamber is one-third to one-half full. If the drip chamber is too full, pinch off tubing below the drip chamber, invert the container, squeeze the drip chamber, hang up the bottle, replace the tubing.
- Regulate flow to prescribed rate.
- Place on bag. (Mark time on label tape or on glass bottle).
- Observe client for signs of overhydration or dehydration to determine response to IV fluid therapy.
- Observe IV system for patency and development of complications.

ADMINISTERING MEDICATIONS BY HEPARIN LOCK

A heparin lock is an IV catheter that is inserted into a vein and left in place either for intermittent administration of medication or as open line in the case of an emergency.

Administering medications by heparin lock is defined as one of IV therapy which can allow being freedom clients while he/she has not received IV therapy.

Purpose

- To provide intermittent administration of medication
- To administer medication under the urgent condition

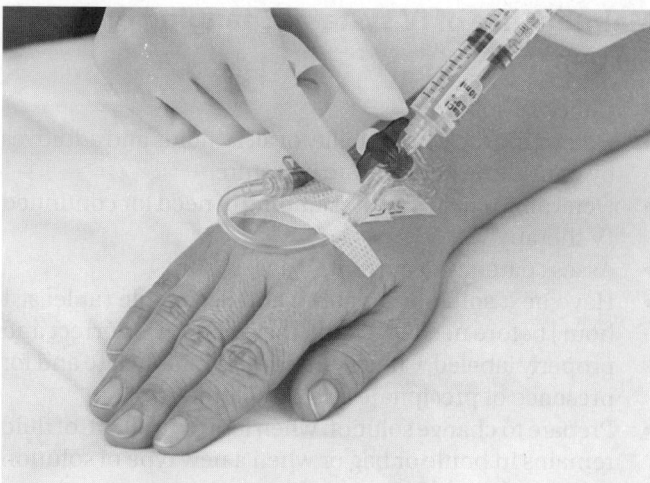

Fig. 21.7: Intravenous bolus dose (medication) administration.

Equipment Required

- Client's chart and Kardex
- Prescribed medication
- Spirit swabs
- Disposable gloves if available (1)
- Kidney tray (1)
- Steel tray (1)

For Flush

- Saline vial or saline in the syringe (1)
- Heparin flushes solution (1)
- Syringe (3-5 mL) with 21-25 gauge needles (1)

For Intermittent Infusion

- IV bag or bottle with 50-100 mL solution (1)
- IV tubing set (1)
- IV stand (1)
- 21-23 gauge needle (1)
- Adhesive tape

Nursing Alert

- A heparin lock has an adapter which is attached to the catheter.
- An anticoagulant, approximately 2mL heparin, is injected into the heparin lock.
- To reduce the possibility of clotting, flush the heparin lock with 2-3 mL of saline 8 hourly (or once in every duty); saline lock.
- Choose heparin lock or saline lock to decrease the possibility of making coagulation according to your facility's policy or doctors order.

Maintenance of IV System: Changing of IV System

- Perform hand hygiene
- Assemble all equipment
- Verify the medication order
- Check the medication's expiration date
- **For Bolus Injection:** Prepare the medication. If necessary, withdraw from an ampoule or a vial
- Explain the procedure to the client
- Identify the client before giving the medication
- Put on gloves
- Cleanse the heparin lock port with a spirit swab
- Steady the heparin lock with your dominant hand
  - Insert the needle of the syringe containing 1 mL of saline into the center of the port
  - Aspirate for blood return
  - Inject the saline
  - Remove the needle and discard the syringe in the sharps container without recapping it
- Cleanse the port again with a spirit swab
  - Insert the needle of the syringe containing the medication
  - Inject the medication slowly
  - Withdraw the syringe and dispose of it properly
- *Cleanse the port with a spirit swab:* Flush the lock with 1 mL heparin flush solution according your hospital/agency policy
- **For intermittent infusion**
  - Use premixed solution in the bag
  - Connect the tubing and add the needle
  - Prepare the tubing with solution
- Follow the former action.
  - Cleanse the port again with a spirit swab
  - Insert the needle or needleless component attached to the IV setup into the port
  - Attach it to the IV infusion pump or calculate the flow rate
  - Regulate drip according to the prescribed delivery time
  - Clamp the tubing and withdraw the needle when all solution has been infused
  - Discard the equipment used safely according to hospital/agency's policy
- Cleanse the port with a spirit swab
  - Flush the lock with 1 mL heparin flush solution according your hospital/agency policy
  - Remove gloves and perform hand hygiene
- Record
  - Record the IV medication administration on the appropriate form
  - Record the fluid volume on the client's balancesheet
- Check the client's response to the medication within the appropriate time.

INTRAVENOUS CUTDOWN

Cut down is a small incision to insert a canula or catheters directly into the vein or artery. Whenever the blood vessels become collapsed and invisible the veins will have to expose opened and a metal canula or a piece of fine polythene tubing is inserted into the vein to start an infusion.

Purpose

- To restore and maintain the child's fluid and electrolytes balance.
- To maintain body homeostasis when the oral intake is inadequate to serve this purpose.
- To measure central venous pressure.
- To administer larger fluid, e.g. cardiac arrest.

Principles

- This procedure should carried out by a doctor assisted by a nurse.
- Aseptic techniques must be adhered to throughout all intravenously procedures to prevent bacterial contamination.
- The single most effective aseptic procedure is good hand washing technique.
- It asepsis is not maintained local infection, septic phlebitis or septicemia may result.

Preliminary Assessment

- Check the physician's order for vein cut down.
- Take written concern from the patient.
- Explain the procedure to the patient.
- Win the co-operation of the patient.
- Arrange all the articles and make sure that it is available in the unit.

Preparation of the Patient

- Explain the procedure to the patient of the patient.
- The site of cut down is prepared as for any major surgery.
- If any hair is present get the site shaved and cleaned.
- The bedding and garments are protected with a Mackintosh and towel.
- Prepare all the articles and strict aseptic technique should be followed.

Equipment

IV Solutions

- Betaline solutions.
- Alcohol solution 70°C.
- Hypoallergenic tape.
- Splint.
- Sterile gauze.
- Sterile cotton wool.
- Sterile drapes.
- Sterile cut down tray.
- Syringes 2 mL and 5 mL.
- Needle 25 and 20 gauge.
- The 4/0 black silk suture.
- Assorted size of stereo polyethylene tubing.
- Local anesthesia as prescribed.
- Normal saline 0.9 percent.
- Sterile gloves according to doctor's size.
- Restraining devices.

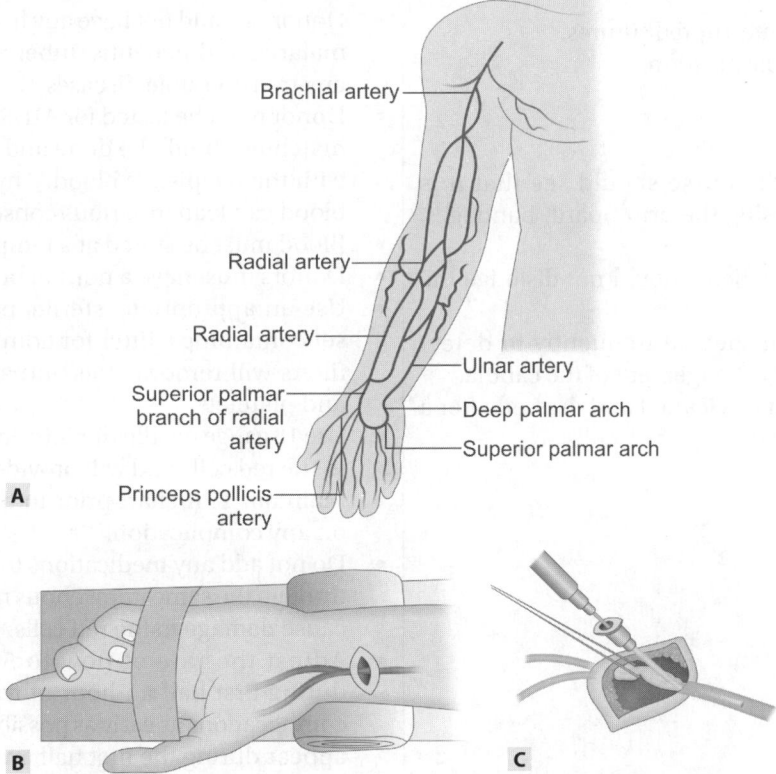

Figs. 21.8 A to C: Intravenous cut down common site and procedure.

- Sterile gown.
- Gallipot.
- Hand towel.
- Window towel.
- Knife handles no. 15 blades.
- Forceps.
- Scissors.
- Gauze and cotton.
- Needle holders.

Procedure

- Ensure that the physician has explained the procedure to the career and to gain consent and cooperation.
- Position the patient.
- Open the cut down set and drop the inner pack into the trolley. Physician scrubs his hands thoroughly up to the elbows for a full 3 minutes.
- Dries his hands and grim on the sterile hand towel provided.
- Don a sterile gown and the appropriate sized gloves.
- Opens the dressing pacts. Pour betadine and spirit directly from the bottle into the gallipots.
- Under local anesthesia and with aseptic precautions, the skin is incised and the vein is exposed.
- The aneurysm needle is passed under it.
- The loop of the threat is cut down two strands and is formed under vein.
- Tie the vein to prevent the blood flow.
- The vein is then cut partially between the two ligatures.
- The canula is passed into the proximal ligature is tied the canula in place.
- Wound is closed with interrupted sutures.
- Leave it on a comfortable position.

After Care

- After the procedure the nurse should see that it is secured carefully by using the arm board, bandages, adhesive plaster, etc.
- The movement of the patient should not dislodge the IV canula.
- The cut down site is inspected frequently to detect infiltration of fluid and dislodgement of the canula.
- The illusion site should be cleaned and dressed after a week sutures are removed.

Complication

- Infiltration.
- Infusion phlebitis.
- Thrombosis.
- Pyrogenic reaction.
- Air embolism.
- Circulatory overload.
- Shock.

BLOOD TRANSFUSION

Blood transfusion (Fig. 21.9) is the transfusion of whole blood or its components such as blood cells and plasma from one person (donor) to another person (recipient).

Purpose

- To replace blood volume and blood pressure during hemorrhage (hemoptysis, hemetemisis, antepartum and postpartum hemorrhage, operations, etc.) trauma or burns.
- To increase the 02 carrying capacity or hemoglobin level in cases of severe anemia which are not corrected by the administrations of vitamins and iron therapy.
- To provide antibodies and leukocytes (immune transfusions) to in severally ill patients and persons having lowered immunity by giving blood or plasma taken from persons who has just recovered from the same disease.
- To correct or treat defiance of plasma proteins clotting factors and hemophilic globulin, etc.
- To combat infection in patients with leukopenia.
- To replace the blood with hemolytic agents with fresh blood (exchange blood transfusions) as in case of erythroblastosis fetalis, hemolytic anemia, etc.
- To improve the leukocyte count of blood as in agranaulocytosis.

General Instructions

- Blood should be fresh.
- Donors should not have any history of jaundice, cancer, malaria, and hepatitis, tuberculosis, syphilis, AIDS or any transmissible diseases.
- Donor must be tested for AIDS. His grouping and cross matching should be done and it should be compatible with the recipient's blood. Any error in the labeling of blood can lead to serious consequences.
- Blood must be stored at a temperature 1-6 °C.
- Donors must have a normal pulse and blood pressure.
- Use an appropriate, sterile, pyrogen free transfusion set containing a fitter for administration of blood one filters will remove clots and aggregates of leukocytes and platelets.
- Use 18 gauge needles for infusion. It will prevent damage to the red cells and will provide adequate rate of flow.
- Maintain TPR chart prior to blood transfusion to find on any complication.
- Do not add any medications to the blood or administer through the same intravenous needle, because they may cause damage to the red cells.
- Adjust the rate of flow to 5 to 10 mL per minute during first half an hour of transfusion to detect any complications as early as possible. Because signs usually appear during the first half an hour of the transfusion.

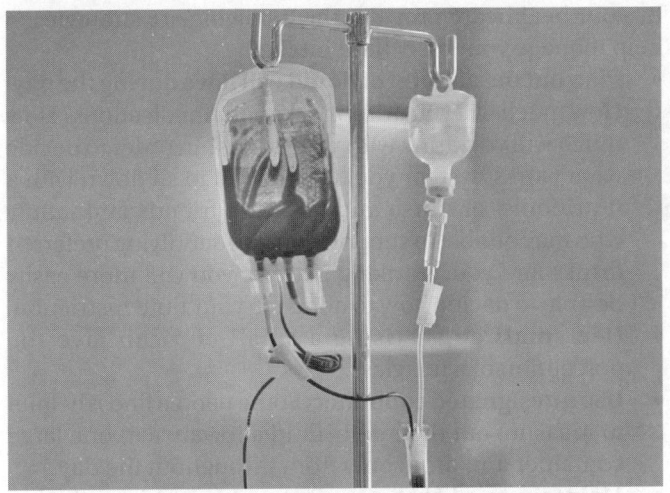

Fig. 21.9: Blood transfusion.

The subsequent flow rate depends upon the condition of the patient and the need for rapid transfusion.
- The blood should be given at a slower rate if the patient is elderly suffering from heart and lung diseases, anemia, etc.
- Whole blood and packed cells are administrated cold. Avoid shaking the container. If needed the blood may be allowed to stand in the room temp for 30 to 45 minutes, before administering to the patient.

Preparation

- Collection of blood from the donor is done in the laboratory by the laboratory technicians.
- All the articles used for the collection of blood should be sterile.
- Each donor unit must be labeled in clear, readable letters.
- The donor blood immediately after it is withdrawn should be placed in the refrigerator.
- Stored blood shall be inspected daily.
- The transportation of the blood in the hospital should be done within 30 minutes.
- Freezing, heating of the blood will destroy the blood cells.
- Where sending the recipient's blood sample for grouping and cross-matching it must be carefully labeled at the bedside of the recipient with identifications.
- Care is to be taken to prevent introduction of air into the apparatus.
- It is recommended to use 18 gauge needles for infusion, to prevent damage of the red cells to provide an adequate rate of flow.
- Medications antibiotics, vitamins, calcium.
- Rinse the infusion set with normal saline before starting the solution.
- Before the administrations of blood the vital signs should be recorded correctly.
- Adjust the rate of flow to 5 to 10 mL per minute during the first 30 minutes of transfusion (raised complications).
- Whole blood and packed cells are administered cold; blood may be allowed to stand in the room temp for 30 to 45 minutes before it is administered.
- Once the blood is exposed to the atmosphere it should be discarded.
- Watch the patient carefully for the onset of any complications any reactions developed, it should be reported to the charge nurse and the physician immediately.
- Keep the patient warm and comfortable with blankets (if necessary).
- Offer bed part before the procedure.
- Record in the nurse's record with date and time (amount of blood administrated, group, rate of flow, any reactions seen, any medications).

Procedure

- Explain the procedure to the patient and his relatives to get co-operation.
- Make him comfortable.
- Take the equipment to the bedside.
- Needle or casual should be inserted in the vein with complete aseptic technique.
- Keep the needle in position with adhesive tape.
- In small children or in case of difficult patient splint must be used. It should be securely placed bandage.
- Regulate the rate of flow from 40 to 45 drops per minute or according to physicians order.
- Observe the patient constantly inspect the bottle frequently, if chill or shivering any other occurs at the time of infusion, stop it immediately and irrigate the tubing with sterile fluid and inform it to the physician.

After Care of Patient

- After the infusions have been started, the nurse should see that it is secured carefully by using the arm board, bandages, adhesive plaster, etc.
- The movement of the patient in bed should not dislodge the IV cannula.
- The cut down site is inspected frequently to detect infiltration of fluid the dislodgement of the cannula, etc.
- The incision site should be cleaned and dressed daily to help in the healing of the wound.
- After a week, the sutures are removed.

Complications

Incompatibility: When the donor's blood is not compatible with the recipient's blood, it is known as hemolytic reactions. In a hemolytic reaction, there is clumping of the erythrocytes which blocks the capillaries. Causes the erythrocytes to disintegrate and release hemoglobin into the blood. It eventually gets into the kidney tubules. Their blockage produces kidney failure. The symptoms of hemolytic reaction are chills, fever, and headache of back pain, then dyspnea, cyanosis, chest pain and oliguria.

Pyrogenic reactions: It is due to bacterial contamination of the blood or of the administration set. The symptoms are fever, shaking chills warm flushed skin, headache, black pain and nausea which progress on to hematemesis, diarrhea and delirium.

Allergic reactions: The patient may be sensitive to substances in the plasma. The symptoms are urticaria, occasional wheezing, joint pain, generalized itching, nasal congestion, and circulatory collapse.

Circulatory overload: It is due to the rapid flow; also it may occur by giving whole blood to the severe chronic anemic patient, a patient with heart failure. The symptoms are bounding pulse, engorged peripheral veins, dyspnea, cough, slow the transfusion or step the transfusion and inform the doctor.

Transmission of infectious diseases: If donors are not carefully screened for diseases like jaundice, syphilis, malaria, filarial and AIDS, the patient may get untoward reactions and may suffer from above diseases.

FLUID RESTRICTION

Although there are many different circumstances where a person may be prescribed to follow a fluid restriction diet, some of the more common medical conditions and associated symptoms requiring fluid restriction are listed below:
- Heart problems, including congestive heart failure (CHF)
- Kidney problems, including end stage renal disease (ESRD) and people undergoing dialysis
- Endocrine system and adrenal gland disorders, including adrenal insufficiency
- Conditions that cause the release of stress hormones
- Treatment with medications called corticosteroids
- Low levels of sodium in your body also known as hyponatremia.

Signs and Symptoms

Fluid overload—too much fluid in your body. Although your healthcare provider will often examine you and test your blood, it is also very important to take charge of your health and monitor yourself. Watch out for:
- Swelling of the hands, ankles, and/or feet
- Increased size of the veins in your neck
- Weight gain
- Rapid heartbeat
- Increased blood pressure
- Increased urination
- Changes in mental status.

Treatment Considerations and Tips: In addition to following a low-sodium diet and taking diuretics ("water pills") as prescribed by your healthcare provider, a fluid restriction can help to achieve your health goals. Depending on the fluid limit outlined for your condition and prescribed by your healthcare provider the following are strategies to help manage your daily fluid intake:
- **Plan out the amount of liquid will have during the day:** How much will you drink to take your medications? How much will you drink with your meals? In order to decide what works best for you, it is helpful to sit down with a nutritionist or nurse and talk with friends and family who may be able to support you. By identifying preferred drinks and your drinking pattern, you will more easily be able to decide how to adjust to your fluid restriction.
- **Use small cups:** Using a small cup can give the perception of a full glass.
- **Use a designated container:** Some people find it helpful to measure out their daily fluid allowance in one large container and drink only from throughout the day.
- **Maintain good oral care:** By brushing your teeth after meals, rinsing with alcohol free mouthwash, chewing sugarless gum or sucking on hard candy you may be able to decrease dry mouth and urges to drink.
- **Avoid foods with high levels of sodium (salt):** These types of foods will increase your thirst.
- **Weigh yourself daily:** It is important to use the same scale around the same time each day to get the most accurate information and report any weight gain of 2 pounds or more in one day to your physician.
- **Record the fluid intake:** Recording your fluid intake will help make sure that you are not taking in more fluids than expected. It is a good idea to write this information on a tracking log/calendar (a sample is attached).

CONCLUSION

The main fluid in the body is water. Sixty percent of the total body weight is water. The water is distributed in three main compartments separated from each other by cell membranes. The intracellular compartment is the area within the cell. The extracellular compartment consists of the interstitial area (between and around cells) and the inside of the blood vessels (plasma). Electrolytes are the chemicals dissolved in the body fluid. The distribution has important consequences for the ultimate balance of fluids. Fluid and electrolyte disorders are volume related, compositional, or both. Diagnosis and therapy focuses on measurements such as blood pressure, pulse, central venous pressure, serum electrolyte values, arterial blood gas partial pressures, and pH. These are, however, gross indicators of what are really important: normal cellular function and satisfactory, if not optimal, metabolic status. Normal compensatory responses to fluid and electrolyte abnormalities preserve volume and composition. In the extreme, however, composition (e.g., electrolyte content) is sacrificed to ensure adequate volume. The "volumes" of importance are blood (plasma), interstitial fluid (functional extracellular fluid [FECV]), and intracellular fluid (ICF). Thus, mechanisms that initially act to maintain oxygen delivery at the cellular level ultimately can result in hyperosmolar or hypo-osmolar states that may be life-threatening. The proper analysis of fluid/

electrolyte problems is a three-dimensional approach. This approach involves assessing: (1) the total mass or total body stores of each electrolyte, which is the product of its concentration and the volume of its distribution; (2) the rate of electrolyte movement in and out of the body, i.e., balance; and (3) the movement of each electrolyte in and out of each compartment, i.e. changes in body composition, in health and various pathophysiologic states. Electrolytes are essential for normal cellular function. Alterations in circulating electrolyte concentrations are common in critically ill patients and occur in most patients admitted to the intensive care unit during their hospital stay. Abnormal electrolyte concentrations reflect altered metabolic status. The most common form of monitoring composition of the body fluids is measuring electrolyte concentrations in fluids, particularly serum.

BIBLIOGRAPHY

1. Alice L Price. The Art, Science and Spirit of Nursing. Philadelphia, WB Saunders Company, 3rd edn, 1968.
2. Kozier, Barbara B, Du Gas, Beverly Witter. Fundamentals of Patient Care: A Comprehensive Approach to Nursing. WB Saunders Company; 1967.
3. McClosky JC, Grace HK. Current Issues in Nursing, 4th edn. St Louis: Mosby Year Book, Inc, 1994.
4. Mitchell PR, Grippando GM. Nursing Perspectives and Issues, 5th edn. Albany, New York: Delmar Publishers, Inc, 1993.
5. Potter P, Perry A. Fundamentals of Nursing: Concepts, Process and Practice, 3rd edn. Mosby Year Book; 1993.
6. Shafer, Kathleen. Medical-Surgical Nursing, 6th edn. Saint Louis, CV Mosby Co, 1975.
7. Shakuntala Sharma 'Birpuri'. Principles and Practice of Nursing. Jaypee Brothers Medical Publishers (P) Ltd, New Delhi, 1997.
8. Sr Nancy. Principles and Practice of Nursing; Vol 1, 3rd edn. NR Brothers, Indore, 1992.
9. Taylor C, Lillis C, LeMone P. Fundamentals of Nursing: The Art and Science of Nursing Care. Philadelphia: JB Lippincott, 1993.
10. Thresyamma CP. Fundamentals of Nursing: Procedure Manual for General Nursing Course. PC Mathew, Kottayam, Kerala, 1992.
11. Virginia Henderson. Principles and Practice of Nursing. New York, MacMillan Publishing Co, 1970.

REVIEW QUESTIONS

Long Essays

1. Explain mechanisms controlling fluid and electrolyte movement.
2. Discuss about fluid volume deficit (FVD).
3. Describe electrolyte imbalances.
4. Enumerate in brief about blood transfusion procedure.

Short Essays

1. Factors affecting fluid movement.
2. Physiology of body fluids.
3. Regulation of fluids and electrolytes or homeostatic mechanism.
4. Fluid volume excess (FVE).
5. Importance of electrolytes.
6. Intravenous catheter insertion.
7. Acid-base imbalances.
8. Hypocalcaemia.
9. Maintenance of IV system.
10. Intravenous cut down.

Short Answers

1. Movement of fluid and electrolytes.
2. Regulation of body fluids.
3. Fluid intake.
4. Facilitated diffusion.
5. Sources of water intake.
6. Fluid pressure.
7. Hyperphosphatemia.
8. Acidosis and alkalosis.
9. Heparin lock.

MULTIPLE CHOICE QUESTIONS

1. **All the following are important electrolytes in the body, except:**
   a. Potassium ions
   b. Carbon ions
   c. Chloride ions
   d. Sodium ions

2. **A base may be defined as a chemical compound that:**
   a. Removes hydrogen ions from a solution
   b. Adds sodium chloride to a solution
   c. Adds hydrogen ions to a solution
   d. Eliminates sodium ions from a solution

3. **Intracellular fluid compartment refers to all the water found in:**
   a. The bones of the body
   b. Areas outside the body cells
   c. Areas within the gastrointestinal tract
   d. All cells of the body

4. **Approximately one-third of the body water exists in the:**
   a. Kidneys and urinary bladder
   b. Blood
   c. Extracellular fluid compartment
   d. Transcellular fluid compartment

5. **The interstitial fluid is generally poor while the plasma is generally rich in:**
   a. Hydrogen ions
   b. Sodium and chloride ions
   c. Protein
   d. Carbohydrates

6. **Water leaves the body by all the following mechanisms, except:**
   a. Through air expired from the lungs
   b. Through metabolic reactions taking place in the cells
   c. Through sweat given off at the skin
   d. From feces eliminated from the intestine

7. **In the process of osmosis:**
   a. Water moves from a region of high solute concentration to a region of low solute concentration
   b. Water moves from a region of low solute concentration to a region of high solute concentration
   c. Sodium ions move through a semipermeable membrane
   d. Chloride ions follow the movement of sodium ions to a region of low concentration

8. **The concentration of solutes is the same on both inside and outside cells, then:**
   a. Water leaves the cells
   b. Water rushes into the cells
   c. Water flows out of the cells into the transcellular environment
   d. The osmotic pressure is zero
9. **Osmoreceptors detect a decreased blood volume and increased blood concentration of salt and stimulate:**
   a. Increased kidney activity
   b. Increased salivary secretions
   c. Thirst
   d. Increased secretion of progesterone
10. **The hormones aldosterone and ADH both have an important function in:**
    a. Fluid balance in the body
    b. The regulation of acid concentration in the body
    c. Stimulation of a conscious desire for water
    d. The activity of buffer systems

ANSWERS

| 1. b | 2. a | 3. d | 4. c | 5. c | 6. b | 7. b | 8. d | 9. c | 10. a |

CHAPTER 22

Administration of Medications

LEARNING OBJECTIVES

- Introduction: Definition of medication, administration of medication, drug nomenclature, effects of drugs, forms of medications, purposes, pharmacodynamics and pharmacokinetics
- Factors influencing medication action
- Medication orders and prescriptions
- Systems of measurement
- Medication dose calculation
- Principles, 10 rights of medication administration
- Errors in medication administration
- Routes of administration
- Storage and maintenance of drugs and nurses responsibility
- Terminologies and abbreviations used in prescriptions and medications orders
- Developmental considerations
- Oral, sublingual and buccal routes: Equipment, procedure
- Introduction to parenteral administration of drugs: Intramuscular, intravenous, subcutaneous; intradermal—location of site, advantages and disadvantages of the specific sites, indication and contraindications for the different routes and sites.
- Equipment: Syringes and needles, cannulas; infusion sets: parts, types, sizes
- Types of vials and ampoules, preparing injectable medicines from vials and ampoules
   - Care of equipment: decontamination and disposal of syringes, needles, infusion sets
   - Prevention of needle-stick Injuries
- Topical Administration: Types, purposes, site, equipment, procedure
   - Application to skin & mucous membrane
   - Direct application of liquids, gargle and swabbing the throat
   - Insertion of drug into body cavity: Suppository/medicated packing in rectum/vagina
   - Instillations: Ear, eye, nasal, bladder, and rectal
   - Irrigations: Eye, ear, bladder, vaginal and rectal
   - Spraying: Nose and throat
- Inhalation: Nasal, oral, endotracheal/tracheal (steam, oxygen and medications)—purposes, types, equipment, procedure, recording and reporting of medications administered
- Other parenteral routes: Meaning of epidural, intrathecal, intraosseous, intraperitoneal, intrapleural, intra-arterial

TERMINOLOGY

- **Pharmacotherapeutics:** It deals with the relative effects of drugs in human systems for various disorders.
- **Pharmacokinetics:** It is the study of genetically induced drug responses that are often responsible for some idiosyncratic (unexplainable) responses.
- **Pharmacodynamics:** It deals with experimental science pertaining to theories of drug action.
- **Pharmacokinetics:** It is the study of how drugs enter in the body, reach their site of action, are metabolized and eliminated from the body.
- **Absorption:** It is the passage of drug molecules into the blood. To exert therapeutic effect, the drugs must depend on the physical properties of the drug, route of administration, presence or absence of food in the stomach and interaction with the drugs.
- **Distribution:** After a drug is absorbed, it is distributed within the body, to tissues and organs and ultimately to its specific site of action.
- **Metabolism:** After a drug reaches its site of action, it is metabolized into an inactive form, detoxified and degraded chiefly by liver. Also the lungs, kidneys, blood and intestines metabolize drugs.
- **Excretion/Elimination:** When drugs are metabolized they exit the body through the kidneys, liver, bowels and exocrine glands.
- **Drug:** It is a substance used in the diagnosis, treatment, cure, relief or prevention of a disease. The terms "medication", medicine, medicinal are used synonymously with the term "drug". A drug repair diseased tissues or organs. It can only facilitate normal cellular functions. Drugs are given to produce a "therapeutic effect" but these may also cause secondary effects and lethal effects. A single medication may have many therapeutic effects. For example, aspirin is an analgesic, antipyretic and anti-inflammatory drug. It reduces platelet count.
- **Side-effects:** Unintended but anticipated secondary effects, which may be harmless or injurious.
- **Adverse reaction:** It is the secondary effect which reflects the drug's action on other areas of the body.
- **Toxic effects:** Usually develop after a prolonged intake of high doses of medication due to accumulation of

drug in the blood because of impaired metabolism or excretion.
- **Lethal effects:** Excess amount of drugs within the body may have a lethal effect.
- **Iatrogenic disease:** Disease caused unintentionally by drug therapy. Hepatic toxicity resulting in biliary obstruction.
- **Idiosyncratic reaction:** When the client over-reacts or under-reacts to a drug or has a reaction different from normal.
- **Allergic reaction:** It is an unpredictable immunological response after exposure to an initial dose of medication. A drug allergy may be mild or severe (anaphylactic reaction). Common allergy symptoms are urticaria, eczema, pruritus and rhinitis.
- **Drug abuse:** It is inappropriate intake of a substance either continually or periodically. It has two main facts: drug dependence and drug habituation.
- **Drug dependence:** It is an individual's physiological or psychological reliance on or need to take a drug or substance.
- **Drug habituation:** It denotes a mild form of psychological dependence. The habituated individual develops the habit of taking the substance and feels better after taking it.
- **Drug tolerance:** An increase in dosage may be needed to cause a therapeutic effect in persons with low metabolism in response to a drug.
- **Drug interaction:** When one drug modifies the action of another drug interaction occurs.
- **Synergistic effect:** When the physiological action of two drugs in combination is greater than the effect of the drugs when given separately. For example, diuretics and vasodilators act together to keep the blood pressure at a desirable level.
- **Antagonist:** Drugs that have no special pharmacological action of their own but inhibit or prevent the action of a drug to produce a response.
- **Bioavailability:** The proportion of the administered dose of a drug, which reaches the circulation.
- **Pharmacological/Chemical name:** It provides an exact description of the drug's composition. An example of its chemical name is acetylsalicylic acid, which is commonly known as aspirin.
- **Trade name/Brand name:** The name under which a manufacturer markets a drug. A drug may have many different trade names.
- **Generic name:** The name that is proposed by the company that first develops the drug.
- **Material Media:** It is a record/book which deal with source, physical and chemical properties, preparations and uses of drugs.
- **Pharmacopeias:** It is an official document containing a list of drugs which have established their uses. It contains a description of physical properties and tests for identification, purification and potency of drugs.
- **Monthly Index of Medical Specialties (MIMS):** It is published in every month. It contains information on drugs, their trade names, along with the name of the manufacturing company with indications and contraindications of the drug, cost of the product.
- **Formulary:** It is a collection of formulas and prescriptions.

INTRODUCTION TO MEDICATION ADMINISTRATION

Definition

- Drug (Drogue means a dry herb in French) is a substance used in the diagnosis, prevention or treatment of a disease. WHO definition "A Drug is any substance or product that is used or intended to be used to modify or explore physiological systems or pathological states for the benefit of the recipient."
- Pharmacokinetics is the study of the absorption, distribution, metabolism and excretion of drugs, i.e. what the body does to the drug (in Greek Kinesis = movement).
- Pharmacodynamics is the study of the effects of the drugs on the body and their mechanisms of action, i.e. what the drug does to the body. Therapeutics deals with the use of drugs in the prevention and treatment of disease.
- Toxicology deals with the adverse effects of drugs and also the study of poisons, i.e. detection, prevention and treatment of poisonings (Toxicon = poison in Greek).
- Chemotherapy is the use of chemicals for the treatment of infections. The term now also includes the use of chemical compounds to treat malignancies. Pharmacy is the science of identification, compounding and dispensing of drugs. It also includes collection, isolation, purification, synthesis and standardization of medicinal substances.

SOURCES OF DRUGS

The sources of drugs could be natural or synthetic.

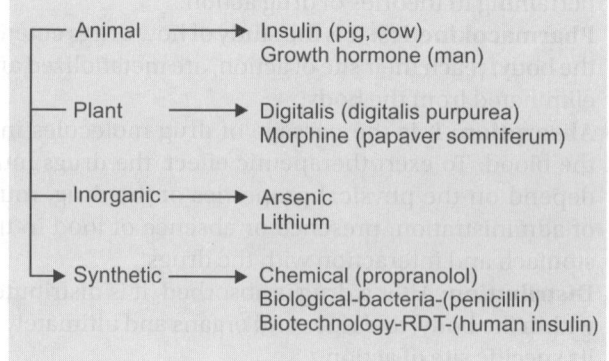

Fig. 22.1: Sources of drugs.

Natural sources drugs can be obtained from:
- **Plants**, e.g. atropine, morphine, quinine, digoxin, pilocarpine, physostigmine.
- **Animals**, e.g. insulin, heparin, gonadotropins and antitoxic sera.
- **Minerals**, e.g. magnesium sulfate aluminum hydroxide, iron, sulfur and radioactive isotopes.
- **Microorganisms:** Antibacterial agents are obtained from some bacteria and fungi. Thus we have penicillins cephalosporins, tetracyclines and other antibiotics.
- **Human:** Some drugs are obtained from man, e.g. immunoglobulin from blood, growth hormone from anterior pituitary and chorionic gonadotropins from the urine of pregnant women. Synthetic, most drugs are now synthesized, e.g. quinolones, omeprazole, sulfonamides, pancuronium, neostigmine.

Many drugs are obtained by cell cultures, e.g. urokinase from cultured human kidney cells. Some are now produced by recombinant DNA technology, e.g. human insulin, tissue plasminogen activator and some drugs by hybridoma technology, e.g. monoclonal antibodies.

DRUG INFORMATION SOURCES

- **Official Compendia:** Official compendia include information sources (or books) on drugs which are recognized by the government of that country as 'legal standard'. Thus Indian Pharmacopoeia, National Formulary, British Pharmacopoeia codex, Pharmaceutical codex, United States pharmacopoeia and such other Pharmacopeias are official compendia.
  Pharmacopoeia: Pharmacopoeia is the official publication containing a list of drugs and medical preparations. In Greek 'Pharmacon' means drug and 'poeia' is to make. It contains list of drugs and related substances, their source, formulae and other information needed to prepare the drugs, their physical properties, tests for their identity, purity and potency. Each country may follow its own pharmacopoeia. We thus have Indian Pharmacopoeia, British Pharmacopoeia, United States Pharmacopoeia, USSR and Japan Pharmacopoeia. The European Pharmacopoeia was published by the Public Health Committee and the European Pharmacopoeia commission. The International Pharmacopoeia is published by WHO in many languages like English, French Spanish and Russian.
  The first pharmacopoeia of India was published in 1868. But later under the British rule, the British Pharmacopoeia was followed. After independence, a committee was set up and Indian Pharmacopoeia was released in 1955. Experts from pharmaceutical industry, drug control laboratories and research and teaching institutions helped the committee. All pharmacopoeias are revised at regular periods to delete old useless drugs and to include newly introduced ones.
  Drug formulary: Also provides information on drugs. The National Formulary is a smaller book that contains information on formulations which are used therapeutically. It is prepared by the National Formulary committee set up by the Ministry of Health Government of India. Expert opinion is also taken from medical associations, hospitals, teaching institutions and pharmaceutical industry in preparing this book.
- **Nonofficial Compendia:** The books other than the official compendia which provide information on drugs are known as nonofficial drug compendia.
  Textbooks: These include the textbooks of pharmacology, journals and periodicals. Textbooks like—*Goodman and Gilman's:* The Pharmacological Basis of Therapeutics, Merck Index, The United States Dispensary, Remington's Pharmaceutical Sciences and others are quite informative. Many Indian textbooks are also available.
  - **Journals:** Several journals are published by local, national and international medical organizations. They provide updated information on drugs with research and review articles.
  - **Local:** Several regional (e.g. southern, northern) and state level medical societies release journals at regular intervals.
  - **National:** Indian Pharmacological Society, Indian Society of Clinical Pharmacology and other similar national level organizations bring out journals at regular intervals.

DRUG ADMINISTRATION

A drug or medicine is a substance used for diagnosis, treatment, cure, relief or prevention of disease.

Purpose of Medicine

- It used for diagnosis.
- It treats the disease condition.
- To prevent health alterations.
- To promote health condition.
- To treat infections allergic and inflammation.
- To relieve pain.

Forms of Medications

- **Capsule:** a solid dosage form in which the drug is enclosed in a hard or soft soluble container, usually of a form of gelatin.
- **Lotion:** Medicine in liquid suspension applied externally to protect skin.
- **Solution:** Liquid preparation that may used orally, parenterally or externally can also be instilled into body organ or cavity (e.g. bladder irrigation) contains water with one or more dissolved compounds, must be sterile for parenteral use.
- **Suppository:** Solid dosage form mixed with gelatin and shaped inform of pellet for insertion into body cavity (rectum or vagina).

- **Suspension:** Finely divided drug particles dispersed in liquid medium.
- **Syrup:** Medication dissolved in concentrated sugar solution, may contain flavoring to make medication more palatable.
- **Tablet:** Powdered dosage form compressed into hard disks or cylinders in addition to primary medication contains binders, integrators, lubricates and filler.

Types of Medication Action

- **Therapeutic effect:** It is the expected or predictable physiological response—a medication cause.
- **Site:** Effect is the unintended secondary effect—a medication predictably will cause. Side effects may be harmless or injurious.
- **Adverse effects:** These are generally considered severe responses to medication. For example, a client maybe becomes comatose when a drug is ingested.
- **Toxic effect:** May develop after prolonged intake of a medication or when a medication accumulation in the blood because of impaired.
- **Idiosyncratic reaction:** Medicine may cause an idiosyncratic effect. This occurs when a patient over react or under reacts to a drug or has a reaction different from the normal.
- **Allergic reaction:** It is an unpredictable reaction of a drug. In this, the drug acts as an antigen and antibodies are produced. Allergy causes antigen, antibody reaction.

FACTORS INFLUENCING MEDICATION ACTION

Some of the factors affecting drug action are: Age, size, sex, genetic inheritance and physical/emotional conditions.

Age

- Standard dosages are based on the amount of a drug that will cause the desired effect in an average adult. The bodies of very young and very old patients do not function exactly like the average adult body.
- In infants, body systems are not fully developed, they may have trouble breaking down or excreting drugs.
- The body systems of the elderly may not function as efficiently as when they were younger—the aging process slows down the work of certain organs.
- Smaller doses or different drugs may be required when treating the very old or the very young.

Size

- The size of the person and whether they are fat or thin have an effect on drug action
- If an average dose of medication is given to a very tall or very obese or very small and thin patient, the concentration of the drug in the bloodstream will not be the right amount to produce the effect you want.

Sex

- Women may react more strongly to certain drugs than men
- Women are generally smaller and have a higher proportion of fat than men.

Genetic Factors

- The individual makeup of each person causes slight differences in processes like biotransformation
- Some people have very unusual drug reactions that may be linked to genetic factors.

Disease Conditions

- Diseases can strongly affect how patients respond to drugs
- The organs necessary for biotransformation and excretion may be impaired
- Diseases of the liver and kidneys can affect the processing and elimination of drugs
- Any disease can change the effectiveness of a drug without warning.

Emotional Conditions

- Mental state can be an important factor in the success or failure of drug therapy
- Negative emotional states and strong feelings such as jealousy, anger, or fear may have a noticeable effect on drug action
- A patients expectations can also affect the drug action, a psychological effect called the placebo effect can add to the effectiveness of medication therapy.

Factors surrounding the administration of medications may also cause differences in people's response to drugs:

Route: Drugs are absorbed, distributed, and excreted at different rates when given by different means or routes (drugs are quickest when injected into the bloodstream, slowest when administered by mouth).

Time of day: Drugs that make a patient sleepy are ordered to be taken at bed-time; stomach-irritating drugs may be taken with meals to avoid discomfort. Normal bodily functions also vary with the time of day, thus affecting drug action.

Drug taking history: Some drugs can collect in the body, so the dosage must be adjusted to avoid overmedicating, repeated doses of the same drug may make the patient less responsive to the drug. Certain combinations of drugs can slow down or speed up the effects or can cause unusual or dangerous reactions.

Environmental factors: Extremes of weather or temperature can affect the action of drugs because heat and cold influence body functions. Heat relaxes the blood vessels and speeds up circulation so drugs act faster. Cold slows their action by constricting the blood vessels and slowing circulation. High altitude makes some drugs ineffective because of the lower levels of oxygen.

Factors Influence the Medication Dosage

- **Age:** Infants, children and the old requires smaller dosage of a drug than that of an adult.
- **Weight:** A person of overweight requires a large dose the usual one.
- **Male requires:** Large dose than females.
- **Cumulative action of the drug:** The frequency and dose of a drug administered depends upon the rate of excretion from the body.
- **Tolerance:** It is a capacity of taking excessive dose without producing toxic effect.
- **Habituation:** When a particular drug used continuously for a long period. The drug is withdrawn, they may stop physical craving for it and show definite organic symptoms.
- **Addition:** Prolonged use of alcohol and narcotics may produce an extreme form of habituation and result in a condition known addiction.
- **Route of administration:** Drugs given by IV route have a very quick and immediate action.

ROUTE OF ADMINISTRATION

The route of a drug depends on its properties desired effect, patient's physical and mental condition.

- **Oral administration:** It is the most common route and the most convenient route for most patients.
- **Sublingual:** The drug is placed under the tongue and letting it slowly dissolve, e.g. nitroglycerine.
- **Inhalations:** The patient inhales the fumes in the lung to have a local and systemic effect, e.g. nitrous oxide (anesthetic effect).
- **Inunctions (topical application):** It is the application of the drug into the skin usually by a friction, e.g. ointment.
- **Instillation:** It is putting a drug in liquid form into the body cavity such as urinary bladder or into body orifices such as ears eyes and nose.
- **Insertions:** Means introducing solid forms of drugs in to the body orifices, e.g. suppositories are introduced into the rectum and vagina.
- **Implantation:** Means planting or putting in of solid drugs into the body tissues.
- **Parenteral administration:** Parenteral means giving of therapeutic agents outside the alimentary tract.

  It is the type of administration accomplished by a needle.
  i. Intramuscular—into the muscle.
  ii. Subcutaneous—into the subcutaneous tissue.
  iii. Intradermal—into the dermis.
  iv. Intravenous—into the vein.
  v. Intra-arterial—into the artery.
  vi. Intracardiac—into the cardiac muscles.
  vii. Intrathecal—into the spinal cavity.
  viii. Intraosseous—into the bone narrow.
  ix. Intraperitoneal—into the peritoneal cavity.

MEDICATION ORDERS AND PRESCRIPTIONS

Prescription medications are dispensed only upon the clear, complete, and signed order of a person lawfully authorized to prescribe. Verbal prescription orders are received only by a licensed pharmacist. Residents shall maintain only those medications prescribed by their physician or authorized prescriber.

Medication orders (prescriptions) contain all of the elements required by law, including:
- Patient name
- Name of medication

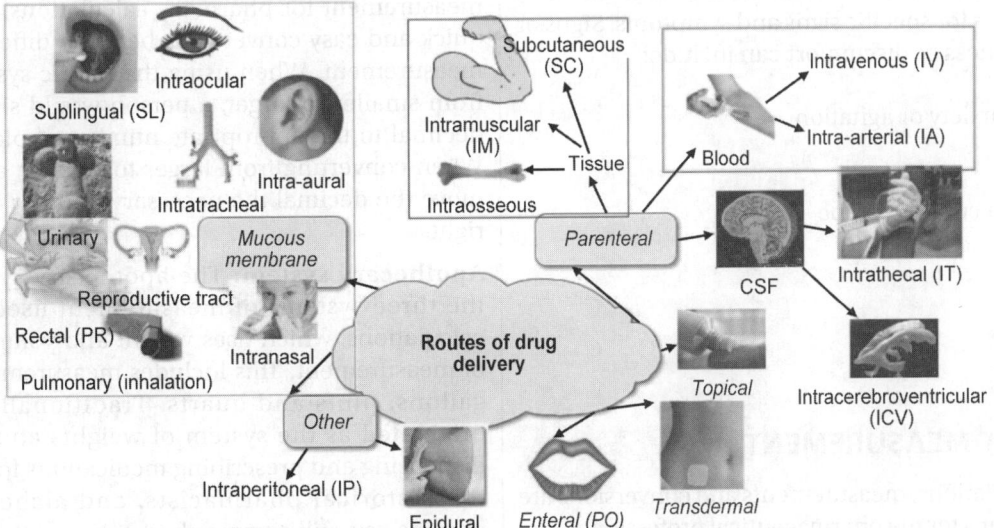

Fig. 22.2: Routes of drug administration.

- Strength of medication
- Dose
- Dosage form
- Time or frequency of administration
- Route of administration
- Quantity to dispense or duration of therapy
- Prescriber name and signature
- Refill authorization
- Date
- PRN (as needed) medication orders should specify the frequency of administration, maximum daily dosage, and condition for which the medication is being administered (e.g., pain, sleep).
  Prescription orders are required for all non-prescription medications for residents who receive medication assistance from the staff.
- Any dose or order that appears inappropriate considering the resident's age, allergies, diagnosis, or current medication regimen is verified with the prescriber.
- Each medication order—prescription and non-prescription—is recorded on the resident's medication information record or medication administration record (MAR).

A medication order is written directions provided by a prescribing practitioner for a specific medication to be administered to an individual. The prescribing practitioner may also give a medication order verbally to a licensed person such as a pharmacist or a nurse. Examples of some different types of medication orders are:
- Copy of a written prescription
- Written order on a consultation form, signed by the practitioner
- Written list of medication orders, signed by the practitioner
- Copy of a pharmacy call—in order, given to you by the pharmacist
- A verbal order given to a licensed person
- Electronic prescriptions signed electronically via a secured system.

PRN medication orders: PRN medications are given on an "as needed" basis for specific signs and symptoms. Signs or symptoms of illness or discomfort can include:
- Tiredness
- Increased anxiety or agitation
- Headache
- Earache
- Redness in a cut or a scrape
- Coughing
- Sneezing
- Fever
- Itching
- Cramping.

SYSTEMS OF MEASUREMENT

Pharmacy calculations, measurements and conversions are essential functions for the pharmaceutical professional. The system of pharmaceutical measurements involves various calculations and conversions of the formulation, ingredients and components of a medication dosage. Many pharmacy calculations use different methods of measurements. There are three measurement systems in pharmacy calculations, which a pharmaceutical professional must learn to carry out the critical functions used in the pharmacy.

Importance of Measurement Systems

One of the most essential functions of a pharmaceutical professional is the ability to perform accurate pharmaceutical measurements, calculations and conversions. Without this ability, a pharmaceutical professional is not able to apply their knowledge of pharmacology in a practical manner during their everyday work functions. This is important as one incorrect calculation, conversion or measurements will affect a dosage, and can potentially harm a patient. Possessing a working knowledge of the pharmaceutical systems of measurement will only benefit a pharmaceutical professional.

Metric Unit of Measure	
Measures of length	
1 meter (m)	= 1000 millimeters (mm)
1 meter (m)	= 100 centimeters (cm)
1 kilometer (km)	= 1000 meters
1 decimeter (dm)	= 1/10 meter
Measure of weight	
1 gram (g)	= 1000 milligrams (mg)
1 kilogram (kg)	= 1000 grams
Liquid measures	
1 liter (L)	= 1000 milliliters (mL)
1 deciliter (dL)	= 1/10 liter

Metric system: The metric system is a decimal system with all multiples and divisions based on a factor of 10. This system is also the most commonly used system of measurement for pharmacy calculations, as it allows for quick and easy conversions between different systems of measurement. When using the metric system to convert from smaller to larger, a person would simply move the decimal to the appropriate number of places to the left. When converting from larger to smaller, a person would move the decimal the necessary number of places to the right.

Apothecary system: The apothecary system is one of the three systems of measurement used in pharmacy calculations, which uses weight and volume as divisions of measurement. This includes measurements of ounces, gallons, pints and quarts. Traditionally, this system originated as the system of weights and measures for dispensing and prescribing medications for apothecaries, the historical pharmacists, and alchemists. Today, pharmacists still commonly use the apothecary system as their main system of measurement.

The common systems

Apothecaries' system:
The apothecaries' system is an obsolete system formerly used by apothecaries (now called pharmacists or chemists) in English-speaking countries

Apothecaries' fluid measure
60 minims (m) = 1 fluidrachm (f ʒ)
8 fluidrachms = 1 fluidounce (f oz)
16 fluidounces = 1 pint (pt or 0)
2 pints = 1 quart (qt)
4 quarts = 1 gallon (gal or C)

Apothecaries' measure of weight
20 grains (gr) = 1 scruple (ɘ)
3 scruples (60 grains) = 1 drachm (ʒ)
8 drachms (480 grains) = 1 ounce (oz)
12 ounces (5760 grains) = 1 pound (lb)

- 1 cm = 10 mm
- 1 tbsp = 15 mL
- 1 cup = 8 fl oz
- 1 pint = 2 cups
- 12 inches = 1 foot
- 1 L = 1.057 qt
- 1 lb = 16 oz
- 1 tbsp = 3 tsp
- 60 minute = 1 hour
- 1 cc = 1 mL
- 2 pints = 1 qt
- 8 oz = 240 mL = 1 glass
- 1 tsp = 60 gtt
- 1 pt = 500 mL = 16 oz
- 1 oz = 30 mL
- 4 oz = 120 mL (Casey, 2018).

Avoirdupois system: The avoirdupois system is similar to the apothecary system, however, the avoirdupois system exclusively measures weight based on 16-ounces equaling 1 lb. This system of measurement is the everyday weight-measuring system most people recognize. In pharmaceutical measurements, the avoirdupois system is useful for measuring bulk quantities when buying or selling, including over-the-counter pharmaceuticals and chemicals.

MEDICATION DOSE CALCULATION

There are 3 primary methods for calculation of medication dosages—Dimensional Analysis, Ratio Proportion, and Formula or Desired Over Have Method. We are going to explore the Desired Over Have or Formula Method, one of these 3 methods, in more detail.

Drug calculations require the use of conversion factors, for example, when converting from pounds to kilograms or liters to milliliters. Simplistic in design, this method allows clinicians to work with various units of measurement, converting factors to find the answer. These methods are useful in checking the accuracy of the other methods of calculation, thus acting as a double or triple check.

Preparation: When clinicians are prepared and know the key conversion factors, they will be less anxious about the calculation involved. This is vital to accuracy, regardless of which formula or method employed.

Conversion Factors

- 1 kg = 2.2 lb
- 1 gallon = 4 quart
- 1 tsp = 5 mL
- 1 inch = 2.54 cm
- 1 L = 1,000 mL
- 1 kg = 1,000 g
- 1 oz = 30 mL = 2 tbsp
- 1 g = 1,000 mg
- 1 mg = 1,000 µg

Technique

There are 3 primary methods for the calculation of medication dosages, as referenced above. These include Desired Over Have Method or Formula, Dimensional Analysis, and Ratio and Proportion.

Drug dosage based on age
- Before the physiologic differences between adult and pediatric patients were clarified, the latter were treated with drugs as if they were merely miniature adults.
- Various rules of dosage in which the pediatric dose was a fraction of the adult dose, based on relative age, were created for youngsters.

Young's rule, based on age:
$$\frac{Age}{Age + 12} \times Adult\ dose = Dose\ for\ child$$

Cowling's rule:
$$\frac{Age\ at\ next\ birthday\ (in\ years) \times Adult\ dose}{24} = Dose\ for\ child$$

Friend's rule for infants:
$$\frac{Age\ (in\ months) \times Adult\ dose}{150} = Dose\ for\ infant$$

Clark's rule, base on weight:
$$\frac{Weight\ (in\ lb) \times Adult\ dose}{150\ (average\ weight\ of\ adult\ in\ lb)} = Dose\ for\ child$$

Desired over have or formula method: Desired Over Have or Formula Method is a formula or equation to solve for an unknown quantity (x) much like ratio proportion. Drug calculations require the use of conversion factors, such as when converting from pounds to kilograms or liters to milliliters. Simplistic in design, this method allows us to work with various units of measurement, converting factors to find our answer. Useful in checking the accuracy of the other methods of calculation as above mentioned, thus acting as a double or triple check.

- A basic formula, solving for x, guides us in the setting up of an equation:
  D/H × Q = x, or Desired dose (amount) = ordered Dose amount/amount on Hand × Quantity.
  For example, a provider requests lorazepam 4 mg IV Push for a patient in severe alcohol withdrawal. The clinician has 2 mg/mL vials on hand. How many milliliters should he or she draw up in a syringe to deliver the desired dose? Dose ordered (4 mg) × Quantity (1 mL)/Have (2 mg) = Amount wanted to give (2 mL)
  Units of measurement must match, for example, milliliters and milliliters, or one needs to convert to like units of measurement. In the example above, the ordered dose was in milligrams, and the have dose was in milligrams, both of which cancel out leaving milliliters (answer called for milliliters), so no further conversion is required.

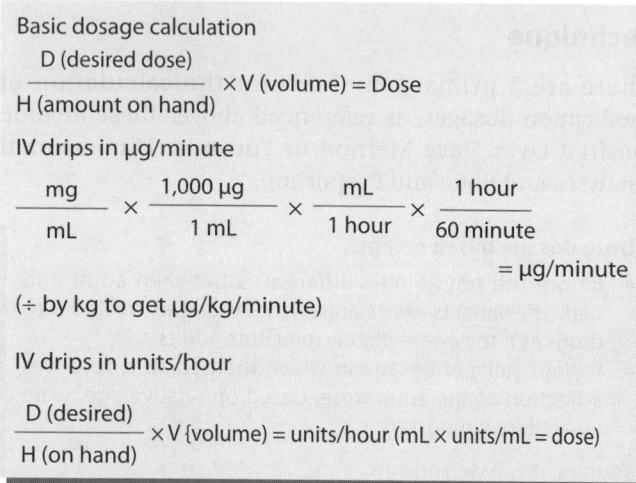

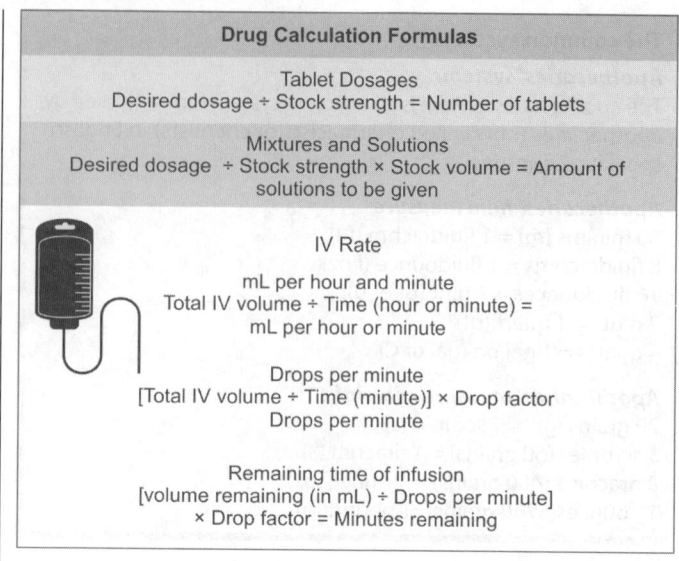

Fig. 22.3: Drug calculation formula.

We have addressed zeros, and now let us look at 1.
- If one multiplies a number by a 1, then the number is unchanged.
- In contrast, if you multiply a number by zero, the number becomes zero.
- Examples listed below are as follows: 18 × 0 = 0 or 20 × 1 = 20.

Ratio and Proportion Method: The Ratio and Proportion Method has been around for years and is one of the oldest methods utilized in drug calculations. Addition principals are a problem-solving technique that has no bearing on this relationship; only multiplication and division are used to navigate through a ratio and proportion problem, not adding. An example listed below will provide a better explanation using a fraction or a colon format:

A provider orders lorazepam 4 mg IV Push now for a CIWA score of 25. There are 2 mg/mL vials on hand. How many milliliters are required to carry out the ordered dose?
- Have on hand / Quantity you have = Desired amount/x
- 2 mg/1 mL = 4 mg/x
- 2x/2 = 4/2
- x = 2 mL
  In colon format, one would use H:V::D:X and multiply means DV and Extremes HX.
- Hx = DV, x = DV/H, 2:1::4:x, 2x = (4)(1), x = 4/2, x = 2 mL

Dimensional analysis method: An order placed by a provider for lorazepam 4 mg IV PUSH for CIWA score of 25 or higher, follow CAGE Protocol for subsequent dosages based on CIWA scoring.
- The clinician has 2 mg/mL vials in the automated dispensing unit.
- How many milliliters are needed to arrive at an ordered dose?
- The desired dose placed over 1 remember, (x mL) = 4 mg/1 × 1 mL/2 mg × (4)(1)/2 × 4/2 × 2/1 = 2 mL, keep multiplying/dividing until the desired amount is reached, 2 mL in this example.
- Notice, the fraction was set up with milligrams and milligrams strategically placed so like units could cancel each other out, making the equation easier to solve for the unit desired or milliliters. The answer makes sense, so work is done.
  Zeros can be canceled out in the same way as like units. For example:
- 1000/500 × 10/5 = 2, the 2 zeros in 1000 and 2 zeros in 500 can be crossed out since like units in numerator and denominator, leaving 10/5, a much easier fraction to solve and the answer makes sense.

TEN RIGHTS OF MEDICATION ADMINISTRATION

Understanding the 10 Rights of Drug Administration can help prevent many medication errors. Nurses, who are primarily involved in the administration of medications, benefit from this simplified memory aid to help guide them administer medications safely.
- **Right drug:** The first right of drug administration is to check and verify if it's the right name and form. Beware

Administration of Medications

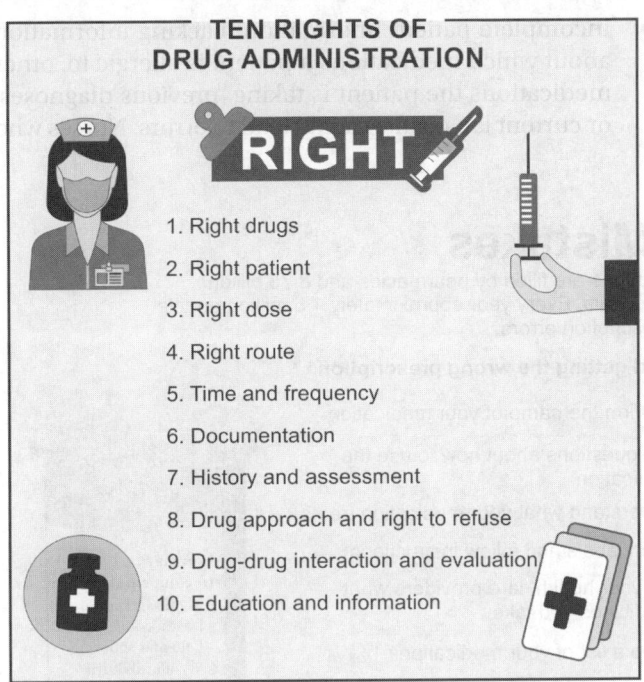

Fig. 22.4: Rights of medication administration.

of look-alike and sound-alike medication names. Misreading medication names that look similar is a common mistake. These look-alike medication names may also sound alike and can lead to errors associated with verbal prescriptions.

- **Right patient:** Ask the name of the client and check his/her ID band before giving the medication. Even if you know that patient's name, you still need to ask just to verify.
- **Right dose:** Check the medication sheet and the doctor's order before medicating. Be aware of the difference between an adult and a pediatric dose.
- **Right route:** Check the order if it's oral, IV, SQ, IM, etc..
- **Right time and frequency:** Check the order for when it would be given and when was the last time it was given.
- **Right documentation:** Make sure to right the time and any remarks on the chart correctly.
- **Right history and assessment:** Secure a copy of the client's history to drug interactions and allergies.
- **Drug approach and right to refuse:** Give the client enough autonomy to refuse the medication after thoroughly explaining the effects.
- **Right drug-drug interaction and evaluation:** Review any medications previously given or the diet of the patient that can yield a bad interaction to the drug to be given. Check also the expiry date of the medication being given.
- **Right education and information:** Provide enough knowledge to the patient of what drug he/she would be taking and what are the expected therapeutic and side effects.

ERRORS IN MEDICATION ADMINISTRATION

The main professional goal of nurses is to provide and improve human health. Medication errors are among the most common health threatening mistakes that affect patient care. Such mistakes are considered as a global problem which increases mortality rates, length of hospital stay, and related costs. This study was conducted to evaluate the types and causes of nursing medication errors.

Types of Medication Errors

Medication errors can occur anywhere along the route, from the clinician who prescribes the medication to the healthcare professional who administers the medication.

The different types of medication errors include (but are not necessarily limited to):

- Prescribing errors, wherein the selection of a drug is incorrect based on the patient's allergies or other indications. Additionally, the wrong dose, form, quantity, route (oral vs intravenous), concentration, or rate of admission could be used.
- Omission errors, in which there is a failure to give a medication dose before the next one is scheduled.
- Wrong time errors, wherein a medication is given outside the predetermined interval from its scheduled time.
- Improper dosing errors, wherein a greater or lesser amount of a medication is delivered than is required to manage the patient's condition.
- Wrong dose errors, wherein the correct dosage was prescribed, but the wrong dose was administered.
- Improper administration technique errors, such as administering a medication intravenously instead of orally.
- Wrong drug preparation errors, wherein a medication is incorrectly formulated (i.e., too much or too little diluting solution added when a medication is reconstituted).
- Fragmented care errors, wherein a lack of communication exists between the prescribing physician and other healthcare professionals.

These are just some of the many possible medication errors that can occur.

Causes of Medication Errors

- Distraction: A nurse who is distracted may read "diazepam" as "diltiazem." The outcome is not insignificant-if diazepam is accidentally administered, it could sedate the patient, or worse (e.g., if the patient has an allergy to the drug).
- Environment: A nurse who is chronically overworked can make medication errors out of exhaustion. Additionally, lack of proper lighting, heat/cold, and other environmental factors can cause distractions that lead to errors.

- Lack of knowledge/understanding: Nurses who lack complete knowledge about how a drug works, its various names (generic and brand), its side effects, its contraindications, etc. can make errors.
- Incomplete patient information: Lacking information about which medications a patient is allergic to, other medications the patient is taking, previous diagnoses, or current lab results can all lead to errors. Nurses who

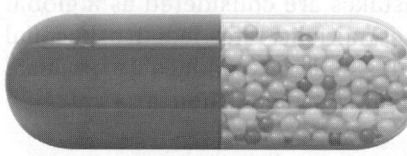

Medication Mistakes

Every year 2.5 billion prescriptions are filled by pharmacies and 3.75 billion drugs are administered at hospitals. Every year approximately 1.5 million people suffer injuries because of prescription errors.

Examples of medication mistakes

- Hospital fails to properly input prescription into computer database
- Wrong medicine or prescription is administered

- Wrong dosage is administered
- Allergic reactions to medicine or prescription
- Negligent prescription

- Failure to recognize drug interactions
- Failure to properly instruct patient on drug dosage and administration
- Mistakes in writing or filling prescriptions
- Failure to know proper uses of drugs

Avoid getting the wrong prescription

- Confirm the name of your medication
- Ask questions about how to use the medication
- Understand what your medication treats

- Read labels and follow instructions
- Tell your health care providers what medicines you take

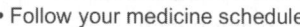
- Keep a list of your medications

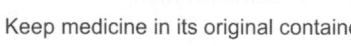
- Follow your medicine schedule
- Keep medicine in its original container

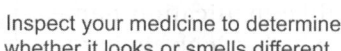
- Inspect your medicine to determine whether it looks or smells different

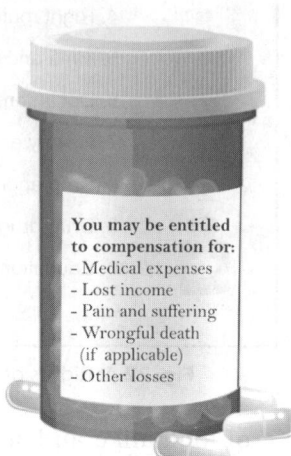

You may be entitled to compensation for:
- Medical expenses
- Lost income
- Pain and suffering
- Wrongful death (if applicable)
- Other losses

Fig. 22.5: Common medication mistakes.

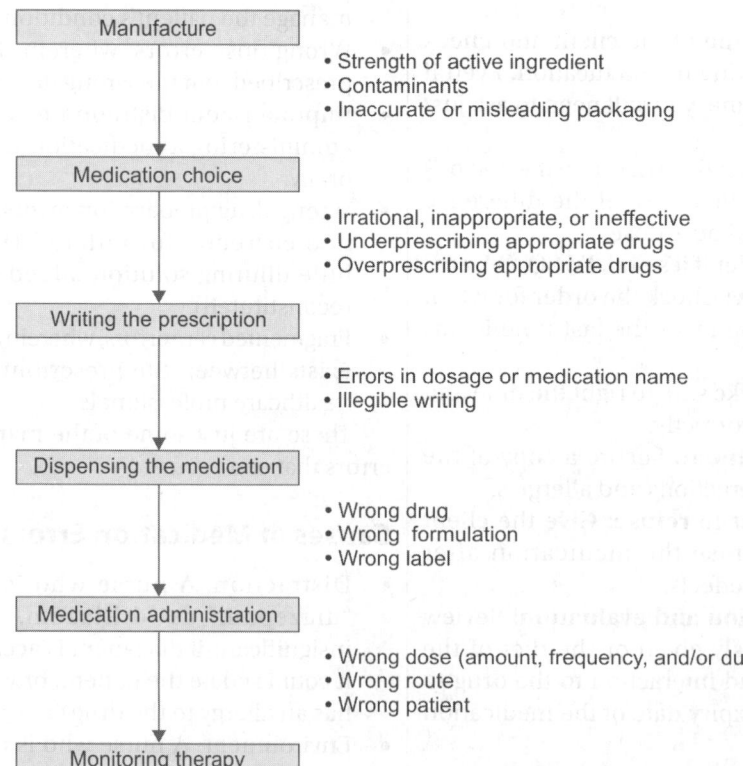

Fig. 22.6: Medication production and delivery system.

aren't sure should always ask the physician or cross-check with another nurse.
- **Memory lapses:** A nurse may know that a patient is allergic, but forget. This is often caused by distractions. Forgetting to specify a maximum daily dose for an "as required" drug is another example of a memory-based error.
- **Systemic problems:** Medications that aren't properly labeled, medications with similar names placed in close proximity to one another, lack of bar code scanning system, and other issues can lead to medical errors.

Preventing Medication Errors

Nurses may not have the authority to make infrastructural changes, but they do have the power to suggest needed changes and take precautions to prevent medication errors, including the following:

Know the patient: This includes the patient's name, age, date of birth, weight, vital signs, allergies, diagnosis, and current lab results. If patients have a barcode armband- use it. The added administration times of using arm band systems have led some nurses to create potentially dangerous "workarounds" to avoid scanning barcodes. Don't make this potentially dangerous mistake—use all of the information at your disposal to ensure patient safety, and avoid shortcuts.

Know the drug: Nurses need access to accurate, current, readily available drug information, whether the information comes from computerized drug information systems, order sets, text references, or patient profiles. If you have any questions or concerns about a drug, don't ignore your instincts-ask. Remember that you are still culpable, even if the physician prescribed the wrong medication, the wrong dose, the wrong frequency, etc.

Keep lines of communication open: Breakdowns in communication among physicians, nurses, pharmacists, and others in the healthcare system can lead to medication errors. The "SBAR" method can help alleviate miscommunications. **SBAR** (**S**ituation, **B**ackground, **A**ssessment, and **R**ecommendation) works like this:

Situation: "The situation is that Mr. Smith is complaining of chest pain."

Background: "He had hip surgery yesterday. About two hours ago he began complaining of chest discomfort. His pulse is 115, and he is short of breath and agitated."

Assessment: "My assessment is that Mr. Smith may be having a cardiac event."

Recommendation: "My recommendation is that you see him immediately, and that we start him on O_2 and administer an analgesic immediately. Do you agree?"

Double check high alert medicines: High-alert medicines such as heparin can have devastating consequences if not administered properly. A tragic case involving the death of three infant patients after receiving massive heparin overdoses happened as a result of misleading packaging. Since this incident, the drug manufacturer now uses larger font sizes, tear-off cautionary labels, and different colors to distinguish drug doses. Medications often look alike and sound alike-this can be a source of errors. Double check high alert medications with another nurse to prevent accidental overdoses and other medication errors.

Document each drug administered: Accurate documentation is essential and should include accurate recording of the drug information, the name of the drug, the dose, route, time, patient response, and any refusal of the drug by the patient.

Take an active role in correcting issues you identify: If you see that look-alike or sound-alike medications are stored next to each other, ask your supervisor to correct the problem, emphasizing the increased risk of medication errors. Request that medications be reconciled (i.e., that the names, dosages, and administration routes of all medications are compared to identify conflicts). Request that a bar coding system be implemented that allows for the verification of the six medication rights (right individual, right medication, right dose, right time, right route, right documentation).

Consequences of errors: Medication errors can have serious and costly consequences, such as increased patient lengths of stay, additional medical interventions, serious harm, or even death.

CARE OF MEDICINE AND MEDICINE CUPBOARD

- All the medicines and drugs must be checked as they are received from the dispensary.
- Dangerous drugs are given by special order and every dose should be accurate.
- Medicine cupboard should be kept in room, near to the ward.
- All poisonous drugs must be kept separately in a separate cupboard and it must be kept locked and the keys should be with ward sister.
- Medicine for external use should be kept in a separate part of the cupboard.
- The cupboard should be kept in well lighted and poison bottles should be clearly labeled.
- There should be separate compartment for mixture, tablets, powders, etc.
- The container should be arranged alphabetically so that it is easy to find them
- A register should be maintained to keep the account of the dangerous drugs.
- Check the expiry date of every drug and make use of it before its expiry date.
- Emergency drugs should be kept in a place where they are easily obtained for emergency use.

Rules for Administration of Medicines

Rules Regarding Labels

- Administer medications only from the properly labeled container.
- Poisonous drugs should be labeled in red ink.
- Read labels of medicine 3 times and check with doctor's order.
- Pour the medicine form the bottle only after shaking the bottle.
- Do not use the medicine that is different in color, taste, odor and consistency.

Rules Regarding Measuring Medicine

- Always use a calibrated ounce glasses or medicine glass to measure the medicine.
- Always give exactly what is ordered by the doctor.
- Make sure that the medicine glasses are clean and dry before pouring medicine.
- Hold the ounce glass at eye level and place thumb nail of the hand at the required level and then pour the medicine.
- Pour the medicine just before the time of administration into the medicine glasses

Rules Regarding Administration

- Observe the five rights in giving each medication right patient, right time, right medicine, right dosage and right method of administration.
- Give medicines only after checking a signed medication order by the doctor.
- Accept verbal orders, only in emergency to save the life of a patient.
- Always identify the patient before giving medication.
- Stay with the patient until he has taken medicine completely.
- An error in medication should be immediately reported to the ward sister.

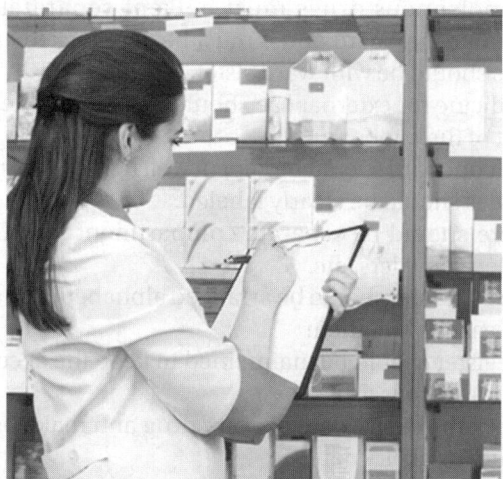

Fig. 22.7: Medication stock checking.

- Use proper light while giving medicines because dim light can cause errors.
- Never give water after giving cough syrups. It leaves a soothing effect to prevent cough.
- Drugs which stimulate appetite should be given before food.

Rules Regarding Recording of Drugs

- Record each dose of medicine soon after it is administered.
- Follow standard observations in recording medicine.
- Record time, dose and route of the medicine give.
- Record only those medicines, which have been administered.
- Record unusual effects such as allergic reactions.

Precautions to be Taken

- Check the doctor's order no medicine should be given without doctor's written order.
- Give the medications only from a clearly labeled container.
- Be sure that the medicine glasses are clean and dry before use.
- Shake the liquid medicine before pouring into the ounce glass.
- Wipe the mouth of the bottle, close it tightly and replace the bottle in the proper place after use.
- Pour the medicine from the bottle on the side opposite to the label.
- Once poured out, the medicine should not be returned to the bottle to prevent contamination of the whole medicine.
- Give medicine at the correct time and see that patient takes it.
- Always give the medicine that you have prepared yourself.
- Do not leave the medicine with the patient.
- Record after drug is given.

Nurses Responsibility in Drug Administration

The nurse should know the following:

- The nature of the drug—that is the name classification, types of preparation, effects, dosage absorption and excretion, routes and time of administration.
- Essential parts of a medication order.
- Abbreviations and symbols used in writing a medication order.
- Weights and measures used.
- Preparation of solutions and calculation of fractional dose.
- Storing of medicines in proper containers.
- Factors of safety in the administration of medicines.
- Rules for administration of medicines.
- Ethical and legal aspects.

Legal Aspects of Drug Administration

- Under the law the nurses are responsible for their work, though there is a written order.
- The nurses must know the minimum and maximum dose every medicine which she gives to the patient and its effect.
- The nurse must know the law about the use of narcotics. These drugs must be kept in a separate cupboard, the cupboard is kept locked and key is kept with the ward sister or senior nurse on duty.
- The special register should be maintained for narcotics drugs, which includes clear detail about the patient nurse and the doctor who ordered the narcotic drug.
- The nurse must observe five rights of giving medications to avoid errors.
- The narcotic drugs should be stocked only persons/Institutions who have licensed to do so.

Scientific Principles

- Almost all drugs are harm producer and are foreign materials that the body producing reactions.
- Additional force of water towards the glass produces a downward curve called meniscus.
- The human tongue presents an irregular surface and so tablets, powders and capsules produce friction and prevent easy swallowing.
- The sense of taste is acute and unpleasant taste may produce nausea and vomiting the taste buds of the tongue can be partially desensitized by cold drinks.
- Well diluted drugs and empty stomach favor absorption of drugs. But certain drugs are irritating to mucous membrane of the stomach.
- Medical record is a legal one and reference for future study and research.
- Using common medicine glasses promote cross infection.
- Volatile liquids when kept open or not tightly corked diffuse through air and get decomposed.
- An element of error is a possibility all human activity and commit or omit a dose of medicine means the existence of the end of life of the person.
- Understanding of how the drug benefits how it is to be given and side effects of the drug will help the patient to take drug regularly and a report to the physician concerned.
- Administration of the medicine is a therapeutic measure it will be therapeutic only, if the patient get the desired effect of the drug.

ORAL MEDICATION

Oral medications are defined as the administration of medication by mouth and ensuring that patient swallows the medicine.

Purpose

- To prevent the disease.
- To cure the disease.
- To promote the health.
- To give palliative treatment.
- To give as a symptomatic treatment.

Nurses Responsibility in Administration of Oral Medication

- Check the diagnosis and age of the patient.
- Check the purpose of medication.
- Check the identification of the patient—the name and bed number.
- Check the physician's orders for the correct name of the drug, dosage and method of administration.
- Check the nurse record for the time at which the last dose was given.
- Check for any contraindications present in the patient for an oral intake of the medicines such as nausea, vomiting unconsciousness, etc.
- Check the character of the drug- whether it can be taken safely by the oral method.
- Check the form of the drug available and the correct method of administration.
- Check the level of consciousness of the patient and ability to follow instructions.
- Check the abilities and limitations in swallowing the medications.

Equipment

A trolley containing:
- A bowel of clean water.
- Ounce glass, medicine glass, dropper teaspoon to measure the medicine.
- Drinking water in a feeding cup.
- Mortar and pestle to crush and powder the table if necessary.

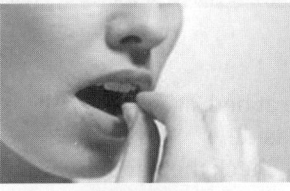

Oral administration

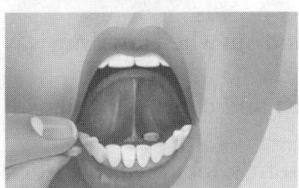

Sublingual administration is where the dosage form is placed under the tongue

Fig. 22.8: Medication administered by oral route.

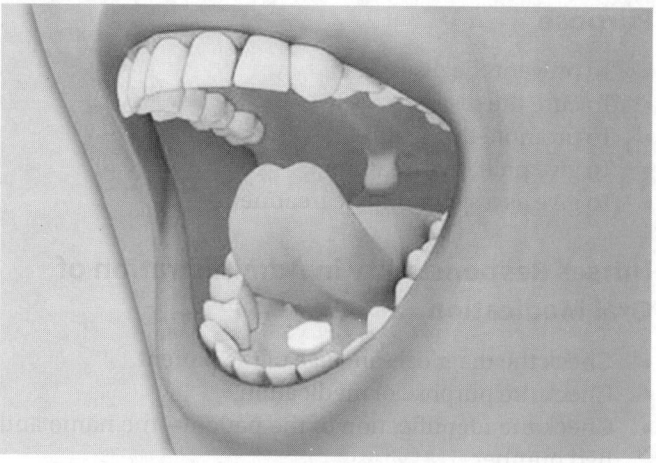

Fig. 22.9: Medication administered by sublingual route.

- Duster/towel to widen the outside the bottle after pouring the medicine ordered.
- Kidney tray and paper bag to discard the waste.
- Medicine cards to write the medication order from patients order sheet.

Preparation of the Patient

- Explain the procedure to the patient. Tell the advantages needs of medication.
- If patient is allowed to sit assist him to sit.
- Never give medication in flat position as there is a danger of aspiration of drug and fluid when swallowed.
- Give a mouth wash, if necessary.
- If medication is ill tasting, prepare a drink to mask the taste of the medication.
- Protect the bed clothes and garments with a towel placed under the chin across the chest.

Technique for administering oral medications

- Follow the medication administration procedure
- Pour the accurate dose: Place the prescribed number of pills or pour the correct amount of liquid into medication cup
- Administer the medication to the client with water or juice
- After administering the medication, perform a check to ensure that the child swallowed the medication

---

Procedure

- Keep the patient comfortable at bed.
- Arrange the articles at the bedside.
- Identify patient by name and check the name board at bedside.
- Check the nurse's record to find out when last drug was administered.
- Check for special instructions and check vital signs if needed.
- Select medicine from patient's locker and check medication label thrice.
- Encourage patient to sit-up and make sure medicines are swallowed.
- First give little water to moisten the mouth and then give medicine one at a time.
- Stay with the patient until the medicine has been swallowed; give him a drink of water after it.

Aftercare of the Patient and Equipment

- Remove the towel and wipe the face with it.
- Position the patient for good body alignment.
- Take all articles to the utility room. Wash and dry all articles and replace them in their proper place.
- Wash hands.
- Record medications given in medication sheet and also nurses record.
- Record any reaction observed after the administration of the drug.
- Report any reaction to the ward sister and doctor incharge.

Contraindications

- Continuous vomiting.
- Gastric or intestinal suction.
- Unconscious patient.
- Patient who are unable to swallow.
- Patient on nil per oral.

Advantages

- This method is safe and convenient.
- It is effective method.
- There is no pain while administering the drug.
- Allergic reaction are very less.

Disadvantages

- Sometimes the patient may not swallow the medicine.
- The drug may only be partially observed.
- It may irritate the gastric mucosa and can cause vomiting or diarrhea and the effect is lost.

SYRINGES AND NEEDLES

Drugs are administered as injections using a needle and a syringe. A syringe consists of a barrel and a plunger (piston). A type of syringe known as Luer-Lock syringe has the advantage that the needle can be locked in position. 'Intravenous injections are given with the help of an infusion set.

Sizes: Syringes are available in various sizes 1, 2, 5, 10, 20 and 50 mL. Syringes may be of two materials-Glass and plastic.

Glass Syringes

Advantages

- The markings are accurate and therefore exact quantity can be drawn.

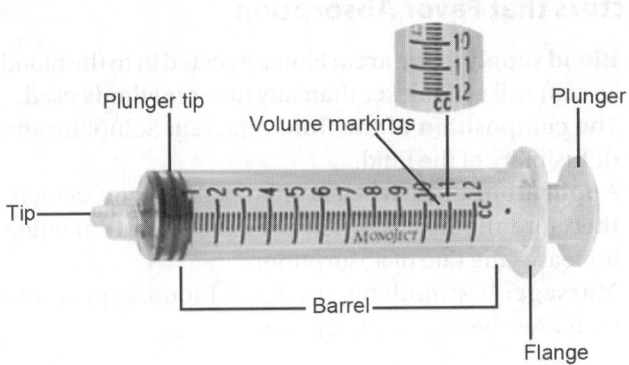

Fig. 22.10: Parts of syringe.

- The fluid level can be clearly seen as the glass is transparent.
- They can be easily sterilized by boiling and reused.
- Glass syringes are resistant to punctures.

Disadvantages

- Glass syringes can break.
- They carry a greater risk of air embolism because they are rigid.
- They are more expensive. Glass syringes are no more preferred because of the risk of spreading dangerous diseases like AIDS when not properly sterilized.

Plastic Syringes

Advantages

- Plastic syringes do not break easily.
- Because they are collapsible, they allow proper emptying of the syringe—hence less risk of air embolism.
- They are cheaper.
- They are disposable.

Disadvantages

- Plastic syringes are not very accurate in scale.
- They cannot be easily sterilized.
- They cannot be reused.

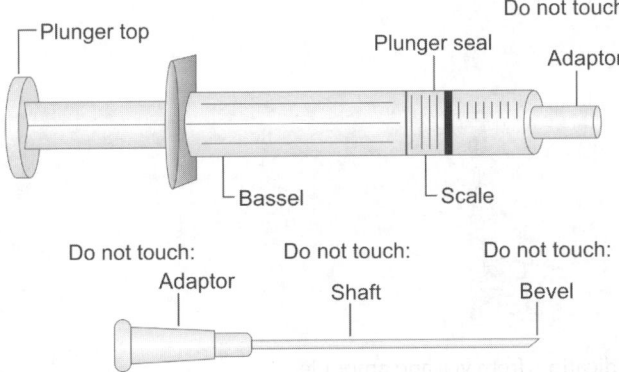

Fig. 22.11: Parts of needle.

Special Syringes

Insulin syringe has markings in units [40 in 1 mL (red) or 80 in l mL (green)] are suitable for administration of insulin.

Tuberculin syringe is a syringe of 1 mL capacity with 0.01 mL markings. It is useful for administration of very small volumes.

Disposable Syringes and Needles

Sterile disposable syringes are made of plastic and are packed with a needle to be fixed at the time of use.

Advantages

They have the following advantages:
- Need no sterilization.
- Injections are less painful as needle is sharp.
- Convenient to use.

Disadvantages

Works out costlier as they are not reusable.

Needles

Needles are made of stainless steel, which is rust proof. The tip which is at the end of the shaft is beveled. The bevelling may be short, very short or regular. Needle is available in different gauge thickness and length. The gauge numbers are from 13 (thickest) to 27 (finest). Depending on the route of administration, size of the patient and the thickness of the solution to be injected, the needle is selected.

INJECTIONS

Injections are parenteral therapy. It means giving of therapeutic agents including food outside the alimentary tract.

An injection is the forcing of a fluid into a cavity, a blood vessel or body tissue through a hollow tube or needle.

Purpose

- To get a rapid and systemic effect of the drug.
- To provide the needed effect even when the patient is unconscious.
- Assures that the total dosage will be administered and the same will be absorbed for the systemic action of the drug.
- Provides the only means of administration for medications that cannot be given orally.
- To obtain a local effect at the sight of the injection.
- To restore blood volume by replacing the fluid, e.g. in shock conditions.
- To give nourishment when it cannot be taken by

Types of Injections (Fig. 22.12)

- Intradermal: Drug introduced into the dermis
- Subcutaneous: Drug introduced into the subcutaneous tissue.

- Intramuscular: Injected into the muscles.
- Intravenous: Introduced into the vein.
- Intraspinal: Introduced into the spinal cavity.
- Intraosseous: Introduced into the peritoneal cavity.
- Venesection: Opening a vein and introducing a tube or wide bore needle and introducing medicines and fluids or taking out blood.
- Infusions: When a large quantity of medicines is fluids are to be introduced into the body.
- Transfusions: It is the introduction of whole blood or plasma into a vein or artery.

Factors that Favor Absorption

- **Blood supply to the area:** Fluids injected in to the blood stream will act quicker than any other methods used.
- **The composition of the fluid injected:** Solubility and diffusibility of the fluid.
- **Application of heat:** Heat dilates the blood vessels; therefore the heat applied over the site of injection increases the rate of absorption.
- **Massage:** It stimulates the local blood supply and increases the rate of absorption.

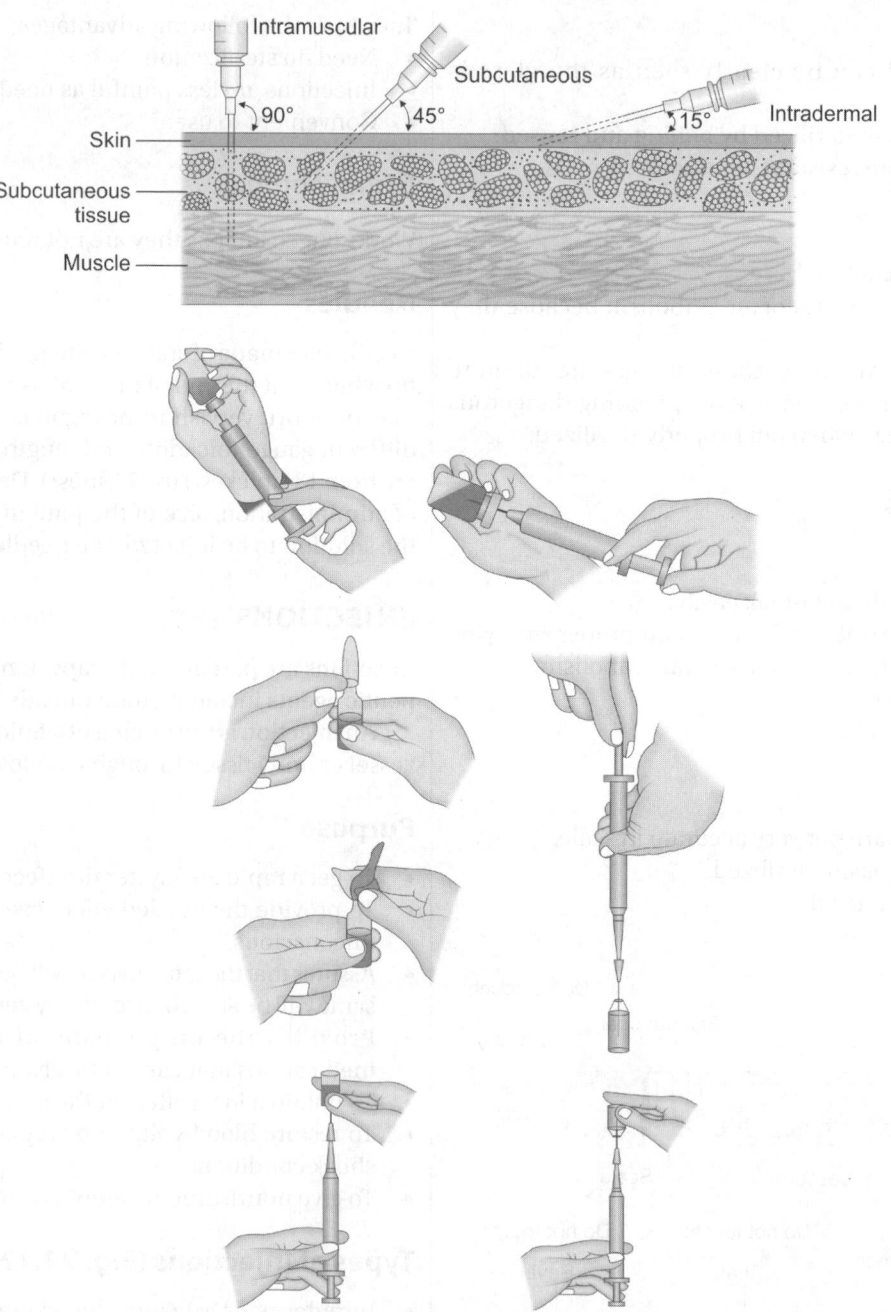

Fig. 22.12: Technique used in loading medication from vial and ampoule.

- **Circulation time of the blood:** Absorption of medicines and fluids injected into the body will diminish in a person who has venous congestion (edema).
- **Physical condition:** The local disease condition of the skin and underlying tissues such as skin lesions, inflammations, etc. delays the absorption of the drug.
- **Addition of the substances:** That tends to breakdown the natural resistance of the tissues can increase the rate of absorption.

Complications of Injections

- Allergic reactions certain drugs, e.g. penicillin.
- Infections (abscess formation).
- Pyrogenic reactions (producing fever).
- Tissue trauma.
- Psychic trauma.
- Pain.
- Accidental intravascular injections.
- Foot drop and persistent paralysis of the limb.
- Air embolism.
- Overdose and under dose of the medication.
- Errors in the administration of the medication.
- Infectious hepatitis.
- Circulatory overload.

Types of Drug and Fluids Administered Drugs

- Preventive action: Antitoxins, toxoids, vaccines and antibiotics.
- Diagnostic acids: Dyes and histamines.
- Remedial action: Antibiotics and quinine.
- Palliative action: Narcotics, sedatives, local anesthetics and general anesthetics.
- Substitution: Hormones, fluids, minerals and vitamins.

Fluids

- D5W: Each 100 mL contains 5 g of glucose
- D10W, D25W, D50W
- DNS: Dextrose 5 percent saline
- NS: Each 100 mL contains 0.9 g sodium chloride
- Sodium lactate: each 100 mL contains 1.866 g sodium ringer lactate.
- Ringer's solution or Hartmann's solution.

Selection of Site for Injection

It depends upon the following:
- Route of administration ordered by doctor.
- Quantity of the drugs.
- Condition of the patient.
- Muscular development.
- Knowledge of anatomical position of the nerves.
- Rotation of the site is necessary to avoid tissue trauma.

Technical Skill Needed

- Arrange the required equipment for the procedure.
- Nurse must be very skillful while giving the injection according to the route ordered by doctor.
- Select correct site for injection.
- Prepare the medication dose accurately.

Criteria for Selection of Syringes and Needles

- **Intradermal:** Tuberculin syringe or 1 mL calibrated in 0.01 mL units. 26 or 27 gauge diameter and 3/8 to 5/8 length size of needle used.
- **Subcutaneous:** Insulin syringe or 1 mL calibrated in 40 or 80 units syringe. 25 gauge and 1/2 to 5/8 inches syringe is used.
- **Intramuscular:** 2.5 mL syringe is used it calibrated in 0.2 ml. 21, 22, 23 gauge 1 to 2 inches in length needles are used.
- **Intravenous:** The size depends upon the amount of fluids to be injected, 18 to 20 gauge 1 to 2 inches needles use.

Golden Rules of Giving Injections

- **Administer the right drug:** To prevent mistakes, take time to check the name and spelling of each drug you administer against the patient's medicine card. Check a drug, at least, twice before giving it. First, when you remove it from the stock cupboard and, second time, before administering it to the patient. Avoid distractions. If you are unfamiliar with the ordered drug, learn about the drug from the pharmacist and the doctor. When in doubt, clear the doubt from the doctor.
- **Administer the drug to the right patient:** Make sure that the name of the patient is correct before you give the medicines. Check the name, diagnosis, and I.P. number. Adopt as a practice to confirm the right patient each time you administer the drug. Never leave a drug at the patient's bedside.
- **Administer the right dose:** You must check and double check the drug dose ordered against the dose you are about to give. Be especially careful when you are administering toxic medications, such as antineoplastic drugs. With these, the margin between a therapeutic and a potentially lethal dose is slim. Use an infusion pump as indicated and monitor the patient closely especially after an initial or loading dose is given or any time a dose is increased.
- **Administer the drug by the right route:** The parenteral route demands more vigilance. Parenteral drugs act so rapidly that a medication error may be very harmful—even fatal. If the order doesn't specify a route, call the doctor immediately for a clarification.
- **Administer the drug at the right time:** Therapeutic blood levels of many drugs depend on consistent,

regular administration times. Never give a drug more than half-an-hour before or after the scheduled time, without checking with the doctor. A hospital drug policy manual is one way to prevent errors associated with administration times. Make sure you coordinate drug administration with the laboratory schedule.

- **Educate your patient about the drug he is receiving:** Take advantage of every opportunity to teach your patient and his family about his prescribed medication. Stress the need for consistent and timely administration. Make sure they understand the importance of taking the medications for the entire prescribed course. Many patients, who begin to feel better after the first few doses, stop taking the drug.
- **Take patient's complete drug history:** It is necessary to know all the drugs your patient has been receiving and all the help he wants. By doing this you ensure his safety. The risk of adverse drug reactions and interactions, of course, rises with the number of drugs being taken.
- **Find out if the patient has any drug allergies:** No drug is completely safe. Any drug may cause an unpredictable reaction producing many different adverse effects - some appearing immediately, others developing over a period of time. Stay alert as you assess your patient's reaction to any drug you give him. Warm him that he should avoid drugs that have caused even a mild allergic response.
- Be aware of potential drug/drug or drug/food interactions.
- **Document each drug you administer:** Never document a drug before administering it but document you must after it is administered.

Commonly Used IV Drugs

- **Antibiotics (Ampicillin, Crystalline Penicillin)**
Indication: Treat mainly gram-positive infection (e.g., otitis media), meningitis, endocarditis, pneumonia. Act by interfering with bacteria cell wall synthesis-well distributed. Poor penetrator to CSF (except in inflamed one). Ineffective against penicillin's producer bacteria. Safe in pregnancy.
Side effect, contraindication (C/I): Serious allergic reactions rarely encephalopathy with high dose or normal dose in renal impairment patients. Never to be given intrathecally. Encephalopathy could be fatal. Accumulation of Na or K for electrolyte restricted patient.
- **Flucloxacillin** of narrow spectrum but effective against pencillinase producer bacteria of good effect against methicillin-sensitive Staphylococcus aureus (MSSA). Piperacillin known as antipseudomonal penicillin. Its activity is extended to cover gram-negative bacteria. Indicated when serious infection by *P. aeruginosa* is suspected.

Drug Interaction of Penicillin
- With probenecid, reduced excretion of penicillin.
- Synergistic effect with aminoglycosides against gram-negative bacteria.
- Reduces excretion of methotrexate, increases toxicity.
- **Cephalosporins** are classified into first, second and third generation and this is determined by the activity against gram-negative bacteria.
They are of broad spectrum (positive, and gram-negative) act by the same way as penicillin dose.
- **Rochin (ceftriaxone)** of longer half-life is given once bacteria and stability against beta-lactamase enzyme. Daily in preoperatively prophylaxis.
- **Fortum (ceftazidime)** of good pseudomonal effect. Side effect and contraindication: Allergic reaction.
- **Amikacin-gentamicin:** Bactericidal acts against gram-negative bacteria including *P. aeruginosa*.

Side Effects

- Damage the 8th cranial nerve leads to deafness, ototoxicity.
- Nephrotoxicity: Excreted via kidneys in renal impairment, accumulation may occur: (i) Never exceed 7–10 days treatment with amikacin-gentamicin. (ii) Never to be given more than TDS/daily. Given in combination with and hemolytic streptococci pneumococci. Contraindicated in pregnancy. Plasma level monitoring is required for peaks and troughs.

Drug Interactions

- With cyclosporin increase the risk of nephrotoxicity.
- With cisplatin increase the risk of nephrotoxicity and ototoxicity.

Erythromycin Injection

Indication: Alternative to penicillin for penicillin hypersensitive patients, good for upper respiratory tract infection, campylobacterenteritis, atypical pneumonia, legionella. Contraindicated, in liver disease (porphyria).

Side effects: If given for more than 14 days—cholestatic jaundice. Avoid concurrent administration of hismanal or Teldane.

Drug interactions: Erythromycin inhibits hepatic microsomal enzyme leads to increase plasma concentration of antiarrhythmic, carbamazepine, terfenadine, and cyclosporin.

Vancomycin

Drug of choice in treatment of pseudomembranous colitis. Methicillin-resistant Staphylococcus aureus (MRSA), prophylaxis for endocarditis.
Side effects/caution: Avoid rapid infusion (anaphylactic shock). Rotate the infusion site. Renal toxicity. History of deafness. Blood disorder should be considered seriously with vancomycin.

Aminophylline

Indication: Indicated alone or in addition to beta-2 agonist to relieve bronchospasm. The drug is metabolized by liver cirrhosis, viral infection—cimetidine, erythromycin, aminophylline half-life decreased with rifampicin, smoking, phentoine carbamazipine. The significance of half-life is important as the therapeutic toxic margin of aminophylline is narrow. When initiating IV therapy with aminophylline we should make sure that the patient was not taking from oral of aminophilline.

Side effects: Arrhythmia due to hypokalemia, convulsion, GIT disturbance. Aminophylline toxicity is treated by correcting the hypokalemia with KCl (60 mmol/1 hour), tachycardia is treated with IV propranolol.

Dopamine/Dobutamine

Are inotropic drugs, cardiac stimulant, exerting their action through beta-1 receptor at the heart. Indicated in case of cardiogenic shock.

Side effects: Tachycardia.

Hypovolemia should be corrected first:

- **Intrathecal injections**

  Definition and purpose: Medicine injected in the subarachnoids space of the spinal canal drugs such as anti-infectious or antineoplastics used for treating meningeal leukemia are injected by this route as they do not travel in the bloodstream. It is also given for anesthesia such as lidocaine hydrochloride (for regional anesthesia).

  Complications
  - Inflammation at the puncture site.
  - Septicemia.
  - Spinal deformities specially while giving anesthesia.

  Note: Care must be taken when preparing this kind of injections to ensure that they do not have any bacterial substance.

- **Epidural analgesia administration**

  This procedure is usually performed by the doctor.

  Purpose
  - It is used for pain in deteriorating condition of joints.
  - To relieve acute pain or chronic in other areas of the body.
  - To relieve intense or severe pain postoperatively.

  Procedure: The medicine is injected into the epidural space, which is situated just outside the subarachnoid space where cerebrospinal fluid flows. Medicine gets spreaded slowly into the subarachnoids space of the spinal canal then goes into the spinal fluid which carries it directly into the spinal area by passing (avoiding) the Blood Brain barrier. However, in some cases medicine may be injected into subarachnoid space Intrathecally.

  Blood brain barrier: It is a barrier membrane between circulating blood and brain. It prevents any damaging substance from reaching the brain tissues and cerebrospinal fluid.

- **Intra-articular injections:** Intra-articular injections are used when drugs are introduced in inflamed joint, hydrocortisone acetate suspensions are used in this way. Care must be taken to ensure sterile technique.

- **Intracardiac injections:** Intracardiac injections are used for cardiac arrests.

  Drugs used are: Adrenaline. They are given in precardial area inside the midclavicular space.

INTRAMUSCULAR INJECTION

Intramuscular injection is defined as introduction of medicine into the muscle in form of solution (**Figs. 22.13A and B**).

Purpose

- To obtain a quick effect of medicine than is obtained by oral administration and subcutaneous administration.
- Assures that the total dosage will be administered and the same will be absorbed for the systemic action of the drug.
- The medicines that is not suitable for intravenous administration.

Principles

- The knowledge of the anatomy and physiology of the body is essential for the safe administration of the injection.
- Injections are means of introducing infection into the body, if carelessly given.
- Drugs that change the chemical composition of the blood will endanger the life of the patient, if not used cautiously.
- Any unfamiliar situation produces anxiety.
- Once a drug is injected it is irretrievable. Antidote may be available for particular medications but the best antidote is prevention.
- Organization and planning results in the economy of time, material and effort.

General Instructions

- Give injections only on the doctors written orders.
- Follow strict aseptic techniques.
- Syringes and needles used for injections should be kept separate from those used for other purpose.
- Always have the syringe and needles in good order.
- Change the needle after withdrawing the drug from a rubber stopped container before giving injection to the patient.
- Observe the five rights of the administration of medicines.
- Never use a drug whose expiry date is over.

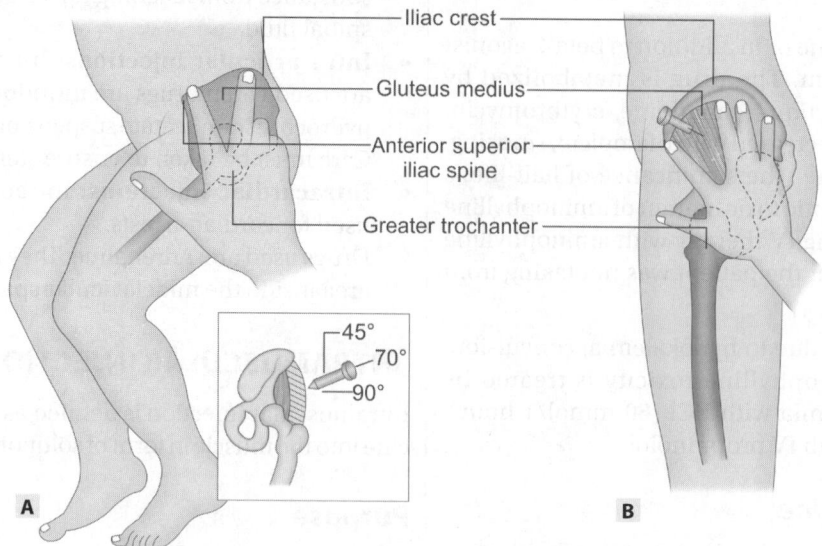

Figs. 22.13A and B: Intramuscular injection administration.

- Always have a patient relaxed and placed in a comfortable position.
- Never allow the patient to walk soon after the injection.
- Always give a test dose in case of penicillin and all types of sera.
- Expel the air from the syringe before the injection.
- Select the appropriate site for giving injections.
- Rotate the site for patients getting insulin to prevent lip dystrophy.
- Use correct technique of injection: The needle inserted gently and quickly, and the drug injected slowly.
- After inserting the needle, always withdraw the piston to make sure that it is not in a blood vessel in case of intramuscular and subcutaneous injections.
- Solution for injection should be clear, sterile, nearly neutral in reaction.
- Massage the area at the site of injection except in case of intradermal injections.
- Injection should be charted immediately.

Site of Intramuscular Injections (Figs. 22.14A to C)

Dorsal gluteal site: Find out the greater trochanter of the femur and the posterior superior iliac spine drawn an imaginary line between these two bony prominences. Site will be upper and outer quadrant.

Vastus lateralis site: The site is at the outer aspect of the thigh. It is the area between mid anterior thigh and mid lateral thigh one hands span from elbow and great trochanter to one hands span above knee.

Ventrogluteal site: Place the tip of the index finger on the anterior superior iliac spine of the patient the middle finger just below the iliac crest.

Mid deltoid site: Locate the lower edge of the acromion process and form a rectangle. The deltoid area is used to inject very small quantities of nonirritating drugs.

Methods of IM Injection Administration

Air lock method: Expel the air from the syringe leaving 0.2 mL, stretch the skin lightly with the index finger. Insert the full needle quickly into the muscle. Withdraw the piston to confirm that the need is not in the blood vessel. Push the piston gently to give the medicine very slowly.

Z-tract method: Expel the air from the syringe, displace the skin laterally using the side of your left hand, Insert the needle aspirate the placement, inject the medicine very slowly, marinating tissue displacement wait for ten seconds to allow the medicine to disperse. Withdraw the needle allowing the displaced tissue to return to its normal position.

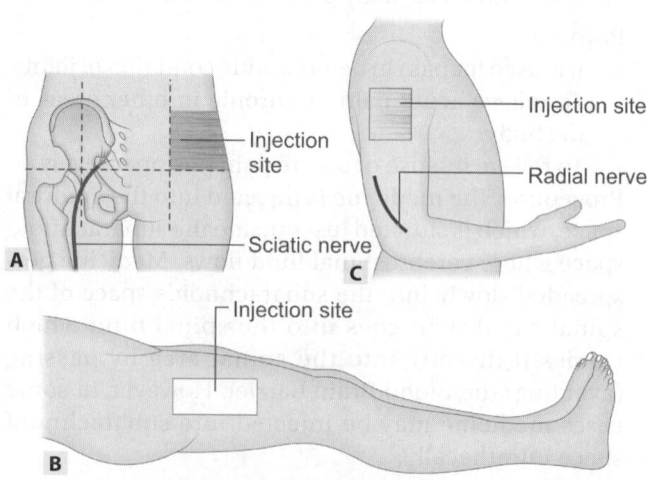

Figs. 22.14A to C: Intramuscular injection site.

Nurses Responsibility Check

- The diagnosis and age of the patient.
- The purpose of injection.
- The doctors order.
- The patient details.
- The nurses record about previous.
- The allergic reactions.
- The necessity for giving test dose.
- The levels of consciousness and follow instructions.
- The site of injection.
- The patient's previous experiences.

Equipment

A tray containing:

- Syringe and needles of various size (sterile).
- Transfer forceps in a jar containing antiseptic solution.
- Sterile cotton swabs and gauze pieces in sterile container.
- Methylated spirit in a container.
- Bowl with water.
- Kidney tray and paper bag
- Drug order sheet.
- Water for injection.
- File to cut upon the ampules.
- Small covered tray (sterile) to carry the prepared injection to the bed side.

Preparation of the Patient and Environment

- Identify the patient correctly.
- Explain the procedure to the patient.
- Provide privacy.
- Keep the patient's attention away from the injection by friendly conversation.
- Place the patient in a comfortable and relaxed position.
- Select a site suitable for the route of administration.

Procedure

- Select the medication.
- Hand wash.
- Prepare the medication.
- Keep the syringe with medications in the sterile tray and cover it.
- Make sure that the medicine taken right and correct dosage.
- Carry medication to the patient in a sterile tray.
- Identify the right patient.
- Prepare the site of injection.
- Inject the medicine by correct technique is essential for the safety of the injection.
- Spread the tissue between the thumb and forefinger to make the skin taut.
- Needle is inserted at a 90 degree angle holding the syringe back the piston with the left hand.
- Using a steady push on the needle and aspirate by pulling back the piston with left hand.
- If no blood comes give the medication slowly by pushing the piston.
- Remove the needle quickly and massage the site for quick absorption of the drug.

Aftercare

- Inspect the area for bleeding.
- Help the patient to dress up.
- Ask the patient to take rest for 15 minutes.
- Check the limb movement to confirm there is no nerve injury.
- Watch for the signs and symptoms of allergic reaction.
- Replace the equipments in the proper place.
- Hand wash.
- Record the procedure on the nurse's record.

SUBCUTANEOUS INJECTION

Subcutaneous injection involves placing medication into the loose connective tissue under the dermis.

Subcutaneous injection means the introduction of medicine into the subcutaneous tissues.

Drug is injected into the layer of fatty tissues beneath the upper layers of the skin.

Purpose

- To administer the medication that is ineffective in the gastrointestinal tract by the action of the digestive juice.
- To administer smaller doses.
- For slow drug absorption.
- To obtain a prompt action of a medicine that is obtained by oral administration.

General Instructions

- A 90 degree angle is normally used with a 5/8 inch needle is used with a 5/8 inch needle for obese patients.
- A 45 degree angle is used with a needle 3/4 inch long or longer for an average patients are in a thin patient.
- The techniques of giving injection for hypodermic injections will be same as in IM injection.
- Use only nonirritating medications.
- Use only small quantity of medication.
- Deposit the medication in a fold formed by picking up a layer of skin and fat.
- Be sure to insert the needle beyond the thickness of the skin (the medication is to be deposited in the subcutaneous tissue).

Equipment

- One mL calibrated in 40 or 80 units, e.g. insulin syringe.
- Hypodermic needles (24 to 25 gauge, 1/2 to 5/8 inches length).
- Sterile cotton swabs.
- Methylated spirit in container.

- Kidney tray with paper bag.
- Drug ordered sheet.
- Small covered tray (sterile) to carry the prepared injections to the bedside.

Criteria for Selection of Site (Figs. 22.15A and B)

- The skin and underlying tissues are free of abnormalities.
- Not over bony prominences.
- Free of large blood vessels and nerves.

Common Sites Subcutaneous Injection

- Outer aspect of the upper arm.
- Posterior chest wall below the scapula.
- Anterior abdominal wall from below breast to iliac crests.
- Anterior and lateral aspect of the thigh.

Procedure

- Read the doctors order and select the medication.
- Wash hands.
- Select appropriate syringe and needle and check whether they are in good working order.
- Recheck the order, medicine card with the label of the medicine, expiry date, etc.
- Mix well and take out the required amount of solution in the syringe.
- Keep in syringe with medication in the sterile tray and cover it.
- Carry medication to the patient and identity the correct medicine.
- Prepare the site for the injection.
- A 90 degree angle is normally used with a 5/8 inch needle for obese patients.
- A 45 degree angle is used with a needle 3/4 inch longer for an average patient or in a thin patient
- The technique of giving injection for hypodermic injections will be same as in IM injections.

Aftercare

- Inspect the area but do not massage.
- Help the patient to dress up.
- Watch for signs and symptoms of any allergic reaction.
- Replace the equipment used for injection.
- Clean all other articles and replace them in their proper place.
- Wash hands.
- Record the procedure on the nurse's record and drug sheet.

INTRADERMAL INJECTIONS

An intradermal injection is the introduction of a hypodermic needle into the dermis. Intradermal medicine when introduced into the dermis (under the epidermis).

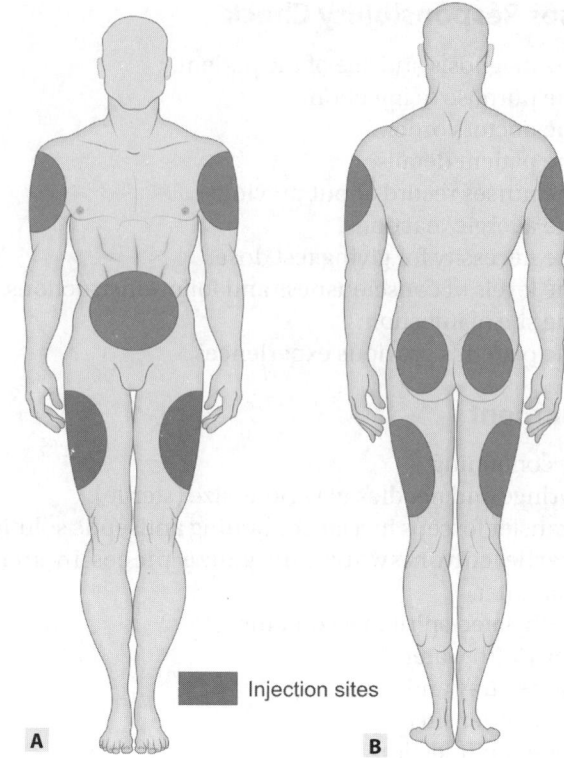

Figs. 22.15A and B: Subcutaneous injection site.

Purpose

- To obtain a local effect at the site of injection of local anesthesia such as xylocaine and novocaine.
- Diagnostic purpose as in sick test, tuberculin test, etc.
- To test for allergic reaction to a drug, e.g. penicillin serum, etc.

Selection of Syringe and Needle

- Size of syringe used for intradermal injections are 1 mL calibrated in 0.01 mL units (tuberculin syringe).
- Size of needle used for intradermal injections are 26 to 27 gauge diameter and 3/8 to 5/8 inch length.

Equipment

A tray containing:
- Syringe and needles of various sizes according to the need in a covered tray (sterile).
- Sterile cotton swabs and gauze piece in sterile containers.
- Methylated spirit in a container.
- Kidney tray and paper bag.
- Drug order sheet.
- Small covered tray (sterile) to carry the prepared injections (syringes and needles with medication) to the bedside.

Preparation of the Patient and Equipment

Identify the patient correctly:
- Explain the procedure to the patient.
- Provide privacy.

- Place the patient in comfortable and relaxed position suitable for the type of injection.
- Select a site suitable for the route of administration, quantity of medication to given to the characteristics of medication.

Procedure

- Read the doctors order and select the medication.
- Wash hands.
- Select appropriate syringe and needle and check whether they are in good working order.
- Recheck the order, medicine card with the label of the medicine, expiry date, etc.
- Mix well and take out the required amount of solution in the syringe.
- Carry medication to the patient and identity the correct patient.

Method of Administration

- This method is used for skin tests to detect allergies.
- Hold the skin tight by grasping it waters the forearm.
- With the bevel of the needle facing up insert the needle at an angle of 10 to 15 degrees to the skin.
- The needle enters between the two layers of the skin. The bevel should be practically visible through the skin.
- Inject the medication slowly to produce wheal on the skin.
- 0.01 to 0.1 mL of medication injected intradermal.
- Take out the needle quickly do not clean or massage the area.

Aftercare

- Inspect the area but do not massage.
- Help the patient to dress up.
- Watch for the sign and symptoms of any allergic reaction.
- Replace the equipment used for injection.
- Clean all other articles and replace them in their proper place.
- Wash hands.
- Record the procedure on the nurse's record and drug sheet.

General Instructions

- As skin contains sensory nerve ending only a small amount of solution can be injected into the skin as it is painful.
- The skin should be healthy free of any skin infection such as edema or irritation the cloths should not irritate the skin.
- Separate syringe and needles should be used for giving injections.

Observation of the Site after Intradermal Injection

Tuberculin Test

- If tuberculin test is done, ask the patient to report after 48 hours.
- Reddened raised area at the site of injection shows a positive reaction.
- If the area is not discolored or raised it is a negative reaction.

Penicillin Test

If the test dose is given for penicillin observes the area for reactionary changes after 20 minutes to 1 hour.

The area will be reddened the wheal will be increase in case of reactionary changes.

If the patient is sensitive to penicillin he may develop the signs and symptoms of anaphylactic shock within few minutes after the injection.

INTRAVENOUS INJECTION

Intravenous Injection is the introduction of a small quantity of drug into the vein by venous puncture. Introduction of drug directly into the blood stream is called intravenous injection.

Purpose

- To have a fast action of the medicine as in emergency.
- To give medicines those are irritating or ineffective when given by other routes.
- To have the action of medicines on the blood stream or the blood vessels.

Common Sites of IV Injection

- Ventral aspect of elbow or forearm median cubical, basilica or cephalic veins.
- Doral aspect of hand—brachial, cephalic or metacarpal veins.
- In the infants, the scalp vein is used.

General Instructions

Expel the air from the syringe before giving the injection by holding it in upright position and gently pressing the piston until a drop of solution comes out to the tip of the needle.

- Always dissolve the drug in correct amount of fluid to minimize the risk of adverse effect of the medicine.
- Observe the patient closely for the signs of adverse reaction of the medicine and have emergency drugs and the antidote in hand while injecting the medicine.
- Do not give the medicine if the injection site shows any edema or intravenous solution is not following properly

to avoid accidental administration of medicine in to the surrounding tissues.
- While giving iron preparation always confirm that the patient is not sensitive to it by giving a test dose.

Types of IV Administration

- Adding the medicine in intravenous solution bottle (intravenous infusion).
- Existing intravenous line for continuous infusion.
- Bolus-Direct intravenous push for immediate or fast action.

Selection of Syringe and Needle

- The size of syringe used for intravenous infusion depends upon the amount of fluids to be injected.
- Size of the needle used are 18 to 21 gauge or 1 to 2 inches.

Preliminary Assessment Check

- The diagnosis and age of the patient.
- The purpose of injection.
- The doctors order for the type, dosage, time and route of administration.
- The patient's name and bed number.
- The nurses record to find out the time at which the last dose was given.
- The symptoms of overdose or allergic reaction.
- The necessity for giving test dose.
- The form of the medicine available and correct method of administration.
- The level of consciousness of the patient.
- The site and previous experience of the patient.

Equipment

A tray containing:
- Syringe and needles of various sizes according to the need in a covered tray (sterile).
- Transfer forceps in a jar containing antiseptic solution.
- Sterile cotton swabs and gauze pieces in sterile containers.
- Methylated spirit in a container.
- Bowl with water.
- Tourniquet.
- Water for injection.
- Drug order sheet.
- File to cut open the ampules.
- Small covered tray (sterile).

Preparation of the Patient and Environment

- Identify the patient correctly.
- Explain the procedure to the patient.
- Provide privacy.
- Place the patient in comfortable and relaxed position suitable of intravenous injection.
- Select a site suitable for the route of administration, quantity of medication to be given and characteristics of medication.

Procedure

- Read the doctors order and select the medication.
- Wash hands.
- Select appropriate syringe and needle and check whether they are in good working order.
- Recheck the order, medicine card with the label of the medicine, expiry date, etc.
- Mix well and take out the required amount of solution in the syringe.
- Carry medicine to the patient.

Method of Administering IV Infection

- Apply a tourniquet on the upper arm.
- Ask the patient to clench and unclench the hand.
- Pull the skin taut and place the needle in line with vein at a 15 to 45 degree angle.
- Insert the needle, a bit below the point where the needle will pierce the vein.
- When the back flow of blood occurs into the syringe release the tourniquet and injects the medicine very slowly.
- Pressure with swab at the puncture site after the needle is withdrawn to prevent bleeding.

Aftercare

- Observe the area for bleeding if bleeding occurs, apply pressure but do not massage.
- Give comfortable position to the patient.
- Ask the patient to take rest at least 15 to 30 minutes so that you can observe him for any reaction.
- Observe the patient for any allergic reaction.
- Replace the equipment used for injection.
- Clean all other articles and replace them in their proper place.
- Wash hands.
- Record the procedure on the nurse record sheet and medication sheet.

Complications

- Allergic reactions.
- Pain.
- Injection abscess.
- Injury of nerves.
- Air embolism.

INTRAVENOUS INFUSIONS

An introduction of a large amount of fluid into body via veins is called as intravenous infusion.

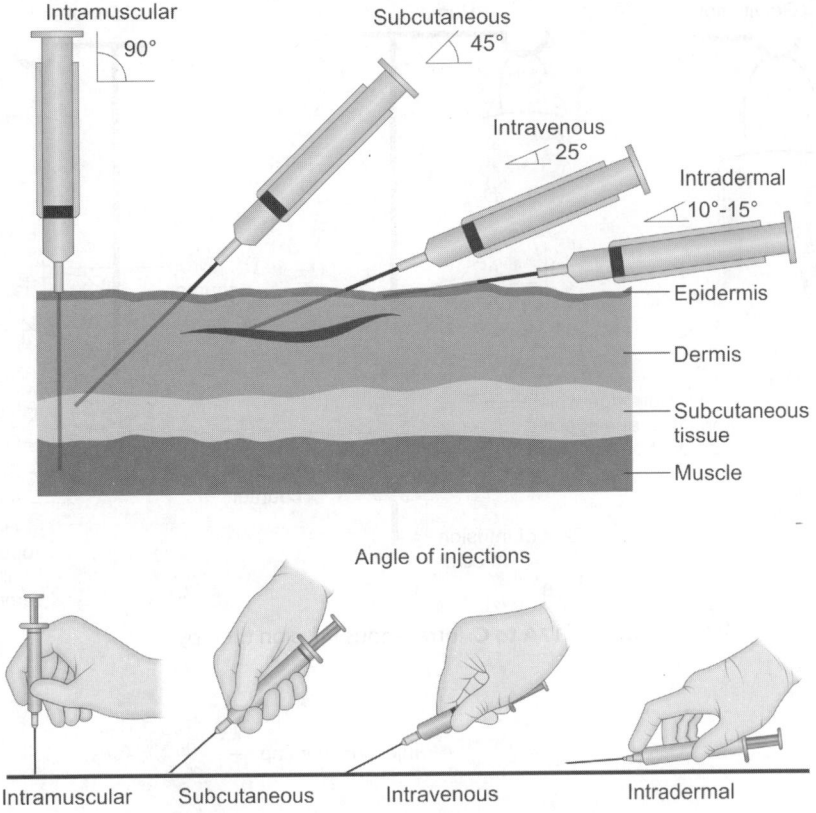

Fig. 22.16: Parentral route of drug administration.

Intravenous infusion is puncturing vein with sterile cannula/needle into a vein to supply the body with fluids, electrolyte, nutrients and medication **(Figs. 22.17A to C)**.

Purpose

- To supply fluids and electrolytes.
- To restore fluid volume due to dehydration, hemorrhage, vomiting, diarrhea, etc.
- To meet patient's basic requirements, e.g. calories, vitamins, etc.
- To maintain homeostatic balance.
- To treat in emergency conditions some medications are given intravenously.
- To prevent and treat shock and collapse.

Indication

- To save the patients in life threatening situations, e.g. and extensive burns.
- To introduce a drug into the circulation for diagnostic purpose, e.g. intravenous pyelogram (IVP).
- To supply fluids and nutrients to the patients who are unable to digest or absorb a diet administered mouth or through the nasal tube.
- To dilute toxins in case of toxemia or septicemia.
- When blood or blood products are to be given, e.g. anemia, hemorrhage.

Solution Used

- Isotonic solutions: Sodium chloride 0.9 percent commonly used.
- Hypotonic solutions or buffer substances sodium/potassium, calcium chlorides and lactic acid.
- Nutrient solutions dextrose 5, 10, 25, 50 percent.
- Alkalinizing and acidifying solutions.
- Blood volume expanders: Plasma substitutes and contain large molecular substances, e.g. dextran, lomodex, hemocoele, etc.

Factors Affecting Fluid Movement

- **Diffusion** molecules move from a solution of higher concentration to solution of lower concentration. Increase in the temperature increases the rate of diffusion.
- **Osmosis:** The diffusion water molecules through a permeable membrane from an area of lesser solute concentration.
- **Hydrostatic pressure:** It is the pressure exerted by a fluid within a closed system. Counter balancing the osmotic pressure of the plasma, which attract fluid into the vascular system.
- **Dialysis:** The diffusion of molecules of soluble constituents through a permeable membrane is known as dialysis.

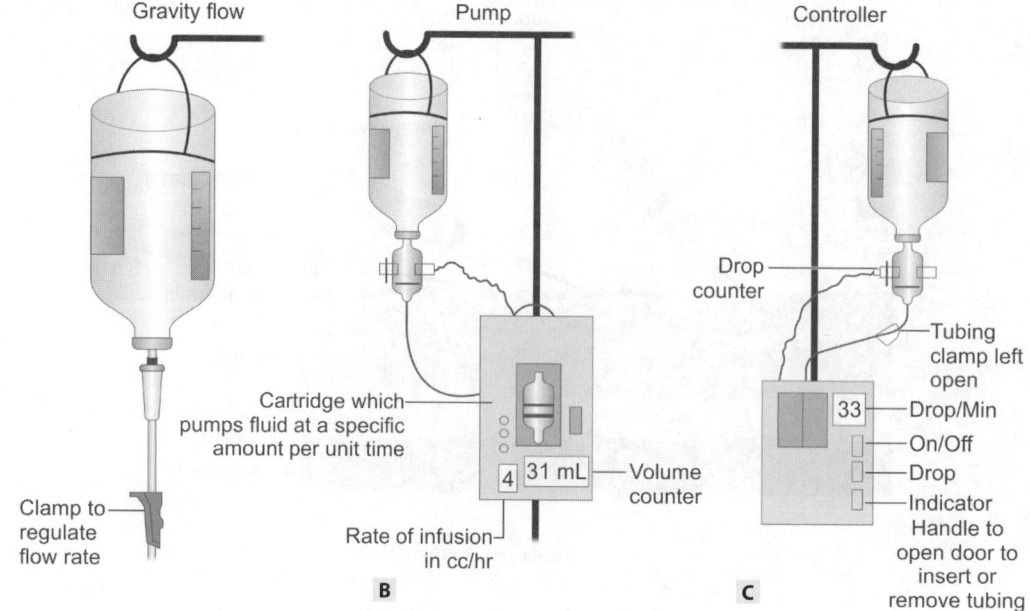

Figs. 22.17A to C: Intravenous infusion therapy.

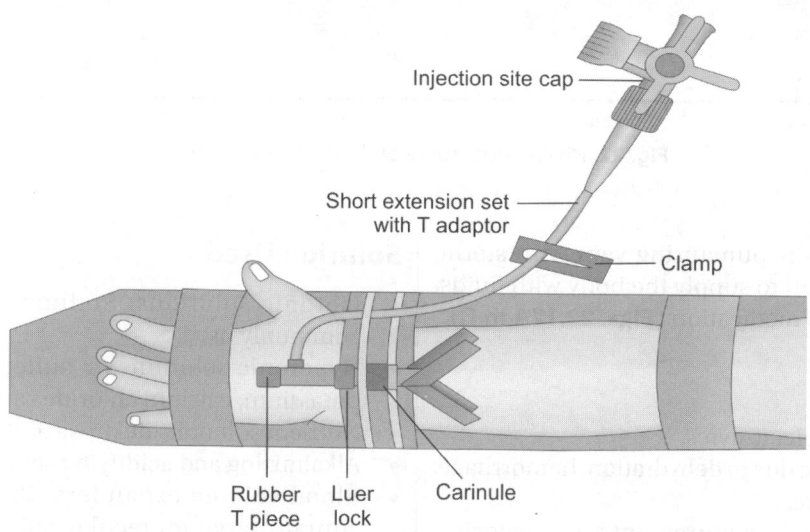

Fig. 22.18: Intravenous catheter connected to three way extension.

- **Filtration:** It may be defined as the passage of fluids and dissolved substances across membranes because of differences in mechanical pressure on two sides of the membrane.
- **Selective permeability of membranes:** In body, the capillary and the cell membranes are described as selective permeable.

Factors that Favor Absorption

- Warmth: Application of heat over the site of injection or the use of warm solution.
- Massaging: Massaging the part gently increases the local supply and increase absorption.
- Diffusibility and solubility of the drug.

Venipuncture Site

The selection of site depends upon following facts:
- The condition of veins.
- The characteristics of tissues over the vein.
- Purpose and durations of infusions.
- The type and amount of IV fluids ordered.
- The diagnosis and general condition of the patient.

The commonly used veins are:
- Basilic and cephalic veins (forearm).
- Median cubital, cephalic and basilica veins (antecubital fossa).
- Radial vein (radial area).
- Dorsal Metacarpel veins (the hand).
- Veins in the foot.

- Femoral and saphenous veins (thigh).
- Veins in the scalp (for infants).

Complications of IV infusion

- **Circulatory overload:** The intra vascular compartment contains more fluid than the normal. Circulatory overload results in cardiac failure and pulmonary edema.
- **Infiltration:** It is the escape of fluid in to the subcutaneous tissues due to dislodgement of needle.
- **Hematoma formation** The walls of blood vessels may be damaged due to careless introduction of the needle into the body.
- **Thrombophlebities:** It is caused by mechanical trauma to the vein or the chemical irritation of some substances introduced into the veins such as potassium chloride.
- **Pyrogenic reactions:** It is characterized by temperature elevation, chills, headache, nausea, vomiting and circulatory collapse in serve cases.
- **Air embolism:** The vascular collapse occurs due to occlusion of the vessel by embolism. The signs of pulmonary embolism are dyspnoea, cyanosis, low blood pressure, shock and collapse, tachycardia and unconsciousness.
- **Infection at the needle site:** Contamination occurs during insertion or left exposed for a long period.
- **Serum hepatitis:** Infectious hepatitis have been attributed to improperly disinfected syringes and needles.
- **Allergic reaction:** This may due to certain drugs administered along with the IV fluids.

Fluid Rate Calculation

$$\text{Flow rate} = \frac{\text{Total volume infused in mL} \times \text{drops/mL}}{\text{Total time of the infusion in minutes}}$$

Total volume infused = 200 mL in 24 hours
Drops per mL = 15
Total time in minutes = 24 × 60 = 1440 minutes

$$\text{Flow rate} = \frac{2000 \times 15}{144} = 16.6 \text{ drops}$$

General Instructions

- Follow strict aseptic technique, thought the procedure.
- Administer IV fluids only with a clearly written prescription.
- Maintain the specified rate of flow to prevent circulatory overload.
- Constant and continuous observation for any unfavorable symptoms.
- Observe the rights during administration.
- Check the expiry date before opening the bottles.
- If fluids are discolored, cloudy in appearance that should not be used for infusion.
- Do not use any site that is tender, red, edematous and inflamed.
- Never allow the bottle to get empty completely to prevent the entry of air into the tissues.
- Keep the patient warm and comfortable with blankets if necessary.
- Immobilize the joints with splints when the needle is placed near a joint.
- Frequent observation of the vital signs throughout the procedure will help to detect many complications.
- Allow the patient to void before the IV infusion is started.

Observation Needed throughout the Procedure

- Flow rate and potency of IV tubing.
- Dislodgement of needle.
- Signs of circulatory over load.
- Urinary output.
- Needle site.
- Fluid level in the bottle.
- Vital signs at frequent intervals.

Preliminary Assessment Check

- Patient's name, age, bed no and diagnosis.
- Purpose of infusion.
- Doctor's order.
- Level of consciousness.
- General conditions.
- Abilities and limitation.
- Need for additional restraints.
- Articles available.
- Previous experience.

Equipment

A tray containing:
- Sterile IV solution.
- Sterile IV infusion set.
- Sterile needle of choice (butterfly or canula).
- Sterile syringe (2 or 5 mL).
- Sterile transfer forceps in a jar.
- Sterile cotton swabs and gauze pieces.
- Surgical spirit.
- Kidney tray and paper bag.
- Bowl with water.
- Tourniquet.
- Adhesive tape and scissors.
- Specimen bottles.
- Mackintosh and towel.
- IV pole.
- Restrainer (splint with roller bandages).

Preparation of the Patient and Environment

- Explain the procedure.
- Sent the visitors outside.
- Provide privacy.

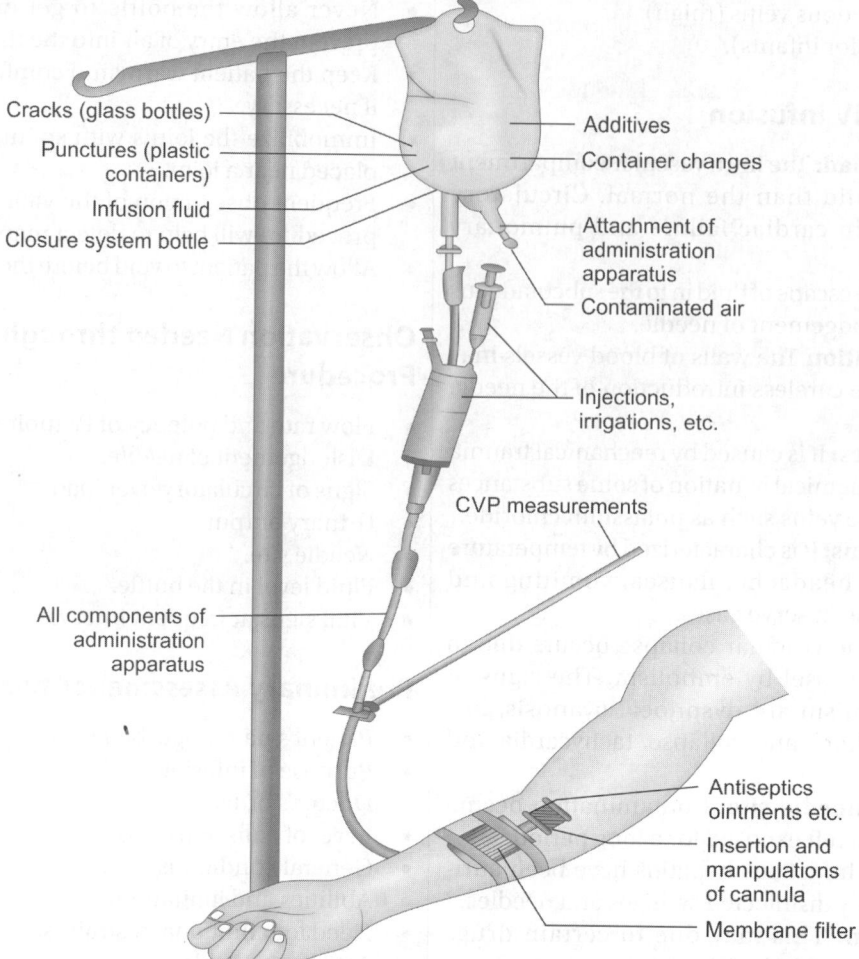

Fig. 22.19: Intravenous fluid administration system.

- Allow the patient to empty the bladder.
- Check the vital signs.
- Adjust the height of the bed.
- Arrange the articles at the bedside.
- Place the patient in comfortable and relaxed position.
- Provide adequate light in the room.

Procedure

- Hand wash.
- Prepare the IV solution; insert the drip set, and the air vent into the bottle openings.
- Hang the bottle on the IV pole about 18 to 24 inches high.
- The patient is placed in supine or sitting position with head tilted back.
- Draw the lower lid and ask the patient to look up.
- Instill the ordered number of drops in the center of the lower lid 2 cm above the eyes.
- After instillation, ask the patient to close the eye and move eye balls from side so that medications will spread all over the sac.
- Wipe of excess medication.

Aftercare

- Dry lids with dry cotton swabs.
- Make the patient comfortable.
- Remove articles from bedside.
- Hand wash.
- Record the procedure in the nurse's record.

Patient Education

- If the patient is on self medication, give him clear instructions and make sure that he is clear of it.
- Ask the patient to consult the doctor regularly.
- Do not massage the eyeball after instillation of medications.

Complication: Improper dressing and procedure may lead to further serious infection.

TRANSDERMAL ROUTE

Highly lipid soluble drugs can be applied over the skin for slow and prolonged absorption, e.g. nitroglycerine ointment in angina pectoris. Adhesive units, inunction, iontophoresis and jet injection are some forms of transdermal drug delivery. Adhesive units (transdermal therapeutic systems) are adhesive patches of different sizes and shapes made to suit the area of application. The drug is held in a reservoir between an outer layer and a porous membrane. This membrane is smeared with an adhesive to hold on to the area of application. The drug slowly diffuses through the membrane and percutaneous absorption takes place. The rate of absorption is constant and predictable and highly potent. Pulmonary epithelium and mucous membranes of the respiratory tract are also absorbed through these membranes. Sites of application are chest, abdomen, upper arm, back or mastoid region, e.g. hyoscine, nitroglycerine fentanyl, estrogen, testosterone transdermal patches.

Advantages

- Duration of action is prolonged.
- Provides constant plasma drug levels.
- Patient compliance is good.

Inunction: In this route of administration the drug is rubbed in to the skin and it gets absorbed to produce systemic effects.

Iontophoresis: In this procedure, galvanic current is used for bringing about penetration of lipid insoluble drugs into the deeper tissues where its action is required, e.g. salicylates. Fluoride iontophores is used in the treatment of dental hypersensitivity.

Jet injection: As absorption of drug occurs across the layers of the skin, dermojet may also be considered as a form of transdermal drug administration.

TRANSMUCOSAL

Drugs are absorbed across the mucous membranes. Transmucosal administration includes sublingual, nasal and rectal routes.

Sublingual: Here, the tablet or pellet containing the drug is placed under the tongue. It dissolves and the drug is absorbed across the sublingual mucosa, e.g. nitroglycerine, nifedipine, buprenorphine.

Advantages

- Absorption is rapid—within minutes the drug reaches the circulation.
- First pass metabolism is avoided.
- After the desired effect is obtained, the drug can be spat out to avoid the unwanted effects.

Disadvantages

- Buccal ulceration can occur.
- Nasal drugs can be administered through nasal route either for systemic absorption or for local effects.

For example;
- Oxytocin spray is used for systemic absorption.
- For local effect—decongestant nasal drops, e.g. oxymetazoline; budesonide nasal spray for allergic rhinitis.

RECTAL RECTUM

It has a rich blood supply and drugs can cross the rectal mucosa to be absorbed for systemic effects. Drugs absorbed from the upper part of the rectum are carried by the superior hemorrhoidal vein to the portal circulation (can undergo first pass metabolism) while that absorbed from the lower part of the rectum is carried by the middle and inferior hemorrhoidal veins to the systemic circulation.

Drugs like-indomethacin, chlorpromazine diazepam and paraldehyde can be given rectally. Some irritant drugs are given rectally as suppositories.

Advantages

- Gastric irritation is avoided.
- Can be administered by unskilled persons.
- Useful in geriatric patients and others with vomiting and those unable to swallow.

Disadvantages

- Irritation of the rectum can occur.
- Absorption may be irregular and unpredictable.
  Drugs may also be given by rectal route as enema.
  Enema is the administration of a drug in a liquid form into the rectum. Enema may be evacuant or retention enema.

Evacuant enema: In order to empty the bowel, about 600 ml of soap water is administered rectum while soap lubricates. Enema is given prior to surgeries, obstetric procedures and radiological examination of the gut.

Retention enema: The drug is administered with about 100 ml of fluids and is retained in the rectum for local action, e.g. prednisolone enema in ulcerative colitis.

TOPICAL

Drugs may be applied on the skin for local action as ointment, cream, gel, powder, paste, etc. Drugs may also be applied on the mucous membrane as in the eyes, ears and nose as ointment, drops and sprays. Drugs may be administered as suppository for rectum, bougie for urethra and pessary and douche for vagina. Pessaries are oval shaped tablets to be placed in the vagina to provide high local concentrations of the drug at the site, e.g. antifungal pessaries in vaginal candidiasis.

SPECIAL DRUG DELIVERY SYSTEMS

In order to improve drug delivery to prolong, the duration of action and thereby improve patient compliance, special drug delivery systems are being tried. Drug targeting, i.e. to deliver drugs at the site where it is required to act is also being aimed at, especially for anticancer drugs. Some such systems are ocusert, progestasert, transdermal adhesive units, prodrugs, osmotic pumps. Computerized pumps and methods using monoclonal antibodies and liposomes as carriers.

Ocusert: Ocusert systems are thin elliptical units that contain the drug in a reservoir which slowly releases the drug through a membrane by diffusion at a steady rate, e.g. pilocarpine ocusert used in glaucoma is placed under the lid and can deliver pilocarpine for 7 days.

Progestasert: It is inserted into the uterus where it delivers progesterone constantly for over one year.

Transdermal Adhesive Units

Prodrug is an inactive form of a drug which gets metabolized to the active derivative in the body. A prodrug may overcome some of the disadvantages of the conventional forms of drug administration, e.g. dopamine does not cross the blood-brain-barrier (BBB); levodopa, a prodrug crosses the BBB and is then converted to dopamine in the CNS. Prodrugs may also be used to have a longer duration of action, e.g. bacampicillin (a prodrug of ampicillin) is longer acting.

Osmotic pumps are small tablet shaped units containing the drug and an osmotic substance in two different chambers. The tablet is coated with a semi permeable membrane in which a minute laser drilled hole is made. When the tablet is swallowed and reaches the gut, water enters into the tablet through the semi permeable membrane. The osmotic layer swells and pushes the drug slowly out of the laser-drilled orifice.

This allows slow and constant delivery of the drug over a long period of time. It is also called gastrointestinal therapeutic system (GITS). Some drugs available in this formulation are iron and prazosin.

Computerized miniature pumps: These are programmed to release drugs at a definite rate either continuously as in case of insulin or intermittently in pulses as in case of GnRH. Various methods of drug targeting are tried especially for anticancer drugs to reduce toxicity.

Monoclonal antibodies: They are antibodies against the tumor specific antigens, are used to deliver anticancer drugs to specific tumor cells.

Liposomes: They are phospholipids suspended in aqueous vehicles to form minute vesicles. Drugs encapsulated in liposomes are taken up mainly by the reticuloendothelial cells of the liver and are also concentrated in malignant tumors. Thus, site-specific delivery of drugs may be possible with the help of liposomes.

Nurses Responsibility

- Ensure that the correct drug is administered by the right route and in the right dose.
- History of allergy should be taken particularly before parenteral administration of drugs.
- Monitor the adverse effects.
- Drugs should be kept in a safe place.
- Check the prescription, drug label and the patient's name before the administration of drugs.

INSTILLATION OF EAR DROPS

Instillation of ear drops into the auditory canal (**Fig. 22.20**).

Purpose

- To clean the ear.
- To remove the foreign body or wax.
- To relieve inflammation, congestion and pain.
- To kill an insect lodged in the ear.
- To anesthetize.

General Instructions

- Explain the procedure clearly to get patients cooperation.
- The auditory canal should be cleaned before instill the ear drops.

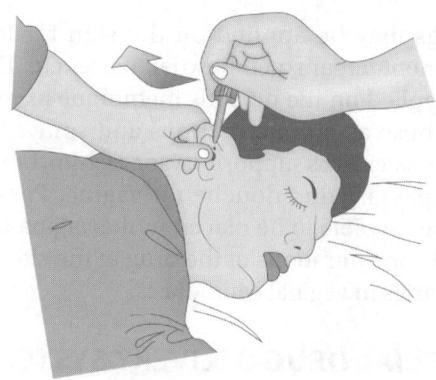 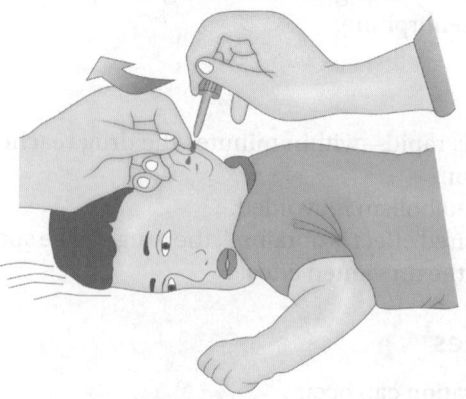

Fig. 22.20: Administration of medication into ear.

- Drops must be warm, when they are instilled into the ear.
- Hold the pinna of the ear upward and backward in case of adults and in children put it down backward to straighten the external auditory canal.
- Plug the ear with a small cotton ball or a small gauze piece.
- Allow 3 or 4 drops trickle down on one side of the canal so that the air may escape from the auditory canal and medication may reach up on the ear drum.
- Do not ignore any complaint by the patient.

Equipment

A small tray containing:
- Medicine with dropper.
- Applicators with cotton tips.
- Normal saline.
- Little cotton.
- Kidney tray and paper bag.

Procedure

- Wash hands and collect the articles and take it to the bedside.
- Explain the procedure to the patient.
- Place the patient in supine or sitting position with head to side and the affected ear up.
- Pull the pinna down and back in case of adult and down and back in case of infant/child. Rest the other hand on patients head to avoid damaging the ear with dropper if the patient moves.
- Instill the medicine drop by drop directing the flow toward the canal do not allow the dropper to touch the ear.
- Place loose cotton in the outer ear absorbs any excess medicine and keeps the patients head turned to the side for 10 to 15 minutes.

Aftercare

- Place the patient comfortably.
- Replace the articles.
- Hand wash.
- Record the procedure in nurse's record sheet.

INSTILLING NASAL DROPS

Instillation of medication into the nose in the form of nasal drops (**Fig. 22.21**).

Purpose

- To diagnose nasal condition.
- To relieve inflammation and congestion in case of rhinitis.
- To prevent and control bleeding.

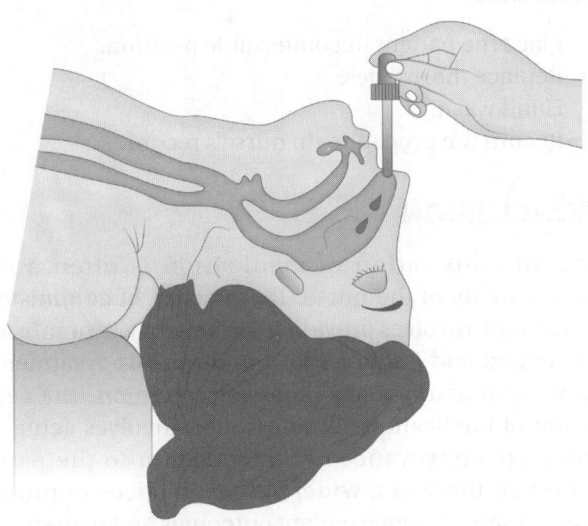

Fig. 22.21: Administration of medication into nose.

General Instructions

- It is a clean procedure.
- Avoid touching the tip of nose with dropper since it may contaminate.
- Avoid touching the inner surface of the nose with dropper since it may cause the patient to sneeze.
- Position the patient as necessary to provide medicine flow to the affected area.
- Do not use oily solution as nasal drops since it interferes with the normal ciliary's action.
- Do not use decongestants excessively or frequently as they become ineffective and may actually worsen the patient's nasal congestion.
- Instruct the patient remain in the same position for sometime following instillation to allow the medicine to act on mucus membrane of anterior nares and then drain in to the posterior nares.

Equipment

A small tray containing:
- Medicine with rubber tipped dropper.
- Handkerchief or little clean cotton and paper bag.

Procedure

- Hand wash.
- Arrange the articles at the bedside.
- Explain the procedure to the patient.
- Draw up the medicine in dropper.
- Position the patient flat supine with head slightly to the affected side to provide flow to the Eustachian tube.
- Insert the tip of dropper just inside the nares and instill the drops as ordered.
- Ask the patient to remain the position for five minutes and avoid blowing the nose.

Aftercare

- Place the patient in comfortable position.
- Replace the articles.
- Hand wash.
- Record the procedure in nurse's record.

CONCLUSION

The administration of medication is often a chief responsibility of the nurse. The practice of administering medication involves providing the patient with a substance prescribed and intended for the diagnosis, treatment, or prevention of a medical illness or condition. The central action of medication administration involves actual and complete conveyance of a medication to the patient. However, there is a wider set of practices required to achieve safe, effective patient outcomes and to prepare for and evaluate the outcome of medication administration. Laws regarding medication administration vary from state to state. Doctors, physicians, physician assistants, nurse practitioners, and nurses are generally trained and authorized to administer medication, while other medical disciplines may have a limited responsibility in this area. In certain circumstances, unlicensed personnel may be trained and authorized to administer medication in residential care settings. State and federal laws also restrict the distribution of and access to medications that can be abused (called controlled substances). Responsibility for controlled substances includes accountability for any discarded substances, double-locked storage, and counting of medication supply at regular intervals by clinician teams. Preparation for medication administration begins with the order for medication, in most circumstances written by the physician.

Nurse practitioners and physician assistants are also often authorized to write prescriptions. State laws vary regarding these privileges. A record of orders for medication and other treatments is kept in the medical chart. Universally accepted safe clinical practice guidelines and state laws govern the components of medication orders in order to ensure consistency and patient safety. All orders should contain the patient's name, the date and time when the order is written, and the signature of the ordering clinician. In addition to the clinician who administers medication, other members of the health care team play vital roles surrounding the medication administration process. Doctors or other prescribing clinicians are responsible for writing clear, legible orders and for monitoring the response of the patient to medication. They are also responsible for responding to potential adverse effects and concerns by the patient or other clinicians. Pharmacists are responsible for evaluating the medication order for potential problems, correctly filling the order, and monitoring the medication supply. All health care professionals are responsible for complying with medication-related policies designed to protect the patient and/or staff and for maintaining current knowledge regarding medication and medication administration.

BIBLIOGRAPHY

1. Alice L Price. The Art, Science and Spirit of Nursing, 3rd edition. Philadelphia, WB Saunders Company, 1968.
2. Carol T, Lillis C, LeMone P. Fundamentals of Nursing: The Art of Science of Nursing, 3rd edition. Philadelphia: Lippincott-Raven Publishers, 1997.
3. Henderson V. Principles and Practice of Nursing, New York, MacMillan Publishing Co, 1970.
4. Kathleen S, et al. Medical-Surgical Nursing, 6th edition. Saint Louis; CV Mosby Co. 1975.
5. Kozier Barbara B Du Gas Beverly Witter. Fundamentals of Patient Care: A Comprehensive Approach to Nursing. WB Saunders Company; 1967.
6. McClosky JC, Grace HK. Current Issues in Nursing, 4th edition. St. Louis: Mosby Year Book, Inc; 1994.
7. Mitchell PR, Grippando GM. Nursing Perspectives and Issues, 5th edition. 1993. Albany, New York: Delmar Publishers, Inc, 1993.
8. Potter PA, Perry AG. Fundamentals of Nursing: Concepts, Process and Practice, 4th edition. St Louis: Mosby-Year Book, Inc, 1997.
9. Shakuntala Sharma 'Birpuri'. Principles and Practice of Nursing. Jaypee Brothers Medical Publishers (P) Ltd, New Delhi, 1997.
10. Sr. Nancy. Principles and Practice of Nursing, vol 1, 3rd edition. NR Brothers, Indore, 1992.
11. Thresvamma CP. Fundamentals of Nursing, Procedure Manual for General Nursing Course. Kottayam, Kerala, 1992.

REVIEW QUESTIONS

Long Essays

1. Explain the factors influencing medication action.
2. Nurses responsibility in administration of oral medication.
3. Discuss in detail about intravenous injection procedure.

Short Essays

1. Forms of medications.
2. Route of administration.
3. Medication dose calculation.
4. Errors in medication administration.
5. Care of medicine and medicine cupboard.
6. Intramuscular injection.
7. Intravenous infusions.
8. Instillation of ear drops.

Short Answers

1. Sources of drugs.
2. Rights of medication administration.
3. Syringes and needles.
4. Golden rules of giving injections.
5. Methods of intramuscular injections administration.
6. Site of intramuscular injections.

MULTIPLE CHOICE QUESTIONS

1. **The most common type of medication error is:**
   a. Wrong drug
   b. Wrong route of administration

c. Administering improper dose
d. Wrong patient

2. **In medicines management, the extent to which patients take medication as prescribed by healthcare professionals is termed:**
   a. Concordance
   b. Adherence
   c. Holistic care
   d. Paternalism

3. **Natural sources drugs can be obtained from:**
   a. Plants, e.g. atropine, morphine, quinine, digoxin, pilocarpine, physostigmine.
   b. Animals, e.g. insulin, heparin, gonadotropins and antitoxic sera.
   c. Minerals, e.g. magnesium sulfate aluminum hydroxide, iron, sulfur and radioactive isotopes.
   d. All of the above

4. **The purpose of drug administration is:**
   a. To prevent health alterations.
   b. To promote health condition.
   c. To treat infections allergic and inflammation.
   d. All of the above

5. **Complications of injections are the following, *except*:**
   a. Allergic reactions certain drugs, e.g. penicillin.
   b. Pulmonary edema
   c. Infections (abscess formation).
   d. Pyrogenic reactions (producing fever).

ANSWERS

1. c   2. b   3. d   4. d   5. b

CHAPTER 23

Sensory Needs

LEARNING OBJECTIVES

- Introduction
- Components of sensory experience: Reception, perception and reaction
- Arousal mechanism
- Factors affecting sensory function
- Assessment of sensory alterations, sensory deficit, deprivation, overload and sensory poverty
- Promoting meaningful communication (patients with aphasia, artificial airway and visual and hearing impairment), care of unconscious patients
- Unconsciousness: Definition, causes and risk factors, pathophysiology, stages of unconsciousness, clinical manifestations
- Assessment and nursing management of patient with unconsciousness, complications

TERMINOLOGY

Sensory neuron: Sends information from sensory receptors (e.g., in skin, eyes, nose, tongue, ears) toward the central nervous system and ultimately the brain.

Interneuron: Sends information between sensory neurons and motor neurons.

Motor neuron: Sends information away from the central nervous system to muscles or glands.

Optic nerve: The cranial nerve that serves the retina - what connects your brain to your eye.

Central nervous system: The nervous system is the highway along which your brain sends and receives information about what is happening in the body and around it.

Anosmia: Loss of the sense of smell; usually the result of physical disruption of the first cranial nerve.

Aqueous humor: Watery fluid that fills the anterior chamber containing the cornea, iris, ciliary body, and lens of the eye.

Audition: Sense of hearing.

Chemoreceptor: Sensory receptor cell that is sensitive to chemical stimuli, such as in taste, smell, or pain.

Cochlea: Auditory portion of the inner ear containing structures to transduce sound stimuli.

Cone photoreceptor: One of the two types of retinal receptor cell that is specialized for color vision through the use of three photopigments distributed through three separate populations of cells.

Equilibrium: Sense of balance that includes sensations of position and movement of the head.

External ear: Structures on the lateral surface of the head, including the auricle and the ear canal back to the tympanic membrane.

Exteroceptor: Sensory receptor that is positioned to interpret stimuli from the external environment, such as photoreceptors in the eye or somatosensory receptors in the skin.

General sense: Any sensory system that is distributed throughout the body and incorporated into organs of multiple other systems, such as the walls of the digestive organs or the skin.

Gestation: Sense of taste.

Gustatory receptor cells: Sensory cells in the taste bud that transduce the chemical stimuli of gustation.

Mechanoreceptor: Receptor cell that transduces mechanical stimuli into an electrochemical signal.

Olfaction: Sense of smell.

Olfactory bulb: Central target of the first cranial nerve; located on the ventral surface of the frontal lobe in the cerebrum.

Olfactory sensory neuron: Receptor cell of the olfactory system, sensitive to the chemical stimuli of smell, the axons of which compose the first cranial nerve.

Opsin: Protein that contains the photosensitive cofactor retinal for photo transduction.

Optic disc: Spot on the retina at which RGC axons leave the eye and blood vessels of the inner retina pass.

Optic nerve: Second cranial nerve, which is responsible for visual sensation.

Osmoreceptor: Receptor cell that senses differences in the concentrations of bodily fluids on the basis of osmotic pressure.

Photoisomerization: Chemical change in the retinal molecule that alters the bonding so that it switches from the 11-*cis*-retinal isomer to the all-*trans*-retinal isomer.

Photoreceptor: Receptor cell specialized to respond to light stimuli.

Proprioception: Sense of position and movement of the body.

Proprioceptor: Receptor cell that senses changes in the position and kinesthetic aspects of the body.

Pupil: Open hole at the center of the iris that light passes through into the eye.

Receptor cell: Cell that transduces environmental stimuli into neural signals.

Retina: Nervous tissue of the eye at which photo transduction takes place.

Rod photoreceptor: One of the two types of retinal receptor cells that is specialized for low-light vision.

Special sense: Any sensory system associated with a specific organ structure, namely smell, taste, sight, hearing, and balance.

Umami: Taste submodality for sensitivity to the concentration of amino acids; also called the savory sense.

Vision: Special sense of sight based on transduction of light stimuli.

Visual acuity: Property of vision related to the sharpness of focus, which varies in relation to retinal position.

INTRODUCTION

A sensorium (plural: sensoria) is the sum of an organism's perception, the "seat of sensation" where it experiences and interprets the environments within which it lives. The term originally entered English from the Late Latin in the mid-17th century, from the stem sens- ("sense"). In earlier use it referred, in a broader sense, to the brain as the mind's organ. In medical, psychological, and physiological discourse it has come to refer to the total character of the unique and changing sensory environments perceived by individuals. These include the sensation, perception, and interpretation of information about the world around us by using faculties of the mind such as senses, phenomenal and psychological perception, cognition and intelligence.

CONCEPT OF SENSORY INTEGRATION

Sensory integration is the body's ability to take in information from the world around us and to make sense of it. Human beings have seven senses—touch, taste, smell, vision, hearing, proprioception and vestibular. Some individuals have difficulties making sense of the sensory information they receive from their environment and this then impacts upon their ability to function and complete activities successfully.

Some of the defining characteristics of impaired and disturbed sensory and perceptual alterations include the client's changes in terms of behavior, problem solving, sensory sharpness and acuity, and decision making which can lead to the client's restlessness, a lack of orientation, confusion, altered communication, poor concentration, hallucinations, and a lack of focus and attention.

DEFINITION

- North American Nursing Diagnosis Association (NANDA) defined as: Impaired and disturbed sensory perception is "a change in the amount or patterning of incoming stimuli accompanies by a diminished, exaggerated, distorted, or impaired response to such stimuli" as those associated with the client's visual, auditory, tactile, gustatory, olfactory and kinesthetic responses to these stimuli.
- Sensorium is the totality of those parts of the brain that receive process and interpret sensory stimuli. The sensorium is the supposed seat of sensation, the place to which impressions from the external world are conveyed and perceived.
- **Altered sensorium:** The term altered sensorium describes limitations on or problems with the brain's ability to receive process or interpret sensory information. Examples of altered sensorium include hallucinatory and confusional states, delirium, coma and sleep.

FUNCTIONING OF SENSORY ORGANS

Specific sensory receptors are contained in specific sense organs. Each of the five senses (sight, hearing, smell, taste,

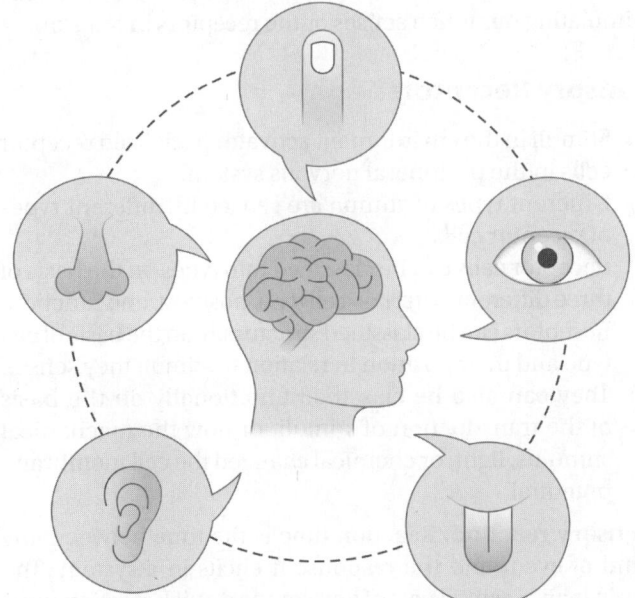

Fig. 23.1: Five senses: Sight, hearing, smell, taste and touch.

and touch) has a specific sense organ associated with it. The most familiar sense organs are the eyes, ears, nose, skin and taste buds. These organs have receptors that can respond to stimuli by producing nerve impulses in a sensory neuron. The receptors convert the energy of a stimulus into electrical energy that can travel in the nervous system.

Normal sensation: Normally the nervous system continually receives thousands of bits of information from sensory nerve organs, relays the information through appropriate channels, and integrates the information into a meaningful response. Sensory stimuli reach the sensory organs to elicit an immediate reaction or present information to the brain to be stored for future use. The nervous system must be intact for sensory stimuli to reach appropriate brain centers and for an individual to perceive the sensation. After interpreting the significance of a sensation, the person is then able to react to the stimulus.

COMPONENTS OF SENSORY EXPERIENCE

Sensory Experience Perception

- Perception simply implies the use of the senses in our possession to gain a better understanding of the world around us.
- This processing happens to be done through the organ, usually called "the senses" like hearing, vision, taste, smell, and touch. The sensory perception involves detecting stimuli and subsequently recognizing and characterizing it.
- There are five different stimulus types involved in sensory processing viz. chemical, mechanical, electrical, light and temperature.

The process of sensory perception begins when something in the real world stimulates our sense organs.

For instance, light reflects off a surface, stimulating our eyes or warmth, emanates from a hot cup of beverage, thereby stimulating our touch senses or the receptors in our skin.

Sensory Receptors

- Stimuli in the environment activate specialized receptor cells in the peripheral nervous system.
- Different types of stimuli are sensed by different types of receptor cells.
- Receptor cells can be classified into types on the basis of three different criteria—cell type, position, and function.
- Receptors can be classified structurally on the basis of cell type and their position in relation to stimuli they sense.
- They can also be classified functionally on the basis of the transduction of stimuli, or how the mechanical stimulus, light, or chemical changed the cell membrane potential.

Sensory reaction: Reaction time is the time between any kind of event and the response it elicits in a system. The brain is an essential part of developing a quick reaction time. This information travels from sensory neurons along the optic nerve from the eye to the brain. The brain processes this information, and then sends a signal through motor neurons down the arm to tell the muscles in the hand to close and catch the ruler.

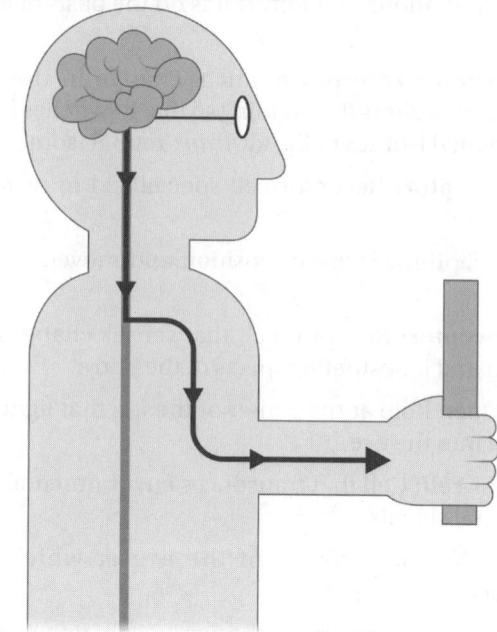

Fig. 23.2: Message transmitted through neural pathway.

FACTORS INFLUENCING SENSORY FUNCTION

Many factors influence the capacity to receive or perceive stimuli. All are conditions or situations that you manage when delivering care. Some of the risk factors associated with impaired and disturbed sensory and perceptual abilities are impaired sensory processing and the absence of the processing of stimuli secondary to disorders such as blindness, deafness, a loss of taste or smell, and an inability to feel things, some of which can occurs as the result of genetics, aging, trauma, biochemical causes, electrolyte imbalances and both excesses of stimulation and deficits in terms of sensory stimulation.

Age: Infants and children are at risk for visual and hearing impairment because of a number of genetic, prenatal, and postnatal conditions. A concern with high-risk neonates is that early, intense visual and auditory stimulation can adversely affect visual and auditory pathways and alter the developmental course of other sensory organs.

Meaningful stimuli: Meaningful stimuli reduce the incidence of sensory deprivation. In the home meaningful stimuli include pets, music, television, pictures of family members, and a calendar and clock. The same stimuli need to be present in health care settings. Note whether patients have roommates or visitors. The presence of others offers positive stimulation.

Amount of stimuli: Excessive stimuli in an environment causes sensory overload. The frequency of observations and procedures performed in an acute health care setting are often stressful. If a patient is in pain or restricted by a cast or traction, overstimulation frequently is a problem.

Social interaction: The amount and quality of social contact with supportive family members and significant others influence sensory function. The absence of visitors during hospitalization or residency in an extended care facility influences the degree of isolation a patient feels. This is a common problem in hospital intensive care settings, where visitation is often restricted.

Environmental factors: A person's occupation places him or her at risk for hearing, visual, and peripheral nerve alterations. Individuals who have occupations involving exposure to high noise levels (e.g., factory or airport workers) are at risk for noise-induced hearing loss and need to be screened for hearing impairments. Hazardous noise is common in work settings and recreational activities. Noisy recreational activities that weakens hearing ability include target shooting and hunting, woodworking, and listening to loud music.

Cultural factors: Certain sensory alterations occur more commonly in select ethnic groups. Cultural disparities in vision impairment are significant, in part because visual impairment may be indirectly associated with an increased risk of suicide through poor self-rated health.

SENSORY ASSESSMENT

- Sensory processing is a broad term that generally refers to the handling of sensory information by neural systems, including the functions of receptor organs and the peripheral and central nervous systems.
- According to Dunn, sensory processing is a complex endeavor.
- Sensory input from the environment and from the body itself provides information to the brain.
- The brain organizes, integrates, synthesizes, and uses this information to understand experiences and organize appropriate responses.
- The processing of information allows individuals to respond automatically, efficiently, and comfortably to the specific sensory inputs received.
- The neurobiological process comprises a series of five stages, registration, modulation, discrimination, integration, and praxis, and is central to cognitive processes such attention, visual perception, memory, and planned action.

Sensory Assessment

Tactile

- Ritualistic behaviors
- Touching/holding objects
- Resisting/seeking touch

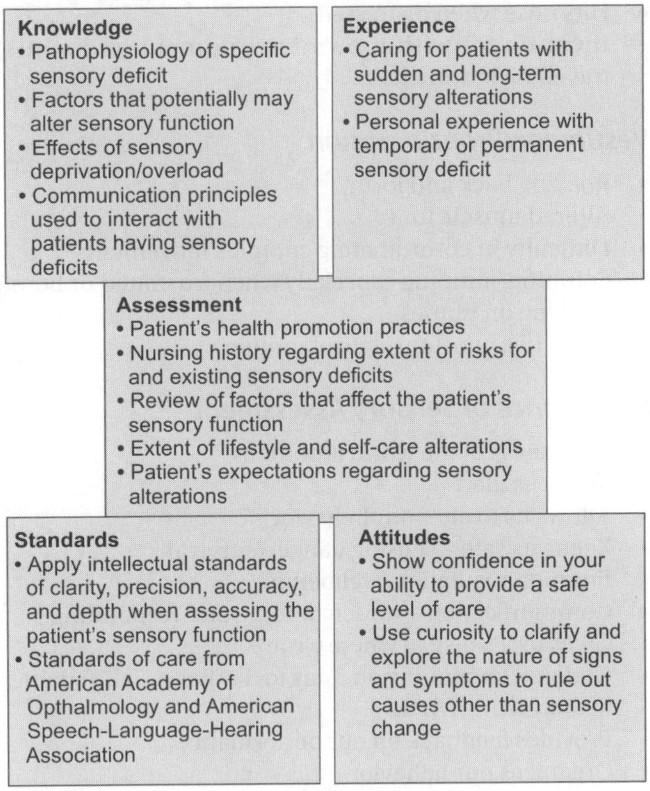

Knowledge
- Pathophysiology of specific sensory deficit
- Factors that potentially may alter sensory function
- Effects of sensory deprivation/overload
- Communication principles used to interact with patients having sensory deficits

Experience
- Caring for patients with sudden and long-term sensory alterations
- Personal experience with temporary or permanent sensory deficit

Assessment
- Patient's health promotion practices
- Nursing history regarding extent of risks for and existing sensory deficits
- Review of factors that affect the patient's sensory function
- Extent of lifestyle and self-care alterations
- Patient's expectations regarding sensory alterations

Standards
- Apply intellectual standards of clarity, precision, accuracy, and depth when assessing the patient's sensory function
- Standards of care from American Academy of Opthalmology and American Speech-Language-Hearing Association

Attitudes
- Show confidence in your ability to provide a safe level of care
- Use curiosity to clarify and explore the nature of signs and symptoms to rule out causes other than sensory change

Fig. 23.3: Sensory assessment.

- Difficulty tolerating clothing
- Dislike wet/sloppy food textures—strong preference for dry foods
- Seeks pressure—squeezing self/pulling clothing over his head
- Low response to temperature and pain
- Self-injurious behavior.

Visual

- Notices small changes in his environment
- Looks at minute particles
- Picks up small pieces of fluff
- Attracted to lights
- Moves fingers/objects in front of his eyes
- Fascination with reflection/bright colored objects
- Studies finer details of objects rather than the whole object
- Can appear startled if approached suddenly
- Hits/rubs own eyes when distressed.

Auditory

- Frustration within crowded/noisy environments
- Banging objects/doors
- Makes loud rhythmic sounds
- Delayed responses to instructions/sounds.

Olfactory—smell

- Smells self/people/objects
- Occasionally smears feces and is fascinated with the smell

- Hits nose when distressed
- Incontinent within own environment and whilst travelling in vehicle.

Vestibular/Proprioception
- Rocking back and forth
- Altered muscle tone
- Difficulty in co-ordinating complex movements
- Spinning/jumping especially when frustrated or bored
- Walking on tiptoes
- Often in a constant state of motion.

Importance of Sensory Assessment
- Awareness of the world around us
- Keeps us alert
- Allows us to alter our behavior
- Keeps us safe—sensing danger/survival
- Emotion regulation/wellbeing
- Communication—understanding and responding
- Gives us a sense of where we are
- General functioning on a day to day basis—all activities of daily living (ADLs)
- Provides feedback on our performance
- Organizes our behavior
- Helps us to look after basic needs (hunger, warmth etc)
- Learning and development
- Assists with future planning/transition/discharge from hospital.

NURSES, RESPONSIBILITY IN SENSORY AND THOUGHT DISTURBANCES

- Provision of safety using, for example, falls risk protocols for those at risk for falls and keeping dangerous cleaning chemicals in a secure and safe place
- Frequent monitoring of the client
- Maintaining of the client's comfort
- Anticipation of the client's needs and then addressing them
- Provision of an environment that is not loaded with extraneous stimuli
- Reorientation of the client to time, place and person as often as necessary
- Explaining procedures to the client in a manner that they can understand while using assistive devices and aids such as pictures and gestures that can be helpful to facilitate the client's understanding
- Maintaining as much consistency in terms of the client's routines and those that provide nursing care to them
- Managing hallucinations with a medication such as a dopamine antagonist
- Using close ended questions that require a simple yes or no answer when necessary
- Communicating with the client at eye level and will maintaining eye contact.

Disturbances Affecting Vision

Impaired sensory and perceptual disturbances affecting vision can be better coped with by the client when the nurse and other health care providers:
- Communicate with low vision clients at eye level and within the client's functioning field of vision
- Insure that the client with low vision has and uses corrective lenses, including eyeglasses, and other devices such as magnifiers
- Greet the client by name and introduce one when entering the client's space
- Use Braille and large print materials for low vision clients
- Maintain a clutter free and organized client environment
- Provide the client with details about the locations items within the client's immediate and extended environment

Auditory Deficits

Clients with auditory deficits can better cope with this deficit when the nurse and other health care providers:
- Provide the client with their assistive devices such as a hearing aid
- Speak slowly while sitting at the client's eye level and clearly pronouncing words to facilitate lip reading
- Use written, rather than oral, communication when indicated
- Eliminate all extraneous environmental noises and distractions when communicating with the client
- Utilize the services of an American Sign Language interpreter when indicated.

SENSORY ALTERATIONS

The most common types of sensory alterations are sensory deficits, sensory deprivation, and sensory overload. When a patient suffers from more than one sensory alteration, the ability to function and relate effectively within the environment is seriously impaired.

Sensory deficits: A deficit in the normal function of sensory reception and perception is a sensory deficit. A person loses a sense of self with impaired senses. Initially he or she withdraws by avoiding communication or socialization with others in an attempt to cope with the sensory loss. It becomes difficult for the person to interact safely with the environment until he or she learns new skills. When a deficit develops gradually or when considerable time has passed since the onset of an acute sensory loss, a person learns to rely on unaffected senses. Some senses may even become more acute to compensate for an alteration. For example, a blind patient develops an acute sense of hearing to compensate for visual loss.

Patients with sensory deficits often change behavior in adaptive or maladaptive ways. For example, a patient with a hearing impairment turns the unaffected ear toward the speaker to hear well, whereas another patient avoids people because he or she is embarrassed about not being able to understand what other people say.

SENSORY DEPRIVATION

Sensory deprivation, on the other hand, occurs when the client is deprived of a normal level of sensory stimulation as can occur among inmates and prisoners in isolation as well as residents in a private room without visitors and socialization.

Signs and symptoms of sensory deprivation: The client who is affected with sensory deprivation may experience abnormal responses to the few stimuli that the client is exposed to, delusions, hallucinations, apathy, and depression, a lack of orientation, lethargy, poor concentration, confusion, memory deficits and somatic complaints.

- The reticular activating system in the brainstem mediates all sensory stimuli to the cerebral cortex; thus patients are able to receive stimuli even while sleeping deeply.
- Sensory stimulation must be of sufficient quality and quantity to maintain a person's awareness.
- Three types of sensory deprivation are reduced sensory input (sensory deficit from visual or hearing loss), the elimination of patterns or meaning from input (e.g., exposure to strange environments), and restrictive environments (e.g., bed rest) that produce monotony and boredom).
- In adults the symptoms are similar to psychological illness, confusion, symptoms of severe electrolyte imbalance, or the influence of psychotropic drugs. Therefore always be aware of a patient's existing sensory function and the quality of stimuli within the environment.

SENSORY OVERLOAD

Sensory overload occurs when the person gets more stimulation than they are able to manage and process; and sensory deprivation occurs when the client does not get enough sensory stimulation to sustain the person in a state of balance. Sensory overload occurs when the client is subjected to an extraordinary amount of internal and external stimuli such as a high level of anxiety and a noisy environment with constant activity as often occurs in emergency departments and critical care areas, respectively.

Signs and symptoms of sensory overload: The client affected with sensory overload may exhibit signs and symptoms of sensory overload like anxiety, restlessness, sleep deprivation, disordered thinking and cognitive processes, fatigue, poor problem solving and decision making skills, poor performance, and muscular tension.

- When a person receives multiple sensory stimuli and cannot perceptually disregard or selectively ignore some stimuli, sensory overload occurs.
- Excessive sensory stimulation prevents the brain from responding appropriately to or ignoring certain stimuli. Because of the multitude of stimuli leading to overload, a person no longer perceives the environment in a way that makes sense.
- Overload prevents meaningful response by the brain; the patient's thoughts race, attention scatters in many directions, and anxiety and restlessness occur.
- The amount of stimuli necessary for healthy function varies with each individual. People are often subject to environmental overload more at one time than another.
- A person's tolerance to sensory overload varies with level of fatigue, attitude, and emotional and physical well-being.
- The acutely ill patient easily experiences sensory overload. The patient in constant pain or who undergoes frequent monitoring of vital signs is at risk.
- Multiple stimuli combine to cause overload even if the nurse offers a comforting word or provides a gentle back rub.
- Some patients do not benefit from nursing intervention because their attention and energy are focused on more stressful stimuli.
- Another example is a patient who is hospitalized in an intensive care unit (ICU), where the activity is constant. Lights are always on.
- Patients can hear sounds from monitoring equipment, staff conversations, equipment alarms, and the activities of people entering the unit. Even at night an ICU is very noisy.
- It is easy to confuse the behavioral changes associated with sensory overload with mood swings or simple disorientation. Look for symptoms such as racing thoughts, scattered attention, restlessness, and anxiety.
- Patients in ICUs sometimes resort to constantly fingering tubes and dressings. Constant reorientation and control of excessive stimuli become an important part of a patient's care.

NURSING PROCESS APPLICATION IN SENSORY PROBLEMS

Apply the nursing process and use a critical thinking approach in your care of patients. The nursing process provides a clinical decision-making approach for you to develop and implement an individualized plan of care for your patients.

Assessment: During the assessment process, thoroughly assess each patient and critically analyze findings to ensure that you make patient-centered clinical decisions required for safe nursing care.

Through the patient's eyes: When conducting an assessment, value the patient as a full partner in planning, implementing, and evaluating care. Patients are often hesitant to admit sensory losses. Therefore start gathering information by establishing a therapeutic rapport with the patient. Elicit his or her values, preferences, and expectations with regard to his or her sensory impairment. Many patients have a definite plan as to how they want their care delivered. Some patients expect caregivers to recognize and appropriately manage and adjust their environment to meet their sensory needs. This includes helping the patient learn and adapt to a changed lifestyle based on the specific sensory impairment.

Persons at risk: Older adults are a high-risk group because of normal physiological changes involving sensory organs. However, be careful not to automatically assume that a patient's sensory problem is related to advancing age. For example, adult sensorineural hearing loss is often caused by exposure to excess and prolonged noise or metabolic, vascular, and other systemic alterations.

Sensory alterations history: The nursing history includes assessment of the nature and characteristics of sensory alterations or any problem related to an alteration. When taking the history, consider the ethnic or cultural background of the patient because certain alterations are higher in some cultural groups.

During the history it is useful to assess the patient's self-rating for a sensory deficit by asking, "Rate your hearing as excellent, good, fair, poor, or bad." Then, based on the patient's self-rating, explore his or her perception of a sensory loss more fully. This provides an in-depth look at how the sensory loss influences the patient's quality of life.

Mental status: Assessment of mental status is valuable when you suspect sensory deprivation or overload. Observation of a patient during history taking, during the physical examination, and while providing nursing care offers valuable data about key patient behaviors and his or her mental status. Observe the patient's physical appearance and behavior, measure cognitive ability, and assess his or her emotional status. The Mini-Mental State Examination (MMSE) is a tool you can use to measure disorientation, change in problem-solving abilities, and altered conceptualization and abstract thinking. For example, a patient with severe sensory deprivation is not always able to carry on a conversation, remain attentive, or display recent or past memory. An important step toward preventing cognition-related disability is education by nurses about disease process, available services, and assistive devices.

Physical assessment: To identify sensory deficits and their severity, use physical assessment techniques to assess vision, hearing, olfaction, taste, and the ability to discriminate light touch, temperature, pain, and position summarizes specific assessment techniques for identifying sensory deficits. You gather more accurate data if the examination room is private, quiet, and comfortable for the patient. In addition, rely on personal observation to detect sensory alterations. Patients with a hearing impairment may seem inattentive to others, respond with inappropriate anger when spoken to, believe people are talking about them, answer questions inappropriately, have trouble following clear directions, and have monotonous voice quality and speak unusually loud or soft.

COMMUNICATING PATIENTS WITH APHASIA

Aphasia is loss of the ability to understand or express spoken or written language. It commonly occurs after strokes or traumatic brain injuries. It can also occur in people with brain tumors or degenerative diseases that affect the language areas of the brain.

People who have aphasia have language problems. They may have trouble saying and/or writing words correctly. This type of aphasia is called expressive aphasia. People who have it may understand what another person is saying. If they do not understand what is being said, or if they cannot understand written words, they have what is called receptive aphasia. Some people have a combination of both types of aphasia.

Good Tips for Better Communication

- Face the patient and establish eye contact.
- Speak in a normal manner and tone.
- Use short phrases, and pause between them to give the patient time to understand what you're saying.
- Limit conversation to practical and concrete matters.
- Use gestures, pictures, objects, and writing.
- As the patient uses and handles an object, say what the object is. It helps to match the words with the object or action.
- Be consistent in using the same words and gestures each time you give instructions or ask a question.

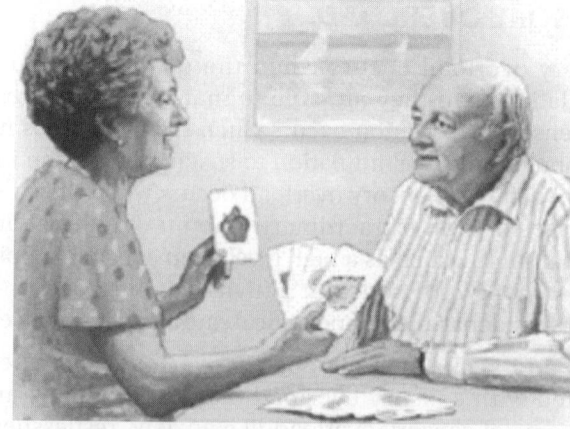

Flash cards may be used to improve naming skills

Fig. 23.4: Communicating patients with aphasia.

- Keep extraneous noises and sounds to a minimum. Too much background noise can distract the patient or make sorting out spoken messages difficult.

Communication Strategies: Some Dos and Don'ts

The impact of aphasia on relationships may be profound, or only slight. No two people with aphasia are alike with respect to severity, former speech and language skills, or personality. But in all cases it is essential for the person to communicate as successfully as possible from the very beginning of the recovery process. Below are some suggestions to help communicate with a person with aphasia:
- Make sure you have the person's attention before you start.
- Minimize or eliminate background noise (TV, radio, other people).
- Keep your own voice at a normal level, unless the person has indicated otherwise.
- Keep communication simple, but adult. Simplify your own sentence structure and reduce your rate of speech. Emphasize key words. Don't "talk down" to the person with aphasia.
- Give them time to speak. Resist the urge to finish sentences or offer words.
- Communicate with drawings, gestures, writing and facial expressions in addition to speech.
- Confirm that you are communicating successfully with "yes" and "no" questions.
- Praise all attempts to speak and downplay any errors. Avoid insisting that that each word be produced perfectly.
- Engage in normal activities whenever possible. Do not shield people with aphasia from family or ignore them in a group conversation. Rather, try to involve them in family decision-making as much as possible. Keep them informed of events but avoid burdening them with day to day details.
- Encourage independence and avoid being over-protective.

COMMUNICATING PATIENT'S ARTIFICIAL AIRWAY

Communication with hospitalized patients is essential to improve the quality and safety of health care. Patients in the ICU are often deprived of speech and their ability to communicate, because of intubation. There is a significant relationship between the loss of speech and severe emotional reactions among ICU patients, such as a high level of frustration, stress, anxiety, and depression. The most commonly used communication methods with critically ill patients, like lip reading, gestures, and head nods, are time-consuming, inadequate to meet all communication needs, and frustrating for both patients and nurses. Current practice in the ICU is to use less sedation in mechanically ventilated patients, which increases the number of patients potentially able to communicate while mechanically ventilated and awake.

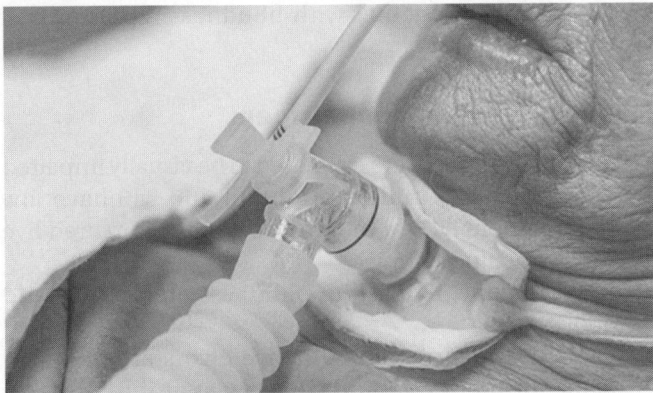

Fig. 23.5: Communicating patients with tracheostomy tube.

The primary objective of this review is to assess the effectiveness of communication aids for patients requiring an artificial airway (endotracheal or tracheostomy tube), defined as the proportion of patients able to:
- Use a non-vocal communication aid to communicate at least one symptom, need or preference; or
- Use a voice enabling communication aid to phonate to produce at least one intelligible word.

Secondary objectives are to assess the effects on:
- Time to communication (non-vocal aid) of a symptom, need or preference or time to phonation of intelligible speech (voice enabling aid);
- Patient and/or communication partner (family, friend, caregiver or healthcare professional with whom a patient may interact) reported perceptions of communication including—ease/difficulty, satisfaction/frustration, aid/technique usability and acceptability/unacceptability;
- Communication frequency, quality, success, and efficiency;
- Health-related quality of life/satisfaction with life;
- Emotional and psychological distress;
- Length of stay and healthcare utilization costs; and
- Adverse events including: respiratory instability (altered respiratory rate; oxygen desaturation); haemodynamic instability (tachy/bradycardia; hyper/hypotension); need for tracheostomy change; use of physical restraints; treatment interference.

COMMUNICATING VISUAL IMPAIRMENT

There are four levels of visual function, according to the International Classification of Diseases-10:
 i. Normal vision
 ii. Moderate visual impairment
 iii. Severe visual impairment
 iv. Blindness.

Moderate visual impairment combined with severe visual impairment are grouped under the term *"low vision"*:

low vision taken together with blindness represents all visual impairment.

Facts about Visual Impairment

- 285 million People are estimated to be visually impaired worldwide—39 million are blind and 246 have low vision. About 90% of the world's visually impaired live in low-income settings.
- 82% of people living with blindness are aged 50 and above.
- Globally, uncorrected refractive errors are the main cause of moderate and severe visual impairment; cataracts remain the leading cause of blindness in middle- and low-income countries.
- The number of people visually impaired from infectious diseases has reduced in the last 20 years according to global estimates work.
- 80% of all visual impairment can be prevented or cured.

The Causes of Visual Impairment

Globally the major causes of visual impairment are:
- Uncorrected refractive errors (myopia, hyperopia or astigmatism), 43 %
- Unoperated cataract, 33%
- Glaucoma, 2%.

People at risk: Approximately 90% of visually impaired people live in developing countries.

People aged 50 and over: About 65 % of all people who are visually impaired are aged 50 and older, while this age group comprises about 20 % of the world's population. With an increasing elderly population in many countries, more people will be at risk of visual impairment due to chronic eye diseases and ageing processes.

Children below age 15: An estimated 19 million children are visually impaired. Of these, 12 million children are visually impaired due to refractive errors, a condition that could be easily diagnosed and corrected. 1.4 million are irreversibly blind for the rest of their lives and need visual rehabilitation interventions for a full psychological and personal development.

Signs of visual impairment: Common signs that a child may have a visual impairment include the following.
- Eyes that don't move together when following an object or a face
- Crossed eyes, eyes that turn out or in, eyes that flutter from side to side or up and down, or eyes that do not seem to focus
- Eyes that bulge, dance, or bounce in rapid rhythmic movements
- Pupils that are unequal in size or that appear white instead of black
- Repeated shutting or covering of one eye (as noticed with Julian)
- Unusual degree of clumsiness, such as frequent bumping into things or knocking things over
- Frequent squinting, blinking, eye-rubbing, or face crunching, especially when there's no bright light present
- Sitting too close to the TV or holding toys and books too close to the face
- Avoiding tasks and activities that require good vision
- If any of these symptoms are present, parents will want to have their child's eyes professionally examined. Early detection and treatment are very important to the child's development.

The global response to prevent blindness: Globally, 80% of all visual impairment can be prevented or cured. Areas of progress over the last 20 years include:
- Governments established national programmes and regulations to prevent and control visual impairment;
- Eye care services increasingly available and progressively integrated into primary and secondary health care systems, with a focus on the provision of services that are high quality, available and affordable;
- Campaigns to educate about visual function importance and raise awareness, including school-based education; and
- Stronger government leadership on international partnerships, with increasing engagement of the private sector.

WHO response: WHO coordinates the international efforts to reduce visual impairments. Its role is to:
- Monitor the worldwide trends of visual impairment by country and by region;
- Develop policies and strategies to prevent blindness appropriate for various development settings;
- To give technical assistance to Member States and partners;
- To plan, monitor and evaluate programmes; and
- To coordinate effective international partnerships in support of national efforts.

Vision Impairment and Nursing Diagnoses

In assisting residents with these kinds of vision impairments, it is important to plan and also apply certain principles in order for the care to be effective. Vision loss is an hindrance in determining who might be entering the room therefore it is important to knock and identify one's self first before entering. This is to keep the resident informed and be able to know the person coming in. When placing the resident in a room, keep them well-versed of the surroundings and the organization of things inside, in order for the resident to visualize where he is and so he knows where to go and get the things he needs.

Nursing Care for Visual impairment

It is really important to pay special attention to impaired vision in **nursing care plan**. Some residents who still have little vision left need less attention; still the nurse should maintain the right lighting in order for them to use their available vision. When giving care or doing a procedure to the resident, explain it to them before doing it, in order to keep them aware of what is happening to them and encourage cooperation.

Keep the bed in the lowest position possible, so that visually impaired residents will not have problems in going out of bed when they want to. Every person has fears of the unknown therefore explain noises that might be heard or sound different.

When feeding a resident with vision impairment describe each food and balance the pace of feeding to ensure safety and maintain appetite of the food. Give assistance while feeding, but also encourage them to be as independent as they can be.

Let the residents feel the light switch before leaving the room so that they will be familiar where to locate it. When walking with the resident and assisting him, stand next to the resident but slightly be behind them in order to be cautious for possible fall of residents and be able hold them.

Use a gait belt in order to securely hold the resident but make sure that the belt is properly placed around them. Use devices that can help improve the vision of residents such as magnifying glass, eyeglasses and other reading devices and keep these equipments clean and in perfect condition. Any damage or loss of the devices should be reported to the nurse immediately.

COMMUNICATING WITH HEARING IMPAIRMENT

Hearing loss can be caused by many different causes, some of which can be successfully treated with medicine or surgery, depending on the disease process.

Causes

- Exposure to loud noise.
- Head trauma.
- Virus or disease.
- Autoimmune inner ear disease.
- Hearing loss that runs in the family.
- Aging (presbycusis).
- Malformation of the inner ear.
- Meniere's Disease.

Three Types of Hearing Loss

i. **Conductive hearing loss:** When hearing loss is due to problems with the ear canal, ear drum, or middle ear and its little bones (the malleus, incus, and stapes).
ii. **Sensorineural hearing loss:** When hearing loss is due to problems of the inner ear, also known as nerve-related hearing loss.
iii. **Mixed hearing loss:** Refers to a combination of conductive and sensorineural hearing loss. This means that there may be damage in the outer or middle ear and in the inner ear (cochlea) or auditory nerve.

Assessment of Hearing

- **Rinne's test:** A vibrating tuning fork is placed on the mastoid process of the patient. Instruct him to tell the clinician when he stops hearing. Immediately bring the tuning fork close to his ear and ask whether he can hear the vibrations now. Normally the person can. This is because air conduction of Sound is better than b' conduction. This is called Rinne's positive (which is normal). In conduction deafness: Bone conduction is better than air conduction (Rinne's negative). In neural deafness: Both air and bone conductions are decreased, but still air conduction is better than bone conduction (Reduced Rinne's positive).
- **Weber's test:** A vibrating tuning fork is kept over the vertex or forehead of the subject. Normally he can hear the vibrations in both ears equally. In conduction deafness: It is better heard in the affected ear or Weber's is lateralized to the affected ear. In neural deafness-It is heard better in the normal ear or Weber's lateralized to the normal ear.
- **Absolute bone conduction (ABC) test:** A vibrating tuning fork is kept over the mastoid process of the patient and instructs him to signal when he stops hearing. Immediately transfer the tuning fork on to the Physician's mastoid process and check whether he can receive any sound. Here it is assumed that the hearing power of the physician is normal.

Investigations

- Assessment of hearing loss includes detailed history, developmental assessment and tests of hearing. If the child does not respond to sounds of a voice, he is completely deaf or mentally retarded.
- Test of hearing includes: Using a tuning fork and an ordinary wrist-watch may also be used for the detection of defective hearing. Audiometer test used after 3 years of age. Labyrinthine test for vestibular functions are carried out satisfactorily by means of caloric tests which are simple, inexpensive and accurate.
- Verbal recognition and speech test, electro psychological test and electronystagmogram (ENG) is especially helpful in the evaluation of nystagmus.

Treatments of Conductive Hearing Loss

Types of **conductive hearing loss** include congenital absence of ear canal or failure of the ear canal to be open at birth, congenital absence, malformation, or dysfunction of the middle ear structures, all of which may possibly be surgically corrected. If these are not amenable to successful surgical correction, then the hearing alternatively may be improved with amplification with a bone conduction hearing aid, or a surgically implanted, osseointegrated device (for example, the Baha or Ponto System), or a conventional hearing aid, depending on the status of the hearing nerve.

Other causes of **conductive hearing loss** are—infection; tumors; middle ear fluid from infection or eustachian tube dysfunction; foreign body; and trauma (as in a skull fracture). Acute infections are usually treated with antibiotic or antifungal medications. Chronic ear infections, chronic middle fluid, and tumors usually require surgery. If there is no response to initial medical therapy, infectious middle ear fluid is usually treated with antibiotics—while chronic non-infectious middle ear fluid is treated with surgery (or pressure equalizing tubes).

Treatment of Sensorineural Hearing Loss

- **Sensorineural hearing loss** can result from acoustic trauma (or exposure to excessively loud noise), which may respond to medical therapy with corticosteroids to reduce cochlea hair cell swelling and inflammation to improve healing of these injured inner ear structures.
- **Sensorineural hearing loss** can occur from head trauma or abrupt changes in air pressure such as in airplane descent, which can cause inner ear fluid compartment rupture or leakage, which can be toxic to the inner ear. There has been variable success with emergency surgery when this happens.
- **Sudden sensorineural hearing loss**, presumed to be of viral origin, is an otologic emergency that is medically treated with corticosteroids.
- **Bilateral progressive hearing loss** over several months, also diagnosed as autoimmune inner ear disease, is managed medically with long-term corticosteroids and sometimes with drug therapy. Autoimmune inner ear disease is when the body's immune system misdirects its defenses against the inner ear structures to cause damage in this part of the body.
- **Fluctuating sensorineural hearing loss** may be from unknown cause or associated with Meniere's disease. Symptoms of Meniere's disease are hearing loss, tinuitis (or ringing in the ears), and vertigo. Meniere's disease may be treated medically with a low-sodium diet, diuretics, and corticosteroids. If the vertigo is not medically controlled, then various surgical procedures are used to eliminate the vertigo.
- **Sensorineural hearing loss from tumors** of the balance nerve adjacent to the hearing nerve, generally are not reversed with surgical removal or irradiation of these benign tumors. If the hearing loss is mild and the tumors are very small, hearing may be saved in 50 percent of that undergoing hearing preservation surgery for tumor removal.
- **Sensorineural hearing loss from disease** in the central nervous system may respond to medical management for the specific disease affecting the nervous system. For example, hearing loss secondary to multiple sclerosis may be reversed with treatment for multiple sclerosis.
- **Irreversible sensorineural hearing loss**, the most common form of hearing loss, may be managed with hearing aids. When hearing aids are not enough, this type of hearing loss can be surgically treated with cochlear implants.

Treatments for mixed hearing loss: Audiologist Mark Ross recommends taking care of the conductive component first. There have been times when the addition of the conductive component made the person a better hearing aid candidate, by flattening out the audiogram for example, while the underlying sensorineural component presented a high-frequency loss. However, still the emphasis would be on treating medically what can be treated.

Management

- The successful management of impaired hearing children lies in early diagnosis. It is important determine the type of hearing defect.
- **Conduction hearing loss** can be treated both medically and surgically. The medical management includes acute infections with antibiotics, respiratory allergy, and surgical management includes myringotomy and adenotonsillectomy.
- **Sensori-neural defects treated in team approach:** It includes physicians, audiologists and speech therapists. Prompt management of bacterial meningitis, judicious use of ototoxic drugs, are very important.
- **Impaired hearing:** The diagnosis and therapy must be started before the age of 3 years. The mother (trained by specialist) must be able to give auditory training to her child in infancy.
- **Speech therapy** has a useful role to play in the training of partially deaf children and this form of service should be utilized.

CARE OF UNCONSCIOUS PATIENT

Unconscious is a lack of awareness of one's environment and the inability to respond to external stimuli. Unconsciousness is a condition where cerebral functions are depressed and patient has inability to respond to sensory stimuli.

A coma is a state of unconsciousness in which the patient cannot be aroused even with powerful stimuli. The major causes of sudden alteration in consciousness include trauma, hemorrhage, infections, metabolic neurotoxins, exogenous neurotoxins, and combined causes.

Causes

- Head injury.
- Cerebral catastrophes.
- Infections.
- Asphyxia.
- Poisons

Types

Unconscious can be classified into:
- Brief, lasting for a few seconds or an hour.
- Sustained, lasting for a few hours.

Investigation

- Blood examination for glucose, urea nitrogen, electrolytes, and pH value.
- Complete blood count.
- Lumbar puncture for cerebrospinal fluid examination.
- Liver function tests.
- X-ray of skull.
- Electroencephalography.

Assessment of Unconscious Patient

Physical Assessment

Glasgow Coma Scale

- Eye opening:
  - Spontaneous—4
  - To speech—3
  - To pain—2
  - No response—1
- Verbal response:
  - Oriented—5
  - Confused—4
  - Inappropriate words—3
  - Incomprehensible sounds—2
  - No response—1
- Motor response:
  - Obeys commands—6
  - Localize—5
  - Withdraws—4
  - Flexes—3
  - Extends—2
  - No response—0
- Total score—3–15

Treatment

- Respiration should be maintained by patent airway. The air passage should be cleared of secretions. If necessary oxygen should be administered. Blood gas studies should be monitored.
- If patient is in the shock, it should be treated.
- The intracranial pressure may be reduced by the followings:
  - Ventricular tapping to remove the cerebrospinal fluid.
  - Burr hole to monitor intracranial pressure
  - Use of osmotic diuretics to relieve tension caused due to cerebral edema. For example, Mannitol is used to reduce intracranial pressure.
- Antibiotics are necessary, to treat infections.
- Sedatives are prescribed for the restless patients.
- Stool softeners may be required to prevent constipation.
- Specific treatment is started as soon as the diagnosis is confirmed.

  For example, antibiotics to treat infections, insulin to treat ketoacidosis, removal of tumor by surgery or decompression of cranial bone in case of depressed fracture of the skull.

Nursing Intervention

- Unconscious children require constant observation to detect any changes in the vital functions or early changes of complications. Therefore, prompt recording and notifying the doctor is necessary.
  The nurse should provide an organized nursing care.
- Adequate respiration should be maintained by keeping the patent airway. The patient should be placed in semi prone position on one side. The suction of the nasopharynx should be done promptly as required. Oxygen should be administered when necessary. Position should be changed every two hours to facilitate ventilation.
- Vital signs should be monitored by keen observation as the following:
  - Level of consciousness, including behavioral signs, 'reflexes,-and responses, should be recorded
  - Hyperthermia can be treated with the cooling measures and tepid sponge.
  - Respiration can he assisted by chest physiotherapy such as, percussion and vibration every two hourly.
  - Blood pressure should be monitored.
- Cerebral edema should be prevented by the accurate use of the prescribed diuretics and fluid intake. Daily weight may help to assess the over hydration or dehydration, by comparing the weight with the intake and output balance. Raising the head end of the bed will help to relieve the cerebral pressure.
- Conical damage should be prevented by providing regular eye care cleaning the eyes with the normal saline, instillation of prescribed eye drops, and proper application of the eye pads helps to protect the eyes from the damage.
- The patient should be protected from the injuries. The side rails of the bed should be up to prevent falls. The padding of the hard surfaces of the bed at the head end and side rails can protect from injuries during the convulsions.
  Timely administration of prescribed sedatives, for the restless patients, may be required.
- The pressure sores can be prevented by regular skin care. The nutrition and the fluid balance should be maintained by monitoring the intravenous fluids and nasogastric feeding.
- The bowels should be kept in regular movement to prevent constipation. The use of the stool softener suppositories may be administered as prescribed.
- General hygiene should be maintained. The oral care should be provided every three to four hours. Cleaning the skin with, the special care to the skin folds, can prevent excoriation.

- Deformities should be prevented. Proper body alignment with the careful positioning to facilitate drainage or the oral secretion, preventing pressure on the dependent extremities.

  The use of a foot board can help to prevent a foot drop. Exercises with normal range of motion of the extremities should be given, regularly, to prevent contractures of joints.
- The sensory stimulation can be provided by touch, cuddling the child, and music played at the bedside.

Nursing Assessment of LOC
- Evaluation of mental status.
- Cranial nerve functioning.
- Reflexes.
- Motor and sensory functioning.
- Scanning, imaging, tomography, EEG.
- Glasgow coma scale.

Nursing Diagnosis
- Ineffective airway clearance related to altered level of consciousness
- Risk for injury related to decreased level of consciousness.
- Risk for impaired skin integrity related to immobility
- Impaired urinary elimination related to impairment in sensing and control.
- Disturbed sensory perception related to neurologic impairment.
- Interrupted family process related to health crisis.
- Risk for impaired nutritional status.

Management
- **Maintaining patent airway**
  - Elevating the head end of the bed to 30 degree prevents aspiration.
  - Positioning the patient in lateral or semi prone position.
  - Suctioning.
  - Chest physiotherapy.
  - Auscultate in every 8 hours.
  - Endo tracheal tube or tracheotomy.
- **Protecting the client**
  - Padded side rails
  - Restrains.
  - Take care to avoid any injury.
  - Talk with the client in-between the procedures.
  - Speak positively to enhance the self esteem and confidence of the patient.
- **Maintaining fluid balance and managing nutritional needs**
  - Assess the hydration status.
  - More amount of liquid.
  - Start IV line.
  - Liquid diet.
  - NG tube.
- **Maintaining skin integrity**
  - Regular changing in position.
  - Passive exercises.
  - Back massage.
  - Use splints or foam boots to prevent foot drop.
  - Special beds to prevent pressure on bony prominences.
- **Preventing urinary retention**
  - Palpate for a full bladder.
  - Insert an indwelling catheter.
  - Condom catheter for male
  - Inducing stimulation to urinate.
- **Providing sensory stimulation**
  - Provided at proper time to avoid sensory deprivation.
  - Effort are made to maintain the sense of daily rhythm by keeping the usual day and night patterns for activity and sleep.
  - Maintain the same schedule each day.
  - Orient the client to the day, date, and time accordingly.
  - Touch and talk.
  - Proper communication.
  - Always address the client by name, and explain the procedure each time.
- **Family needs**
  - Family support.
  - Educate the needs of client.
  - Care to be provided.
- **Potential complications**
  - Respiratory distress.
  - Pneumonia.
  - Aspiration.
  - Pressure ulcer.

NURSING CARE PLAN FOR UNCONSCIOUS PATIENT

- Ineffective airway clearance related to upper airway obstruction by tongue and soft tissues, inability to clear respiratory secretions as evidenced by unclear lung sounds, unequal lung expansion, noisy respiration, presence of stridor, cyanosis, or pallor.

  Client expected outcome: The client maintains patent airway as evidenced by clear lung sounds, equal lung expansion and absence of stridor, cyanosis and pallor.

  Nursing interventions
  - Assess respiratory rate pattern, lung sounds, lung expansion, signs of tissue hypoxia, cyanosis, pallor; presence of airway secretions; occlusion of oropharynx by epiglottis or tongue; aspiration of vomitus or oral secretions.
    Rationale: Provides data for planning care.
  - Elevate had of bed to 30 degree angle or place client in lateral or semiprone position.
    Rationale: Head elevation prevents aspiration. Lateral position permits the jaw and tongue to fail forward, thus promoting drainage of secretions.
  - Insert oral airway (if tongue is paralyzed or is obstructing the airway).

- Rationale: Prevents obstruction of airway; obstructed airway leads to cerebral hypoxia which increases ICP.
- Suction airway intermittently.
  Rationale: In the absence of cough and swallowing reflexes, secretions rapidly accumulate in the posterior pharynx and upper trachea and can lead to aspiration. Intermittent suctioning prevent this.
- Administer humidified oxygen to the airway before and after suctioning.
  Rationale: Prevents hypoxia which may be caused by sucking out of air while suctioning.
- Initiate chest physiotherapy and postural drainage (unless contraindicated)
  Rationale: Promotes pulmonary hygiene
- Prepare for endotracheal intubation or tracheostomy
  Rationale: Allows efficient removal of tracheo-bronchial secretions and protects the airway from aspiration.
- Connect the client to mechanical ventilator as needed.
  Rationale: Helps maintaining oxygenation when spontaneous respiration is not possible.
- Increase amount of fluids administered at least 2.5 litre per day.
  Rationale: Loosens airway secretions promoting easy removal.
- Auscultate chest at least every 8 hours.
  Rationale: Helps detect adventitious breath sounds or absent breath sounds.
- Monitor ABG measurements.
  Rationale: Help detect complications of respiratory problems at the earliest.

- **Ineffective cerebral tissue perfusion related to effects of increased ICP as evidenced by papilledema, Cushing's traid, vomiting.**
  Client expected outcome: The client maintains optimum cerebral perfusion as evidenced by absence of signs of increased ICP (papilloedema, projectile vomiting, Cushing's triad, pupillary changes).
  Plan of action
  - Assess signs of increased ICP, cerebral edema.
    Rationale: Provides baseline data.
  - Maintain head of the bed elevated to 30 degree angle.
    Rationale: Promotes venous return through jugular veins thus preventing cerebral edema.
  - Maintain head and neck aligned.
    Rationale: Hyperextension, rotation, or hyperflexion of neck causes decreased venous return which will lead to cerebral edema formation.
  - Administer low flow oxygen and maintain oxygen therapy.
  - Suction airway when needed.
    Rationale: These measures prevent hypoxia.
  - Monitor ABG values
    Rationale: Rapidly increasing blood flow to the brain causing cerebral edema.
  - Maintain $PaCO_2$ (normally 35–45 mm Hg) through hyperventilation.
    Rationale: Decreased $PaCO_2$ presents vasodilation and thus reduces cerebral blood volume.
  - Administer osmotic diuretics e.g., mannitol or corticosteroids: Dexamethasone, as prescribed.
    Rationale: Osmotic diuretics promote venous return, corticosteroid manage inflammatory response. Both these are used to prevent cerebral edema.
  - Administer stool softness as prescribed.
    Rationale: Soft bowel involvements prevent straining or valsalva maneuver because it will increase intra-abdominal pressure and thereby increasing ICP.

- **Risk for injury related to unconscious state.**
  Client expected outcome: The client remains free of injury
  Nursing interventions
  - Assess risk factors for injury—lack of side rails, seizures, loss of corneal blink reflex, invasive lines and equipment, restraints, tight dressings, environmental dressings, environmental irritants, damp bedding or dressings, nail not cut.
    Rationale: Help obtain data to plan care.
  - Keep side rails up and bed in lowest position whenever the client is not receiving direct care.
    Rationale: Prevent fall and injury.
  - Observe seizure precautions for client with history of seizure episodes.
    Rationale: Seizure without maintaining safety is a common safety hazard among unconscious clients.
  - Use padded side rails.
    Rationale: Prevents injury during seizure activity.
  - Keep client's nail short.
  - Administer prescribed seizure drugs.
    Rationale: Helps prevent seizure episodes by maintaining high seizure threshold.
  - Use caution when moving the client.
    Rationale: Unconscious client cannot voice pain.
  - Give adequate support to the limbs and head when moving or turning the unconscious client.
    Rationale: Limbs without tone may dislocate if they are allowed to fall unsupported.
  - Always turn the client toward the nurse
    Rationale: Prevent falls.
  - Protect from external sources of heat such as hot water bags.
    Rationale: Unconscious clients cannot voice pain.
  - Release restraints (if used) every 2 hours.
    Rationale: Helps in providing range of motion exercises; prevents complication of immobility.
  - Avoid restraints as far as possible, allow one family member/significant other to be with the client.
    Rationale: Restraints may worsen the client's condition if he is confused.
  - Keep bed and bedding free of moisture, dust and debris.

Rationale: Prevents skin excoriation.
- Avoid over sedation.
Rationale: Over sedation alters respirations, which increases ICP and masks changes in level of consciousness.
- Avoid speaking negatively about the client or his condition.
Rationale: The last sense to go is the sense of hearing for psychological integrity.

- **Risk for fluid volume deficit related to inability to ingest fluids, dehydration from osmotic diuretics.**

  Client expected outcome:
  The client maintains optimum fluid volume state.

  Nursing interventions:
  - Assess hydration status by examining tissue turgor, mucus membranes, assessing intake and output changes and analyzing laboratory data (blood urea and nitrogen, creatinine, S.Na, S.K, S.Cl, CO_2)
  Rationale: Help plan care.
  - Hydrate the client with use of IV fluids initially.
  Rationale: Meet fluid needs rapidly.
  - Avoid over hydrating the client with IV fluids or blood transfusions.
  Rationale: Excessive or rapid administration of fluid may lead to cerebral edema and increased ICP.
  - Administer fluids slowly.
  - Continue fluid administration with use of Ryle's tube.
  Rationale: For long-term fluid administration in unconscious clients.
  - Administer corticosteroids and diuretics in suspected cerebral edema.
  Rationale: Maintain normal volume of fluids.
  - Monitor intake and output and urine specific gravity.
  Rationale: Helps detect abnormality from normal.
  - Evaluate peripheral pulses and BP at regular intervals; in severe cases, hemo-dynamic parameters (CVP, PAP, PAWP, CO measurement).
  Rationale: These are parameters to measure circulatory adequacy/inadequacy.

- **Ineffective thermoregulation related to damage to hypothalamic center as evidenced by persistent elevation of body temperature, warm and dry skin, flushed appearance of skin.**

  Client expected outcome: The client maintains thermoregulation as evidenced by normal body temperature.

  Plan of action
  - Assess body temperature, look for possible sites of infections (respiratory, CNS, urinary tract, wound, blood, IV sites).
  Rationale: Provides baseline data. Unconscious clients may have controlled fever because of hypothalamic involvement of infection.
  - Monitor temperature frequently or continuously.
  Rationale: Helps detect changes in temperature and to administer prompt treatment.
  - Control persistent elevation of temperature with use of
    - Antipyretics
    - Cooling blankets adequate fluid intake
    - Tepid sponge
    - Cold compress
    - Well-ventilated room
  Rationale: Fever increases metabolic demands of brain, decreases circulations and oxygenation resulting in cerebral deteriorations.
  - Control shivering in fever with use of
    - Blankets
    - Warm environment
    - Heat applications
    - By avoiding rapid over-cooling
  Rationale: Shivering increases metabolic demands ICP.

- **Risk for impaired tissue integrity cornea related to absence of corneal blink reflex, dryness of eyes.**

  Client expected outcome: The client maintains intact corneal tissue integrity as evidenced by moist corneal tissues, absence of corneal ulceration.

  Plan of action
  - Assess signs of impaired corneal integrity (corneal drying, irritation, ulceration) look for presence of corneal blink response.
  - Rationale: Data help plan care.
  - Protect eyes with an eye shield.
  Rationale: If eyes remain open for long periods corneal ulceration will develop.
  - Make sure the client's eye is not rubbing against anything such as bedding or client's own clothing.
  Rationale: In conscious clients, usually blinking and corneal reflexes are absent; can result in injury.
  - Inspect the condition of eyes with a flash light at regular intervals.
  Rationale: Helps detect corneal irritation at the earliest stage.
  - Remove contact lenses if worn.
  Rationale: Prevents corneal dryness and injury.
  - Irrigate eyes with sterile saline or prescribed solution as ordered.
  Rationale: Remove discharge and debris, prevents inflammation.
  - Instill prescribed ophthalmic ointment in each eye.
  Rationale: Prevents glazing and corneal ulceration.
  - Instill artificial tears as prescribed.
  Rationale: Keep eyes moist thereby preventing corneal dryness.
  - Apply eye patches when indicated.
  Rationale: Ensures that eyes remain closed under patch.
  - Prepare for temporary tarsorrhaphy (suturing of eyelids in closed position).

Rationale: Keeps eyes closed in case unconscious state is prolonged.

- **Altered oral mucous membrane related to mouth breathing, absence of pharyngeal reflex, inability to ingest fluid as evidenced by dryness, inflammation crusting and halitosis.**

  Client expected outcome: The client maintains intact oral mucous membrane as evidenced by absence of dryness, inflammation, crusting and halitosis and presence of pink, moist mucous membranes.

  Plan of action:
  - Assess oral mucous membrane for dryness, cracks, encrustation, and signs of inflammation.
    Rationale: Helps plan appropriate care.
    Parotitis is common in unconscious client whose mouth is unclean.
  - Inspect mouth every 8 hours using flashlight and tongue depressor; if dentures present, remove them and then inspect.
    Rationale: Helps detect problems in earlier stage.
  - Cleanse and rinse mouth carefully with appropriate solution every 2 to 4 hours.
  - Rationale: Keep mucous membranes clean, moist and free of inflammation (e.g., parotitis).
  - Apply thin coat of petrolatum on lip after oral care.
    Rationale: Prevents drying, cracking and encrustation.
  - Avoid use or lemon or alcohol-containing agents clearing.
    Rationale: Cause dryness.
  - Gently swab nose with wet cotton applicator and apply water-soluble lubricant.
    Rationale: Remove encrustations from nose and facilitates nose breathing preventing dryness of mouth from mouth breathing.

- **Imbalanced nutrition—less than body requirement, related to inability to eat and swallow as evidenced by weight and other nutritional parameters less than normal.**

  Client expected outcome: The client maintains optimum nutrition as evidenced by stable weight, adequate calories for age, height and weight, balanced intake and output, normal Hb, BUN, total lymphocytes, total proteins and serum albumin.

  Plan of action:
  - Assess nutritional status and requirements height-weight, laboratory tests, signs of malnutrition dry and loose skin and mucous membrane emaciated appearance.
    Rationale: Provides baseline data to plan the care.
  - Administer fluids intravenously, meeting nutritional requirement, with careful monitoring of fluid intake and output.
    Rationale: Intravenous administration meets nutritional requirements rapidly; too rapid administration of fluids lead to cerebral edema formation.
  - Administer fluid diet in the form of juice, shake, soup, porridge, water via Ryle's tube.
    Rationale: Unconscious client cannot take oral feeds. These feeds meet nutritional requirement. Unconscious clients have increased metabolic needs (immunodeficiency, proteins wasting, lung tissue, catabolism, negative nitrogen state).
  - Initiate TPN, if the client cannot tolerate Ryle's tube feeds (excessive vomiting, regurgitation, decreased peristalsis, absent bowel movement).
    Rationale: Meets nutritional requirements of coma clients.
  - Monitor nutritional parameters (height, weight, laboratory test, clinical examinations) at regular intervals.
    Rationale: Help determine nutritional adequacy or inadequacy.

- **Self-care deficit (bathing, feeding, grooming, toileting) related to unconscious state as evidenced by unkempt and poorly nourished look, constipation, bed soiling.**

  Client expected outcome: Client's self-care needs are met as evidenced by neat and groomed appearance; nourished look, absence of soiling of bed and constipation.

  Plan of action:
  - Assess self-care needs; self-care deficits of the client, availability of care given to perform self-care activities.
    Rationale: Provides baseline data to plan care.
  - Perform bed bath daily and as required (upon soiling of bed with stool, urine, sweat or dirt).
    Rationale: Clean skin prevents bacterial growth. Promotes overall well-being
  - Provide oral hygiene 4 hourly.
    Rationale: Unconscious clients suffer from problems of neglected mouth such as inflammation. Oral and nasal mucosa dryness, halitosis, spread of infection to adjacent structures.

- **Risk for complications—pressure sores, contractures, deep vein thrombosis, hypostatic pneumonia, constipation—related to immobility**

  Client expected outcome: The client remains free of complications associated with immobility

  Plan of action:
  - Give skin care to pressure prone areas hourly
    Rationale: Massage increases circulation; skin cleanliness is needed to prevent pressure sore by moisture and excessive dryness.
  - Avoid vigorous massage of bony prominences.
    Rationale: Vigorous massage causes skin excoriation over bony prominences.
  - Provide high calorie, high protein, vitamin-rich diet with more amounts of fluids (diet in the form of fluids such as porridge, soup, shake, juice).

Rationale: Adequate nutrition and fluid intake keep the skin nourished, thus prevents pressure sore formation.

Contractures and joint deformity, muscle wasting:
- Keep the body in the anatomical position with use of devices like footrest, trochanteric rolls, sand rags, rolled cloth, waterfilled gloves, etc.
  Rationale: Keeping the body aligned helps prevent joint deformity and contractures.
- Give protein-rich diet.
  Rationale: Maintain positive nitrogen balance. Keeps muscles straightened.
- Perform range of motion exercises 4 hourly after removing the support devices.
  Rationale: Passive exercise helps straightened weak muscles; looses spastic muscles; promote joint flexibility and increase overall well-being of the client.

DVT
- Elevate lower extremities above the heart level intermittently for 20 minutes.
  Rationale: Helps increase venous return, thus preventing thrombus formation.
- Perform passive range of motion exercises to extremities 4 hourly.
- Use elastic stockings as required.
- Monitor and compare the circumference of both legs at regular intervals.
  Rationale: Difference in leg circumference indicates DVT.
- Monitor for presence of redness, swelling and increased temperature of legs.
  Rationale: The signs of inflammation indicates DVT.

Hypostatic pneumonia/aspiration pneumonia
- Suction the airway at regular intervals.
  Rationale: Unconscious clients are unable to remove oral and airway secretions.
- Accumulation of secretion leads to pneumonia.
- Change position 2 hourly.
  Rationale: Prevents pooling of secretions in the lungs thus preventing hypostatic pneumonia.
- Initiate chest physiotherapy and postural drainage unless contra-indicated.
- Feed the client in head elevated position.
  Rationale: Prevent aspiration of oral secretions and content, thereby pneumonia.
  Aspirate Ryle's tube before feeding.
- Watch for regurgitation and vomiting.
- Keep head turned to one side.
- Give fluids (compatible with output)
  Rationale: Helps loosen airway secretions facilitating easy removal.

Constipation
- Provide adequate fluids.
  Rationale: Increased fluids required for softening the feces.
- Administer stool softness and enema as indicated.
  Rationale: Helps in easy bowel evacuation.
- Change position 2 hourly.
  Rationale: Change of position increases the bowel movements.
- Administer commercially available bowel evacuation powders (given in the form of liquid) as ordered.
  Rationale: These preparations help form stools and facilitate bowel evacuation.

- **Interrupted family process related to chronic illness of a family member as evidenced by anger, grief, non-participation in client care.**

  Client expected outcome: The family demonstrates increased coping as evidences by showing an ability to solve problem, not neglecting the needs of family members.

  Plan of action:
  - Assess family's response towards the client's illness-severe anxiety, denial, anger, remorse, grief, reconciliation-then usual use of coping mechanisms, role of client in the family, communication pattern, social support available, financial status, relationship between family members.
    Rationale: Provides baseline data which helps to plan care.
  - Develop a supportive and trusting relationship with the family or significant others.
    Rationale: High establish interpersonal relationship which is the keystone for care.
  - Provide information and frequent updates on client's condition and progress.
    Rationale: Helps alleviate anxiety and to cope better with client's condition.
  - Involve family in routine care, teach procedures that they can perform at home.
    Rationale: A sense of responsibility helps to reduce anxiety; promotes continuity of care.
  - Demonstrate and teach methods of sensory stimulation to be used frequently.
    Use physical touch and reassuring voice
  - Talk in a meaningful way even when client does not seem to respond.
  - Orient person periodically to person, place and time.
    Rationale: These interventions help family to understand that the client is having internal awareness of what is going on around, through he is not responding to stimuli. This understanding will help them to better cope with client's condition; and reduce their anxiety to a greater extent and increase their participation in client care.
  - Teach family to recognize and report unusual restlessness of the client
    Rationale: Restlessness may indicate cerebral hypoxia or metabolic imbalance.

- Enlist help of social worker, home health agency or other resources.
  Rationale: assist family with such issues as financial concerns, need for medical equipment in home and respite care.

BIBLIOGRAPHY

1. Campbell VA, Crews JE, Moriarty DG, Zack MM, Blackman DK. Surveillance for sensory impairment, activity limitation, and health-related quality of life among older adults–United States, 1993-1997. MMWR CDC Surveill Summ. 1999;48(8):131-56.
2. Dandona L, Dandona R. Revision of visual impairment definitions in the International Statistical Classification of Diseases. BMC Med. 4:7. 2006.
3. Davis A. The prevalence of hearing impairment and reported hearing disability among adults in Great Britain. Intl J Epidemiol. 1989;18: 911-917.
4. Dobkin BH. Rehabilitation and recovery of the patient with stroke. In: Grotta JC, Albers GW, Broderick JP, et al. (Eds). Stroke: Pathophysiology, Diagnosis, and Management, 6th edition. Philadelphia, PA: Elsevier; 2016: chap 58.
5. Kirschner HS. Aphasia and aphasic syndromes. In: Daroff RB, Jankovic J, Mazziotta JC, Pomeroy SL (Eds). Bradley's Neurology in Clinical Practice, 7th edition. Philadelphia, PA: Elsevier; 2016: chap 13.
6. Vitale S, Cotch MF, Sperduto RD. Prevalence of visual impairment in the United States. JAMA. 2006;295(18):2158-63.
7. Weber PC, Cass SP. Clinical assessment of postural stability. Am J Otol. 1993;14:566-9.

REVIEW QUESTIONS

Long Essays

1. Describe the factors influencing sensory function.
2. Explain the nurses responsibility in sensory and thought disturbances.
3. Discuss the care of unconscious patient.
4. Describe the nursing process application in sensory problems.

Short Essays

1. Functioning of sensory organs.
2. Components of sensory experience.
3. Sensory assessment.
4. Sensory alterations.
5. Sensory deprivation.
6. Sensory overload.
7. Communicating patients with aphasia.
8. Communicating patient's artificial airway.
9. Nursing care for visual impairment.

Short Answers

1. Sensorium.
2. Altered sensorium.
3. Auditory deficits.
4. Causes of visual impairment.
5. Communicating visual impairment.
6. Types of hearing loss.

CHAPTER 24
Care of Terminally Ill, Death and Dying

LEARNING OBJECTIVES

- Loss: Types
- Grief, bereavement and mourning
- Types of grief responses
- Manifestations of grief
- Factors influencing loss and grief responses
- Theories of grief and loss: Kübler-Ross five stages of dying
- The R process model (Rando's)
- Death: Definition, meaning, types (brain and circulatory deaths)
- Signs of impending death
- Dying patient's Bill of Rights
- Care of dying patient
- Physiological changes occurring after death
- Death declaration, certification, autopsy, embalming
- Last office/death care
- Counseling and supporting grieving relatives
- Placing body in the mortuary
- Releasing body from mortuary
- Overview: Medicolegal cases, advance directives, do-not-intubate/do-not-resuscitate (DNI/DNR), organ donation

TERMINOLOGY

Advance care planning: Making plans about the care you would want if you could no longer speak for yourself while you are healthy enough to consider options, make choices and discuss with your family; making a living will and naming a healthcare surrogate are part of advance care planning.

Advance directive: A document that describes the healthcare you would and would not want if you were seriously ill and unable to speak for yourself.

Anticipatory grief: Mourning the death of a loved one before that person has died, common when the patient is terminally ill.

Bereavement: Grief following the death of a loved one.

Assisted death: This is also known as "physician-assisted suicide", "physician-assisted dying" or "aid in dying" and is legal the US states of Oregon and Washington. It permits mentally competent, terminally-ill adult patients to request a prescription for life-ending medication from their physician.

Autonomy: This is the exercise of self-determination and choice among alternatives, based on the individual's values and beliefs.

Continuum of care: This relates to a course of therapy during which a patient's needs for comfort care and symptom relief is managed comprehensively and seamlessly. Hospice provides a continuum of care to terminally-ill patients, and aid-in-dying is assumed as the option of last resort at the end of that continuum.

Coma: "It is a profound or deep state of unconsciousness. An individual in a state of coma is alive but unable to move or respond to his or her environment." Coma can result from chronic illness or severe injury/trauma.

Comfort care: This medical specialty, also referred to as palliative care, is often associated with hospice; however, it can also be used independently and alongside curative treatments. Palliative care is available in every state, appropriate for anyone at any stage of life suffering with a debilitating illness–terminal or not–and focuses on pain management and providing comfort.

DNR/DNI: DNR/DNI stands for do-not-resuscitate/do-not-intubate and is a specific physician order. Do-not-resuscitate means that in the event of cardiac arrest, no cardiopulmonary resuscitation (CPR) or electric shock will be performed to re-start the heart.

Double effect: This is the doctrine established by St. Thomas Aquinas in the 13th century in which an action that has two effects. The doctrine is often used to describe the impact of administering high doses of morphine or terminal sedation—treatments intended to relieve suffering but that often hasten death.

Durable power of attorney: This is a document appointing a surrogate to make medical decisions in the event that an individual becomes unable to make those decisions on their own. It is also sometimes referred to as a "health care proxy."

Euthanasia: This is translated literally as "good death" and refers to the act of painlessly but deliberately causing the death of another who is suffering from an incurable, painful disease or condition.

Active euthanasia: This is generally understood as the deliberate action of a medical professional or layperson to hasten a patient's death.

Passive euthanasia: This is generally understood as a patient's death due to actions *not taken* by a medical professional or layperson—actions that would normally keep the patient alive.

Voluntary euthanasia: This occurs at the request of the person who dies.

Non-voluntary euthanasia: This refers to when a patient is unconscious or otherwise mentally unable to make a meaningful choice between living and dying, and a legal surrogate makes the decision on the patient's behalf.

Involuntary euthanasia: This occurs when a patient's death is hastened without the patient's consent. While generally viewed as murder, there are some instances in which the death may be viewed as a "mercy killing."

Futile measures: This generally refers to the medical care of patients in which the care will have little or no effect on the patient's outcome or prognosis.

Guardian ad litem (GAL): A Latin term for a court-appointed representative who makes decisions in a legal proceeding on behalf of a minor or an incompetent or otherwise impaired person.

Hospice; Hospice is an organization or institution that provides comfort (also-known-as palliative) care for dying individuals when medical treatment is no longer expected to cure the disease or prolong life. Hospice sometimes also applies to an insurance benefit that pays the costs of comfort care usually at home for patients with a prognosis or life expectancy of six months or less.

Intent: This is a concept used to draw a moral distinction between aid-in-dying and other acts/omissions that cause death—such as terminal sedation and withdrawing life-sustaining therapy. "Intent" assumes the ability to draw a clear distinction between *knowledge* of a certain outcome and an *intention* to produce that outcome.

Life-sustaining treatment: This is any treatment, the discontinuation of which would result in death. Such treatments include technological interventions like dialysis and ventilators. They also include such simpler treatments as feeding tubes and antibiotics.

Living will: A "living will" is a type of advance directive containing instructions about future medical treatment in the event the individual is unable to communicate specific wishes due to illness or injury. Each state has its own regulations concerning the use of living wills.

Palliative care: This medical specialty is often associated with hospice; however, it can also be used independently and alongside curative treatments. Palliative care is available in every state, appropriate for anyone at any stage of life suffering with a debilitating illness–terminal or not– and focuses on pain management and providing comfort.

Surrogate decision making: This is a procedure that allows a loved one to make medical-care decisions in accordance with a patient's known wishes. If the patient's wishes are not known, the decisions are generally said to be made in the patient's "best interests."

Terminal sedation: Generally practiced during the final days or hours of a dying patient's life, this coma-like state is medically induced through medication when symptoms such as pain, nausea, breathlessness or delirium cannot be controlled while the patient is conscious. Patients generally die after of the sedation's secondary effects of dehydration or other intervening complications.

Withholding/withdrawing treatment: This refers to omitting or ending such life sustaining treatments as ventilators, feeding tubes, kidney dialysis or medication that would otherwise prolong the patient's life. This legal act may be upon the patient's request, as the result of an advance directive or based upon the medical determination of futility.

INTRODUCTION

Life is a series of losses and gains. Everyone experiences losses at various points in the life continuum. Birth, loss and death are universal and individually unique events of the human experience. At any stage of one's life, there is the potential for loss, grief and death. The goals of nursing focuses on health maintenance and health restoration, with an emphasis on facilitating maximum potentials in wellness.

Birth and death are two aspects of life, which will happen to everyone. Dying and death are painful and personal experiences for those that are dying and their loved ones caring for them. Death affects each person involved in multiple ways, including physically, psychologically, emotionally, spiritually, and financially. Whether the death is sudden and unexpected, or ongoing and expected, there is information and help available to address the impact of dying and death.

LOSS

A person experiences loss in the absence of an object, person's body part or function, or emotion that was formerly present. Loss is an inevitable part of life, and grief is a natural part of the healing process. The reasons for grief are many, such as the loss of a loved one, the loss of health, or the letting go of a long-held dream. Dealing with a significant loss can be one of the most difficult times in a person's life.

Five Categories of Loss

i. **Loss of external object:** It involves any possession that is worn-out, misplaced, stolen or ruined by disaster, e.g. jewellery, to money, etc.
ii. **Loss of a known environment:** It is a loss associated with separation from a known environment, includes

familiar setting for a period or relocating permanently and transfers from place to place, hospitalization.
iii. **Loss of significant others:** It includes loss of parents, spouses, children, siblings, teachers, friends, neighbors and colleagues. And also entertainment figures and well known persons like cine actors, athletes, cricketers, popular figures of a particular field.
iv. **Loss of an aspect of life:** It includes loss of a body part, physiological function, or psychological function, e.g. loss of limb, eye, hair teeth, breast, etc., loss of urinary or bowel control, loss of memory, humor of self-esteem, of self-confidence, of power, of respect, of love, self-concept, self-identity, of job.
v. **Loss of life:** Each person responds differently to death. Some will welcome death as a relief; some will have fear of separations, abandonment, loneliness, or mutilation, etc.

Other Classifications of Loss

Actual loss: It is easily identified and can be recognized by others as well as person sustaining the loss, loss of a limb, of a spouse, of a object and of a job.

Perceived loss: It is felt by the person but is intangible or less intangible to others. For example:
a. **Makirational loss,** i.e. loss resulting from normal life transitions (loss of youth, of financial independence).
b. **Situational loss,** i.e. loss occurring suddenly in reference to a specific external event (sudden death of loved one). Other example of actual or perceived loss are physical loss, and psychological loss, e.g. losing limb from accident, losing limb leads to loss of self-image.

Factors Influencing Loss, Grief, and Coping Ability

- The individual's current stage of development
- Interpersonal relationships and social support networks
- Type and significance of the loss
- Culture and ethnicity
- Spiritual and religious beliefs and practices
- Prior experience with loss
- Socioeconomic status
- Factors that may increase an individual's risk for dysfunctional grieving include:
  - Having a great deal of dependence on the deceased
  - The deceased dying unexpectedly at a young age, through violence, or by a socially unacceptable manner
  - Inadequate coping skills or lack of social supports
  - Lack of hope or pre-existing mental health issues, such as depression or substance abuse

GRIEF

Grief is a normal response to any loss, grieving is the emotional reaction to loss. It occurs with loss caused by separation as well as with loss caused by death. Sometimes the terms, grief, mourning and bereavement are often used interchangeable. Grief is a subjective state of emotional, physical and social response to the loss of a valued entity. The loss may be real, in which case it can be substantiated by others (e.g. death of a loved one), or perceived by the individual alone, in which case it cannot be perceived or shared by others (e.g. loss of feeling of femininity following mastectomy).

Definition

- **Grief:** It is a form of sorrow that follows the perception or anticipation, loss of one or more valued or significant objects. These responses often include helplessness, loneliness, hopelessness sadness, guilt and anger.
- **Bereavement:** It is the state of grieving during which a person goes through grief reaction. It is the state of thought, feeling, and activity that follows loss, or includes grief and mourning. It is the experience of having lost something or someone by death.
- **Mourning:** It is the period of acceptance of loss and grief during which the person learns to deal with loss. It is the process that follows, a loss and includes working through grief. The process of grief and mourning are intense, internal, painful and lengthy. Mourning refers to culturally defined patterns of expressions of grief. Mourning patterns include funerals, wakes, memorials, black dress and defined time of social withdrawal.

TYPES OF GRIEF

There are several different types of grief reactions that people can have. Some of these are considered to be normal while others signify an alteration in coping with the loss.

Normal or uncomplicated grief: This type of grief symbolizes the most desirable and universal reaction to loss and is considered to be normal Corless (2010). The individual will have physical, emotional, cognitive, and behavioral reactions following the loss and will eventually move toward adjusting to it. The period of time for this can vary from person to person and is dependent on the type of relationship, type of loss and individual factors related to the bereaved. The nurse should support the family to take the time that they need for this normal grief processes to happen.

Chronic grief	Normal grief reactions that continue for an extended period of time.
Delayed grief	Normal grief reactions which are suppressed or postponed because the survivor avoids the pain of loss (consciously or unconsciously).
Exaggerated grief	An intense reaction to the loss that can include thoughts of suicide, phobias or nightmares.
Masked grief	Survivor is not aware that their behaviors are a result of the loss.

Anticipatory grief: Anticipatory grief is grief that occurs before the loss of a loved one. Sometimes anticipatory grief starts at the time of a terminal diagnosis and can proceed until the person dies. Both patients and family members can feel anticipatory loss. For the patient, they can anticipate the loss of independence, function or comfort. This can cause a lot of pain and anxiety if not given the proper support. For the family, they often start grieving for the loss of their loved one before they die. Perhaps it is because they bear witness to the pain or suffering they see their loved one go through or maybe they are also envisioning their own life without their loved one in it. They start to think about all the things that they still wanted to share with their loved one, who will likely not live long enough to do. This type of grief has been shown to help cushion a person's bereavement reaction.

Complicated grief: Complicated grief may require professional assistance depending on its severity. Individuals could be at risk for complicated grief if they experience losses that are sudden or traumatic or resulting from suicide/homicide. If the person has already had recent losses or previous losses from which they did not resolve their grief, it can contribute to developing complicated grief reaction with the new loss. Lack of a support network or concurrent stressors such as ailing health or relationships, also can contribute to this type of grief.

Disenfranchised grief: This type of grief is defined as grief that has not been validated or recognized. This type of grief often develops in individuals who have lost loved ones to stigmatized illnesses, such as AIDS, or through socially unacceptable ways, such as abortion. The loss of a previously severed relationship, such as with divorce, can also contribute to this type of grief because the individual may not be able to mourn as openly for that loved one due to the circumstances surrounding their relationship.

Unresolved grief: In this type of grief, the bereaved has failed to move through the stages of grief and accomplish the work needed to come to terms with the loss. Many factors can contribute to the manifestation of this type of grieving and can include—lack of formal closure (loved one's body never found or laid to rest), multiple or concurrent losses, or social isolation.

MANIFESTATIONS OF GRIEF

Feelings

Sadness is a common feeling experienced after the loss of a loved one. This is often demonstrated by crying, a gesture that evokes a sympathetic and protective reaction from others. Not allowing sadness to be experienced with or without tears has the potential to lead to complicated grief.

Numbness or shock is often experienced immediately after a loss. This serves as a defense to block pain and to protect the bereaved from being overwhelmed. It allows opportunity to be gradually introduced to the reality of the loss.

Anger is frequently associated with loss. It is not uncommon for the anger experienced to be directed at either the deceased of the bereaved, the bereaved themselves – or both. Worden (2005) suggests that anger comes from a sense of frustration due to an inability to prevent the death and as a regressive experience that occurs after losing someone close. Anger experienced by the bereaved needs to be appropriately identified in order to bring it to a healthy conclusion.

Guilt is also common in the process of grief. The bereaved might feel guilty about being alive while the loved one is dead. Guilt is often manifested over something that occurred during the time of death that the bereaved individual feels they could have prevented somehow.

Anxiety is a common feeling associated with loss and it comes primarily from; a fear that they will not be able to take care of themselves and a heightened sense of personal death awareness. The anxiety experienced may vary from mild anxiety to more extreme panic attacks. In this sense, being confronted with the reality of death can be a little frightening. Other feelings associated with grief include loneliness, fatigue, helplessness, yearning and emancipation.

Cognitions: The most common cognitive response to death is a preoccupation with the deceased, which occurs as a form of obsessional thinking. Some preoccupation may be in the form of intrusive thoughts that may be related to guilt or other unresolved issues. This commonly occurs in the early stages of grief and disappears after a short while.

Prolonged experience of these thoughts may trigger depression. Hallucination (visual and auditory) of the deceased loved one is also a frequent experience of the bereaved. Other cognitive responses may include confusion, disbelief, and passive suicidal thoughts.

Physical Sensations

In addition to feelings and cognitions associated with grief, there are also physical sensations that transpire during the grieving process. Although often overlooked, they may be key indicators of the individual's grief reaction. Examples of commonly reported physical sensations are listed in the table below.

Physical Sensations of Grief

- Hollowness in the pit of the stomach
- Tightness in the chest and throat
- Oversensitivity to noise
- Breathlessness
- Lack of energy
- Dry mouth
- Muscular weakness.

Behaviors: There are a number of behaviors associated with a normal grief reaction too. These are often experienced immediately after a loss and correct themselves over time. Disturbances in sleep and eating patterns are very common during times of grief. Absent mindedness and social withdrawal are also common behaviors that are evident in the grieving process. Behaviors such as dreams of the deceased and avoiding reminders of the deceased are also reported in the early stages following loss.

STAGES OF GRIEF

Kubler-Ross (1969) having done extensive research with terminally ill patients identified five stages of feelings and behavior that individuals experience in response to a real, perceived or anticipated loss:

Stage I: Denial: This is a stage of shock and disbelief. The response may be one of "No, it cannot be true!" Denial is a protective mechanism that allows the individual to cope within an immediate timeframe while organizing more effective defense strategies.

Stage II: Anger: "Why me?" and "It is not fair!" are comments often expressed during the anger stage. Anger may be directed at self or displaced on loved ones, caregivers, and even God. There may be a preoccupation with an idealized image of the lost entity.

Stage III: Bargaining: "If God will help me through this, I promise I will go to church every Sunday and volunteer my time to help others". During this stage, which is generally not visible or evident to others, a bargain is made with God in an attempt to reverse or postpone the loss.

Stage IV: Depression: During this stage the full impact of the loss is experienced. This is a time of quiet desperation and disengagement from all associations with the lost entity.

Stage V: Acceptance: The final stage brings a feeling of peace regarding the loss that has occurred. Focus is on the reality of the loss and its meaning for the individuals affected by it.

All individuals do not experience each of these stages in response to a loss, nor do they necessarily experience them in this order. Some individuals grieving behavior may fluctuate, and even overlap between stages.

Grief Process (Reactions to Grief and Death)

Grief is the emotional pain caused by a loss. Reactions to both grief and dying are similar. The stages of these reactions overlap and vary among individuals. Engel (1954) proposed that grieving process has six phases as given below:

i. **Shock and disbelief:** Here the person usually refuses to accept the fact of loss, followed by a stunned or numb responses; 'No''not me' etc.
ii. **Developing awareness:** It is characterized by physical and emotional responses such as anger, feeling empty, and crying: 'why me?'
iii. **Restitution:** It involves the rituals surrounding loss and with death includes religious, cultural, and social expressions of mourning such as funeral service.
iv. **Resolving the loss:** It is dealing with the void left by the loss.
v. **Idealization:** It is the exaggeration of the good qualities of the person or object lost, followed by acceptance of loss and lessened need to focus on it.
vi. **Outcome:** It is the final resolution of the grief process, including dealing with loss as a common life occurrence.

Treatment: Normal grief does not require any treatment while complicated grief requires medication depending on the prevailing behavior responses.

Nursing Intervention

- Provide an open accepting environment.
- Encourage ventilation of feelings and listen actively.
- Provide various diversional activities.
- Provide teaching about common symptoms of grief.
- Reinforce goal-directed activities.
- Bring together similar aggrieved persons, to encourage communication, share experiences of the loss and to offer companionship, social and emotional support.

GRIEF PROCESS

Every step of the process is natural and healthy. It is only when a person gets stuck in one step for a long period of time that the grieving can become unhealthy, destructive and even dangerous. Going through the grieving process is not the same for everyone, but everyone does have a common goal; acceptance of the loss and to keep moving forward. This process is different for every person but can be understood in four or more stages, depending upon the theory that is being used.

Shock and denial: Shock is the initial reaction to loss. Shock is the person's emotional protection from being too suddenly overwhelmed by the loss. The person may not yet be willing or able to believe what their mind knows to be true. This stage normally lasts two or three months.

Intense concern: Intense concern often manifests by being unable to think of anything else. Even during daily tasks, thoughts of the loss keep coming to mind. Conversations with one at this stage always turn to the loss as well. This period may last from six months to a year.

Despair and depression: Despair and depression is a long period of grief, the most painful and protracted stage for the griever (during which the person gradually comes to terms with the reality of the loss). The process typically involves a wide range of feelings, thoughts, and behaviors. Many behaviors may be irrational. Depression can include feelings of anger, guilt, sadness and anxiety.

Recovery: The goal of grieving is not the elimination of all the pain or the memories of the loss. In this stage, one shows a new interest in daily activities and begins to function normally day to day. The goal is to reorganize one's life, so the loss is an important part of life rather than its center.

THEORIES OF GRIEF AND LOSS

Grief models can help people to work through the grieving process, reassured that what they are going through is 'normal.' The following grief theories are among the best-known models exploring how people grieve and learn to heal, living with loss.

The five stages of grief: The five stages of grief is one of the best-known grief theories. Psychiatrist Dr Elisabeth Kubler-Ross identified denial anger, bargaining, depression and acceptance as the key 'stages' our minds go through after someone dies. Some people have said that the five stages of her grieving process are too orderly to reflect just how messy grief can be. Dr Kubler-Ross later said that her theory was never intended as a linear journey, but a series of points we may often revisit, as we adjust to life without someone we loved.

Tonkin's model of grief: Dr Lois Tonkin's model of grief is based on the principle that grief is a wound we gradually heal around. Growing around our grief means that the loss of someone will always be a part of us, but that this void and sadness will eventually not dominate our capacity to truly live.

The four tasks of grieving: Dr J William Worden's four tasks of grieving, offers four things we can strive to do, in order to live with the loss of someone: Accept the reality of what's happened, process the pain, adjust to a life without someone's physical presence and create a new connection with them, in our memory.

The six Rs of mourning: The six Rs of mourning is clinical psychologist Dr Therese Rando's theory about how actively grieving is in itself, a healing act.

The six tasks she identifies aim to work through four grief phases: recognizing the reality of a death, reacting to the separation, 're-experiencing' good and bad memories, letting go of how things were and accommodating memories of someone, in your changed world.

The dual process model: Clinical psychologists Professor Margaret Stroebe and Dr Henk Schut's dual process model of grief, works around to ways of journeying through bereavement. It allocates time to think about how much you miss your loved one and time also to take on practical activities that can give you respite, for short a while, from your pain. The idea is to go back and forth, or 'oscillate' between these stages, as you work to accommodate someone's physical absence from your life.

The reconstruction of meaning: This grief theory, the reconstruction meaning explores how to adjust to the alien place you find yourself in, when someone dies. Bereavement can turn your world upside down, making it difficult to find meaning in it. Perhaps your own sense of identity has changed and your sense of 'place.' This grief model can help you in 'meaning-making', through assimilating (adjusting to a loss) and accommodating.

KUBLER-ROSS FIVE STAGES OF DYING

The stages of mourning and grief are universal and are experienced by people from all walks of life. Mourning occurs in response to an individual's own terminal illness, the loss of a close relationship, or to the death of a valued being, human or animal. There are five stages of normal grief that were first proposed by Elisabeth Kübler-Ross in her 1969 book:

i. **Denial and isolation:** The first reaction to learning of terminal illness or death of a cherished loved one is to deny the reality of the situation. It is a normal reaction to rationalize overwhelming emotions. It is a defense mechanism that buffers the immediate shock. We block out the words and hide from the facts. This is a temporary response that carries us through the first wave of pain.

ii. **Anger:** As the masking effects of denial and isolation begin to wear, reality and its pain re-emerge. We are not ready. The intense emotion is deflected from our vulnerable core, redirected and expressed instead as anger. The anger may be aimed at inanimate objects, complete strangers, friends or family. Anger may be directed at our dying or deceased loved one. Rationally, we know the person is not to be blamed. Emotionally, however, we may resent the person for causing us pain or for leaving us. We feel guilty for being angry, and this makes us angrier.

iii. **Bargaining:** The normal reaction to feelings of helplessness and vulnerability is often a need to regain control–
   - If only we had sought medical attention sooner...
   - If only we got a second opinion from another doctor...
   - If only we had tried to be a better person toward them...
   - Secretly, we may make a deal with God or our higher power in an attempt to postpone the inevitable. This is a weaker line of defense to protect us from the painful reality.

iv. **Depression:** Two types of depression are associated with mourning. The first one is a reaction to practical implications relating to the loss. Sadness and regret predominate this type of depression. We worry about the costs and burial. We worry that, in our grief, we have spent less time with others that depend on us. This phase may be eased by simple clarification and reassurance. We may need a bit of helpful cooperation and a few kind words. The second type of depression is more subtle and, in a sense, perhaps more private. It is our quiet preparation to separate and to bid our loved one farewell. Sometimes all we really need is a hug.

v. **Acceptance:** Reaching this stage of mourning is a gift not afforded to everyone. Death may be sudden and unexpected or we may never see beyond our anger or denial. It is not necessarily a mark of bravery to resist the inevitable and to deny ourselves the opportunity to make our peace. This phase is marked by withdrawal and calm. This is not a period of happiness and must be distinguished from depression.

SIX 'R'S OF MOURNING

Rando divides mourning into six separate tasks to be completed and groups those tasks into three stages. The three stages are avoidance, confrontation and accommodation. Rando uses it to be the active process of dealing with that grief. Bear this in mind as you read about the six 'R's.

Phase 1: Avoidance

The avoidance phase is when you may be unable or unwilling to fully understand what has happened. Though you might understand the fact that your loved one has died, a part of you can still not accept this as reality. The avoidance phase has one task:
  i. **Recognise the loss:** According to Rando, fully recognising the loss means understanding what happened and really accepting it, knowing in your heart, that your loved one has gone.

Phase 2: Confrontation

The confrontation phrase involves dealing with your grief and finding ways to process what you are experiencing. There are three tasks in this phase:
  i. **React to the separation:** This means understanding and embracing all the complex, powerful emotions you are feeling. It also means acknowledging something known as 'secondary losses'. For example, the death of a spouse may also mean the loss of financial security, the loss of your idea of the future, the loss of romantic intimacy. These are all secondary losses for which you may also be grieving.
  ii. **Recollect and re-experience:** Recollecting means remembering your time with your loved one, through the good and bad. These memories will become an important way of maintaining a relationship with your loved one, as they will continue being an important influence in your life.
  iii. **Relinquish old attachments:** This may sounds harsh at first, but 'relinquishing old attachments' does not necessarily mean moving on or forgetting your loved one. It's a long and very gradual process where you slowly begin to process the impact of your loved one's absence.

Phase 3: Accommodation

The accommodation phase is all about finding meaning in life again. This doesn't mean you won't still have feelings of sadness or longing, but you will be able to have moments of happiness again. There are two tasks in this phase:
  i. **Readjust:** Readjusting to the new world without forgetting the old world. Readjusting can mean becoming more comfortable with new roles and responsibilities, but also accepting who you are now and how the death of your loved one may have changed you.
  ii. **Reinvest emotional energy:** This is another way of describing the act of enjoying life again, finding new friends or projects, and rediscovering a sense of purpose. This should not be interpreted as 'replacing' your loved one, as Rando very much emphasises the continuation of your love for them.

FACTORS INFLUENCING LOSS AND GRIEF RESPONSES

In each situation in which an individual (or group) experiences a death, funeral, or loss, the responses may differ greatly from previous responses to similar losses. No two losses are the same. No two relationships are the same. No two points in time are the same. Many factors vary, and so our grief responses vary also.
- Current health situation
- Relationship with person who has died/thing which has been lost
- Age of person grieving
- Previous experience of grief
- Cultural background
- Belief system
- Financial situation
- Knowledge around cause of loss/death
- Personality
- Concurrent losses/changes occurring
- Support systems—family/friends/community
- Cause of death (i.e. expected or not expected)
- Expectation of death
- Recognition of loss by others (i.e. disenfranchised grief)
- Social 'acceptability' of cause of death
- Social 'acceptability' of relationship of bereaved to deceased
- Ability to communicate feelings
- Language levels.

There are many other factors also. It can assist us, when supporting others, to recognise the cumulative effect of changes and transitions in a person's life journey. A major loss rarely occurs in isolation, and to be capable of assessing the overall impact of grief on an individual is one of the first steps to appropriate support.

GRIEF, BEREAVEMENT AND MOURNING

Grief and bereavement are universal experiences that people go through when they are dealing with a loss in their lives. In end-of-life care, nurses must understand the fundamentals about grief, loss, and bereavement on the part of patients and families, and also within themselves. Individuals each express and cope with losses differently and a nurse should expect to see that when working with patients and families at the end of life.

  i. Bereavement includes grief and mourning and has been considered to be the "time period in which the survivor adjusts to their life without their loved one".
  ii. This period can include the time right after the loss or death occurs, during the funeral proceedings, and during the grieving process afterward.
  iii. Different individuals respond to this period in various ways. A person's age, physical and emotional health, culture, and previous experience with loss can all affect the way that they grieve during this period of time.
  iv. Bereavement differs from grief in that it includes the period of time from the beginning of the loss until acceptance has been reached.
  v. Mourning takes place during this time and can differ based on personal and cultural factors.

The role of the nurse includes three things:
- The nurse must facilitate the grieving process by assessing the grief;
- The nurse must assist the patient with issues and concerns related to the grief; and
- The nurse must support the survivors. The purpose of this chapter is to identify the main components related to grief, bereavement and mourning in the context of end-of-life care, to describe the various types of grief, and to explore the support needed to help individuals cope and live with the loss.

Support for the Bereaved

- Both informal and formal support can be utilized to help bereaved individuals cope with the loss of their loved one.
- The kind of support a person requires will differ and it is important for the nurse to conduct a thorough grief assessment.
- Grief should be assessed frequently in the bereavement period in order for the nurse to be able to develop an effective plan to assist the bereaved in coping with their loss.
- Bereavement follow-up with families is part of most hospice programs and can include formal activities and events to promote closure and acceptance.
- Many hospices have non-denominational memorial services to honor those patients who have been lost.
- Family members and staff are invited to participate, and these can be effective at helping both parties find closure. Other formal types of support can include support groups.
- Most organizations and/or health care systems have various support groups for individuals, some of which are specific to a particular type of illness (i.e., cancer).
- Individual or group counseling or psychotherapy are other methods that can assist the bereaved in coping with their loss.

- Nurses are in the ideal position to assist patients with identifying and expressing their feelings related to the loss.
- One of the biggest facilitators of this process which nurses can engage in is active listening. By actively listening to the bereaved, it helps them express their feelings and feel as though they are being heard.
- Developing a strong nurse-patient-family relationship in the beginning of the health care encounter can help with the support needed during the bereavement period.

Nursing Interventions: Facilitate Mourning

- Grant time for the grieving process.
- Identify expected grieving behaviors, such as crying, somatic symptoms, and anxiety.
- Use therapeutic communication. Name the emotion the client is feeling. For example, say, "You sound as though you are angry. Anger is a normal feeling for someone who has lost a loved one. Tell me about how you are feeling."
- Avoid communication that inhibits the open expression of feelings, such as offering false reassurance, giving advice, changing the subject, and taking the focus away from the grieving individual.
- Assist the grieving individual to accept the reality of the loss.
- Support efforts to "move on" in the face of the loss.
- Encourage the building of new relationships.
- Provide continuing support; encourage the support of family and friends.
- Assess for signs of ineffective coping, such as refusing to leave the home months after the client's spouse has died.
- Share information about mourning and grieving with the client, who may not realize that her feelings, such as anger toward the deceased, are expected.
- Encourage attendance at bereavement or grief support groups. Provide information about available community resources.
- Initiate referrals for individual psychotherapy for clients who are having difficulty resolving grief.
- Ask the client if contacting a spiritual advisor would be acceptable or encourage the client to do so.
- Participate in debriefing provided by professional grief/mental health counselors.

COUNSELING AND SUPPORTING GRIEVING RELATIVES

Grief counseling is a form of psychotherapy that aims to help people cope with the physical, emotional, social, spiritual, and cognitive responses to loss. These experiences are commonly thought to be brought on by a loved person's death, but may more broadly be understood as shaped by any significant life-altering loss (e.g., divorce, home foreclosure, or job loss).

- Grief counseling becomes necessary when a person is so disabled by their grief; and, so overwhelmed by their loss that their normal coping processes are disabled or shut down.
- Grief counseling facilitates expression of emotion and thought about the loss, including their feeling sad, anxious, angry, lonely, guilty, relieved, isolated, confused, or numb.
- It includes thinking creatively about the challenges that follow loss and coping with concurrent changes in their lives.
- Often people feel disorganized, tired, have trouble concentrating, sleep poorly and have vivid dreams, and they may experience the change in appetite.
- Grief counseling facilitates the process of resolution in the natural reactions to loss. It is appropriate for reaction to losses that have overwhelmed a person's coping ability.
- Grief counseling may be called upon when a person suffers anticipatory grief, for example, an intrusive and frequent worry about a loved one whose death is neither imminent nor likely.
- Anticipatory mourning also occurs when a loved one has a terminal illness. This can handicap that person's ability to stay present whilst simultaneously holding onto, letting go of, and drawing closer to the dying relative.

Five stages to rebuild a shattered life:
i. **Impact:** Shock, denial, anxiety, fear, and panic.
ii. **Chaos:** Confusion, disbelief, actions out of control, irrational thoughts and feelings, feeling despair, feeling helpless, desperate searching, losing track of time, difficulty sleeping and eating, obsessive focus on the loved one and their possessions, agony from imagining their physical harm, shattered beliefs.
iii. **Adapting:** Bringing order back into daily life while you continue to grieve—take care of basic needs (personal grooming, shopping, cooking, cleaning, paying bills), learn to live without the loved one, accept help, focus on helping children cope, connect with other grieving families for mutual support, take control of grieving so that grief does not control you, slowly accept the new reality.
iv. **Equilibrium:** Attaining stability and routines: reestablish a life that works alright, enjoy pleasant activities with family members and good times with friends, do productive work, choose a positive new direction in life while honoring the past, learn how to handle people who ask questions about what you've been through.
v. **Transformation:** Rethinking your purpose in life and the basis for your identity; looking for meaning in tragic, senseless loss; allowing yourself to have both painful and positive feelings about your loss and become able to choose which feelings you focus on; allowing yourself to discover that your struggle has led you to develop a stronger, better version of yourself than you expected could exist; learning how to talk with others about your heroic healing journey without exposing them to your pain; becoming supportive of others trying to deal with their losses.

CARE OF DYING

Cassen (1991) suggests seven essential features in the management of the dying patient:
i. **Concern:** Empathy, compassion, and involvement are essential.
ii. **Competence:** Skill and knowledge can be as reassuring as warmth and concern. Patients benefit immeasurably from the reassurance that their providers will not allow them to live or die in pain.
iii. **Communication:** Allow patients to speak their minds and get to know them.
iv. **Children:** If children want to visit the dying, it is generally advisable; they bring consolation to dying patients.
v. **Cohesion:** Family cohesion reassures both the patient and family. The clinician who gets to know the family maximizes patient support and is prepared to help the family through bereavement.
vi. **Cheerfulness:** A gentle, appropriate sense of humor can be palliative; a somber or anxious demeanor should be avoided.
vii. **Consistency:** Continuing, persistent attention is highly valued by patients who often fear that they are a burden and will be abandoned; consistent physician involvement mitigates these fears.

Signs of Dying

This includes the following changes:
- Loss of appetite
- Decreased oral fluid intake and decreased thirst.
- Increasing weakness and/or fatigue
- Decreasing blood perfusion, including decreased urine output, peripheral cyanosis and cool extremities.
- Neurologic dysfunction, including delirium, lethargy and coma and changes in respiratory patterns.
- Loss of ability to close eyes.
- Noisy breathing as pharyngeal muscle relax.
- In particular, neurologic dysfunction can sometimes result in terminal delirium. Which can include a mounting syndrome of confusion, hallucinations, delirium, myocardial jerks and seizures prior to death?
- Pitting edema develops, especially of the extremities and sa crum.
- Movement and sensation are gradually lost.
- Temperature elevation will be there, but the skin feels cold and clammy.
- Pulse becomes irregular, weak and fast.
- BP falls as the peripheral circulation decreases.
- The skin cyanosed as circulation decreases.
- Respiration become noisy.

- Reflexes disappear.
- Urine decreases.
- Pain usually subsides.
- Mental alertness varies.
- Jaw and facial muscles relax with the expression becoming peaceful.

Nursing Care of Dying Patient

- Creating a peaceful environment to the patient's liking.
- Preparing instructions about whom to call (usually not all) when death occurs.
- Give the relatives time to witness what is happening.
- Creating and using rituals that can help mark the occasion in the respectful way.
- When death occurs, families should encouraged to take whatever time they need to feel what has happened, and say their goodbyes. There is no need to rush the body to a funeral home, and some families want to stay with the body for a period of time after death.

Meeting Physical Needs

A patient in the terminal stages of a disease, is given all the nursing care possible to ensure the most comfort and freedom from pain. Physical comfort is important as well as emotional and spiritual comfort.

Meeting Nutritional Needs

- Patients suffer discomfort due to decreased gastrointestinal activity.
- Nutrients and fluids are given intravenously when they are not tolerated orally.
- Sips of water is given as long the swallowing reflex is present.
- When there is problem gauze soaked with water may be placed in the patient's mouth for him to suck and moisten the mouth.

Meeting Special Needs

- Mucus that collects in the throat is removed by placing the patient in a lateral position, wiping it way, or by suctioning.
- Frequent oral hygiene is done to keep the mouth free of dried secretions, and feeling fresh to the patient.
- Vaseline or cream is applied to the lips to keep them soft.
- The nostrils are kept cleans and lubricated as necessary.
- The eyes are cleaned with cotton balls miostened with normal saline.
- Lubricating drops or ointment may be applied to the eyes.
- The patient may perspire profusely even though the skin feels cool.
- Bath the patient and change the linen needed.
- Light weight bed covering should be used. Heavy covering seems to be uncomfortable to dying patients.

- Urinary and fecal incontinence often occur due to relaxing of the sphincter muscles. Pads are used to keep the bed linen from being soiled. The patient is checked frequently and pads or linen changed as necessary. The patient's skin is washed and dried each time it is soiled.
- Frequent change of position (make sure the position permits each breathing).
- Pain is a great problem in some diseases. The doctor orders sufficient medication to control pain. It must be given as frequently as permitted. If it does not adequately control the pain, inform the doctor.
- Nursing measures for pain are used to make the patient comfortable on a minimum of medication.
- Dimness and shadows are confusing and increase a sense of loneliness. So we have to provide adequate light facility to the patient.

Meeting Emotional Needs

- Touch is an important method of communication with a dying person. The patient appropriates someone holding his hand or playing a hand on an arm, his head or some other part of the body. It conveys a feeling of caring and concern. Quiet, encouraging conversation to the patient is helpful.
- Speak in a normal voice to the patient or to others in his presence.
- Do not speak in a whisper in the patient's presence. It is very distressing to most sick people.
- Hearing is believed to the last sense to disappear. Weeping is disclosed in the patient's presence or nearby.

Signs of Death

- Absence of heartbeat and respirations.
- Fixed pupils.
- Skin color turns to a waxen pallor and extremities may darken.
- Body temperatures drops.
- Muscles and sphincters relax, sometimes resulting in release of stool or urine.

Existential Approaches in Management of Death Anxiety

- Death anxiety is inversely proportional to life satisfaction.
- When an individual is living authentically, anxiety and fear of death decrease.
- Recognition of death plays a significant role in psychotherapy, for it can be the factor that helps us transform a stale mode of living into a more authentic one (Yalom, 1980). Confronting this realization produces anxiety.
- Frankl (1969) also contends that people can face pain, guilt, despair and death in their confrontation, challenge their despair and thus triumph. It also postulates that a distinctly human characteristic is the struggle for a sense of significance and purpose in life.

- Existential therapy provides the conceptual framework for helping the client challenge the meaning in his or her life.

Management of Dying Patient

Cassen (1991) suggests seven essential features in the management of the dying patient:
i. **Concern:** Empathy, compassion, and involvement are essential.
ii. **Competence:** Skill and knowledge can be as reassuring as warmth and concern.
iii. **Communication:** Allow patients to speak their minds and get to know them.
iv. **Children:** If children want to visit the dying, it is generally advisable; they bring consolation to dying patients.
v. **Cohesion:** Family cohesion reassures both the patient and family.
vi. **Cheerfulness:** A gentle, appropriate sense of humor can be palliative; a somber or anxious demeanor should be avoided.
vii. **Consistency:** Continuing, persistent attention is highly valued by patients who often fear that they are a burden and will be abandoned; consistent physician involvement mitigates these fears.

DEATH

Death is present when an individual has sustained either irreversible cessation of circulatory and respiratory functions or irreversible cessation of all functions of the entire brain, including the brain stem. The supportive nursing care during death is as follows: To give compassionate nursing care and support to the family and patient during the grieving and dying process, the nurse should consider the five aspects of human functioning. By using the nursing process, the nurse does an assessment of each aspect; physical, emotional, intellectual, sociocultural, and spiritual to fully understand and adequately provide interventions in these areas.

Five Aspects of Human Functioning

i. **Physical:** While interviewing and observing the patient, the nurse should assess such areas as sleeping patterns, body image, activities of daily living (ADLs) mobility, general health, medications and pain. The nurse also should address the basic needs of nutrition, elimination oxygenation, activity, rest, sleep and safety.
ii. **Emotional:** Preparing for one's death is a personal endeavor filled with anxiety and fear. Assessing the patient and family's anxiety level, guilt, anger, level of acceptance and identification is important. Major fears of the dying patient include fears of abandonment, loss of control, pain and discomfort and the fear of the unknown. The nurses can intervene appropriately when they are able to accept the patient's family's individual feelings, offer encouragement and support, and give the patient's "permission to die".
iii. **Intellectual:** Intellectual assessment includes an evaluation of the patient and family's educational level, their knowledge and abilities, and expectations they have in regard to how and when death will occur. Some aspects of the intellectual dimension can be altered during the dying process because of physiological changes, medications the patient's emotional state, or the disease process. Being alert, to these changes will avert problems if the patient's memory or sensations are decreased.
iv. **Social:** Assessing the patient and family's support systems is valuable. Ascertaining if family members desire to assist in the patient's daily care will not only lessen the family's sense of loss of control but also will clarify what tasks the family will do and what will be done by nursing staff.
v. **Spiritual:** The nurse assesses the spiritual dimension by gaining insight into the patient's philosophy of life, his religious resources, and how the rituals of his faith group have significance in dealing with his death. Interventions in this area can come from clergy, friends, family, healthcare providers, and significant others. Supporting the patient and family belief system and values is important.

Signs of Approaching Death

- **Central nervous system:** Reflexes gradually disappear, signs of anxiety or distress may be shown by restlessness, tossing movements occur, pulling or pricking of bed clothing, crying and talking incoherently take place.
- **Circulatory system:** Circulation slows gradually. So, there is an alteration in temperature, pulse and respiration. Hands, feet, ears and nose become cold.
- **Respiratory system:** Respiration becomes irregular, Cheyne-Stokes, rapid or very slow. It becomes stertorous due to secretions in the mouth. Pulse becomes weak irregular and fast.
- **Gastrointestinal system:** Hiccoughs, vomiting, abdominal distension are seen. Normal activities of gastrointestinal tract decrease. The gag reflex disappears. The patient is unable to swallow.
- **Genito-urinary system:** Retention of urine, distension of bladder, incontinence of urine and stool due to loss of sphincter control are seen.

Physiological Changes after Death

- **Rigor mortis:** Stiffening of the body that occurs about 2-4hrs after death. Results from a lack of ATP, which causes the muscles to contract, which in turn immobilize the joints It starts in the involuntary muscles (heart, bladder) then progress to head, neck, trunk, extremities.
- **Algor mortis:** Gradual decrease of the body temperature after death. When blood circulation terminates and

hypothalamus ceases to function, body temperature falls down.
- **Livor mortis:** Discoloration of body after death. After blood circulation has ceased, the RBC broken down, leads to discoloration of surrounding tissues.
- **Decomposition:** Tissues after death become soft and eventually liquefied by bacterial fermentation. The hotter the temperature, the more rapid the change. So bodies are stored in cool places/embalming.

Physiological Changes

- **Skin musculoskeletal system:** Perspiration is increased; skin becomes cold and clammy, and it becomes pale or mottled due to congestion of blood in the vein loss of muscle tone.
- **Facial appearance:** Sagging of jaws takes place, cheeks become flaccid and breathing takes place through mouth. Generally, checks are sucked in and blowout. With each respiration, facial muscles are relaxed.
- **Sight, speech and hearing:** Eyes have a sunken appearance and the lids may drop, half-closed. A film appears over the eyes. They do not react to light. Speech becomes mumbled and confused. Hearing becomes dulled, but it is not known when it completely disappears.
- **Absence of pulse,** heart beat and respiration is noted. Pupil of the eye become fixed and does not react to light. There is absence of all reflexes.
- **Rigor mortis sets in.** It is the stiffening of the body after death due to fixation of muscles.

Signs of Clinical Death

- Absence of pulse hearts beat and respiration.
- Red blood cells rolling to a drop or forming rouleaux in retinal vessels.
- Pupils fixed and non reactive to light.
- Absence of all reflexes.
- Rigor mortis.
- Postmortem hypostasis.
- Autolysis.

Care of Dying Person

The Psychological Needs

- Relied from loneliness, fort and depression.
- Maintenance of security self-confidence and dignity.
- Maintenance of hope.

Symptomatic Management

- **Problems associated with breathing:** Shortness of breaths give oxygen interactions to cage his discomfort.
- **Problems associated with eating and drinking:** Anorexia nervosa and vomiting are commonly seen in the dying patient. Provide IV floods, sips of fluids which help the patient to keep the mouth moist.
- **Problems associated with elimination:** Constipation urinary retention, etc. occurs. The problems should be prevented or treated if possible.
- **Problems associated with immobility:** Patients about be comfortably and their position frequently changed.
- **Problems associated with sense organs:** Since the patient lags sight before giving any care, the nurse showed touch the patient and say what she went to do.

Phsical Changes after Death

Rigor Mortis
- Stiffening of the body that occurs about 2-4 hours after death.
- Results from a lack of ATP, which causes the muscles to contract, which in turn immobilize the joints.
- It starts in the involuntary muscles (heart, bladder) then progress to head, neck, trunk, extremities.

Algor Mortis
- Gradual decrease of the body temperature after death.
- When blood circulation terminates and hypothalamus ceases to function, body temperature falls down.

Livor Mortis
- Discoloration of body after death.
- After blood circulation has ceased, the RBC broken down—leads to discoloration of surrounding tissues.

Decomposition
- Tissues after death become soft and eventually liquified by bacterial fermentation.
- The hotter the temperature, the more rapid the change.
- So bodies are stored in cool places/embalming

Dead Body Care

Care of dead body often depends upon the customs and religious beliefs. Nurses provide dignity and sensitivity to the client and family:
- Check orders for any specimens.
- Ask for special requests to family (e.g. shaving, a special gown, Bible in hand.
- Remove all equipments, tubes, supplies and dirty linens.
- Cleanse the body thoroughly, apply clean sheets.
- Brush and comb the hairs.
- The eyelids are closed and held in place for a few seconds, so they remain closed.
- Dentures should be in the mouth to maintain facial alignment.
- Mouth should be closed.
- Remove all the ornaments.
- Absorbent pads are placed under the buttocks to take up any feaces and urine released because of muscle sphincter relaxation.
- All the orifices should be closed.
- Cover with a clean sheet up to the chin.
- Spray a deodorizer to remove unpleasant odor.
- Apply name tag (wrist, right big toe).
- Allow the family members to view the dead body.

- The body is wrapped in a large piece or plastic or cotton material used to enclose a body after death. Identification is then applied outside of the wrapper.
- Hand over all the belongings to the relatives.
- Do complete documentation in the nursing notes. Time of death and actions taken to prevent the death. Who pronounced the death? Any organ donation. Personal articles left on the body. Personal items given to family. Time of discharge and destination of the body. Location of name tags on the body. Special request by family
- Hand over the dead body to the relatives/sent to the mortuary.

HYGIENIC CARE OF DEAD BODY

Family members or close friends may choose to be involved in washing and dressing the body after death has occurred. Caring for a body is not easy and can stir up strong emotions. Washing the person's body after death is much like giving the person a bath during his or her illness.

- **Wash the person's face,** gently closing the eyes before beginning, using the soft pad of your fingertip. If you close them and hold them closed for a few minutes following death, they may stay closed on their own. If they do not, close again and place a soft smooth cloth over them. Then place a small soft weight to keep the eyes in position. To make a weight, fill a small plastic bag with dry uncooked rice, lentils, small beans or seeds. After you have washed the face, close the mouth before the body starts to stiffen. If the mouth will not stay shut, place a rolled-up towel or washcloth under the chin. If this does not provide enough support to keep the mouth closed, use a light-weight, smooth fabric scarf. Place the middle of the scarf at the top of the head, wrapping each end around the side of the face, under the chin and up to the top of the head where it can be gently tied. These supports will become unnecessary in a few hours and can be removed.
- **Wash the hair** unless it has been washed recently. For a man, you might shave his face if that would be his normal practice. .
- **Clean the teeth and mouth.** Do not remove dentures because you may have difficulty replacing them as the body stiffens.
- **Clean the body using a facecloth with water and a small amount of soap.** Begin with the arms and legs and then move to the front and back of the trunk. You may need someone to help you roll the person to each side to wash the back. If you wish, you can add fragrant oil or flower petals to your rinse water. Dry the part of the body you are working on before moving to another. Some families or cultures may also choose to apply a special lotion, oil or fragrance to the person's skin.
- **Dress or cover the body according to personal wishes or cultural practices**. A shirt or a dress can be cut up the middle of the back from the bottom to just below but not through the neckline or collar. Place the arms into the sleeves first and then slipping the neck opening over the head, tucking the sides under the body on each side.
- **Position the arms alongside his or her body and be sure the legs are straight**. If the person is in a hospital bed with the head raised, lower the head of the bed to the flat position.

CARE OF THE BODY AFTER DEATH

After death the body undergoes many physical changes. So care must be provided as early to prevent tissue damage / disfigurement of body parts.

Purpose of Dead Body Care

- To prepare the body for the morgue.
- To prevent discoloration or deformity of the body.
- To protect the body from postmortem discharge.

Nursing Care

- It is the function of the physician to declare the death of the patient. Patients are not legally dead until the physician has certified death and nothing should be done that would interfere with life. The physician fills the death certificate before the body is taken to home.
- Nurses should know whether there is an autopsy or an inquest, and she should get a written permission for autopsy.
- When the death occurs following certain communicable diseases, special attention should be given to prevent it.
- Custom varies in relation to the care of the body after death. Bodies are embalmed or preserved to look as natural as possible.
- The eyes are closed immediately as in sleep and the body is straightened with the arms laid at the sides. Dentures removed are replaced and the mouth is closed. The body should be handled with reverence.
- Remove all appliances used for the care of the patient.
- Remove the ornaments of any type from the dead body. All jewelleries should be removed and entrusted to the closest relative and receipt should be obtained for their delivery.
- Send the body as clean and neatly dressed as possible to the mortuary.
- Proper identification should be done, such as patient's name, age, address, ward number, bed number, date and time, etc.
- Patient's cause of death must be sent to record section for filing.
- After the dead body is removed from the room, the room should be treated as in case of "discharge of patient".

Care of Dead Body

- Check orders for any specimens.
- Ask for special requests to family (e.g. shaving, a special gown, Bible in hand, rosary at the bedside).

- Remove all equipments, tubes, supplies and dirty linens.
- Cleanse the body thoroughly, apply clean sheets.
- Brush and comb the hairs.
- The eyelids are closed and held in place for a few seconds, so they remain closed.
- Dentures should be in the mouth to maintain facial alignment.
- Mouth should be closed.
- Remove all the ornaments, except wedding bands (in some instances).
- Absorbent pads are placed under the buttocks to take up any faces and urine released because of muscle sphincter relaxation.
- All the orifices should be closed.
- Cover with a clean sheet up to the chin.
- Spray a deodorizer to remove unpleasant odor.
- Apply name tag (wrist, right big toe).
- Allow the family members to view the dead body.
- The body is wrapped in a "shroud" a large piece or plastic or cotton material used to enclose a body after death. Identification is then applied outside of the shroud.
- Hand over all the belongings to the relatives.
- Do complete documentation in the nursing notes.
    - Time of death and actions taken to prevent the death.
    - Who pronounced the death?
    - Any organ donation
    - Personal articles left on the body
    - Personal items given to family
    - Time of discharge and destination of the body
    - Location of name tags on the body
    - Special request by family
- Handed over the dead body to the relatives/sent to the mortuary.

Last offices: Last offices—also known as the 'laying out of the dead' refers to the care of a patient's body after they have died. It is an ancient ritual providing an opportunity for people to offer a final mark of respect to the deceased person. Historically, it was a procedure carried out by family members (and this may still be the preference in some religions e.g. Islam) but, in more recent times, it has become the responsibility of the nurse/healthcare worker.

DOCUMENTATION OF DEATH

- Document the date and time of the patient's death and the name of the health care provider who pronounced the death.
- If resuscitation was attempted, indicate the time it started and ended, and refer to the code sheet in the patient's medical record.
- Note whether the death is being referred to the medical examiner and whether an autopsy is being performed.
- Include all postmortem care given, noting whether medical equipment was removed or left in place.
- List all belongings and valuables and the name of the family member who accepted and signed the appropriate valuables or belongings list. Record any belongings left on the patient.
- Document the disposition of the patient's body and the name, telephone number, and address of the funeral home.
- List the names of family members who were present at the time of death.
  If they weren't present, note the name of the family member notified and who viewed the body.
- Be sure to document any care, emotional support, and education given to the family.

MEDICOLEGAL ISSUES

- **Do not resuscitate order (DNR):** Sudden death from cardiac arrest requires CPR by competent persons. This is the life saving measures according to the agency policy unless the primary physician has written a "do not resuscitate order" in the client's medical record. Health care agencies are required to have policies for a DNR decision. The principles of informed consent respected by physician who writes a DNR order. When the client is either comatose or near death there should be knowledge by the physician and the client's family about the actions to prolong the client's life.
- **Wills of the patient:** Various countries have laws regarding the legal requirements for written and oral wills. Nurses are usually required to notify the physician and nurse supervisor before acting as a witness and signing a will. Nurses should refrain from assisting the client with the wording of the will at this should be done with legal advice from an advocate.
- **Pronouncement of death:** The government has formed laws to protect the public when dealing with issues of death. The various definitions of death are as follows: The absence of awareness of external stimuli, lack of movement or spontaneous breathing, absent reflexes, a flat brain wave or EEG and definition of brain death which requires irreversible cessation of all functioning of the brain. It is usually within the scope of practice of medicine to pronounce a client dead.
- **Care of deceased:** When a client dies, the nurse is responsible to treat the deceased with respect and dignity. The nurse should prepare the body for removal to the mortuary according to the agency polices, the nurse is responsible for properly identifying the body could result in severe distress for the family as well as legal ramifications for both hospital and the nurse.
- **Autopsy:** An autopsy is performed to determine the cause of death. In case of suspicious death or the presence of communicable disease. The cause of death also has to do with payment from insurance policies and the workers compensation. It requires consent in writing and nurse is responsible for ensuring that all documentation is in place before releasing a body for autopsy.

- **Organ donation:** The donation of organs for transplantation is a matter that requires compassion and sensitivity from the care givers. It is important that family of the deceased know the importance of and process for organ donation. In some countries, any person of age 18 or older may become an organ donor by written consent. In the absence of proper documentation, a family member or legal guardian may authorize donation of the organs. It requires the collaborative efforts of the nurse with physician. social workers and clergy (priest) to ensure timely removal of the organs.
- **Euthanasia:** It is merci-killing. This means easy or painless death. This word was derived from Greek word meaning "Good death."
    Two types
    i. **Active euthanasia:** It is to take delibrate action to end the patient's life. A physician who administers a lethal dose commits active Euthanasia.
    ii. **Passive euthanasia:** It is stopping from treatment that would prolong a person's life such as chemotherapy, surgery. NG feeding, antibiotic therapy but taking no steps to end his life.
- **Advanced directives:** The concept has to develop as a mechanism for dealing with some of the decisions that arise when caring for terminally ill. When there is no hope for recovery. Their purpose is to speak for an incapacitated patient who cannot speak for himself for his treatment and wishes. Advanced directives incorporate, the concept of living will, the patient's right to refuse unwanted life support such as CPR, antibiotics, food an fluids.
- **Advance directives:**
    - An advance directive tells the health care team what kind of care the patient would like to have if he is unable to make medical decisions (e.g., if in coma)
    - A good advance directive describes the kind of treatment the patient would want depending on the sickness.
- **Counseling for organ donation:**
    - Organ transplantation is truly one of the miracles of modern medicine, saving the lives of many patients and improving the quality of life for many more.
    - Given the ever-increasing gap between the number of organs needed and the supply, nurses have an ethical obligation to help ensure that the desires of people who want to donate organs are respected.
    - Nurses have to ensure that the consent process is informed and voluntary.
    - Information to the patient should consist of a balanced discussion of the available options and counseling to help patients or their families reach the choice that is best for them, including the provision of information about the urgent need for organs and the consolation that many families derive from knowing that their loved one was able to help others.

- **Other medicolegal issues:**
    - Abuse of children, elderly, and spouse
    - Drug-related injury
    - Unknown cause of death
    - Suicide
    - Violent death
    - Poisoning
    - Accidents
    - Suspicion of criminal action.

Nurses Responsibility in Medicolegal Issues

- Obtain death reports.
- Do investigation—the natural death and infant/child death.
- Conduct postmortem, sexual assault/child abuse examinations.
- Collaborate with organ/tissue procurement agencies.
- Provide link between pathologists and lay investigative staff.
- Normally, only uniformed officers attend the natural death scene.
- Understand subtle signs of abuse and neglect.
- Collaborate with pathologist to determine the appropriate medical records.
- Review medical records once received.
- Obtain follow-up information.

ADVANCE DIRECTIVES: EUTHANASIA, WILL, DYING, DECLARATION, ORGAN DONATION, ETC.

An advance directive is a document by which a person makes provision for health care decisions in the event that, in the future, he/she becomes unable to make those decisions. There are two main types of advance directive—the "Living Will" and the "Durable Power of Attorney for Health Care." There are also hybrid documents which combine elements of the Living Will with those of the Durable Power of Attorney.

Living Will

A living will is the oldest type of health care advance directive. It is a signed, witnessed (or notarized) document called a "declaration" or "directive." Most declarations instruct an attending physician to withhold or withdraw medical interventions from its signer if he/she is in a terminal condition and is unable to make decisions about medical treatment. Since an attending physician who may be unfamiliar with the signer's wishes and values has the power and authority to carry out the signer's directive, certain terms contained in the document may be interpreted by the physician in a manner that was not intended by the signer. Family members and others who are familiar with the signer's values and wishes have no legal standing to interpret the meaning of the directive.

Euthansia

The act or practice of killing hopelessly sick or injured individuals (as persons or domestic animals) in a relatively painless way for reasons of mercy; *also*: the act or practice of allowing a hopelessly sick or injured patient to die by taking less than complete medical measures to prolong life—called also *mercy killing*.

Types: Euthanasia can be classified in different ways, including:

- **Active euthanasia:** Where a person deliberately intervenes to end someone's life—for example, by injecting them with a large dose of sedatives.
- **Passive euthanasia:** Where a person causes death by withholding or withdrawing treatment that is necessary to maintain life, such as withholding antibiotics from someone with pneumonia.

Euthanasia can also be classified as:

- **Voluntary euthanasia:** Where a person makes a conscious decision to die and asks for help to do this.
- **Non-voluntary euthanasia:** Where a person is unable to give their consent (for example, because they are in a coma or are severely brain damaged) and another person takes the decision on their behalf, often because the ill person previously expressed a wish for their life to be ended in such circumstances.
- **Involuntary euthanasia:** Where a person is killed against their expressed wishes.

Organ Donation

A person 18 years or older and of sound mind can donate all or any part of their own body for the following purposes: For medical or dental education, research, advancement of medical or dental science, therapy, transplantation.

- The request for organ donation should be done by patent in the presence of a physician or a nurse
- Organs removed from the body following the death cannot be sold.
- All organ donations are voluntary and there should not be any compulsion for the patient/family members.
- Organs usually donated: kidney, heart, lungs, liver, bone, cornea.
- Organ donation should take place within 2-6 hours after the death.

AUTOPSY

Tue term "autopsy" derives from the Greek word "to see for oneself". "Necropsy" is from the Greek for seeing a dead body". Necropsy is the term for a postmortem examination on an animal. An autopsy also knows as a postmortem examination, necropsy or obduction.

Definition: Autopsy is a medical procedure that consists of a thorough examination of a dead body to determine the cause and manner of death and to evaluate any disease or injury that may be present. It is usually performed by a specialized medical doctor called a pathologist.

Classification

- **Forensic:** This is done for medical legal purposes. No family permission is required to complete this type of autopsy. This is carried out when the cause of death may be a criminal matter such as accident, bums.
- **Clinical/academic:** This is usually performed in hospitals for research and study purposes. For a clinical autopsy to take place a cause of death must have already been established & a death certificate completed. To complete this type of autopsy, permission from the deceased's legal next of kin is required.
- **Coroner's:** This type of autopsy involves cases where no medical cause of death is readily available. Cause, manner and mechanism of death are in question. Eventually, the prospectors will identify whether the cases deserve comprehensive forensic autopsy or a routine postmortem.

POSTMORTEM CARE

Nurses are responsible for following federal and state laws regarding requests for organ or tissues donation, obtaining permission for autopsy, ensuring the certification and appropriate documentation of the death, and providing postmortem (after-death) care.

Nursing Interventions

Care of the Body

- Provide care with respect and compassion while attending to the desires of the client and family per their cultural, religious, and social practices.
- **Recognize that the provider certifies death** by pronouncing the time and documenting therapies used, and actions taken prior to the death.
- **Preparing the body for viewing includes:**
  - Maintaining privacy.
  - Shaving facial hair if applicable and/or desired by the family.
  - Removing all tubes and soiled linens (unless organs are to be donated or this is a medical examiner's case).
  - Removing all personal belongings to be given to the family.
  - Cleansing and aligning the body with a pillow under the head, arms outside the sheet and blanket, dentures in place, and eyes closed.
  - Applying fresh linens and a gown.
  - Brushing/combing the client's hair, replacing any hair pieces.
  - Removing excess equipment and linens from the room.

- Dimming the lights and minimizing noise to provide a calm environment.
- **Viewing considerations include:**
  - Asking the family if they would like to visit with the body, honoring any decision.
  - Clarifying where the client's personal belongings should go—with the body or to a designated person.
  - Adhering to the same procedures when the client is an infant, with the exception of:
    - Swaddling the infant's body in a clean blanket.
    - Transporting the infant in the nurse's arms or in an infant carrier.
    - Offering mementos of the infant (identification bracelets, footprints, the cord clamp, a lock of hair, photos).
- **Post-viewing**
  - Apply identification tags according to facility policy.
  - Complete documentation.
  - Remain aware of visitor and staff sensibilities during transport.

Organ Donation

- Recognize that requests for tissue and organ donations must be made by specially trained personnel.
- Provide support and education to family members as decisions are being made. Use private areas for any family discussions concerning donation.
- Be sensitive to cultural and religious influences.
- Maintain ventilatory and cardiovascular support for vital organ retrieval.

Autopsy Considerations

- The provider typically approaches the family about performing an autopsy.
- The nurse's role is to answer the family's questions and support its choices.
- Autopsies can be conducted to advance scientific knowledge regarding disease processes, which can lead to the development of new therapies.
- The law may require an autopsy to be performed if the death is due to homicide, suicide, or accidental death, or if death occurs within 24 hr of hospital admission.
- Most facilities require that all tubes remain in place for an autopsy.

Cultural/Religious Beliefs

- Identify cultural/religious beliefs of family members.
- Be sensitive to these practices when providing postmortem care.

Documentation and Completion of Forms following Federal and State Laws Typically Includes

- Who pronounced the death and at what time
- Consideration of and preparation for organ donation
- Disposition of personal articles
- Who was notified and any decisions made
- The location of identification tags
- The time the body left the facility and the destination.

Care of Nurses who are Grieving

- Caring long-term for clients can create personal attachments for nurses.
- Nurses can use coping strategies such as:
  - Going to the client's funeral.
  - Communicating in writing to the family.
  - Attending debriefing sessions with colleagues.
  - Using stress management techniques.
  - Talking with a professional counselor.

EMBALMING

Embalming is the art and science of preserving human remains by treating them (in its modern form with chemicals) to forestall decomposition. The intention is to keep them suitable for public display at a funeral, for religious reasons, or for medical and scientific purposes such as their use as anatomical specimens. The three goals of embalming are sanitization, presentation and preservation (or restoration). Embalming has a very long and cross-cultural history, with many cultures giving the embalming processes a greater religious meaning.

Concept of Embalming

- It is the process of preserving dead body from decay.
- Injection of chemicals into the body to destroy the bacteria ; thereby prevents rapid decomposition of tissues.
- Embalming fluid contains a mixture of formaldehyde, methanol, ethanol and other solvents.

Definition: Embalming is the process of sanitizing and preserving human remains to render them as safe as possible for handling while retaining naturalness of tissue for funeral viewing purposes. An embalmer is one who is trained in the art and science of embalming.

Steps of Embalming Process

- **Arterial embalming:** Which involves the injection of embalming chemicals into the blood vessels, usually via the right common carotid artery? Blood is displaced from the right jugular vein. The embalming solution is injected with a centrifugal pump and the embalmer massages the corpse to break up clots as to ensure the proper distribution of the embalming fluid. In case of poor circulation, other injection points are used.
- **Cavity embalming:** The suction of the internal fluids of the corpse and injection of embalming chemicals into body cavities, using an aspirator and trocar. The embalmer makes a small incision just above the navel and pushes the trocar in the chest and stomach cavities to

puncture the hollow organs and aspirate their contents. He then fills the cavities with concentrated chemicals that contain formaldehyde. The incision is either sutured closed or a "trocar button" is screwed into place.
- **Hypodermic embalming:** The injection of embalming chemicals under the skin as needed.
- **Surface embalming:** Which supplements the other methods, especially for visible, injured body parts? Atypical embalming takes one or two hours. An embalming case that requires more attention could take longer.

Embalming chemicals: These are variety of preservation, sanitizers, disinfectant agents and additives used in modern embalming. The purpose is to temporarily delay decomposition and restore a natural appearance for viewing a body after death. A mixture of these chemicals is known as embalming fluid and is used to preserve deceased, sometimes only until the funeral, other times indefinitely. Typical embalming fluid contains a mixture of formaldehyde, glutaraldehyde, methanol, ethanol, and other solvents. The formaldehyde content generally ranges from 5 to 35 percent and ethanol content may range from 9 to 56 percent.

BIBLIOGRAPHY

1. Anderw KJ. Critical thinking and nursing education: Perplexities and insights. Journal of Nursing Education. 1991;30(4):152-7.
2. Banjamine JV. Biofeedback Principles and Practice for Clinicians, 3rd edition. Williams and Wikins, Baltimore, 1981.
3. Corless IB. Bereavement. In BR Ferrell, Coyle N. Oxford Textbook of Palliative Nursing. New York: Oxford University Press. 2010; 597-611.
4. Dower B. Developing analytic thinking skill in early undergraduate education. Journal of Nursing Education, 1993.
5. Dugas BW, Knor ER. Nursing Foundations. Ontario. 1995;843-6.
6. Feist J, Linda B. Health Psychology an Introduction to Behavior and Health, 4th edition. International Headquarters, USA, 2000.
7. Kramer MK. Concept clarification and critical thinking: integrated processes. Journal of Nursing Education. 1993;32(9):406-14.
8. Labbe EE, et al. Skin temperature biofeedback tramm. Cognitive developmental factors in noncommercial children. Perception Motor Skills April. 1995;80(2):466.
9. Miller KM, Perry PA. Relaxation technique and postoperation pain in patients undergoing cardiac surgery. Heart Lung. 1990;19:36-46.
10. Newton-John TR, et al. Cognitive behavior therapy versus EMG biofeedback in the treatment of low back pain. Behavioral Research Therapy. 1995;33(6);691-7.
11. Pless BS. Clarifying the concept of critical thinking in nursing. Journal of Nursing Education. 1993;32(9):425-8.
12. Potter PA, Perry AG. Fundamentals of Nursing, 5th edition. Harcourt Health Sciences Company. St. Louis. 2001;1305-08.
13. Sharmas, Kaur J. Hypnosis and pain management. Indian Journal of Nursing, 2006.
14. Tanner A. More thinking about critical thinking and clinical decision making. Journal of Nursing Education. 1993.

REVIEW QUESTIONS

Long Essays

1. Define grief, explain the types and manifestations of grief.
2. Explain the nursing care of dying patient and discuss the physiological changes after death.
3. Define advance directives, explain euthanasia, will, dying, declaration, organ donation in brief.

Short Essays

1. Five categories of loss.
2. Stages of grief.
3. Reactions to grief and death.
4. Theories of grief and loss.
5. Kubler–Ross five stages of dying.
6. Factors influencing loss and grief responses.
7. Counseling and supporting grieving relatives.
8. Signs of approaching death.
9. Steps of embalming process.
10. Postmortem care.
11. Nurses responsibility in medicolegal issues.
12. Care of the body after death.

Short Answers

1. Euthanasia.
2. Advance directive.
3. Withholding/withdrawing treatment.
4. Physical sensations of grief.
5. Signs of dying.
6. Hygienic care of dead body.
7. Medicolegal issues.
8. Autopsy.
9. Organ donation.
10. Living will.

CHAPTER 25

Self-concept

LEARNING OBJECTIVES

- Components (personal identity, body image, role performance, self-esteem)
- Factors affecting self-concept
- Nursing management

TERMINOLOGY

Self-concept: It is an individual's perception of self, including self-esteem, body image, and ideal self.

Emotional intelligence (EI): It refers to the ability to perceive, understand, control/manage, and evaluate emotions.

Identity: It is an individual's conscious description of who he is. A client's identity is assessed by asking the person to describe oneself.

Self-awareness: It involves consciously knowing how the self thinks, feels, believes, and behaves at any specific time

Body image: An individual's perception of physical self, including appearance, function, and ability, is known as one's body image.

Self-esteem: It is a personal opinion of oneself and is shaped by individuals' relationships with others, experiences, and accomplishments in life. A healthy self-esteem is necessary for mental well-being and a positive self-concept.

Role: An individual's role is defined as an ascribed or assumed expected behavior in a social position or group. Specific behaviors that a person exhibits within each role make up role performance.

Self-injury: Self-injury involves intentional self-inflicted tissue damage, such as cutting, burning, skin picking, or pulling one's hair out.

Eating disorders: Anorexia nervosa, bulimia, and binge eating are the three most common eating disorders. Anorexia nervosa and bulimia can lead to life-threatening conditions, resulting in permanent damage to major organs of the body.

INTRODUCTION

Self-concept is our personal knowledge of who we are, encompassing all of our thoughts and feelings about ourselves physically, personally, and socially. Self-concept also includes our knowledge of how we behave our capabilities, and our individual characteristics. Our self-concept develops most rapidly during early childhood and adolescence, but self-concept continues to form and change over time as we learn more about ourselves.

DEFINITION

- Social psychologist Roy Baumeister says that self-concept should be understood as a knowledge structure. People pay attention to themselves, noticing both their internal states and responses and their external behavior. Through such self-awareness, people collect information about themselves. Self-concept is built from this information and continues to develop as people expand their ideas about who they are.
- Self-esteem is defined as the way an individual thinks about himself or herself, and how good he or she feels. Positive self-esteem develops when a person feels good and capable of responding to challenges and stressors. Nevertheless, when a person exhibits mild to a remarkable shift in the view of him or herself such as negativity about self, low self-esteem develops. Low self-esteem can reduce the quality of a person's life in many different ways, including negative feelings, fear, relationship problems, or low resilience. This change in self-esteem is a temporary phase in response to feeling helpless to control the current situation.

CONCEPT OF SELF-CONCEPT

Self-concept, the individual's perception of self, affects relationships, functional abilities, and health.
- Self-concept is unique to the individual;
- It can be positive or negative;
- It has emotional, intellectual, and functional dimensions;
- It changes with the environmental context;

- It changes over time; and
- It has a powerful influence on one's life.

A person's self-esteem is influenced by (and may also influence) his or her ability to function in the society and associate to others within it. Cultural norms, gender, and age are variables that affect how an individual sees himself or herself. Some of the common causes of low self-esteem include unhappy childhood, poor academic performance in school resulting in a lack of confidence, ongoing stressful life events, and poor treatment from a partner, parent or career, ongoing medical problems, or mental illness such as anxiety or depression.

DOMAINS OF SELF-CONCEPT

Psychologist Dr. Bruce A. Bracken suggested in 1992 that there are six specific domains related to self-concept:
- Social domain—the ability to interact with others.
- Competence domain—the ability to meet basic needs.
- Affective domain: the awareness of emotional states.
- Physical domain—feelings about looks, health, physical condition, and overall appearance.
- Academic domain—success or failure in school.
- Family domain—how well one function within the family unit.

POSITIVE HEALTH CONCEPT

- A positive self-concept is an important part of a client's happiness and success.
- Individuals with a positive self-concept have self-confidence and set goals they can achieve.
- Achieving their goals reinforces their positive self-concept. A client with a positive self-concept is more likely to change unhealthy habits (such as sedentary lifestyle and smoking) to promote health than a client with a negative self-concept.
- A person's self-concept is composed of evolving subjective conscious and unconscious self-assessments.
- Physical attributes, occupation, knowledge, and abilities of the person will change throughout the life span, contributing to changes in one's self-concept.

Characteristics of a Positive Self-concept

Characteristics of a client with a positive self-concept include:
- Self-confidence
- Ability to accept criticism and not become defensive
- Setting obtainable goals
- Willingness to take risks and try new experiences.

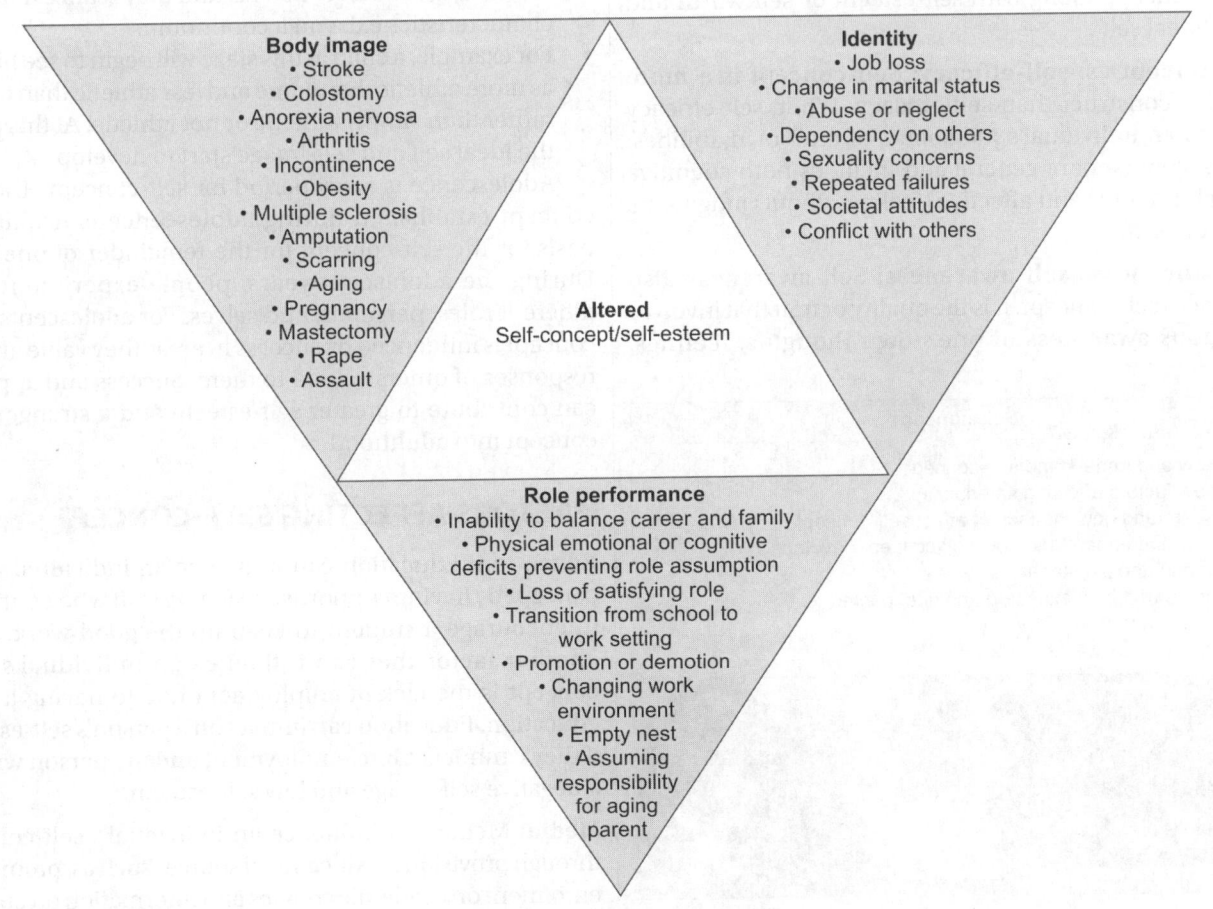

Fig. 25.1: Domains of self-esteem.

Positive Self-talk

Positive self-talk can be used to change negative inner messages to positive ones.
- Send yourself positive thoughts.
- Say the positive thoughts out loud.
- Remind yourself of your positive attributes and accomplishments.
- Recall memories of success.
- Tell yourself out loud something new that you learned or something good that you did today.

Self-concept vs. self-esteem: Self-concept is an overarching idea we have about who we are—physically, emotionally, socially, spiritually, and in terms of any other aspects that make up who we are (Neill, 2005). We form and regulate our self-concept as we grow; based on the knowledge we have about ourselves. It is multidimensional, and can be broken down into these individual aspects.

Self-concept vs. self-image: Self-image is related to self-concept but is less broad. Self-image is how an individual sees themselves, and it does not have to align with reality. A person's self-image is based on how they see themselves, while self-concept is a more comprehensive evaluation of the self, largely based on how a person sees themselves, values themselves, thinks about them, and feels about them. Carl Rogers posited that self-image is a component of self-concept, along with self-esteem or self-worth and one's "ideal self".

Self-concept vs. self-efficacy: Self-concept is a more complex construct than self-efficacy. While self-efficacy refers to an individual's judgments of their own abilities, self-concept is more general and includes both cognitive (thoughts about) and affective (feelings about) judgments about oneself.

Self-concept vs. self-awareness: Self-awareness also influences self-concept. It is the quality or trait that involves conscious awareness of one's own thoughts, feelings, behaviors, and traits. To have a fully developed self-concept (and one that is based in reality), a person must have at least some level of self-awareness.

DEVELOPMENT OF SELF-CONCEPT

- Self-concept begins to develop in early childhood. This process continues throughout the lifespan. However, it is between early childhood and adolescence that self-concept experiences the most growth.
- By age 2, children begin to differentiate themselves from others.
- By the ages of 3 and 4, children understand that they are separate and unique selves. At this stage, a child's self-image is largely descriptive, based mostly on physical characteristics or concrete details.
- Children increasingly pay attention to their capabilities, and by about 6 years old, children can communicate what they want and need. They are also starting to define themselves in terms of social groups.
- Between the ages of 7 and 11, children begin to make social comparisons and consider how they're perceived by others.
- At this stage, children's descriptions of themselves become more abstract.
- They begin to describe themselves in terms of abilities and not just concrete details, and they realize that their characteristics exist on a continuum.
- For example, a child at this stage will begin to see himself as more athletic than some and less athletic than others, rather than simply athletic or not athletic. At this point, the ideal self and self-image start to develop.

Adolescence is a key period for self-concept. The self-concept established during adolescence is usually the basis for the self-concept for the remainder of one's life. During the adolescent years, people experiment with different roles, personas, and selves. For adolescents, self-concept is influenced by success in areas they value and the responses of others valued to them. Success and approval can contribute to greater self-esteem and a stronger self-concept into adulthood.

FACTORS AFFECTING SELF-CONCEPT

Education: Education can influence an individual's self-concept by having supportive teaching staff who continues to encourage a student to keep up the good work. Also, another factor that can influence an individual's self-concept is the lack of employment due to having a poor education. Education can impact on a person's self-esteem if they cannot get into employment and the person will get a negative self-image and low self-esteem.

Media: Media can influence an individual's self-concept through provision of educational sources such as, promoting enrolment on academic courses and information on current situation happening in our society. A further reason that

Self-concept
• To know and understand self-concept
• To know factors affecting self-concept
• To understand how the factors affect self-concept
• To know and understand how self-concept develops throughout the life stages
• To understand how expected and unexpected life events affect self-concept
Name:..

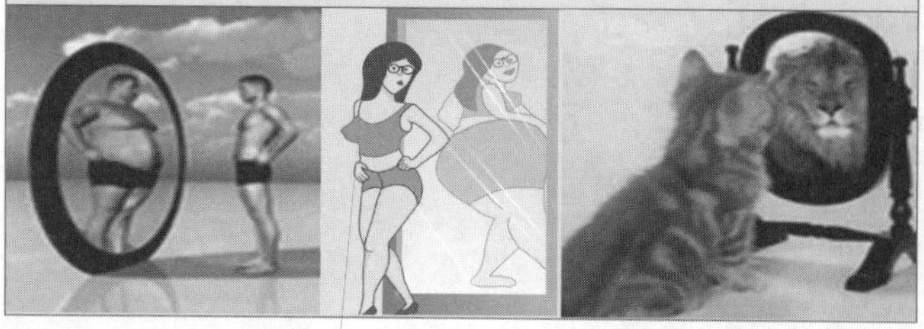

Fig. 25.2: Concept of self and image.

can influence an individual's self-concept is displaying of images of models or celebrities being underweight.

Appearance: Appearance can affect an individual's self-concept both constructively and harmfully. For example, appearance constructive influence will be pictures displayed by sports encouraging individual's to keep up a healthy lifestyle. Further to point, appearance can have a negative influence on a person's life through advertising photos of underweight models and this can influence young women to try to seem very thin.

Culture: Culture is a belief that you have or self values. This can influence our self-concept if we do not endorse other individual's culture. Cultural diversity can have a positive influence if we embrace the differences of others, but if differences are used to discriminate against others, its harmful. Also, this can be the way you were brought up by your parents or a guardian.

Abuse: There are different types of abuse; they are physical, emotional, neglect and sexual. These or any type of abuse can be detrimental to a person, however, abuse can influence a person if they have been neglected and they will develop a low self esteem. In addition, a person has been neglected may feel socially excluded and may suffer from mental health conditions.

Relationships: Relationship can influence an individual's self concept if you do not have a supportive family, peers. This will may lead the individual to have a negative self concept with socialization. Furthermore, having high expectations can also have a negative self concept of an individual, additionally if the person has been compared to other peer groups or siblings can have a negative influence.

Gender: Gender is characterized by being a man or woman. This categorization can influence a person's self-concept of stereotyping job roles for both genders. For example, men should play football and women should stay at home and cook the meals also take care of the children. Finally, I believe that these factors may influence an individual's self-concept everyone should be treated equally regardless of their gender.

Income: Income can influence individual self concept if they do not have enough income they may be despair that they cannot afford to live a normal life. For example, with insufficient low income a person cannot maintain their lifestyle factors, such as paying their rent, afford heating facilities within their home plus have a balance diet.

Age: It can be said that self-concept can fluctuate throughout different life stages, for example also, age can influence a person's self concept during childhood and adolescent development. Through comprehending his ideal self receiving peer pressure. Self-concept is the way an individual visualize them self. For example, Self-concept can be very influential in the way we see ourself; by receiving critical comments by peers or family member, which can cause low self esteem. Self-concept is made up of factors such as self image, ideal self and self esteem.

Health-related factors that may affect body image include stroke, spinal cord injury, amputation, mastectomy, burns, surgical and/or procedural scarring, and loss of a body part or function. Other common physical changes that affect body image involve the development of acne and weight gain and/or loss. According to the Centers for Disease Control and Prevention, approximately 66% of American adults are overweight or obese. These physical issues may add stress and anxiety on the client, lowering their self-esteem and self-confidence.

Illness, injury, and aging can lead to alterations in a person's role. Additional alterations may include pregnancy, loss of a job, retirement, or death of a significant other. How the individual views these changes or losses will determine the impact on one's self-concept. Individuals who view these alterations negatively are at risk for ineffective role performance and a decreased self-concept.

SELF-CONCEPT THEORY

The self-concept theory holds many assumptions about our personal judgment towards our selves. Here are some of them:

- **Self-concept is learned:** One of the very basic assumptions of this theory is that no person is born with a self-concept. Self-concept is believed to develop as a person grows old. This means that our perceptions towards our selves can be shaped and can be altered, and can also be affected by environmental factors. In this sense, self-concept is actually a product of socialization and development. A person may have a perception of himself different from what other people thinks of him. For example, an individual feels that he is generous while others see him as a selfish person.

- **Self-concept is organized:** A person may have numerous views of himself. He may think that he is kind, patient, loving and caring, or selfish, cruel, rude and stubborn. No matter how many different perceptions you have on yourself, still, there is one perception that facilitates all of these insights, causing one organized self-concept. When a person believes something that is congruent to his self-concept, it is more likely that he would resist changing that belief. He tends to stick to his present view of himself for quite a long time, and

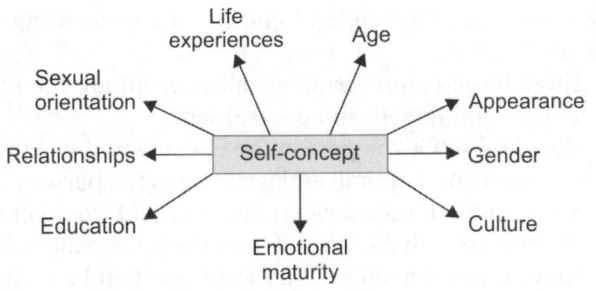

Fig. 25.3: Influences to self-concept.

changing this perception of his self may take too long, but change is feasible.
- **Lastly, self-concept is dynamic:** As a person faces different situations and new challenges in his life, his insight towards himself may constantly change depending on the way he responds to such life changes. We see things depending on our self-concept. We behave according to how we see ourselves in a situation. Therefore, self-concept is a continuous development wherein we tend to let go of the things and ideas that are not congruent to our self-concept, and we hold on to those that we think are helpful in building a more

CARL ROGERS AND THE SELF-CONCEPT THEORY OF PERSONALITY

Famed psychologist, theorist, and clinician Carl Rogers posited a theory of how self-concept influences and, indeed, acts as the framework for, one's personality. The image we have of who we are contributes to our personality, and our actions—combined with our personality—create a feedback loop into our image of ourselves. Rogers believed that our personality is driven by our desire for self-actualization. This is the condition that emerges when we reach our full potential and our self-concept, self-worth, and ideal self all overlap.

Self-image or how you see yourself: Each individual's self-image is a mixture of different attributes including our physical characteristics, personality traits, and social roles. Self-image doesn't necessarily coincide with reality. Some people might have an inflated self-image of themselves, while others may perceive or exaggerate the flaws and weaknesses that others don't see.

Self-esteem or how much you value yourself: A number of factors can impact self-esteem, including how we compare ourselves to others and how others respond to us. When people respond positively to our behavior, we are more likely to develop positive self-esteem. When we compare ourselves to others and find ourselves lacking, it can have a negative impact on our self-esteem.

Ideal self or how you wish you could be: In many cases, the way we see ourselves and how we would like to see ourselves do not quite match up.

ERIKSON'S THEORY

Erikson's (1963) psychosocial theory states that an individual's development proceeds throughout life. Each of his eight developmental stages includes psychosocial tasks that need to be mastered

Newborn and infant: At birth, the newborn does not differentiate itself from the parents. As the parents begin to care for the newborn, their feelings and attitudes toward the newborn will begin to develop the baby's self-concept. The parents will experience a change in their own self-concept. Parental roles are being established, body images are formed in the mother before and after giving birth, and emotional changes will affect the parents' self-concept.

Toddler and preschooler: The toddler needs a supportive environment for body image and self-esteem to develop positively. The parents should provide the toddler with an environment to practice his newly learned skills. The toddler needs to be encouraged to try his skills again (such as learning to walk or potty training) if not successful at first. Praising the toddler for mastery of learning his new skill is important in developing a positive self-concept.

School age and adolescence: The school experience has a major impact on a child's development of self-concept, identity, body image, self-esteem, and role. Parents, teachers, and peers have a direct influence on the child's developing feelings, views, and sense of self. Children compare their physical appearance, academic and athletic abilities, and social status to those of their peers and seek approval and acceptance from this group. Bullying by verbal, emotional, or technological methods (e-mail, chatting, blogging, texting, or twittering) is common in this age group and negatively affects a child's developing self-concept. The school-age child places importance on receiving acceptance and approval by one's peer group to feel included and positive about one.

Adulthood: The natural process of aging will lead to significant changes in a person's self-concept. Over the course of a lifetime, an adult will experience changes in one's roles, body, and identity. Young adults strive to develop relationships, careers, and often a family. Older adults attempt to define themselves by their accomplishments. Major life events in adulthood will continuously shape a person's self-concept, such as obtaining a college degree, getting a job, marriage, divorce, losing a job, retirement, and the death of a significant other. How the individual views and copes with these changes will determine the influence and impact they have on the person's self-concept.

COMPONENTS OF SELF-CONCEPT

The components of self-concept are identity, body image, self-esteem, and role performance. Personal identity is the sense of what sets a person apart from others. It may include the person's name, gender, ethnicity, family status, occupation, and roles. Personal identity develops during childhood from self-reflection and feedback from others. Erikson's psychosocial theory stresses the importance of the family, peer group, and community in forming the personal identity.
- Three basic components of self-concept are the ideal self, the public self, and the real self.
- The ideal self is the person the client would like to be, such as a good, moral, and well-respected person.
- Sometimes, this ideal view of how a client would like to be conflicts with the real self (how the client really thinks about oneself, such as "I try to be good and do what's right, but I'm not well respected").

The three components of "self-concept"
Embodies the answer to the question "Who am I"

Self-image   Self-esteem

Ideal self

Fig. 25.4: Components of self-concept.

- This conflict can motivate a client to make changes toward becoming the ideal self. However, the view of the ideal self needs to be realistic and obtainable or the client may experience anxiety or be at risk for alterations in self-concept.
- Public self is what the client thinks others think of him and influences the ideal and real self.
- Positive self-concept and good mental health results when all three components are compatible.

BODY IMAGE

- The attitude about one's physical attributes and characteristics, appearance, and performance changes as the body changes over time.
- The way one perceives the body is affected by personal identity and self-esteem.
- Self-esteem is the judgment of personal performance compared with the self-ideal.
- The self-ideal is based on personal standards and self-expectations. Self-esteem is most threatened during adolescence.
- Self-esteem is associated with locus of control. People with an internal locus of control perceive that they affect their own destiny, as opposed to people with an external locus of control, who perceive that others affect their destiny.
- Normal growth and developmental changes may influence and alter body image, such as the physical and hormonal changes that occur during puberty and adolescence.
- The onset of puberty involves the emergence of secondary sex characteristics in the female and male client.
- While these are normal expected physical changes that occur during the adolescent stage, these changes will impact an adolescent's body image, thus affecting self-concept.
- In later adulthood, physical and hormonal changes present as thinning and graying of hair, wrinkling and loss of skin elasticity, weight gain, decrease in hearing and vision, and decrease in mobility.
- While some adults accept these changes as the normal process of aging, others may find themselves resisting or feeling negatively about them.
- These changes will naturally cause the adult to reevaluate the image they have of their body and how they feel about it.
- A person's body image will continue to change throughout the growth and developmental life span stages.

ROLE PERFORMANCE

- Role is a set of expected behaviors that are determined by familial, cultural, and social norms.
- People express their self-identity through their roles. Some people take on a "sick role," a set of social expectations met by an ill person, such as being exempt from role responsibilities, being obligated to get well and seeking help.
- Self-concept develops throughout life.
- An infant whose needs are met develops a positive self-concept and develops a sense of self distinct from the primary caregiver.
- Toddlers develop a sense of autonomy and self-image and are self-centered. Positive and negative self-concept develop based on feedback from significant others.
- Adolescents are quite interested in appearances and social status. They cannot separate their body image from their self-concept and are usually self-critical.

Developing positive self-concepts
• Appreciate the abilities and talents one possesses • Positive self-concepts evolves with the moral values that should be emphasised among students • Activities that help: Group/individual presentation, musical performances, stage performances

- Adults gradually adapt to the changes in self-image resulting from physical changes and health challenges, at the same time developing and introducing new roles.

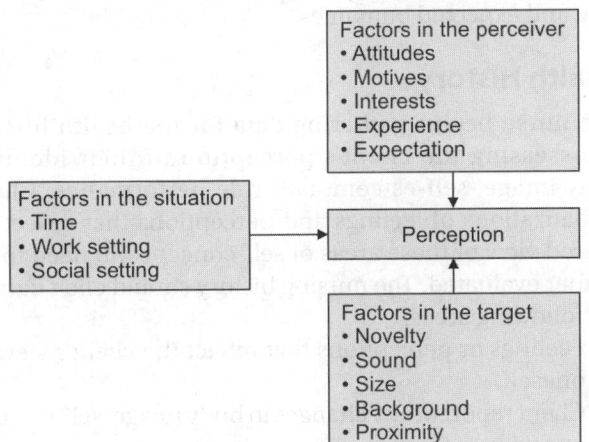

Fig. 25.5: Factors affecting body image.

- The factors affecting self-concept are altered health status from the loss or disruption of a body part; developmental processes, such as pregnancy or menopause; and experience, such as frequently failing.
- Illness, injury, and aging can lead to alterations in a person's role. Additional alterations may include pregnancy, loss of a job, retirement, or death of a significant other.
- How the individual views these changes or losses will determine the impact on one's self-concept.
- Individuals who view these alterations negatively are at risk for ineffective role performance and a decreased self-concept.

SELF-ESTEEM

- Self-esteem is a personal opinion of oneself and is shaped by individuals' relationships with others, experiences, and accomplishments in life.
- A healthy self-esteem is necessary for mental well-being and a positive self-concept.
- This is achieved by setting attainable goals and successfully accomplishing the goals, resulting in an increase in self-confidence, assertiveness, and feeling valued. Since self-esteem impacts all aspects of life, it is important to establish a healthy, realistic view of oneself
- Individuals with low self-esteem put little value on themselves and their accomplishments.
- They feel that they are not good enough and that they are worth less than others and often feel ashamed of themselves.
- They engage in negative self-talk, frequently apologize, and seek constant reassurance. Often this type of person is a perfectionist who struggles with failure.

IDENTITY

- Identity is an individual's conscious description of who he is. A client's identity is assessed by asking the person to describe oneself.
- This description of oneself provides the nurse with insight into whether the client is comfortable with one's identity.
- A client who uses positive self-descriptions will exhibit a healthy self-identity.
- An individual's identity is developed over time, constantly evolving, and influenced by self-awareness.
- Self-awareness involves consciously knowing how the self thinks, feels, believes, and behaves at any specific time.
- According to Burkhardt and Nathaniel (2008), we can enhance self-awareness by developing the ability to step back and look at any situation while being aware of ourselves and how we are reacting to the situation.
- A client needs to be able to identify one's personal and emotional feelings of a situation without judging oneself.

ASSESSMENT OF SELF-CONCEPT

- Assessment of self-concept is often subtle, depending upon the client's developmental level and chronological age.
- The nurse should attend to the client's verbal and nonverbal clues when discussing self-concept, personality, body image, self-esteem, or role changes.
- Determining the client's strengths to better understand the person's ability to form relationships, care for self, and adapt to stressors is also important.
- Possible nursing diagnoses related to self-concept are disturbed body image, parental role conflict, disturbed personal identity, ineffective role performance, chronic low self-esteem, situational low self-esteem, disturbed personal identity, anxiety, social isolation, hopelessness, and powerlessness.
- The major goal of clients with altered self-concept is to gain a sense of well-being and to facilitate growth.
- Interventions to use are supporting healthy defense mechanisms, examining the client's options and resources, ensuring the satisfaction of physical and psychosocial needs, and promoting success.

NURSING PROCESS

The nursing process facilitates providing nursing care to clients at risk for alterations in self-concept, body image, self-esteem, and role performance.

Assessment

Assessment data are the basis for prioritizing the client's problems and the nursing diagnoses. Clients at risk for alterations in self-concept, identity, body image, self-esteem, and role performance require a health history and physical examination. Frequent reassessment may be necessary to facilitate appropriate changes in the plan of care and expected outcomes.

Health History

The nurse begins gathering data for the health history by assessing the client's perception of their identity, body image, self-esteem, and role performance. Client verbalizations of feelings and perceptions that reflect an altered view of these areas of self-concept will need to be further evaluated. The nursing history should elicit data in the following areas:

- Feelings or perceptions that reflect the client's view of oneself
- Client report of any changes in body image, self-esteem, or role

- Feelings of powerlessness and/or hopelessness related to any of these changes.

Physical Examination

A complete health assessment includes a physical examination to obtain objective data relative to the client's health status and presenting problems. When assessing the client's self-concept, identity, body image, self-esteem, and role performance, the nurse should focus the physical examination on:
- Nonverbal actions and behaviors
- Withdrawal
- Lack of appetite
- Wanting to sleep all the time
- Not participating in care
- Intentional hiding, not touching, or not looking at the body part involved
- Isolation
- Interaction with others.

SELF-CONCEPT DISTURBANCE: LOW SELF-ESTEEM

Low Self - Esteem is feeling negative about them, including loss of self-confidence, worthless, useless, helpless, pessimistic there is no hope and despair.

Etiology

- Retarded ego development.
- Reduced role models.
- Shortage of positive feedback.
- Recurrent feedback resulted in reduced self worth.
- Parent child relationship is not satisfactory.
- Environmental disorganized and chaotic.
- And treatment of child maltreatment.
- Family system dysfunction.

Characteristic behavior

- Negative feelings about themselves.
- said self worthless, useless and incapable.
- Saying negative things against the state of the body.
- Complaining is not able to perform the role and function as it should.
- Withdraw from social life.
- Critical to self or others.
- Destructive to others and themselves.
- Talks chaotic.
- Preparing the presence of role strain.
- Easily offended.
- Productivity declined.
- Extreme view of life.
- Rejection of self.
- Pulling away from reality.

- Saying pessimistic in the face of life.
- Themselves not feel adequate.
- Physical complaints.

Predisposition factor: Factors predisposing to chronic low self-esteem is the refusal of parents who are not reality, repeated failures, have less personal responsibility, dependence on others, the ideal self is not realistic.

Precipitation factors: Factors precipitation occurrence of chronic low self-esteem is the loss of some members of the body, appearance or body shape, have failed, and declining productivity.

Disorders of self-concept: Chronic low self-esteem can occur situational or chronic.
a. **Situational:** Chronic low self esteem can occur situationally caused by trauma that appear suddenly, for example, have surgery, an accident, a victim of rape or becoming prisoners and should go to jail. In addition, hospitalized also can cause the lace on the person's self-esteem because of physical illness, installation tool that makes the client uncomfortable, expectations were not achieved will be the structure, shape and function of the body, and treatment of health workers who lack respect the client and family.
b. **Chronic:** Chronic low self esteem usually been going on since long before the pain felt by the client or before treated. The client already had before being treated and negative thoughts become more frequent while being treated.

Both predisposing factors and precipitation above, if someone has a good influence in thinking, being and acting, it is considered to have influenced the individual coping so menjdai ineffective (ineffective coping mechanisms). If the condition of the client is left without any further intervention can lead to a condition where the client does not have the will to get along with others (social isolation). Clients who experience social isolation can make cool clients with the world and his own mind that the risk of violent behavior can emerge.

Nursing Diagnosis

- Chronic low self esteem.
- Ineffective individual coping.
- Social isolation.
- Disturbed sensory perception: Hallucinations.
- Risk for violent behavior.

SITUATIONAL LOW SELF-ESTEEM

Situational low self-esteem is defined as the development of a negative perception of self-worth in response to current situation. These problems can be demoralizing and lead to self-esteem issues. The emotional struggle that patients do to improve self-esteem demands weeks, months, or even years and may require professional guidance beyond the range of the bedside or community nurse. Nurses, due to the nature of the job, have confined and more frequent interactions with patients than other health care professionals. Nursing care can have a huge impact on the patient's attitude and treatment efficacy.

Related factors: Factors or etiology that may be related to the nursing diagnosis:
- Actual or anticipated loss
- Academic or employment challenges
- Behavior inconsistent with personal values
- Belief systems
- Body image
- bullying
- Change in social roles (e.g., hospitalization, assumption of the "sick role")
- Disturbed body image
- Functional impairment
- Lack of recognition
- Rejections
- Society (e.g., social media, peer pressure)
- Teen pregnancy
- Trauma (e.g., Physical, emotional, sexual abuse).

Defining Characteristics

Situational low self-esteem is characterized by the following signs and symptoms. Listed below are the common subjective and objective data or nursing assessment cues for this nursing diagnosis:
- Acts out
- Dependent
- Depressed
- Expressions of helplessness or uselessness
- Hostile
- Indecisive, nonassertive behavior
- Insecure
- Lacks self-confidence
- Negative attitude
- Poor communication
- Poor self-image
- Non-risk-taker
- Self-negating statements
- Shy
- Socially inept
- Underachieving
- Unhappy
- Unmotivated
- Verbally reports current situational challenge to self-worth
- Verbally reports feeling of unable to deal with situation
- Withdrawn.

Goals and Outcomes

The following are the common goals and expected outcomes for situational patient reports progress in current situation.
Patient verbalizes positive self-acceptance.

Nursing assessment for situational low self-esteem: Gather your subjective and objective data in this nursing assessment guide for the nursing diagnosis:

Assessment	Rationale
Invite the patient to record past and current achievements—emotional, social, interpersonal, intellectual, vocational, and physical.	This approach is beneficial in presenting the patient with a more realistic view of his or her capabilities. Patients undergoing situational stress often lose sight of their past accomplishments in handling related circumstances.
Welcome statements the patient reveals about himself or herself.	The feeling of being unloved, unworthy, and incompetent is often expressed by patients with low self-esteem. The patient often presents himself or herself unable to manage the current situation.
Encourage the patient to express if he or she is able to associate these changes to a specific event in his or her life.	The patient may be knowledgeable of up-to-date situations that negatively change his or her self-concept.
Evaluate the degree to which the patient believes he or she is "in control" of his or her own behavior.	Patients may be taken in a vicious cycle of behaviors intended to cover the primary self-esteem dilemma. The acting-out fosters a sense of unworthiness and undermines efforts to esteem-building.
Assess the patient's feelings of comfort and content with his or her own performance.	Patients with self-esteem issues may appear as though their actions are not in keeping with their own personal, moral, or ethical values; they may also deny these behaviors, project blame, and rationalize personal failure.
Assess for presence of unfinished grief.	Ongoing grief may hinder the patient's ability to move forward in life.
Evaluate recent variations in the patient's behavior.	Patients may be able to compensate for low-esteem through exceptional performance in work or areas of special interest while still having dilemmas with how he or she envisions self. Some patients may withdraw from engagement in work or family situations in an attempt to lessen the impact of the situation of self-esteem. Low self-esteem will not be fixed without weighing these issues into the care plan.
Evaluate the extent to which the patient feels loved and respected by others.	Lack of recognition of achievements or rejection by others may contribute to feelings of unworthiness. Care and support by others will be essential in developing the patient's self-esteem.
Assess how competent patients feel about their ability to perform and carry out their own and others' expectations.	The patient may have developed the ability to carry out personal responsibilities despite low self-esteem. This may be a positive indicator of the patient's potential for successful improvement of self-esteem.

Nursing Interventions for Situational Low Self-esteem

The following are the therapeutic nursing interventions for nursing diagnosis:

Nursing Interventions	Rationale
Act as a role model for the patient or significant others in healthy expression of feelings or concerns. Assume responsibility for own thoughts and actions by using "I think" language in conversations.	Patients may want an example of positive measures to display feelings. Self-awareness enables the nurse to show authentic behavior.
Present an environment favorable to the expression of feelings:	
• Spend time with the patient; set aside enough time so that the encounter is calm and deliberate.	Having enough time for the patient conveys the nurse's interest in and acceptance of the patient's feelings. A trusting relationship is an important factor in building self-esteem.
• Provide privacy.	Private discussions need to take place in a setting where the patient is free to express feelings without being overheard.
• Apply active listening and open-ended questions.	These communication methods permit the patient to verbalize interests, concerns, worries, and thoughts without interruption. This technique will convey a sense of respect for the patient's abilities and strengths in addition to recognizing problems and concerns.
Consider the "normal" impact of change on self-esteem. Reassure the patient that such modifications often occur in a variety of emotional or behavioral responses.	Disturbances in self-esteem are natural responses to important changes. Reconstitution of the patient's self-esteem occurs as part of the patient's adjustment to change.
Support the patient in his or her attempts to secure autonomy, reality, positive self-esteem, sense of capability, and problem-solving.	The patient needs continuous positive feedback and support to manage behaviors to promote self-esteem. The patient will benefit from feedback that provides a realistic appraisal of his or her development and strengthens the effective change made by the patient.
Give anticipatory direction to reduce anxiety and fear if interference in self-esteem is an expected part of the process of adjustment to changes in health status.	The patient requires a view that places the change in self-esteem within the context of the normal recuperative process.

Contd...

Nursing Interventions	Rationale
Educate the patient to join in activities anticipated to result in healthy self-esteem.	The patient needs to explore options to improve self-esteem by substituting negative behaviors with positive actions.
Present referral information about community resources, self-help groups, and professional counseling.	Professional and community sources of support provide the patient with more resources to sustain the work of rebuilding positive self-esteem.
Educate the patient about the harmful effects of negative self-talk.	Recognition of unfavorable thoughts can lift the patient to develop new techniques for coping. The patient must replace negative beliefs and ideas with positive thoughts about self.

DISTURBED BODY IMAGE

Confusion in mental picture of one's physical self.

Body image is how a person feels about his or her body and what they do about those feelings. Some may feel inferior about their bodies and try to improve them through a variety of means called appearance management behaviors. As a significant component of one's self-concept, body image disturbance can have an intense impression on how individuals see their overall selves.

A person begins forming his or her perceptions of body's attractiveness, health, acceptability and functionality in early childhood. This body image continues throughout the lifespan and receives feedback from peers, family member, and coaches. For example, a woman may experience Disturbed Body Image during pregnancy. Physical changes associated with aging may result in body image disturbance for the older adult. Personality traits such as perfectionism and self-criticism can also affect the development of a negative internalized image of the body.

Appropriate care for distorted body image is a significant step to recovery. Cognitive behavioral therapy, an approach where irrational thoughts are recognized, analyzed and restructured to more rational self-talk, is frequently used in planning care to address body image disturbance.

Related Factors

Here are some factors that may be related to disturbed body image:
- Permanent alteration in structure and/or function (e.g., mutilating surgery, removal of body part [internal or external])
- Situational changes (e.g., temporary presence of a visible drain or tube, dressing, attached equipment; pregnancy).

Defining Characteristics

Disturbed body image is characterized by the following signs and symptoms:

- Actual change in structure or function
- Alteration in social function (e.g., withdrawal, isolation, flamboyance)
- Focusing behavior on changed body part/function
- Intentional hiding of body part
- Refusal to discuss or acknowledge change
- Refusal to look at, touch, or care for altered body part
- Verbal preoccupation with changed body part or function
- Verbalization about altered structure or function of a body part.

Goals and Outcomes

The following are the common goals and expected outcomes for Disturbed Body Image:
- Patient incorporatess changes into self-concept without negating self-esteem.
- Patient verbalizes acceptance of self in situation.
- Patient discusses with family about situation, changes that have occurred.
- Patient develops realistic goals/plans for the future.

Nursing Assessment

The nurse's assessment of the perceived alteration and importance placed by the patient on the altered structure or function will be very important in planning care to address body image disturbance.

Assessment	Rationales
Assess meaning of loss or change to patient, including future expectations and impact of cultural or religious beliefs.	The extent of response is more related to the value or importance the patient places in the part or function than the actual value or importance. This necessitates support to work through to optimal resolution.
Assess the perceived impact of change in ADLs, social participation, personal relationships, and occupational activities.	Alteration in body image can have an effect on the patient's ability to carry out daily roles and responsibilities.
Assess the result of body image disturbance in relation to the patient's developmental stage.	Adolescents and young adults may be individually affected by changes in the structure or function of their bodies at a time when developmental changes are normally rapid and at a time when developing social and intimate relationships is particularly important.
Evaluate the patient's behavior regarding the actual or perceived changed body part or function.	There is a broad range of behaviors associated with body image disturbance, ranging from totally ignoring the altered structure or function to preoccupation with it.
Evaluate the patient's verbal remarks about the actual or perceived change in body part or function.	Negative statements about the affected body part may indicate limited ability to integrate the change into the patient's self-concept.

Nursing Interventions

The following are the therapeutic nursing interventions for *disturbed body image*:

Interventions	Rationales
Acknowledge and accept expression of feelings of frustration, dependency, anger, grief, and hostility. Note withdrawn behavior and use of denial.	Acceptance of these feelings as a normal response to what has occurred facilitates resolution. It is not helpful or possible to push patient before ready to deal with situation. Denial may be prolonged and be an adaptive mechanism because patient is not ready to cope with personal problems.
Recognize the normalcy of response to the actual or perceived change in body structure or function.	Experiencing stages of grief over loss of a body part or function is normal and typically involves a period of denial, the length of which varies among individuals.
Set limits on maladaptive behavior. Maintain nonjudgmental attitude while giving care, and help patient identify positive behaviors that will aid in recovery.	Patient tend to deal with this crisis in the same way in which they have dealt with problems in the past. Staff may find it difficult and frustration to handle behavior that is disrupting and not helpful to recuperation but should realize that the behavior is usually directed toward the situation and not the caregiver.
Support verbalization of positive or negative feelings about the actual or perceived loss.	It is worthwhile to encourage the patient to separate feelings about changes in body structure or function from feelings about self-worth. Expression of feelings can enhance the patient's coping strategies.
Assist the patient in incorporating actual changes into ADLs, social life, interpersonal relationship, and occupational activities.	The more noticeable the change in body structure or function, the more anxious the patient may have about the response of others to the change. Opportunities for positive feedback and success in social situations may hasten adaptation.
Exhibit positive caring in routine activities.	Positive remarks by the nurse may encourage the patient develop more positive responses to the changes in his or her body.
Be realistic and positive during treatments, in health teaching, and in setting goals within limitations.	This enhances trust and rapport between patient and nurse.
Provide hope within parameters of individual situation; do not give false reassurance.	This promotes positive attitude and provides opportunity to set goals and plan for future based on reality.
Give positive reinforcement of progress and encourage endeavors toward attainment of rehabilitation goals.	Words of encouragement can support development of positive coping behaviors.
Encourage family interaction with each other and with rehabilitation team.	A good conversation provides ongoing support for patient and family.

Contd...

Contd...

Interventions	Rationales
Provide support group. Give information about how can be helpful to patient.	Support groups promote ventilation of feelings and allows for more helpful responses to patient.
Provide thorough teaching and complete aftercare instructions for the patient.	Reinforcing teaching can help patient achieve self-care.
Discuss with patient about the normalcy of body image disturbance and the grief process.	The patient experiencing a body image change needs new information to support cognitive appraisal of the change.
Teach the patient adaptive behavior (e.g., use of adaptive equipment, wigs, cosmetics, clothing that conceals the altered body part or enhances remaining part or function, use of deodorants).	Adaptive behaviors help the patient compensate for the actual changed body structure and function.
Support the patient in identifying ways of coping that has been beneficial in the past.	These may help the patient adjust to the current issue.
Refer the patient and caregivers to support groups composed of individuals with similar alterations.	Lay people in similar situations offer a different type of support, which is perceived as helpful.
Refer to physical and occupational therapy, vocational counselor, psychiatric counseling, clinical specialist psychiatric nurse, social services, and psychologist, as needed.	These are helpful in identifying ways/devices to regain and maintain independence. Patient may need further assistance to resolve persistent emotional problems.

CONCLUSION

Self-concept is an overarching idea we have about who we are—physically, emotionally, socially, spiritually, and in terms of any other aspects that make up who we are (Neill, 2005). We form and regulate our self-concept as we grow, based on the knowledge we have about ourselves. It is multidimensional, and can be broken down into these individual aspects. Self-concept is the way people think about themselves. It is unique, dynamic, and always evolving. This mental image of oneself influences a person's identity, self-esteem, body image, and role in society. As a global understanding of oneself, self concept shapes and defines who we are, the decisions we make, and the relationships we form. Self-concept is perhaps the basis for all motivated behavior.

BIBLIOGRAPHY

1. Ackley BJ, Ladwig GB, Msn RN, Makic MBF, Martinez-Kratz M, Zanotti M. Nursing Diagnosis Handbook E-Book: An Evidence-Based Guide to Planning Care. Mosby. 2019.
2. Barrios V, Kwan VSY, Ganis G, Gorman J, Romanowski J, Keenan JP. Elucidating the neural correlates of egoisstic and moralistic self-enhancement. Consciousness and Cognition: An International Journal. 2008;17(2):451-6.
3. Baumeister RF, Zell AL, Tice DM. How emotions facilitate and impair self-regulation. In: Gross JJ, Gross JJE (Eds). Handbook of Emotion Regulation. New York, NY: Guilford Press. 2007; 408-26.
4. Burkhardt M, Nathaniel A. Ethics and Issues. Clifton Park, NY: Delmar Cengage Learning. 2008.
5. Cappeliez P. An explanation of the reminiscence bump in dreams of older adults in terms of life goals and identity. Self and Identity. 2008;7(1):25-33.
6. Carpenito-Moyet LJ. Handbook of Nursing Diagnosis. Lippincott Williams and Wilkins. 2006.
7. Crocker J. Social stigma and self-esteem: Situational construction of self-worth. Journal of Experimental Social Psychology. 1999;35(1), 89-107.
8. Fisher ME, Moxham PA, Bradshaw BW. U.S. Patent No. 4,813,422. Washington, DC: U.S. Patent and Trademark Office. 1989.
9. Hermann A, Lucas G. Individual differences in perceived esteem across cultures. Self and Identity. 2008;7(2):151:67.
10. Huelskoetter M, Murray R. Psychiatric Mental Health Nursing: Giving Emotional Care. C & E Publishing Co. 1991.
11. Koch E, Shepperd J. Testing competence and acceptance explanations of self-esteem. Self and Identity. 2008;7(1):54-74.
12. Rosenberg M. Society and the Adolescent Self-image. Princeton, NJ: Princeton University Press. 1965.
13. Shives LR. Basic Concepts of Psychiatric-Mental Health Nursing, 7th Edition. Lippincott Williams and Wilkins. 2008.
14. Urden LD, Stacy KM, Lough ME. Thelan's Critical Care Nursing: Diagnosis and Management. Maryland Heights, MO: Mosby. 2006;918-66
15. Wilburn V, Smith D. Stress, self-esteem, and suicidal ideation in late adolescence. Adolescence. 2005;40(157):33.
16. Wright J, Basco M. Getting Your Life Back: The Complete Guide to Recovery from Depression. Simon and Schuster, Inc. 2001.

REVIEW QUESTIONS

Long Essays

1. Define self-concept and explain development of self-concept.
2. Self-concept theory, explain the components of self-concept.

Short Essays

1. Concept of self-concept.
2. Domains of self-concept.
3. Characteristics of a positive self-concept.
4. Factors affecting self-concept.
5. Carl Rogers and the self-concept.
6. Theory of personality.
7. Erikson's theory.
8. Assessment of self-concept.
9. Self-concept disturbance: low self-esteem

Short Answers

1. Self-concept.
2. Emotional intelligence.
3. Body image.
4. Positive health concept.
5. Self-concept vs self-esteem.
6. Self-concept vs self-image.
7. Role performance.

CHAPTER 26

Sexuality

LEARNING OBJECTIVES

- Sexual development throughout life
- Sexual health
- Sexual orientation
- Factors affecting sexuality
- Prevention of STIs, unwanted pregnancy, avoiding sexual harassment and abuse
- Dealing with inappropriate sexual behavior

TERMINOLOGY

Abortionl: Ending a pregnancy.

Abortion pill: Describes the process of medication abortion, which includes the use of two medications, mifepristone and misoprostol, to safely end a pregnancy.

Abstinence: Not having sex with anyone.

Abstinence-only programs: A form of "sex education" that teaches abstinence (not having sex) as the only morally correct option for unmarried people. They don't include information about protection from STDs or pregnancy.

Ace: Short for asexual, meaning the sexual orientation, or spectrum of identities, associated with experiencing no sexual attraction towards anyone.

Acquaintance rape: Sexual assault by someone the victim knows.

Afterbirth: The placenta and other tissue that empty out of the uterus following childbirth.

Age of consent: The age at which state law considers a person old enough to decide to have sex with someone.

Balanitis: An inflammation of the glans and foreskin of the penis that can be caused by infections (including STDs), harsh soaps, poor hygiene, etc. It is the most common in uncircumcised penises.

Barrier methods of birth control: Birth control that blocks sperm from passing through the cervix (the barrier between the vagina and uterus). These include the condom, female condom, diaphragm, cervical cap, spermicide, and sponge.

C-section: Giving birth when a doctor surgically removes the baby from the uterus.

Calendar method: A fertility awareness-based method for predicting fertility in which users chart their menstrual cycles on a calendar. Can be used to plan a pregnancy or as birth control if cycles are tracked over many months.

Conception: The beginning of pregnancy. The moment when the pre-embryo attaches to the lining of the uterus and pregnancy begins.

Condom: Thin, stretchy pouches worn on the penis during sex. Mostly made from latex or plastics (like polyurethane and polyisoprene). Sometimes made from lambskin. Condoms are an over-the-counter barrier method of birth control that also provides protection from STDs with one exception-lambskin condoms don't protect against STDs.

D & C (dilation and curettage): The use of a curette-a metal medical instrument with a narrow loop-to gently scrapes away the uterine lining, and the use of suction to remove tissue from the uterus. Can be used for abortion care or for treatment of a miscarriage.

D & E (dilation and evacuation): The use of suction and medical tools to remove tissue from the uterus during an abortion.

Infatuation: Intense, usually short-lived, emotional or sexual attraction to another person.

Infertility: The inability to become pregnant or to cause a pregnancy.

Infibulation: The most severe form of female genital mutilation. It includes removing the outside clitoris and labia, and sewing the opening of the vagina closed.

Insemination: Putting sperm into the vagina, cervix, uterus, or fallopian tubes to cause a pregnancy.

Intact penis: A penis with a foreskin, also called uncircumcised.

Intercourse: Sexual activity in which the penis goes into the vagina (vaginal intercourse) or the anus (anal intercourse).

Sex: A label assigned at birth of female, male, or sometimes intersex. Also, the act of vaginal, anal, or manual (using hands) intercourse, or oral-genital stimulation, with a partner.

Sex addiction: A compulsion to have frequent sex that gets in the way of daily life, such as work, school, and spending time with family and friends.

Sex assignment: The designation of biological sex-female, male, or intersex -usually made by a doctor at the birth of a child.

Sex cell: A reproductive cell—egg or sperm.

Sex change operation: Outdated and offensive term for "gender affirming surgery."

Sex chromosomes: The cell structures that carry hereditary information that typically differentiate female from male in humans and other mammals. XX chromosomes are typically associated with females. XY chromosomes are typically associated with males.

Sex drive: The urge and desire to have sex.

Sex flush: The temporary reddening or darkening of the skin that may happen from sexual arousal during the plateau stage of the sexual response cycle. It may occur on the belly, breasts/chest, face, hands, and soles of the feet.

Sex selection: The attempt to control the sex of your future children.

Sex therapy: Treatment to resolve a sexual problem or dysfunction, such as premature ejaculation, inability to have orgasm, or a low level of sexual desire.

Sex worker: A person who's paid for providing sex or sexually arousing activities, including phone or camera sex, erotic massage, lap dancing, or striptease.

Sex-negative: Believing that sex and sexuality are bad or dangerous.

Sex-positive: Accepting sex and sexuality as a natural, good part of life.

Sexism: Systemic and individual discrimination against women.

Sexology: The scientific study of sex and sexuality through many disciplines including, but not limited to, anthropology, biology, history, law, medicine, psychology, and sociology.

Sexophobia: Fear of sex/sexuality.

Sexual abuse: Sexual activity that's harmful, exploitative, or not consensual.

Sexual arousal: Erotic excitement.

Sexual assault: The use of force or coercion, physical or psychological, to make a person engage in sexual activity.

Sexual dysfunction: A psychological or physical disorder that affects sexual anatomy, behavior, health, or well-being.

Sexual harassment: Unwanted sexual advances from someone. Includes suggestive gestures, language, or touching.

Sexual health: Enjoying emotional, physical, and social well-being in regard to one's sexuality, including free and responsible sexual expression that enriches one's life. (sexual health is not only the absence of sexual dysfunction or disease.)

Sexual identity: Your understanding of your own sex, gender identity, sexual orientation, and sexual expression/preferences.

Sexual intercourse: Usually, sex that includes penetration of the vagina with a penis. Can also describe penetration of the anus with a penis.

Sexual minority: An individual or group whose gender identity, sexual behavior, sexual orientation, or sexual preference is thought to be outside socially accepted norms. Generally any group/identity that is outside of heterosexual, cisgender, or monogamous.

Sexual norms: Social standards based on a society's attitudes, customs, and expectations regarding sex and sexuality.

Sexual orientation: Identities that describe what gender(s) a person is romantically and/or sexually attracted to. There are many sexual orientations. Some common sexual orientations include gay, lesbian, straight, and bisexual.

Sexual preference: People, activities, or other things that you like, sexually.

Sexual response cycle: A long researched and commonly used framework of human response to sexual stimulation, originally mapped by Masters & Johnson. The 5 stages of the cycle are desire, excitement, plateau, orgasm, and resolution.

Sexuality: Sex, gender identity, sexual orientation, sexual preference, and the way these things interact with emotional, physical, social, and spiritual life. Sexuality is shaped by your family and the social norms of your community.

Sexually transmitted disease (STD): Infections that are passed from one person to another during vaginal, anal, or oral sex, or sexual skin-to-skin contact. More accurately called sexually transmitted infection.

Sexually transmitted infection (STI): Infections that are passed from one person to another during vaginal, anal, or oral sex, or sexual skin-to-skin contact. Commonly known as sexually transmitted disease.

Skene's glands: 2 glands on either side of the opening to the urethra that release fluid during female ejaculation. Also called paraurethral glands or female prostate glands.

Smegma: A sticky, white, unpleasant-smelling substance produced under the foreskin at the glans of the penis and clitoris. It's formed by dead skin cells, oils, and genital fluid secretions/sweat.

Sodomy: An outdated term for oral sex, anal sex, or other genital contact that isn't vaginal sex.

Sonogram: An image produced by an ultrasound that shows the inside of the body. Used to view the fetus during pregnancy.

Speculum: A plastic or metal instrument used to separate the walls of the vagina so a doctor or nurse can examine the vagina and cervix.

Sperm: A reproductive cell that combines with an egg to cause a pregnancy. Made in the testes.

INTRODUCTION

Sexuality is an integral part of human life. Sexual health is an important indicator of both physical and mental health and is an essential component of general health. Sexual health is negatively affected by many factors including physical/mental health status, chronic illnesses, and surgery, changes in body structure or function. The impairment of sexual health paves the way for the emergence of sexual dysfunctions. Sexual dysfunctions lead to disruptive problems that lower self-confidence and self esteem and impair interpersonal relationships. They can also develop as a secondary co morbid condition due to an illness or treatment process whereas they can be a major health problem. For this reason, regardless of their diagnosis, it is important to create a setting in which the problems related to sex can be easily expressed by the patients / individuals who need care, to take sexuality seriously into consideration during the caring process, and to allocate more time for the protection of sexual health in patient education.

SEXUAL HEALTH CONCERNS

Sexual health is a state of physical, mental and social well-being in relation to sexuality. It requires a positive and respectful approach to sexuality and sexual relationships, as well as the possibility of having pleasurable and safe sexual experiences, free of coercion, discrimination and violence.

- **Sexual health concerns related to body integrity and to sexual safety**
    - Need for health-promoting behaviors for early identification of sexual problems (e.g. regular check-ups and health screening, breast and testicular self-scans).
    - Need for freedom from all forms of sexual coercion and sexual violence (including rape, sexual abuse and harassment).
    - Need for freedom from body mutilations (e.g. female genital mutilation).
    - Need for freedom from contracting or transmitting STIs (including HIV).
    - Need for reduction of sexual consequences of physical or mental disabilities.
    - Need for reduction of impact on sexual life of medical and surgical conditions or treatments.
- **Sexual health concerns related to eroticism**
    - Need for knowledge about the body, as related to sexual response and pleasure.
    - Need for recognition of the value of sexual pleasure enjoyed throughout life in safe and responsible manners within a values framework that is respectful of the rights of others.
    - Need for promotion of sexual relationships practiced in safe and responsible manners.
    - Need to foster the practice and enjoyment of consensual, non-exploitative, honest, mutually pleasurable relationships.
- **Sexual health concerns related to gender**
    - Need for gender equality.
    - Need for freedom from all forms of discrimination based on gender.
    - Need for respect and acceptance of gender differences.
- **Sexual health concerns related to sexual orientation**
    - Need for freedom from discrimination based on sexual orientation.
    - Need for freedom to express sexual orientation in safe and responsible manners within a values framework that is respectful of the rights of others.
- **Sexual health concerns related to emotional attachment**
    - Need for freedom from exploitative, coercive, violent or manipulative relationships.
    - Need for information regarding choices or family options and lifestyles.
    - Need for skills, such as decision-making, communication, assertiveness and negotiation that enhance personal relationships.
    - Need for respectful and responsible expression of love and divorce.
- **Sexual health concerns related to reproduction**
    - Need to make informed and responsible choices about reproduction.
    - Need to make responsible decisions and practices regarding reproductive behavior regardless of age, sex and marital status.
    - Access to reproductive health care.
    - Access to safe motherhood.
    - Prevention of and care for infertility.

DEFINITIONS

- Sex is an essential part of person's health. WHO has defined as "Sexual health is an integration of the somatic, emotional, intellectual and social aspects of sexual-being, in ways that positively enrich and enhance the personality, communication and love".
- Sexuality has been defined as the part of life that has to do with being male or female. Sexuality in individual evolves and matures as an interactional process in a biologic environment influenced by family members, friends, and church, and culture, social and school factors.
- Sexual health as defined by the World Health Organization (WHO) is "... a state of physical, emotional, mental and social well-being in relation to sexuality..." (WHO) suggesting a whole child approach to sexual

health education and not merely the absence of unplanned pregnancy or sexually transmitted infections.

SEXUAL DEVELOPMENT THROUGHOUT LIFE

Childhood and adolescence is a time of burgeoning sexuality. Each stage has its own developmental sexual milestones and problems. Understanding of the biological and psychological aspects of sexuality informs of understanding among children, adolescents and adults.

Sexuality in Childhood (Birth to Age 2)

- The capacity for a sexual response is present from birth. Male infants, for example, get erections, and in fact, boy babies are sometimes born with erections.
- Vaginal lubrication has been found in female infants in the 24 hours after birth.
- Infants and young children have many other sensual experiences, including sucking on their fingers and toes,
- The first intimate relationship that children experience is with the mother or the primary caretaker.
- This relationship involves many of the tactile senses and includes being rocked and cuddled, being bathed, cleaned and diapered.
- These experiences may establish preferences for certain kinds of stimulation that persist throughout life

Freud's Oral Stage of Development

- The experiences noted in this section form the basis of the first stage of Freud's psychosexual stages: the oral stage of development.
- This stage begins at birth. During the oral stage, the mouth the primary focuses of libidal energy.
- Nursing infants derive pleasure from sucking and accepting things into the mouth. Should difficulties occur at this stage, such as problems with nursing, the adult may develop an oral character?
- The oral stage culminates in the primary conflict of weaning, which concludes the sensory pleasure of nursing. This stage lasts approximately one and one-half years.

Freud's Anal Stage of Development

- At one and one-half years, the child enters the anal stage. This stage generally coincides with the beginning of toilet training.
- According to Freud, the child becomes preoccupied with the erogenous zone of the anus and with the retention or expulsion of the feces.
- There is a conflict between the id-driven compulsion and pleasure connected with the expulsion of bodily wastes,

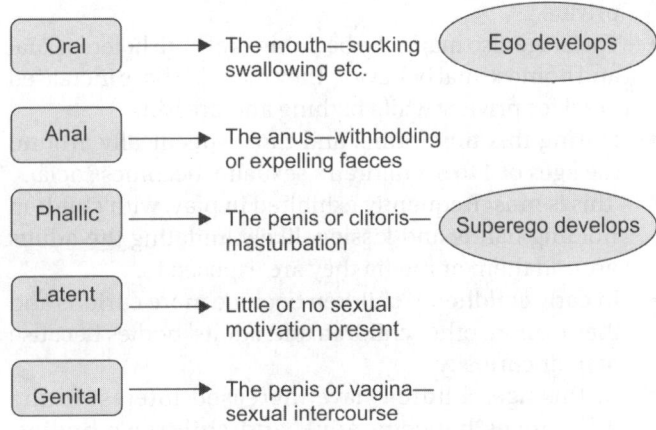

Fig. 26.1: Sexual development throughout life.

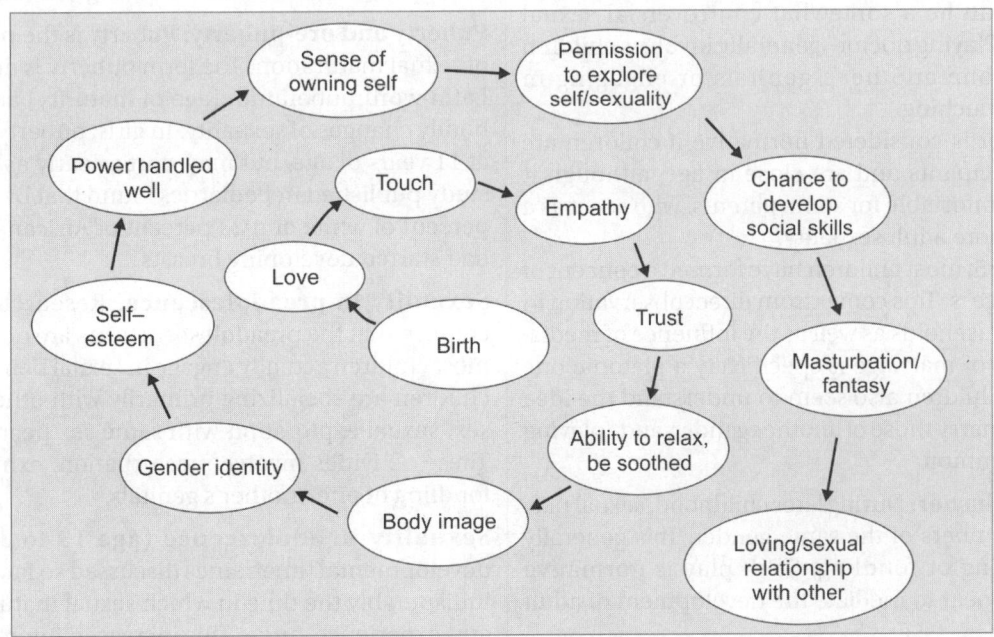

Fig. 26.2: Milestones in sexual development.

and the ego and superego, which represent parental and societal pressures to control bodily functions.
- Struggles around toileting may result in an anal fixation, leading to anal character traits. This stage lasts from one and one-half to two years.

Sexuality in Early Childhood (Ages 3 to 7)

- The early childhood years are marked by an increased interest in the environment as well as an increase in sexual exploration.
- As children become more social beings, their sexual interactions expand from self-focused activities, such as genital stimulation and masturbation, to other-focused activities.
- By interacting socially, children begin to what is socially acceptable and to learn privacy boundaries.
- For example, although the incidence of masturbation continues in frequency, children begin to learn that that masturbation is something that is done in private.
- This stage also marks the beginnings of both heterosexual and homosexual behavior. They may also have increased need for privacy while bathing and dressing
- During this timeframe, and most specifically around the ages of 4 to 5, children's sexuality becomes social. This is most frequently exhibited in play, with children holding hands and kissing, likely imitating the adults around them or media they are exposed to.
- In early childhood, children become more curious and they explore other children and adults' bodies because of their curiosity.
- At this age children have increased interest in the differences between adult and children's bodies. Pretending to be mommy or daddy and "playing doctor" and become more common activities.
- The latter can be a somewhat controversial sexual milestone. "Playing doctor" generally involves children examining one another's genitals or engaging in fondling or touching.
- This behavior is considered normative if children are willing participants and are close in age, although it can be uncomfortable for some parents, who see it as a prelude to more adult sexuality.
- By about age 5, most children have formed a concept of what marriage is. This comes from direct observation in their own households as well as the influence of media. The concept of marriage is specifically a platonic one at this age. Children also seem to understand the idea that people marry those of another gender, and "playing house" is common.

Homosexual behavior: During later childhood, sexual play may involve members of the same gender. This generally involves touching or fondling. Such play is normative and does not appear to mediate the development of adult sexuality.

Freud's phallic stage of development The phallic stage (ages 3–6) of development is probably the most well-known of Freud's stages due to his theory of the Oedipus/Electra complex. In this stage, the child's erogenous zone is the genital region. It is within the context of the child's natural curiosity about his and other people's genitals that the essential conflict (the Oedipus complex) arises. The Oedipus complex involves the child's unconscious desire to possess the opposite-sexed parent and to eliminate the same-sexed one.

According to Freudian theory, the child's identification with the same-sex parent is the successful resolution of the Oedipus complex and of the Electra complex. This is also a key psychological experience in developing a mature sexual role and identity. Freud thought that fixation at the phallic stage causes a person to be afraid or incapable of close love or a cause of homosexuality.

Sexuality in Preadolescence (Ages 8 to 12)

- The ages of 8 to 12 reflect a transition from childhood to adolescence. For most children, it is during this timeframe that puberty occurs. While once thought to be a stage of latency in which sexual drive is dormant.
- Freud saw latency as a period of repression of sexual desires and erogenous impulses.
- According to the psychosexual theory, children transfer this repressed libidal energy into asexual pursuits such as school, athletics, and same-sex friendships.
- Freud thought that it was only with the onset of puberty that sexuality reawakens and the genitals once again become a central focus of libidal energy.
- Although many parents would like to believe that preadolescence is a latency period, this does not actually seem to be the case. Children's interest in sexuality appears to remain active during this time.

Puberty and pre-puberty: Puberty is the physical process of sexual maturation. The term puberty is derived from the Latin word puberatum (age of maturity) and refers to the bodily changes of sexuality. In girls, puberty usually begins at 11 years of age, but may start as early as age 7. A recent study published in Pediatrics found that by age 7, about 10 percent of white and 23 percent of African-American girls had started developing breasts.

Sexuality in preadolescence: Research continues to confirm that the preadolescent years are not ones in which most children actually engage in sexual behaviors. Because children are socializing primarily with others of the same sex, sexual exploration with same sex peers is normative. These activities involve masturbation, exhibitionism and fondling of one another's genitals.

Sexuality in adolescence (age 13 to 19): Of all the developmental timeframes discussed so far, adolescence is indisputably the time in which sexual maturation, interest and experience surge. This increased interest is caused by continued focus and awareness of body changes and rising hormone levels. There is also the cultural expectation that teens begin to prepare for more adult roles through dating and some degree of more intimate contact, which may or may not be sexual intercourse. For both young men and young women testosterone level seems to have an affect on sexual activity. For young men this relationship is very strong. For young women it appears that testosterone levels, rather than levels of estrogen or progesterone levels, was related to sexuality. For girls, pubertal development also had an effect on sexuality

Freud's genital stage of development (puberty onwards): In the genital stage libidinal energy once again focuses on the genitals and interest turns to relationships, specifically to romantic and sexual relationships with peers. This stage spans both adolescent and adult years.

CIRCLES OF SEXUALITY MODEL

A useful model for understanding the various components of sexuality is the circles of sexuality model developed by Dennis Dailey. This model depicts sexuality as having 5 main components: sexualization, identity, health and reproduction, intimacy, and sensuality. Each component consists of several subtopics related to its characteristics and influences on human sexuality. One component of the model is equalization, which is the use of the body to influence, control, and manipulates others.

Sexualization: Sexualization includes sexual teasing, flirting, seduction, sexual harassment, rape, and sexual misuse.

Sexual identity: Another component of the model is sexual identity. As defined by Dailey, sexual identity is one's sense of self as a sexual being and how one may live or is identified. This component of the model includes gender identity, sexual orientation, and gender roles.

Health and sexual reproduction: A third component of the model is health and sexual reproduction, which is often the foundation of sexuality education. The circles of sexuality model expand beyond the basic understanding of sexuality for procreation and include contraception, fertility management, infertility, abortion, menopause, and sexually transmitted diseases.

Intimacy: The fourth component of the circles of sexuality model is intimacy, which Dailey describes as the need and ability to experience emotional closeness to another human being and to have this closeness reciprocated.

Sensuality: Finally, this model includes sensuality, which is the need and ability to accept one's body as an erotic possibility and sexual entity. The components of sensuality include body image, anatomy, skin hunger, the sexual response cycle, and attraction.

The circles of sexuality model are a fairly encompassing model, but discussions of female sexuality should also consider culture, values, beliefs, and historical social constructs. Despite the existence of many positive constructs of healthy sexuality.

COMPONENTS OF SEXUALITY

Its components are biological gender, gender identity, gender role and sexual orientation. Sexual health and reproduction relates to attitudes and behaviors toward our health and the consequences of sexual activity.

- **Biological:** Biological component of all those structural and physiological aspects are included which determine the sex of the baby in the womb.
- **Gender identity:** It is an internal sensation which makes one feels, of being a man or women. It also influenced by social, cultural and psychological factors.
- **Gender role:** It is a behavior, which expresses the feeling of being a man or woman, sexual behavior or sexual relationship.

Four components of sexual identity: biological sex, gender identity, social sex-role, and sexual orientation. Theories about the development of each component and how they combine and conflict to form the individual's sexual identity are discussed. As defined here, social sex-role includes the individual's femininity and masculinity. Sexual orientation includes the individual's physical and affectional sexual preferences for relationships with members of the same and/or opposite biological sex.

CHARACTERISTICS OF SEXUAL HEALTH

From a holistic perspective, sexual health includes emotional, psychological, physical, intellectual and spiritual dimensions. The following are characteristics of sexually healthy adults however sexual health is developed over a life-span, from cradle to grave. Integrating sexuality into one's life in a balanced way is a life-time endeavor.

- Maintains balance between lifestyle and sexual behavior.
- Keeps healthy and comfortable attitude towards different types of sexual behavior.
- Accepts the responsibility of sexual pleasure and reproduction.
- Suitable behavior with reference to biological sex, gender identity and gender behavior.
- Capable of physical and psychosexual responses.

Communication

- Interact with all genders in appropriate and respectful ways
- Communicate effectively with family and friends
- Ask questions of other adults about sexual issues, when necessary
- Are able to communicate and negotiate sexual limits
- Communicate respectfully their desires to have sex and not to have sex

- Accept refusals of sex without hostility or feeling insulted
- Can physically express feelings of attraction and desire in ways that do not focus on the genitals (e.g. holding, caressing, kissing, etc.)
- Talk with a partner about sexual activity before it occurs, including limits, contraceptive and condom use, and meaning in the relationship
- Communicate with partners their intentions for the relationship (e.g. only dating, want marriage)
- Listen to and respect others' boundaries and limits
- Are sensitive to non-verbal cues of others' boundaries and limits.

Relationships

- Develop friendships that do not have a sexual agenda
- Avoid exploitative relationships
- Choose partners who are responsible, trustworthy, safe and giving
- Can be sexually intimate without being physical (ex: talk about sexual feelings, verbally express attraction, do things that awaken desire in partner)
- Can express themselves in ways other than genitally (e.g. holding, caressing, kissing, etc.)
- Take personal responsibility for their own boundaries.

Self-esteem and Self-worth

- Appreciate their own bodies
- Are sensually aware and able to stay conscious in their bodies
- Can touch their own bodies without feeling shame or disgust
- Allow they to experience pleasurable sensual and sexual feelings
- Have the capacity to nurture themselves and others, and accept nurturing from others
- Feel joy in sexual experiences of their choosing
- Know when they need touch rather than sex and try to get their needs for touch met appropriately
- Have a developed sense of self, an understanding of who they are
- Enjoy sexual feelings without necessarily acting upon them
- Accept refusals of sex without hostility or feeling personally insulted
- Allow they to be vulnerable
- Are comfortable with their sexual identity and orientation
- Are becoming aware of the impact of negative sexual experiences such as sexual abuse, and the impact of negative cultural messages on their sexual development
- Are taking steps to address issues that have arisen as a result of past experiences
- Feel confident in their ability to set appropriate boundaries

- Realize that, by working through sexual issues, individuals may heal psychological and emotional wounding from past experiences and damaging beliefs.

Education

- Realize the consequences of sexual activity
- Comprehend the impact of media messages on thoughts, feelings, values, and behaviors related to sexuality
- Understand that the drive for sex is powerful and can be integrated into one's life in positive and healthy ways
- Respect the right of all people to enjoy and engage in the full range of consensual, non-exploitive sexual behaviors.

Values

- Decide on what is personally "right" and act on these values
- Demonstrate tolerance for people with different values
- Are not threatened by others with sexual orientation different from theirs
- Show respect to others whose cultural values, ethnic heritage, age, socioeconomic status, religion, and gender are different from theirs.

Contraception, Protection, and Body Integrity

- Take responsibility for their own bodies and their own orgasms
- If sexually active, use contraception effectively to avoid unplanned pregnancy and use condoms and safer sex to avoid contracting or spreading a sexually transmitted disease
- Practice health-promoting behaviors, such as regular checkups, breast or testicular self-exams, regular and routine testing for STDs.

Spirituality

- Honor the sacred aspect of sexual union
- Understand that sexual energy is not separate from being human
- Understand that sexual union is one way human beings connect body and soul.

CHARACTERISTICS OF A SEXUALLY HEALTHY PERSON

The American Sexual Health Association defines someone who is sexually healthy as possessing the following characteristics, behaviors, and belief systems around sex and relationships:
- They understand that sexuality is a natural part of someone's life, and sexuality involves more than just sexual behavior.

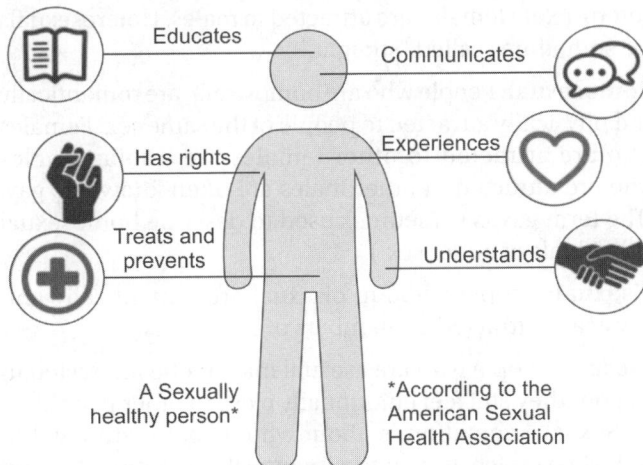

Fig. 26.3: Characteristics of a sexually healthy person.

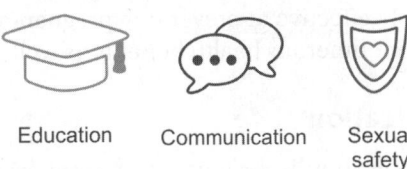

Fig. 26.4: Need of sexual health.

- A person who is sexually healthy can recognize that everyone has sexual rights.
- Sexually healthy people make safe, reliable efforts to prevent unintended pregnancy, STIs, and also seek care and treatment when they are needed.
- Sexually healthy people have access to sex education, information, and resources to care for sexual health issues.
- A sexually healthy person can experience sexual pleasure, satisfaction, and intimacy when they desire those experiences.
- People who are sexually healthy can openly communicate about their sexual health and needs with intimate partners and healthcare providers when needed.

These are worthy goals to set and obtain for people who want to make sexual health a priority in their lives. Not everyone will be able to check off each item from the list, and that's not necessarily an indicator that a person is lacking in sexual health or is otherwise unhealthy. Each person has different ideas and standards for sexual health, and it is an incredibly personal part of a person's identity and behavior. But generally, safety, both physical and emotional, and happiness for everyone in a sexual relationship are the keys to living a sexually healthy, authentic life.

IMPORTANCE OF SEXUAL HEALTH

There are several paths to becoming sexually healthy, and they include education, safety, and also communication with healthcare providers and intimate partners.
- Adequate and appropriate knowledge is essential for healthy practices in sexuality.
- It helps to adopt and modify suitable behavior with reference to biological sex, gender identity and gender behavior.
- It helps to understand and get conscious about one's own sexual feeling and qualities.
- It helps to keep the health in comfortable attitude toward different types of sexual behavior.
- It helps to develop effective interpersonal relations with both sexes.
- It protects and prevents the occurrence of sexually transmitted diseases.

Sexual health is important because it enables people to take charge of their reproductive health, and their emotional well-being surrounding their intimate relationships.

Education

- They will learn about the risks of unintended pregnancy and unprotected sex, and how to prevent STIs and unwanted pregnancy.
- Most likely, they will also learn about sexual abuse, and consensually versus non-consensual sexual acts.
- It's crucial that people continue to learn about sex and sexuality as they age so that they can make informed, healthy decisions about romantic relationships and their reproductive health.

Sexual Safety

- Safety can refer to preventing pregnancy and STIs. It can also refer to staying safe from sexual abuse, assault, rape, or sexual exploitation.
- While many birth control methods are incredibly effective at preventing unintended pregnancy, most forms of birth control do not prevent against the spread of STIs.
- Over half of all adults will contract an STI at some point in their lives. STIs can be spread through vaginal, anal, and oral sex.
- Unfortunately, some STIs do not even cause any symptoms. It's possible to spread an asymptomatic STI to an unsuspecting partner if a person does not use an effective barrier method during sex.
- Latex condoms and abstinence are the only effective methods for preventing the spread of STIs during sexual activity.
- It is important to use barrier methods and get regularly tested for STIs if someone is sexually active. Untreated STIs can cause pain, infertility, and they can even kill.
- Women who are sexually active may want to consider a hormonal birth control method in addition to condoms to prevent unintended pregnancy.

- Birth control pills, patches, shots, implants, and rings are incredibly effective at preventing pregnancy, and they also offer numerous health benefits as well.

Communication

- Communication is a significant part of sexual health. When a person becomes sexually active, it is vital that they communicate with their doctors and healthcare team.
- A doctor can inform of their risks, what types of safety measures to take, and how to prevent sexual health risks.
- Supportive, knowledgeable healthcare officials can also answer questions relating to sexual health, and prescribe birth control if it fits a person's lifestyle and is safe to take.
- Sometimes, people may have a sexual restriction or a sexual health issue. An informed doctor can prescribe medications to help with any problems that may limit a person's sexual functioning and lower their quality of life.
- Relationships thrive when both partners are respectful, and communicate their needs, expectations, and their boundaries.
- A sexually healthy person is someone that is respectful of their partner's boundaries.
- It is vital for their sexual health to be in a relationship with someone who does not pressure them into doing something that makes them uncomfortable.
- For healthy sexual relationships, both partners need to have open lines of communication about pregnancy, and safe sex practices.
- Sexually healthy people will tell their partners if they have been diagnosed with an STI so that their partners can get tested and receive treatment.
- Being in good sexual health means that someone is informed, respectful to themselves and others, and practices safe sex.
- Sexual health also means that someone can enjoy a sexual relationship without fear or coercion.

SEXUAL ORIENTATION

During the teen years, the hormonal and physical changes of puberty usually mean people start noticing an increase in sexual feelings. It's common to wonder and sometimes worry about new sexual feelings. It takes time for many people to understand who they are and who they're becoming. Part of that involves better understanding of their own sexual feelings and who they are attracted to.

Sexual orientation: Sexual orientation is the emotional, romantic, or sexual attraction that a person feels toward another person. There are several types of sexual orientation; for example:

Heterosexual: People who are heterosexual are romantically and physically attracted to members of the opposite sex. Heterosexual males are attracted to females, and heterosexual females are attracted to males. Heterosexuals are sometimes called "straight."

Homosexual: People who are homosexual are romantically and physically attracted to people of the same sex. Females who are attracted to other females are lesbian; males who are attracted to other males are often known as gay. (The term gay is sometimes used to describe homosexual individuals of either sex.)

Bisexual: People who are bisexual are romantically and physically attracted to members of both sexes.

Asexual: People who are asexual may not be interested in sex, but they still feel emotionally close to other people.

Sexual orientation is about whom you're attracted to and who you feel drawn to romantically, emotionally, and sexually. It is different than gender identity. Gender identity is not about who you're attracted to, but about whom you ARE — male, female, gender queer, etc. This means that being transgender (feeling like your assigned sex is very different from the gender you identify with) isn't the same thing as being gay, lesbian, or bisexual. Sexual orientation is about who you want to be with. Gender identity is about who you are.

There are a bunch of identities associated with sexual orientation:

- People who are attracted to a different gender (for example, women who are attracted to men or men who are attracted to women) often call themselves straight or heterosexual.
- People who are attracted to people of the same gender often call themselves gay or homosexual. Gay women may prefer the term lesbian.
- People who are attracted to both men and women often call themselves bisexual.
- People whose attractions span across many different gender identities (male, female, transgender, gender queer, intersex, etc.) may call themselves pansexual or queer.
- People who're unsure about their sexual orientation may call themselves questioning or curious.
- People who don't experience any sexual attraction for anyone often call themselves asexual.

CONSEQUENCES OF POOR SEXUAL HEALTH

Poor sexual health can lead to a host of adverse consequences. Coercion, and also a lack of education or sexual health resources can lead to unintended pregnancy and STIs. Failing to communicate with doctors can also cause long-term physical health consequences. An unknown, untreated STI can cause the disease to spread, and even cause permanent health issues in the patient. Being unable to communicate in sexual and romantic relationships can cause emotional pain and distress, and severely impact the quality of someone's life.

Sexual Health Problems

- Sexual health problems are the result of conditions, either in an individual, a relationship or a society, that require specific action for their identification, prevention and treatment.
- The expert working group of Pan American Health Organization/World Health Organization (PAHO/WHO) proposed a syndromic approach to classification that makes problems easier to identify by both health workers and the general public, and easier to report for epidemiological considerations.
- All of these sexual health problems can be identified by primary health workers. Some can be addressed by trained health workers at a primary level, but for others referral to a specialist is necessary.
- Clinical syndromes that impair sexual functioning (sexual dysfunction) such as sexual aversion, dysfunctional sexual arousal and vaginismus in females, and erectile dysfunction and premature ejaculation in males.
- Clinical syndromes related to impairment of emotional attachment or love (paraphilias) such as exhibitionism, paedophilia, sadism and voyeurism.
- Clinical syndromes related to compulsive sexual behavior such as compulsive sexual behavior in a relationship.
- Clinical syndromes involving gender identity conflict such as adolescent gender dysphoria.
- Clinical syndromes related to violence and victimization such as clinical syndromes after being sexually abused as a child (including post-traumatic stress disorder); clinical syndromes after being sexually harassed; clinical syndromes after being violated or raped; clinical phobia focused on sexuality; patterns of unsafe sexual behavior placing self and/or others at risk for HIV infection or/and other STIs.
- Clinical syndromes related to reproduction such as sterility, infertility, unwanted pregnancy, abortion complications.
- Clinical syndromes related to sexually transmitted infections such as genital ulcers, urethral, vaginal or rectal discharge, lower abdominal pain in women, asymptomatic STIs.
- Clinical syndromes related to other conditions such as clinical syndromes secondary to disability or infirmity, secondary to mental or physical illness, secondary to medication.

IMPROVE THEIR SEXUAL HEALTH

- Education and communication are the keys to leading a sexual health life. There are many self-help books and resources available, and it is important to speak to a romantic partner about boundaries and needs.
- Sometimes, it can be difficult to speak about sensitive subjects to a sexual partner. Shame and negative social conditioning can cause people to ignore their needs or the needs of their partner. In some cases, it can be beneficial to speak to a therapist or counselor who is knowledgeable and supportive of sexual health.
- Talk therapy or one-on-one therapy, and even couples counseling can help people wade through these issues and come out the other side in better sexual health. Therapy can give people the tools they need to communicate their boundaries and expectations respectfully, and in a safe, judgment-free environment.
- It is also important to speak to a doctor about sexual health needs. Many different organizations are primarily geared toward serving the patient's sexual needs. These organizations can help someone choose the right type of birth control for their lifestyle, and also offer STI and pregnancy testing.
- Sexual health is an integral part of living an authentic life. Making sexual health a priority can significantly improve a person's emotional, physical, and mental well-being, as well as enhance their intimate relationships and quality of life.

SEXUAL RESPONSE CYCLE

The sexual response cycle is the physiologic manifestation of the interplay of sexual interest, culture and psychology. it can be initiated by an individual alone as in masturbation or through a relationship with another person.

Masters (1966, 1970) Johnson, and kolodny (1986): Emphasized that the entire human body including the nervous system is involved in the sexual arousal. Two particular responses are during the sexual response cycle:
- Myotonia
- Vasocongestion.

Myotonia: Myotonia or muscle tension, increases throughout the body during sexual stimulation and is controlled by the peripheral nervous system (PNS). During sexual arousal, there is a link between the sense organs of the PNS, Central nervous system, and the output branches, the somatic and the autonomic branches. The facial, abdominal, pelvic, back, leg and arm muscles, which are controlled by the somatic branch of the PNS, all show increased activity and tension during the sexual response cycle.

Vasocongestion: In the circulatory system, vasocongestion, or blood pooling, increase the size of many parts of the body. Vasocongestion occurs in the erectile tissue, where the blood fills specially constructed spaces in the nipples, clitoris, and penis. The shaft of the penis is made up of spaces and cavities like sponge. The blood vessels leading to the tissues dilate, permitting an increased inflow of blood, thereby filling the spaces in the erectile tissue with blood.

Another type of vasocongestion occurs when existing blood vessels engorge with blood these results in increased size of breasts and labia. Vaginal lubrication occurs because there is increased pressure in the vaginal capillaries therefore its size is increased which leads to high flow of fluid in the vagina.

PHYSIOLOGICAL AND SEXUAL RESPONSE IN WOMEN

The sexual response in the women has been divided into four phases:
i. Excitement phase
ii. Plateau phase
iii. Orgasm phase
iv. Resolution phase

Excitement

Vagina: Vaginal lubrication occurs, inner two third of the vagina lengthen and distend, change to purple color, outer third of the vagina fills with blood.

Labia: Labia minora enlarge and became more deeply colored, labia majora flatten and thin, move away from midline.

Uterus: Uterus elevates, pulling on vagina and making a tent or open area at inner third of the vagina.

Breasts: Breasts increase in size, nipples become erect.

Cardiovascular/heart rate: Slows early, then increases in rate, blood pressure respiratory system elevates as the phase progresses, breathing may increase in rate.

Skin: Sexual flush-measles like rash seen on the chest and the abdomen.

Plateau Phase

Vagina: Vaginal opening decreases by one third.

Labia: Labia minora turn from pink to bright red in nulliparous women and from red to deep wine in multiparous woman.

Clitoris: Skin retracts from unstimulated position to inaccessible place under clitoralhood.

Orgasm Phase

Vagina: Contractions begin in the outer third of the vagina at 0.8 second intervals and recur from 3 to 15 times; time between the contractions lengthens and the strength of the contractions decreases.

Uterus: Contracts similar to labor.

Rectum: Rectal contractions linked 1st time with the vaginal contractions.

Muscular system: Release of muscle spasm, some loss of voluntary control, with spasms and contractions of many muscle groups.

Cardiovascular/heart rate: Two times normal, blood pressure increases by one respiratory system third, breathing rate three times normal.

Resolution Phase

Breasts: Loss of nipple erection, slower loss of breast volume, sex flush and swelling around the nipples disappear.

Skin: Film of perspiration covers the body.

Vagina: Congestion in the outer third of the vagina and the vaginal walls disappear in 15 minutes.

Labia: Labia majora return to its unstimulated size, labia minora return to prestimulation color in 15 seconds and pre-stimulation size slowly.

Clitoris: Within 15 seconds clitoris returns to normal position, loss of vasocongestion is slower.

Uterus: Uterus descends to unstimulated position.

Cardiovascular/blood pressure: Breathing and heart rate return to prestimulated respiratory system condition. There is an urge to urinate, particularly in nulliparous woman.

PHYSIOLOGICAL CHANGES AND SEXUAL RESPONSE IN MEN

Excitement Phase

Penis: Erection caused by the blood engorgement, increase in size.

Scrotum/testes: Scrotal skin tenses becomes congested and thick, testes rise higher in scrotum, size increase about 50 percent.

Breasts: Nipple erection and swelling.

Muscular system: Increasing spasm of long muscles of legs, arms and abdominal muscles

Rectum: Voluntary contractions occur, late in this phase.

Cardiovascular/heart rate: Slows initially, and then quickens, breathing may respiratory increase late in this phase.

Plateau Phase

Skin: Sex flush occurs over the chest, neck, and face.

Muscular system: Increased muscular tension in the face, neck, abdomen, and limbs.

Penis: Glans penis enlarges.

Testes: Increase in size about 50 to 100 in size, elevation of testes fully accomplished.

Cardiovascular system: Blood pressure elevates as the phase progresses.

Orgasm Phase

Penis: There is penile muscle and urethral contractions result in actual ejaculation of the seminal fluid out of the penis.

Testes: Contractions of testes, prostate gland, and the seminal vesicles as they collect sperm and seminal fluid and expel them into the entrance of the urethra.

Muscular system: Release of muscular spasm, loss of some voluntary control with spasms and contractions of many muscle groups.

Rectum: Contractions are linked to genital contractions.

Cardiovascular/heart rate: Blood pressure, and breathing increase, generally respiratory higher than in woman.

Resolution Phase

Penis: After ejaculation ½ erections is lost quickly; second stage slower.

Scrotum/testes: Scrotal wall reverts to uncongested state.

Testes: Descends rapidly, loss of swelling.

Skin: Skin flush disappears, perspiration usually confined to the palms and soles of the feet.

Breasts: Nipple erection is lost.

Muscular system: Loss of muscle tension over a 5 minute period.

Cardiovascular system: Heart rate, blood pressure and breathing return to normal The above depict the physiologic sexual responses of both male and female according to Masters and Johnson's phases in the sexual response cycle who has explained clearly about these phases. Subjectively the orgasmic phase is the peak pleasurable experience in both the sexes. Woman has the potential for multiple orgasms and may experience the second third orgasm as the most pleasurable. In man, the orgasm with the largest ejaculate is experienced as the most pleasurable and this is the first orgasm. The orgasms in woman have been described as twice as long as the men's and with greater intensity. Individual variations, of course, do result in difference from these generalizations. The vasocongestion in female is generalized to the entire pelvic area, in contrast to the male's more localized congestion, total volume of the blood is removed by muscle contraction, is greater in female. Another unique feature of the female sexual response is that the uterine contractions in the woman during orgasm show the same-recorded pattern as the first stage of labor, but they differ in amplitude. The sexual arousal in woman occurs more readily during the Luteal phase or the last 14 days of the menstrual cycle. This result in increased pelvic congestion, increased vaginal fluid, and subsequent increased 'interest'.

According to masters and Johnson (1966) interpreted sexual functioning as an interaction between the biophysical and psychosocial system. These systems could rein force or inhibit each other. In an individual who has acquired positive attitudes and values about the gender, sex role, and the characteristics of masculinity and femininity and has the positive image as a sexual being, the biologic and sexual response cycle will be enhanced.

Certain cultural characteristics of femininity and masculinity may inhibit or enhance the biophysical response cycle. Feminine characteristic of affection and affiliation may enhance the sexual relationship, whereas passivity and submissiveness may contribute to denial and suppression of individual sex needs. Similarly, a masculine identity of assertiveness and activity may contribute to healthy acknowledgement and pursuit of a sexual relationship, but competitiveness and independence may inhibit underlying sexual relationship.

NURSE'S RESPONSIBILITY IN COLLECTING THE SEXUAL HISTORY

Taking a sexual history is a skill that the nurse should develop with experience:

- Develop a warm, open, trusting relationship with the client.
- The problems that have been shared by the clients to the nurse should be valued and treated as confidential.
- The individuals need for self worth must be respected.
- The nurse needs to collect a thorough sexual history if a sexual problem is suspected or identified.
- Once the sexual problem is revealed by the nurse from the client, nurse needs to help the client to solve the problem.
- The nurse can do a proper referral to the client after collecting the complete information.
- Effective communication skill, adequate knowledge about his or her own self on the healthy sexual continuum are needed for the nurse to establish a trusting relationship with the clients.

The main important points to be remembered before taking a sexual history include the following:

- Assume everyone does everything.
- Give positive feedback to the individual.
- Follow the lead of the client, that is, listen carefully to the clients' messages about what concerns her or him.
- Avoid using ambiguous expressions like "making love" for vaginal intercourse and be familiar with and use when appropriate the special vocabularies of cultural or economic groups like "prick" (for penis) or "cunt" (vagina).
- Be aware of particular sexual customs and norms that predominate in specific groups.
- Use eye-to-eye contact
- Validate the client's responses by clarifying and restating the question or response.
- Avoid statements like "everyone does that".

The important sexual history components, which must be collected and documented—general, physical, developmental and lifestyle factors:

- Ask for any past history of systemic illness. Example— diabetes, history of STD, e.g. vaginitis, syphilis
- Collect the history of progression of physical sexual maturity, onset of menarche, regularity of the menses, any menstrual problems in female, age of first ejaculation of semen, any history of masturbation.
- Check for any past history of use of contraceptives, abortions, and fetal loss.
- Review of the present illness, duration, onset of the problem and its severity.

- Dietary history: Veg/non-veg, and any tobacco/smoking/drugs, alcohol abuse.
- Past history of drugs abuse (opium/brown sugar/abin/kanja/marjuvana) Any treatment taken for the drug abuse.

Psychosocial factors the nurse should ask for the following:

- Progression through and accomplishment of age-appropriate psychosocial tasks.
- Body image, satisfaction with the physical appearance.
- Self-concept, self-evaluations about gender, femininity or masculinity, etc.
- Past-parent-child relationship, attitudes and values conveyed toward sex.
- Quality of current intimate relationship.

Past Sexual Activity

- Age of first sexual intercourse.
- Frequency of the intercourse.
- Types of sexual contact.
- Number of partners, ages, sex.
- Problems, satisfaction, and orgasmic competency.
- History of sexual abuse.

Current Sexuality Related to Childbearing

- Attitudes, myths, or knowledge related to sexuality and childbearing.
- Change in frequency.
- Change in sexual interest.
- Techniques of intercourse.
- Satisfaction and problems.
- Spouse agreements or differences.

Infection of the reproductive system may be classified as: Non-specific usually caused by a mixture of microbes, e.g. staphylococci, streptococci, coliform bacteria, *Clostridium perfringens*. Specific, caused by sexually transmitted microbes, the most common of which being *Neisseria gonorrhoeae, Trichomonas vaginalis*, chlamydia, herpes viruses, human immunodeficiency virus (HIV) and hepatitis B. Microbes that cause sexually transmitted infections are unable to survive outside the body for long periods and have no intermediate host.

- **Chlamydia:** The microbe *Chlamydia trachomatis* causes inflammation of the female cervix. Infection may ascend through the reproductive tract and cause pelvic inflammatory disease. In the male, it may cause urethritis, which may also ascend and lead to epididymitis. Chlamydia infection is often present in conjunction with other sexually transmitted diseases. The same organism causes trachoma, an eye infection that is the primary cause of blindness worldwide.
- **Gonorrhea:** This is caused by *Neisseria gonorrhoeae*, which affects the mucosa of the reproductive and urinary tracts. In the male, suppurative urethritis occurs and the infection may spread to the prostate gland, epididymis and testes. In the female the infection may spread from vulvar glands, vagina and cervix to the body of the uterus, uterine tubes, ovaries and peritoneum. Healing by fibrosis in the female may cause obstruction of the uterine tubes, leading to infertility. In the male it may cause urethral stricture. Non-venereal transmission of gonorrhea may cause neonatal ophthalmia in babies born to infected mothers. The eyes are infected as the baby passes through the vagina.
- **Syphilis:** This disease is caused by *Treponema pallidum*. There are three clearly marked stages although the third is now rarely seen in Britain. After an incubation period of several weeks, the primary sore (chancre) appears at the site of infection, e.g. the vulva, vagina, perineum, penis or round the mouth.

  In the female the primary sore may be undetected if it is internal. After several weeks the chancre subsides spontaneously. Secondary lesions appear 3 to 4 months after infection. They consist of skin rashes and raised papules (condylomata lata) on the external genitalia and vaginal walls. These subside after several months and are followed by a latent period of a variable number of years. Tertiary lesions (gurnmas) then develop in many organs, and may involve the nervous system, leading to general paralysis.

  Sexual transmission occurs during the primary and secondary stages when discharge from lesions contains microbes. Congenital transmission occurs when microbes from an infected mother cross the placenta to the fetus, often with fatal consequences. Accidental spread of infection may occur by blood transfusion if a donor's blood is taken during the incubation period after microbes have spread to the blood from the site of infection.
- *Trichomonas vaginalis:* These protozoa cause acute vulvovaginitis. It is usually sexually transmitted and is commonly present in women with gonorrhoea.
- **Candidiasis:** The yeast *Candida albicans* is frequently a commensal in the normal vagina and causes no problems. It is normally prevented from flourishing by vaginal acidity, but in certain circumstances it proliferates, causing candidiasis (thrush). Common precipitating factors include:
    - Antibiotic therapy, which kills the bacteria that keep vaginal pH low
    - Pregnancy
    - Reduced immune function.
- **Acquired immune deficiency syndrome (AIDS) and hepatitis B infection:** These viral conditions may be sexually transmitted, but there are no local signs of infection.

NURSE'S RESPONSIBILITY

- Obtain a detailed sexual history.
- Include both partners while collecting the history

- If the any one of the partners is absent at the time of history collection careful attention to be taken about his/her perspective about the present pregnancy.
- Collect a complete history, which will help the nurse to identify the specific problem.
- The nurse should always respect and consider the sexual attitudes and the taboos of the client.
- By giving adequate information the couple will be benefited about the factor affecting the sexuality in pregnancy, postpartum period and about the safe sexual practice during the child bearing period (e.g. comfortable sexual positions).
- The nurse can educate the couple to do the proper grooming and hygiene which needs to be modified during pregnancy to enhance the sexual self.
- Advise to take 2 times baths, adequate mouth care, and use of deodorant since there is increased vaginal discharge, heat sensitivity, nausea and vomiting during the pregnant period.
- Advise the pregnant mothers to wear the attractive feminine clothes will highlight the woman's increased voluptuousness.
- Educate the couples if they wish, to adapt different positions for the sexual intercourse which may reduce the discomfort of the mother for example: side-by-side, rear entry, or female—superior positions may be suggested as an alternative male upright missionary position. The rear entry position (knee chest position) will shift the pelvic contents up it avoids the direct pressure on the abdomen and frees the hands for manual
- Manual fondling and mouth stimulation may be suggested as the alternative to penile-vaginal intercourse
- Touching, caressing, and holding are important alternatives if the orgasm and the intercourse are contraindicated.
- Suggest back rubs; full body massage, sensual stroking, hugging and use of the vibrators are important forms of the sexual communication.
- The nurse should educate the penilevaginal intercourse can be considered safe for the pregnant couples except in the following situations: History of: a. Repeated miscarriage, b. Uterine abnormalities or cervical incompetence, c. Premature onset of labor, d. Premature rupture of membranes, d. Unexplained vaginal bleeding, e. Unexplained abdominal pain.

PREVENTION OF SEXUALLY TRANSMITTED DISEASES

Sexually transmitted infections (STIs) are infections that are spread by sexual contact. STIs can cause severe damage to your body—even death. Except for colds and flu, STIs are the most common contagious (easily spread) infections in the United States, with millions of new cases each year. Although some STIs can be treated and cured, others cannot.

STIs transmitting: A person with an STI can pass it to others by contact with skin, genitals, mouth, rectum, or body fluids. Anyone who has sexual contact—vaginal, anal, or oral sex—with another person may get an STI. STIs may not cause symptoms. Even if there are no symptoms, your health can be affected.

Causes STIs: STIs are caused by bacteria or viral infections. STIs caused by bacteria are treated with antibiotics. Those caused by viruses cannot be cured, but symptoms can be treated.

Preventing Measure of STIs

There are several ways to avoid or reduce your risk of sexually transmitted diseases (STDs) or sexually transmitted infections (STIs).

- **Abstain.** The most effective way to avoid STIs is to not have (abstain from) sex.
- **Stay with one uninfected partner:** Another reliable way of avoiding STIs is to stay in a long-term mutually monogamous relationship in which both people have sex only with each other and neither partner is infected.
- **Wait and test:** Avoid vaginal and anal intercourse with new partners until you have both been tested for STIs. Oral sex is less risky, but use a latex condom or dental dam to prevent direct (skin-to-skin) contact between the oral and genital mucous membranes.
- **Get vaccinated:** Getting vaccinated early, before sexual exposure, is also effective in preventing certain types of STIs. Vaccines are available to prevent human papillomavirus (HPV), hepatitis A and hepatitis B.
- **Use condoms and dental dams consistently and correctly:** Use a new latex condom or dental dam for each sex act, whether oral, vaginal or anal. Never use an oil-based lubricant, such as petroleum jelly, with a
- **Don't drink alcohol or use drugs:** If you are under the influence, you're more likely to take sexual risks.
- **Communicate:** Before any serious sexual contact, communicate with your partner about practicing safer sex. Be sure you specifically agree on what activities will and won't be OK.
- **Consider male circumcision:** There's evidence that male circumcision can help reduce a man's risk of acquiring HIV from a woman who is infected (heterosexual transmission) by as much as 60%. Male circumcision may also help prevent transmission of genital HPV and genital herpes.
- **Consider preexposure prophylaxis:** The Food and Drug Administration (FDA) has approved the use of the combination drugs emtricitabine plus tenofovir disoproxil fumarate (Truvada) and emtricitabine plus tenofovir alafenamide (Descovy) to reduce the risk of sexually transmitted HIV infection in people who are at very high risk.

Nurses Role

- Sexually active adolescents have high rates of STIs and many barriers to prevention and treatment because of

- developmental immaturity, difficulty with access to health care, and need for confidential care.
- Serious health consequences of STIs may occur many years after infection, further compounding adolescents' ability to link cause and effect.
- Nurses who are committed to the challenge of providing services for adolescents to prevent STIs can help by providing access to confidential care and promoting sexual health.
- High-risk youth require intensive preventive efforts. Nurses are in an ideal position to meet this challenge in their roles as providers, counselors, and sexuality educators in individual health care encounters and in prevention programs in clinics, schools, and community centers.
- Effective STI prevention programs should apply theories of behavior change, incorporate adolescents' attitudes and beliefs, and solicit input from the adolescents themselves.

PREVENTION OF UNWANTED PREGNANCY

Unintended pregnancy, defined as mistimed or unplanned pregnancy,1 is associated with significant personal and societal costs.

The role of nurses in primary prevention of unintended pregnancy:

- Nurses has a long tradition of provision of SRH care to a large proportion of underserved and economically vulnerable people.
- Nurses are in an ideal position to initiate primary prevention methods such as engaging women in dialogue about a lifetime reproductive plan, including strategies to avoid unplanned or mistimed pregnancy.
- Additional forms of primary prevention of unplanned pregnancy offered by nurses include education and counseling regarding implantable devices (e.g., subcutaneous or intrauterine), as well as lifestyle modifications aimed at optimizing general and reproductive health and protecting future fertility.

Nurses as providers of secondary prevention of unintended pregnancy: Secondary prevention includes assessment of a mistimed or undesired pregnancy, counseling regarding pregnancy options specific to the stage of the pregnancy, support of the woman's choice to terminate or maintain the pregnancy, referral or provision of the appropriate services, care coordination, and prevention of future unintended pregnancies.

Nurses providing tertiary prevention of unintended pregnancy: Assessment of pregnancy status, including determining gestational age and ascertaining whether the pregnancy is unintended, is the nurse's initial focus. If the pregnancy is mistimed or undesired and the gestational age is later than the first trimester, the nurse or midwife would then discuss the range of available options, including options for termination as well as pregnancy continuation with the goal of adoption and/or pregnancy with the goal of parenthood.

PREVENTION OF SEXUAL HARASSMENT

The most effective weapon against sexual harassment is prevention. Harassment does not disappear on its own. In fact, it is more likely that when the problem is not addressed, the harassment will worsen and become more difficult to remedy as time goes on.

- Anti-harassment policies explain what harassment is, tell all employees that harassment will not be tolerated, and set out how employers and employees should respond to incidents of harassment. Anti-harassment policies should also set forth a detailed mechanism by which employees can make complaints when sexual harassment occurs.
- Provide education and information about harassment to all staff on a regular basis. The circulation of information, open communication and guidance is of particular importance in removing the taboo of silence which often surrounds cases of sexual harassment.
- Develop an anti-harassment policy together with employees, managers, and union representatives.
- Communicate the policy to all employees.
- Make sure that all managers and supervisors understand their responsibility to provide a harassment-free work environment.
- Ensure that all employees understand the policy and procedures for dealing with harassment—new and long-term employees alike—this involves training, information and education.
- Show you mean it—make sure the policy applies to everyone, including managers and supervisors.
- Promptly investigate and deal with all complaints of harassment.
- Appropriately discipline employees who harass other employees.
- Provide protection and support for the employees who feel they are being harassed.
- Take action to eliminate discriminatory jokes, posters, graffiti, e-mails and photos at the work site.
- Monitor and revise the policy and education/information programs on a regular basis to ensure that it is still effective for your workplace.

PREVENTION SEXUAL ABUSE

Sexual abuse can lead to long-lasting, even life-long, consequences and is a serious problem on an individual, familial and societal level. Therefore, prevention measures on different levels are a public health issue. Minors as well as adults should be involved in prevention work in order to prevent sexual abuse of minors in a sustainable way. Besides norms, structures and values in society, the respective laws as well as attitudes and structures should be changed and amended in such a way that abusers and the abuse are clearly confronted everywhere.

- Rescue women and children from unsafe or violent environments and rehabilitate them at a safe temporary or permanent shelter.
- Provide vulnerable women with financial support or vocational training and help them become financially and socially self-reliant.
- Provide legal advice to help victims of sexual or physical violence understand her rights and initiate the judicial process to attain justice.
- Provide counseling and psychological rehabilitation
- Prevention measures are directed primarily at adults and only secondarily at children and youth; this puts the responsibility for the protection of minors from sexual abuse squarely in the hands of adults.
- Prevention measures are implemented in frequent, short, and regular intervals.
- Prevention measures employ appropriate language; it is important to provide compact information that is easily understandable, specific and comprehensive and which does not ask too much of the target group.
- In the case of children, relevant questions include if and to what extent they have had sex education.
- Both girls and boys are equally and equivalently seen as potential victims.
- Prevention programs are implemented by a team representing both genders.
- Prevention measures confront the day-to-day complexities of a specific target group; this means that besides gender and language, culture, religion, politics, status as well as the legal system of the respective state is taken into account.

SEXUAL HEALTH EDUCATION

Sexual healthcare is as important as the care of physical and mental health, yet many primary care nurses are ill prepared to address these needs. A fundamental factor is how you conduct the consultation as this can affect whether the patient takes on board any advice given, and whether they feel able to return for future discussions. The principles apply to all nursing consultations, but the following are particular areas to consider for a sexual health consultation:

- **Confidentiality and privacy**—even to those less than 16 years of age if they are competent according to Fraser guidelines and for each patient if a partner is a member of the same practice.
- **Non-verbal skills**—both yours and the patient's. Avoid appearing shocked or judgmental. Body language is imperative; ensure you appear welcoming. Have a relaxed seating position and let the patient see that you are listening by nodding your head and recapping.
- **Give a friendly, welcoming greeting**. Introduce yourself and ask 'how can I help?'. Advise the patient you may need to ask some very personal questions to assist you in the consultation, and ask if they agree to this.
- **Use demonstration models** where necessary (e.g. when teaching correct use of condoms).
- **Always be aware of potential safeguarding** issues for all ages, particularly patients at risk, domestic violence, child sexual exploitation, patients with learning disabilities and mental capacity issues. Ensure you are aware of the local safeguarding policy and escalation and your surgery's reporting mechanism.

Factors to include in the Consultation and Rationale

- Onset and duration of symptoms—to enable consideration of differential diagnosis.
- Characteristics of discharge—color, odor, consistency - to clarify what is normal for the patient.
- Any associated symptoms (itching, dysuria, postcoital bleeding, intermenstrual bleeding, pelvic pain, deep dyspareunia) to identify if referral is required.
- Current contraception—hormonal methods of contraception are known to increase vaginal discharge.
- Condom use—to assist the risk assessment for STIs.
- First day of last menstrual period—to exclude pregnancy.
- Date of last episode of sex—to identify incubation periods for infection. In the under 25s the most common STI is chlamydia which has a two-week incubation period.
- Does she have a current partner? If yes, is it male or female? This will assist with risk assessment.
- Apart from her current partner is she having sex with anyone else—again, this will assist with risk assessment.
- How many sexual partners has she had in the past six months? For risk assessment.
- History of previous STIs and participation in National Chlamydia Screening Programme—to assist with risk assessment
- Comorbidities including epilepsy, diabetes, whether she is immunocompromised—to explore non sexual reasons for discharge.
- Current medication—to exclude drug interactions.
- Exclude possibility of non-infective causes including retained tampons, condoms, foreign bodies, cervical ectopy, polyps or dermatological disease.
- A comprehensive sexual health history was taken and provided the following information.
- Patient was symptomatic for two weeks with a white-grey discharge. Only when asked about its odour did she confirm it had a 'fishy smell'. She reported no other symptoms. When asked about hygiene and bathing she said she performed vaginal douching. This demonstrates how effective communication skills and appropriate questions will often provide further depth.
- Her current contraception was a subdermal contraceptive implant inserted 10 months previously, and she reported no condom use.

- She had amenorrhea—a common side-effect with this contraceptive method.
- Her last episode of sex was two weeks ago with her current male partner. She has no other sexual partners. She has had this one sexual partner in the past six months.
- She had no previous episodes of infection and no comorbidities or medication, and no reports of possibility of foreign objects.
- She had a negative chlamydia test result 12 months ago when she was with her previous sexual partner.

National Sexuality Education Standards

The National Sexuality Education Standards recommend that an evidence-based sexual health education program include the following characteristics:
- Focuses on specific behavioral outcomes;
- Addresses individual values and group norms that support health-enhancing behaviors;
- Focuses on increasing personal perceptions of risk and harmfulness of engaging in specific health risk behaviors, as well as reinforcing protective factors;
- Addresses social pressures and influences;
- Builds personal and social competence;
- Provides functional knowledge that is basic, accurate and directly contributes to health—promoting decisions and behaviors;
- Uses strategies designed to personalize information and engage students;
- Provides age and developmentally appropriate information, learning strategies, teaching methods and materials;
- Incorporates learning strategies, teaching methods, and materials that are culturally inclusive;
- Provides adequate time for instruction and learning;
- Provides opportunities to reinforce skills and positive health behaviors;
- Provides opportunities to make connections with other influential persons; and
- Includes teacher information and plan for professional development and training to enhance effectiveness of instruction and student learning.

ADVANTAGES OF NURSES IN SEXUAL HEALTH SERVICES

The arena of sexual health services provides an ideal specialty in which nurses can unlock their potential and take on more advanced clinical roles, formerly associated with care by doctors. Some of the underlying reasons are listed below:
- Almost 90% of the nursing workforce is female– clients within sexual health services show a preference for care delivered by females. Nurse-led services can achieve clinical outcomes that are equally as effective as medical care.
- Patient satisfaction with care delivered by nurses has been shown to be equal, or superior, to satisfaction with care delivered by doctors.
- The availability of nurse prescribing enables nurses to deliver the full range of contraceptive care and to provide a range of treatments for sexually acquired infections.
- Nursing emphasizes concordance as opposed to compliance—this increased patient involvement in decision-making helps to empower clients.
- Nursing places strong emphasis on patient education and preventative health care (both of which are important features within sexual health care).

NURSES RESPONSIBILITY IN SEXUAL HEALTH

Nurses are responsible for strengthening the sexual health of the individuals they care for, encouraging them to express their sexual problems, identifying the causes of these problems, making appropriate initiatives to resolve these identified problems, and raising their quality of life. It is necessary for nurses to have the knowledge and skills to evaluate patient sexuality and to be supported on these skills in clinical practice. It is recommended that nurses participate in field-specific courses/in-service training programs and the use of the model be encouraged.

CONCLUSION

Sexuality is inseparable from sexual health and can refer to sex, gender identities, orientation, pleasure, intimacy, expression, and reproduction. While each element of human sexuality is important, all of these components interconnect to make us complete sexual beings. Educators and other human service providers thus require professional preparation to ensure they can meet the needs of their learners, effectively manage programming, and successfully implement strategies that allow individuals to embrace or manage their sexual existence. An inclusive approach to sexual health is best to meet the sexual health needs of all women, while ensuring their agency and control of their own bodies.

BIBLIOGRAPHY

1. Basson R, Brettos LA, Laan E, Redmond G, Utian WH. Assessment and management of women's sexual dysfunctions: problematic desire and arousal. J Sex Med. 2005;2(3):291-300.
2. French K. Sexual Health, 1st edition. United Kingdom: Blackwell Publshing Ltd, 2009;1-7.
3. Haboubi N, Lincoln N. Views of Health Professionals on Discussing Sexual Issues with Patients. Disability and Rehabilitation. 2003;25(6):291-6.
4. Higgins A, Barker P, Begley CM. Sexuality: The challenge to espoused holistic care. International Journal of Nursing Practice. 2006;12(6):345-51.

5. Kinsey AC. Sexual behavior in the human male. Philadelphia: W.B. Saunders; Bloomington, IN: Indiana U. Press. 1948/1998.
6. Magnan M, Reynolds K, Galvin E. Barriers to addressing patient sexuality in nursing practice. Medsurgical Nursing. 2005;14(5):282-9.
7. Martinson FM. The sexual life of children. Westport, CT: Bergin and Garvey, 1994.
8. Masters WH, Johnson VE, Kolodny RC. Human Sexuality. Boston: LittleBrown, 1982.
9. Mick J. Sexuality assessment: 10 strategies for improvement. Clinical Journal of Oncology Nursing. 2007;11(5):671-5.
10. Mick J. Using The Better Model to Assess Sexuality. Clinical Journal of Oncology Nursing. 2004;8(1):84-6.

REVIEW QUESTIONS

Long Essays

1. Define sexuality; explain sexual development throughout life.
2. Describe the characteristics of a sexually healthy person.
3. Explain the physiological and sexual response in women and men.

Short Essays

1. Importance of sexual health.
2. Circles of sexuality model.
3. Components of sexuality.
4. Freud's anal stage of development.
5. Sexual orientation.
6. Consequences of poor sexual health.
7. Sexual response cycle.
8. Nurse's responsibility in collecting the sexual history.
9. Prevention of sexually transmitted diseases.
10. Sexual health education.

Short Answers

1. Sexual safety.
2. Homosexual
3. Sexual health problems.
4. Orgasm phase.
5. Preventing measure of STIs.
6. Prevention of unwanted pregnancy.
7. Prevention of sexual harassment.
8. Prevention sexual abuse.
9. National Sexuality education standards.

CHAPTER 27
Stress and Adaptation

LEARNING OBJECTIVES
- Sources, effects, indicators and types of stress
- Types of stressors
- Stress adaptation: General adaptation syndrome (GAS), local adaptation syndrome (LAS) manifestation of stress—physical and psychological coping strategies/mechanisms
- Stress management
  - Assist with coping and adaptation
  - Creating therapeutic environment
- Recreational and diversion therapies

TERMINOLOGY

Eustress or positive stress: Manageable stress which can lead to growth and enhanced competence.

Distress or negative stress: Uncontrollable, prolonged, or overwhelming stress is destructive.

Adaptation: It is the change that takes place as a result of the response to a stressor.

Coping: A balancing act between biological, psychological, and social process.

Stress: It is a condition in which the human system responds to changing in its normal balanced state. Stress results from a change in the environment that is presided as a challenge a threat or a danger and can have both negative and positive effects.

Stressor: Stressor is they neither positive nor negative but they can have positive and negative effects as the persons responds to the changes.

Adaptation: When person is in a threatening situation immediate response occur. Those responses are often involuntary, are called coping response. The change that takes places as a result of the responses to a stressor is adaptation.

Homeostasis: The various physiologic mechanisms within the body responses to internal changes to maintain relative constancy in the internal environment is called homeostasis.

Negative stress: It is a contributory factor in minor conditions, such as headaches, digestive problems, skin complaints, insomnia and ulcers. Excessive, prolonged and unrelieved stress can have a harmful effect on mental, physical and spiritual health.

Positive stress: Stress can also have a positive effect, spurring motivation and awareness, providing the stimulation to cope with challenging situations. Stress also provides the sense of urgency and alertness needed for survival when confronting threatening situations.

Adaptive coping: Contribute to resolution of the stress response.

Maladaptive coping: Strategies that cause further problems.

Active coping: Actively seeking resolution to the stress.

Homeostasis: It refers to a steady state within the body and various physiologic mechanisms within the body respond to internal changes to maintain a relative constancy in the internal environment.

Resilience: Resistant quality that permits a person to recovery quickly and thrives in spite of adversity.

Alarm reaction: First stage of the general adaptation syndrome; characterized as the body's immediate physiological reaction to a threatening situation or some other emergency; analogous to the fight-or-flight response

Fight-or-flight response: Set of physiological reactions (increases in blood pressure, heart rate, respiration rate, and sweat) that occur when an individual encounters a perceived threat; these reactions are produced by activation of the sympathetic nervous system and the endocrine system.

General adaptation syndrome: Hans Selye's three-stage model of the body's physiological reactions to stress and the process of stress adaptation—alarm reaction, stage of resistance, and stage of exhaustion.

Primary appraisal: Judgment about the degree of potential harm or threat to well-being that a stressor might entail.

Secondary appraisal: Judgment of options available to cope with a stressor and their potential effectiveness.

Stage of exhaustion: Third stage of the general adaptation syndrome; the body's ability to resist stress becomes depleted; illness, disease, and even death may occur.

INTRODUCTION

Stress is a fact of everyday life and it can be defined either as a reaction or as a stimulus. Over the years and with the progress of science many factors have been identified as sources of stress, such as biological, chemicals, microbial, psychological, developmental, socio-cultural and environmental. Stress is normal and, to some extent, a necessary part of life. Despite it being something everyone experiences, what causes stress can differ from person to person. For instance, one person may become angry and overwhelmed by a serious traffic jam, while another might turn up their music and consider it a mild inconvenience. A fight with a friend might follow one person around for the rest of the day, while another might easily shrug it off.

MEANING OF STRESS

The term stress means pressure and in human life it represents an uneasy experience. It is an unpleasant psychological and physiological state caused due to some internal and or external demands that go beyond our capacity.

Body coping mechanism with stress: Each person has his own normal (homeostatic) level of arousal at which he functions best. If something unusual in the environment occurs, this level of arousal is affected.

SOURCES OF STRESS

- **Environmental stressors:** Noise, pollution, traffic and crowding and weather.
- **Physiological stressors:** Illness, injuries, hormonal fluctuations, inadequate sleep or nutrition.
- **Social stressors:** Financial problems, work demands, social events, losing a loved one etc.
- **Thoughts:** Negative self talk, catastrophizing and perfectionism.
- **Change of any kind can induce stress:**
  - Fear of the new, the unknown
  - Feelings of personal insecurity
  - Feelings of vulnerability
  - Fear of rejection
  - Need for approval
  - Fear of conflict
  - Fear of taking a risk
  - Fear of inability to cope with changed circumstances
- **Individual personalities that can induce stress:**
  - Low self-esteem
  - Feelings of over-responsibility
  - Fear of loss of control
  - Fear of failure, error, mistakes
  - Chronic striving to be perfect
  - Chronic guilt
  - Chronic anger, hostility or depression
- **Interpersonal issues that can induce stress**
  - A lack of adequate support within the relationship
  - A lack of healthy communication within the relationship
  - A sense of competitiveness between the people involved
  - Threats of rejection or disapproval between people
  - Struggle for power and control in the relationship
  - Poor intimacy or sexuality within the relationship
  - Over dependency of one person on another
- **System (family, job, school, club, organization issues that can induce stress)**
  - Lack of leadership
  - Unco-operative atmosphere
  - Competitive atmosphere
  - Autocratic leadership
  - Lack of team work
  - Confused communication.

SYMPTOMS OF STRESS

Symptoms of stress appear in many forms. Some symptoms only impact the person who is directly experiencing stress, while other symptoms may have an impact on our relationship with others.

Physical Symptoms

- Muscle tension
- Colds or other illnesses
- High blood pressure
- Rapid breathing or pounding of the heart
- Indigestion
- Ulcers
- Difficulty in sleeping
- Fatigue
- Headaches back or neck problems
- Increased smoking or drinking alcohol
- Backaches
- Being more prone to accidents.

Cognitive Symptoms

- Forgetfulness
- Unwanted or repetitive thoughts
- Difficulty in concentration
- Fear of failure
- Self criticism.

Emotional Symptoms

- Irritability
- Depression
- Anger

- Fear or anxiety
- Feeling overwhelmed
- Mood swings.

Behavioral Symptoms

- Eating more or less
- Sleeping too much or too little
- Withdrawing from others
- Procrastinating or neglecting responsibilities
- Using alcohol, cigarettes, or drugs to relax
- Nervous habits (e.g. nail biting, pacing).

TYPES OF STRESS

Acute stress: Sometimes stress can be brief, and specific to the demands and pressures of a particular situation, such as a deadline, a performance or facing up to a difficult challenge or traumatic event. This type of stress often gets called acute stress.

Episodic acute stress: Some people seem to experience acute stress over and over. This is sometimes referred to as episodic acute stress. These kind of repetitive stress episodes may be due to a series of very real stressful challenges, for example, losing a job, then developing health problems, followed by difficulties for a child in the school setting. For some people, episodic acute stress is a combination of real challenges and a tendency to operate like a 'stress machine'. Some people tend to worry endlessly about bad things that could happen, are frequently in a rush and impatient with too many demands on their time, which can contribute to episodic acute stress.

Chronic stress: The third type of stress is called chronic stress. This involves ongoing demands, pressures and worries that seem to go on forever, with little hope of letting up. Chronic stress is very harmful to people's health and happiness. Even though people can sometimes get used to chronic stress, and may feel they do not notice it so much, it continues to wear people do.

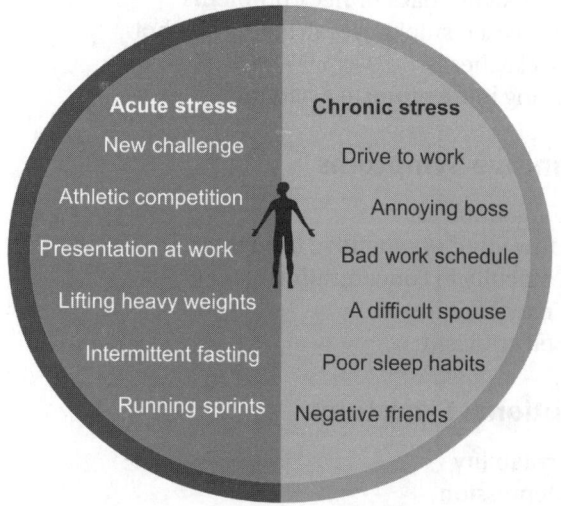

Fig. 27.1: Difference between acute and chronic sex.

Physical stress: A common type of stress is physical stress, which refers to actual physical activities and events that wreak havoc on the human body. One good example is travel. Traveling frequently can send you to different time zones, which makes sleeping and waking difficult. Physical stress also includes stress brought on by sleeping too much, not getting enough sleep, spending too many hours on your feet or working long hours. If you ever spent a day chasing your kids around an amusement park or stuck in an airport and dealing with flight delays, you have likely experienced physical stress.

Emotional stress: Out of all the different kinds of stress, emotional stress is the most common. This can occur after you go through an intense break up or divorce, lose a loved one, have a fight with your spouse or experience any other problem that causes you to feel depressed or anxious. Emotional stress often manifests in the same way that depression does. You may experience weight changes, changes in how you fall asleep or how long you sleep, feelings of isolation and mood swings. Emotional stress can also occur when you feel overwhelmed at home or at work.

Traumatic stress: When thinking about the types of stress, many people don't think about traumatic stress. Traumatic stress is a type of stress that occurs because of some type of trauma to the human body and may lead to intense pain, coma or even death. It often relates to some kind of physical change that occurs. If you went through an operation, your body may experience stress until you recover from that surgery. A car accident, second or third degree burns or even a case of pneumonia may all cause traumatic stress.

TYPES OF STRESSORS

A stressor is anything that causes the release of stress hormones. There are two broad categories of stressors: physiological (or physical) stressors and psychological stressors.

Physiological (or physical) stressors: These are stressors that put strain on our body (i.e.: very cold/hot temperatures, injury, chronic illness, or pain).

Psychological stressors: These are events, situations, individuals, comments, or anything we interpret as negative or threatening (i.e.: not being able to find a babysitter for your sick child when you cannot take time off work).

Absolute stressors: These are stressors that everyone exposed to them would interpret as being stressful. These are objective stressors that are universal (i.e.: earthquakes, a tsunami, or the events of September 11th 2001).

Relative stressors: These are stressors that only some exposed to them would interpret as being stressful. These are subjective stressors that cause different reactions in different people (i.e. time pressure at work, traffic, paying taxes, writing an exam).

Acute time-limited stressors: Acute time-limited stressors are ones given in a controlled environment such as a lab.

If you are part of a study, the tech may present you with a stimulus that causes some level of anxiety for you. This could be presenting you with something that you have a phobia of or making you do something you don't feel comfortable doing. The stressor sparks intense stress but only for the time it takes to illicit a response.

Brief naturalistic stressors: Brief naturalistic stressors are ones that occur naturally in your environment such as taking a test. The stress you experience usually only lasts for the time you are in the stressful situation.

Stressful events sequences: Stressful events sequences happen when there is a traumatic event that causes additional stressors. An example of this is if you are a victim of a natural disaster and then have to deal with the loss of loved ones, belongings, and pulling your life back together.

Chronic stressors: Chronic stressors are situations that happen that force you to change your identity or social roles. If you become disabled, you will need to adjust your life to accommodate your disabilities.

Distant Stressors: Distant stressors are stress that happened a long time ago but continue to affect your immune system negatively because of emotional and cognitive issues. Some examples of distant stressors include—child abuse, prisoner of war and loss of a loved one.

GENERAL ADAPTATION SYNDROME (HANS SELYE, 1945)

Homeostatic mechanisms are aimed at counteracting the everyday stress of living. If they are successful, the internal environment maintains normal physiological limits of temperature, chemistry and pressure. If stress is extreme or long lasting, the normal mechanisms may not be sufficient. In this case, the stress triggers a wide-ranging set of bodily changes called general adaptation syndrome (GAS). When stress appears, it stimulates the hypothalamus to initiate the GAS through two pathways:
- The first pathway is stimulation of the sympathetic division of the autonomic nervous system and adrenal medulla. This produces an immediate set of responses called the alarm reaction.
- The second pathway, called the resistance reaction involves the anterior pituitary gland and adrenal cortex; the resistance reaction is slower to start, but its effects last longer.

Alarm reaction: The alarm reaction or fight-or-flight response is the body's initial reaction to a stressor. It is a set of reactions initiated when the hypothalamus stimulates the sympathetic division of the autonomic nervous system, and the adrenal medulla. The alarm reaction is meant to counteract a danger by mobilizing the body's resources for immediate physical activity. The stress responses which characterize the alarm reaction include the following:
- Heart rate and strength of cardiac muscle contraction increases; this circulates blood quickly to areas where it is needed to fight the stress.
- Blood vessels supplying skin and viscera, except heart and lungs, constrict; at the same time blood vessels supplying skeletal muscles and brain dilate; these responses route more blood to organs active in the stress responses, thus decreasing blood supply to organs which do not assume an immediate active role.
- RBC production is increased leading to an increase in the ability of the blood to clot. This helps control bleeding.
- Liver converts glycogen into glucose and releases it into the bloodstream; this provides the energy needed to fight the stressor.
- The rate of breathing increases and respiratory passages widen to accommodate more air; this enables body to acquire more oxygen.
- Production of saliva and digestive enzymes reduces. This reaction takes place as digestive activity is not essential for counteracting stress.

Resistance Reaction

- The resistance reaction is the second stage in the stress response. It is initiated by regulating hormones secreted by the hypothalamus, and is a long-term reaction. These regulating hormones are corticotropin releasing hormone (CRH), growth hormone releasing hormone (GHRH) and thyrotropin releasing hormone (TRH).
- CRH stimulates the anterior pituitary to increase its secretion of Adrenocorticotropic hormone (ACTH). ACTH stimulates the adrenal cortex to secrete more of its hormones. The action of these hormones helps to control bleeding, maintain blood pressure, etc.
- GHRH stimulates the anterior pituitary to secrete human growth hormone (HGH). TRH causes the anterior pituitary to secrete thyroid-stimulating hormone (TSH). The combined actions of (HGH) and TSH help to supply additional energy to the body.
- The resistance reaction allows the body to continue fighting a stressor for a long time. Thus it helps us to meet emotional crisis, perform strenuous tasks, fight infection, or resist the threat of bleeding to death.
- Generally, the resistance reaction is successful in helping us cope with a stressful situation, and our bodies then return to normal. Occasionally it fails to fight the stressor, especially if it is too severe or long-lasting. In this case, the general adaptation syndrome (GAS) moves into the stage of exhaustion.

Exhaustion stage: At this stage, the cells start to die, and the organs weaken. A long-term resistance reaction puts heavy demand on the body, particularly on the heart, blood vessels and adrenal cortex, which may suddenly fail under the strain. In this respect, ability to handle stressors is to a large extent determined by the general health.

LOCAL ADAPTATION SYNDROME

According to Selye's theory, a local adaptation syndrome (LAS) occurs and includes the inflammatory response and repair processes that occur in the local site tissue injury. The syndrome occurs in small, topical injuries, such as contact dermatitis. If the local injury is severe enough, the general adaptation syndrome is activated as well. Local adaptation syndrome involves only in specific body part only, or the local site injury.

Selye emphasized that stress is the nonspecific response common to all stressors, whether they are physiologic, psychological or social design. For example, if you put your hand on a hot stove, a reflex causes you to immediately remove your hand before a "Hey, this is hot!" message even gets to your brain.

Physiologic homeostasis: Local adaptation system (LAS) involves only one specific body part:
- Reflex pain response
- Inflammatory response
- Reflex response occurs when the body responds to a stimulus without the involvement of the brain.
- Is an involuntary or automatic, action that your body does in response to something-without you even having to think.

STRATEGIES OF STRESS MANAGEMENT

- **Take a deep breath:** When you feel 'uptight' try taking a minute to slow down and breathe deeply. Breathe in through your nose and out through your mouth. Try to inhale enough so that your lower abdomen rises and falls. Count as you exhale slowly.
- **Practice specific relaxation techniques:** Relaxation techniques are extremely valuable tools in stress management. Most of the techniques like meditation, self hypnosis, and deep muscle relaxation work in a similar fashion. In this state both the body and the mind are at rest and the outside world is screened out for a time period. The practice of one of these techniques on a regular basis can provide a wonderfully calming and relaxing feeling that seems to have a lasting effect for many people.
- **Manage time:** One of the greatest sources of stress is poor time management. Give priority to the most important ones and do those first. If a particularly unpleasant task faces you, tackle it early in the day and get over with it; the rest of your day will include much less anxiety. Most importantly, do not overwork yourself, schedule time for both work and recreation.
- **Connect with others:** A good way to combat sadness, boredom and loneliness is to see out activities involving others.
- **Talk it out:** When you feel something, try to express it. Share your feelings. "Bottled up" emotions increase frustration and stress. Talking with someone else can help clear your mind of confusion so that you can focus on problem solving. Also consider writing down thoughts and feelings. Putting problems on paper can assist you in clarifying the situation and allow you a new perspective.
- **Take a "minute" vacation:** Imagining a quiet country scene can take you out of the turmoil of a stressful situation. When you have the opportunity, take a moment to close your eyes and imagine a place where you feel relaxed and comfortable. Notice all the details of your chosen place, including pleasant sounds, smells and temperature or change your mental "channel" by reading a good book or playing relaxing music to create a sense of peace and tranquility.
- **Monitor your physical comfort:** Wear comfortable clothing. If it is too hot, go somewhere where it is not. If your chair is uncomfortable, change it. If your computer screen causes eye-strain or backaches, change that, too. Don't wait until your discomfort turns into a real problem. Taking five minutes to arrange back support can save you several days of back pain.
- **Get physical:** When you feel nervous, angry or upset, release the pressure through exercise or physical activity. Running, walking or swimming are good options for some people, while others prefer dance or martial arts. Working in the garden, washing your car, or playing with children can relieve that "uptight" feeling, relax you and often will actually energize you. Remember, your body and mind work together. Most experts recommend doing 20 minutes of aerobic activity daily will reduce stress.
- **Take care of your body:** Healthy eating and adequate sleep fuels your mind as well as your body. Avoid consuming too much caffeine and sugar. Take time to eat breakfast in the morning, it really will help keep going through the day. Well-nourished bodies are better prepared to cope with stress, if you are irritable and tense from lack of sleep or not eating right, you will be less able to "go the distance in dealing with stressful situations". Increase the amount of fruits and vegetables in daily diet. Take time for personal interests and hobbies. Listen to one's body.
- **Laugh:** Maintain your sense of humor, including the ability to laugh at yourself.
- **Know your limits:** There are many circumstances in life beyond your control, consider the fact that we live in an imperfect world. Know your limits. If a problem is beyond your control and cannot be changed at the moment, don't fight the situation. Learn to accept what is, for now, until such time when you can change things.
- **Think positively:** Refocus the negative to be positive. Make an effort to stop negative thoughts.
- **Clarify:** Clarify your values and develop a sense of life meaning. Clarify your values and deciding what you really want out of your life, can help you feel better about yourself and have that sense of satisfaction and centeredness that helps you deal with the stresses of life. A sense of spirituality can help with this.
- **Compromise:** Consider cooperation or compromise rather than confrontation. A little give and take on both sides may reduce the strain and help you feel more comfortable.

- **Have a good cry:** A good cry during periods of stress can be a healthy way to bring relief to your anxiety, and it might prevent a headache or other physical consequences of "bottling" things up.
- **Avoid self-medication:** Alcohol and other drugs do not remove the conditions that cause stress. Although they may seem to offer temporary relief, these substances only mask or disguise problems. In the long run, alcohol use increases rather than decreases stress, by changing the way you think and solve problems and by impairing your judgment and other cognitive capacities. Medications should be taken only on the advice of a doctor.
- **Look for the "pieces of gold" around you:** Pieces of gold are positive or enjoyable moments or interactions. These may seem like small events but as these "pieces of gold" accumulate they can often provide a big lift to energy and spirits and help you begin to see things in new, more balanced way.

ROLE OF NURSE IN STRESS MANAGEMENT

Assessment of the person: Assess for the following characteristics in the individual. Such individuals are at high risk of developing stress-related disorders:
- Rigid and self-punishing moral standards
- High and unrealistic expectations
- Too much dependence on others for love and affection and approval
- Inability to master change or learn new ways of dealing with frustration
- Easily prone to extreme emotional responses of fear, anxiety and depression
- Type A personality persons

In addition, the presence of stressful life events such as births, deaths, marriages, divorces, retirement, economic success or failure, etc can predispose the person to stress-related illnesses.

Assessment of the family: Assess the family's perception of the problem, and whether it is supportive of the client's efforts at coping.

Assessment of the environment: Occupations with a high degree of stress; adverse environmental influences like too much of lighting, temperature, etc.

Nursing Intervention for Stress Management

Interventions are directed towards relief of acute or chronic stress. A nurse can help the person to examine the situation, identify possible solutions and accept his feelings without guilt or fear. People suffering from acute stress-related illnesses often need to change their lifestyles and ways of relating to others. The initial work of the nurse involves helping the client to recognize that change is essential, and develop clear personal objective in relation to the change. Some clients may show resistance to a necessary change. In such cases, nursing measures include:

- Increasing the client's awareness as an actual or potential health problem exists.
- Helping him realize that the health problem can increase if personal changes do not occur.
- Identifying all possible resources (his family, friends etc.). To support the client through the process of change, and cooperation with the treatment.
- When the client becomes aware of the nature of the health problem and is told of the change needed, he often experiences a feeling of anxiety, depression and anger. The client is encouraged to talk about the losses that have resulted from the behavior change. Recognizing this grieving process provides the nurse with clear direction as to how she can help the client.
- Family members also need accurate information about the nature of the disorder, and how they can help the client in coping with stress. The client and families also need to be informed about various alternatives such as meditation, yoga, relaxation training etc. These techniques have a valuable role to play in helping individuals cope with stressful life events.
- In all this, the nurse must always bear in mind that they are only facilitators of the change process, and the clients have the rights and responsibilities in relation to change.

ADAPTATION

Adaptation is the process by which an organism makes itself suitable to live in a particular environment. Human beings are the most intelligent of all organisms, and due to his high degree of intelligence, and other capacities, he is able to make better adaptation to the environment.

Levels of adaptation: There are three levels of adaptation namely:

1. **Physical adaptation:** By physical adaptation is meant adjustment to the physical environment. This adaptation is not voluntary because, physical conditions are inevitable and organism has to make adjustment in order to survive. Physical adaptation remains with all its compulsions.
2. **Biological adaptation:** Every organism is adapted to live in a particular environment. If they are taken out of the environment, life or even survival may be difficult. Human beings are capable of making adaptation in this area also. For example, a person adapted to hot climate will try to make adjustments even in cold climate by making adaptations.
3. **Social adaptation:** Social adaptation is the process of adjusting to sociocultural environment. Human beings are capable of not only adapting to the environment, but also making adaptations to suit his needs.

Every human being is continuously involved in this process of social adaptation. Social adaptation begins with a newborn has first to adapt himself to the new environment the child learns the meaning of gestures. The skill of language is slowly acquired. He learns to communicate with others around.

Environment and adaptation: The environment in which human beings live may be favorable or unfavorable. For example, fertile land, availability of water, moderate climate, presence of natural resources, etc. are favorable conditions in the natural environment, whereas mountainous land, extreme climate, natural calamities like flood, famine and earthquake, lack of natural resources, etc. are un-favorable natural conditions. Similarly, in the social situation also, a person may find favorable or unfavorable conditions. A happy home, responsible parents, healthy neighborhood, good friends, etc. are all favorable social situations, whereas poverty, death of parents, slum dwelling/Criminal neighborhoods are unfavorable social conditions.

CONCEPT OF CRISIS AND RESOLUTION

Crisis can be viewed as an integral component of everyday life situations. A crisis may influence people's lives in different ways. As a consequence of a crisis experience, the individual may go down to a lower or less healthy level of functioning than what was before, the crisis, or he may resume the same level of functioning by repressing the crisis and the related emotions. On the other hand, he may function at a healthier level than prior to the crisis, because the challenge of a crisis can bring out new strengths, skills and coping mechanisms.

Intervention at a crisis is extremely important to prevent mental illness, because long-standing problems make the person totally incapable of handling the situation. If proper guidance is provided at the correct time, the victim will come out of it better equipped to handle future problems in life.

Definition: Crisis is a state of disequilibrium resulting from the interaction of an event with the individual's or family's coping mechanisms, which are inadequate to meet the demands of the situation, combined with the individual's or family's perception of the meaning of the event (Taylor 1982).

Crisis response: Hendricks (1985) suggests that certain individuals are more prone to crisis than others. The following are characteristics often found in individuals who are regarded as being more susceptible to crisis:
- Dissatisfaction with employment or lack of employment.
- History of unresolved crisis.
- History of substance abuse.
- Poor self-esteem, unworthiness.
- Superficial relationship with others.
- Difficulty in coping with everyday situations.
- Under utilization of resources and support systems.
- Aloofness and lack of caring.

It is important to note that individual personality traits must also be considered in conjunction with these characteristics. Crisis is defined by the individual; what is a crisis for one is merely an occurrence for another. This factor is a critical component that must be evaluated in relation to crisis prone characteristics as well as personality traits.

Types of Crisis

- **Maturational crisis:** A maturational crisis is a stage in a person's life where adjustment and adaptation to new responsibilities and life patterns are necessary. The transition points where individuals move into successive stage often generate disequilibrium. Individuals are required to make cognitive and behavioral changes and to integrate those physical changes that accompany development. The extent to which individuals experience success in the mastery of these tasks depends on previous successes, availability of support systems, and influence of role models and acceptability of new role by others.

  The transitional periods or events that are most commonly identified as having increased crisis potential are adolescence, marriage, parenthood, midlife and retirement.

- **Situational crisis:** A situational crisis is one that is precipitated by an unanticipated stressful event that creates disequilibrium by threatening one's sense of biological, social or psychological integrity. Examples of events that can precipitate situational crises are premature birth, status and role changes, death of a loved one, physical or mental illness, divorce, change in geographic location and poor performance in school.

- **Social crisis:** Social crisis is accidental, uncommon, and unanticipated and results in multiple losses and radical environmental changes. Social crises include natural disasters like floods, earthquakes, violence, nuclear accidents, mass killings, contamination of large areas by toxic wastes, wars, etc. This type of crisis is unlike maturational and situational crisis because it does not occur in the lives of all people. Because of the severity of the effects of social crisis coping strategies may not be effective. Individuals confronted with social crisis usually do not have previous experience from which to draw expertise. Support systems may be unavailable because they may also be involved in similar situations. Mental health professionals are called upon to act quickly and provide services to large numbers of people and in some cases, the whole community.

Phases of Crisis

Caplan (1964) has described four phases of crisis as described below:

Phase I: Perceived threat acts as a precipitant that generates increased anxiety. Normal coping strategies are activated, and if unsuccessful, the individual moves into Phase II.

Phase II: The ineffectiveness of the Phase I coping mechanisms leads to further disorganization. The individual experiences a sense of vulnerability. The individual may attempt to cope with the situation in a random fashion. If the anxiety continues and there is no reduction, the individual enters Phase III.

Phase III: Redefinition of the crisis is attempted and the individual is most amenable to assistance in this phase. New problem solving measures may also affect a solution. Return to pre-crisis level of functioning may occur. If problem solving is unsuccessful, further disorganization occurs and the individual is said to have entered Phase IV.

Phase IV: Severe to panic levels of anxiety with profound cognitive, emotional and physiological changes may occur. Referral to further treatment resources is necessary.

Signs and Symptoms of Crisis

- The major feeling in a crisis situation is anxiety. The individual experiences a heavy burden of free-floating anxiety.
- The anxiety may be manifested through depression, anger and guilt. The victim will attempt to get rid of the anxiety using various coping mechanisms, healthy or unhealthy.
- The individual may become incapable of even taking care of his daily needs and may neglect his responsibilities.
- The individual may become irrational and blame others for what has happened to him.

Resolution of Crisis

There are three ways by which the individual may resolve the crisis:

- **Pseudo-resolution:** In this, the individual uses repression and pushes out of consciousness the incident and the intense emotions associated with it, so there will not be any change in the level of functioning of the individual. But in future, if and when a crisis occurs, the repressed feelings may surface and influence the feelings aroused by the new crisis. In such a situation, the particular crisis may be more difficult to resolve because the feelings associated with the earlier crisis are neither expressed nor handled at that time.
- **Unsuccessful resolution:** In this, the victim uses pathological adaptation at any phase of crisis, resulting in a lower level of Healthy resolution of a crisis depends upon the following three factors:
  i. Realistic appraisal of the precipitating event, i.e. recognition of the relationship between the event and feelings of anxiety is necessary for effective problem-solving to occur.
  ii. Availability of support systems.
  iii. Availability of coping measures over a lifetime: A person develops a repertoire of successful coping strategies that enable him to identify and resolve stressful situations functioning. The victim, rather than accepting the loss and reorganizing his life, keeps ruminating over the loss. An example is prolonged grief reaction, which results in depression.
- **Successful resolution:** In this, the victim may go through the various phases of crisis, but reaches Phase III where various coping measures are utilized to resolve the crisis situation. The individual develops better skills and problem solving ability, which can be and will be used in various crisis situations in future.

CRISIS INTERVENTION

Crisis intervention is a technique used to help an individual or family to understand and cope with the intense feelings that are typical of a crisis. Nurses function as part of the interdisciplinary team in the use of crisis intervention as a therapeutic modality. Nurses may employ crisis techniques in their work with high-risk groups such as clients with chronic diseases, new parents and bereaved persons. Nurses may also use crisis intervention in dealing with intra-group staff issues and client management issues. The term crisis was defined by Caplan (1964). In crisis intervention is a situation, the therapist becomes a part of the individuals life situation because the individual unable to solve problem.

Common Problems

- Loss. Health, physical integrity, financial.
- Change problems. Adjustment to new social role e.g. marital status, parenthood, work.
- Interpersonal problems.
- Conflict problems. Individual faces difficult to choose.

Characteristics

- Occurs in all individual at one time or another.
- Precipitated by specific identifiable events.
- Personal by nature.
- Acute not chronic.
- Potential for psychological growth or deterioration.

Phases in Crisis Development

Phase 1: The individual is exposed to a precipitating stressor.

Phase 2: When previous problem-solving techniques do not relieve the stressor, anxiety increases further.

Phase 3: All possible resources both internal and external are called upon to resolve the problem and relieve the discomfort.

Phase 4: If resolution does not occur in previous phase, Caplan stats that the tension mounts beyond a further threshold or its burden increases over time to a breaking point. Major disorganization of the individual with drastic results often occurs.

Types of Crisis

Class 1: Dispositional crisis: Acute responses to an external situational stressor.

Class 2: Crisis of anticipated life transitions: Normal life cycle transitions that may be anticipated but over which the individual may feel a lack of control.

Class 3: Crisis resulting from traumatic stress: These crises are precipitated by unexpected, external stresses over which the individual has little or no control and from which he or she feels emotionally overwhelmed and defeated.

Class 4: Maturational/development crisis: These crisis are internal origin and reflect underlying development issues that involve depending, value conflict, sexual identity, control and capacity for emotional intimacy.

Class 5: Crisis reflecting psychopathology: Psychopathology that may precipitate crisis includes borderline personality disorder, severe neuroses schizophrenia.

Class 6: Psychiatric emergencies: Crisis situation in which general functioning has been severely impaired and the individual incompetent or unable to assume personal responsibility.

Techniques

- Reassurance
- Suggestion
- Environmental manipulation.
- Psychotropic medication.

Crisis Intervention

Individuals experiencing crisis have an urgent need for assistance.

Crisis intervention takes place in both inpatient and outpatient:
- Helping the individual to gain mastery of the situation.
- Dealing with excessive use of the defense of denial.

Initial Assessment

Detailed enquiry about the event of the last 48 hours:
- Current problems.
- Level of coping ability.
- Degree of support from the family and friends.
- Degree to which home situation is helpful or the opposite.
- Mental state.

Intensive Care

- Organization of immediate practical task.
- Removal of patient from stressful environment which may involve admission to hospital.
- Lowering arousal and distress by psychological support. Important to ensure adequate sleep.
- Reinforcing appropriate communication.
- Showing concern and warmth and encouraging hope.

Crisis Counseling

Which defines the patient-therapist relationship and extent of the intervention?

- Facilitating the expression of effect.
- Facilitating communication.
- Facilitating the patient understands of both his/her problems and feelings.
- Showing concern and empathy and bolsteng self-esteem.
- Facilitating problem solving behavior.

Problem-solving Therapy

- Identify and define problem.
- Identify alternative method of coping with that problem.
- Cognitively rehearse each alternative and become clear about its implications.
- Choose one alternative to follow.
- Define the behavioral step required to carry out that alternative.
- Carry out the alternative step by step.
- Check the effects of this behavior to ensure that the choice of alternative has been a suitable one.

Role of the Nurse

- Explain the principles of the technique.
- Help with problem definition.
- Suggest additional coping methods.
- Remind patient where his/her strengths and weaknesses lie.
- Help patient to confront reality if necessary.
- Help patient to breakdown action in to manageable steps.
- Help in evaluation of coping behavior.

Pharmacological Management

- Minor tranquilizer to lower arousal.
- Hypnotic to ensure adequate sleep.
- Antidepressant if depression in inhibiting coping behavior.

Aims of Crisis Intervention Technique

- To provide a correct cognitive perception of the situation.
- To assist the individual in managing the intense and overwhelming feelings associated with the crisis.

Steps to Provide a Correct Cognitive Perception

Assessment of the situation:
- This may be achieved by direct questioning with the purpose of identification of the problem and the people involved.
- It is necessary to identify the support systems available and to know the depth in which the individual's feelings are affected.

- Assessment should also be done to identify the strengths and limitations of the victim.

Defining the Event

- The victim at times may not be able to identify the precipitating event because of possible denial, or due to reluctance to talk about it.
- It may be necessary for the therapist to review the details of the incidents in the past 2 to 4 weeks in order to identify the event that precipitated the crisis. Such a review will help the victim becoming aware of the precipitating event.
- Develop a plan of action.
- The victim and the people closely associated with him should have active involvement in developing the plan of action.
- The therapist must be aware that the victim may not be in a condition to mentally comprehend complicated information due to the overwhelming anxiety experienced by him. The instructions given by the therapist must be simple and clear, and too much information should not be given at a time. The instructions may have to be written down, as the victim may not be able to retain all the information.

Steps to Assist the Victim in Managing the Intense Feelings

Helping the Individual to be Aware of the Feelings

- The victim needs help in identifying his own feelings, which is the first step in handling them.
- The therapist should use appropriate communication technique so that the victim will feel comfortable to express his feelings without the fear of being judged or criticized.
- The therapist should also be efficient in observing verbal and non-verbal behavior of the victim, so that he will be able to make a careful assessment of his feelings. Help the individual to attain mastery over the feelings
- The individual should be given adequate support and guidance through therapeutic process in order to handle feelings associated with crisis but special care should be taken not to give any false reassurance.
- He should not in any way be encouraged to blame others, as this will only let him escape from taking any responsibility.
- Care must be taken to ensure that the individual does not develop too much dependency on the therapist, which is unhealthy.
- After the victim and the support groups prepare the plan of action under the guidance of the therapist, it should be discussed with the victim and the concerned others, so that they will have a clear understanding of the methods of implementation of the plan.
- To improve coping with the situation necessary environmental manipulation must be done in physical or interpersonal areas.
- It is advisable to have another appointment for the victim to visit the therapist within a week, in order to assess how the plan is working out, and if needed, to revise and modify the plan.

NURSING PROCESS APPLICATION IN CRISIS INTERVENTION

Nurses respond to crisis situations on a daily basis. Crisis can occur in any unit e.g. in general hospitals, home settings, community health centers, schools, offices, and in private practice. Indeed, nurses may be called upon to function as crisis helpers in any situation. Knowledge of crisis intervention techniques is thus an important clinical skill of all nurses, regardless of the setting or practice specialty.

Nursing assessment: The first step of crisis intervention is assessment.

During this phase the nurse collects data regarding the following factors:

- Precipitating event or stressor.
- Patient's perception of the event or stressor.
- Nature and strength of the patient's support systems, coping resources.
- Level of psychological stress patient is suffering from and the degree of impairment he is experiencing.
- Patient's previous strengths and coping mechanisms.

During this phase the nurse begins to establish a positive working relationship with the patient.

Nursing diagnoses: The primary nursing diagnoses in crisis intervention are:

- Ineffective individual coping
- Ineffective family coping
- Altered family process
- Post-trauma response
- Ineffective individual coping refers to the inability to ask for help, problem solving or meet role expectations
- Ineffective family coping occurs when the family's support systems are not successful and family's economic or social well being is threatened
- Altered family processes result when family members are unable to adapt to the traumatic experience constructively
- Post-traumatic response is a sustained painful response to an overwhelming traumatic event.

Planning: In planning the previously collected data is analyzed and specific interventions are proposed.

During this phase the nurse will undertake the following activities:

- Dynamics underlying the present crisis are formulated
- Alternative solutions to the problem are explored

- Steps for achieving the solutions are identified
- Environmental support needed to help the patient is decided upon, coping mechanisms that need to be developed and those which need to be strengthened are identified.

Implementation: The following interventions are carried out to resolve crisis:

Environmental manipulation: Environmental manipulation includes interventions that directly change the patient's physical or interpersonal situation. These interventions may remove stress or provide situational support. For example a patient having difficulty in his job may take a week of sick leave so that he can be removed temporarily from that stress.

General support: The nurse uses warmth, acceptance, empathy and reassurance to provide general support to the patient.

Generic approach: The generic approach is designed to reach high risk individuals and large groups as quickly as possible. It applies a specific method to all individuals faced with a similar type of crisis (e.g. in social disasters). Debriefing is a method of generic approach. In debriefing method, disaster victims are helped to recall events and clarify traumatic experiences. It attempts to place the traumatic event in perspective, allows the individual to relive the event in a factual way, encourages group support, and provides information on normal reaction to critical events. The goal of debriefing is to prevent the maladaptive responses that may result if the trauma is suppressed.

Individual approach: The individual approach is a type of crisis intervention similar to the diagnosis and treatment of a specific problem in a specific patient. It is particularly useful in combined situational and maturational crises and also beneficial when symptoms include homicidal and suicidal risk. The nurse must use the intervention that is most likely to help the patient develop an adaptive response to the crisis.

Techniques of Crisis Intervention

- **Catharsis:** The release of feelings that takes place as the patient talks about emotionally charged areas.
- **Clarification:** Encouraging the patient to express more clearly the relationship between certain events.
- **Manipulation:** Using the patient's emotions, wishes or values to benefit the patient in the therapeutic process.
- **Reinforcement of behavior:** Giving the patient positive reinforcement to adaptive behavior.
- **Support of defenses:** Encouraging the use of healthy, adaptive defenses and discouraging those that are unhealthy or maladaptive.
- **Increasing self-esteem:** Helping the patient to regain feelings of self worth.
- **Exploration of solutions:** Examining alternative ways of solving the immediate problem.

Evaluation: The nurse and patient review the changes that have occurred. The nurse should give credit for successful changes to patients so that they realize their effectiveness and understand that what they learnt from crisis may help in coping with future crisis. If the goals have not been met, the patient and nurse can return to the first step- assessment and continue through the phases again.

Modalities of crisis intervention: Community-based crisis intervention modalities have recently been developed. They are based on the philosophy that the health care team must be active and go out to the patients rather than wait for the patients to come to them. Nurses working in these modalities intervene in a variety of community settings, ranging from patients homes to street corners.

Mobile crisis programs: Mobile crisis teams provide front-line interdisciplinary crisis intervention to individuals, families and communities. The nurse, who is a member of a mobile crisis team, should be able to provide on-site assessment, crisis management, treatment, referral and educational services to patients, families and the community at large. Nurses are thus able to ensure mental health care for even the most under-served populations efficiently and cost effectively.

Telephone contacts: Crisis intervention is sometimes practiced by telephone rather than through face-to-face contacts. The nurse should have effective listening skills to provide crisis intervention to victims.

Group work: People who have common traits on stressors will form a group. The group provides an opportunity for members to express common concerns and experiences, foster hope and build mutual support. The nurse's role in the group is active, focal and focused on the present. The nurse and the group help the patient solve the problem and reinforce new problem solving behavior.

Disaster response: As part of the community, nurses are called on when an adventitious or social crisis strikes the community. Floods, earthquakes, airplane crashes, fires, nuclear accidents etc. precipitate large number of crises. The nurse has an important role in dealing with psychosocial problems of disaster victims. The nurse participates in crisis operations and acts as a case-finder for persons suffering from psychosocial stress. It is important that nurses in the immediate post disaster period go to places where victims are likely to gather, such as hospitals, shelters, morgues. During this period nurses use the generic approach of crisis intervention so that as many people as possible can receive help in a short duration of time.

Victim outreach programs: Victim outreach programs use crisis intervention techniques to identify the needs of victims and then to connect them with appropriate referrals and other resources. Nurses often work in victim outreach programs, where victims are often seen immediately after the crisis. These victims need thorough evaluation, empathic support, and information and help with the large system and social networking system.

Crisis Intervention Centers

Crisis intervention centers provide emergency psychiatric care and counseling to victims, experiencing extreme stress or conflict, often involving suicide attempts or drug or alcohol abuse. These centers, which are usually self-contained units within a hospital or community health care center, provide services 24 hours a day. The services may be delivered directly on the premises, or counseling may be provided over the telephone. The primary objective of crisis intervention centers is to help the person cope with immediate problem and to offer guidance and support for long-term therapy.

Health education: Nurses are involved in identifying people who are at high risk for developing crisis and in teaching coping strategies to avoid the development of crisis. The public also needs education so that they can identify those needing crisis services, be aware of available services, change their attitude so that people will feel free to seek services, and obtain information about how others deal with potential crisis producing problems.

GRIEF AND RESOLUTION OF GRIEF

Grief is a subjective state of emotional, physical and social response to the loss of a valued entity. The loss may be real, in which case it can be substantiated by others (e.g. death of a loved one), or perceived by the individual alone, in which case it cannot be perceived or shared by others (e.g. loss of feeling of femininity following mastectomy).

Stages of Grief

Kubler-Ross (1969) having done extensive research with terminally ill patients identified five stages of feelings and behavior that individuals experience in response to a real, perceived or anticipated loss:

- **Stage I-Denial:** This is a stage of shock and disbelief. The response may be one of "No, it can't be true!" Denial is a protective mechanism that allows the individual to cope within an immediate time-frame while organizing more effective defense strategies.
- **Stage II-Anger:** "Why me?" and "It is not fair!" are comments often expressed during the anger stage. Anger may be directed at self or displaced on loved ones, caregivers, and even God. There may be a preoccupation with an idealized image of the lost entity.
- **Stage III-Bargaining:** "If God will help me through this, I promise I will go to church every Sunday and volunteer my time to help others". During this stage, which is generally not visible or evident to others? a bargain is made with God in an attempt to reverse or postpone the loss.
- **Stage IV-Depression:** During this stage the full impact of the loss is experienced. This is a time of quiet desperation and disengagement from all associations with the lost entity.
- **Stage V-Acceptance:** The final stage brings a feeling of peace regarding the loss that has occurred. Focus is on the reality of the loss and its meaning for the individuals affected by it. All individuals do not experience each of these stages in response to a loss, nor do they necessarily experience them in this order. Some individuals grieving behavior may fluctuate, and even overlap between stages.

Resolution of grief: Resolution of the process of mourning is thought to have occurred when an individual can look back on the relationship with the lost entity and accept both the pleasure and the disappointments (both the positive and negative aspects) of the association. Preoccupation with the lost entity is replaced with energy and desire to pursue new situations and relationships. The length of the grief process may be prolonged by a number of factors: If the relationship with the lost entity had been marked by ambivalence, reaction to the loss may be burdened with guilt, which lengthens the grief reaction.

In anticipatory grief where a loss is anticipated, individuals often begin the work of grieving before the actual loss occurs. Most people experience the grieving behavior once the actual loss occurs, but having this time to prepare for the loss can facilitate the process of mourning, actually decreasing the length and intensity of the response. The number of recent losses experienced by an individual also affects the length of the grieving process and whether he is able to complete one grieving process before another loss occurs.

MALADAPTIVE GRIEF RESPONSES

Maladaptive grief responses to loss occur when an individual is not able to satisfactorily progress through the stages of grieving to achieve resolution. Several types to grief responses have been identified as pathological These are prolonged, delayed/inhibited, and distorted responses.

Prolonged response: It is characterized by an intense preoccupation with memories of the lost entity for many years after the loss has occurred.

Delayed or inhibited response: The individual becomes fixed in the denial stage of the grieving process. The emotional pain associated with loss is not experienced, but there may be evidence of anxiety disorders or sleeping disorders. The individual may remain in denial for many years until the grief response is triggered by a reminder of the loss or even by another unrelated loss.

Distorted response: The individual who experiences a distorted response is fixed in the anger stage of grieving. The normal behaviors associated with grieving, such as helplessness, hopelessness, sadness, anger and guilt are exaggerated out of proportion to the situation. The individual turns the anger inward on the self and is unable to function in normal activities of daily living. Pathological depression is a distorted grief response.

Treatment: Normal grief does not require any treatment while complicated grief requires medication depending on the prevailing behavior responses.

Nursing Intervention

- Provide an open accepting environment.
- Encourage ventilation of feelings and listen actively.
- Provide various diversional activities.
- Provide teaching about common symptoms of grief.
- Reinforce goal-directed activities.
- Bring together similar aggrieved persons, to encourage communication, share experiences of the loss and to offer companionship, social and emotional support.

RECREATION AND DIVERSIONAL THERAPIES

Recreation is an activity of leisure, leisure being discretionary time. The "need to do something for recreation" is an essential element of human biology and psychology. Recreational activities are often done for enjoyment, amusement, or pleasure and are considered to be "fun".

Indoor Recreational Options

Reading: The benefits of reading cannot be stressed enough. I feel that people who love reading, can never get bored when they are alone. Reading is not only a great source of entertainment, but also a vast source of knowledge and inspiration. Reading can be one of the best activities you can enjoy indoors.

Writing: What better way to spend a lazy afternoon, then pour heart and allow creative juices to flow with a pen and a paper! Well, writing cannot just be fun, but it can be great stress buster as well.

Internet surfing: Well, if there is nothing else to do, you can always log on to the Internet. The Internet provides you an endless number of options for recreation, which include online games, online shopping, online chatting, video surfing, blogging, social networking, online dating or even reading the online news.

Dance: Dancing is not just an art, it also a great exercise and hence an effective stress buster! Although, it is always an added advantage if you take formal training in this art, it certainly isn't a prerequisite! Anyone and I mean, absolutely anyone can dance.

Music: Just like dance, music is just as leisurely - you don't have to be a great singer or a musician to enjoy music. I listen to music while I am driving to and from work, and I can't tell you the number of times I just start singing while listening to these songs.

Indoor games: A game of snooker, pool, table tennis, indoor tennis, badminton, racquetball or squash can be a great way to spend your time indoors and enjoy yourself!

Outdoor Recreational Options

Hiking: If it is a crisp sunny day with fresh fragrant winds, then what better thing to do than to go hiking in the lap of nature? Load your backpack and go hiking, either with a bunch of friends or by yourself! Hiking is a wonderful experience that will help you forget your stress and get rid of all your negativity.

Camping: Well, have a great camping place nearby? How about going camping? Enjoy nature's bounty as you camp at a verdant camping site, light up a fire and sit around with a sumptuous barbecue meal and refreshing drinks!

Fishing: Fishing is a favorite recreational sport for many ardent fishing lovers and yes, before all the animal right issues start coming into the picture, let me tell you that most of the fishing lovers allow their catch to go back to the water bodies once trapped in the nets. There are various types of fishing like trout fishing, sport fishing, bass fishing, fly fishing or even ice fishing.

Sailing: Imagine a pleasant day at a lake nearby, your boat gliding over the azure waters as you stand against the humid breeze and feel the wind in your hair. Sounds wonderful doesn't it? Well, sailing is exciting, and no matter with whom you want to go sailing; this can be a fun experience. Make it a lively family picnic at the sea on a bright sunny day or a quiet rendezvous with your lover in the evening, while you watch the orange-red sun melt in the waters. In addition to this, you can also pick out other activities like boating, kayaking or rafting.

Scuba diving: Well, if you have always been a water lover, and would love to experience the flora and fauna of the deep waters, then scuba diving might be your thing! For beginners, it is advised to have a professional instructor with you. It is truly exhilarating to watch the beautiful shoals of fish pass right by your side or even grab bits of fish food from your hands! For adventure lovers, this is one must-do activity!

Skateboarding: Who said only kids should try skateboarding? But having said that I must add that no matter how old you are, you need to be physically fit to try out such sports! Skateboarding might be a fun way to spend time and enjoy the beauty of your lovely neighborhood or even meet your friends around the corner!

Skydiving: Having recently tried skydiving I can vouch for the fact that this is one adventure sport that you don't wanna miss! The excitement of the free-fall and the heavenly experience of the view that you enjoy during the parachute ride after the free fall, are truly blissful! The initial jump from about 12,000 feet is enough to give you the adventurous rush or kick that adventure-sports enthusiasts always talk about!

Skiing: Skiing or Snow Skiing is a collective term used for a number of sports that make use of skis as the primary equipment. There are several styles of skiing, some of which include Nordic skiing, Alpine skiing and Telemark skiing. If you are planning to visit the snowy mountains or are fortunate to have them close by, then skiing is something you must definitely try out. Another snow sport which is an amalgamation of skating and skiing is snowboarding.

Swimming: Swimming is also a favorite activity amongst water lovers. Swimming is an excellent way to relax yourself as well as a fun workout to keep you healthy. For people who just hate exercising in the gym, regular swimming might be a great way to stay in shape.

BIBLIOGRAPHY

1. Beck AT. Cognitive therapies and the emotional disorder. International University Press, New York, 1976.
2. Campbell C. Crisis in care – stress survey, disturbing findings. Nursing Mirror. 1985;160:16-24.
3. Holmes TS. Life situations and disease. J Acad Psychosom Med. 1978;19:747.
4. Johnson M, Maas M, Moorhead S. Nursing outcomes classification (NOC) 2nd edition. St. Louis. MO: Mosby, 2000.
5. Loupasakis A. Laugh the best treatment. Kedros 2nd edition. Athens, 2002.
6. Manos N. Basics of Clinical Psychiatry. University Studio Press. Thessaloniki, 1988.
7. Marttin P., Long MV, Poon LW. Age changes and differences in personality traits and states of the old and very old. The Journals of Gerontology 2002;(57B):144-52.
8. Peplau H. A working definition of anxiety. In: Burd SF., Marshall MA (Eds). Some Clinical Approaches to Psychiatric Nursing. New York: Macmillan, 1968.
9. Plati C. Specific clinical problems: Nursing approach. Athens, 1998.
10. Raya A. Mental Health Nursing and Psychiatric Nursing. Athens, 1993.
11. Reynaud SN. Meeker BJ. Coping styles of older adults with ostomies. Journal of Gerontological Nursing. 2002;28(5):30-6
12. Selye H. Stress in health and disease. Reading, MA: Butterworth, 1976.
13. Selye H. The Stress of Life revised edition. New York: McGraw-Hill, 1976.
14. Smeltzer SC, Bare BG [Eds]. Brunner and Suddarth's Textbook of Medical-Surgical Nursing, 10th edition. Philadelphia: Lippincott Williams & Wilkins, 2004.
15. Yurkovich E. (1989) Patient and nurse roles in the therapeutic community. Perspect Psychiatric Care. 1989;15(3):18-22.

REVIEW QUESTIONS

Long Essays

1. Define stress, explain the sources and symptoms of stress.
2. Define stressors, explain the types of stressors.
3. Discuss the strategies of stress management.
4. Describe the role of nurse in stress management.

Short Essays

1. Types of stress.
2. General adaptation syndrome (Hans Selye, 1945).
3. Local adaptation syndrome.
4. Concept of crisis and resolution.
5. Crisis intervention.
6. Nursing process application in crisis intervention.
7. Techniques of crisis Intervention.
8. Recreation and diversional therapies.

Short Answers

1. Chronic stress.
2. Absolute stressors.
3. Resistance reaction.
4. Phases of crisis.
5. Resolution of crisis.
6. Types of crisis.
7. Stages of grief.

CHAPTER 28
Cultural Diversity and Spirituality

LEARNING OBJECTIVES

- **Cultural diversity**
  - Cultural Concepts: culture, subculture, multicultural, diversity, race, acculturation, assimilation
  - Transcultural nursing
  - Cultural competence
  - Providing culturally responsive care
- **Spirituality**
  - Concepts: faith, hope, religion, spirituality, spiritual wellbeing
  - Factors affecting spirituality
  - Spiritual problems in acute, chronic, terminal illnesses and near-death experience
  - Dealing with spiritual distress/problems

TERMINOLOGY

Culture lag: The gap of time between the introduction of material culture and nonmaterial culture's acceptance of it.

Diffusion: The spread of material and nonmaterial culture from one culture to another discoveries things and ideas found from what already exists.

Globalization: The integration of international trade and finance markets.

High culture: The cultural patterns of a society's elite innovations.

Popular culture: Mainstream, widespread patterns among a society's population.

Subcultures: Groups that share a specific identification, apart from a society's majority, even as the members exist within a larger society.

Acculturation: Cultural modification of an individual, group, or people by adapting to or borrowing traits from another culture; a merging of cultures as a result of prolonged contact. It should be noted that individuals from culturally diverse groups may desire varying degrees of acculturation into the dominant culture. Assimilation: To assume the cultural traditions of a given people or group; the cultural absorption of a minority group into the main cultural body.

Culturally appropriate: Exhibiting sensitivity to cultural differences and similarities, and demonstrating effectiveness in translating that sensitivity to action through organizational mission statements, communication strategies, and services to diverse cultures.

Cultural awareness: Recognition of the nuances of one's own and other cultures.

Cultural competence: The ability of individuals to use academic, experiential, and interpersonal skills to increase their understanding and appreciation of cultural differences and similarities within, among, and between groups.

Afterlife (or life after death): A generic term referring to a continuation of existence, typically spiritual and experiential, beyond this world, or after death. This article is about current generic and widely held or reported concepts of afterlife.

Agnosticism: The view that the existence of God or the supernatural is unknown or unknowable.

Animism: The religious belief that all objects, places, and creatures possess a distinct spiritual essence.

Asceticism: Denotes a life which is characterized by refraining from worldly pleasures (austerity). Those who practice ascetic lifestyles often perceive their practices as virtuous and pursue them to achieve greater spirituality.

Atheism: In the broadest sense, is the absence of belief in the existence of deities. Less broadly, atheism is the rejection of belief that any deities exist.

Faith healing: The use of solely spiritual means in treating disease, sometimes accompanied with the refusal of modern medical techniques. Another term for this is spiritual healing. Faith healing is a form of alternative medicine.

Fasting: The act of willingly abstaining from all food and in some cases drink, for a period of time. Depending on the tradition, fasting practices may forbid sexual intercourse, (or any sexual desire), masturbation, as well as refraining from eating certain types or groups of food (e.g. meat).

Spirituality: In a narrow sense, is a concern with matters of the spirit, however that may be defined; but it is also a wide term with many available readings. It may include belief in supernatural powers, as in religion, but the emphasis is on personal experience.

Cultural diversity: Differences in race, ethnicity, nationality, religion, gender, sexual identity, socioeconomic status, physical ability, language, beliefs, values, behavior patterns, or customs among various groups within a community, organization, or nation.

Cultural humility: It is a lifelong process of self-reflection and self-critique. Cultural humility does not require mastery of lists of "different" or peculiar beliefs and behaviors supposedly pertaining to different cultures, rather it encourages to develop a respectful attitude toward diverse points of view.

Cultural sensitivity: Understanding the needs and emotions of your own culture and the culture of others.

Ethnic: Of or relating to large groups of people classed according to common racial, national, tribal, religious, linguistic, or cultural origin or background.

Ethnocentrism: The emotional attitude that one's own ethnic group, nation, or culture is superior; an excessive or inappropriate concern for racial matters.

Homophobia: Irrational hatred or fear of homosexuals or homosexuality.

Power: The ability to control others; authority, sway, influence; a person or thing having great influence, force, or authority.

Prejudice: It implies a preconceived and unreasonable judgment, or opinion, usually an unfavorable one marked by suspicion, fear, or hatred.

Racism: A doctrine or teaching, without scientific support, that claims to find racial differences in character, intelligence, etc.; that asserts the superiority of one race over another or others, and that seeks to maintain the supposed purity of a race or the races; any program or practice of racial discrimination, segregation, etc. based on such beliefs.

Segregation: The policy or practice of compelling racial groups to live apart from each other, go to separate schools, use separate social facilities, etc.

Sexism: Discrimination against people on the basis of sex; specifically discrimination against, and prejudicial stereotyping of, women.

Supremacist: A person who believes in or promotes the supremacy of a particular group, race, etc.

Bigotry: The behavior, attitude, or beliefs of a person who holds blindly and intolerantly to a particular creed, opinion, etc.; intolerance; prejudice.

Discrimination: The act of discriminating or distinguishing differences; the ability to make or perceive distinctions, perception, and discernment; a showing of partiality or prejudice in treatment; specific action or policies directed against the welfare of minority groups.

Diversity: A quality, state, fact, or instance of being different or dissimilar; difference; variety.

INTRODUCTION

Psychosocial support involves the culturally sensitive provision of psychological, social and spiritual care. Nurses play a unique role in supporting patients; by building dialogue with patients nurses can begin to understand how patients view themselves as individuals, what is important to them, and how their relationship with others may affect their decisions and their ability to live with those decisions during their treatment and beyond (Ellis et al 2006). Good communication and assessment skills are essential to building a rapport with patients and can help the nurse develop a clinical relationship with the patient and their family.

CONCEPTS: CULTURE, SUBCULTURE AND MULTICULTURAL

Culture

An integrated pattern of human behavior that includes thoughts, communications, languages, practices, beliefs, values, customs, courtesies, rituals, manners of interacting, roles, relationships and expected behaviors of a racial, ethnic, religious or social group; the ability to transmit the above to succeeding generations; culture is always changing.

Subculture

Smaller cultural groups that exist within but differ in some way from the prevailing culture interest sociologists. These groups are called subcultures. Examples of some subcultures include "heavy metal" music devotees, body-piercing and tatoo enthusiasts, motorcycle gang members, and Nazi skinheads. Members of subcultures typically make use of distinctive language, behaviors, and clothing, even though they may still accept many of the values of the dominant culture.

- A subculture is a group of people within a culture that differentiates itself from the parent culture to which it belongs, often maintaining some of its founding principles.
- Subcultures develop their own norms and values regarding cultural, political and sexual matters.
- Subcultures are part of society while keeping their specific characteristics intact.
- The concept of subcultures was developed in sociology and cultural studies. Subcultures differ from counter cultures.
- First, it's important to understand the concept of a subculture.
- A subculture is a unique culture shared by a smaller group of people who are also a part of a larger culture.
- A larger culture often contains many subcultures, and an individual can be part of several of them.

- Each subculture has distinct norms and customs that aren't a part of the broader culture in which it is enveloped. Think of the Amish, or bikers, or hippies, or Whovians. Each of these groups has unique cultures, yet they all exist within the broad culture of the United States.

Multicultural

- The term "multicultural" relates to the presence of multiple cultural groups within a single society; multicultural nursing involves an awareness of the different cultural groups that make up our society in a healthcare setting.
- Together, transcultural (connecting different cultures) and multicultural (awareness of different cultures) skills allow you to grow as a person and as a professional.
- Patients' cultural views often influence their decisions about healthcare.
- Being able to recognize these cultural concerns can help you overcome obstacles with patients and deliver the best care possible.
- This perspective of multiculturalism respects cultural variations rather than requiring that the dominant culture assimilate the various cultures.
- It holds that certain shared cultural tenets are important to society as a whole, but that some cultural differences are important, too.
- For example, children in schools today are being taught that the United States is not the only culture in the world, and that other viewpoints may have something to offer Americans.

Acculturation

- Acculturation is a process of social, psychological, and cultural change that stems from the balancing of two cultures while adapting to the prevailing culture of the society.
- Acculturation is a process in which an individual adopts, acquires and adjusts to a new cultural environment.
- Individuals of a differing culture try to incorporate themselves into the new more prevalent culture by participating in aspects of the more prevalent culture, such as their traditions, but still hold onto their original cultural values and traditions.
- The effects of acculturation can be seen at multiple levels in both the devotee of the prevailing culture and those who are assimilating into the culture
- Acculturation is also a two-way process because both cultures will still change and be affected by each other.

Cultural Assimilation

- Cultural assimilation is the process in which a minority group or culture comes to resemble a dominant group or assume the values, behaviors, and beliefs of another group.
- A conceptualization describes cultural assimilation as similar to acculturation while another merely considers the former as one of the latter's phases.
- Assimilation could also involve the so-called additive acculturation wherein, instead of replacing the ancestral culture, an individual expands their existing cultural repertoire.

CULTURAL COMPETENCE

Cultural competence in nursing practice focuses on knowledge, attitude, and skill. Consistently working towards being culturally competent is an exercise in compassion and respect. Employ these techniques on a regular basis to grow your level of competency:

- Ask questions and take time to learn about what the answers mean in different cultures.
- Use clear, descriptive communication that aligns with the communication practices of your patient's culture.
- Keep an open mind and employ the skills you practice when the occasional conflict arises.
- Acknowledge and be aware of any situations in which you may portray a lack of sensitivity, and work to keep from doing so.
- Actively seek out colleagues and peers of different cultures to learn more about interacting and respecting your differences.

Increasing cultural competence in nursing practice: Through years of research and education, many medical scholars have shared knowledge and techniques that nurses can employ to practice cultural competence. Cultural competencies for nurses these techniques are built upon three pillars:

1. Knowledge
2. Attitude
3. Skills

- **Knowledge:** Learning about the culture base of those in your area is the first step to strengthening your cultural competence. Depending on your location, the number of cultures you encounter will vary. Seek out information on topics such as shared traditions and values of each cultural group. Berlin and Fowkes designed the mnemonic, **LEARN**, in conducting a cultural assessment. This mnemonic stands for 5 steps outlined below:

Listen: Listen to the patient's perception of the presenting problem.
Explain: Explain your perception of the patient's problem. Is it physiological, psychological, spiritual, and/or cultural? It can and often will be more than one.
Acknowledge: Acknowledge the similarities and differences between the patient's perception and your perceptions. In certain cases, it may be easier to focus on the similarities while working towards bridging the gap between the differences.
Recommend: Recommendations are built upon the knowledge gained from the first three steps. It is

inevitable that culture will affect the recommendations, and the patient must be involved in this process.

Negotiate: In some instances, the patient may require negotiating a treatment plan. It is imperative that nurses are sensitive to the cultural practices of each patient while still providing the best care possible.

Cultural competency in nursing is an ongoing practice. Having the ability to execute an analysis ensures you can handle each unique situation as it arises.

- **Attitude:** Attitude plays a large role in the ability to become and serve as a culturally competent caregiver. In this case, "attitude" refers to a level of awareness in yourself and your patients in regards to stereotypes, rules of interaction and communication customs. A caregiver will likely identify most with the culture in which they were raised. With that comes a need to identify and debunk stereotypes from other cultures. There are situations in which we may portray a lack of sensitivity without knowing how our actions may affect others. Reflect on your own cultural attitude, so that even the most subtle of stereotypical tendencies do not affect the level of care provided to your patients.
- **Skills:** Developing a skill set based on increasing your cultural competency can be accomplished by focusing on skills like communication and conflict-resolution. Communication is a key component of skilled nursing. It also involves learning to adapt to new and different situations in a flexible way. Remember that the hospital environment may not be familiar ground for your patients.

PROVIDING CULTURALLY RESPONSIVE CARE

Cultural competency, cultural safety, cultural respect, cultural awareness and cultural sensitivity are all terms that have (often interchangeably) been used to describe the training and/or attributes required by health professionals. Culture can be defined as complex beliefs and behaviors acquired as part of relationships within particular families and other social groups and can predispose people to view and experience health and illness in ways that can influence decisions, attitudes and beliefs around access and engagement in healthcare.

Definition

Culturally responsive care can be defined as an extension of patient centered-care that includes paying particular attention to social and cultural factors in managing therapeutic encounters with patients from different cultural and social backgrounds

Culturally responsive care: The word "responsiveness" places emphasis on the capacity to respond. Examples include finding out about the patient's history of present illness, their health beliefs and use of alternative treatments, expectations of care, linguistic challenges, and culturally-based family dynamics that guide decision-making processes. A basic premise of culturally sensitive care is that health care professionals must be able to recognize the client's culture, their own culture, and how both affect the patient-provider relationship. The following are key in addressing this important premise:

- Everyone has a culture.
- There is an American medical culture and it is very different from many of the cultures that our patients and their families come from.
- We need to understand where our American medical culture differs from other cultures in significant ways that impact communication and influence health outcomes for patients.
- Resistance to cultural difference is part of being human, and reactions to cultural difference are automatic, often subconscious, and can have strong influence on the patient-provider relationship.
- A provider's culture is influenced by his/her own personal values and beliefs, as well as those of the western medical culture.
- A provider's ability to communicate effectively in cross-cultural interactions is greatly enhanced by his/her grasp of cross-cultural communication skills.
- Culturally sensitive care requires a broad understanding of how culture affects health beliefs and behaviors.
- Providing linguistically appropriate care requires being able to assess the need for interpreters in the clinical setting and interact with interpreters effectively.

Culturally responsive healthcare professional by the following characteristics:

- Has the knowledge to make an accurate health assessment, one which takes into consideration a patient's background and culture.
- Has the ability to convey that assessment to the patient, to recognize culture-based beliefs about health and to devise treatment plans which respect those beliefs.
- Is willing to incorporate models of health and health care delivery from a variety of cultures into the biomedical framework.

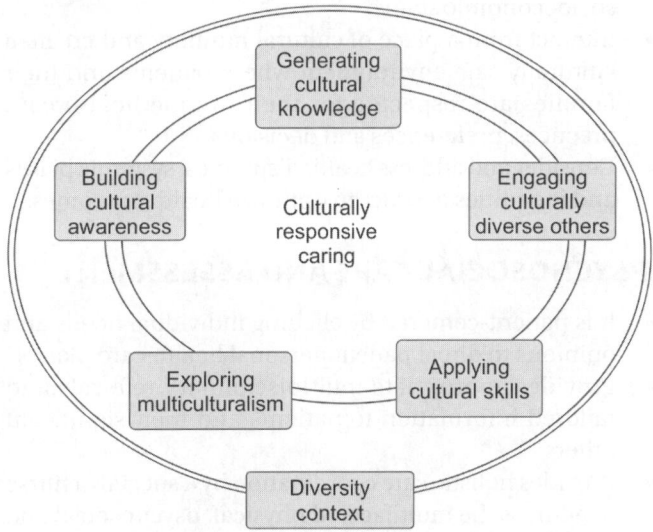

Fig. 28.1: Cultural progressive care model.

- To be culturally competent, a healthcare professional should acknowledge culture's profound effect on health outcomes and should be willing to learn more about this powerful interaction.

Role of Professionals

- It is the responsibility of the health professional to deliver culturally responsive healthcare.
- Being culturally responsive places the onus back onto the health professional to appropriately respond to the unique attributes of the person, family or community they are working with.
- Self-reflection and reducing power differences are central to being culturally responsive; therefore making assumptions based on generalizations about a person's ethnic, cultural or social group is unacceptable.
- Part of the challenge of becoming culturally responsive health professionals is learning to reach beyond personal comfort zones and being able to comfortably interact and work with people, families and communities who are both similar and markedly different.
- Assess; don't assume. Assess the influence of the family's cultural background on the child's behavior specific to health and illness. Don't assume that this child will act the same as the last child you took care of from the same cultural or ethnic group.
- Humbly acknowledge yourself as a learner and consider that the child and family members have unique personal experiences in the healthcare system.
  Confirm if the information that you have about a cultural group is accepted or practiced by your patient and their family.
- Identify the family's culturally influenced practices, strengths and beliefs that you can include or support within what will be a mutually agreed upon plan.
- Recognize that a family's cultural background will influence health-related behaviors as will previous experiences, level of education, language skills and socioeconomic status.
- Interact from a place of cultural humility and create a culturally safe environment where patients and their families are respected for their unique health care practices, preferences and decisions.
- Consider and address health disparities, systemic biases and inequities in order to optimize health outcomes.

PSYCHOSOCIAL CARE AND ASSESSMENT

- It is patient-centered by eliciting individual needs and opinions to direct patient personal health care plan
- Provides appropriate multidisciplinary referrals and tailored information to patients and their significant others
- Provides holistic care coordination by a specialist nurse to address the multifaceted physical, psychosocial and sexual needs of this patient group and their significant others efficiently at critical points in the illness trajectory
- Provides instruction in evidence based self-care, including psychosexual rehabilitation and stress reduction strategies to assist women to actively achieve optimal health status
- It is cost-effective because the engagement of peers means minimal, if any, additional nursing time thus increasing the likelihood of sustainability. This intervention package is likely to result in improved psychological and physical wellbeing, which are recognized as critical clinical outcomes.

Psychosocial assessment: Psychosocial assessments are often overlooked as a portion of the physical examination. However, a person's psychological well-being has much to do with physical health. The following guide to psychosocial assessment can be remembered by the acronym "SELF PACING". The findings from this assessment in addition to the physical findings will provide a comprehensive view of the patient's status.

S – Self-esteem: Include information pertaining to hygiene, grooming, eye contact, statements about oneself and any other characteristics that provide information about the patient's self esteem.

E – Energy level: Patient's with psychological problems often have an alteration in level of activity.

L – Lifestyle: Living arrangements, significant relationships, occupation, hobbies or lack of interest in leisure activities, education, and any other data that provides information about the patient's personal situation.

F – Family system: This refers to the patient's contact and support from family members or significant others, family stressors, crisis events, and usual coping skills.

P – Physiological: This area relates to the results of the physical assessment.

A – Affect: Include information about the patient's mood or emotional feelings. It may be described as happy, euphoric, flat, inappropriate, and other descriptive terms.

C – Culture: This refers to all cultural, racial, or anthropological variables that influence one's lifestyle and mental health. This may refer to issues of homelessness. Assess religious and spiritual preferences, if any. Discuss any related food needs and other areas of impact spirituality will have on their health status.

I – Interests: As expressed by the patient.

N – Needs: As expressed by the patient (as opposed to those identified by the health care worker).

G – Goals: As expressed by the patient (as opposed to those identified by the health care worker).

CULTURAL DIVERSITY

Cultural diversity in nursing practice derives its conceptual base from nursing, other cross-cultural health disciplines, and the social sciences such as anthropology, sociology and psychology. Culture is conceptualized broadly to encompass the belief systems of a variety of groups. Cultural diversity refers to the differences between people based on a shared ideology and valued set of beliefs, norms, customs, and meanings evidenced in a way of life. Culture consists of patterns of behavior acquired and transmitted symbols, constituting the distinctive achievement of human groups, including their embodiment in artifacts; the essential core of culture consists of historically derived and selected ideas and especially their attached values.

Six Prominent Models from Transcultural Nursing

Model	Essential lesson for the culturally responsive health care encounter
Leininger's sunrise model	To be culturally congruent, providers must collaborate with the patient by sharing power and respecting the patient's culture as well as theri own.
Purnell model for cultural competence	To be consciously compentent, a provider must acquire relevant culture-specific information about the patient.
Compinha-Bacote's process of cultural competence in the delivery of health care services	To be culturally responsive, the provider must begin with cultural desire, that is, have the attitude that reflects " I want to do " not " I have to " do so.
Jeffreys' cultural competence and confidence (CCC) model	To continue to develop cultural responsiveness, providers should exhibit moderate levels of self-efficacy, defined as a balance between confidence and concern about their skill set, which is most likely to motivate further learning.
Andrews and Boyle's transcultural concepts in nursing practice	Culturally responsive care is dependent on the strength of the provider's verbal and nonverbal cross-cultural communication skills.
Giger-Davidhizar transcultural assessment model (GDTAM)	Culturally responsive care requires that the provder evaluate how the following six cultural phenomena may affect cultural responsiveness in the health care encounter—communication, space, social organization, time, environmental control, and biological variations.

Impact of Cultural Diversity

- The impact of culture as a causative influence on the perceptions, interpretations and behaviors of persons in specific cultural groups is important.
- Issues such as cultural differences in defining health and in designing treatments are also important.
- As knowledge of specific cultures is gained, cross cultural comparison can lead to recognition of possible universal aspects as well.
- Ideology is comprised of the ideas of a group, their nature and source, and the doctrines, opinions or ways of thinking of a group.
- These are attached to an agreed upon set of beliefs or a creed. Value(s) refer to the especially favorable way of regarding the ideas, behaviors, customs, and institutions of a group as desirable, useful, estimable, important, or truthful.
- Ethnocentrism is the belief that one's own culture is superior to all others. This belief is common to all cultural groups; all groups regard their own culture as not only the best but also the correct, moral and only way of life.
- This belief is pervasive, often unconscious and is imposed on every aspect of day-to-day interaction and practices including health care.
- It is this attitude which creates problems between nurses and clients of diverse cultural groups.

TABLE 28.1: Components of model for cultural competence.

Component	Definition
Cultural awareness	Self-examination and in-depth exploration of one's own cultural and professional background; identification of biases and possible prejudices when working with specific groups of clients
Cultural knowledge	The proces of seeking and obtaining an information base on different cultural and ethnic groups, as well as understanding the groups' world views, which will explain how members of a group interpret their illness and how being a member guides their thinking, doing, and being
Cultural skill	Ability to collect relevant cultural data about patients' immediate problem and accurately perform culturally specific assessments; involves how to perform cultural assessments and culturally based physical assessments
Cultural encounter	The process that encourages nurses to engage directly in cross-cultural interactions with patients from culturally diverse backgrounds; directly interacting with such patients will refine or modify existing beliefs about a cultural group and prevent possible stereotyping that may have occurred
Cultural desire	Motivation to want to engage in the process of becoming culturally aware, knowledgeable, and skillful and to seek cultural encounters, as opposed to being reqired to seek such encounters; includes a genuine passion to be open to others, accept and respect differences, and be willing to learn from others as cultural informants

Cultural Diversity in Nursing Practice

- Knowledge of cultural diversity is vital at all levels of nursing practice. Ethnocentric approaches to nursing practice are ineffective in meeting health and nursing needs of diverse cultural groups of clients.
- Knowledge about cultures and their impact on interactions with health care is essential for nurses, whether they are practicing in a clinical setting, education, research or administration.
- Cultural diversity addresses racial and ethnic differences, however, these concepts or features of the human experience are not synonymous.

- Knowledge and skills related to cultural diversity can strengthen and broaden health care delivery systems.
- Other cultures can provide examples of a range of alternatives in services, delivery systems, conceptualization of illness, and treatment modalities.
- Cultural groups often utilize traditional health care providers, identified by and respected within the group.
- Concepts of illness, wellness, and treatment modalities evolve from a cultural perspective or world view.
- Concepts of illness, health, and wellness are part of the total cultural belief system. Culture is one of the organizing concepts upon which nursing is based and defined. Nurses need to understand:

Nurses can increase their own cultural competencies by following a few guidelines:

- Recognizing cultural differences and the diversity in our population.
- Building your own self-awareness and examining your own belief systems.
- Describing and making assessments based on facts and direct observation.
- Soliciting the advice of team members with experience in diverse backgrounds.
- Sharing your experiences honestly with other team members or staff to keep communication lines open, acknowledging any discomfort, hesitation, or concern.
- Practicing politically correct communication at all times – avoid making assumptions or stereotypical remarks.
- Creating a universal rule to give your time and attention when communicating.
- Refraining from making a judgment based on a personal experience or limited interaction.
- Signing up for diversity and inclusions seminars.
- Becoming involved in your agencies diversity programs—find out what your resources are—most institutions have something in place.

Nurse's Role in Cultural Diversity

- Nurses bring their personal cultural heritage as well as the cultural and philosophical views of their education into the professional setting.
- It is important for the nurse to understand that nurse-patient encounters include the interaction of three cultural systems—the culture of the nurse, the culture of the client and the culture of the setting.
- Access to care can be improved by providing culturally-relevant, responsive services. Individuals need choices of delivery systems in seeking health care.
- Nurses in clinical practice must use their knowledge of cultural diversity to develop and implement culturally sensitive nursing care. Nurses take pride in their role as client advocates.
- Recognizing cultural diversity, integrating cultural knowledge, and acting, when possible, in a culturally appropriate manner enables nurses to be more effective in initiating nursing assessments and serving as client advocates.
- All nursing curricula should include pertinent information about diverse health care beliefs, values, and practices. Such educational programs would demonstrate to nursing students that cultural beliefs and practices are as integral to the nursing process as are physical and psycho-social factors.
- Nurse administrators need to foster policies and procedures that help ensure access to care that accommodates varying cultural beliefs.
- Nurse administrators need to be knowledgeable about and sensitive to the cultural diversity among providers and consumers.
- Nurse researchers need to utilize the cross-cultural body of knowledge in order to ask pertinent research questions. Through exploration of other cultures, nurse researchers and practitioners find that while cultures differ, there are also many similarities among groups.
- Nurses are in a position to influence professional policies and practice in response to cultural diversity.

TRANSCULTURAL NURSING

Transcultural nursing is an essential aspect of healthcare today. The ever-increasing multicultural population poses a significant challenge to nurses providing individualized and holistic care to their patients. This requires nurses to recognize and appreciate cultural differences in healthcare values, beliefs, and customs. Nurses must acquire the necessary knowledge and skills in cultural competency.

Definition

- Leininger defined transcultural nursing as: "A legitimate and formal area of study, research, and practice focused on culturally based care, values, and practices to help cultures and sub-cultures maintain or regain their health and face difficulties or death in a culturally congruent and beneficial caring ways".
- Transcultural Nursing is a comparative study of cultures to understand similarities (cuture universal) and differences (culture-specific) across human group.

Goals

The goals of transcultural nursing is to give culturally congruent nursing care, and to provide culture specific and universal nursing care practices for the health and well-being of people or to aid them in facing adverse human conditions, illness or death in culturally meaningful ways.

Concept of Transcultural Nursing

- Transcultural nursing is a distinct nursing specialty which focuses on global cultures and comparative cultural caring, health, and nursing phenomena.

- The transcultural nurse looks to respond to the imperative for developing a global perspective within the nursing field in an increasingly globalized world of interdependent and interconnected nations and individuals.
- The primary aim of this specialty is to provide culturally congruent nursing care.
- To be an effective transcultural nurse, you should possess the ability to recognize and appreciate cultural differences in healthcare values, beliefs, and customs.
- Transcultural nurses shouldn't only be familiar with the religious customs, values, and beliefs of patients, but also how someone's way of life, their modes of thought, and their unique customs can immensely affect them in how they deal with illness, healing, disease, and deaths.
- Culturally competent nursing care helps ensure patient satisfaction and positive outcomes.
- The need for transcultural nursing will continue to be an important aspect in healthcare. Additional nursing research is needed to promote transcultural nursing.

Factors Influencing Transcultural Nursing Care

- Folk medicine practices.
- Refers to the nursing care of all patients, taking into consideration their religious and sociocultural backgrounds
- Specific anatomical characteristics
- Attitudes about mental illness and retardation.

Variables related to Transcultural Nursing

- Environmental factors and related disorders (e.g., ghetto living, lead poisoning)
- Attitudes toward health care, relationships, and interactions (e.g., personal space, eye contact).

Major Factors

- Reactions to pain, aging, and death.
- Attitudes about physical appearance and obesity
- Religious belief about illness and death

Principles: Basic principles related to culturally sensitive nursing practices are described below.
- The importance and influence of the culture should be considered,
- Cultural differences should be valued and respected,
- Cultural influences in the manners of individuals should be understood,
- An empathic approach should be put into action towards individuals with cultural diversity,
- Individuals' cultures should be respected,
- Health professionals should be patient with individuals in cultural issues,
- Individuals' behaviors should be thoroughly analyzed,
- Cultural knowledge should be increased and enhanced,
- Adaptation and orientation programs about cultural diversity should be offered.

The Scope of Cultural Nursing Practice

The scope of cultural nursing practice can be:
- Identification of cultural needs
- Understanding the cultural connections of the individual and the
- Using emotional strategies for the caregivers and the patients to reach the reciprocal goals.

Culturally congruent care: The care that is beneficial and meaningful to the people being served.

Culturally diverse nursing care: An optimal mode of health care delivery. It refers to the variability of nursing approaches needed to provide culturally appropriate care that incorporates an individual's cultural values, beliefs and practices including sensitivity to the environment from which the individual comes and to which the individual ultimately return.

Transcultural Healthcare

- It is vital that health services are also appropriate for the target cultures to the extent that they are compatible with contemporary medical understanding.
- People's beliefs and practices are part of the culture of the society in which they live.
- Cultural characteristics should be seen as a dynamic factor of health and disease.
- In order to be able to provide better health care, it is necessary to at least understand how the group receiving care perceives and responds to disease and health, and what cultural factors lie behind their behaviors.

Importance of Transculture

- Nurses connect with countless patients throughout their careers, and no two patients are alike. Transcultural nursing is the ability to connect with people from different cultures and to bring those cultures together to improve their health.
- The term "multicultural" relates to the presence of multiple cultural groups within a single society; multicultural nursing involves an awareness of the different cultural groups that make up our society in a healthcare setting.
- Cultural perspectives play a big role in shaping patients' beliefs about their health and healthcare. As a nurse, your job is to provide the very best care for each patient. That means taking patients' cultural backgrounds into consideration when helping them make decisions about their care.

Roles and Duties of a Transcultural Nurse

Transcultural nurses seek to provide culturally congruent and competent care to their patients. Providing culturally congruent care means providing care that fits the patient's valued life patterns. Since this will vary from culture to culture, transcultural nurses are expected to be familiar with a wide variety of cultures and their corresponding values. Providing culturally competent care refers to the ability of the transcultural nurse to bridge cultural gaps in caring, as well as working with cultural contrast to enable clients and families to bring about meaningful care. The functions and obligations of transcultural nurses include, but aren't limited to, the following:

- Communicate with foreign patients and their loved ones
- Educate families on patients' medical status
- Act as a bridge between a particular patient's culture and healthcare practice
- Determine the patient's cultural heritage and language skills
- Determine if any of the patient's health beliefs relate to the cause of their illness or problem
- Collect information on any home remedies the person is taking to treat their symptoms
- Understand the influence of culture, race, and ethnicity on the development of social and emotional relationships, child rearing practices, and attitude toward health
- Collect information about the socioeconomic status of the family and its influence on their health promotion and wellness.

Overcoming Barriers to Communication

Establishing an environment where cultural differences are respected begins with effective communication. This occurs not just from speaking the same language, but also through body language and other cues, such as voice, tone, and loudness.

- Greet the patient using his last name or his complete name. Avoid being too casual or familiar. Point to yourself, say your name, and smile.
- Proceed in an unhurried manner. Pay attention to any effort the patient or his family makes to communicate.
- Speak in a low, moderate voice. Avoid talking loudly. Remember, we all have a tendency to raise the volume and pitch of our voice when a listener appears not to understand. But he may think that you're angry and shouting.
- Organize your thoughts. Repeat and summarize frequently. Use audiovisual aids when feasible.
- Use short, simple sentences and speak in the active voice.
- Use simple words, such as "pain" rather than "discomfort." Avoid medical jargon, idioms, and slang.
- Avoid using contractions, such as *don't, can't, or won't*.
- Use nouns instead of pronouns. For example, ask your patient's parent, "Does Juan take this medicine?" rather than "Does he take this medicine?"
- Pantomime words, using gestures such as pointing or drinking from a cup, and perform simple actions while verbalizing them.
- Give instructions in the proper sequence. For example, rather than saying, "Before you take the medicine, get into bed," you should say, "Get into your bed, and then take your medicine."
- Discuss one topic at a time and avoid giving too much information in a single conversation. For example, instead of asking, "Are you cold and in pain?" separate your questions and gesture as you ask them: "Are you cold?" "Are you in pain?"
- Validate whether the patient understands by having him repeat instructions, demonstrate the procedure you've taught him, or act out the meaning.
- Use any appropriate words you know in the person's language. This shows that you're aware of and respect his native language.

MODELS OF TRANSCULTURAL NURSING

- **Leininger's sunrise model:**
  - The "Culture Care Diversity and Universality" theory developed by Leininger in 1960, the first nurse who made the first work in this field and received the title of anthropologist, is the first theory developed in the field of transcultural nursing and still used worldwide.
  - This theory focuses on exploring different and universal cultures and providing comparative care.
  - It adopts a multi-factorial approach affecting health and care such as environmental conditions, ethnography, language, gender, class, racism, social structuring, belief, politics, economics, kinship, technology, culture and philosophy.
  - This model includes technological, religious and philosophical, kinship and social factors, cultural values and lifestyle, political and legal, economic and social factors, which have been used in many studies in the west and in other countries since 1960.
- **Narayanasamy's ACCESS model:** Narayanasamy described the model in 1998 with the letters ACCESS (Assessment, Communication, Cultural negotiations and compromise, Establishing respect, Sensitivity and Safety) to form the framework of cultural care practices.

TABLE 28.2: ACCESS model for transcultural nursing.

Assessment	Focus on cultural aspects of clients' lifestyle, health beliefs, and health practices
Communication	Be aware of variations in verbal and non-verbal responses
Cultural negotiation and compromise	Become more aware of aspects of other people's culture as well as understanding clients' views and explaining their problems
Establishing respect and rapport	A therapeutic relation which portrays genuine respect for clients' cultural beliefs and values is required
Sensitivity	Deliver diverse culturally sensitive care to culturally diverse groups
Safety	Enable clients to derive a sense of cultural safety

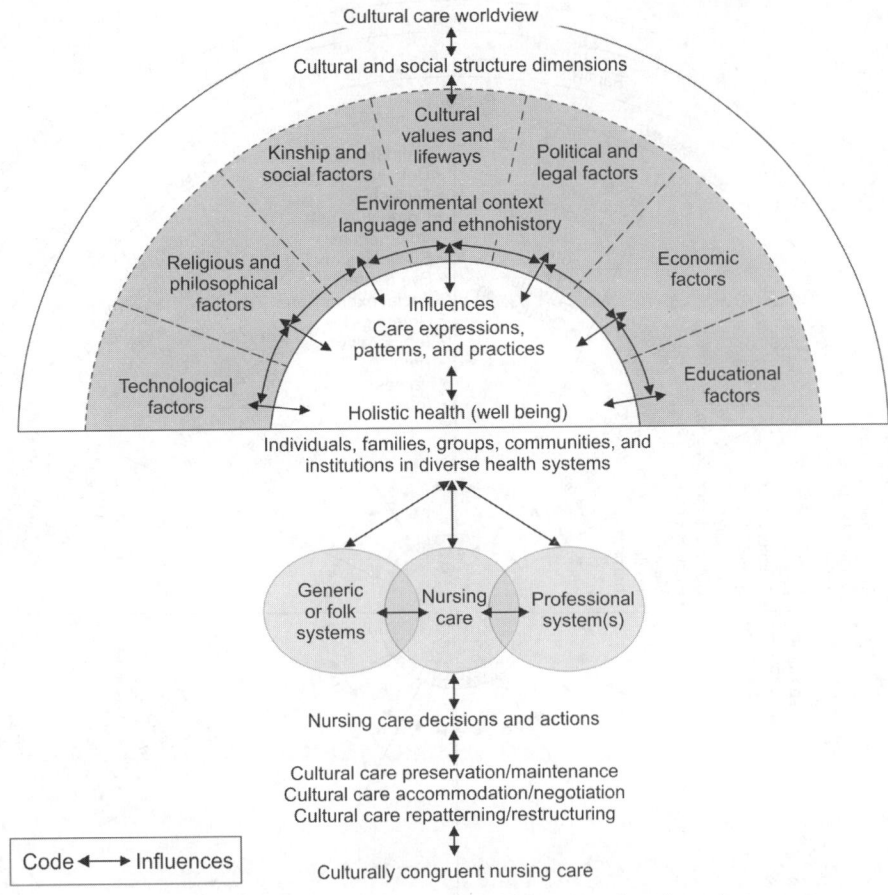

Fig. 28.2: Leininger's sunrise model for transcultural nursing.

- **Giger and Davidhizar's transcultural assessment model:** The model developed in 1988 was first published in 1990. This model is a tool developed to assess cultural values and their effects on health and disease behavior.
- **Purnell's cultural competence model:** This ethnographic model created to promote cultural understanding of people's status in the context of health promotion and illness is based on ethical perspectives of individual, family and community. It can be used in primary, secondary and tertiary protection stages.

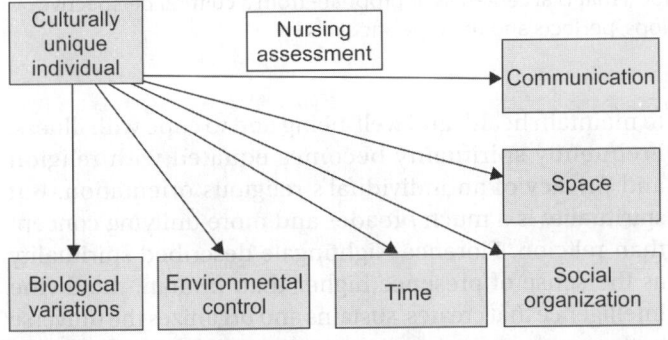

Fig. 28.3: Giger and Davidhizar's transcultural assessment model.

NURSES' COMPETENCES TO PROVIDE TRANSCULTURAL CARE

- Having the ability to understand complex cultural dimensions,
- Assuming a holistic approach to care instead of biophysical approach,
- Showing efforts to reach rapidly increasing cultural beliefs and activities that are unique to distinct groups and individuals
- Being able to change the idea of believing that individuals' own race is superior to others,
- Being able to make cultural evaluations,
- Developing communicative and scientific language skills,
- Being able to deal with cultural differences in real terms and make interpretations,
- Being able to use appropriate cultural teaching techniques
- Compromising cultural beliefs and studies with the general state of provision of health care,
- Respecting for the sociocultural diversity of women, newborn babies and their families.

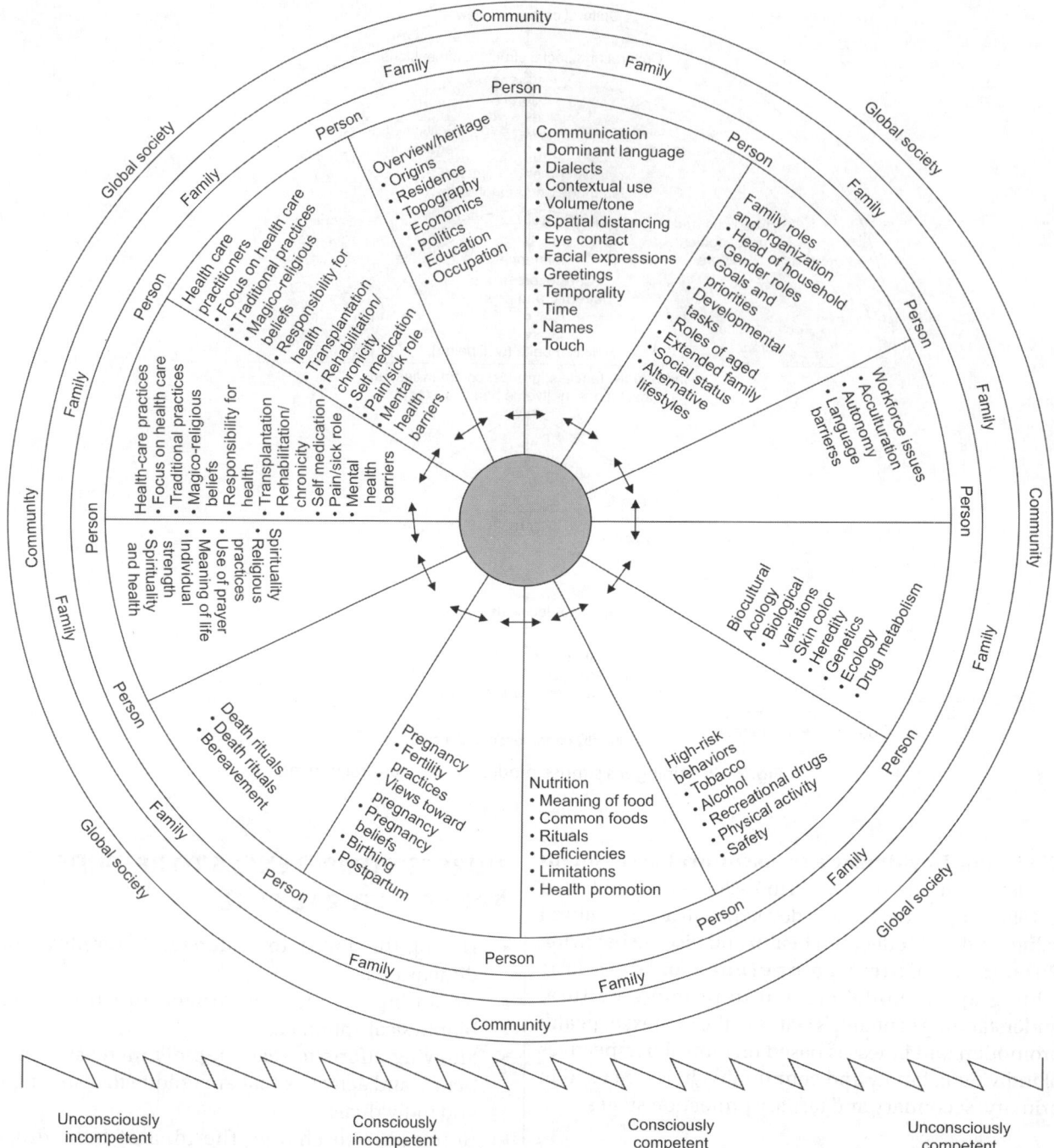

Fig. 28.4: Purnell's model for cultural competence. A care preparation that is accepted as appropriate from a cultural perspective requires that the nurse personally develops, perfects and uses specific skills.

SPIRITUALITY AND NURSING

The word "spirituality" derives from the Latin word spiritus, which refers to breath or wind. The spirit gives life to, or animates, a person. It signifies whatever is at the center of all aspects of a person life. A person's health depends on a balance of physical, psychological, sociological, cultural and spiritual factors. Spirituality is often identified as the important factor that helps to achieve the balance needed to maintain health and well-being and to cope with illness. Frequently spirituality becomes equated with religion and privacy of an individual's religious orientation. But spirituality is a much broader and more unifying concept than religion. Florence Nightingale described spirituality as the sense of presence higher than human, the divine intelligence that creates, sustains and organizes the universe and an awareness of our inner connection with this higher reality.

TABLE 28.3: FICA spiritual history tool.

Category	Sample questions
Faith and belief	Do you have spiritual beliefs that help you cope with stress? If the patient responds "no," consider asking: what gives your life meaning?
Importance	Have your beliefs influenced how you take care of yourself in this illness?
Community	Are you part of a spiritual or religious community? Is this of support to you, and how?
Address in care	How would you like me to address these issues in your health care?

MEANING AND DEFINITION

Spirituality is a concept that is unique to each individual. Individual's definitions of their own spirituality are influenced by their culture, life experiences, beliefs and ideas about life. There are two important characteristics of spirituality about which most authors agree:

- It is a unifying theme in people's lives
- It is a state of being atheist search for meaning in life through their work and their relationships with other individuals.

Because atheists feel they are alone, they sense a strong responsibility for themselves. They also tend to believe in a joint responsibility for others. In acting for themselves, they feel they should also act for all of mankind.

Spirituality and Religion

- Religion and nature are two vehicles that people use to connect themselves with God or a high power; however bonds to religious institutions, beliefs or dogma are not required to experience the spiritual sense of self.
- Faith, considered the formulation of spirituality, is a belief in something that a person cannot see.
- Spirituality is also a component of hope, and especially during chronic, serious or terminal illness, patients and their families often find comfort and emotional strength in their religious traditions or spiritual beliefs.
- Recently, nurse researchers as well as pastoral care professionals, physicians, social workers, and others have proposed that spirituality has special importance as the integrating theme that unifies all aspects of an individual's health.
- It is a force intrinsic to human nature and is one of the deepest and most potent resources for healing.
- Religion is commonly associated with the state of doing or a specific system of practices associated with a particular domination, sect, or form of worship.
- Religion is defined as a system of organized beliefs and worship that a person practices to outwardly express his or her spirituality.

- Many clients practice a faith or belief in the doctrines, and expressions of a specific religion or sect, such as protestant catholic, orthodox, Jehovah's Witness, Judaism, Buddhism, Islam, and Hinduism.
- A person's religion influences the manner in which an individual exercises a faith of belief and action.
- Religion serves different purposes in people's lives. For some, religion is a set of rules and rituals used to worship a supreme being.
- For others religion is a way of life providing nourishment and a connectedness to all of life. When providing spiritual care to clients it is important to understand the difference between religion and spirituality.

LIFESPAN CONSIDERATION IN SPIRITUAL HEALTH

- A person's level of growth and development influences his or her spiritual expression.
- Building on the theories of Erickson and Piaget, Fowler (1981) formulated a theory of faith development as the person's integrating center of valuing.
- Fowler's theory does not address the content of a person's faith such as a specific religious belief system, but views faith as another way of knowing the world, a spiritual knowing based on a particular phase of psychological and cognitive development.
- The following explanation integrates faith stage concepts with growth and development and identifies spiritual needs arising from these stages.

Newborn and Infant

- Trust in caregivers is the basis not only for development of a sense of safety, security of self in the world, and interpersonal relationship but also for faith development.
- Human beings' initial knowledge of the world is through relationship. If parents who are secure and have a sense of meaning and commitment meet basic trust needs, infants will sense this kinesthetically and incorporate this feeling into their "inner most being".

TABLE 28.4: HOPE spirirul assessmem.

H
Sources of hope, strength, comfort, meaning, peace, love and connection
O
The role of organized religion for the patient
P
Personal spirituality and practice
E
Effects on medical care and end-at-lite decisions

TABLE 28.5: FICA spiritual assessment.

F—faith and beliefs
 What are your spiritual or religious beliefs?
 Do you consider yourself spiritual or religious?
 What things do you believe in that give meaning to your life?

I—importance and influence
 Is it important in your life?
 How does it affect how you view your problems?
 How have your religion/spirituality influenced your behavior and mood during this illness?
 What role might your religion/spirituality play in resolving your problems?

C—community
 Are you part of a spiritual or religious community?
 Is this supportive to you and how?
 Is there a person or group of people you really love or who are really important to you?

A—address
 How would you like me to address these issues in your treatment?

Toddler and Preschooler

- The first stage of faith development, intuitive-projective, is characterized by a continuing differentiation of self from others and an awakening of consciousness and memory.
- The introduction of language and gestures facilitates the child's ability to participate in some faith rituals of family's religion.
- Children will respond to routines such as grace before meals, bedtime stories and prayers, special celebration, and holidays if they are offered as a consistent, natural part of family life.
- Children also respond positively to those who treat seriously their questions about the world, life and death. Though and an awakening of consciousness and memory.
- The introduction of language and gestures facilitates the child's ability to participate in some faith rituals of family's religion.
- Children will respond to routines such as grace before meals, bedtime stories and prayers, special celebration, and holidays if they are offered as a consistent, natural part of family life.
- Children also respond positively to those who treat seriously their questions about the world, life and death. Though children do not know about such matters rationally, they intuitively sense the deeper spiritual questions of existence.

School Age Child and Adolescent

- Children notice the difference between themselves as individuals and others in similar or different groups.
- They continue to be sensitive to good-bad issues, often trying to "make up" for wrong doing in concrete, literal ways.
- Children can now think in a historical perspective and see themselves as part of their family tree. The use of "story" is a major strategy for giving meaning to experience.
- Childhood is the period when the lore, legends, language and symbols of a particular religious group are best presented.
- Wishes, needs, facts and fantasy may appear somewhat confused, but children are attempting to make sense of the world. This period is the mythic-literal period.
- The major change in adolescence is the beginning of the ability to think abstractly, to conceptualize, and to synthesize.
- Adolescents can ask more sophisticated, philosophic questions, test the truth, evaluate others behavior, and note incongruities. They develop their own personal style, based on their beliefs, attitudes and values. Although adolescents they carry out this function mainly within the peer group.
- Mutuality and interpersonal relationships have major effects, making the development process both individualistic and conventional.
- Although the spiritual need is the same, faith is now centered within the peer group, synthesized differently from the parents.
- Authority has moved from the parents to the peer group. Thus the name for this stage is synthetic-conventional.

Disease	Spirituality
Denial	Acceptance
Violence	Peace
Dishonesty	Honesty
Isolalion	Communication
Anger/rage	Serenity
Shame	Self-esteem
Guilt	Freedom
Family dysfunction	Healthy relationships
Tiredness	Energy
Attempted suicide	Desire to live

Adult and Older Adult

- In the individualize-reflective stage, young adults move away from the conforming peer group and clarify boundaries of self hood and commitment.
- An encounter with people or groups other than those that provided support in the previous stage often precipitates this shift.
- Values, beliefs and attitudes change a result of interacting in more diverse, pluralistic settings, which can be stressful and frightening.
- Some situations precipitating this shift include new jobs, international travel, advanced study or education, or new religious affiliations possibly intertwined with

achieving intimate relationships, choosing careers and starting families.
- The challenge during this stage is to establish one's own sense of faith and commitment based on personal experience and reflection on meaning in life.
- The middle years are fulfilled through productive activity in Erickson's term, generativity. This time is of growth and renewed questioning, in some ways very similar to adolescence.
- Adults, however, deal with a broader world view rather than with group conformity.
- Older adults notice the polarities or extremes in life such as young and old, rich and poor, masculine and feminine, war and peace, constructive and destructive, and self-awareness and self-denial.
- These tensions enhanced or precipitated by personal and environmental situations, demand integration and resolution. This is referred to as conjunctive faith.
- Most people do not achieve the final stage of faith, universalizing. Usually only great leaders such as Mahatma Gandhi, Martine Luther King and Mother Teresa appear to have achieved this world view.
- Terms such as justice, love and compassion describe the goals of the person in the universalizing stage.

CHARACTERISTICS OF SPIRITUALITY

The major characteristics of spirituality include a sense of wholeness and harmony within one's self, with God or a higher power as one defines it. It does not mean that individuals are totally satisfied with life or have all the answers. Assisting clients with the ensuring spiritual struggle is a valid and important aspect of maintaining health and giving health care.

- **Holism:** Holism, the position of viewing the universe as a system of harmonious interconnectedness rather than sum of isolated parts, integrates the mind and body and emphasizes spirit. A holistic approach recognizes the spiritual struggle as valid and important aspects of health and health care. It is the integrating factor of "previously compartmentalized constructs of physical body, rational mind, emotional psyche, and intuitive spirit".

Characteristics of spiritual well being	
• Sense of inner peace	• Humor
• Compassion for others	• Wisdom
• Reverence for life	• Generosity
• Gratitude	• Ability to transcend self
• Appreciation for unity and diversity	• Capacity for unconditional love

The concept of a spiritual wellness program has been introduced in some long-term care facilities. In this program, a spiritual wellness staff uses a holistic approach to care in order to address the needs of older residents, their family members, and the staff. Sigmund Freud's early disciple Carl Lung expanded the concept of the unconscious to make it include good emotions and even spiritual urges.

- **Spiritual need:** Definitions of spiritual need vary according to each author's belief system. In summarizing the various definitions, spiritual need represents a normal expression of a person's inner being that seeks meaning in all experience and a dynamic relationship with self, others and to the supreme other as the person defines it. Spiritual needs include trust, forgiveness, love and relatedness, faith, creativity and hope, meaning and purpose and grace.

  Spiritual needs are identified, as an individual's desire to find meaning and purpose in life, pain and death. The spiritual realms are often considered a very private area. In order to provide a holistic care, however, the nurse must pay attention to the spiritual dimension of each client, recognizing spiritual needs and assisting the client in meeting them.

- **Spiritual quest:** Life may be viewed as a spiritual quest, not only to answer life's philosophic questions but also to seek a higher level of consciousness or a deeper awareness of spiritual life. For example, the recovery as a spiritual journey; group members practice a spiritual discipline to live more meaningfully day-by-day. Recovery begins through a "leap of faith" which lays that there is no meaning to be found other than that which is beyond one's self.

  A common question asked by spiritual seekers is, to what extent they should pay attention to their health. For some seekers this question arises because interest in spiritual life, which is primarily a quest for the eternal, immutable, ever pure, immortal, infinite spirit, seems to be incompatible with interest in the ever changing, impure, limited, perishable physical body.

- **Spiritual well-being:** Spiritual wellness manifests as inner strength and peace. Spiritual well-being is a condition marked by an affirmation of life, peace, harmony, and a sense of interconnectedness with God, self, community and environment that nurtures and celebrates wholeness. In the hierarchy of human needs, spiritual well-being appears to connote fulfillment of needs beyond the self-actualization level. All the subjects expressed a belief in a supreme being, had some means of communication with that entity through prayer and worship, and had an extensive social support system of meaningful personal relationships.

FACTORS AFFECTING SPIRITUAL HEALTH

A number of factors affect expression of spiritual needs. Such things include culture, gender and previous experience. Individual reactions vary depending on personality and past coping styles. Other factors contributing to spiritual health include appropriate religious education, a firm spiritual identity, a dynamic and adaptable belief system, and maintenance of belief system in times of adversity or under questioning by others, recognition of spiritual assistance

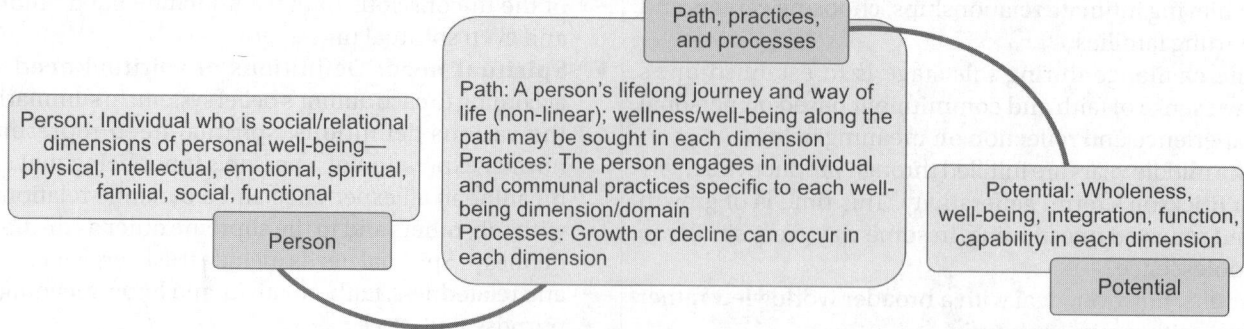

Fig. 28.5: Factors affecting spiritual health.

when needed, empathy for other's beliefs and values, and a sense of spiritual fulfillment.

Other factors, such as crises, moral issues, and separation, can affect changes in spiritual health and well-being, placing individuals at risk for altered spiritual function. These factors, however, are subjective and mean different things to different people.

- **Religious problems:** Client's religious problems can affect their spirituality. Customary religious practices, if interrupted or changed, may affect the structure or support that religion contributes to the person's sense of well-being.
- **Change in denominational membership or religious conversion:** Marrying a person with a different religious background or moving to a new community that does not have a branch of a particular religious group, will create, at least initially, loss for an individual. If a loss is felt, the individual experiences separation from a previously valued religious community. The extent of the loss is influenced by the choice the individual had in the change, how flexible the person's religious expression is, and what communities of faith are available to the individual.
- **Loss or questioning of faith:** A person often finds a way to express his or her faith through religious practices. Persons who are at an early stage of development of their faith who find their faith challenged by an event such as acute or chronic illness, terminal disease, or loss of a loved one may become vulnerable to loss of or doubt about their faith. This can also occur when one is shunned by one's religious community or when one is seriously a question the position one's religious denomination takes on a public issue. A loss or questioning of faith can cause serious guilt and a sense of loneliness even when it can lead to more mature faith and stronger conviction.
- **Culture:** Altitudes, beliefs and values arise from one's sociocultural background. Usually, but not always, people follow the spiritual and religious tradition of their families of origin. In inter faith marriages; children may follow the practices of one parent over the other. Many times, religious preference is tied to the ethnic background.
- **Gender:** Spiritual expression also depends on societies and the religious group's beliefs and teachings about gender or expected behaviors for males and females. A person's organized religion may prescribe how each sex dresses and if one wears a head covering. In some cases, the spiritual leader is always male.
- **Previous experience:** It would appear that if one's faith and values are confronted, then deeper spiritual needs would arise. During a crisis, past coping styles or learned ways of handling situations are likely to be evident. Life experiences in general are influences. Such experiences may or may not be related to age.
- **Crisis and change:** A crisis may strengthen a person's spirituality, which often happens when people face death. Just as crisis may strengthen one's faith, it may also weaken it. Crisis may be related to pathophysiologic changes, required treatments, or situations affecting the person. Personal changes that result from the death or illness of a loved one, opposition to personal religious beliefs by significant others, or change in personal status can become other sources of spiritual distress. Being hospitalized can interrupt usual religious practices at a time when they are most needed, which can add to spiritual distress.
- **Separation from spiritual ties:** Experience of being hospitalized or becoming a resident in a retirement or nursing home can initially be shattering. To some extent, such individuals are isolated from personal freedom, personal privileges, and social support systems. This separation from spiritual ties places people at risk for altered spiritual function.
- **Moral issues regarding therapy:** Many religions view healers and the healing process as evidence of God at work in the world. Certain groups, however, object to some modern medical interventions. For example, some Christians oppose abortion because of their belief that the soul enters the body at conception. Religious teachings influence attitudes toward many other medical procedures such as right-to-die decisions, organ transplantation, circumcision, birth control, sterilization, autopsies and handling of the diseased. The choice to treat may be difficult to make if the religious beliefs say "no" and the health care system says "yes".

Many health care agencies have ethics committee to clarify and review such situation so more adequate and informed decisions are made.

- **Inadequate or inappropriate care:** When dealing with spiritual care, nurses must be careful neither to avoid assisting clients with such care nor to involve themselves without desire on the client's part. Doing nothing or jumping in too quickly may result in inadequate or inappropriate care.

  Grandstorm (1985) elaborates on these reasons when she identifies five fairly complex values issues between nurses and clients.

- **Pleuralism:** Nurses and clients embrace a wide spectrum of beliefs and creeds.
- **Fear:** Related to not being able to handle situations, intruding on client's privacy, or becoming confused in one's own belief and value system.
- **Awareness of own spiritual quest:** What gives meaning, purpose, hope and sense of love in one's own life.
- **Confusion:** Confusion over difference between religious and spiritual concepts.
- **Basic attitudes:** Attitudes relative to illness, aging and suffering. The nurses need opportunities to reflect on their own philosophies and belief systems.

SPIRITUAL DIMENSIONS OF NURSING

Spiritual dimension of nursing is the form of knowledge, attitude and skills from the above exposition on self-awareness and spirituality to nursing practice.

- **Practice:** As guidance, an outline of the salient points related to the spiritual dimensions of the patient's needs is given for consideration when preparing nurses in the four stages of nursing process—assessment, planning, implementation, and evaluation an applied to spiritual care.
- **The learning process:** Experiential and student centered learning could be used to develop nurse's communication and counseling skills. The teacher could act as facilitator to enable nurses to develop knowledge and awareness of patient's spirituality.

The Person and Spiritual Well-being

Human beings, who are body-mind-spirit entities, have five dimensions with needs specific to each dimension:

- The physical—with needs, for example, for food and fluids;
- The social—with needs, for example, to relate, to love and be loved, to experience mutuality and friendship;
- The emotional—with needs, for example, to experience and express feelings;
- The psychological—with needs, for example, of security, comfort, safety; and
- The spiritual—with needs to find a sense of purpose and meaning, hope, and peace of mind.

AGE-SPECIFIC SPIRITUAL INTERVENTIONS

- **Newborn and infant:** Hospitalization and illness potentially disrupt infant's basic trust in parents; the nurse can support the spiritual needs of parents by listening, offering support and promoting stability. Encourage parents to be present and involved in the caring process with infants as much as possible.
- **Toddler and preschooler:** Support families to carry out rituals of faith. If the family is unavailable to do this, nurses can carry out these rituals for them.

  Young children are sensitive to good or bad issue. Do not tell them that painful or scary treatments are in any way a punishment.
- **School age child and adolescent:** Nurses continue to provide major support to families by carrying out familiar religious rituals in the health care setting. For children, classify fact and fantasy when it comes to all medical interventions and procedures. Acceptance and classification of the experience are the effective models to offer meaning to children. For adolescents, development of a personal style and interaction with peers remain priorities even during illness. Involve the adolescent's peers by encouraging them to remain available either through visits, letter or telephone. Adolescents are capable of conceptualizing personal relationship with God. In times of illness, they may question the meaning of the experienced, trying to integrate into their lives, much as adults would do under similar circumstances. These issues can often be discerned during a nursing history and assessment.
- **Adult and older adult:** Young adult's faith challenge is to establish and to reflect on personal faith and life's meaning. At the very least, all nurses must understand that young adults have the need for spiritual mentoring. Continue to be supportive of each client's family and social network because these relationships give meaning to the client's life. During the middle year, adults become more concerned with a broader worldview and

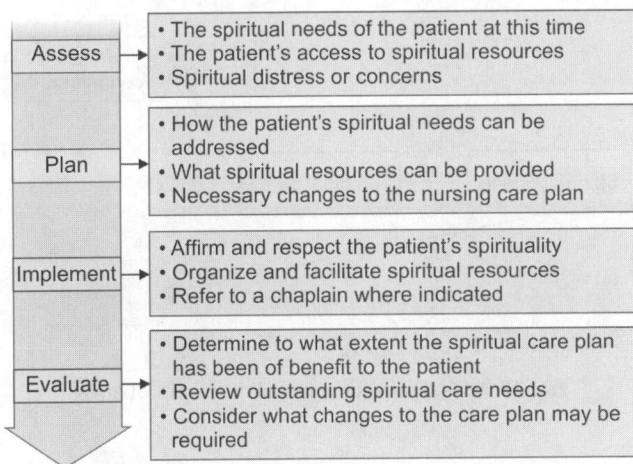

Fig. 28.6: Spiritual assessment process in nursing.

polarities. By accepting the possibility of mutuality in the relationship, the nurse has the opportunity to give new meaning and hope to the client. As with other age groups, listening and support are essential as clients deal with health illness.

Using a life review strategy, in which clients recollect past experiences and come to the understanding of them, is helpful. As infirmity increases, older adults may be less able than previous years to participate in their faith communities. At this point, facilitate connection with people or groups in the community who can either visit regularly or assist with transportation. Providing answers is not important. Rather the focus is giving clients the opportunity to discuss death and to make their own choices about how arrangement should be handled.

- **Special population:** There are differences in the spiritual concerns of persons with acute illness, persons living with pain, or persons facing surgery. For example, persons living with mental illness often have spiritual question because the mental illness can be in a form expressed in terms of religious delusion or hallucinations. Often, though, health care providers including nurses avoid spiritual issues for fear of "supporting" the symptoms of the mental illness. There are new views of "recovery" as the spiritual need for ope. Hope is the "turning" point in a person's illness. So instead of avoiding spiritual care, several articles suggest way) if incorporating into care.

DEALING WITH SPIRITUAL DISTRESS/PROBLEMS

Spiritual distress is a disturbance in a person's belief system. As an approved nursing diagnosis, spiritual distress is defined as "a disruption in the life principle that pervades a person's entire being and that integrates and transcends one's biological and psychological nature."

Definition: Spirituality has been defined as "more of a journey and religion may be the transport to help us in our journey" (Narayansamy, 2004). Patients who are dying often think about their own spirituality. For some, it is a time to become more in touch with one's spirituality, and for others it is a time for their spirituality to become even stronger. Still, there are patients who do not want to discuss spiritual issues and are often angry at their situation and angry at any higher powers which they feel responsible for their impending death. As a nurse who cares for patients nearing the end of their lives, spirituality is something that needs to be taken into consideration.

Meaning of spiritual distress: Spiritual pain or distress happens if you have questions and become upset about your belief and value systems. It occurs when a person is unable to find sources of meaning, hope, love, peace, comfort, strength, or connection in life. This may happen when something happens in our life those conflicts with our beliefs about ourselves and how we are in the world. Spiritual pain or distress can be normal feelings for someone who is living with illness. Spiritual distress most often occurs when a person is experiencing change, challenges, physical and emotional pain, other symptoms, and losses associated with serious illness.

Signs and symptoms of spiritual distress include:
- Feelings of anger or hopelessness.
- Feelings of depression and anxiety.
- Difficulty sleeping.
- Feeling abandoned by God.
- Questioning the meaning of life or suffering.
- Questioning beliefs or sudden doubt in spiritual or religious beliefs.
- Asking why this situation occurred.

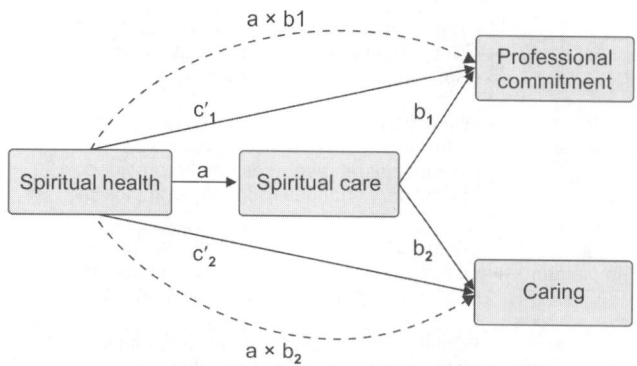

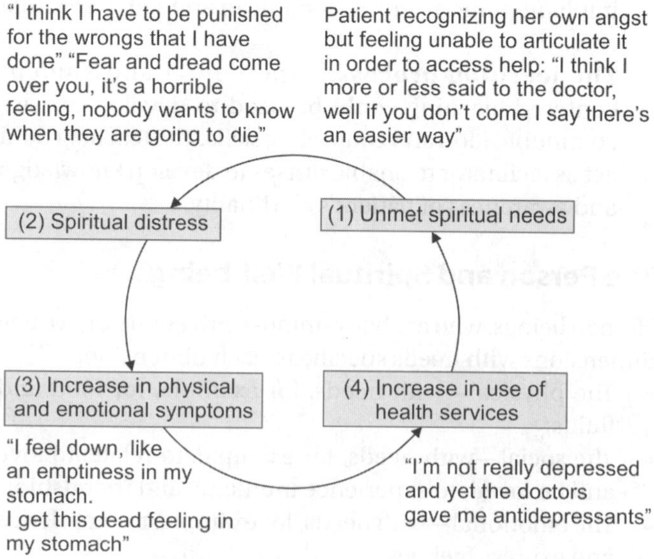

Fig. 28.7: Dealing with spiritual distress/problems.

Fig. 28.8: Indicators spiritual distress.

Indicators spiritual distress: The indicators (pain, alienation, anxiety, guilt, loss, and despair) must or may be present in defining the characteristics of spiritual distress. The use of indicators in diagnosing alterations in spiritual health is controversial because indicators may appear related to both spiritual and psychosocial problems.

Seven manifestations of spiritual distress: The diagnosis of spiritual distress is defined by indicators that are present—spiritual pain, spiritual alienation, spiritual anxiety, spiritual guilt, spiritual anger, spiritual loss, and spiritual despair.

i. Nursing diagnoses: Spiritual pain, as evidenced by expressions of discomfort of suffering relative to one's relationship with God, verbalization of feelings of having a void or lack of spiritual fulfillment, and/or a lack of peace in terms of one's relationship to one's creator.

ii. Nursing diagnoses: Spiritual alienation, as evidenced by expressions of loneliness or the feeling that God seems very far away and remote from one's everyday life, verbalization that one has to depend upon one's self in times of trial or need, and/or a negative attitude toward receiving any comfort or help from God.

iii. Nursing diagnoses: Spiritual anxiety, as evidenced by expression of fear of God's wrath and punishment; fear that God might not take care of one, either immediately or in the future; and/or worry that God is displeased with one's behavior.

iv. Nursing diagnoses: Spiritual guilt, as evidenced by expressions suggesting that one has failed to do the things which he should have done in life and/or done things which were not pleasing to God; articulation of concerns about the "kind" of life one has lived.

v. Nursing diagnoses: Spiritual anger, as evidenced by expression of frustration or outrage at God for having allowed illness or other trials, comments about the "unfairness" of God, and/or negative remarks about institutionalized religion and/or its ministers or spiritual care givers.

vi. Nursing diagnoses: Spiritual loss, as evidenced by expression of feelings of having temporarily lost or terminated the love of God, fear that one's relationship with God has been threatened, and/or a feeling of emptiness with regard to spiritual things.

vii. Nursing diagnoses: Spiritual despair, as evidenced by expressions suggesting that there is no hope of ever having a relationship with God or of pleasing Him and/or a feeling that God no longer can or does care for one."

CONCLUSION

Spirituality is defined as connectedness with self, others, a life or God that allows people to experience, self-transcendence and find meaning in life. Spirituality helps people discover a purpose in life, understand the vicissitudes of life and develop their relations with God or a high power. Within the framework of spirituality a person discovers the truth about self, about the world and about the concepts such as love, compassion, wisdom, honesty, commitment, imagination, reverence, and morality. Often, spiritual behavior is expressed through sacrifice, self-discipline and spending time in activities that focus on the inner self or soul.

BIBLIOGRAPHY

1. Cassell EJ. Recognizing suffering. Hastings Center Report, 1991;21(3), 24-31.
2. Curtis JR, Engelberg R, Young JP, Vig LK, Reinke LF, Wenrich, MD. et al. An approach to understanding the interaction of hope and desire for explicit prognostic information among individuals with severe chronic obstructive pulmonary disease or advanced cancer. Journal of Palliative Medicine. 2008;11, 610-20.
3. Eliott JA, Olver IN. Hope and hoping in the talk of dying cancer patients. Social Science & Medicine. 2007;(64):138-49.
4. Ersek M, Cotter V. The meaning of hope in the dying. In: Ferrell BR, Coyle N (Eds). Oxford Textbook of Palliative Nursing. New York: Oxford University Press. 2010; 579-95.
5. Felder BE. Hope and coping in patients with cancer diagnoses. Cancer Nursing. 2004;(27):320-4.
6. Narayansamy A. The puzzle of spirituality for nursing: A guide to practical assessment. British Journal of Nursing. 2004;13(19):1140-44.
7. Oberg Kalervo. Cultural shock: Adjustment to new Cultural environments." Practical Anthropology. 1960;7:177-82.
8. Ogburn William F. "Cultural Lag as Theory." Sociology & Social Research. 1957;41(3):167-74.
9. Powell LH, Shahabi L, Thoresen CE. Religion and spirituality: Linkages to physical health. Am Psychol. 2003;58(1):36-52.
10. Smith Dorothy. The Everyday World as Problematic: A Feminist Sociology. Toronto: University of Toronto Press. 1987.
11. Sumner William G. Folkways: A Study of the Sociological Importance of Usages, Manners, Customs, Mores, and Morals. New York: Ginn and Co. 1906.
12. The World Health Organization Quality of Life assessment (WHOQOL): position paper from the World Health Organization. Soc Sci Med. 1995; 41(10):1403-9.
13. Zerwekh JV. Nursing Care at the End of Life: Palliative Care for Patients and Families. Philadelphia: F.A. Davis Company, 2006.

REVIEW QUESTIONS

Long Essays

1. Explain providing culturally responsive care.
2. Discuss about cultural diversity.
3. Describe about lifespan consideration in spiritual health.
4. Explain in detail about transcultural nursing.

Short Essays

1. Cultural competence.
2. Culturally responsive care.
3. Psychosocial care and assessment.
4. Impact of cultural diversity.

5. Cultural diversity in nursing practice.
6. Transcultural healthcare.
7. Roles and duties of a transcultural nurse.
8. Models of transcultural nursing.
9. Nurses' competences to provide transcultural care.
10. Spirituality and nursing.
11. Factors affecting spiritual health.
12. Spiritual dimensions of nursing.
13. Dealing with spiritual distress/problems.

Short Answers

1. Culture.
2. Subculture.
3. Multicultural.
4. Acculturation.
5. Cultural assimilation.
6. Cultural awareness.
7. Cultural competence.

CHAPTER 29

Nursing Theories

LEARNING OBJECTIVES

- Introduction
- Meaning and Definition
- Purposes
- Types of theories with examples
- Overview of selected nursing theories—Nightingale, Orem, Roy
- Use of theories in nursing practice

TERMINOLOGY

Philosophy: Beliefs and values that define a way of thinking and are generally known and understood by a group or discipline.

Theory: A belief, policy, or procedure proposed or followed as the basis of action. It refers to a logical group of general propositions used as principles of explanation. Theories are also used to describe, predict, or control phenomena.

Concept: Concepts are often called the building blocks of theories. They are primarily the vehicles of thought that involve images.

Models: Models are representations of the interaction among and between the concepts showing patterns. They present an overview of the thinking behind the theory and may demonstrate how theory can be introduced into practice.

Conceptual framework: A conceptual framework is a group of related ideas, statements, or concepts. It is often used interchangeably with the conceptual model and with grand theories.

Proposition: Propositions are statements that describe the relationship between the concepts.

Domain: Domain is the perspective or territory of a profession or discipline.

Process: Processes are a series of organized steps, changes or functions intended to bring about the desired result.

Paradigm: A paradigm refers to a pattern of shared understanding and assumptions about reality and the world; worldview or widely accepted value system.

Metaparadigm: A metaparadigm is the most general statement of discipline and functions as a framework in which the more restricted structures of conceptual models develop. Much of the theoretical work in nursing focused on articulating relationships among four major concepts: person, environment, health, and nursing.

INTRODUCTION

Nursing theories are organized bodies of knowledge to define what nursing is, what nurses do, and why do they do it. Nursing theories provide a way to define nursing as a unique discipline that is separate from other disciplines (e.g., medicine). It is a framework of concepts and purposes intended to guide the practice of nursing at a more concrete and specific level. Nursing theories are the basis of nursing practice today. In many cases, nursing theory guides knowledge development and directs education, research, and practice. Historically, nursing was not recognized as an academic discipline or as a profession we view it today. Before nursing theories were developed, nursing was

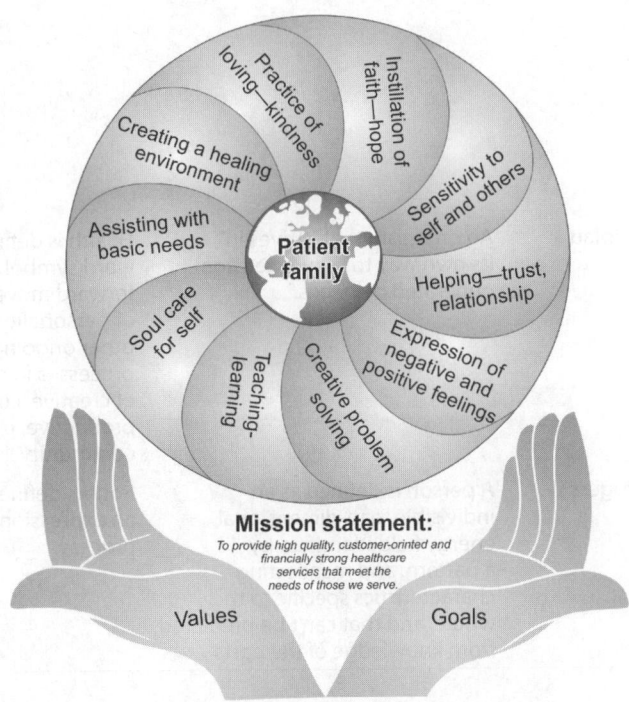

Fig. 29.1: Values and goals of nursing theories.

considered to be a task-oriented occupation. The training and function of nurses were under the direction and control of the medical profession.

HISTORY OF NURSING THEORIES

The first nursing theories appeared in the late 1800s when a strong emphasis was placed on nursing education.

- In 1860, Florence Nightingale defined nursing in her "Environmental Theory" as "the act of utilizing the environment of the patient to assist him in his recovery."
- In the 1950s, there is a consensus among nursing scholars that nursing needed to validate itself through the production of its own scientifically tested body of knowledge.
- In 1952, Hildegard Paplau introduced her Theory of Interpersonal Relations that puts emphasis on the nurse-client relationship as the foundation of nursing practice.
- In 1955, Virginia Henderson conceptualized the nurse's role as assisting sick or healthy individuals to gain independence in meeting 14 fundamental needs, thus her Nursing Need Theory was developed.

Nursing Metaparadigm of Different Nurse Theorists

	Person	Health	Nursing	Environment
Nightingale	Human beings were not defined by Nightingale specifically	Nightingale (1859/1992) did not define health specificilly	"What nursing has to do is to put the patient in the best condition for nature to act upon him" (Nightingale, 1859/1992)	Nightingale's writings reflect a community health model in which all that surrounds human beings is considered in relation to their state of health.
Orem	Humans are defined as "men, women, and children cared for either singly or as social units," and are the "material object" of nurses and others who provide direct care	Health is "being structurally and functionally whole or sound."	Nursing is an art through which the practitioner of nursing gives specialized assistance to persons with disabilities which makes more than ordinary assistance necessary to meet needs for self-care	The environment has physical, chemical and biological features. It includes the family, culture, and community
Henderson	Individuals have basic needs that are component of health and require assistance to achieve health and independence or a peaceful death	Health was taken to mean blance in all realms of human life	"The unique function of the nurse is to assist the individual, sick or well, in the performance of those activities contributing to health or its recovery that he would perform unaided if he had the necessary strength, will or knowledge. And to do this in such a way as to help him gain independence as rapidly as possible."	No explicit definition of the environment, though she stated that: "maintaining a supportive environment conducive for health is one of the elements of her 14 activities for client assistance."
Peplau	An organism that "strives in its own way to reduce tension generated by needs."	Health is defined as "a word symbol that implies forward movement of personality and other ongoing human processes in the direction of creative, constructive, productive, personal, and community living."	Hildegard Peplau considers nursing to be a "significant, therapeutic, interpersonal process."	Although Peplau does not directly address society/environment, she does encourage the nurse to consider the patient's culture and mores when the patient adjusts to hospital routine.
Rogers	A person is defined as an indivisible, pan-dimensional energy field identified by a pattern, and manifesting characteristics specific to the whole, and that can't be predicted from knowledge of the parts	Rogers defines health as an expression of the life process	Nursing aims to assist people in achieving their maximum health potential.	It is the study of unitary, irreducible, indivisible human and environmental fields: people and their world.

Contd...

Contd...

	Person	Health	Nursing	Environment
King	Individuals are social beings who are rational and sentient. Humans communicate their thoughts, actions, customs, and beliefs through language.	Health is a dynamic life experience of a human being, which implies continuous adjustment to stressors in the internal and external environment through optimum use of one's resources to achieve maximum potential for daily liying.	Environement is the bacground for human interactions. It is both external to, and internal to, the individual.	Nursing is a process of action, reaction, and interaction whereby nurse and client share information about their perceptions in the nursing situation.
Watson	Human being is a valued person to be cared for, respected, nurtured, understood, and assisted; in general a philosophical view of a person as a fully functional integrated self.	Health is the unity and harmony within the mind, body, and soul; health is associated with the degree of congruence between the self as perceived and the self as experienced	Society provides the values that determine how one should behave and what goals one should strive toward	Nursing is a human science of persons and human health iliness experiences that are mediated by professional, personal, scientific, esthetic, and ethical human care transactions

- In 1960, Faye Abdullah published her work "Typology of 21 Nursing Problems" that shifted the focus of nursing from a disease-centered approach to a patient-centered approach.
- In 1962, Ida Jean Orlando emphasized the reciprocal relationship between patient and nurse and viewed the professional function of nursing as finding out and meeting the patient's immediate need for help.
- In 1968, Dorothy Johnson pioneered the Behavioural System Model and upheld the fostering of efficient and effective behavioral functioning in the patient to prevent illness.
- In 1970, Martha Rogers viewed nursing as both a science and an art as it provides a way to view the unitary human being, who is integral with the universe.
- In 1971, Dorothea Orem states in her theory that nursing care is required if the client is unable to fulfill biological, psychological, developmental, or social needs.
- In 1971, Imogene King 's Theory of Goal attainment states that the nurse is considered part of the patient's environment and the nurse-patient relationship is for meeting goals towards good health.
- In 1972, Betty Newman in her theory states that many needs exist, and each may disrupt client balance or stability. Stress reduction is the goal of the system model of nursing practice.
- In 1979, Sr. Callista Roy viewed the individual as a set of interrelated systems who strives to maintain the balance between these various stimuli.
- In 1979, Jean Watson developed the philosophy of caring highlighted humanistic aspects of nursing as they intertwine with scientific knowledge and nursing practice.

DEFINITION

- A theory is a statement that purports to account for or characters some phenomenon and that it pulls out the salient parts of a phenomenon so that one can separate the critical and necessary factors or relationships from the accidental or unessential factors or relations- 1990.
- A model is analogous to an equation in mathematics. Nursing models usually describe person, environment, health, and nursing.
- A theory is a set of concepts interrelated to from proposition that are useful for prediction and control.
- A theory is a conceptual system or the framework invented for some purpose.
- A theory is a set of interrelated constructs (concepts adapted for a scientific purpose), definitions and propositions that present new systematic phenomena by specifying relations among valuables with the purpose of emplaning and predicting the phenomena.

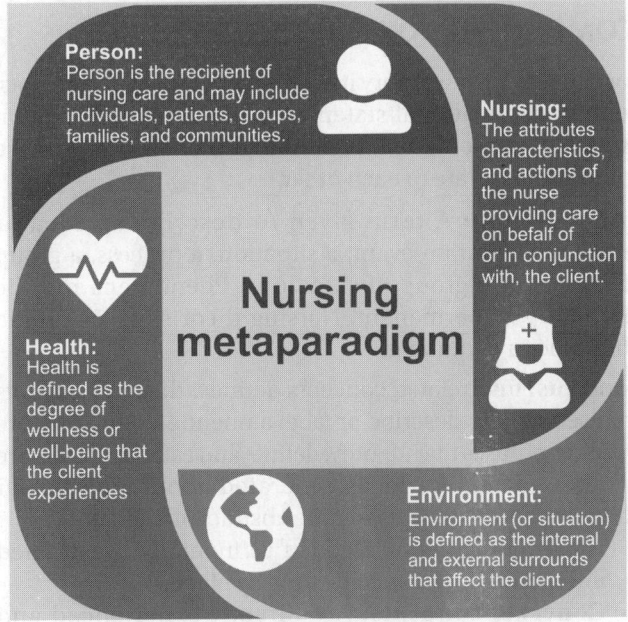

Fig. 29.2: Components of nursing metaparadigm.

- A theory is a systematic abstraction means that theory is a representation of reality, and purposes include description explanation and prediction of phenomena, and control of some reality.
- Nursing theory is a set of concepts, depositions and propositions that project a systematic view of phenomena by designating specific interrelationship among concepts for the purposes of describing, explaining, predicting and or controlling phenomena.

NURSING METAPARADIGM

There are four major concepts that are frequently interrelated and fundamental to nursing theory: person, environment, health, and nursing. These four are collectively referred to as metaparadigm for nursing.

Person: Person (also referred to as Client or Human Beings) is the recipient of nursing care and may include individuals, patients, groups, families, and communities.

Environment: Environment (or situation) is defined as the internal and external surrounds that affect the client. It includes all positive or negative conditions that affect the patient, the physical environment, such as families, friends, and significant others, and the setting for where they go for their healthcare.

Health: Health is defined as the degree of wellness or well-being that the client experiences. It may have different meanings for each patient, the clinical setting, and the health care provider.

Nursing: The attributes, characteristics, and actions of the nurse providing care on behalf of or in conjunction with, the client. There are numerous definitions of nursing, though nursing scholars may have difficulty agreeing on its exact definition, the ultimate goal of nursing theories is to improve patient care.

COMPONENTS OF NURSING THEORIES

For a theory to be a theory it has to contain a set of concepts, definitions, relational statements, and assumptions that explain a phenomenon. It should also explain how these components relate to each other.

Phenomenon: A term given to describe an idea or responses about an event, a situation, a process, a group of events, or a group of situations. Phenomena may be temporary or permanent. Nursing theories focus on the phenomena of nursing.

Concepts: Interrelated concepts define a theory. Concepts are used to help describe or label a phenomenon. They are words or phrases that identify, define, and establish structure and boundaries for ideas generated about a particular phenomenon. Concepts may be abstract or concrete.
- **Abstract concepts:** Defined as mentally constructed independent of a specific time or place.
- **Concrete concepts:** Are directly experienced and related to a particular time or place.

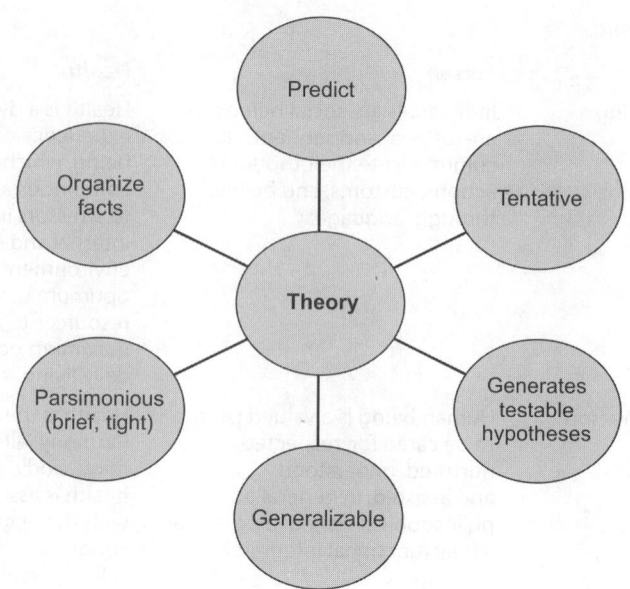

Fig. 29.3: Components of nursing theories.

Definitions: Definitions are used to convey the general meaning of the concepts of the theory. Definitions can be theoretical or operational.

Theoretical definitions: Define a particular concept based on the theorist's perspective.

Operational definitions: States how concepts are measured.

Relational statements: Relational statements define the relationships between two or more concepts. They are the chains that link concepts to one another.

Assumptions: Assumptions are accepted as truths and are based on values and beliefs. These are statements that explain the nature of concepts, definitions, purpose, relationships, and structure of a theory.

PURPOSES OF THEORIES AND CONCEPTUAL MODEL

- Theoretical and conceptual framework plays a several interrelated roles in the progress of science.
- This enables the researchers in his research findings meaning full and generalizable.
- Theories allows the researchers to knit together the observations and fact into an orderly scheme.
- Theoretical frameworks and efficient mechanisms for drawing together and summarizing accumulated facts.
- Sometimes if helps in separating and isolating investigations. The leakage of 'finding into coherent studies.' This makes the body of accumulated knowledge more accessible and thus more useful to both to practitioner, who have seek to implement findings and to research her, who seeks to extend the knowledge base.
- Theories and conceptual models help to simulate research and the extension of knowledge by providing both direction and impetus.

GOALS OF THEORETICAL NURSING MODELS

- Identify domain and goals of nursing.
- Provide knowledge to improve nursing administration practice, education, and research.
- Guide research to establish empirical knowledge based on nursing.
- Identify area to be studied.
- Identify research technique and tools that will be used to validate nursing interventions.
- Identify nature of contribution that research will make to advancement of knowledge.
- Formulate legislation for governing nursing practice, research and education.
- Formulate regulations, interpreting nurse practice acts that nurses and others better understand laws.
- Develop curriculum plans for nursing education.
- Establish criteria for measuring quality of nursing care, education and research.
- Guide development of nursing care delivery system.
- Provide systematic structure and rationale for nursing activities.

BASIC CHARACTERISTICS OF A THEORY

- Theories can interrelate concepts in such a way as to create a different way of looking at a particular phenomenon.
- Theories must be logical in nature.
- Theories should be relatively simple yet generalizable.
- Theories can be the bases for hypotheses that can be tested.
- Theories contribute to and assist in increasing the general body of knowledge within the discipline though the research implemented to validate them.
- Theories can be utilized by the practitioners to guide and improve their practice.
- Theories must be consistent with other validated theories laws and principles but will leave open unanswered questions that need to be investigated.

NURSING THEORIES IMPORTANT

The importance of nursing theory and its significance to nursing practice:
- Nursing theories help recognize what should set the foundation of practice by explicitly describing nursing.
- By providing a definition of nursing, nursing theory also helps nurses to understand their purpose and role in the healthcare setting.
- Theories serve as a rationale or scientific reasons for nursing interventions and give nurses the knowledge base necessary for acting and responding appropriately in nursing care situations.
- Nursing theories provide the foundations of nursing practice; helps generate further knowledge, and indicate in which direction nursing should develop in the future.
- By providing nurses a sense of identity, nursing theory can help patients, managers, and other healthcare professionals to acknowledge and understand the unique contribution that nurses make to the healthcare service.
- Nursing theories prepare the nurses to reflect on the assumptions and question the values in nursing, thus further defining nursing and increasing knowledge base.
- Nursing theories aim to define, predict, and demonstrate the phenomenon of nursing.
- It can be regarded as an attempt by the nursing profession to maintain and preserve its professional limits and boundaries.
- In many cases, nursing theories guide knowledge development and directs education, research, and practice although each influences the others.

THEORETICAL MODELS OF NURSING PRACTICE

Model is a symbolic representation of the interrelations exhibited by a phenomenon within a system or a process. The model is presented as a conceptual framework or a theory that explains a phenomenon and allows predictions to be made about a patient or a process By examining the following situation, one can identify how a theoretical approach can be used in nursing practice.

Situation: Mrs. Mary Dolphin is nine months pregnant and is expecting her first child within a week. She is visiting her obstetrician for an examination. The office nurse has been requested to do health teaching either during the office visits or in Mrs. Dolphin's home. Mrs. Dolphin is an executive career woman of Irish descent who has been married for one year. Mr. Dolphin is in governmental service and travels a great deal, frequently leaving Mrs. Dolphin alone. During the entire pregnancy Mrs. Dolphin has been co-operative and enthusiastic. No complications or unusual problems (other than morning sickness which lasted for six weeks during her 1st trimester) have occurred during the pregnancy.

KINDS OF THEORIES

- **Stress theories:** The nurse needs to assess Mrs. Dolphin's previous ability to deal with stress theories that give clues as to how individuals deal physiologically and psychologically with stress, will assist the nurse in understanding how people can be expected to react.
- **Developmental theories:** Theories relating to the development of each member of the family will give

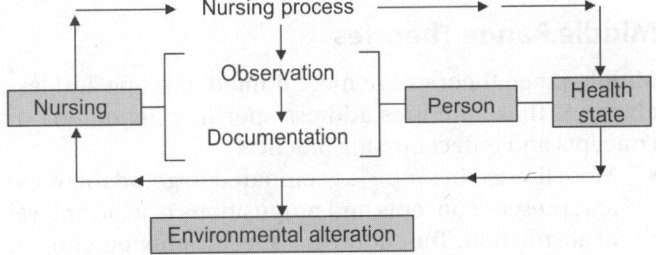

Fig. 29.4: Conceptual framework/Models.

the nurse an appropriate knowledge base on which to assess specific developmental levels and tasks for each member of the family.
- **Family theory:** The structure and functions of the family unit and the interrelationships of a family group are reflected in theories relating to the family.
- **Interactive theories:** The professional nurse must have a sound base of theoretical. Knowledge about interactions since the base of health teaching relates to the nurse's ability to interact with Mrs. Dolphin and Mr. Dolphin ability to interact with others.
- **Adoptive theories:** Mrs. Dolphin needs to be assessed in terms of her ability to adapt to both her pregnancy and the birth of a child. The nurse needs to be able to explain and hypothesize physical and emotional changes in Mrs. Dolphin.
- **Other theories:** Other theories can also be identified that will offer the nurse insight into both assessing and planning care. For example: Role theories will assist in explaining both the role of the nurse and Mrs. Dolphin's role as a mother. Change theory will offer insight into the expected behaviors that evolve when significant change occurs within an environment. Nursing theories that explain phenomena and guide the nurse in giving care would be instrumental as guidelines to care.

TYPES OF THEORY (BY ABSTRACTION)

There are three major categories when classifying nursing theories based on their level of abstraction: grand theory, middle-range theory, and practice-level theory.

Grand Theory

Grand theories are broad in scope and complex. These theories require further specification through research before they can be fully tested. A grand theory is not intended to provide guidance for specific nursing interventions but to provide the structural framework for broad, abstract ideas.
- Grand theories are abstract, broad in scope, and complex, therefore requiring further research for clarification.
- Grand nursing theories do not provide guidance for specific nursing interventions but rather provide a general framework and ideas about nursing.
- Grand nursing theorists develop their works based on their own experiences and the time they were living explaining why there is so much variation among theories.
- Address the nursing metaparadigm components of person, nursing, health, and environment.

Middle Range Theories

Middle range theories are more limited in scope and less abstract. These theories address specific phenomena or concepts and reflect nursing practice.
- More limited in scope (as compared to grand theories) and present concepts and propositions at a lower level of abstraction. They address a specific phenomenon in nursing.
- Due to the difficulty of testing grand theories, nursing scholars proposed using this level of theory.
- Most middle-range theories are based on the works of a grand theorist but they can be conceived from research, nursing practice, or the theories of other disciplines.

Descriptive Theories

Descriptive theories are the first level of theory development. They delineates phenomena speculate on why phenomena occur and describe the consequences of phenomena.
- Descriptive theories are the first level of theory development. They describe the phenomena and identify its properties and components in which it occurs.
- Descriptive theories are not action oriented or attempt to produce or change a situation.
- There are two types of descriptive theories: factor-isolating theory and explanatory theory.

Factor-isolating Theory

- Also known as category-formulating or labeling theory.
- Theories under this category describe the properties and dimensions of phenomena.

Explanatory Theory

Explanatory theories describe and explain the nature of relationships of certain phenomena to other phenomena.

Perspective Theories

Prescriptive theories address nursing therapeutics and the consequences of interventions. These types of theories predict the consequence of a specific nursing intervention.
- Address the nursing interventions for a phenomenon, guide practice change, and predict consequences.
- Includes propositions that call for change.
- In nursing, prescriptive theories are used to anticipate the outcomes of nursing interventions.

Practice-level Nursing Theories

- Practice nursing theories are situation specific theories that are narrow in scope and focuses on a specific patient population at a specific time.

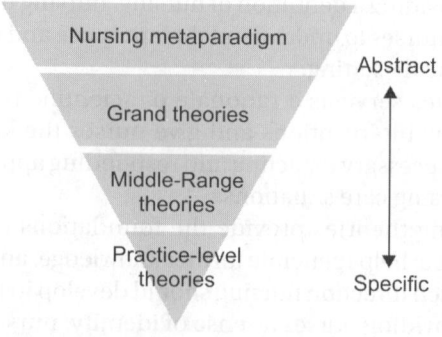

Fig. 29.5: Levels of nursing theory.

- Practice-level nursing theories provide frameworks for nursing interventions and suggest outcomes or the effect of nursing practice.
- Theories developed at this level have a more direct effect on nursing practice as compared to more abstract theories.
- These theories are interrelated with concepts from middle-range theories or grand

DEVELOPMENT OF NURSING THEORIES

- The development of nursing science and theory is a scholarly activity.
- Developing this science involves generating knowledge; although this knowledge can be used with knowledge from other disciplines, it is designed to advance and support nursing practice and healthcare.
- As nursing continues to evolve, nurses theorize about the nature of nursing practice, the principles on which practice is based, and the proper goals and functions of nursing in society.
- Conceptional and theoretical nursing models are used to provide knowledge to improve practice, guide research and curricular and identify domain and goals of nursing practice.
- Nursing theories provide the nurse with goals of assessment, nursing diagnosis and intervention; common ground for communication; and professional autonomy and accountability.
- They also guide future directions for nursing research; practice, education, and administration.
- Theories of nursing can help the nursing student to understand how the roles and actions of nurses fit together in nursing. The brief descriptions of selected nursing theories are as follows.

PAPLAU'S THEORY (1952)

Hildegard E Paplau was born on September 1, 1909, and graduated from Pottstown, Pennsylvania hospital, school of nursing in 1931. The nature of science and nursing refers to the body of verified knowledge found within the discipline of nursing, i.e. mainly knowledge from the biological and behavioral sciences.

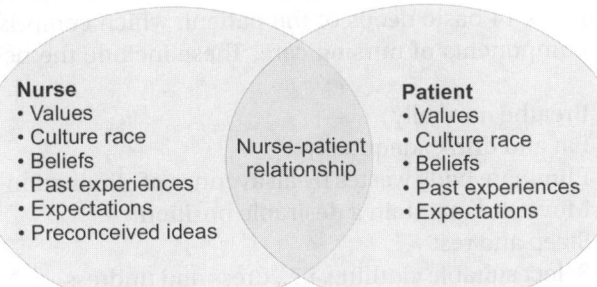

Fig. 29.6: Paplaus interpersonal relationship model.

The synthesis, reorganization, or extension of concepts drawn from the basic and applied sciences, which is their reformation tend to become new concepts have led to the growth of nursing science. Then the evolution of Paplau's theory of interpersonal relations resulted. Paplau's theory focuses on the individual nurse and the interaction process; the result is the nurse-client relationship. The major concepts defined/viewed are as follows.

Psychodynamic nursing: Psychodynamic nursing is being able to understand one's own behavior to help others identify felt difficulties, and to apply principles of human relations to the problems that arise at all levels of experience. She describes the structural concepts of interpersonal process and both the nurse-patient relationship to be based on psychodynamic nursing.

Interpersonal Theory and Nursing Process

Assessment
- Data collection and analysis (continuous)
- May not be a felt need

Nursing diagnosis
Planning
- Mutually set goals

Implementation
- Plans initiated toward achievement of mutually set goals
- May be accomplished by patient, nurse or family.

Evaluation
- Based on mutually expected behaviors.
- May lead to termination and initiation of new plans

Orientation
- Non-continuous data collection
- Felt need
- Define needs

Identification
- Interdependent goal setting

Exploitation
- Patient actively seeking and drawing help
- Patient initiated

Resolution
- Occurs after other phases are completed successfully
- le'lds to termination.

Nurse-patient Relationship

Nurse-patient relationship described by the Paplau in four phases, i.e. orientation, identification, exploitation, and resolution:

- **In orientation phase,** the individual has a felt need and seeks professional assistance. The nurse helps the patient recognize and understand his problem and determine his need for help
- **In identification phase,** the patient identifies with those who can help him (relatedness). The nurse permits exploration feelings to aid the patient in undergoing illness as an experience that reorients feelings and strengthens positive forces in the personality and provides needed satisfaction
- **In exploitation phase,** the patient attempts to derive full value from what is offered him through the relationship. Now goals to be achieved through personal efforts can be projected and power shifted from the nurse to the patient as the patient delays gratification to achieve the newly formed goals

- **In the phase of resolution,** old goals are gradually put aside and new goals are adopted. This is a process in which the patient frees himself from identification with the nurse.

Nursing roles: Paplau describes six different nursing roles that emerge in the various phases of the nurse-patient relationship as given below: Role of the stranger In this role both nurse and patient are stranger to each other, the patient should be treated as he is and with ordinary courtesy. This coincides with the identification phase.

Role of resource person In this role nurse provides specific answers to questions, especially health information, and interprets to the patient the treatment or medical plan of care. Here the nurse also determines what type of response is appropriate for constructive learning, either straight forward factual answers or providing counseling.

Teaching role: It is a combination of all roles. Paplau separates teaching into two categories, i.e. instructional which consists largely of giving information and is the form explained in educational literature and practical which is using the experience of the learner as a basis from which learning products are developed.

Leadership role: It involves the democratic process. The nurse helps the patient meet the tasks at hand through a relationship of cooperation and active participation.

Surrogate role: The patient casts the nurse in the surrogate role. The nurse's attitudes and behaviors create 'feeling tones' in the patient that reactivate feelings generate in a prior relationship. The nurse's function is to assist the patient in recognizing similarities between herself and the person recalled by the patient. She then helps the patient see the differences in her role and that of the recalled person. In this phase, nurse and patient defines areas of dependence, independence and finally interdependence.

Counseling role: Paplau believes the counseling role has the greatest emphasis on psychiatric nursing. Counseling functions in the nurse-patient relationship by the way nurses response to patient demands.

Nursing: Nursing is described by Paplau as a significant, therapeutic, interpersonal process. It functions comparatively with other human processes that make health possible for individuals in communities. When professional health teams offer health services, nurses participate in the organization of conditions that facilitate natural ongoing tendencies in human organism.

Nursing is an educative instrument, a maturing force that aims to promote forward movement of personality in the direction of creative constructive, productive, personal, and community living.

Person: Person refers to man. Man is an organism that lives in an unstable equilibrium.

Health: Health is defined by Paplau as 'a word symbol that implies forward movement of personality and other ongoing human processes in the direction of creative, constructive, productive, personal and community living'.

Environment: Environment is defined in terms of 'existing forces outside the organism and in the context of cultures', from which morals, customs, and beliefs are acquired. However, general conditions that are likely to lead to health always include the interpersonal process.

According to this theory the client is an individual with a felt need, and nursing is an interpersonal and therapeutic process. Nursing goal is to educate the client and family and to help the client reach mature personality development. Therefore nurse strives to develop a nurse-patient relationship in which the nurse serves as a research person, counselor and surrogate. This theory creates a 'making force' through which interpersonal effectiveness assists in meeting the client needs.

HENDERSON'S THEORY (1955)

Virginia Henderson was born in 1897, a native of Kansas city, Missouri, spent her developmental years in Virginia because her father practiced law in Washington DC. During World War I, she developed an interest in nursing. The major concepts defined by Henderson are as follows:

Nursing: Henderson defines nursing in functional terms, i.e. 'the unique function of the nurse is to assist the individual, sick or well, in the performance of those activities contributing to health or its recovery (or to peaceful death) that he would perform unaided if he had the necessary strength, will or knowledge. And to do this is such a way as to help him gain independence as rapidly as possible'.

Health: Henderson did not define health, but looking into several definitions of health. She views health in terms of patient's ability to perform unaided the 14 components of nursing care. She says it is 'the quality or health rather than life itself, that margin of mental physical vigor that allows a person to work most effectively and to reach his highest potential level of satisfaction of life'.

Environment: By using Webster's definition, Hendersons defines 'environment as the aggregate of all the external conditions and influence affecting the life and development of an organism'.

Person (patient): Henderson views the patient as an individual who requires assistance to achieve health and independence or peaceful death. The mind and body are inseparable. The patient and his family are viewed as a unit.

Needs: Henderson did not define a need, but she identifies 14 basic needs of the patient, which comprises the components of nursing care. These include the need to:
i. Breathe normally
ii. Eat and drink adequately
iii. Eliminate body wastes by all avenues of elimination
iv. Move and maintain a desirable position
v. Sleep and rest
vi. Select suitable clothing, i.e., dress and undress
vii. Maintain body temperature within the normal range by adjusting clothing and modifying the environment

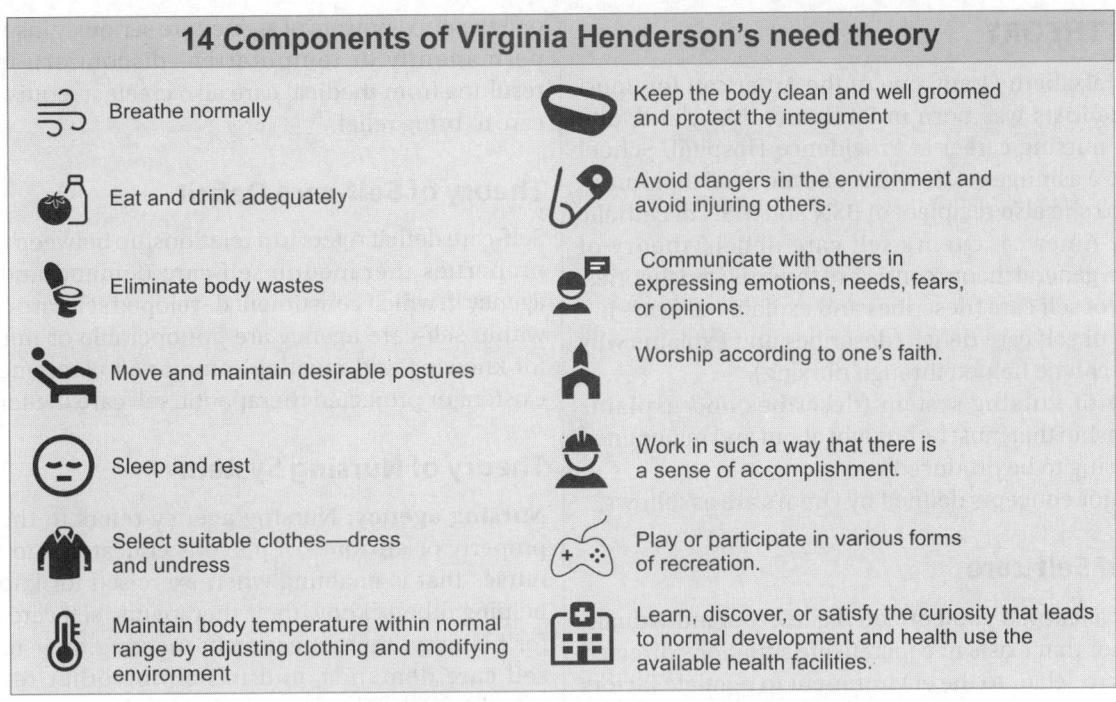

Fig. 29.7: Components of Henderson's theory.

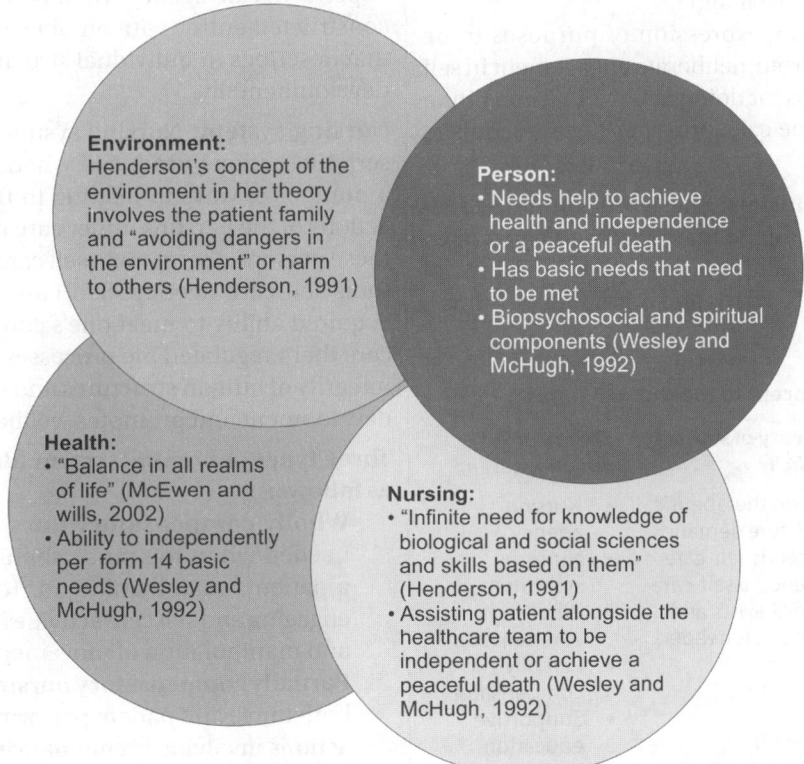

Fig. 29.8: Application of Henderson's theory.

viii. Keep the body clean and well groomed and protect the integument
ix. Avoid dangers in the environment and avoid injuring others
x. Communicate with others in expressing emotions, needs, fears or opinions
xi. Worship according to one's faith
xii. Work in such a way that there is a sense of accomplishments
xiii. Play or participate in various forms of recreation, and
xiv. Learn, discover or satisfy the curiosity that leads to normal development and health and use the available health facilities.

Henderson viewed nursing as an art and a discipline separate from medkine, and viewed the nurse's role as that of a substitute for the patient, a helper to the patient, and a partner with the patient. The fourteen basic needs compose Henderson's components of nursing care.

OREM'S THEORY

Dorothea Elizabeth Orem, one of the American foremost nursing theorists was born in Baltimore, Maryland. She began her nursing career at Providence Hospital, School of Nursing, Washington DC, where she received diploma in nursing and she also recipient of BSN and MSN of catholic University America. Orem's self care deficit' theory of nursing as a general theory consists of three related theories:
- Theory of self care (describes and explains self care).
- Theory of self care deficit (describes and explains why people can be helped through nursing).
- Theory of nursing system (describes and explains relationship that must be brought about and maintained for nursing to be produced).

The major concepts defined by Orem's are as follows.

Theory of Self-care

Self care is a learned good oriented activity of individuals. It is behavior that exists in concrete life situations directed by persons to self or to the environment to regulate factors that affects their own development and functioning in the interests of life, health, or wellbeing.

Self care requisites are expression of purposes to be attained, results desired from-deliberate engagement in self care. They are the reasons for doing actions that constitute self care. There were three categories of self care requisite as given below.

Universal self care requisites: These are common to all human beings and include the maintenance of air, water, food elimination, activity and rest, and solitude and social interaction, prevention of hazards and promotion of human functioning.

Relationship of Orem's concept to the three theories

Theory of self-care	Theory of self-care deficit	Theory of nursing system

• Self-care
• Self-care agency
• Self care requisites
  – Universal
  – Developmental
  – Health
  – Deviation
• Therapeutic self-care demand
	When therapeutic self-care demand exceeds self-care agency, a self-care deficil exists and nursing is needed.	• Nursing agency
		• Nursing systems
		• Wholly compensatory
		• Partially compensatory
		• Supportive education

Development self-care requisites: These are self-care requisites that they promote processes for life and maturation and prevent conditions deleterious to maturation or mitigate those effects.

Health deviation self-care requisites: These are defined by Orem that disease or injury affects not only specific structures and physiologic or psychological mechanisms, but also integrated human functioning. When integrated functioning is seriously affected the individuals' developing or developed powers of agency are seriously inspired either permanently or temporarily—discomfort, frustration resulting from medical care also create a requisites for self care to bring relief.

Theory of Self-care Deficit

Self-care deficit refers to a relationship between the human properties therapeutic self care demand and self-care agency in which constituent developed self care capabilities within self-care agency are nonoperable or not adequate for knowing and meeting some or all components of the existent or projected therapeutic self care demand.

Theory of Nursing System

Nursing agency: Nursing agency refers to the complex property or attribute of persons educated and trained as nurses that is enabling when exercised for knowing and helping others, know their therapeutic self care demands, for helping others meet or in meeting their therapeutic self care demands, and in helping other regulate the exercise or development of their self care agency or their dependent care agency. Therapeutic demand is a humanly constructed entity, with an objective basis in information that describes in individual structurally, functionally, and developmentally.

Nursing system: Nursing system refers to a continuing series of actions produced when nurses link one way or a number of ways in helping to their own actions or the actions of the persons under care that are directed to meet these persons' therapeutic self care demands or to regulate their self care agency. Self care agency is the complex acquired ability to meet one's continuing requirement for care them regulated life processes, maintains or promotes integrity of human structures and functioning, and human development and promotes wellbeing.

Three types of nursing system (described by Orem) are as follows:
 i. **Wholly compensatory nursing systems:** These are needed when the nurse should be compensating for a patients total inability for (or prescription against) engaging and self care activities that require ambulation and manipulation of movements.
 ii. **Partially compensatory nursing system:** It exists when both nurse and patient perform care measures or other actions involving manipulative tasks or ambulation.
 iii. **Supportive educative nursing system:** These are for situations when the patient is able to perform or can and should learn to perform required measures for externally or internally oriented self care but cannot do so without assistance. The methods of assistance will include acting or doing for guidance, i.e. teaching, supporting, and providing a developmental environment.

In Orem's self care deficit theory, nursing care becomes necessary when client is unable to fulfill biological, psychological, developmental and/or social needs. The

Nursing Theories

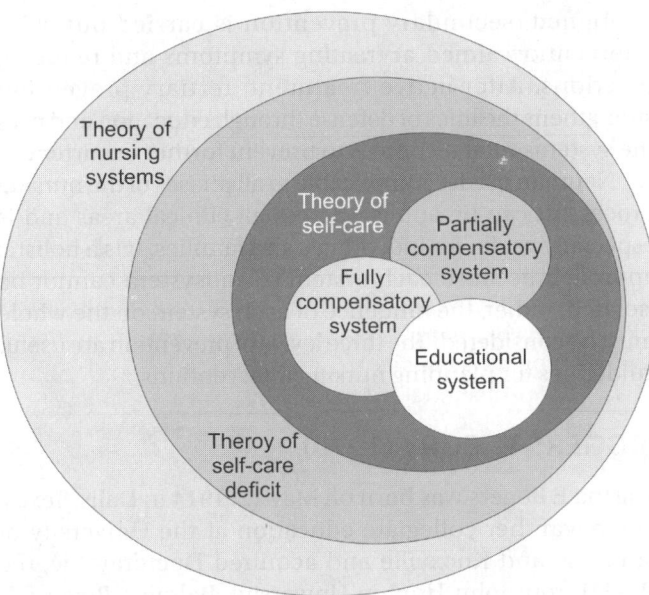

Fig. 29.9: Orem's theory of self care and deficit.

goal of nursing is to care for and help client within total self care. She viewed person/patient in an individual unable to continuously maintain self care in sustaining life and health, in recovering from disease or injury or in coping with their effects.

Universal Self-care Requisites

Air	Breaths without difficulty, no pallor cyanosis
Water	Fluid intake is sufficient. Edema present over ankles. Turgor normal for the age
Food	Hb—9.6 gm %, BMI = 14. Food inlake is not adequate or the diet is not nutritious.
Elimination	Voids and eliminates bowel without difficulty.
Activity/rest	Frequent rest is required due to pain. Pain not oompletely relieved, Activity level has come down. Deformity of the joint secondary to the disease process and use of the joints.
Social interaction	Communicates well with neighbors and calls the daughter by phone. Need for medical care is oommunicated to the daughter.
Prevention of hazards	Need instruction on care of joints and prevention offalls. Need instruction on improvement of nutritional status. Prefer to walk bare foot.
Promotion of normacy	Has good relation with daughter

According to Orem, health is an ability to meet self care demands that contribute to the maintenance and promotion of structural integrity, functioning, and development. Illness occurs when a individual is incapable of maintaining self-care as a result of health related limitations. She perceived environment that any setting in which a patient has unmet self care needs. And nursing is service of deliberately selected and performed actions to assist individuals to maintain self care, including structural integrity, functioning, and development. Accordingly nursing care is necessary when the client is unable to fulfill biological, psychological, developmental and/or social needs. The nurse determines why a client is unable to meet these needs, what must be done to enable the client to meet them and how much self care the client is able to perform.

Orem describes her philosophy of nursing as follows: Action and the provision and management of it on continuous basis in order to sustain life and health, recover from disease or injury, and cope with their effects. Self care is a requirement of every person — man, women, and child. When self care is not maintained, illness, disease or death will occur. Nurses sometimes manage and maintain required self care continuously for persons who are totally incapable. In other instance, nurses help persons to maintain required self care by performing some but not all care measures, by supervising others who assist patients and by instructing and guiding individuals as they gradually move toward self care.

Orem suggests that a person needs nursing when the person has a health related self care deficit. The areas of nursing practice are:
- Entering into and maintaining nurse-client relationships with individuals families or groups.
- Determining if and how clients can be helped through nursing.
- Responding to clients' requirements and needs.
- Giving direct help to clients and families.
- Coordinating and integrating nursing with the clients' daily living, other health care activities, and social or educational services required.

NEUMAN'S THEORY (1972)

Betty Neuman was born on 1924, completed her initial nursing education at Akron, Ohio in 1947, then earned master degree in mental health in 1966 and received doctorate degree in clinical psychology in 1985. She was a pioneer of nursing involvement in mental health.

The major concepts identified in her model are; holistic client approach, open system, basic structure, environment, created environment, stresses, lines of defence and resistance, degree of reaction, prevention as intervention, and reconstruction. Further included the concepts of scholastic approach, content, process input and output, negontrophy, entropy, stability, wellness and illness.

To Neuman, the persons are dynamic composite of physiological, socio-cultural, and developmental variables that function as an open system. As an open system, the person interacts with adjusts to and it adjusted by the environment, which is viewed as stressor. Stressors disrupt the system. She includes intrapersonal, interpersonal and extra personal stressor.

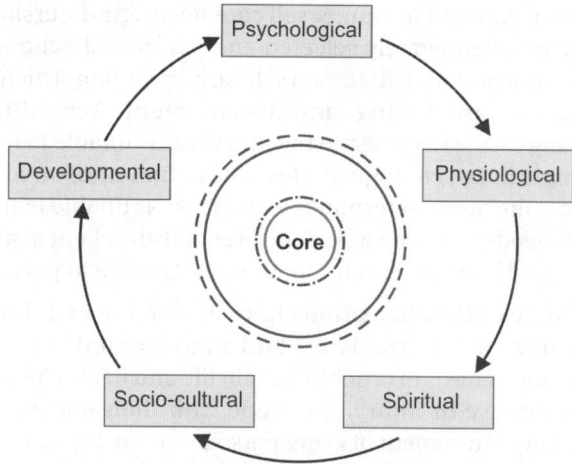

Fig. 29.10: Betty Neuman systems model.

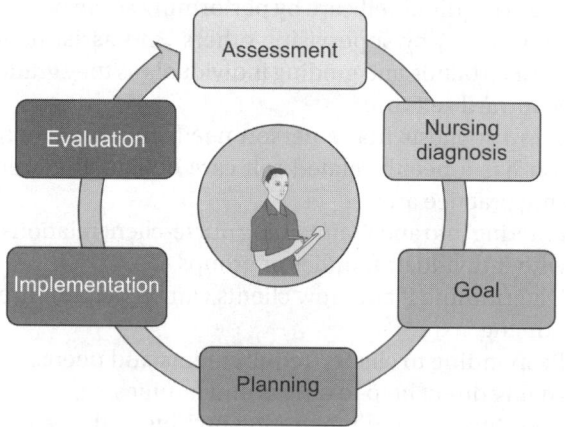

Fig. 29.11: Application of system theory in nursing.

Neuman believes that nursing is concerned with the whole person. She views nursing as a 'unique profession in that it is concerned with all of the variables affecting an individual response to stress'. Because the nurses perception influences the care program. Neuman equates health to wellness and defines health and/or wellness as 'the condition in which all parts and subparts (variables) are in harmony with the whole of the client. So health is a dynamic equilibrium on the normal line of defence. Illness occurs due to reaction to stressor with lines of resistance, internal and external stressors and restrictive factors are the environment. The reduction of the stressors through prevention acts at three levels of nursing.

The goal of nursing is to assist individual, families, and groups in attaining and maintaining maximal level of total wellness. The nurse assesses managers and evaluates client systems. Nursing focuses on the variables affecting the client response to the stressor. Nursing action are earned out on three levels. When the stressor is identified but no reaction has occurred; interventions can decrease the degree of reaction or increase the line of defense. This is called primary prevention. When the reaction has already happened, secondary prevention is carried out, with intervention aimed at treating symptoms and reducing reactions. After active treatment, tertiary prevention strengthens the lines of defense through education and uses the systems total resources to prevent further occurrence.

Neuman model is applicable to all phases of the nursing process. It can be applied across all clinical areas and is especially useful for individuals and families. It is a holistic approach because each system or subsystem cannot be isolated; rather, the influence of each system on the whole must be considered. The three levels of prevention are useful guidelines for planning nursing interventions.

ROGERS THEORY (1970)

Martha E Rogers was born on May 12, 1914 in Dalls, Texas. She began her collegiate education at the University of Jannesse and Knoxville and acquired Doctorate degree (Ed.D) from John Hoplun University, Balmier. Roger felt that historically the term 'nursing' most often has been used as a verb simplifying 'to do' when nursing is perceived as a science. The term 'nursing' being a noun, signifies body of knowledge. She describes nursing as a learned profession that is both a science and an art.

'Nursing is a humanistic science dedicated to compassionate concern for maintaining and promoting health, preventing illness and caring for and rehabilitating the sick and disabled'. Nursing seeks to promote symphonic interactions between the environment and man, to strengthen the coherence and integrity of the human beings and do direct and redirect patterns of interaction between man and his environment for the realization of maximum health potential.

Rogers considers man (unitary fuliman being) as an energy field co-existence within the universe. An energy field constitutes the fundamental unit of both the living and nonhiving. Field is unifying concept and energy signifies the dynamic nature of the field. Energy fields are infinite, so she identified only two, i.e. the human field and the environment field:

- The unitary human being (human field) is defined as an irreducible, indivisible, pandimensional energy field identified by pattern and manifested characteristics that are specific to the whole and which cannot be predicted from knowledge of the parts

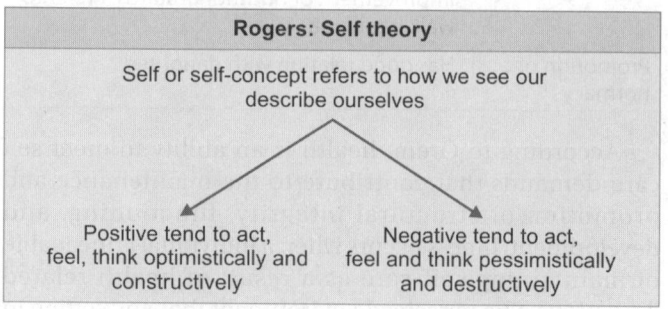

Fig. 29.12: Rogers theory on self concept.

- The environment field is defined as an irreducible pandimensional energy field identified by pattern and integral with human field. Each environmental field is specific to its given human field. Both change continuously and creatively. Unitary man evolves along life process. Client continuously changes and coexists with environment.

Rogers viewed the terms health and illness as value leader, arbitrarily defined but as part of the same continuum, i.e. health occurs when patterns of living are in harmony with environmental change and illness occurs when patterns of living conflicts with environmental change and are deemed unacceptable.

Transzendence	Spiritual needs to feel as one with the univers
Self realization	The need to fulfill one's own potential and to have imponant goals to reilch
Aesthetic needs	Needs of order and beauty
Cognitive needs	Needs of knowledge, understanding and new coherences
Self worth	Needs of trust, the feeling of to be someone and to obtain respect by others
Relationship	Needs of affiliation, relation to others, to love and to be loved
Safeness	Needs of safeness, cosiness, ease and to be free of anxieties
Biological needs	Needs of nutrition, water, oxygen, relaxation, and sexuality

The four dimension used in Rogers theory of energy fields, openness (universe of open system) pattern and organization and to derive principles about how human beings develops. Her views on nursing primarily as a science and is committed to nursing research. Nursing, therefore, corporate knowledge of the basic sciences and physiology, as well as nursing knowledge. The science of nursing aims to provide a body of abstract knowledge growing out, of scientific research and logical analysis and capable of being translated into nursing practice. Nursing body of knowledge is a new product specific to nursing.

According to this theory the goal of nursing is to maintain and promote health, prevent illness and care for and rehabilitate ill and disabled client through humanistic science of nursing.

ROY'S THEORY (1979)

Sister Callista Roy, a member of the Sisters of St Joseph of Carondeler, was born on October 14, 1939 in Losangles, California. She was the receiver of BA in Nursing, M.Sc Nursing, and MA in Sociology and PhD in Sociology.

The major concepts defined by Roy are as follows:
- **Person:** According to Roy, a person is a biopsychosocial being in constant interaction with a changing environment. She defined the person, the recipient of nursing care, as a living complex, adaptive system with internal processes (the cognator and regulator) acting to maintain adaptation in the four adaptive modes, i.e. physiological needs, self-concept, role functions, and interdependence. The person as a living system is 'a whole' made up of parts or subsystems that function as a unity for some purpose, patient is a person or family with unusual stressor or ineffective coping mechanism.

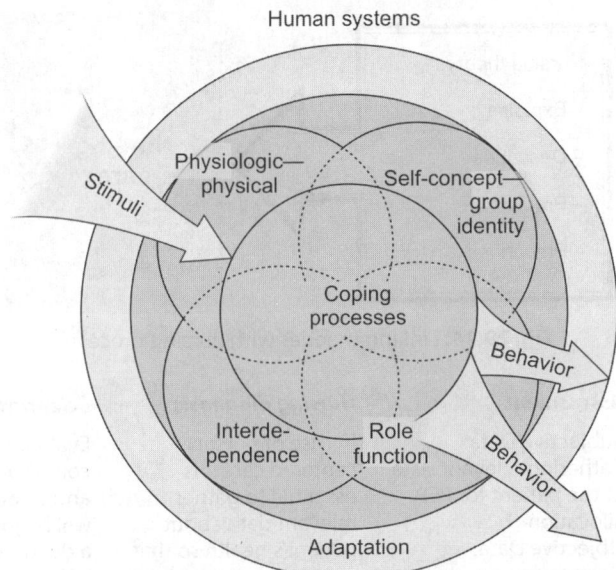

Fig. 29.13: Roy's adaptation model.

- **Health:** It is a state and a process of being and becoming an integrated and whole person. Lack of integration represents lack of health.
- **Environment:** According to Roy environment is all the conditions, circumstances, and influences surrounding and affecting the development and behavior of persons or groups. Factors in the environment that affect the person are categorized as focal, contextual, and residual stimuli.

Nursing: It is defined broadly as 'a theoretical system of knowledge which prescribes a process of analysis and action related to the care of the ill or potentially ill person.

Roy differentiates nursing as a science from nursing as a practice discipline. Nursing science is a developing system of knowledge about person that observes, classifies, and relates the processes by which persons positively affect their health status. Nursing as practice discipline is nursing scientific body of knowledge used for the purpose of providing an essential service to sick.

LINKING THEORIES WITH NURSING PROCESS

Theories are general explanations which scholars use to explain, control and understand commonly occurring events. Theories are best understood as preliminary explanations that reflect the current understanding of events. "Theory is defined as a set of propositions used to

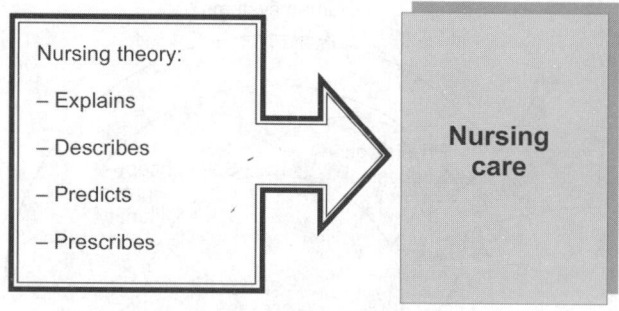

Fig. 29.14: Linking theories with nursing process.

describe, explain, predict and control events". Here set refers to a group of circumstances, situations, and so on, joined and treated as a whole; propositions refers to statements about how two or more concepts are related; concepts refers to an abstract classification of data, temperature; describe means of tell about in details; explain means to offer reasons for; predict means to foretell/forecast; control means to exercise as regulating influence over; and phenomena refer to theory includes the joint functions of theory, i.e. description explanation, prediction and control.

Assessment	Nursing diagnosis	Scientific rationals	Intervention	Evaluation
Subjective Data: Cathering relevant data of the patient for PEP allocation Objective Data: Demonstrating knowledge and integration of safety and quality principle of patient care	In case of person centered care it is essential to gather relevant data about patient's health so that proper diagnosis can be prepared.	Evaluating patient's condition, his history and treatment methods will be jotted down in a document with the help of the information on the paper nursing intervention will be planned	Nursing interventions are used to reduce rialc and improve patient's present condition	Mapping improvement of patients will help nurses to decide whether to stop or continue with nursing intervention

Nursing intervention may take place at any point on the continuum. Nursing diagnosis may focus on behavior associated with a medical diagnosis or other health behavior that the patient wishes to change. A nurse may practice primary prevention by intervening in a potential health problem, secondary prevention by intervening in an actual acute health problem or tertiary prevention by intervening to limit the disability caused by actual chronic health problems.

The nursing assessment of the patient includes presenting complaints, past history, family history, personal history, occupational history, sexual history, physical examination and mental status examination. Additional data may be collected from significant other sources and by reviewing the systems. A nursing diagnosis is then formulated and based on this diagnosis; planning and interventions, is carried out. Finally, evaluation will be done to find out the effectiveness of nursing interventions. Providing nursing care is a collaborative effort, with both the nurse and the patient contributing ideas and energy to the therapeutic process.

USE OF THEORIES IN NURSING PRACTICE

In Practice

- Assist nurses to describe, explain, and predict everyday experiences.
- Serve to guide assessment, interventions, and evaluation of nursing care.
- Provide a rationale for collecting reliable and valid data about the health status of clients, which are essential for effective decision making and implementation.
- Help to describe criteria to measure the quality of nursing care.
- Help build a common nursing terminology to use in communicating with other health professionals.
- Ideas are developed and words are defined.
- Enhance autonomy (independence and self-governance) of nursing through defining its own independent functions.

In Education

- Provide a general focus for curriculum design
- Guide curricular decision making.

In Research

- Offer a framework for generating knowledge and new ideas.
- Assist in discovering knowledge gaps in the specific field of study.
- Offer a systematic approach to identify questions for study; select variables, interpret findings, and validate nursing interventions.
- Approaches to developing nursing theory.
- Borrowing conceptual frameworks from other disciplines.
- Inductively looking at nursing practice to disc over theories/concepts to explain phenomena.
- Deductively looking for the compatibility of a general nursing theory with nursing practice.
- Questions from practicing Nurse about using Nursing theory.

Practice

- Does this theory reflect nursing practice as I know it?
- Will it support what I believe to be excellent nursing practice?

- Can this theory be considered in relation to a wide range of nursing situation?
- Personal interests, abilities and experiences.
- What will it be like to think about nursing theory in nursing practice?
- Will my work with nursing theory be worth the effort?

CONCLUSION

Theory helps in providing knowledge to improve practice by describing, explaining, predicting, and controlling phenomena. Nurses power is increased through theoretical knowledge because systematically developed more likely to be successful. In addition, nurses will know why they are doing, what they are doing if challenged. Theory provides professional autonomy by guiding the nursing practice, education and research functions of profession. And also there has been interest in identifying a body of nursing knowledge that is essential to professional nursing practice. Theory development contributes to knowledge building and is seen a means of establishing 'nursing as a profession'.

BIBLIOGRAPHY

1. Alligood M, Tomey A. Nursing Theorists and Their Work, 7th edition. Maryland Heights: Mosby-Elsevier. 2010.
2. Alligood MR, Tomey AM. Nursing Theory Utilization and Application, 2nd edition Mosby, Philadelphia, 2002.
3. Alligood MR. Nursing Theorists and their Work-E-Book. Elsevier Health Sciences. 2017.
4. Barnard KE. Nursing research related to infants and young children. Annual Review of Nursing Research. Springer, Berlin, Heidelberg. 1984; 3-25.
5. Becker MH, Radius SM, Rosenstock IM. Compliance with a medical regimen for asthma: a test of the health belief model. Public Health Reports. 1978;93:268-77.
6. Becker MH. The Health Belief Model and Personal Health Behavior. Health Education Monographs. Vol. 2 No. 4.
7. Botha ME. Theory Development in perspective: The role of conceptual frameworks and models in theory development". Journal of Advanced Nursing. 1989;14(1):49-55.
8. Brown HI. Perception, theory, and commitment: The new philosophy of Science. University of Chicago Press. 1979.
9. Brown M. Research in the development of nursing theory: the importance of a theoretical framework in nursing research. Nursing Research. 1964.
10. Champion VL. Instrument development for health belief model constructs. Advances in Nursing Science. 1984;6:73-85.
11. Chinn PL, Jacobs MK. A model for theory development in nursing. Advances in Nursing Science. 1978;1(1):1-12.
12. Colley S. Nursing theory: its importance to practice. Nursing Standard (through 2013). 2003;17(46):33.
13. Conner M, Norman P. Predicting Health Behavior. Search and Practice with Social Cognition Models. Open University Press: Ballmore: Buckingham, 1996.
14. Dewey, John. Logic: The Theory of Inquiry. New York: Hold Rinehart and Winston, 1938.
15. Donaldson SK, Crowley DM. The discipline of nursing. Nursing Outlook. 1978;26:113-20.
16. Eisen M et al. A health belief model-social learning theory approach to adolescents' fertility control: Findings from a controlled field trial. Health Education Quarterly, Vol. 19, 1992.
17. Fawcett J. (2005). Criteria for evaluation of theory. Nursing Science Quarterly, 18(2), 131-5.
18. Fitzpatrick JJ, Whall AL. (Eds). Conceptual Models of Nursing: Analysis and Application. Connecticut, Norwalk: Appleton & Lange. 1996.
19. George B Julia. Nursing Theories: The Base for Professional Nursing Practice, 3rd edition. Norwalk, Appleton and Lange.
20. Glanz K, Marcus Lewis F, Rimer BK. Theory at a Glance: A Guide for Health Promotion Practice. National Institute of Health, 1997.
21. Glanz K, Rimer BK, Lewis FM. Health Behavior and Health Education: Theory, Research and Practice. San Fransisco: Wiley & Sons, 2002.
22. Kaplan A. The Conduct of Inquiry: Methodology for Behavioural Science. Routledge, 2017.
23. Kaplan Abraham. The Conduct of Inquiry: Methodology for Behavioral Science. Scranton, PA: Chandler Publishing Co.(1964).
24. Meleis AI. Theoretical Nursing: Development and Progress. Lippincott Williams & Wilkins. 2011.
25. Meleis Ibrahim Afaf. Theoretical Nursing: Development and Progress 3rd edition. Philadelphia, Lippincott, 1997.
26. Potter A Patricia, Perry G Anne. Fundamentals of Nursing – Concepts Process and Practice, 3rd edition. London Mosby Year Book, 1992.
27. Rosenstock I. Historical Origins of the Health Belief Model. Health Education Monographs. 1974;(2):4.
28. Smith MJ, Liehr PR. Middle Range Theory for Nursing. New York: Springer Publishing, 2008.
29. Taylor Carol, Lillis Carol. The Art and Science of Nursing Care, 4th edition. Philadelphia, Lippincott, 2001.
30. Tomey AM, Alligood MR. Nursing theorists and their Work, 5th edition Mosby, Philadelphia, 2002.
31. Wills M Evelyn, McEwen Melanie. Theoretical Basis for Nursing. Philadelphia. Lippincott Williams and Wilkins, 2002.

REVIEW QUESTIONS

Long Essays

1. Define nursing theory. Explain the four major concepts of metaparadigm.
2. Explain theoretical models of nursing practice.
3. Describe linking theories with nursing process.

Short Essays

1. History of nursing theories.
2. Components of nursing theories.
3. Goals of theoretical nursing models.
4. Descriptive theories.
5. Theory of self-care.

Short Answers

1. Philosophy.
2. Theory.
3. Models.
4. Conceptual framework.
5. Phenomenon.
6. Characteristics of a theory.
7. Grand theory.
8. Middle range theories.

CHAPTER 30
First Aid and Emergencies

LEARNING OBJECTIVES

- Definition, basic principles, scope and rules
- First aid management
  - Wounds, hemorrhage and shock
  - Musculoskeletal injuries: Fractures, dislocation, muscle injuries
  - Transportation of injured persons
  - Unconsciousness
- Respiratory emergencies and basic CPR
- Foreign bodies—skin, eye, ear, nose, throat and stomach
- Burns and scalds
- Poisoning, bites and stings
- Frostbite and effects of heat
- Community emergencies

TERMINOLOGY

Abdominal thrusts: Maneuver to relieve airway obstructions in adults and children.

Advanced life support (ALS): The ALS units have a minimum of one paramedic and one emergency medical technique (EMT), can administer certain medications, and have advanced airway equipment, cardiac monitors, advanced cardiac life support equipment and blood glucose testing equipment.

Asystole: When the heart has no contractions due to a lack of electrical impulses. Characterized by the lack of a heartbeat, which creates a flat line on a heart monitor. Colloquially called a flat line.

American heart association: It is a non-profit organization that fosters appropriate cardiac care to reduce disability and deaths caused by cardiovascular disease and stroke. It was founded by six cardiologists in 1924 and is headquartered in Dallas.

Airway: The protection and maintenance of a clear passageway for gases (principally oxygen and carbon dioxide) to pass between the lungs and the atmosphere.

Breathing: Inflation and deflation of the lungs (respiration) via the airway.

Basic life support (BLS): Emergency procedures performed to sustain life that includes cardiopulmonary resuscitation (CPR), control of bleeding, treatment of shock, stabilization of injuries and wounds, and first aid.

BLS CPR algorithm: This illustrates the components of high quality cardiopulmonary resuscitation that should be learned by everyone. CPR is a science and requires properly performing the actions as instructed.

Circulation: Providing an adequate blood supply to tissue, especially critical organs, so as to deliver oxygen to all cells and remove metabolic waste, via the perfusion of blood throughout the body.

CPR: It stands for cardiopulmonary resuscitation. It is an emergency lifesaving procedure that is done when someone's breathing or heartbeat has stopped. This may happen after an electric shock, heart attack, or drowning. Rescue breathing provides oxygen to the person's lungs.

Abrasion: A medical term used to refer to the damage to the skin through to scraping or wearing away.

Acetaminophen: An analgesic pain reliever that is used to reduce fever as well as treat arthritis, headaches and minor pain.

Airbag: A safety device in a vehicle that inflates rapidly when there's an automobile collision to protect the occupant from striking into objects that may cause injuries.

Airway: The respiratory tract where air passes in and out of the lungs. The nose and the mouth are the normal entry and exit ports of the airway.

Anaphylaxis: An acute or serious allergic reaction to a chemical or an allergen, potentially life-threatening. For possible serious allergic reaction/anaphylaxis cases, make sure anaphylaxis first aid is administered.

Anaesthetic: A substance that causes a person to be insensitive to pain or lack of feeling/awareness to pain especially during surgery and other painful procedures.

Angina: A medical term that refers to the chest pain or discomforts that is caused by reduced blood flow to the heart.

Avulsion: Soft tissue injury; a tearing away of a section of skin or other soft tissue from the deeper layers causing severe bleeding.

Basic life support (BLS): This is a level of medical care for victims of life-threatening injuries until a full medical care is given to them at the hospital. It can be provided by a BLS trained person, a paramedic or emergency medical technician.

Breathing: The process of which air is inhaled through the mouth or nose, and then air is expelled from the lungs due to muscle contraction and relaxation, respectively.

Bruise: An injury caused by an impact that damages soft tissues and underlying blood vessels. Discoloration appears on the area of the body affected; another term for contusion.

Burn: An injury that gives a feeling of discomfort caused by exposure to heat, flame, chemical agents, radiation, or electricity. In case you get caught or find the need to help another person who had burns.

Cardiopulmonary: A medical term referring to or relating to the heart and the lungs.

Cardiopulmonary resuscitation (CPR): A life-saving first aid procedure of chest compressions given to patients who is in cardiac arrest. This medical process helps patient's body pump blood when the heart fails.

Chest pain: A feeling of tightness, heavy pressure, or crushing pain around the chest area—between the neck and upper abdomen. It can be a result of angina, heart attack, and other important diseases. Chest pain is a warning to seek medical attention.

Choking: It is the inability to breathe because the trachea is blocked, constricted, or obstructed. This is caused also by lack of air. It is a common cause of an accident to young children that may lead to death.

Collision: Collision is an event when two or more moving bodies collide through an exertion of very strong forces. The term often relates to vehicular accidents.

Concussion: A brain injury that is caused by a sudden blow to the head that shades the brain inside the skull. It can result to confusion, loss of memory with/without headache.

Contusion: The medical term for bruise. It is caused by injury to the skin tissues or broken blood vessels that usually results in bleeding beneath the skin.

Cuts: Cuts or laceration is a wound caused by a tear or a deep cut in the flesh or skin. It can be minor or major depending on the different types of curt and its severity.

Cyanosis: Refers to the bluish discoloration near the surface of the skin usually to the hands and feet. This occurs when there's low oxygen level in red blood cells.

Defibrillator: A device that uses electrical shocks to restore normal heartbeat and correct abnormal heart rhythm.

Dislocation: Also known as luxation. This happens when there's an undesirable separation in the joint at the end of the bone; usually moved out of its normal connection with another bone. Dislocation is usually caused by sudden impact or fall.

Emergency: A serious or dangerous situation that requires immediate or urgent action to avoid worsening of the scenario. A situation is considered to be an emergency if it poses an immediate threat to life, property, health or the environment.

Emergency code: Codes used by hospitals to quickly alert staff to different emergencies and relay essential information without causing stress and panic among visitors and patients in the hospital.

Emergency department: It is a medical treatment facility that accommodates emergency cases and provides medical care to patients without prior appointments.

Emergency oxygen: A portable oxygen unit, available in different sized cylinders, that increases a person's oxygen level internally during emergency cases.

Fainting: It occurs when there is a little amount of oxygen supply to the brain, a person loses its consciousness for a short period of time.

Febrile convulsion: A seizure that occurs in children associated with very high temperature causing the child to overheat.

Fracture: A medical term for a broken bone. Bone fractures usually require immediate hospital care.

Frostbite: A feeling of numbness or freezing of the skin or other tissues due to extremely low temperatures. Skin turns pale at the start then turns red and cold.

Heart attack: Occurs when the flow of oxygen-carrying blood to the heart is blocked often due to fat build-up, cholesterol or other substances.

Hemorrhage: Another term for bleeding. A forceful escape of blood from a ruptured blood vessel, especially when there's excessive discharge. Hemorrhage may be external (visible outside) and internal (no sign of bleeding outside the body).

Hyperglycaemia: The medical term for 'high blood sugar', often associated with diabetes (diabetes mellitus). When there is an excess blood sugar (glucose) in the blood and the body fails to convert it into energy.

Hypoglycaemia: The medical term for 'low blood sugar'. The most common cause is when a person is taking Hyperglycaemia (diabetes mellitus) medications to lower down the blood sugar level.

Incision: A surgical wound, clean-cut caused by a sharp-edged object usually, made with a knife.

Injury: A term that refers to harm or damage to the body due to accidents, falls, hits or weapons.

Overdose: Taking an excessive dose of drugs, whether prescribed by the doctor, legal or illegal and over the counter drugs, which leads to a serious health condition, or worse, death.

Poison: Any substance or toxin that is harmful to the body. It can be in chemical form or gas form. Severe cases of poisoning can be life-threatening.

Puncture: A wound or injury that has a small entry, which is in contrast to an open cut. This is caused by a pointed object such as nail that you accidentally stepped on which penetrated the skin. This wound carries danger of tetanus.

Shock: A condition where in the body is not getting enough blood flow which can be life-threatening as the body will not be able to function properly due to lack of oxygen and nutrients supplied to the body.

Sore: A term that refers to something painful or aching.

Sprain: An injury to the tissues surrounding a joint where ligaments are either stretched or torn that causes pain and swelling but not dislocated. Ankle sprain is the most common.

Stroke: Medical emergency when there is not enough oxygen or nutrients in a person's brain because of a blood clot or bleeding in the brain.

Trauma: Can be a physical or emotional injury resulting from a terrible event or accident.

Unconscious: The part of the mind that is not aware of the surroundings and oneself. This is due to lack of oxygen, shock, or injury.

Vertigo: The feeling where you sense that your environment is moving or spinning. It is a form of dizziness including a sensation of disorientation.

Vomit: Is an act of involuntary ejection of contents of the stomach back into the mouth and outside the body. Other terms for vomit are emesis or throwing up.

Wound: An injury to living tissues usually characterized as skin cut or broken, typically open or closed.

INTRODUCTION TO FIRST AID

First aid is the immediate and temporary care given to the victim of an accident or sudden illness. A person trained in first aid can very often save a life, help the patient towards recovery and prevent the injury or illness from becoming worse, by prompt arid correct action until the services of a doctor can be obtained. In order to become a good first aider, knowledge of anatomy and Physiology is needed, and it is recommended that the study of first aid and bandaging should go along with the study of anatomy and physiology in the Auxiliary Nurse-Midwife Course.

Aims of First Aid

- To save life, for example by giving artificial respiration, or stopping severe bleeding, and by treating shock.
- To prevent further injury, by removing the cause or the patient from the danger, where possible, and giving only such treatment as is immediately needed.
- To arrange for removal to hospital or the care of a doctor as soon as possible.

Objectives of First Aid

The objectives of the first aid will include the following:
- To preserve life
- To prevent further injury and deterioration of the condition
- To prevent complications related to injury or illness or conditions
- To make the victim as comfortable as possible to conserve the strength
- To put the injured person under professional medical care at the earliest.

Principles of First Aid

(Dos in Giving First Aid)	(Don'ts in Giving First Aid)
• Do stay calm • Do reassure and comfort the victim • Do check for a medical bracelet indicating a condition, such as epilepsy or diabetes • Do loosen any tight clothing • Do keep the victim covered to reduce shock	• Don't give food and drink to an unconscious person • Don't move an injured person unless you need to place him/her in the recovery position.

Scope of First Aid

- To determine the nature of the case requiring attention so far as is necessary for intelligent and efficient treatment—diagnosis.
- To decide on the character and extent of the 'treatment' to be given and to apply the treatment most suited to the circumstances until medical aid is available.
- To arrange for the 'disposal' of the casualty by removal either to his home or other suitable shelter, or to hospital.

Qualities of Good First-aider

- Promptness—quick thinking and quick action.
- Skill acquired through practice.
- Calm confidence.
- Commonsense and ability to improvise.
- Tact.
- Keen observation.

General Rules for First Aid

- Go quickly and confidently to the person or persons needing first aid, and decide what needs to be done without delay.
- If breathing has stopped, immediately start artificial respiration. Every second counts.

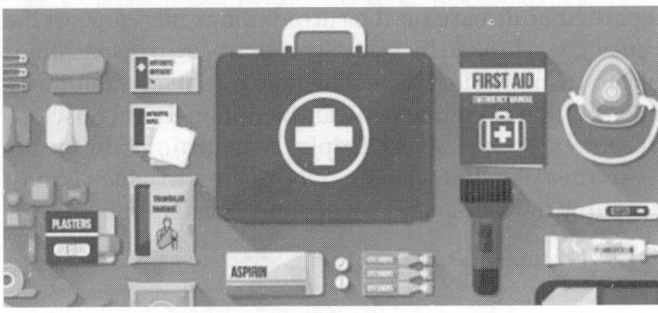

Fig. 30.1: Introduction to first aid.

- If there is bleeding, control it.
- Reassure the patient and others present, and so help to lessen anxiety.
- Do not allow a crowd around the patient, who needs fresh air. Enlist the help of one or two.
- See that the patient is in the best position to recovery, usually lying down.
- Loosen any tight clothing, but do not remove clothes unnecessarily.
- Arrange for medical aid as soon as possible, and for informing the patient's relatives.
- Do not attempt too much-Do the minimum that is required to save life and prevent the condition from worsening.
- Stay with the patient, continuing to observe and care for her until handing over to a doctor.

Principles of First Aid

When any person comes across another seriously injured person he should follow the following principles:
- Make sure that victim's airway is not blocked by the tongue, secretions or some foreign body—restore respiration.
- Make sure that the person is breathing, if not administer artificial respiration—restore respiration.
- Make sure that the patient has a pulse or no pulse if no pulse is felt, administer cardiopulmonary resuscitation (CPR)—restoration of circulation.
- Check for bleeding—take measures to control bleeding.
- Act fast if the victim is bleeding severely or if he has swallowed poison or if his heart or breathing has stopped every second counts for his survival.
- Arrange without delay for shifting of the victim to hospital for medical attention, although most injured persons can be safely moved. It is vitally important not to move a person with serious neck and/or back injuries unless taking proper measure to ensure and have to save him from further danger.
- Keep the victim/patient lying down and quieted. If he has vomited and there is no danger that his neck is broken, turn him on his side to prevent choking.
- Have someone called for medical assistance while applying first aid. The person who summons help should explain the nature of the emergency and ask what should be done if the arrival of the ambulance in pending.
- Examine the victim gently, cut clothing, if necessary to avoid abrupt movements if added pain. Do not pull clothing away from burns unless it is still smouldering.
- Reassure the victim, try to remain calm yourself. Your calmness can allay his fear and panic.
- Do not give fluids to an unconscious or semi conscious persons by slapping or shaking.
- Look for an emergency identification card for medical information related to victim.

Importance of First Aid

To give efficient first aid, one should have good knowledge of human anatomy and physiology of the human body and common sense and experience. The main importance of first aid is:
- The immediate objective of first aid at a given situation is to save the life of the individual.
- It is the first objective of first aid to reduce pain and prevent further injury or complication.
- First aid should help to avoid further injury. It should correct situations which tend to increase the original injury.
- The first aid should form a basis for subsequent treatment by the doctor or the hospital staff.
- It can be done by supplying details of accident, injury and the first aid treatment given etc. The ultimate aim of First aid is to prevent disability and death.

Transport of Injured or Sick Person

The transport must be safe, steady and quick. The method used will depend on the nature and severity of the injury, the distance, and the number of helpers and nature of transport available.
- **If only one helper and injury not severe:**
  - **Cradle method** may be used for a child or light person: The arms must be passed well beneath the patient's knees and his back.
  - **Human crutch:** Stand at patient's injured side, pat your arm around his waist. Place his arm around your neck, and grasp his hand with your free hand.
  - **Pick-a-back:** Put the patient bearer's back, with legs astride the back. The legs are held by the bearer. The patient holds on to the bearer's shoulders.
  - **Fireman's lift:** Taking the patient's weight on your shoulders, place your right arm round his legs, and grasp his right arm.
- **If two helpers:**
  Hand seats: Four-handed seat (see picture) when the patient can hold on with both arms round helpers' necks. Three-handed or two-handed seats may be used if the patient needs hack support.

Diagnosis

In deciding the nature of the case, the 'first aider' must consider its 'history, symptoms and signs'. The 'history' is the story of how an accident or sudden illness occurred. This may be obtained from the casualty (if conscious) or from witnesses. It may be information that a person is subject to a particular disease on the surroundings may suggest the cause, e.g. a broken bicycle. 'Symptoms' are the sensations of the casualty such as feeling cold or shivery, faintness, nausea, thirst pain, which can be obtained, if conscious describes. Pain is a very helpful diagnostic point for the 'first aider' as it draws his attention to the part which is most probably in trouble and saves a great deal of time during

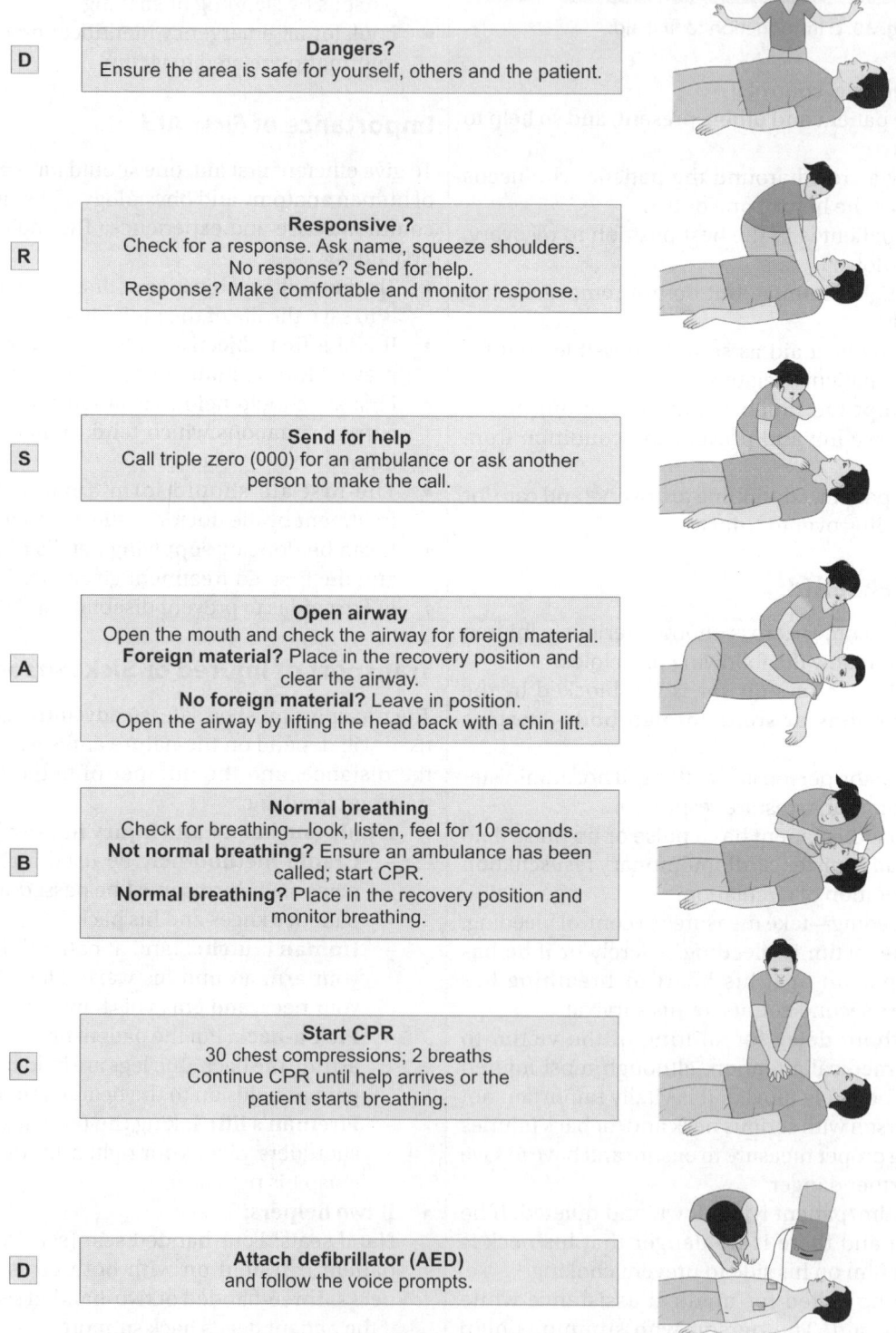

Fig. 30.2: DRSABCD technique of resuscitation.

his examination of the casualty. 'Signs' are any variations from the normal conditions of the casualty such as pallor, congestion, swelling and deformity, which can be observed by the first aider. Signs are the most reliable indications on which to base diagnosis, but the circumstances of each particular case will determine the relative importance of history, symptoms and signs.

Treatment: If the cause of the condition is still active remove the cause if possible, e.g. log of wood on leg, or remove the casualty from the cause of the conditions, e.g. gas-filled room. Give treatment to preserve life, promote recovery and prevent the condition becoming worse. Pay special attention to the treatment of failure of breathing, severe bleeding and shock. When there is the slightest doubt as to whether a casualty is dead or alive, continue treatment until medical aid has been obtained.

Disposal: The speed with which a casualty is brought under medical care is of tremendous importance in his recovery.

Unless the casualty is examined by a doctor on the spot, it is the responsibility of the first aider to see that he is conveyed to his home (or other suitable temporary shelter) or to hospital as soon as possible in the manner most suitable in the circumstances. A tactful message should be sent to the casualty's home or relatives indicating in a general way what has happened and the casualty's destination.

THE MANAGEMENT OF THE CASE

The first aider must always:
- Respond quickly to calls for assistance, the saving of a life may depend on promptness of action.
- Adopt a calm and methodical approach to the casualty quick and confident examination and treatment will relieve pain and distress, lessen the effect of the injury and may save life. Time spent on long and elaborate examination of a casualty may be time lost in his ultimate recovery.
- Treat obvious injuries and conditions endangering life such as failure of breathing, severe shock, before making a complete diagnosis.
- Take first aid material if this is immediately available. If standard equipment is not available the first aider must depend on material to hand which will have to be provided as required.
- Study the surroundings carefully. These may influence the action to be taken and therefore require careful consideration for example:
  - Danger from falling building, moving machinery, electric current, fire, poisonous gases and similar hazards.
  - Weather: If the accident occurs out-of-doors, the casualty may be treated in the open if the weather is fine; if the weather is bad, he must be removed to shelter as soon as is reasonably possible.
  - Shelter note houses and buildings near at hand, whether occupied or unoccupied and whether likely to be particularly useful, such as a chemist's shop, otherwise, temporary shelter may be provided by means of umbrellas, rugs and the like.

Characteristic of a Good First-aider

- **Observant**—notice all signs
- **Resourceful**—make best use of all things
- **Gentle**—shouldn't cause pain
- **Tactful**—shouldn't be alarming
- **Sympathetic**—should be comforting

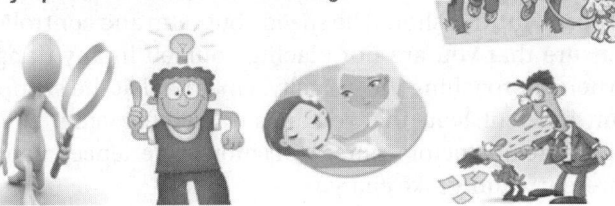

- Light it is impossible to treat a patient satisfactorily without sufficient light and the first aider must provide for this.
- Assistance crowds must be tactfully controlled. If a doctor is present, work under his direction, If not, ask if anyone with a knowledge of first aid is present. If neither is available make use of bystanders to the best advantage.
- Reassure the casualty by speaking encouragingly to him. Warn him to be still and tell him that he is in trained hands.

GOLDEN RULES OF FIRST AID

- Do "first things first quickly", and without fuss or panic.
- "Give artificial respiration" if breathing has stopped-every second counts.
- Stop any bleeding.
- "Guard against or treat for shock" by moving the casualty as little as possible and handling him gently.
- "Do not attempt too much" do the minimum that is essential to save life and prevent the condition from worsening.
- "Reassure the casualty" and those around and so help to lessen anxiety.
- Do not allow people to crowd round as fresh air is essential.
- Do not remove clothes unnecessarily.
- Arrange for the removal of the casualty to the care of a doctor (or) hospital as soon as possible.

Action at an emergency: The basic principles of first aid apply to all injuries or illnesses regardless of severity. Whatever the incident, it is the first aider's responsibility to act quickly, calmly and correctly in order to:

- Preserve life
- Prevent deterioration in the casualty's condition
- Promote recovery.

These objectives are best achieved by:
- A rapid but calm approach.
- A quick assessment of the situation and the casualty.
- A correct diagnosis of the condition based on the history of the incident, and the casualty's history, symptoms and signs.
- Immediately and appropriate treatment of any conditions diagnosed.
- Proper disposal of the casualty according to the injury or condition.

Approach: This should be speedy but calm and controlled. Ensure that you are not placing yourself in any danger when approaching the casualty. On arrival at the scene of any incident, state that you are a trained first aider and, if there are no doctors, nurses (or) more experienced people present, calmly take charge.

General rules: Whenever and wherever you come across an emergency, use your common sense, know your limitations and do not attempt to do too much.

Assisting the situation: As soon as you have taken control at an incident, it is crucial that you make an accurate assessment of the situation and decide on the priorities of action, to do this you must consider:
- Whether you and the casualty are in any danger.
- If the casualty has any life threatening conditions.
- If any bystanders can help you.
- Whether you need to call for assistance.

Safety: The first aider must minimize the risk of danger to him, the causality and by standers, and guard against any further causality.

FIRST AID KIT

First aid kits of different sizes can be brought at a chemists shop.

Alternatively, individual items may be brought and kept in a compact metal box. Supplies should not be kept in different places. It is important that everything be ready for immediate use. The following items should be included in the first aid kit.
- Gauze dressing 5 and 10 cm square in individual sterile package.
- Rolls of gauze bandages 5 and 8 cm wide.
- Adhesive bandages in assorted sizes.
- Roll of absorbent cotton.
- Adhesive tape.
- Mild antiseptic.
- Scissors, tweezers, safety pins.
- Tube of petroleum jelly.
- Laundered ironed and sheets of cotton about 1 meter square for making slings and bandages.

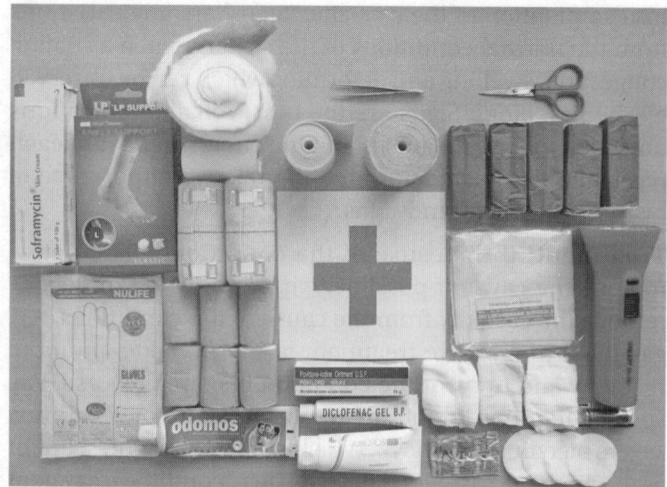

Fig. 30.3: First aid equipment.

- Paper and pencil to record clues including patients pulse rate.
- Tongue depressor.
- Airway.
- Splints.
- Thermometer.
- Rubber catheter, tourniquet.
- Mackintosh.
- Matchbox.

Gauze dressing and bandages come in sterile packages. Supplies left over from opened packages do not remain sterile should be replaced. Items other than those mentioned above may be added to the kits, e.g. baking soda, salt, potassium permanganate crystals, milk of magnesia and a medicine dropper.

In an emergency, one should not hesitate to use nonsterile supplies such as ironed sheets, torn strips or pads made from clean clothing, etc. When first aid is to be given to a large number of people, e.g. victims of a disaster, a large number of drugs, syringes, needles and infusion sets are required. The drugs to be included are glucose saline, normal saline, 5% dextrose in water, 25% dextrose in water, 50% dextrose in water, 7.5% sodium bicarbonate, adrenaline, atropine, nikethamide, phenobarbitone, diazepam, promethzine, antitetanus serum, tetanus toxoid 2% lignocaine distilled water for injection, etc.

Some of the disinfectants and antiseptics commonly used are as follow:
- **Dettol:** It is used to clean wounds and surrounding area (2-4 teaspoonfuls in 500 mL of water). It is also used to sterilize instruments that cannot be sterilized by heat.
- **Savlon:** It is used to wash hospital equipment, disinfect soiled linen and spray patients room (1/2 measure in 2 liters of water). It is also used to clean wounds.
- **Potassium permanganate:** It is used for throat gargles, bladder wash (1:60). It is also used in snake bites. It can be used for purification of water.
- **Spirit** it is used for disinfection of skin, instruments and ampoules. It should not be applied to wounds or

raw surfaces because it removes coagulum formed on the raw area.

- **Boric acid:** It is used in solution form (5%) as mouthwash and for irrigation of the urinary bladder, skin and mucosal inflammation like eczema, burns, bedsores, etc. It can be used in ointment form and as dusting powder.
- **Iodine:** It is used in the form of tincture (2%) for disinfection of skin, treatment of wounds, etc.
- **A crifla vine:** It is an aniline dye used as an antiseptic (1:1000) for dressing wounds. Glycerin acriflavine is useful for edematous and infected wounds.
- **Nitrofurazone:** It is used as an antibacterial agent for dressing wounds.
- **Hydrogen peroxide:** It is used for cleaning wounds on contact with tissues, it releases nascent oxygen which oxidizes necrotic material, and the tissue debris and necrotic material float on the bubbles formed.
  Some heat is generated in the process.
- **Gention violet:** It is used (1% solution) such application to infected wounds, mucous membranes and serous surfaces. It is used for treatment of monilial infections of throat and vagina.
- **Carbolic acid:** It is used to cauterize dog bites, snake bites, etc. It is, also used to sterilize sharp instruments like scissors and scalpels.

WOUNDS

The skin is normally intact. A break (or) tear in the skin may occur following an accident. The result is a wound. The deeper the wound, the more likely it is to get infected as it cannot be properly cleaned. The appearance of the wound and its likelihood of infection depend on what causes the wound. Aims of the first aider when dealing with wounds are—(i) to stop the bleeding (ii) to prevent infection.

Injury to the skin may be caused by the following:
- A cut with a sharp instrument, e.g. knife, glass, stone, etc.
- A blow with a blunt instrument, e.g. stick, stone, etc.
- A broken bone whose sharp pierces the skin from inside, usually when open fracture occurs.

The degree of injury to the skin ranges from an abrasion to a deep wound.

Abrasions

An abrasion (or) gauze is a scraping away of the superficial layer of the skin. Abrasions are actually very superficial cuts in the skin.

Signs
- Superficial scraping of the skin.
- Slight bleeding.

Treatment
- Wash the site with clean boiled water and soap.
- Remove any girt (or) other foreign matter.
- Wash with antiseptic lotion and apply G.V. paint.
- Apply clean gauze covered with cotton wool padding and bandage.

Follow-up
Tell the patient to come and see you if he gets fever.

Types of Wound

Incised Wound
An incised wound is caused by a sharp cutting instrument. It edges are straight and it is usually accompanied by profuse bleeding, which helps to wash away any germs that might

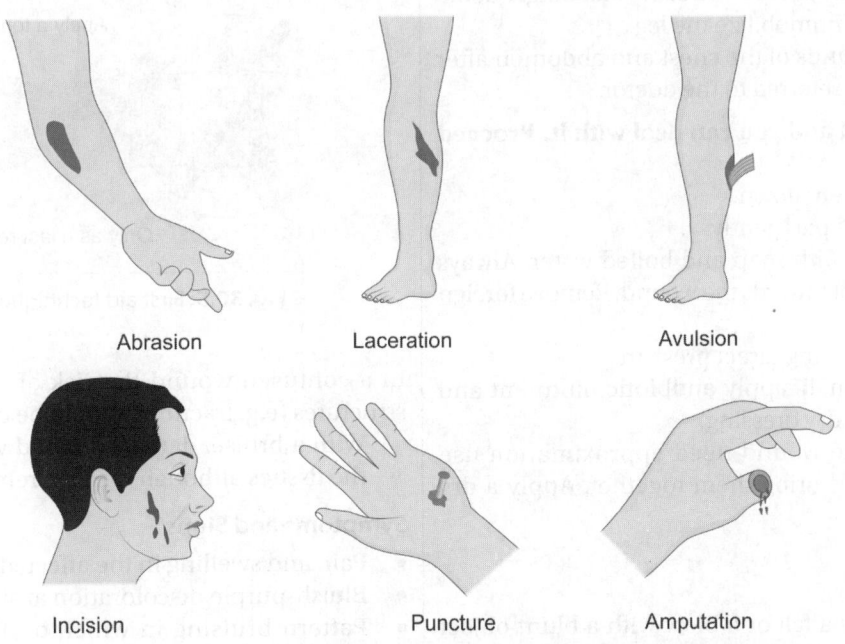

Fig. 30.4: Types of wounds.

have entered the wound. A deep incised wound may cut through tendons and or arteries.

Lacerated Wound

A lacerated wound is caused by a blunt instrument. Its edges are ragged and bruising surrounds the wound. Usually lacerated wounds do not bleed much and any dirt which may have entered the wound is not thoroughly flushed out.

Punctured Wound

A punctured wound is caused by a stab from as knife, needle, nail, bullet, etc. and is often small and deep. There is usually little bleeding so that the germs and dirt introduced to the bottom of the wound by the stabbing instrument are not washed out. These wounds are likely to become easily infected and the risk of tetanus is high. Also, because of the depth of these wounds, injury to important structures may be caused.

Signs

- The appearance of the wound edges depends on type of wound.
- Bleeding is present to a varying extent.
- Signs of shock may be present depending on the severity of the wound and the amount of bleeding.

Treatment

You should proceed with the treatment of a wound as follows:

- Handle the injured part as gently and as little as possible.
- Sit (or) lay the patient down and raise the wounded limb.
- Stop the bleeding.
- Treat for shock.
- If the wound is large and will require suturing, apply a dry dressing and transfer the patient to hospital after applying a firm bandage to control the bleeding. Put the arm in a sling (or) immobilize the leg.
- All punctured wounds of the chest and abdomen after first aid should be referred to the doctor.

If the wound is small and you can deal with it. Proceed as follows:

- Sit (or) lay the patient down.
- Handle the injured part gently.
- Clean the wound with soap and boiled water. Always clean away from not towards the wound. Remove foreign matter.
- Stop the bleeding using direct pressure.
- If the wound is small, apply antibiotic ointment and cover with a clean dry dressing.
- If the edges of the wound need approximation use adhesive plaster to bring them together. Apply a dry sterile dressing.

Contused Wound

This can be caused by a fall or a blow with a blunt object which splits the skin and bruises the surrounding tissues.

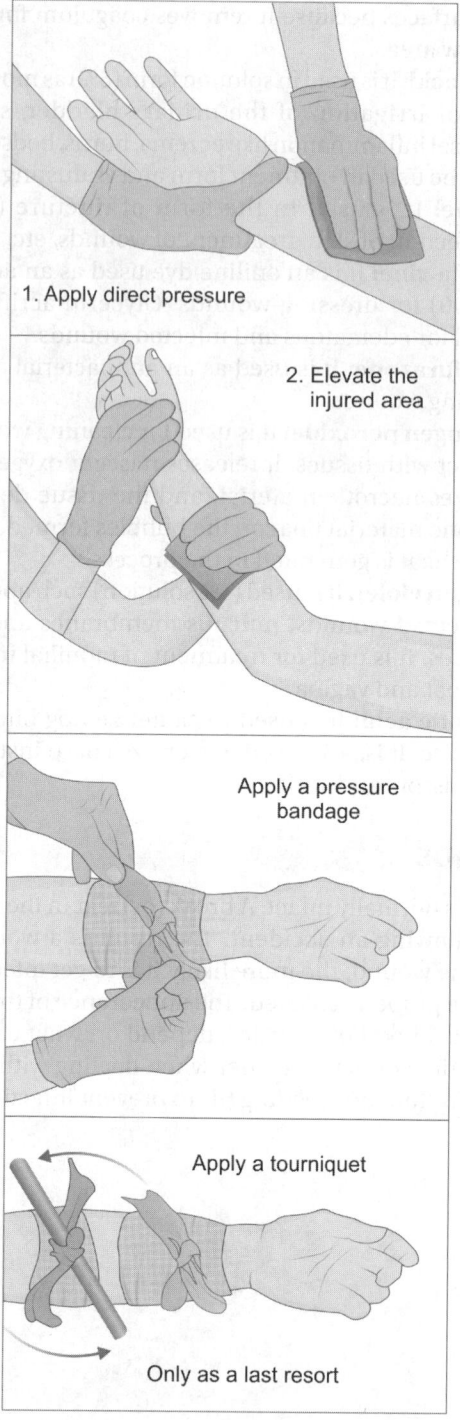

Fig. 30.5: First aid techniques for wounds.

In a contused wound the risk of damage to underlying structures (e.g. fracture) should be considered.

With a bruise, damaged blood vessels leak blood into the tissues although the skin remains unbroken.

Symptoms and Signs

- Pain and swelling in the affected area.
- Bluish-purple discoloration at site of injury.
- Pattern bruising in which outlines of the casualty's clothing are seen in the bruise. This is a potentially

dangerous sign as it may indicate damage to internal organs.

Aim

Slow down blood flow by cooling and gentle compression.

Treatment

- Raise and support the injured part in the position the casualty finds most comfortable.
- Apply a cold compress to the injured area to restrict bleeding and reduce swelling.
- If in doubt about the severity of the injury, seek medical aid.

Gunshot Wound

This wound is caused when a missile strikes the body at high speed and can result in serious internal injury. There will be a wound where a missile enters the body and often a much larger exit wound. Internal organs, tissues and blood vessels may be damaged during the missile passage through the body. In addition external bleeding, there may be internal bleeding.

Eye Wounds

All eye injuries are potentially serious. Even superficial grazes can lead to scarring of the surface of the eye (cornea) on infection, with possible deterioration of eye sight and even permanent blindness.

The eye can be cut (or) bruised by direct flows, broken spectacles, (or) sharp, clipped fragments of metallic materials, girt (or) glass which fly into it. (For treatment of foreign bodies in the eye, refer the topic on Foreign Bodies in the Eye).

Symptoms and Signs

- Partial or total loss of vision of the affected eye, even with no visible injury.
- Painful, blood shot eye, possibly with a visible wound of eyeball (or) eyelid.
- Loss of blood (or) clear fluid from the eye wound, possibly with flattening of the normal round contour of the eyeball as the contents leak.

Aim

Protect the eye by preventing movement and seek medical aid.

Treatment

- Lay the casualty down on his back. Support his head and keep it as still as possible.
  Do not attempt to remove embedded foreign bodies.
- Ask the casualty to close his injured eye and gently cover it with an eye pad or a sterile dressing.
  Secure it with a bandage (or) adhesive plaster.
- Advise the casualty to keep his sound eye still because movement will cause the injured eye to move. If necessary, bandage both eyes to prevent unnecessary movement. Reassure the casualty before blindfolding.
- Arrange removal to hospital, maintaining the treatment position.

Wound to the Palm of the Hand

Wounds in the palm can occur when a person handles broken glass or sharp tools or falls on to sharp objects. Such wounds may bleed profusely and can be accompanied by fractures. If the wound is deep, the nerves and tendons in the hand may be damaged.

Symptoms and Signs

- Pain at the site of the wound.
- Bleeding which may be profuse.
- Loss of sensation and movement in the fingers and hand if the underlying nerves and tendons are severed.

Aim

Control bleeding and arrange urgent removal to hospital without attempting to remove any embedded foreign bodies.

Treatment

- To control bleeding, place a sterile dressing (or) gauze and a clean pad over the wound and apply direct pressure with your fingers (refer topic on Controlling Blood Loss-Direct Pressure) (or) thumbs (or) by casualty if able.
  If no dressing (or) pad is available, use an improvised dressing, e.g. a clean handkerchief, a freshly laundered towel, a piece of or a pad of clean paper handkerchief can be used. Improvised dressing should be covered and held in position using whatever materials are available at the time, e.g. a folded scarf.
- Elevate the injured arm above the level of the heart.
- Ask the casualty to maintain pressure by clenching her fist over the dressing (or) pad. If the casualty cannot do this tell her to grasp the fist of her injured hand with her other hand.
- Bandage the fist firmly, using the loose ends of the dressing or a folded triangular bandage. Tie off firmly across the bent fingers to maintain pressure.
- Support the arm in an elevation sling (refer topic on Elevation Sling) and arrange removal to hospital.

Bruises

A bruise consists of internal bleeding which seeps through the tissues, and appears as a discoloration under the skin. A heavy fall on fleshy parts of the body, e.g. the buttocks, can result in considerable bruising. A bruise may follow blows, sprains (or) fractures.

Symptoms and Signs

- Pain and swelling in the affected area.
- Bluish-purple discoloration at site of injury.
- Pattern bruising, in which outlines of the casualty's clothing are seen in the bruise. This is a potentially dangerous sign as it may indicate damage to internal organs.

Aim

Slow down blood flow by cooling and gentle compression.

Treatment

- Raise and support the injured part in the position the casualty finds most comfortable.
- Apply a cold compress to the injured area to restrict bleeding and reduce swelling.
- If in doubt about the severity of the injury, seek medical aid.

Infected Wounds

All open wounds will be contaminated by germs which either come from the cause of the injury, from the air or from the first aider's breath (or) fingers. Some particles of dirt may be carried away from the damaged tissue by bleeding. Any harmful germs which remain are usually destroyed by the white cells in the blood and the wound then stays clean and healthy.

Normal first aid for wounds includes prevention of infection. However, any wound which has not begun to heal properly after about 48 hours may be infected because dirt, dead tissue, foreign bodies and/or bacteria may still be present. If infection develops, it can have serious consequences. It may enter in the blood system and subsequently spread to other parts of the body, permanently destroying tissue and occasionally leading to death.

Symptoms and Signs

- Increasing pain and soreness in the wound.
- Increased surrounding parts with a feeling of heat.
- Pus may ooze from the wound.
- Fever, sweating, thirst, shivering and lethargy if the infection is severe.
- Swelling and tenderness in the glands, in the neck, armpits (or) grain.
- Faint read trails may see on the surface of the inside of the arms (or) legs leading towards lymph glands.

Aim

Seek medical aid.

Treatment

- Dress wound with a prepared sterile dressing (or) similar clean, preferably sterile, material and secure with a bandage.
- Elevate the injured part and immobilize especially if swollen.
- Seek medical aid.

Penetrating Chest Wounds

The rib cage protects not only the heart, lungs and major blood vessels in the chest cavity above the diaphragm, but also the liver and spleen below the diaphragm in the upper abdominal cavity.

A wound to the front (or) back of the chest which penetrates into the chest allows air to enter the space

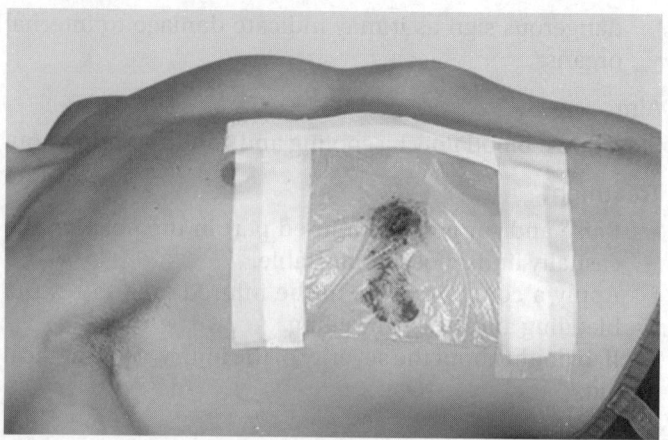

Fig. 30.6: Penetrating chest wounds.

occupied by the lungs, this interfering with breathing. In these injuries, the lung on the affected side collapses, even if it is not punctured. Air in the chest cavity impairs the action of the sound lung and, sometimes, of the heart. The amount of oxygen reaching the bloodstream may be insufficient and asphyxia may result. A wound to the front (or) back of the lower chest may penetrate into the abdominal cavity and give rise to severe internal bleeding.

Symptoms and Signs

- Casualty may have pain in the chest.
- May have an acute sense of alarm.
- Difficulty in breathing; breaths are shallow due to air in the chest cavity.
- Blueness of the mouth, nail beds and skin (cyanosis) indicating the onset of significant asphyxia.
- Bright red, frothy blood may be coughed up.
- The sound of air being sucked into the chest may be heard when the casualty is breathing in.
- Blood-stained liquid bubbling from the chest wound during breathing out.
- Symptoms and signs of shock.

Aim

Ease breathing by immediately sealing the wound. Arrange urgent removal to hospital.

Treatment

- Immediately seal open wound with your palm (or) the casualty's if possible.
- Place the casualty in a half sitting position with his head and shoulders supported; turn the body towards the injured side so the sound lung is upper most.
- Pressure the casualty.
- Gently cover the wounds with a sterile dressing as soon as possible.
- If possible, form an airtight seal by covering the dressing with a plastic sheet (or) metal foil. Secure and seal the edges of the dressing with layers of adhesive tape, strapping and/or bandage.

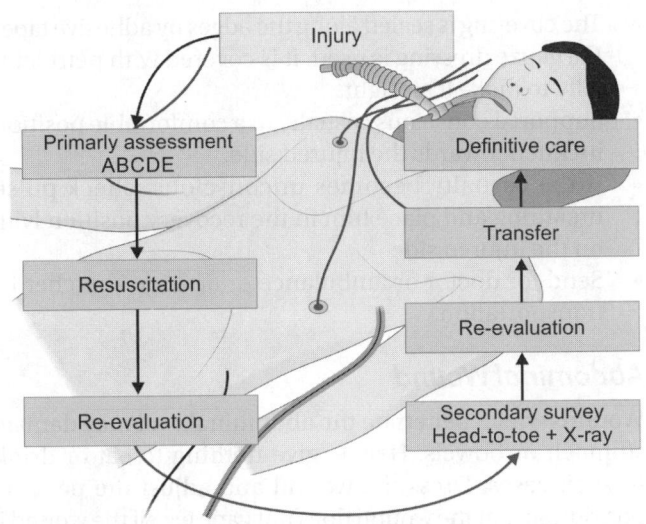

Fig. 30.7: Management of penetrating chest wounds.
(ABCDE: airway, breathing, circulation, disability, exposure).

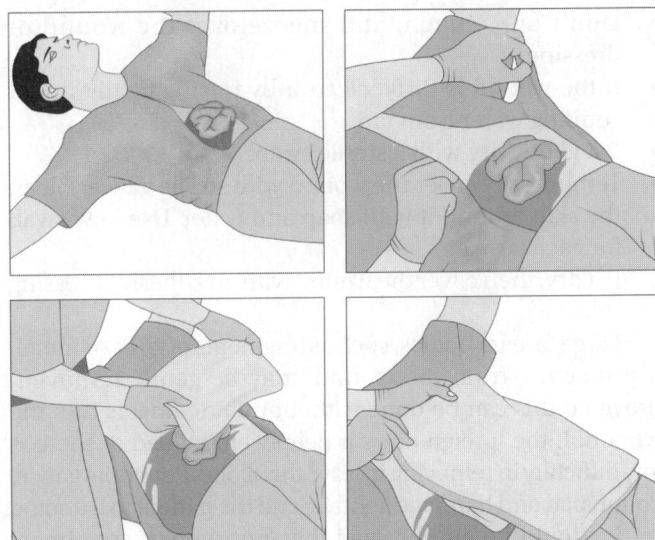

Fig. 30.8: First aid for abdominal trauma.

- Support the arm on the injured side in an elevation sling and make the casualty as comfortable as possible.
- Check breathing rate (refer topic on How We Breath), pulse (refer topic on the Pulse) and level of responsiveness (refer topic on Assessment of Level of Responsiveness) at 10 minute intervals. Look for evidence of internal bleeding (refer topic on External Bleeding).
- If the casualty becomes unconscious, open his airway and check breathing. Complete airway, breathing, circulation (ABC) of resuscitation (refer topic on Resuscitation) if requires and place him in the Recovery Position with his uninjured side upper most.
- Arrange urgent removal to hospital. Transport as a stretcher case, maintaining the treatment position.
  If a foreign body is present (refer a topic on Foreign Bodies) give first aid as for foreign body.

Abdominal Wounds

Wounds of the abdominal wall may be caused by sharp instruments (or) by missiles. A deep wound of the abdominal wall is serious not only because of the external bleeding, but also because the underlying organs may have been punctured (or) lacerated, leading to severe internal bleeding and possible infection. Part of the intestine may also be protruding from the wound.

Symptoms and Signs

- General abdominal pain.
- Bleeding and associated wounds (which may only be a small puncture) in the abdominal area.
- Part of the intestine may be visible in (or) protruding from the wound.
- Casualty may be vomiting.
- Symptoms and signs of shock.

Aim

Protect wound to minimize infection and arrange urgent removal to hospital.

Treatment

i. Lay the casualty on her back with her knees bent up to prevent the wound gaping and to reduce strain on the injured area. Support her knees.
ii. Apply sterile dressing (or) gauze and a clean pad over the wound and secure with a bandage (or) adhesive strapping.
iii. To minimize shock. If shock present-Treatment to shock. Note: Do not remove protruding objects (or) do not give the casualty anything by mouth.
iv. Check breathing rate and pulse at 10 minute intervals. Look for evidence of internal bleeding.
v. If the casualty coughs (or) vomits, support her abdomen by pressing gently on the dressing to prevent protrusion of the intestines from the wound.
vi. If she becomes unconscious, open her airway and check breathing. Complete the ABC of resuscitation if required, and support her abdomen when placing her in Recovery Position.
vii. Arrange urgent removal to hospital. Transport as a stretcher case, maintaining the treatment position. If part of the intestine protrudes from the wound. Do not touch the protruding intestines.
   - Cover with a sterile dressing (or) clean cloth secured with a bandage.
   - If the casualty coughs (or) vomits, support the wound as in Step V.
   - Position and treat the casualty as above.

First Aid Measures in Minor Wounds

Minor bleeding is easily controlled by pressure and elevation. A small adhesive dressing is normally adequate. If bleeding does not stop, then seek medical help.

- Wash your hands thoroughly in soap and warm water
- Avoid touching the wound with your fingers (use disposable gloves, if possible).

- Don't talk, cough, and sneeze over the wound or dressing.
- If the wound is dirty, clean it by rinsing lightly under running water from tap.
- Pat gently dry with a sterile swab.
- Temporarily cover the wound with sterile gauze. Clean the skin around it with soap and water. Use new swab for each stroke.
- Pat dry, then cover the wound with an adhesive dressing (plaster).

Large foreign bodies, such as fragments of glass or metal, if projecting from the wound, may be gently removed, provided this can be done without putting fingers into the wound. If the foreign body is deeply embedded or there is any difficulty in removing it, leave this alone. Put sterile gauze, cotton pad and bandage lightly. Send the patient to a doctor.

It should be emphasized that 'antiseptics' are almost completely ineffective in killing or removing germs embedded in a wound. The chief result of introducing these strong chemicals into or on a wound.

For a small household scratch, antibiotic creams like Soframycin, Furacin or antiseptic solutions like Dettol or Savlon can be used but not for large wounds.

Contusion is wound in which the deep tissues are torn without the overlying skin being broken. Bleeding beneath the skin leads to the 'black and blue' color changes. A dressing is not necessary as germs cannot penetrate the intact skin. Ice packs or cold compresses, if promptly applied, may diminish the amount of bleeding and relieve the pain.

First Aid Measures in Major Wounds

Many serious and major wounds do not bleed profusely, e.g. chest wounds, wounds to the abdomen, eye wounds, etc. but may cause considerable internal damage.

Chest Wounds

The heart and lungs and the major blood vessels around them, lie within the chest. A penetrating wound may cause severe internal damage. The lungs are subject to injury as the air may enter the pleural space and exert pressure on the lungs for its subsequent collapse.

The Signs and Symptoms
- Breathing difficult and painful
- Signs of shock
- Frothy blood on coughing
- Mouth, nails and skin appears blue
- Blood bubbles out of the wound.

The first aid measures for chest wound include the following:
- Cover the open wound by palm of your hand.
- Cover the wound by sterile dressing or pad, then cover the pad by plastic wrap, which should be non-porous. Aluminium foil or plastic covering of a cigarette pack are also useful.
- The covering is sealed along the edges by adhesive tapes. If a gauze dressing is used, it is covered with petroleum jelly to make it air tight.
- Support a conscious casualty in a comfortable position, inclined towards the injured side.
- If the casualty becomes unconscious, check pulse, breathing and place him in the recovery position lying on the injured side.
- Send for doctor or ambulance or arrange stretcher for transportation.

Abdominal Wound

Wounds which penetrate the abdominal wall may damage stomach or bowels. Hence, give nothing to eat or drink. In such cases. Dress the wound and adjust the patient's position so that the wound does not gape e.g., if the wound is horizontal, place him on his back with heads and shoulders raised and a pillow under his knees. Send to hospital on stretcher.

If the intestines have come out:
- Cover with clean pads
- Don't give anything to eat or drink
- Obtain medical aid; till then give casualty rest in bed
- He has to be transported to a hospital. There may be severer hemorrhage when patients pulse becomes feeble and he goes in shock. In that case he should be sent to hospital as a priority case.

If there is an open abdominal wound, evisceration of abdominal organs may occur, with resultant drying and subsequent necrosis of the organs. Any abdominal organs lying outside the abdominal cavity must therefore be kept moist. If sterile dressings and sterile water are not available, it is preferable to cover the organs with a clean moist cloth and risk infection than to risk necrosis and loss of tissue.

HEMORRHAGE

Hemorrhage or bleeding: It is a flow of blood from an artery, vein or capillary.

Types of Hemorrhage

- **Arterial bleeding:** Blood is bright red in color. It spurts at each contraction.
- **Venous bleeding:** Blood in dark red in color. It does not spurt. Steady flow.
- **Capillary bleeding:** Blood is red in color. It does not spurt. Slow in flow.

Effects of Hemorrhage

The loss of red blood cells causes a lack of oxygen to the tissues of the body. A decrease in blood volume causes decrease in blood pressure. The heart's pumping rate increases to compensate for reduced blood pressure. The force of the heart beat is reduced since there is less blood to pump.

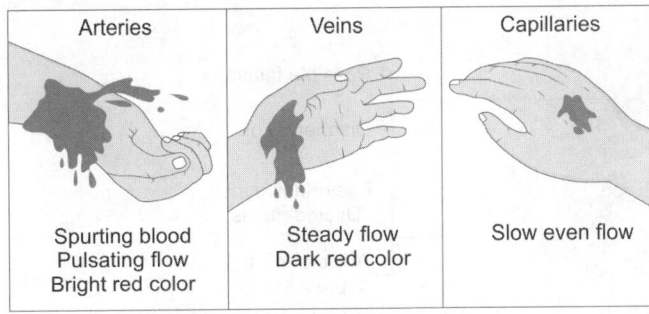

Fig. 30.9: Types of hemorrhage.

How to recognize external bleeding: Evidence of major external blood loss. Symptoms and signs of shock: Causality complains of thirst. Blurring vision, fainting, giddiness. Face and lips become pale. Skin feels cold and clammy. Pulse faster and weaker. Restlessness. Breathing shallow (air hunger). Unconsciousness may occur.

Internal bleeding: Wounds that have penetrated skull. Wound that have penetrated the chest on abdomen.

Signs and symptoms of shock: Blood may appear from one of the body orifices like nose, ear, mouth rectum, urethra, and vagina.

Management: Control bleeding as soon as possible. Keep the wound clean and dress it to minimize blood loss and prevent infection. Quickly transfer the causality to hospital.

How to Control Bleeding

Direct pressure: Place your hand directly over the wound and apply pressure, firm and steady until the bleeding stops. Tie a bandage firmly enough to control bleeding but not so tight to cut off the circulation. Immobilize the injured part. Never replace any dressing once it is applied. If the dressing is soaked, place another dressing and hold both in place with firm pressure.

Elevation: Elevate the bleeding part of the body above the level of the heart so that the flow of blood will slow down in that part and blood clothing take place.

Pressure points: Applying pressure over the pressure points pressing over the underlying bone pressure points on the arms (brachial pressure point) on the groin (femoral pressure point).

Applying a tourniquet: A standard tourniquet is a piece of web belting about 36" long with a buckle device to hold it tightly in place when applied. This is used to stop bleeding. Care to be taken not to cut off the circulation.

Management: Apply direct pressure over the wound with your fingers and palms, with clean pad/cloth you can ask the causality to apply direct pressure herself. Elevate and support the injured part above the level of the casualty's heart to reduce blood loss. If you suspect the causality is going into shock, raise and support her legs so that they are above the level of her heart. Secure the dressing with bandage. Tie it with pressure not too tightly to cut off the circulation. Further bleeding still occurs, put on the bandage over the previous one. Monitor the vital signs. Watch for the signs for shock. Dial for an ambulance and transport the causality to hospital till then the first aider should not leave the causality until taken over by doctor or nurse.

SHOCK

Shock is a clinical syndrome in which, the blood flow to the body is disturbed. The brain will not get enough blood and sudden depression of vital functions may occur. Sudden collapse of circulation is called shock.

Types of Shock

- Hypovolemic shock.
- Cardiogenic shock.
- Neurogenic shock.
- Septic shock.
- Anaphylactic shock.

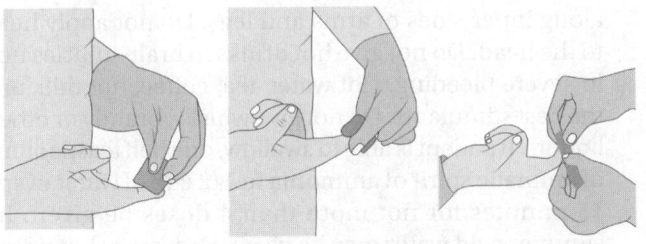

Fig. 30.10: Method of controlling bleeding.

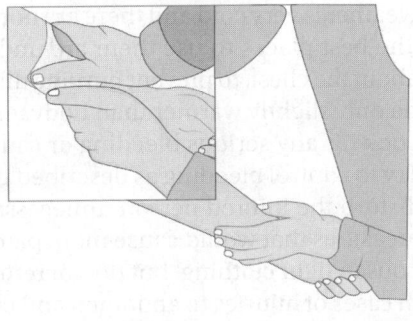
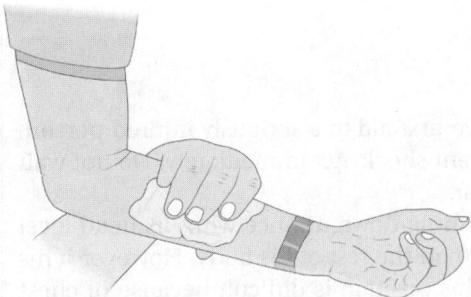

Fig. 30.11: Application of direct pressure helps to control hemorrhage.

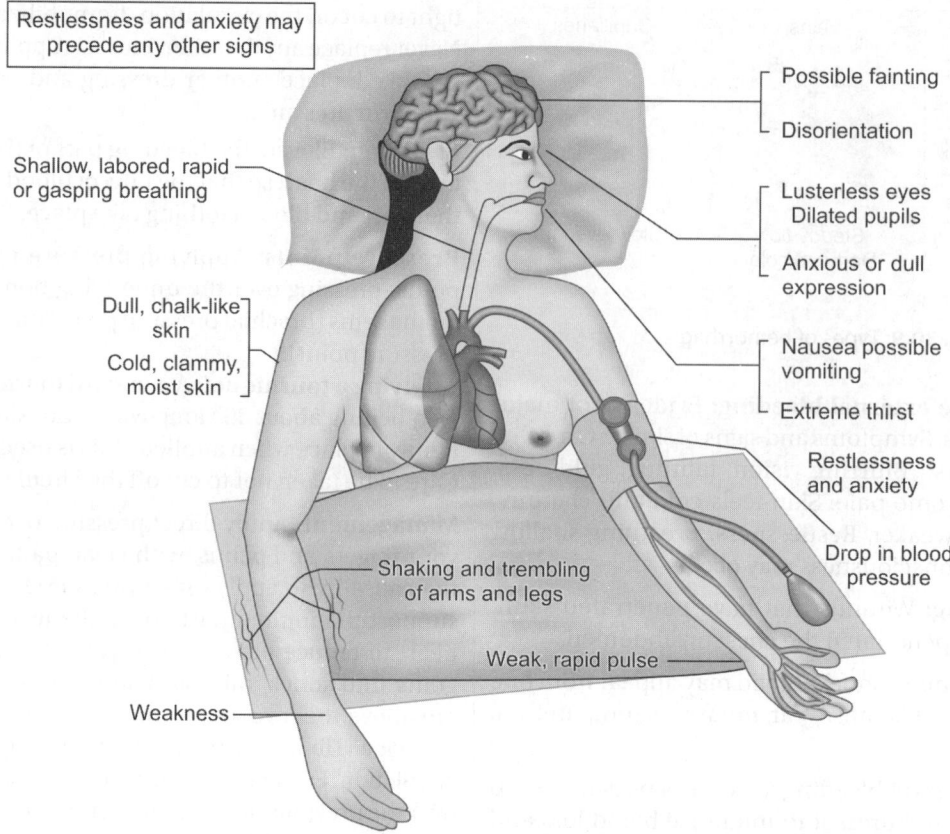

Fig. 30.12: Clinical features of shock.

Causes of Shock

- Accidents.
- Severe bleeding.
- Severe burns.
- Heart attacks.
- Dehydration.
- Bacterial infection.

Clinical Symptoms

- Cold and clammy skin.
- Cyanosis.
- Pallor.
- Weak and rapid pulse.
- Sighing and irregular breathing.
- Sweating.
- Dilatation of pupil.
- Blurring of vision.
- Coma.

First Aid

Whenever you give first aid to a seriously injured person, always try to prevent shock. Act immediately. Do not wait for shock to appear.
- Make the victim lie down at once with his head level with or lower than the rest of his body. However if his breathing in this position is difficult because of chest injuries, raise the head and shoulders by placing pillows under them.
- Cover him properly. Carefully place a blanket under him. If the weather is not hot, place a coat or blanket over him. If the weather is very cold, use several blankets. But do not make him sweat; too much covering is undesirable. Use bottles of hot water, rubber water bags, hot bricks, blankets, etc. in fact anything hot and convenient. Be careful that applications are not too hot. Apply heat along inner sides of arms and legs. Do not apply heat to the head. Do not give hot drinks in brain injuries not in severe bleeding. Hot water, tea, coffee, hot milk are the best stimulants. Do not give whisky, brandy or other liquors. If patient is able to swallow, one half teaspoonful of aromatic spirit of ammonia in 1/2 cup of water every 15 minutes for not more than 4 doses be given. In summer cold water may be given. Ordinarily hot water bottles or electric heating pads should not be used on accident victims. However, they may be used if the weather is very cold and there are not enough blankets. The best places to use them are under the armpits or about the chest, to prevent burning the skin; they should be only slightly warmer than body temperature.
- Look for any serious bleeding or cause of severe pain. Try to control bleeding as described previously. Do not disturb the injured person unnecessarily. Try to avoid measures that would cause more pain.
- Loosen tight clothing, but do not remove them.
- In cases of injuries to abdomen and chest, give nothing by mouth for he may require an operation later on.
- Under no circumstances fluids be given by mouth to an unconscious casualty.

- Do not let a crowd gather round the patient.
- Do not let him see his own injuries.
- Reassure the casualty if he is conscious.
- Arrange for transportation to a hospital or institution on a top priority basis.

First Aid in Shock

Shock occurs with every accident or sudden illness. The nervous system is affected and later if the condition of shock continues, the circulation of blood gradually fails and the patient dies. Prompt first aid treatment is needed to prevent shock increasing and to help the patient to recover from the primary shock. A shocked person may only feel a little faint, weak and cold, and look pale, or he may collapse with the pulse very weak and respirations shallow.

First Aid Treatment

- Reassure the patient.
- Lay him on his back with the head low. If shock is severe, raise the lower part of the body unless there is injury to the head or chest.
- Loosen tight clothing about the neck, chest and waist.
- Wrap him in a blanket or rug.
- Offer him a warm sweet drink, e.g. tea or coffee, unless there is internal injury.
- Keep the patient quiet and undisturbed, giving only essential first aid treatment for injures. Avoid causing pain.
- If there are severe injuries, or shock increases, get the patient to hospital as quickly as possible.
- Bandages of head and neck.
- For these, use 4 to 5 cm bandages, and stand behind the patient.
- The neck bandage may be used in a case of carbuncle. Start the bandage round the head.

The capeline bandage may be used after an operation on the head. To do the capeline bandage, stitch or pin together the ends of two bandages.

A triangular bandage may also be used to cover the head, as in treatment of pediculosis, and to cover the hair in the operating theater. Apply the base of the bandage to the forehead. Take the ends to the back and cross them on top of the point but under the occiput. Tie the ends under the occiput or on the forehead, and bring the point on top of the head and pin it neatly.

MUSCULOSKELETAL INJURIES: FRACTURES, DISLOCATION, MUSCLE INJURIES

Fracture

A fracture is a break in the continuity of a bone.

A complete fracture involves a break across the entire cross section of the bone which is frequently displaced. In an incomplete fracture, the break occurs only through a part of the cross section of the bone which is usually undisplaced.

An open fracture is one that extends through the skin and mucous membrane.

A closed fracture does not communicate with the outside area.

Causes of Fractures

Direct force: A bone can be fractured at the point where the force of a blow is applied.

Indirect force: The bone breaks away from the spot of application of force, e.g., fracture of the clavicle without a stretched hand while falling open and closed fractures. In an open fracture, one of the broken bone ends may pierce the skin surface or there may be a wound at the fracture site. An open fracture carries a high risk of infection. In closed fracture, the skin above the fracture in intact. However bones may be displaced causes damage to the internal organs.

May cause bleeding (internal) and suffer shock.

Types of Fracture

- **Simple (closed) fracture:** The broken ends of the bone do not cut open the skin and show on the outside.
- **Compound (open) fracture:** It extends through the skin and mucous membrane.
- **Complicated fracture:** In addition to the fracture, an important internal organ like brain or major blood vessels, spinal cord, lungs, liver spleen, etc. may also be injured.
- **Greenstick:** A fracture in which one side of a bone is broken and the other side is bent.
- **Transverse:** The fracture is straight across the bone.
- **Spiral:** It is a fracture twisting around the shift of the bone.
- **Communicated:** It is a fracture in which bone has splintered into several fragments.
- **Depressed:** It is a fracture in which fracture fragments are in-driven.
- **Compression:** In this, the fractured bone is compressed by another bone (seen in vertebral fracture).

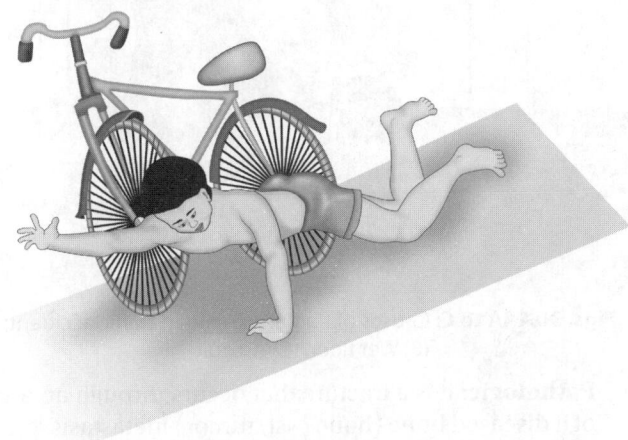

Fig. 30.13: Fall from bicycle.

- **Epiphyseal:** In this, separation of the epiphysis from the rest of the bone.

A fracture is diagnosed by:
- Pain at or near the site of fracture.
- Tenderness on palpation at the site of fracture.
- Swelling at the site of fracture.
- Deformity.
- Crepitus on palpation at the site of fracture.
- Abnormal mobility at the site of fracture.
- Loss of function.
- Shock in severe fracture.
- First aid measures for any fracture.
- Reassure the patient.
- Control hemorrhage.
- Cover any wound with sterile dressing.
- Immobilize the injured part immediately so that no movement is possible.
- Do not apply bandage over the area of fracture.
- Do not give the patient anything orally.

Transfer to a Hospital

Fracture of skull: In most cases, the patient becomes unconscious. There are other features like vomiting, slow pulse rate, paralysis of limbs, disturbance of eye movements, distortion of face, and speech disorders.

The signs of fracture of the base of skull include flow of blood; sometimes, cerebrospinal fluid comes from nose, ear or mouth, and bleeding around eyes is seen.

First aid measures: Place the patient in supine position. Elevate the head with a pillow under it. Turn the head to one side. If there is bleeding from an ear, turn the head to that side. If there is wound on the scalp, trim hair around it and cover the wound with sterile dressing.

Fracture of Face

- Cover the wound with clean cloth.
- Support the broken lower jaw with a bandage, looped under the jaw, and over the top of the head.
- Tilt the head forward over a bowl as blood and fluid may be falling to the back of the throat.
- Keep the air way clean.
- Put the patient in supine position with head turned to one side if he is unconscious.
- Transport the patient to a hospital.

Spinal Fracture

Paralysis is a complication of spinal fracture.
- Check whether the patient can move aides and joints.
- Check the loss of sensations in the lower limb.
- Make the patient lie still on a flat surface.
- Get a doctor immediately.

If a doctor is not available, place a pad between the patient's ankles and bandage the feet together with figure of eight bandage. Place the pad between knees and thighs. Tie the legs together, using broad bandage. Transfer the

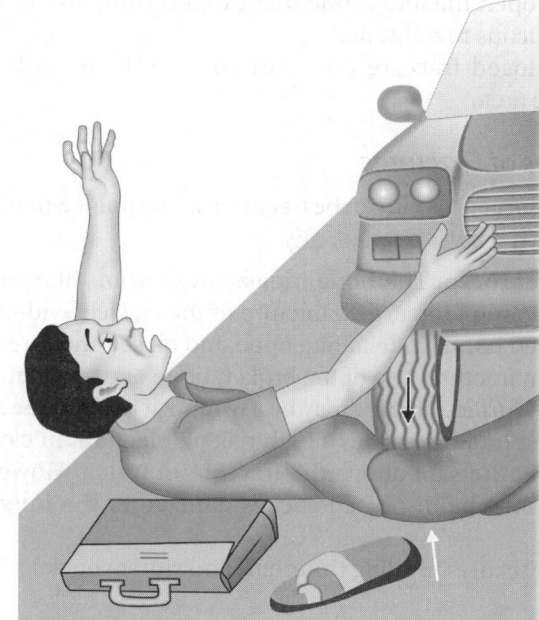
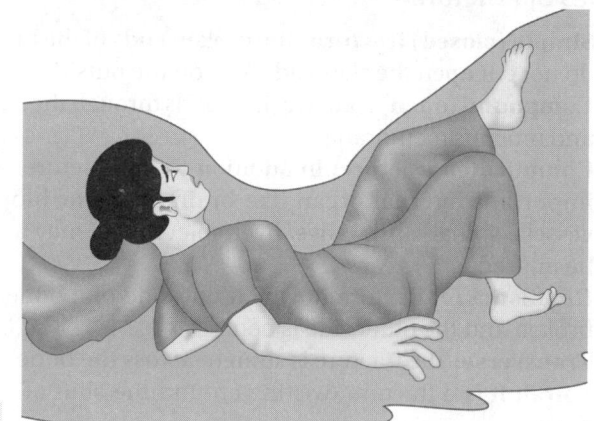
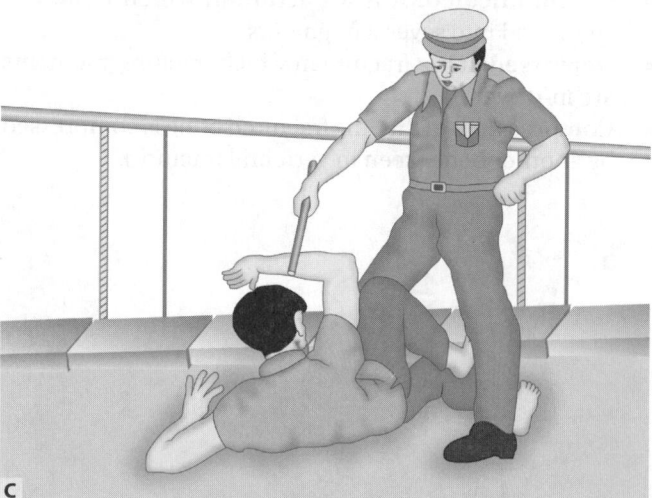

Figs. 30.14A to C: Causes of fracture: (A) Road traffic accident; (B) Wet floor; (C) Assault.

- **Pathologic:** It is a fracture that occurs through an area of a diseased bone (bone cyst, tumor) metastasis, etc.
- **Avulsion:** In this, a fragment of bone is pulled off by ligament or tendon and its attachments.

patient to a hospital. While moving the patient, take the help of four persons.

Lift and move the patient as one piece in a stretcher.

Fracture of Humerus

Place a pad of rolled handkerchief, towel or small clothes in the armpit. Lightly tie the arm to the chest. Bend the elbow and place the hand on the opposite shoulder and apply a collar and cuff sling. Fracture of ribs: If the fracture is not complicated, apply two broad bandages round the chest.

- The center of the first bandage should be below the area of pain and the center of the second above it.
- Do not tie knots too tight. Keep knots on the using side.
- Support the arm, in a large arm sling, on the affected side.
- Shift the patient to hospital.

Colle's Fracture

It is the fractures of the lower end of the radius. It results from a fall on the outstretched hand.

First Aid

- Do not remove casualty's shirt.
- Do not apply a collar and cuff sling.
- Bend his elbow and lay the injured limb against his chest, the fingers just touching the opposite shoulder. Apply adequate padding between the limb and the chest. Secure the limb firmly to the chest by two broad bandages.
- The first with its upper border, level with the top of the shoulder.
- The second with its lower border, level with the tip of the elbow. Tie both bandages at the opposite side of the body.

Feel pulse on the injured side to ensure that there is no interference with the circulation of the limb.

Transport to hospital as a sitting or walking case.

Fracture of Pelvis

This is always the result of direct forces, e.g. a heavy fall. When pelvis is fractured the pelvic organs, especially, the bladder and urinary passages may be injured.

Signs and Symptoms

- Pain in the region of hips and loins increased by moving and coughing.
- Inability to stand.
- Internal hemorrhage may occur, which may be severe.
- There may be desire to pass urine frequently though with difficulty or inability to do so. If passed, the urine may be of dark color from blood.

Treatment

Lay the patient in the position which gives the greatest comfort. This should be preferably on his back, with knees straight. Bind the pelvis with a towel at the level of the iliac bones. Place a wooden board on the canvas of the stretcher to provide a rigid, strong, unbending surface. Keep pads between knees and ankles and tie broad bandages around both the legs. Transport the patient in this position on a stretcher to hospital.

Fracture of Femur

Signs and Symptoms

- Leg appears short.
- Pain and swelling over the site of fracture.
- The foot on that side lies flat and turned to the outer side.
- Shock due to internal hemorrhage.

First Aid

- If shock is present, treat for shock.
- Make two splints, an inner one from the groin to the heel, and an outer one from the armpit to the head. Apply seven broad bandages at the following places.
    - Chest, below armpit.
    - At the level of hip joints.
    - Both ankles and feet.
    - Both thighs above fracture if the shaft is broken.
    - Below the fracture including both thighs.
    - Both legs.
    - Both knees.

Fracture of Patella

Signs and Symptoms

- Swelling, pain and, sometimes, bleeding.
- Muscles above the knee, which move the knee, become helpless.

First Aid

- Place the causality in a Fowler's position.
- The injured leg should be raised to a comfortable position.
- Tie the injured limb to the other limb from thigh to below knee, after padding knees.
- Apply a broad bandage around the upper part of thigh, and a narrow figure of eight bandage around ankle and foot.
- Tie the bandage over the broken piece of the knee cap.
- Elevate the injured limb, on a blanket, and, then, transport the patient to hospital.

Fracture of Tibia and Fibula

Signs and symptoms: Pain, swelling, deformity, if both bones are broken. If only fibula is broken, only minimal deformity is observed.

First aid: The broken limb should be tied to the sound limb, after proper padding. Apply bandage at the upper part of the thigh, on the knee, above the fracture and below the fracture. Transport the patient to hospital in a stretcher.

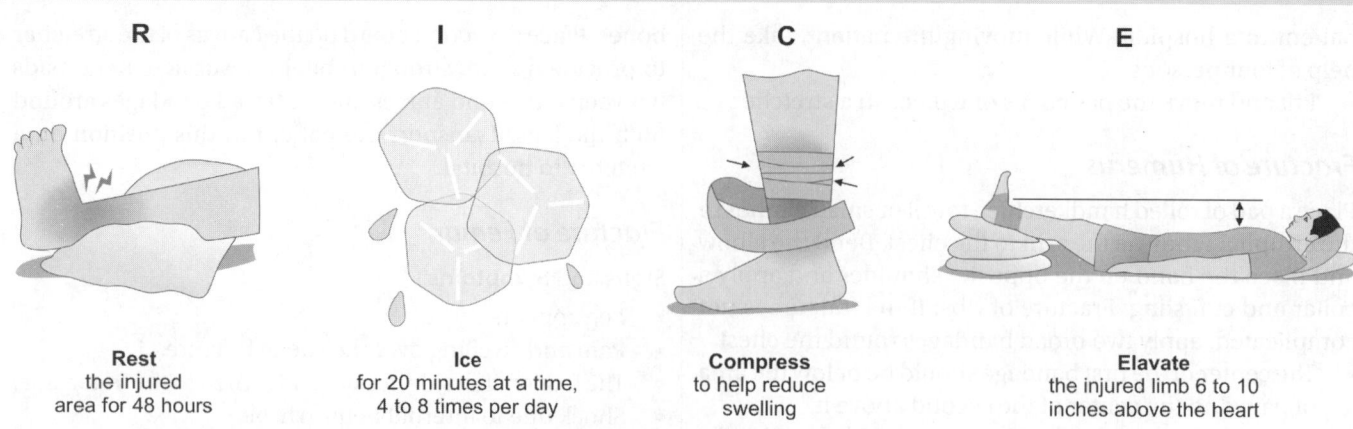

Fig. 30.15: RICE method of fracture management.

Fracture of Ankle

Signs and symptoms: Pain, swelling and sharp restriction of movements in the ankle joint and inability to stand. Immobilize the ankle using an L-shaped splint and transport to hospital.

Sprains and Dislocations of Joints

Sprains

A sprain is the tearing of ligaments of a joint or tissues around the joint.

Causes

Sudden twist Wrench or slip.

Signs and Symptoms

Bruising at the site, pain and swelling; severe pain on movement.

First Aid

- Place the limb in a comfortable position.
- Do not move the limb unnecessarily.
- Apply a firm bandage to the joint.
- Keep the bandage wet with cold water.

Dislocation

In dislocation, there is tearing of tissues around the joints and dislocation of bones.

Signs and Symptoms

- Severe pain around the joint.
- Inability to move the joint.
- Swelling, deformity.

First Aid

Support the joint. In case dislocation occurs in arm, put it in a sling and arrange a stretcher. In the case of leg, after immobilizing the limb, take the causality to hospital immediately.

Crush Injuries

These injuries commonly occur in earthquakes, bomb incidents, mining accidents and demolition work. Prolonged crushing of a mass of muscles, e.g. in the thigh, leads to shock because of the blood loss into the tissues after the casualty has been freed. Toxic substances released by the damaged muscles are:

Introduced into the casualty's circulation and may lead to kidney failure. This sequence is known as 'the Crush Syndrome'.

Because of the danger of kidney failure in all cases where a casualty has been trapped for longer than one hour, call the emergency services immediately and do not attempt to release him (or) her.

Sign and Symptoms

- Crushed limb may be tingling (or) numb.
- Swollen and hard tissue around injured part because serum has poured into the area.
- Bruising and formation of blisters at the site of injury.
- Crushed (or) trapped limb will be cool, pale and pulseless if arteries are compressed.
- Symptoms and signs of fracture.
- Symptoms and signs of shock.

Aim: Prevent damage to the kidneys, arrange urgent medical assistance if the casualty has been trapped for more than one hour.

Treatment

If trapped for less than one hour:
- Release the casualty as quickly as possible.
- Elevate the limb if the injuries allow you to do so.
- Control any bleeding and treat any wounds.
- Immobilize any fractures if present (refer topic on Fractures).

- Position as for treatment of shock (refer topic on Shock) and remove to hospital if necessary.

RICE TREATMENT FOR ACUTE MUSCULOSKELETAL INJURY

The RICE treatment is recommended by health professionals for the early treatment of bone injury or acute soft tissue injuries such as a sprain or strain. It can be helpful for sports injuries, closed fractures, and degenerative joint problems.

The acronym RICE stands for:
- Rest
- Ice
- Compression
- Elevation.

It should be started as soon as pain and swelling occur and used until there is healing of minor injuries or until another treatment has been initiated for more complex problems. Here are the basics of RICE.

Rest

Rest is needed for the healing of injured tissue. Without rest, movement and weight bearing can continue to aggravate an injury and cause increased inflammation and swelling. You should initially reduce using or stop using the injured area for 48 hours. If you have a leg injury, you may need to stay off of it completely and not bear any weight on it. You may need to use assistive devices or mobility aids to keep off of the injured joint or limb.

Ice

Ice is useful for reducing pain and inflammation associated with an acute injury. Icing is believed to be most effective if done the first couple of days after the injury has occurred. You can apply ice for 20 minutes at a time and as frequently as every hour. If you prefer, apply it four to eight times a day.

You can use a cold gel packs or a plastic bag filled with ice, but do not apply a bag of ice directly to the skin.[4] Instead, wrap the bag of ice in a towel or make sure there is some layer of material between the ice and your skin. Often, gel packs or cold packs sold for this purpose have a cover provided.

Compression

Compression of an injured or painful ankle, knee, or wrist helps to reduce the swelling. Elastic bandages, such as all cotton elastic (ACE) wraps, are most commonly used. Special boots, air casts, and splints can serve a dual purpose of compression and support. Your doctor should make a recommendation and discuss your options. Be sure not to apply excessive compression which would act as a tourniquet and interfere with your blood circulation. If you feel throbbing, the bandage is probably wrapped too tight; take it off and put it back on a little looser.

Elevation

Elevate the injured part of the body above heart level. This provides a downward path for draining fluid back to the heart, which may reduce swelling and pain. Try to elevate the entire limb 6 to 10 inches above the heart so there is a complete downhill path. Lie down and use a pillow to help elevate the injured limb.

DISLOCATION

A dislocation is a displacement of the bones which form a joint. Joints most commonly dislocated are the shoulder (in adults), elbow (in children), lower jaw, thumb and fingers. There will be severe pain in the joint, which feels useless and fixed. There will be some deformity (difference in shape when compared with the other limb) and swelling occurs later.

Signs and Symptoms

- Severe pain at or near the joint.
- Loss of normal joint movements.
- Deformity when compared with the other joint.
- Swelling caused by the collection of blood.

Treatment

- Do not try to put the bone back in place.
- Support the limb in the position most comfortable for the patient.
- Immobilize the part as in treating a fracture.
- Take the patient to a doctor quickly.

Shoulder Dislocation

In a healthcare setting, medications are used to relax the patient, but sometimes on an athletic field or in the wilderness that may not be possible. If the muscles around the shoulder are tense, reducing the joint becomes a near-impossible task. The most important step to reducing a dislocated shoulder is helping to get an individual with this injury to relax.

Reducing a shoulder is not accomplished well if there is anxiety, commotion, and chaos. Creating a quiet setting, where a patient with a dislocated shoulder can relax, is by far the most effective way to begin the job of repositioning the joint:

- Have the patient lie down. The patient should lie down in a comfortable position. Allowing the muscles around the shoulder joint to relax is the key to reducing the joint. If anesthesia is unavailable, the patient must be kept as comfortable as possible to allow the muscles to relax.
- Take some deep breaths and relax. Again, the key is to relax. Take a few minutes to allow the injured person to rest. Take a few deep breaths and relax as best possible.

1. Lie down, allowing the muscles around your shoulder to relax

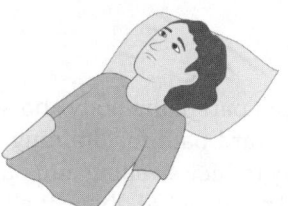

2. Slowly reach the dislocated arm out to the side and over your head

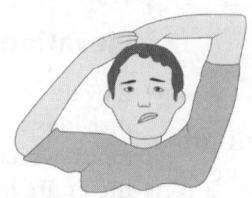

3. Slowly rotate your hand behind your head, as if scratching the back of your neck

4. Reach for your opposite shoulder

5. As you reach, your shoulder should pop back into place

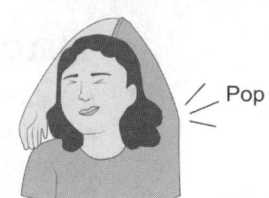

6. Seek medical attention

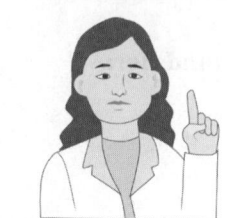

Fig. 30.16: Cervical fracture management.

Patients who are crying, writhing, or upset need to relax before proceeding with treatment.

- Reach the dislocated arm out to the side. Start by reaching the injured arm out to the side and over your head. The elbow should move away from your side. The arm can be supported by a helper, although this is not necessary. This should be a slow movement, and pain should be a sign to slow down. This does not need to be painful.
- Rotate your hand behind your head. Once the arm is over the level of your shoulder, rotate the hand behind your head. The movement should be similar to scratching the back of your neck. Make sure this is done slowly and try to keep relaxed.
- Reach for your opposite shoulder. Once your hand is behind your head, reach for your opposite shoulder. As you are reaching, the shoulder will, hopefully, pop back into place. You should feel a sudden relief of your pain although it is normal to have continued discomfort in the injured shoulder. Shoulder movements should be much less painful once it is in the proper position.
- Seek help when possible. Potentially serious problems are associated with shoulder dislocations and treatment to reposition the shoulder. That is why these should be treated by trained personnel if possible. If a shoulder dislocation must be reduced "in the field," seek medical attention as soon as possible.

Tips for Fixing a Shoulder Dislocation

- The technique should be done slowly. It is important to move slowly and relax, avoiding the temptation to tense your muscles.
- A helper can assist you, but it is not necessary. The helper should gently support your arm through these movements.
- If you forget the movements, think of a baseball pitcher winding up to throw a ball—that's a general movement.
- Always seek medical attention first, if possible. These maneuvers should only be done if medical assistance is unavailable.

Elbow Dislocation

An elbow dislocation occurs when the upper arm and forearm get separated from their normal position. The bone of the upper arm (humerus) normally touching the bones of the forearm (the radius and ulna). When an elbow dislocation occurs, these bones are separated from their normal alignment. Elbow dislocations are the second most common joint dislocation, following shoulder dislocation:

There are two basic types of elbow dislocations:

- **Simple elbow dislocation:** A simple elbow dislocation means there is no fracture of the bones around the elbow joint. The prognosis of simple elbow dislocation is better, as often surgery is not required for treatment.
- **Complex elbow dislocation:** A complex elbow dislocation means that there is a fracture, usually of the forearm, that has occurred along with the elbow dislocation. In a complex elbow dislocation, surgery is often needed to fix the broken bone in order to maintain the elbow joint in a normal position.

Assessment

If someone has injured their elbow, a dislocated elbow joint should be considered as a possible cause of elbow pain. Symptoms of a dislocated elbow include pain, swelling, and inability to bend the elbow.[3] In some elbow dislocations, nerve or blood vessel damage can occur. All elbow dislocations require prompt medical attention, but those with nerve or vascular (blood vessel) injury require special attention.

Prior to putting the elbow back into position (called "reducing" the elbow), an X-ray should be done to view the position of the elbow dislocation and look for any associated fractures.

Treatment

An elbow dislocation is treated by repositioning the bones. Most often the reduction is performed under anesthesia; however, if the patient is able to relax, the reduction may be performed without anesthesia. Often the elbow joint will simply, "pop" back into position, but there can be difficulty achieving normal alignment in more complex injuries. After reducing the elbow, another x-ray must be done to ensure the appropriate alignment of the joint.

If a simple elbow dislocation has occurred, after the joint is reduced, the examiner should determine the stability of the elbow joint. If the elbow will not stay in position, and continually pops back out, surgery will likely be necessary. In most cases, the elbow can be immobilized in a position where the joint is stable. The position of most stability is with the elbow bent, and the hand turned palm down.

Immobilization is limited, as prolonged immobilization can cause significant stiffness of the joint. Patients are started with early elbow motion, usually within days or a week after the injury. Mobility is started in a range where the elbow was stable and gradually increased. Patients with simple elbow dislocations generally achieve a return to work within 1 to 3 weeks of the injury.

INJURIES TO THE JOINT AND MUSCLES

First Aid in Injuries to Joints and Muscles

A strain is the over-stretching of a muscle due to a sudden effort or twisting of the part. There is sudden sharp pain in the muscle, and movement causes more pain. There may be swelling.

Treatment: Rest and support in the most comfortable position using slings, bandages or adhesive plaster. A Sprain is a joint injury with tearing of ligaments caused by sudden twisting of the joint. The ankle is the most common joint to be sprained, the external ligament being torn due to falling with the foot turned inwards. There will be severe pain, and the joint some becomes very swollen.

The tear may be a complete tear or tear of part of the ligament.

Signs and Symptoms

- Severe pain at the time of injury. The pain becomes less lately, but as the bruise increases the pain also increases and is maximum after about four hours.
- Swelling of the joint.
- Discoloration around the joint (bruising) due to the collection of blood.
- Loss of movement at the joint. Unnatural movement, creaking and deformity are absent; this excludes a fracture.

Treatment

Apply a firm bandage before swelling occurs, if possible. Get the patient or a helper to hold the foot up at right angles to the leg. Place a pad of cotton wool or cloth on the outer side, then start the bandage first round the lower part of the leg just above the ankle. Then under the heel, and up on the outer side to give support, and again covering the first turn. Repeat these turn alternately, gradually working towards the point of the heel. Wet the bandage with cold water and keep it wet. This will tighten the bandage and help prevent swelling. Encourage the patient to walk on the ankle or at least to keep moving the joint in all those directions which do not cause acute pain. The patient should be taken to a doctor, if you are doubtful about whether it is a sprain or a fracture, treat it as a fracture.

TRANSPORTING CASUALITIES

Transport of Injured Persons

An injured person may be removed to shelter by the following methods:
- Support by a single helper.
- Hand seats.
- Stretcher.
- Wheeled transport.

The method or methods adopted will depend upon the following factors:
- The nature of the injury.
- The severity of the injury.
- The number of helpers available.
- The distance to shelter.
- The nature of the route to be traversed.

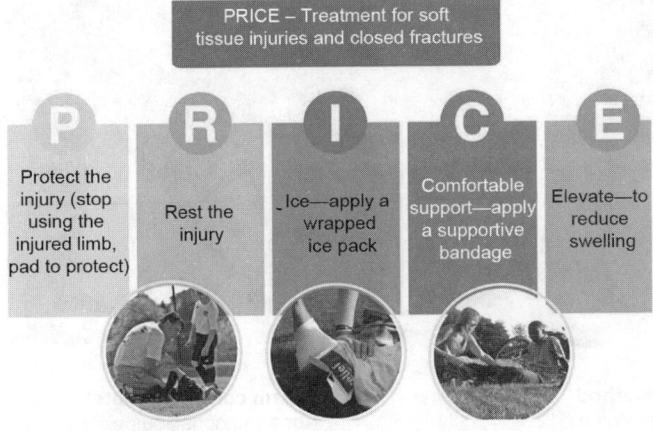

Fig. 30.17: PRICE method of soft tissue management.

Support by a Single Helper

- Cradle method.
- Human crutch.
- Pick a back.
- Fireman's Lift and carry.

Support by Two Helper

- Four handed seat: Grip for four handed seat.
- Two hand seat: Bearer rise together step off right hand-Bearer right foot.
- Bearer right foot left hand Bearer left foot.

Stretcher Exercise

- Preparing and blanketing stretcher.
- Blanketing stretcher with one blanket.
- Blanketing stretcher with two blankets.
- Blanket lift.

Loading Stretcher

Place the blanket or rug on the ground in line with the casualty and roll it lengthwise for half its width. No. 2, 3, 4 will turn the casualty carefully on the uninjured side. No. 1 will place the rolled portion of the blanket or rug close to the casualty's back and all the bearers will gently roll the casualty over until he is lying on his opposite side on the blanket or rug.

When the casualty is not lying on a blanket or rug and none is available.

- No. 4, 3, and 2 will place themselves on the left of the casualty.
- No. 4 facing the shoulder.
- No. 3 facing the hips.
- No. 2 facing the knees.
- No. 1 will place himself on the right of the casualty facing no. 3. All will go down on their left knees and place their forearms beneath the casualty. Paying particular attention to the site of the injury. The fore-and-aft Method.

Loading Stretcher when No Blanket is Available

No. 1 joins his left hand with the left hand No. 4. Right hand with the right hand of No. 3, No. 4 supports the head and shoulders, No. 2 the lower limbs. When No. 1 gives the order 'lift' the casualty must be filled gently and slowly and placed on the knees.

Adjusting: No. 4, 3, and 2. No. 1 will disengage, take hold of the stretcher (left hand across, resting the near pole on his left hip) and place the stretcher under the casualty so that when he is lowered on to it. When no. 1 gives the order 'Lower' the casualty will be raised slightly from the knees of Nos. 4, 3, and 2 lowered gently and carefully on to the stretcher and covered with coats. Bearers then rise and turn to face the foot of the stretcher. If it is necessary to lift the casualty from the right side, bearers will go down on their right knees.

Standing to stretcher: Command 'stand to stretcher' no. 1, will take up a position level with the handles at the foot of the stretcher. No. 2 will step forward opposite No. 1 and No. 3 will double round the head of the stretcher opposite No. 4. When standing to stretcher the positions No. 1 and

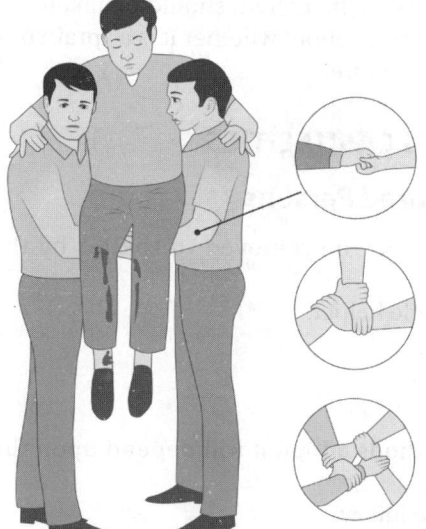
Handed seat or swing carry
for back or leg injury victim

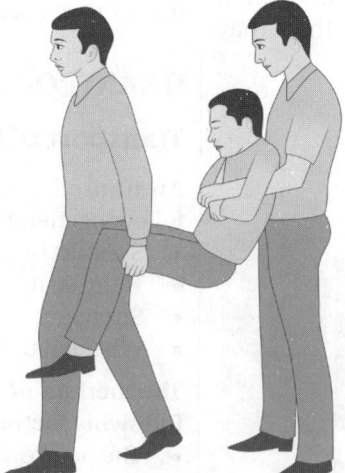
The fore-and-aft method
for an unconscious victim

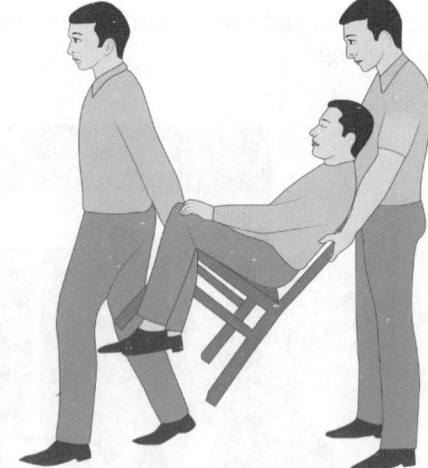
Arm carry (alternate)
for an unconscious victim

Fig. 30.18: Two rescuer handling techniques.

3 bearers will be on the right and those of Number 2 and 4 on the left of the stretcher.

Carrying a Loaded Stretcher

- Hand carriage by four bearers.
- Hand carriage by two bearers.

After the appropriate first aid treatment has been given the following principles of transport must be kept in mind:
- The position assumed by the casualty or in which he has been placed, must not be disturbed unnecessarily.
- Throughout the transport a careful watch must be kept on:
  - The general condition of the casualty.
  - Any dressings, etc. that may have been applied.
  - Any recurrence of hemorrhage.
- The transport must be safe, steady and speedy.

Methods of Carrying

If only one Bearer is Available

Cradle: (to be used only in the case of light casualties or children) lift the casualty by passing one of your arms well beneath his two knees, and the other round his back.

Human Crutch

Standing at his injured side, except where there is injury to an upper limb, assist the casualty by putting your arm round his waist, rasping the clothing at his hip and placing his arm round your neck, holding his hand with your free hand. If his upper limbs are injured and his other hand is free, the casualty may gain additional help from a staff or walking-stick.

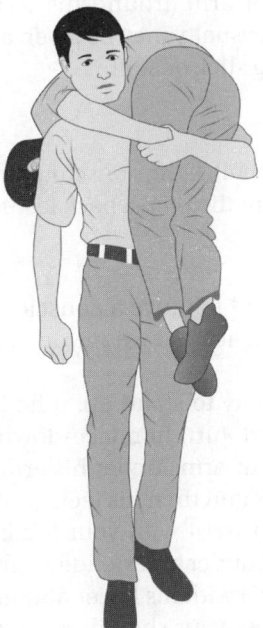

Fig. 30.19: Pick-a-back method of handling the casualty.

Pick-a-back

If the casualty is conscious and able to hold on, he may be carried in the ordinary 'Pick-a-back' fashion.

Fireman's Lift and Carry

(To be used only when the casualty is not too heavy for the bearer). Help the casualty to rise to the upright position. Grasp his right wrist with your left hand. Bend down with your head under his extended right arm so that your right shoulder is level with the lower part of his abdomen and place your right arm between or round his legs. Taking his weight on your right shoulder rise to the erect position. Pull the casualty across both shoulders and transfer his right wrist to your right hand, so leaving your left hand free.

If two or More Bearers are Available

Hand Seats

Four handed seat: This seat is used when the casualty can assist the bearer by using one or both arms.
- Two bearers face each other behind the casualty and grasp their left wrists with their right hands and each other's right wrists with their left hands and stoop down.
- The casualty is instructed to place one arm round the neck of each bearer so that he may raise himself to sit on their hands and steady himself during transport.
- The bearers rise together and stop off, the bearer on the right hand side of the casualty with the right foot, and the left hand bearer with the left foot.

The two handed seat: This seat is mostly used to carry a casualty who is unable to assist the bearers by using his arms.
- Two bearers face each other and stoop (not kneel) one on each side of the casualty. Each bearer passes his forearm nearest to the casualty's head his back just below the shoulders, and, if possible, takes hold of his clothing. They slightly raise the casualty's back and then pass their other forearms under the middle of his thigh and clasp their hands; the bearer on the left of the casualty with his palm upwards and holding a folded handkerchief to prevent hurting by the finger nails; the bearer on the right of the casualty with his palm downwards, as shown in the figure.
- The bearers rise together and step off, the right hand bearer with the right foot and the left hand bearer with the left foot. In all cases of carrying by hand seats the bearers walk with the cross over step and not by side paces.

The Fore-and-aft Method

This method of carrying should be used only when space does not permit of a hand seat. One bearer stands between the casualty's legs, facing the left, bends down and grasps the casualty under his knees. The other bearer takes a position behind the casualty and after raising his trunk passes his hands under the casualty's armpits and grasps his own wrists. The casualty is then lifted. The bearer walks in step.

Stick method: Two bearers can move a patient by means of a stick also. The stick is held horizontally by the two bearers. The patient sits on the stick between the two bearers his arms around the shoulders of the bearers.

Stretchers

Stretchers are of two patterns viz., ordinary and 'telescopic handled'. In general principle they are alike, the component parts being designated the poles, handles, jointed traverses, runners, bed, pillowsack and slings. The 'Head' and 'Foot' of a stretcher correspond to the head and feet of the casualty.

At the head of the stretcher there may be a canvas overlay (the pillow-sack) which can be filled with straw, hay, clothing, etc. to form a pillow. The pillow-sack opens at the head, and its corners can therefore be adjusted without due disturbance of the casualty. The traverses are provided with joints for opening (or) closing the stretcher. The telescopic handled pattern is similar but its length can be reduced to 6 feet by sliding the handles underneath the poles. This is of a great value when working in confined spaces, or when a casualty has to be taken up or down a narrow staircase with sharp turns.

When closed, the pole of the stretcher lie close together, the traverse bars being bent inwards, the canvas bed neatly folded on the top of the poles and held in position by the slings, which are laid along the canvas and secured by a strap which is placed transversely at the end of each sling and passed through the large loop of the other, and round poles and bed.

Carrying sheets which are made of canvas and have eyelet holes at intervals, to which rope handles are attached, are also useful in similar circumstances.

LIFTING CASUALTIES

This is a skill and, if it is done correctly, even a very heavy casualty can be lifted without undue strain. However, it is important that you should not attempt to lift too heavy a weight and that you always obtain assistance from any available bystanders in order to avoid injury to yourself. There are two principles of lifting first you should always use the most powerful muscles those of the thigh, hip and shoulder; second, the weight should be kept as close to your body as possible.

It is very important that the correct posture for lifting is adopted; feet should be placed comfortably apart to ensure a stable, balanced posture and a firm stance. Keep your back straight head erect and hold the casualty close to your body using your shoulders to support the weight. Use your whole hand to strengthen the grasp. If the casualty begins to slip, do not injure your own by trying to prevent him or her falling. Let the casualty slide slowly and gently to the ground without causing more damage to the injured area.

Lifting Technique

When lifting anything it is important to keep your back straight and bend at the knees if necessary.

Carries for one First Aider

If help is available, do not attempt to move a seriously ill or injured casualty on your own.

Cradle Method

To carry light weight casualties or children pass one arm under the casualty's thighs and the other around the trunk above the waist and lift.

Drag Method

This method involves pulling the casualty along the ground without lifting. It should only be used where a casualty is unable to stand and must be moved quickly from a source of danger.

- Fold the casualty's arms across her chest and crouch behind her head place your hands under her shoulders, grasp her armpits and cradle her head on your forearms.
- **Pull her along the ground:** If the casualty is wearing a jacket or coat, unbutton it and pull it back up under her head. Pull her along the ground in the same way with her head supported on the coat.

Human Crutch

This is used to support a conscious casualty who is able to walk with assistance. It should not be used if an upper limb is injured.

- Stand at the casualty's injured side, if any. Place his nearest arm around your neck and hold his hand with your free hand.
- Put your other arm around his waist and grasp his clothing. The casualty may be given additional support from a walking stick or staff.

Pick-a-Back

If the casualty is small, light, conscious and able to hold on to you, carry him in the pick-a back fashion.

Fireman's Lift

This method is used to move a conscious or unconscious child or a light weight adult when you need to keep a hand free.

- Help the casualty to stand up. If he is unconscious or unable to stand, turn him face-down and stand at his head. Place your arms under his armpit and raise him on to his knees and then his feet.
- Grasp his right wrist with your left hand. Bend down with your head under his extended right arm so that your shoulder is level with his lower abdomen; allow him to fall gently across your shoulders. Place your right arm between or around his legs.

- Taking the weight on your right shoulder stand up and gently pull him across both shoulders. Transfer his right wrist to your right hand, leaving your left hand free.

Carries for Two First Aiders

There is a variety of lifts suitable for transporting a casualty with two first aiders.

Four Handed Seat

This method is used to carry a conscious casualty who can assist the bearers by using one or both arms to hold on.
- **Stand facing each other behind the casualty.** Make a seat by grasping your own left wrists with your right hands and your partner's right wrist with the free hand; then squat down beside the casualty.
- **Instruct the casualty to place an arm around** each of you at the neck, to sit back on to your hands and to steady him during transport.
- **Rise together, step off with your outside** feet and walk with cross-over steps and not by side paces, i.e. the bearers rise together and step off the right hand bearer with the right foot and left hand bearer with left foot.

Two Handed Seat

This method is used to carry a casualty who is unable to assist the bearers.
- Squat facing each other on either side of the casualty. Pass your arms nearest the casualty's body under and around her back just below her shoulders and, if possible grasp each other's forearms or the casualty's clothing at the waist.
- Raise the casualty's legs slightly, pass your other arms under the middle of her thighs and grasp each other's wrists.
- Rise together, step off with your outside feet and walk with cross-over steps.

Fore-and-aft Carry

This method can be used to place the casualty on a chair or a carrying chair.
- Supporting the casualty on both sides, both first aiders should help the casualty to it up and fold her arms across her chest.
- One person should move around behind her and place the arms through and under her armpits and grasp her forearms.
- The other bearer should remain at her side and place one arm around her back and the other under her thighs.
- Working together, lifts the casualty on to the chair or stretcher.

Chair Method

When a conscious casualty with no serious injuries is to be moved up or downstairs or along passage ways, the casualty can be seated on an ordinary chair and carried by two people. However, the passages must be cleared of any obstructions or dangers such as loose matting before you start.
- Test the chair to ensure that it is strong enough to support the casualty, then sit her down and secure her in position with broad bandages. Stand facing each other, one in front of the chair and one behind.
- The person behind the chair should support the back of the chair and the casualty; the other should hold the chair by the front legs. Slowly tilt the chair backwards to seat the casualty securely, and then lift together.
- With the casualty facing forwards, move slowly along the passage or stairs.

If space permits, you can both stand facing the side of the chair each supporting the back and the top of a front leg.

Lifting a Casualty in a Wheelchair

Wheelchair bound casualties can be transported where they sit by adapting the chair method.
- Locate the brakes (ask the casualty) and apply securely.
- Make the casualty to sit well back in the chair.
- Examine the wheelchair to find out which parts are fixed. Arm rests and side supports are often removable and will detach if you use them to lift the chair. Supporting the chair from either side, lift by holding the fixed parts, never by the wheels.
- Carry the chair as described above.

Stretchers

These are used to carry a seriously ill or injured casualty to an ambulance or similar sheltered to minimize the risk of further injury. The stretchers in general use include:
- The standard stretcher
- The scoop stretcher
- The trolley bed
- The utila folding stretcher
- The Pole and canvas stretcher
- The carrying sheet
- The carrying chair
- The Neil Robertson stretcher
- The paraguard stretcher.

Most stretchers can be used to transport casualties with any injury and should be rigid enough to carry casualties with a suspected spine fracture without additional boards. All equipment must be tested before it is used.

Testing a Stretcher

To ensure that a stretcher is capable of taking the weight of a casualty, one person should lie on the stretcher and each end of the stretcher should be lifted in turn. Then both ends should be lifted at the same time.

The Standard Stretcher

The 'standard' or Furley stretcher consists of poles, handles, traverses, runners and a canvas bed. The traverses are joined so that the stretcher can be opened and closed. When closed, the poles, i.e. close together with the canvas bed folded on top. This is then kept in position by two transverse straps. If slings are carried they are laid along the canvas held by the straps.

Opening the Stretcher

Place the stretcher on its side with its runners towards you and the studs or buckles securing the straps upper most. Unfasten any straps. Push the traverses fully pen with your foot. Whilst placing the stretcher upright on either end.

Closing the Stretcher

- Turn the stretcher on its side with it runners towards you and the studs or buckles which secure the straps upper most. Push the joints of the traverses inwards with your heel to release them.
- Push the poles together, pulling the canvas out from between them. Fold the canvas neatly on to the poles and secure with the straps.

Scoop Stretcher

The scoop, or orthopedic stretcher is an adjustable stretcher used to lift casualties on to an ambulance trolley bed without altering the position in which they were found. It is not used to carry a casualty any distance. The length can be adjusted to suit any size of casualty and because he or she does not have to be moved, it is particularly useful for picking up a casualty with a suspected spinal fracture or internal injuries. Remove hard objects from the casualty's pocket.

- Bring the stretcher to the casualty's side and adjust the length.
- Uncouple both ends of the stretcher and gently slip each half of the stretcher under the casualty; rejoin the head sections.
- Place the head pad in position.
- While one first aider stays at the head, the other should rejoin the foot section. Secure the head pad to the stretcher.
- Working from either side of the stretcher, lift it and the casualty and place on the trolley bed. Uncouple the stretcher and remove it.

Trolley Bed

This fully adjustable stretcher bed on wheels is made of light metal and is carried in many ambulances.

Trolley beds should always be kept prepared for immediate use. A canvas sheet from a pole and canvas stretcher is laid on the stretcher bed and two blankets are placed on top.

UNCONSCIOUSNESS

Unconsciousness is a term used widely to denote a state of unresponsiveness of an individual to external stimuli. It can be a transient feature or it can be with no observable response to even deep stimuli which is called coma.

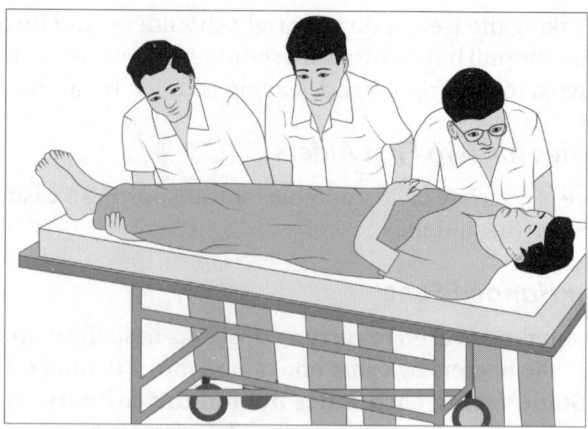

Fig. 30.20: Unconscious patient.

Unconsciousness can be defined as a state in which the cerebral functions are decreased; the individual is unresponsive to sensory stimuli.

Unconsciousness is a lack of awareness of one's environment and the inability to respond to external stimuli. To produce unconsciousness, a disorder must:

- Disrupts the ascending reticular activating system, which extends the length of the brainstem and up into the thalamus.
- Significantly disrupt the function of both cerebral hemispheres.
- Metabolically depress overall brain function. As in a drug over dose.

Causes of Unconsciousness

- **Trauma**
  - To the brain
  - To any other organ which can cause hypovolemia
- **Vascular condition**
  - Cerebral thrombosis
  - Cerebral embolism

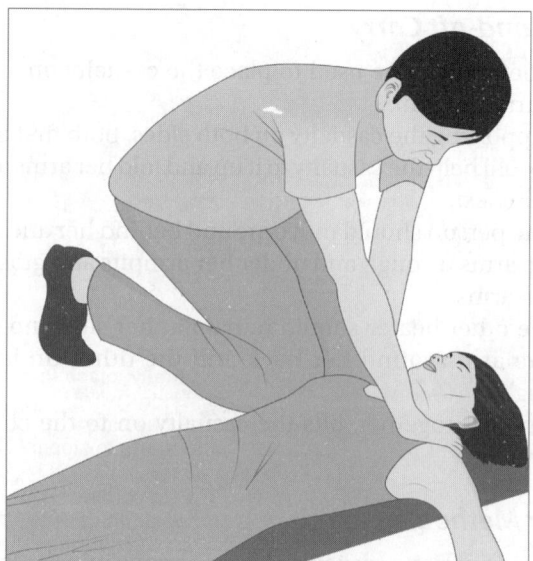

Fig. 30.21: Assessment of response.

- Ruptured aneurysm
- Intracranial hemorrhages
- **Space occupying lesions**
  - Tumor
  - Abscess
  - Subdural hematoma
  - Severe concussion of brain
  - Contusion of brain
  - Extradural hematoma
  - Epilepsy
- **Systemic conditions**
  - Uremia
  - Diabetes
  - Alcoholism
  - Overdosage of drugs
- Any organic condition in brain
- Psychogenic shock: Any unexpected incidents.

Types

Unconsciousness can be classified into:
- Brief, lasting for a few seconds or an hour
- Sustained, lasting for a few hours (coma).

Classification of Coma

- Supratentorial coma
- Infratentiorial coma
- Metabolic coma.

Clinical Manifestation

Clinical manifestations of brief unconsciousness are:
- Weakness.
- Unawareness of self, environment and time clinical manifestations of coma.

Early Symptoms of Supratentorial Coma

- Headache
- Localized sensor motor defect
- Aphasia
- Visual toss
- Seizures.

Later Symptoms

- Lesson expands.
- Pronounced unilateral.
- Changes in neurological status.

Infratentorial Coma, Manifestations

- Changes in CO_2 and O_2 levels.
- Changes in acid base balance.
- Irregular breathing depth and pattern.
- Abnormal eye movements.
- Loss of papillary reactivity to light.

Manifestations of Metabolic Coma

- Tremor.
- Asterisus (flapping tremors of hand).
- Myoclonus.
- Acid base imbalance.

Administer first aid: If you see a person who has become unconscious, take these steps:
- Check whether the person is breathing. If they're not breathing, have someone call 911 or your local emergency services immediately and prepare to begin CPR. If they're breathing, position the person on their back.
- Raise their legs at least 12 inches above the ground.

1. **Check for injuries**
   - If hurt, don't move them and get emergency help
   - If the are vomiting without waking up, get emergency help.

2. **Call 000 (112 on mobiles)**
   Immediately if someone needs help and ask for an ambulance.

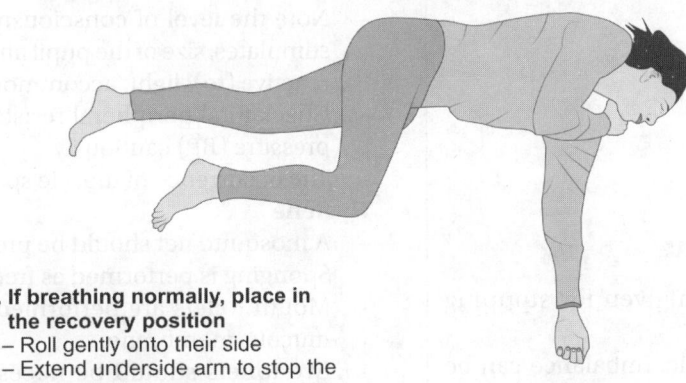

3. **If breathing normally, place in the recovery position**
   - Roll gently onto their side
   - Extend underside arm to stop the person rolling over
   - Bend top leg to support their position
   - Place rolled towel or peice of clothing behind to prevent them rolling onto their back
   - Tilt head back, place upper hand under chin

4. **Stay with them**
   or make sure someone else can to ensure they don't choke on their vomit

Fig. 30.22: Immediate first aid for unconscious patient.

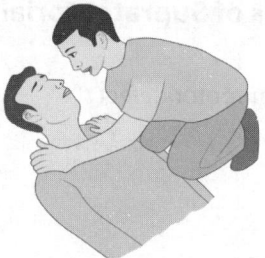
1. Shake and shout

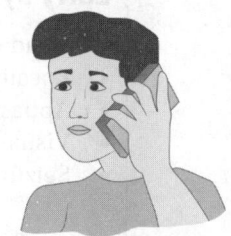
2. Call 911

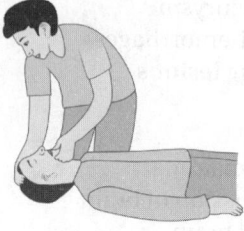
3. Check for breathing

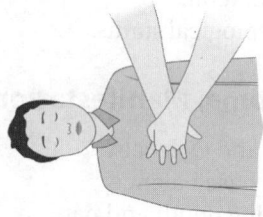
4. Place your hands at the center of their chest

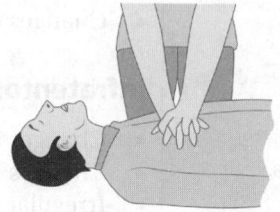
5. Push hard and fast— about twice per second

6. If you have had training, repeat cycles of 30 chest pushes and 2 rescue breaths

Fig. 30.23: Step-by-step CPR guide.

- Loosen any restrictive clothing or belts. If they don't regain consciousness within one minute, call 911 or your local emergency services.
- Check their airway to make sure there's no obstruction.
- Check again to see if they're breathing, coughing, or moving. These are signs of positive circulation. If these signs are absent, perform CPR until emergency personnel arrive.
- If there's major bleeding occurring, place direct pressure on the bleeding area or apply a tourniquet above the bleeding area until expert help arrives.

Diagnosis

- History collections
- Physical examinations
- CT scan
- MRI
- ECG
- Test for abnormal ocular reflex
- Invasive
- Blood test.

Pharmacological Management

- IV diazepam or lorazepam can given for stopping seizures
- Acid base unbalance and isotonic. Imbalance can be treated by giving solution (IV)
- Coma from drug overdose may be reversed by giving proper antidotes, e.g. opium overdose may be reversed by nalaxone.

Nursing Management

The points of nursing case include:
- Position of the patient
- Airway
- Observation and charting
- Hygiene
- Care of Pressure area and preventions of foot drop
- Nutrition
- Eliminations
- Relative.

Position: The patient is nursed in the prone, lateral or sim's position.

Airway: An adequate airway must be manufactured at all times. It may be necessary to hold the patient's jaw forward.
- **Observation and charting**
  - Note the level of consciousness, reaction to vocal stimulates, size of the pupil and pupils, equal, round, reactive (to), light, accommodation (PERRLA)
  - Check total peripheral resistance (TPR) and blood pressure (BP) cautiously
  - The occurrence of muscle spasm is recorded.
- **Hygiene**
  - A mosquito net should be provided.
  - Sponging is performed as frequently as possible.
  - Mouth toilets are performed to prevent drying of mucous membrane.
  - Eye toilets should be necessary to keep the bid margins.

Care of pressure and prevention of foot drops:
  - The patient should be nursed on a stipule matters.
  - Bed lines must be kept taut and dry.

- A bed cradle may be used to take the weight of the bed clothes.
- Patient's position should be changed every hour.
- The fleet should be kept light angle to the leg.
- Passive physiotherapy will help to keep the ankles and feet is good conditions.
- **Nutrition**
  - The diet must be containing adequate supply of all the nutrients.
  - It should be given as IV infusion or gastric tube feedings.
- **Eliminations**
  - The patient is observed for any signs of urinary retention and constipation.
  - If the patient is constipated, a glycerin suppository may be given.
  - Incontinence of urine may occur is which case a bedpan or divided matters may be used for female patient, for a male patient usual may be used.
  - Apply gentle pressure on bladder if three is any urinary retention.
  - Maintain intake output chart.
- **Maintain airway**
  - Patient is kept in lateral position.
  - Airway is inserted to prevent the tongue from falling.
  - Suctioning is done to clear the throat.
  - Endotracheal tube is inserted if needed.
  - O_2 is administered by mask or through endotracheal tube
  - Artificial ventilator is connected if indicated.
  - Tracheotomy is indicated in some conditions.
  - Adjust the ventilators and maintain synchrony or asynchrony on respirator.
- **Observation of vital signs**
  - Monitor vital signs frequently
  - Document arrhythmias
  - Do not make the patient sit if the blood pressure is low and pulse rate is high.
  - Elevate the extremities to prevent local edema.
  - Observe and monitor the neurological signs frequently and report if there is any detonation.
- **Maintain personal hygiene**
  - Mouth care to be given at least twice a day.
  - Eye care is given at least twice a day.
  - Eyes to be protected with pad or with eye ointment to prevent injury and infection.
  - Modified bed (water bed) is used to prevent pressure sores
  - Body bath is given daily with special care to pubic, axila and groin.
  - Skin care is given frequently by turning the position of patient every 2 hours and giving care to the bony prominent/dependant areas of the body.
  - Hair is to be combed and tied at least every day.
  - Finger nails and toe nails are cut at least weekly. Provide sufficient nutrition
  - Nutrition is taken care by giving tube feeding or IV fluids.
- **Maintain urinary and bowel movement**
  - Intake and output chart is maintained.
  - Watch for any urinurea, dysuria.
  - Watch for incontinence and use condom drainage/urinary catheter.
  - Condom/catheter to be changed frequently.
  - Clean the area of condom or catheter daily.
  - Irrigate the catheter if needed.
  - Urine routine investigation is done frequently to look for any infection.
  - Avoid constipation.
  - Give enough fluids.
  - Use suppositories if needed.
- **Prevention of contractures**
  - Passive exercises are given to prevent contractures.
  - Keep the body in proper alignment to prevent any disuse syndrome.
  Special nursing care to be carried out according to the diagnosis, drugs used and surgery if done. Nursing care should also aim at the early rehabilitation of the patient with minimum complication.
- **Care of pressure areas and the prevention of foot drop**
  - The patient should, if possible, be nursed on a ripple mattress.
  - The bed linen must be kept taut and dry.
  - A bed cradle may be used to take the weight of the bedclothes.
  - Pillows protected by plastic covers may be used to separate the bony prominences between the knees and ankles.
  - The patient's position should be changed every hour and pressure areas massaged every two hours. Any sign of reddening or injury to the skin must be reported and the treatment intensified.
  - Foot drop occurring during hospitalization can be prevented by careful nursing.
  The feet should be kept at right ankles to the legs. Foot drop is liable to occur if the bedclothes are tucked in, tightly, causing constant pressure over the toes and feet.
  - A foot board or pillow at the bottom of the bed may be used to prevent the pressure and weight of clothes on the feet.
  - Passive physiotherapy will help to keep the ankles and feet in good condition.

Padded splints may be used to maintain the correct position. If splints are used they must be removed for pressure area care, sponging and physiotherapy and then carefully replaced. The hands and wrists may also need splinting to prevent wrist drop.

RESPIRATORY EMERGENCIES AND BASIC CPR

Choking

- Chocking occurs when the airway is partially or totally obstructed by something which, in the act of swallowing,

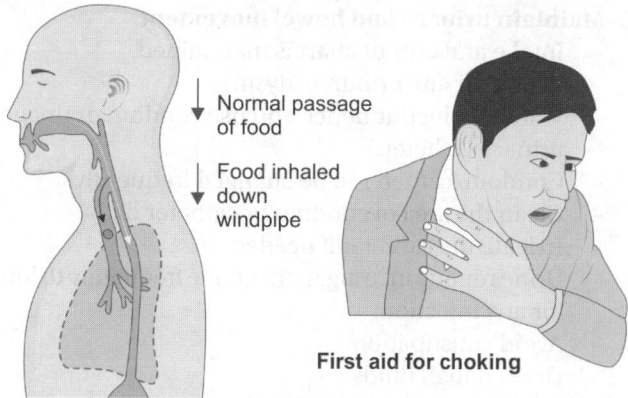

Fig. 30.24: Chocking.

goes into wind pipe rather than down the food passage. However, choking can also be caused by muscular spasm.

- Adults may choke on places of food which have been inadequately chewed and hurriedly swallowed; children are at risk because they like putting objects inside the mouths. It is imperative that any obstruction be removed as soon as possible.
- Encourage a conscious choking casualty to cough the obstruction out. If this does not work, attempt to dislodge it by bending the casualty over and back slapping. Only if this fails, try to force the remaining air out of the lungs by abdominal thrust.
- Both these techniques can be used by any first aider on any casualty (infant, child or adult) in any position (sitting, standing or lying down).
- Administer both back slaps and abdominal thrusts up to four times in a sequence but if the technique is successful the full series does not have to be completed.
- Always treat a casualty in the position found (unless he or she is unconscious). If standing or sitting, treat as opposite; if the casualty is lying down or if you are smaller than the casualty, treat as described for an unconscious casualty.
- If the casualty becomes unconscious, you will have to perform artificial ventilation in order to try to blow air pass the obstruction and into the lungs, in an unconscious casualty the throat may relax sufficiently to allow air pass the obstruction.

Symptoms and Signs

- General symptoms and signs of asphyxia
- Casualty will be unable to speak or breathe and may be gripping the throat.
  The most remarkable features is that he or she will be completely silent.
- Congestion of the face and neck with the veins becoming prominent, blueness of the lips and mouth.
- Possible unconsciousness.

First Aid in Choking

In case of conscious casualty

- Position yourself behind the casualty.
- Bend the casualty forward and give slaps between the shoulder blade.
- If the above fails, hold the casualty from the middle of the abdomen making a fist with one hand and holding it with the other.
- Give rapid and upward push.
- Continue pushing in this manner till the obstruction is cleared.
- Do not give the force if the casualty becomes unconscious.

Note: These pictures are downloaded from the net, kindly redraw the diagram and place it.

Abdominal Thrusts

- Giving abdominal thrusts to a choking victim can dislodge the foreign body from the airway.
- To give abdominal thrusts to a choking victim who is sitting or standing, position yourself behind the victim.
- Place your arms around the victim's waist and form a fist with one hand. Place the thumb side of the fist with the knuckles up against the victim's abdomen slightly above the navel.
- With your other hand, grasp and hold your fist, then give up to five quick upward and inward thrusts to the victim's abdomen.
- If the victim is sitting in a chair, you probably will have to turn the victim, since reaching around the victim and the back of the chair usually is not practical.
- To give abdominal thrusts to a victim who is lying down, kneel and straddle the victim's thighs.

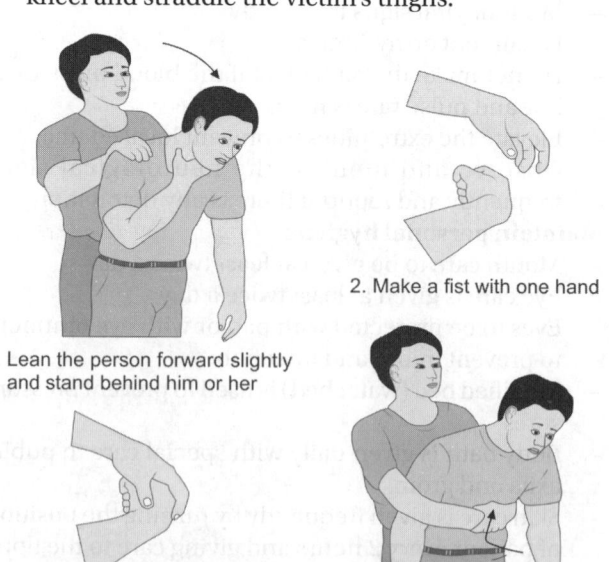

Fig. 30.25: Heimlich maneuver.

- Place the heel of one hand against the victim's abdomen slightly above the navel. Place the other hand over the first hand.
- Point the fingers of the bottom hand toward the victim's head. Then give five quick inward, upward thrusts. Use this method, too, if you are unable to reach around the waist of a conscious victim.
- A conscious choking victim who is alone can self-administer abdominal thrusts. The victim places the thumb side of a closed fist in the same position described above, covers the first with the other hand, then gives inward, upward thrusts.
- Also, if a firm object such as a chair or table is available, the victim can lean over the back of the chair or a corner of the table, pressing the abdomen upward and inward.

If the choking victim is extremely obese or in an advanced stage of pregnancy, give chest thrusts. Position yourself behind the victim and place the thumb side of a fist on the middle of the victim's sternum. Then thrust straight back for five thrusts. If the pregnant or obese victim is lying down, kneel at the victim's side and position your hands the same as for external chest compressions.

In case of unconscious casualty:
- Lay down the victim on the floor.
- Open the mouth holding tongue with the thumb and try to remove the obstruction by sweeping, if anything is observable.
- While giving finger sweeping, the finger curved just like a hook.
- Do not use your finger to take out the foreign body blinding down the throat.
- Call for ambulance. Shift the casualty as soon as possible.

First Aid for Child

- To give abdominal pushes to an unconscious child, sit over the thighs of the casualty and place your hands at the middle of the abdomen with fingers point upwards.
- Press the hands over the abdomen by pushing the hands upwards.

First Aid for Choking Infants (Conscious)

- If the infant is not breathing clear the airway obstruction.
- Place the head of the infant lower than chest.
- Give 5 back blows between the shoulders of the infant.
- If this fails, turn baby face up on the lap.
- Give 5 chest thrusts on breast bone using
- Place your two fingers and give chest6 compression.
- Check oral cavity, if anything is observable, try to take it out.
- Repeat the whole cycle till medical aid is available.

First Aid in Unconscious Infant

- Give rescue breathing by tilting the head of the infant
- Open the airway and give two rescue breathe.
- To check the obstruction, open the mouth of the infant, press the tongue towards the lower jaw and remove the object with finger sweep.
- Monitor the breathing and pulse.

Asphyxia

Asphyxia is a deficiency of oxygen in the blood and an increase of carbon dioxide in the blood and tissues. It occurs due to an interruption in the normal exchange of oxygen and carbon dioxide between the lungs and outside air. Lungs do not get sufficient supply of oxygen for breathing. If this condition continues for some minutes, breathing and heart action stops and death occurs.

The cause of asphyxia will be as follows:
Electric shock, foreign body in the air passages (choking), inhalation of smoke and poisonous gases, Suffocation under bed, earth, etc, hanging, strangulation by tight rope

I. Causes affecting the respiratory tract:
- Fluid in the air passages as in drowning.
- Harmful gases or fumes in the air passages e.g. coal gas, motor exhaust fumes, after damps smoke, sewere gas, and ammonia.

Note: Some gases affect the respiratory centre in addition.
- Foreign bodies in the air passages causing choking, e.g., portions of food, artificial teeth, vomited matter in the case of an unconscious person (owing to failure of the action of the epiglottis) tongue falling back in the case of unconscious person blood collecting from a fractured jaw.
- Compression of wind pipe, e.g. hangings strangulation or throttling.
- Smothering, e.g. overlaying an infant, an unconscious person lying face downwards on a pillow.
- Swelling of the tissues within the throat as a result of burns, scalds, corrosive, stings (wasp or bee), or from some diseases affecting the throat.

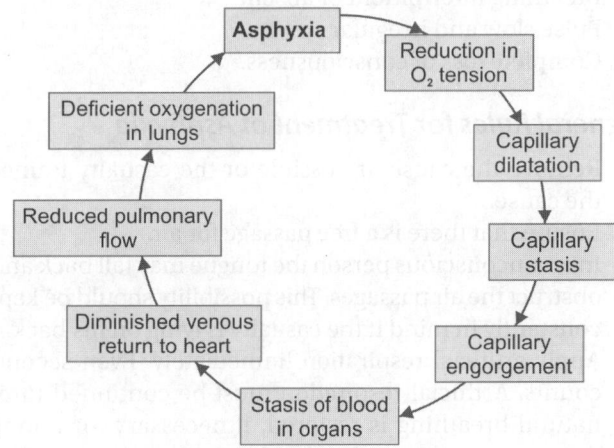

Fig. 30.26: Vicious cycle of asphyxia.

II. Causes affecting the respiratory mechanism:
- Pressure on (or) crushing of the chest resulting from accidents in mines, quarries sand pits or demolition, or from pressure in a crowd.
- Spasm of respiratory muscles in the case of certain poisons e.g. strychnine or diseases, e.g. tetanus lock jaw.
- Nervous-system diseases causing paralysis of the muscles of the chest wall or the diaphragm, e.g. poliomyelitis.
- Electric shock

III. Causes affecting the respiratory centre
- Electric shock
- Stroke by lightning.
- Poisons such as prussic acid and morphine
- Some gases.

The different types of asphyxia are:
- Suffocation by toxic gases.
- Drowning.
- Choking due to the entry of a foreign substance.
- Strangulation.
- Asthma.
- Severe infections of the throat.
- Artificial respiration.
- Fetal asphyxia.

Signs and Symptoms of Asphyxia

Early Stages
- Dizziness and weakness
- Shortness of breath
- Rapid pulse
- Partial loss of consciousness
- Swelling of the veins of the neck.
- Congestion of the face with blueness of cheeks and lips
These signs and symptoms may vary with degree of asphyxia present.

Later Stages
- The lips, nose, ears, fingers and toes are bluish-grey.
- Breathing intermittent or absent
- Pulse slow and irregular
- Complete loss of consciousness.

General Rules for Treatment of Asphyxia
- Remove the cause, if possible or the casualty frames the cause.
- Ensure that there is a free passage for air.
  In an unconscious person the tongue may fall back and obstruct the air passages. This possibility should be kept constantly in mind if the casualty is lying on his back.
- Apply artificial respiration immediately. Even second counts. Artificial respiration must be continued until natural breathing is restored, if necessary for a long time unless a doctor decides that further efforts will be of no avail.
- Utilize any help available to: a. Provide warmth, e.g. blankets; b. Provide shelter from the elements.

First Aid in Special Cases
- **Drowning:** While artificial respiration is being performed instruct by standers to remove wet clothing as far as practicable and wrap the casualty in dry blanket or other dry clothing.
- **Strangulation:** Cut and remove the band constricting the throat.
- **Hanging:** Grasp the lower limbs and raise the body. Free the neck by loosening or cutting the rope. Do not wait for a policeman.
- **Choking:** To dislodge the obstruction bend the casualty's head and shoulder forward, or in the case of a small child hold him upside down, and thump his back hard between the shoulder blades. If this is not successful, encourage vomiting by passing two fingers right to the back of the casualty's throat,
- **Swelling of the tissues within the throat:** If breathing has not ceased or when it has been restored give ice to suck, or failing, ice cold water to sip. Butter, olive oil or medicinal paraffin may also be given.
- **Suffocation by smoke:** Protect yourself by tying a towel, handkerchief ef or cloth, preferable wet, over your mouth and nose. Keep low and remove the casualty as quickly as possible.
- **Suffocation by poisonous gas:** Before entering any closed space known or suspected to contain poisonous gas of any kind, take a deep breath and hold it.

Ensure a free circulation of air by opening or if necessary by breaking doors or windows.

Suffocation

This results when air is prevented from reaching the air passages by an external obstruction such as a plastic bag, soft pillow or a fall of sand. A baby may be suffocated through lying face down on a pillow or cushion.

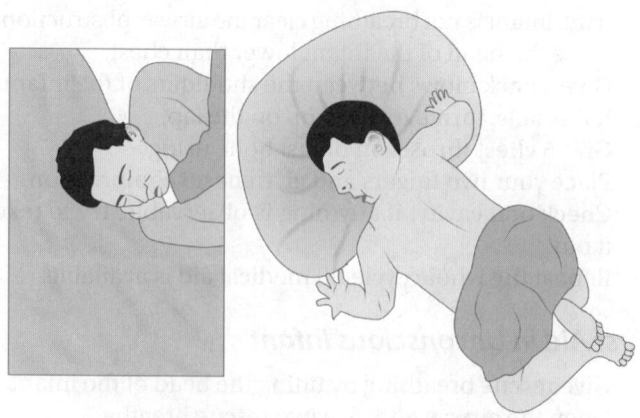

Fig. 30.27: Removing the causality.

General Symptoms and Signs

- Difficulty in breathing: The rate and depth of breathing increases.
- Breathing may become noisy with snoring or gurgling.

Aim

Restore supply of air to the casualty and seek medical aid.

First Aid for Suffocation

- Firstly ensure a patent airway.
- Check for the respiratory rate.
- Check for the level of cyanosis.
- In case of drowning, tilt the client to one side with head down.
- If strangulation is the cause then remove the band that is constricting the throat.
- Asphyxia caused due to swelling of the throat or asthma make the victim sit upright and ensure fresh air.
- In case of suffocation by gases remove the victim as soon as possible to fresh air.
- For all the victims loosen the clothing surrounding the neck.
- If breathing gets restored give sips of cold water.
- If breathing does not restore then start artificial respiration.

The artificial respiration followed is mouth-to-mouth respiration. Follow the procedure given below:

Firstly place the victim on his/her back:

- Tilt his head at the back.
- Pinch the nostrils.
- Cover the mouth of the casuality.
- Blow into his lungs until his chest expands.
- Repeat it 15–20 times.
- Blowing of air should be done with an open mouth, covering both the mouth and nose.
- On the other hand, ensure medical help.
- If you cannot give two effective breaths, start chest compressions.
- The first-aider should give 15 chest compressions, then give 2 inflations to the lungs and then again start 15 chest compressions.
- The cycle should be continued until the patient recovers or till medical aid is called for.

Treatment

- Immediately remove any obstruction or remove the casualty to fresh air.
- If she is conscious and breathing, reassure and observe.
- If she is unconscious, open her airway and check breathing. Complete the ABC of resuscitation if required and place her in the recovery position.
- Seek medical aid, if in doubt about her condition, arrange removal to hospital.
    - Possible frothing at the mouth.
    - Blueness of face, lips and finger nails (cyanosis).
    - Confusion.
    - Lowering of level of responsiveness.
    - Possible unconsciousness.
    - Breathing may stop.

FIRST AID FOR FOREIGN BODIES IN THE EYE, EAR, NOSE, AND THROAT

A "foreign body" means any extraneous matter that enters the body either through a wound in the skin (penetrating) or via one of the natural openings of the body (inserted (or) swallowed), or that enters the eye. A penetrating foreign body can be anything that enters the body, from a tiny splinter of wood (or) glass to a large wooden stake or piece of metal. It may be loose and easily removed without causing further pain or injury (or) it can be embedded.

The latter may in addition, be acting as a plug preventing blood loss. Large embedded foreign bodies may produce a deep wound but small splinters cause little more than minor lacerations. The main problem with injuries involving penetrating foreign bodies is that foreign bodies are rarely clean so there is a high risk of infection.

Splinters

Wood and metal splinters which have become embedded in the skin are probably the most common foreign bodies. They can generally be removed with tweezers. However, if the splinter is deeply embedded or over a joint, seek medical aid as soon as possible.

Symptoms and Signs

- Known contact with pieces of wood, metal or glass.
- An embedded foreign body may be visible.
- Pain and tenderness in the area.

Aim

Gently remove the splinter.

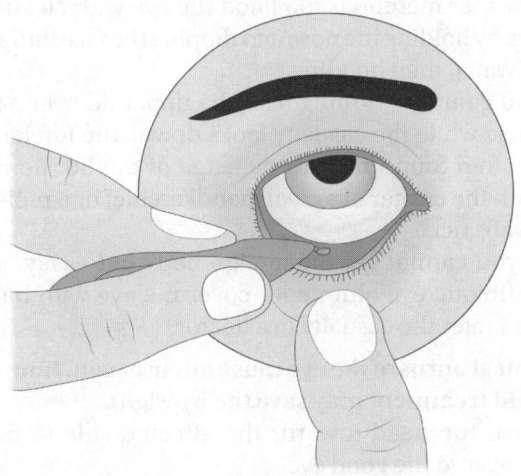

Fig. 30.28: Foreign body removal from the eye done by the ophthalmologist.

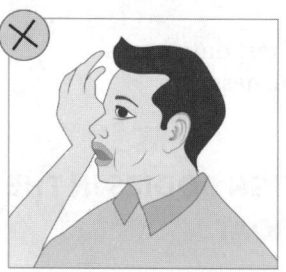 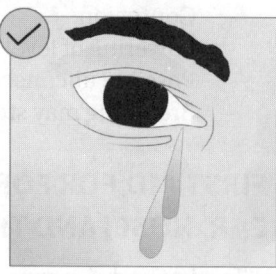 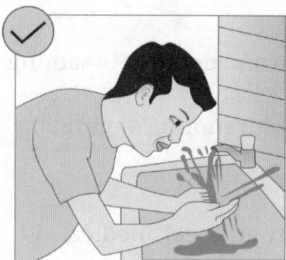 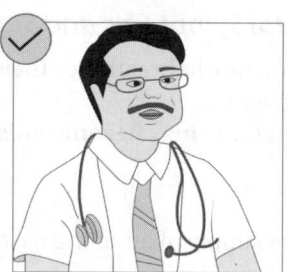

Do not rub the eye | Try to let tears wash the foreign body out or use an eyewash | Wash eye with clean water | Consult your eye specialist if foreign body sensation persists

Fig. 30.29: First aid and medical care for foreign body in the eye.

Treatment

- If the area around the splinter is dirty, cleanse it using soap and water.
- Sterilize a pair of tweezers by passing them through flame.
- Gently try to pull the splinter out of the wound with tweezers. Hold the tweezers as near to the skin as possible and grasp the splinter. Pull the splinter out in the opposite directions to that in which it entered the skin.
- If the splinter does not come out easily (or) begins to break up, treat as an embedded foreign body and seek medical aid.

Foreign Body in the Eye

Dust, grit, insects (or) loose eyelashes may get into the eye, causing great discomfort. If not quickly removed, they may cause serious trouble.

Treatment

- Avoid rubbing the eyes. Blink the eyes rapidly a few times. This may help to dislodge the foreign body.
- If you think the foreign body is under the upper lid, grasp the lid by the lashes and pull it forward over the lower lid, then released it. This may dislodge the foreign body.
- Another method is too flood the eye with clean water, e.g. by holding the nose and dipping the face into a basin of water, then bending.
- You could try turning back the upper lid over a match stick, while the casualty looks down. The foreign body is often found near to the edge of the lid. Remove it with the corner of a clean handkerchief or a moistened swabs tick.
- If you cannot get the foreign body out easily, supply antibiotic eye ointments, cover the eye with bandage and refer the casualty to a doctor.

Chemical burns of the eye cause intense pain. Immediate first aid treatment may save the eyesight.

- Turn the head towards the affected side to prevent danger to the good eye.
- Start immediately pouring clean water over the eye. Separate the eyelids with your fingers, and continue pouring from the inner corner of the eye out, for 10 to 15 minutes.
- Cover the eye with a pad and bandage.
- Send the casualty to hospital as soon as possible.

Hygiene of the Eye

Eyes are very precious, yet very delicate organs and they are easily damaged or affected by disease or malnutrition. Blindness is common in India, and some of the causes areas, follows:

- Infection by gonococcus, especially in newborn babies (ophthalmia neonatorum).
- Smallpox, caused by a virus.
- Trachoma, a virus infection of the eyelids.
- Injury such as foreign body, chemicals, sparks from a fire.
- Deficiency of vitamin A.
- Cataract.

Foreign Body in the Eye

Dust, grit, insects or loose eyelashes may get into, the eye causing great discomfort. If not quickly removed, they may cause serious trouble.

Treatment

- Do not let the patient rub the eye.
- Examine the eye. Pull down the lower lid. If the foreign body can be seen, remove it gently with the corner of a clean handkerchief, moistened in clean water, or with a moistened swab stick.
- If you think the foreign body is under the upper lid, grasp the lid by the, lashes and pull it forward over the lower lid, then release it. This may dislodge the foreign body.
- Another method is, to get the patient to hold his nose, and immerse the eye in water and then blink it.
- You could try turning back the upper lid to look for the foreign body.
- If the foreign body is not dislodged, and especially if it seems embedded in the eyeball, apply a pad and bandage and get the patient to a doctor as quickly as possible.

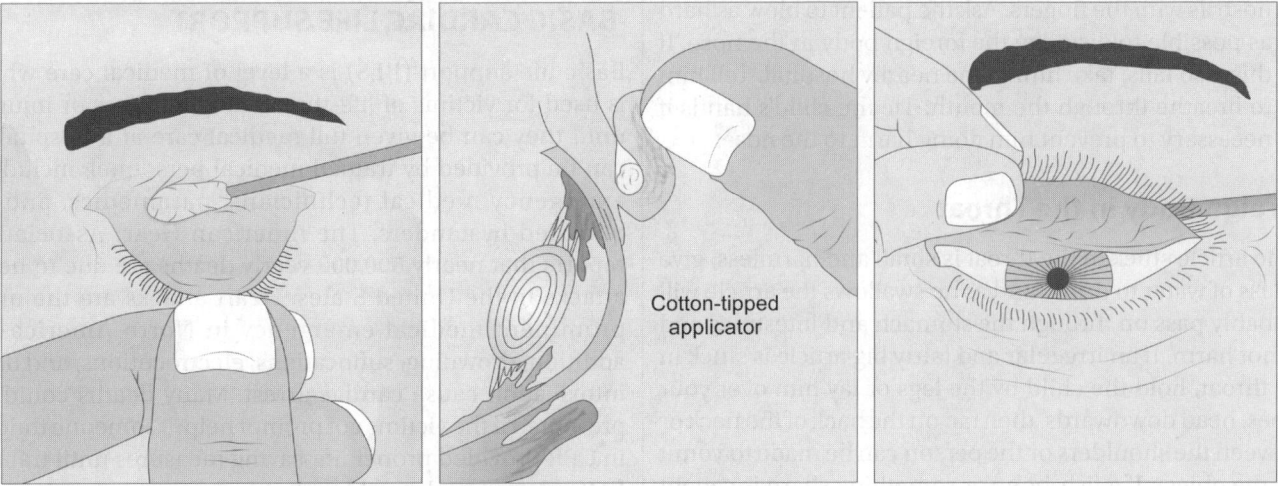

Fig. 30.30: Medical method of foreign body removal from the eye.

- If a corrosive has splashed into the eye, get the patient to blink under water, or wash out the eye with plenty of water. If acid has got into the eye, add some sodium bicarbonate to the water. Apply a pad and bandage, and take the patient to a doctor.

Foreign Body in the Ear

Children often put beads, peas or other small things into the ear or nose. Insects sometimes get into the ear.

Treatment: If you are sure an insect is in the ear, it may be floated out by pouring oil or spirit into the ear.

All other foreign bodies must be left alone and the patient taken to a doctor. Beware of the danger of pushing a foreign body further into the ear or nose.

Foreign Body in the Nose

When this happens you will be faced with a highly excited child who is both frightened and suffering from a sore nose. It is important therefore that you will show both tact and skill in dealing with this emergency.
- Take the history and establish how the accident happened and what the foreign body is.
- Calm down the patient and assure him so that you can get his or her cooperation.
- Examine the nose to see how deep the foreign body has gone. If the foreign body is not too far in the nose.
- Put thick wick made of cloth or take a feather try to tickle the unaffected nostril and make the child to sneeze. Sneezing will help the foreign body in the nose to come out. If this fails, block the ears, mouth and normal

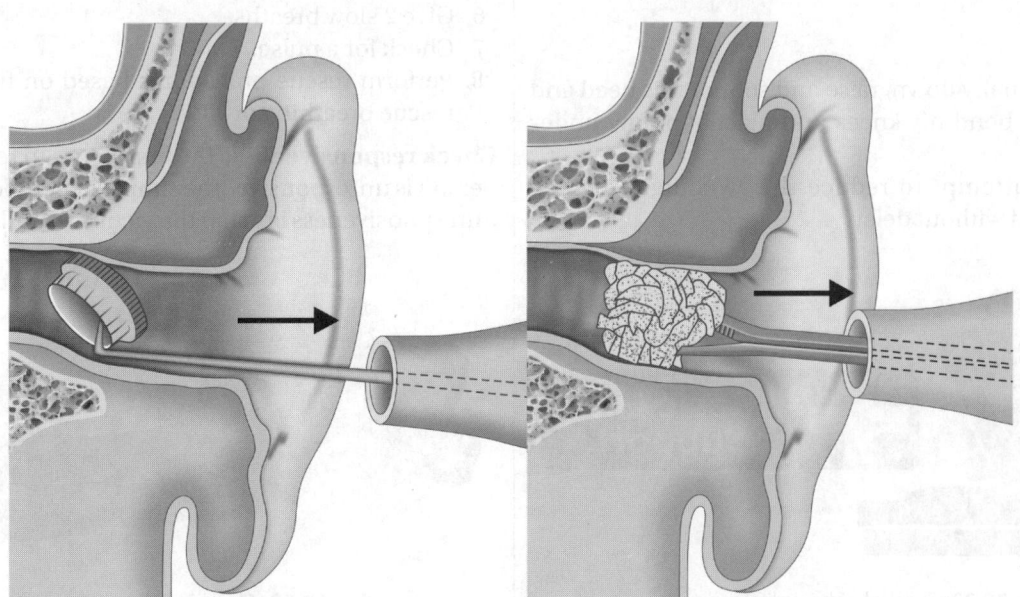

Fig. 30.31: Hospital-based foreign body removal from the ear.

nostrils with the fingers. Ask the patient to blow as hard as possible to dislodge the foreign body in the nose. If this also fails, take him to the nearby hospital. Tell him to breathe through the mouth. Tie the child's hands if necessary to prevent him doing harm to the nose.

Foreign Body in the Throat

If the article stuck in the throat is small and harmless, give a glass of water to drink, and as he swallows the article will probably pass on through the stomach and intestines and do not harm. If an irregular and fairly big article is stuck in the throat, hold the child by the legs or lay him over your knees, head downwards, then tap on the back of the neck or between the shoulders or the person can be made to vomit out the object. If a fish-bone or something sharp is caught in the throat, reassure the person and the relatives, and refer to the health center or hospital at once.

Foreign Body in the Stomach

When smooth objects such as coins or buttons are swallowed, they usually pass through the stomach and intestines out of the body. There is no need for panic, not for any treatment. The case may be shown to a doctor.

Abdominal Hernia or Rupture

Abdominal hernia, commonly referred to as a 'rupture' consists of a protrusion of some part of the abdominal content, usually the bowel through the muscular wall of the abdomen under the skin. It occurs most frequently at the groin, but it is not uncorrupting at the navel or through the scar of an abdominal operation. It may appear in babies or persons of any age. The condition may come on suddenly or gradually, if the onset is sudden there may be swelling and pain, followed sometimes by vomiting.

Treatment

- Lay the casualty down, raise and support his head and shoulders, bend his knees and place a pillow under them.
- Make no attempt to reduce the swelling, but seek medical aid without delay.

BASIC CARDIAC LIFE SUPPORT

Basic life support (BLS) is a level of medical care which is used for victims of life-threatening illnesses or injuries until they can be given full medical care at a hospital. It can be provided by trained medical personnel, including emergency medical technicians, paramedics, and by qualified bystanders. The American Heart Association reports that nearly 500,000 yearly deaths are due to heart attacks in the United States. Heart attacks are the most prominent medical emergency in North America. In addition, drowning, suffocations, electrocutions, and drug intoxication cause cardiac arrest. Many deaths could be prevented if the victims got prompt help-if someone trained in CPR provided proper life-saving measures until trained EMS professionals could take over.

Objectives

- Recognize and prevent cardiac arrest.
- Understand the concept of cardiac arrest and the importance of the time component.
- Early recognition of the emergency and activation of the emergency medical services (EMS)
- Know basic life support in adults with CPR (ventilation and chest compressions).
- Use of automated external defibrillator.

Steps of Basic Life Support

Essentially, there are eight steps for performing adult basic life support:
1. Check victim's responsiveness.
2. Activate the emergency medical service (EMS).
3. Position the unresponsive victim.
4. Open the victim's airway
5. Check for breathing.
6. Give 2 slow breaths.
7. Check for a pulse.
8. Perform rescue procedures based on findings: either rescue breathing or CPR.

Check responsiveness: The first step is to recognize that a person is unresponsive. The simplest method to determine unresponsiveness is to tap the victim's shoulder and shout,

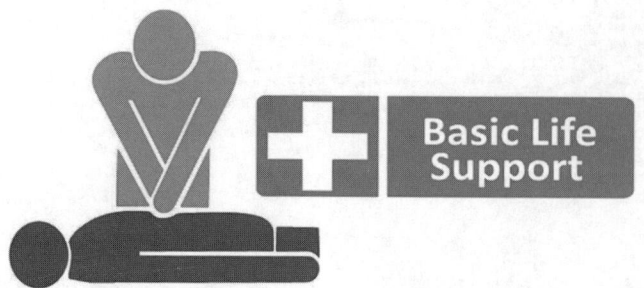

Fig. 30.32: Symbol of basic life support.

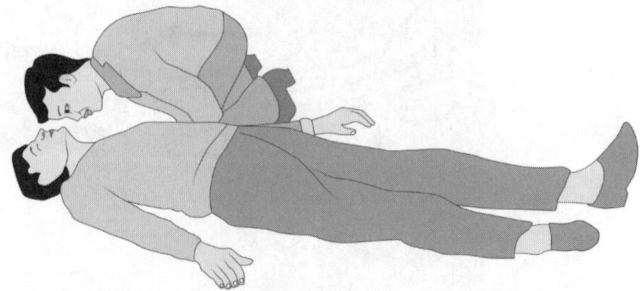

Fig. 30.33: Checking the responsiveness.

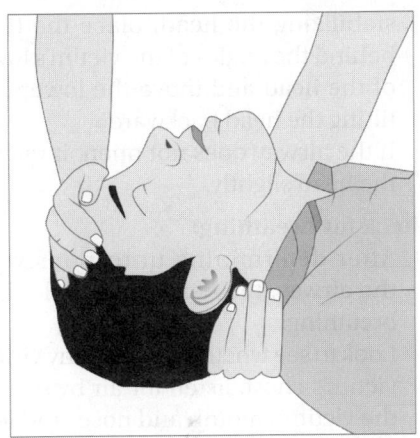 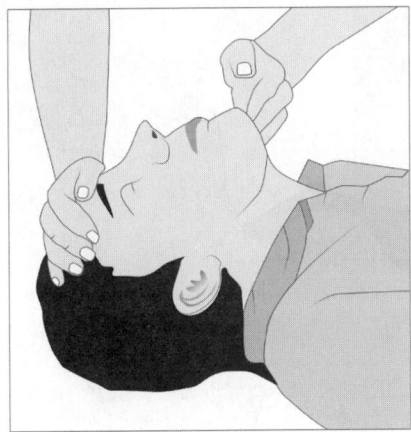

Fig. 30.34: Head tilt-chin lift position.

"Are you okay?" Do not forcefully shake the victim, since he or she may have a spine injury

Activate emergency medical services (EMS): If the victim is unresponsive, activate the EMS immediately, to avoid unnecessary loss of time in acquiring advanced cardiac life support. Direct a bystander to activate the EMS. If no bystanders are present, activate the EMS yourself.

Position the unresponsive victim: An unresponsive victim lying face down must be turned over so CPR can be given, if necessary. If you must turn the victim over, keep the head, neck, and shoulders aligned to avoid any twisting of the body.

Open the victim's airway:
- The most important maneuver in performing rescue breathing is opening the victim's airway.
- The most common cause of airway obstruction in an unconscious person is blockage by the tongue.
- When a victim's airway is opened, the lower jaw is moved forward, bringing the base of the tongue (which is attached to the lower jaw) forward also and away from the back of the throat.
- The easiest way to open an injured person's airway is by tilting the head and lifting the chin.
- To perform the head-tilt/chin-lift, place one hand, palm down, on the victim's forehead and push downward so the head tilts back.
- Then place the index and middle fingers of your other hand under the lower edge of the chin to lift the jaw.
- Simply opening the victim's airway sometimes results in restoration of breathing.
- If you suspect a spine injury, first try to open the airway by lifting the chin without tilting the head back. If the airway remains blocked, tilt the head slowly and gently until the airway is open enough to allow breaths to go in.
- Another technique for a victim with a possible spine injury is to use a jaw thrust without a head tilt. While

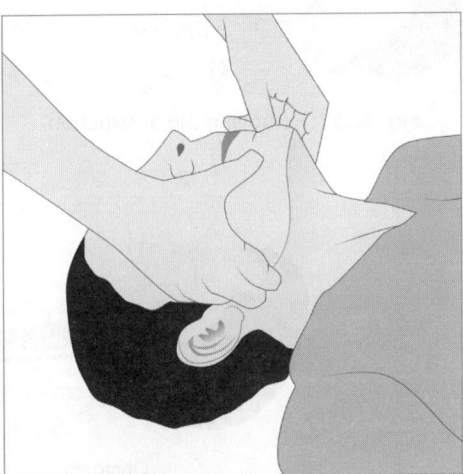

Fig. 30.35: Open the airway.

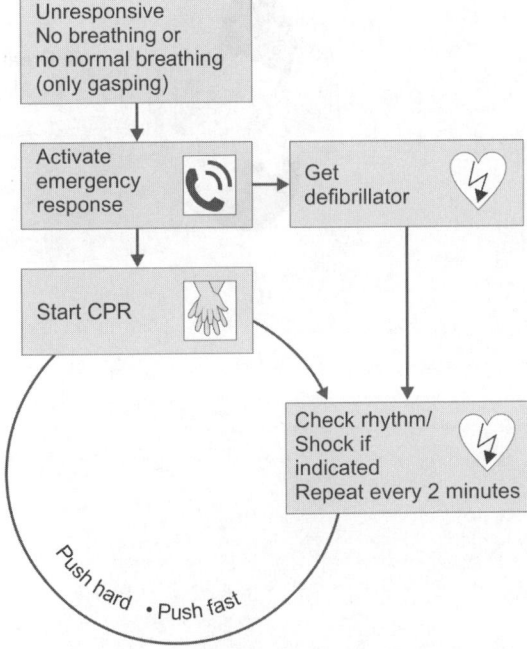

Fig. 30.36: Simplified adult BLS.

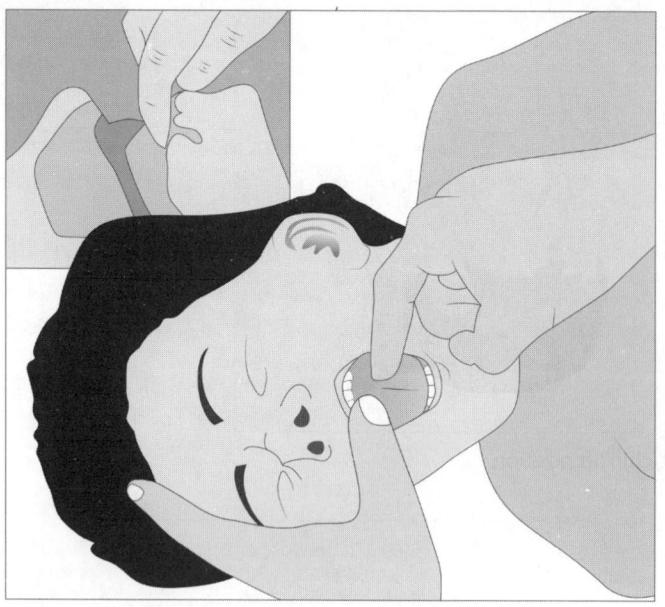

Fig. 30.37: Removing the obstruction.

stabilizing the head, place the fingers of each hand behind the angles of the victim's lower jaw on each side of the head and move the lower jaw forward without tilting the head backward.
- If the airway does not open, it may be necessary to tilt the head slightly.

Check for breathing:
- After determining unresponsiveness and opening the airway, the next step is to look, listen, and feel for breathing.
- Look to see whether there is any visible movement of the victim's chest, listen for air by placing your ear next to the victim's mouth and nose, and feel for air by placing your cheek next to the victim's mouth and nose.
- If breathing is present, you will see the victim's chest rise and fall, hear air coming from the victim's mouth and nose, and feel air against your cheek.
- This process should take only three to five seconds. Place a breathing unconscious victim in the recovery position.

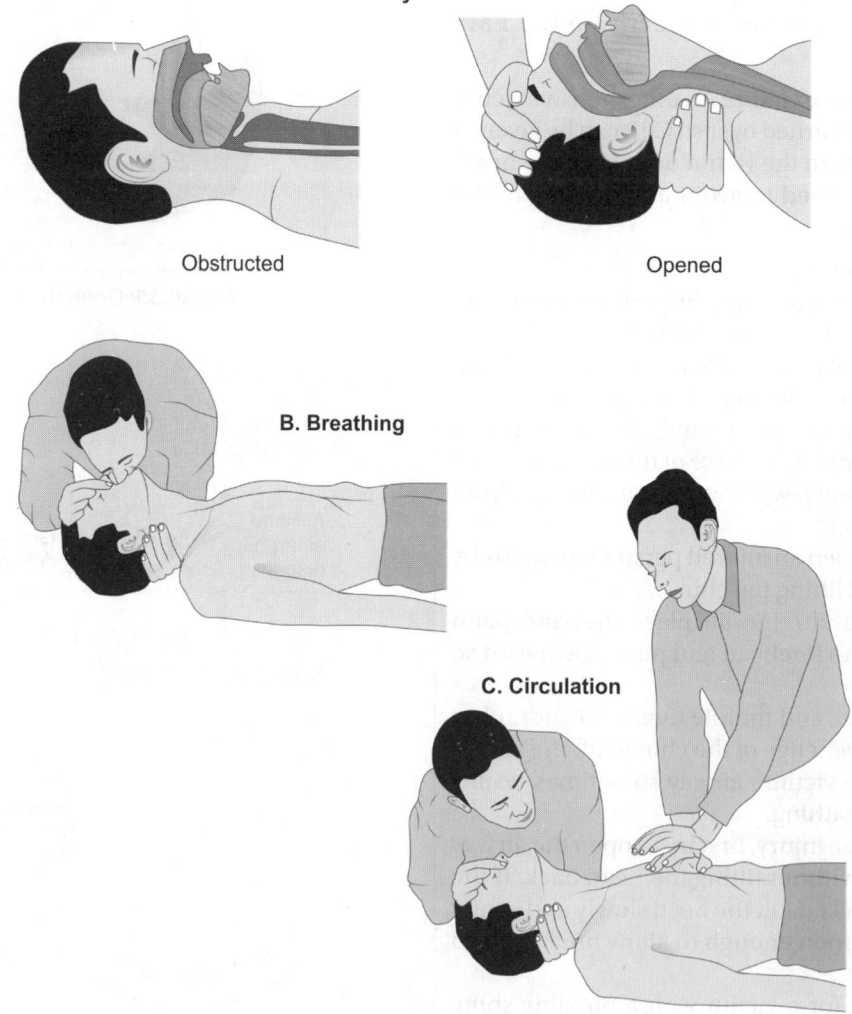

Fig. 30.38: ABC in basic life support.

Perform rescue breathing: If a victim is not breathing, perform rescue breathing.

BURNS AND SCALDS

Skin plays key roles in protecting the body from injury, infection and in maintaining body temperature. The skin consists of two layers. The outer layer (epidermis) and the inner layer (dermis) and fatty tissue (subcutaneous fat) the epidermis is protected by an oily substance called sebum secreted from sebaceous glands which keeps the skin supple and water proof.

Causes of Burns

A burn is an injury caused by:
a. Dry heat such as fire, a piece of hot metal or the sun.
b. Contact with any object charged with a high tension electric current, or by lightning.
c. Friction for example, by contact with a revolving wheel (brush burn) or fast moving rope or wire.
d. Corrosive chemicals:
   - Acids, such as sulphuric, nitric, hydrochloric.
   - Alkalis: such as caustic soda, caustic potash, strong ammonia (or) quick line.

A scald is an injury caused by moist heat, such as boiling water, steam, hot oil (or) tar, improperly applied poultice.

The effects of a burn or scald are the same. There may be reddening of the skin (or) blister formation (or) destruction of the skin (or) destruction of the deeper tissues. Pain is very severe.

There is immediate danger from shock which may be severe and made worse by the intense pain and by loss of plasma into the burnt area. Later there is danger from septic infection. The dangers of a burn increase with its surface area (even if it is only superficial) and if one-third (or) more of the skin area is involved, the patient may become dangerously ill. In small children and especially in infants even small burns should be regarded serious injuries and Medical aid sought without delay.

When a person's clothing catches fire, approach him holding a rug, blanket, coat (or) table cover in front of you for protection, wrap it round him, lay him flat and so smother the flames. If a person's clothing catches fire when alone, he should roll on the floor, smothering the flames with the nearest available wrap and call for assistance, on no account should be rush into the open air. The use of fire-guards will prevent many calamities in the home.

Clothing may be set on fire by standing too close to an electric fire or by carelessness in the kitchen. You should lay the casualty down with the burning side up as soon as possible to prevent flames sweeping upwards, and quickly put out the flames by dousing the casualty with water or other nonflammable liquid.

Alternatively, wrap the casualty tightly in a coat, curtain, blanket (not the cellular type), rug or other heavy fabric, then lay him (or) her flat on the ground. This starves the flames of oxygen and puts, them out.

Do not use nylon, or other inflammable materials to smother the flames.

Do not roll the casualty along the ground as this can cause burning of previously unharmed areas.

If your own clothes catch fire and help is not immediately available, extinguish the flames by wrapping yourself up tightly in suitable material and lying down.

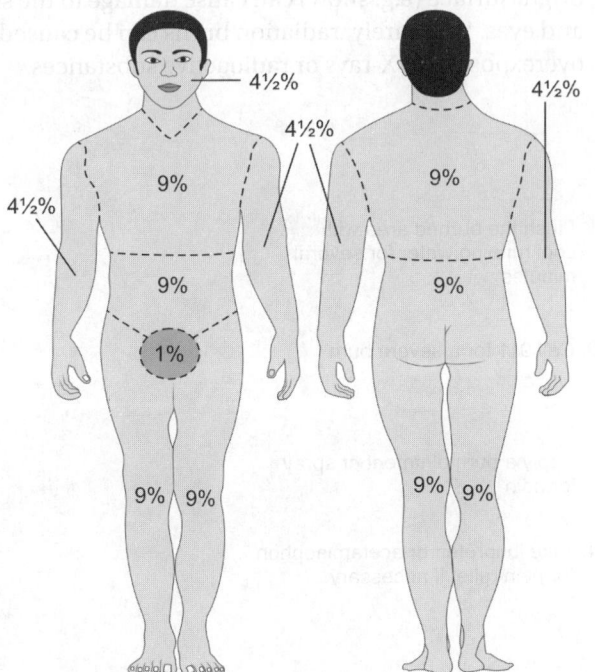

Fig. 30.39: Rule of nines in burn's assessment.

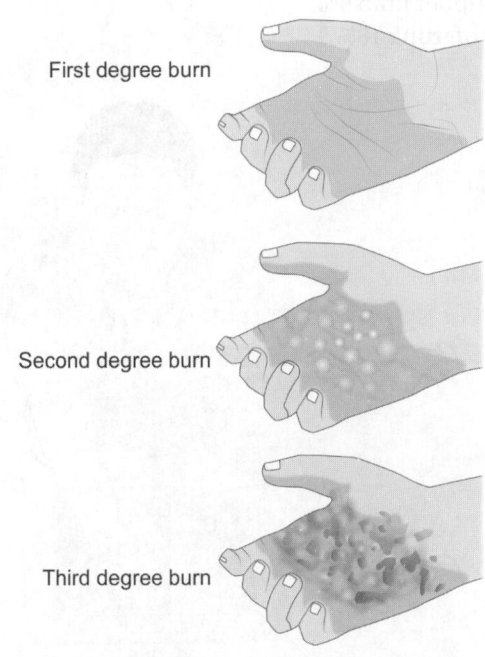

Fig. 30.40: Degrees of burn injury.

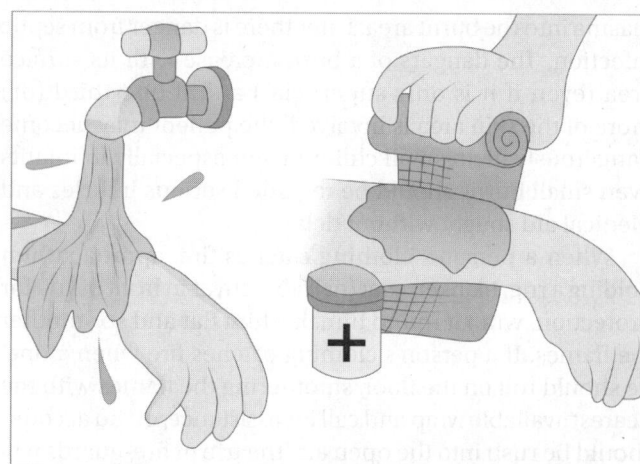

Fig. 30.41: Immediate measures for burn injury.

Burns occur due to:
- Dry heat like fire.
- Contact with hot metals.
- Chemicals, acids, ammonia, caustic soda.
- Electricity.
- Radiation.

Scalds are caused by moist heat due to
- Boiling water.
- Steam.
- Hot oil and coaltar.

Burns may be superficial or deep. Superficial burns involve skin and blister formation takes place. All other burns are deep burns. The simplest way to find out the extent of burns is to apply Wallace's rule of nine.

Rule of Nines

- Head and neck 9%
- Each upper limb 9%
- Front of trunk 18%
- Back of trunk 18%
- Each lower limb 18%
- Perineum 1%

Signs and Symptoms

- Intense burning and pain in the affected area.
- Enhanced thirst.
- Skin is reddened and blisters form in superficial burns.
- Skin is black in color in deep burn.
- Shock.

Types of Burn

Burns can be categorized according to the cause of the injury.

- **Dry burns:** Flames, lighted cigarettes and hot electrical equipment such as irons are all common causes of dry burns fast moving objects rubbed against the skin produce dry friction burns. Alternatively, they may be caused by the skin rubbing against an object. The most common example of this is 'rope burn'.
- **Scalds:** Wet heat such as steam, hot water or fat produces scalds.
- **Cold burns:** These may result from contact with metals in freezing conditions. Freezing agents such as liquid oxygen and liquid nitrogen can also cause cold burns.
- **Chemical burns:** Acids and alkalis found in domestic cleaning products as well as in industry may cause burns if in contact with the skin.
- **Electrical burns:** Electric currents and lightning generate heat and burn skin and underlying tissues.
- **Radiation burns:** Sunrays and light reflected from a bright surface (e.g. snow) can cause damage to the skin and eyes. Very rarely, radiation burns can be caused by overexposure to X-rays or radioactive substances.

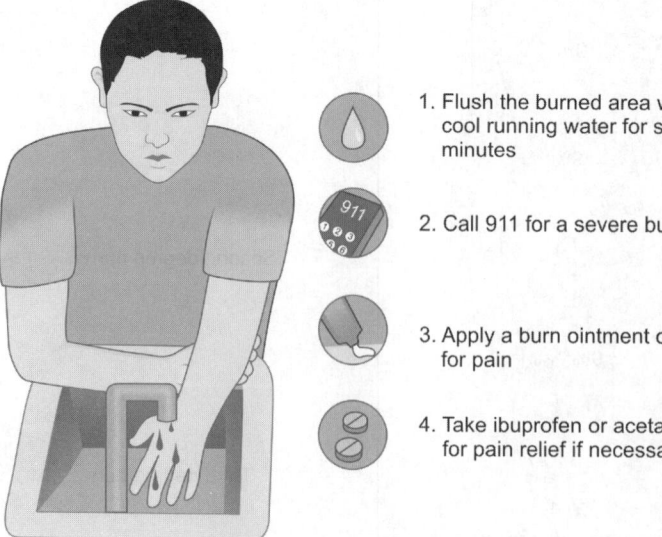

1. Flush the burned area with cool running water for several minutes
2. Call 911 for a severe burn
3. Apply a burn ointment or spray for pain
4. Take ibuprofen or acetaminophen for pain relief if necessary

Fig. 30.42: First aid for burn injury.

Classification of Burns

Burns are classified according to the area and depth of the injury. Any casualty with burns covering an area greater than 2 to 3 cm (1 inch) diameter, or burns deeper than the surface of the skin, or burns arising from electrical contact, must be referred to a doctor or hospital.

Area: The area of a burn gives a rough guide as to whether or not a casualty is likely to suffer stock. The greater the area involved, the greater the possibility of shock, because of greater fluid loss. For example another wire fit adult casualty with a superficial burn covering nine percent or more of the body's surface will need hospital treatment.

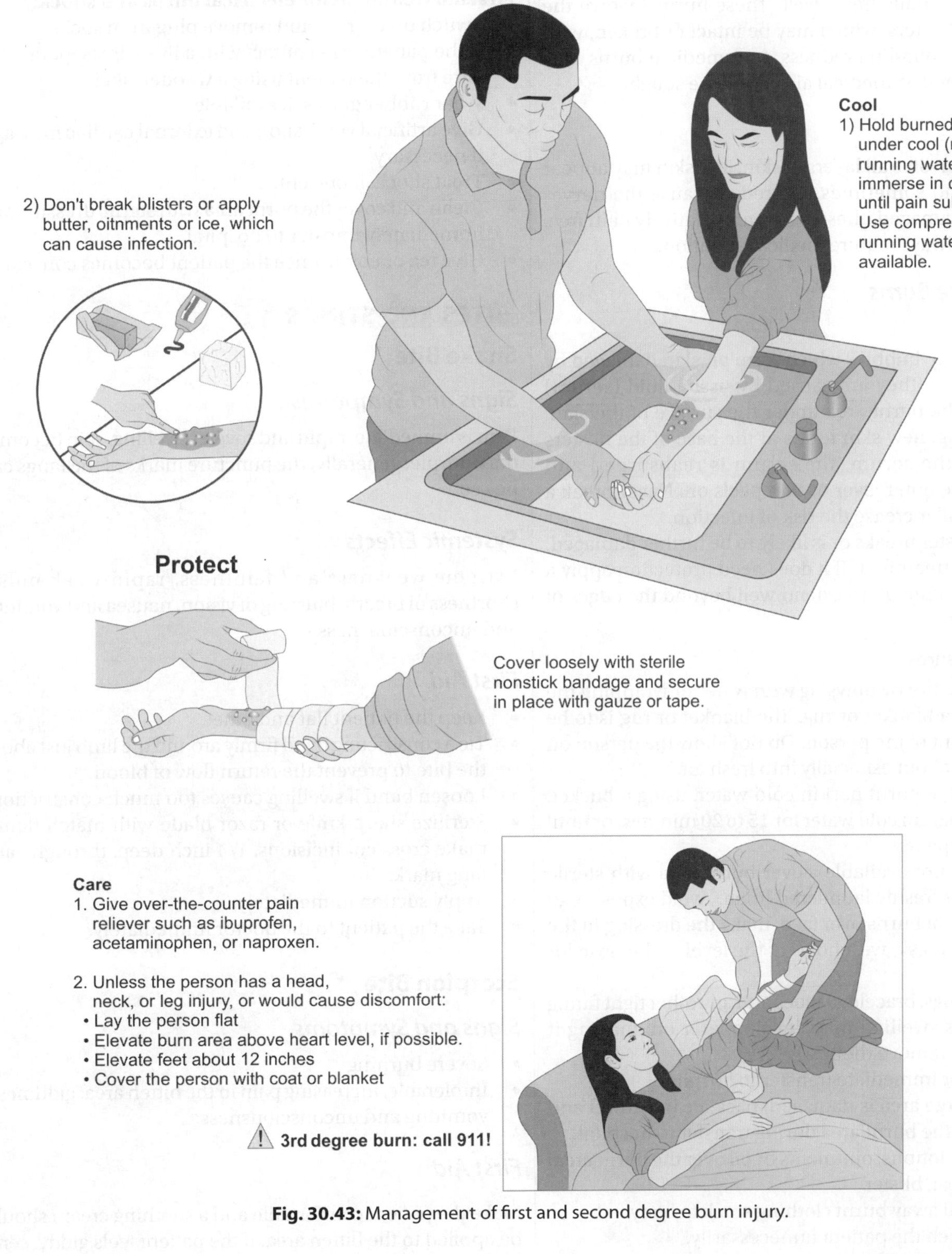

Cool
1) Hold burned skin under cool (not cold) running water or immerse in cool water until pain subsides. Use compresses if running water is not available.

2) Don't break blisters or apply butter, oitnments or ice, which can cause infection.

Protect

Cover loosely with sterile nonstick bandage and secure in place with gauze or tape.

Care
1. Give over-the-counter pain reliever such as ibuprofen, acetaminophen, or naproxen.

2. Unless the person has a head, neck, or leg injury, or would cause discomfort:
 • Lay the person flat
 • Elevate burn area above heart level, if possible.
 • Elevate feet about 12 inches
 • Cover the person with coat or blanket

⚠ 3rd degree burn: call 911!

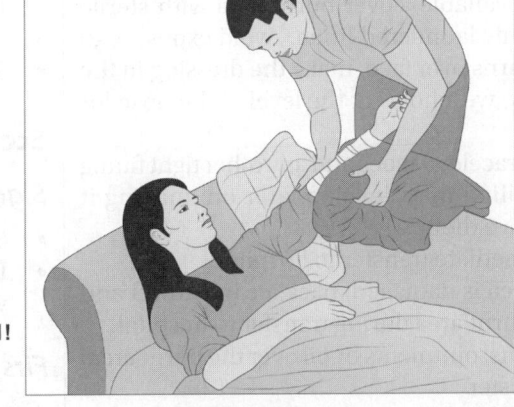

Fig. 30.43: Management of first and second degree burn injury.

Depth of Burns

There are three levels of burning: superficial intermediate and deep or full thickness burns. Note: The severity of a burn depends upon both the area it covers and its depth.

Superficial Burns

These burns involve only the outer layers of skin and result in general redness, swelling and extreme tenderness. This type of burn usually heals well. These burns involve the formation of blisters, which may be intact or broken, with an area of surrounding redness. Intermediate burns may become infected so medical aid should be sought.

Deep Burns

These burns involve all layers of skin. The skin may appear pale, waxy and sometimes charred. Because the nerve-endings are damaged, these burns are relatively pain free. Deep burns always require medical attention.

Intermediate Burns

Blisters

Blisters are thin 'bubbles which form on skin damaged by friction or heat. They are caused by tissue fluid (serum) leaking into the burnt area under the surface of the skin. During healing, new skin forms at the base of the blisters underneath the serum, the serum is reabsorbed and eventually, the outer layer of skin peels off. Never break a blister; you will increase the risk of infection.

Unless blister breaks or is likely to be further damaged, it requires no treatment. If it does need protection apply a dressing large enough to extend well beyond the edges of the burnt area.

First Aid Measures

- Put out the fire by dowsing with water or wrapping the person in a blanket or rug. The blanket or rug is to be held in front of the person. Do not allow the person on fire to run about especially into fresh air.
- Immerse the burnt part in cold water, using a bucket. Keep the part in cold water for 15 to 20 minutes. or until pain disappears.
- If water is not available, cover burnt area with sterile dressing or freshly laundered linen. Avoid exposure to air. In case of burns over face, make the dressing in the shape of a mask, with holes at the level of the nose for breathing.
- Remove rings, bracelets, shoes and any other tight fitting articles, as swelling may develop later on, making it difficult to remove them.
- Arrange for immediate transfer to hospital.
- When a large area is damaged, pack ice in a towel and apply it to the burnt area during transfer to hospital.
- Do not put lotions, ointments or oil over the burnt area.
- Do not break blister.
- Do not pull away burnt clothing stuck to body.
- Do not touch the patient unnecessarily.

In chemical burns, take the following steps:
- Remove the contaminated cloth carefully after soaking it in water.
- Wash the affected area with cold water for 10 to 15 minutes by flooding.
- Use sodium bicarbonate solution to wash acid burns, and vinegar to wash alkali burns, before washing with water.

First aid treatment for electrical burns and shock:
- Switch off current and remove plug from socket.
- If the patient is in contact with a live wire, separate the wire from the patient using a wooden stick.
- Wear rubber gloves, if available.
- Give artificial ventilation and external cardiac massage, if necessary.
- Treat shock, if present.
- Clean and cover the burnt area with sterile dressing and immediately transfer to hospital.
- Give tea or coffee once the patient becomes conscious.

BITES AND STINGS

Snake Bite

Signs and Symptoms

Pain is immediate, rapid and severe, swelling, skin becomes dark purple; generally, the puncture marks of the fangs can be seen.

Systemic Effects

Extreme weakness and faintness, rapid weak pulse, shortness of breath, blurring of vision, nausea and vomiting and unconsciousness.

First Aid

- Keep the patient flat and quiet.
- Tie a constricting band firmly around the limb just above the bite to prevent the return flow of blood.
- Loosen band if swelling causes too much constriction.
- Sterilize sharp knife or razor blade with match flame, make cross cut incisions, 1/4 inch deep, through each fang mark.
- Apply suction immediately.
- Take the patient to the doctor immediately.

Scorpion Bite

Signs and Symptoms

- Severe burning
- Intolerable, increasing pain in the bitten area, giddiness, vomiting and unconsciousness.

First Aid

Make the patient comfortable and a soothing cream should be applied to the bitten area. If the patient feels giddy, send him immediately to the hospital. If blister formation occurs, dress the wound with an antibiotic ointment.

Dog Bite

- The bitten area should be washed immediately with soap and water.
- An antibiotic cream should be applied after cleaning the wound with disinfectants.
- Send the patient immediately to hospital.

Scorpion Sting

In many parts of India scorpions are common and scorpion stings are likely to occur. The person stung, usually a child who is unaware of the dangers of scorpion lurking in dark places, complains of severe pain at the site of the sting and shows signs of shock. The scorpion sting is poisonous and if the child is small or physically weak it may produce serious results. If severe the patient may have cramps, sweating and possibly convulsions.

What to do when you see a patient who has been stung by a scorpion. As a rule, you will be told that the sting is by a scorpion because the patient or some relative has actually seen the scorpion. Proceed as follow:
- Examine the site of the sting.
- Look for signs of shock, particularly in small children.

Treatment
- Apply a cold compress to the site of the sting (or) sodium bicarbonate paste (cooking soda paste).
- Treat for shock.
- Give hot drink and keep the patient warm.

Bee, Wasp and Hornet Stings

Bee, wasp and hornet stings occur frequent in rural areas, especially if their nests are disturbed. The insects have a sting which is left at the site of puncture and has to be removed. If a person is prone to allergies, a bee, wasp or hornet sting may be a serious condition because of the shock produced.

Signs
The site of the sting looks red, swollen and painful.

First Aid Treatment
- Remove the sting with a pair of forceps.
- Apply cold compresses to the site.
- A paste with sodium bicarbonate (cooking soda) or washing soda can be applied or if available antihistamine ointment.
- Treat for shock.

Jellyfish Sting

The effects of jellyfish sting vary from minor local reactions to large wheals, severe pain and sometimes death.

First Aid Measures
First aid measures are:
- A paste of sodium bicarbonate in water
- Seek medical aid urgently if symptoms are severe

Sting of Portuguese Man of War

The effects vary from slight stinging to cramps nausea and difficulty in breathing.

First Aid Measures

The first aid is as follows: Swab the area with methylated spirit to which a little vinegar has been added to acidify it. Do not rub or apply fresh water or sand. Remove any gelatinous strands present in the flesh using cloth or soft paper, once symptoms subside.

Seek medical aid in severe cases.

Sea Urchin Sting

The spine of the sea urchin cans break off into the skin causing local burning and numbness. The wounds heal slowly and the rate of infection is high.
- Wear gloves while handling the sting
- Remove the pine
- Cover the wound with dry dressing
- Get medical aid.

Cone-shaped Shells

A snail like creature is found in such shells. It injects a very potent poison through a minu te hollow barhed harpoon. It can be fetal and there is no antidote such a shell must not be handled. In case a patient is bitten. Watch the patients pulse and respiration, and give external cardiac massage and artificial respiration when necessary. Get medical aid urgently.

POISONING

A poison is any substance which when taken into the body in sufficient quantity is capable of injuring health or destroying life. It may be taken either accidentally or intentionally.

A. Through the lungs, by breathing poisonous gases or fumes. This is put first because gas poisoning causes more deaths then all other poisons combined.
B. By the mouth, i.e. swallowed.
C. By injection under the skin.
- **Gas poisoning:** It occurs mainly from breathing household gas or the fumes of fires, stoves, motor exhausts or the smoke generated from large fires or explosions. Life is endangered by asphyxia.
  Sufferers may appear deceptively well unless severely poisoned when they will be unconscious with difficult breathing.
- **Swallowed poisons exert their dangerous effects:** Either (i) directly on the food passages causing retching,

vomiting, pain and often diarrhea poisons in this class include metallic poisons, poisonous fungi and barnes and contaminated decomposing food. Particularly severe symptoms are caused by the corrosives (strong acids, alkalis and disinfectants) which burn the lips, mouth, gullet and stomach and cause intense pain or (ii) on the nervous system after absorption into the blood usually causing deep unconsciousness (coma) and sometimes asphyxia. The most important of these poisons are alcohol (spirits, wine, beer) taken in excessive amount, and the many drugs taken as tablets, or draughts, to relieve pain (e.g. aspirin and preparations containing opium derivatives) or to produce sleep (e.g.) the barbiturate drugs). All persons unconscious from poisoning by drugs are seriously ill; this also applied to individuals who are insensible from alcoholic intoxication (dead drunk). A few poisons act on the nervous system by causing delirium (e.g. Belladonna) or fits (e.g. strychnine, prussic acid).

- **Infected poisons:** These poisons are infected by hypodermic' syringe, by bites from poisonous septiles or rabid animals or by stings from certain insects. As a result life may be in dangered through coma and asphyxia.

General Rules for the Treatment of Poisoning

- Send for medical aid at once giving brief particulars including, if possible, the suspected cause. Preserve for examination:
  - Any remaining poisons.
  - Any box, carton, bottle or other container which may help to identify the poison.
  - Any vomited matter.
- If the casualty is unconscious:
  - Place him in the recovery position or prone position with the head turned to one side and not resting on a pillow. This will help to prevent vomited matter from entering the wind pipe and keep the tongue clear of the airway. It also makes it easier to apply artificial respirations at once should this be necessary. If, however, there is much retching and vomiting the three quarter prone position (recovery position) may be better, i.e. the casualty is on his side with the upper most leg bent at hip and knee or a pad supporting the chest.
  - Start artificial respiration instantly if the breathing is feeble or unduly slow. Keep it up till the doctor takes charge.
- When poison has been swallowed and the casualty is conscious:
  - Get rid the poison by making him vomit. Tickle the back of the throat with a spoon or two fingers, or if this method fails, give emetics, i.e. two tablespoons of salt to a tumbler of water, preferably tepid. Do not induce vomiting:
    - When the casualty is unconscious.
    - When the lips and mouth are burned. Corrosive acids and alkalis cause yellow or grey stains on the skin, lips and mouth, which are easily recognizable.
  - Neutralize the poison by giving an antidote. An antidote is a substance when reacts with the poison and makes it harmless. For example, when an acid has been swallowed an alkali such as chalk or milk of magnesia should be given. For some poisons there are special antidotes. These are shown in the following table. In certain factories there may be particular hazards and in these cases special antidotes are usually kept readily available. Instructions for their administration should be prominently displayed.
  - Dilute the poison by giving copious draughts of water. This will help to lessen the irritating effect and to delay absorption in strong concentrations, it will also replace fluid host by vomiting.
  - Give soothing drinks such as milk (at least one pint), barely, water, raw eggs or flour beaten up with water.

The More Common Poisons and Antidotes

The quantities mentioned below be reduced by a half for children between two and eight years of age and reduced to a quarter for infants less than two years. Where instructions are given to make the casualty vomit, it is assumed that he is conscious and is able to swallow.

Agricultural Poisons

Certain weed killers and insecticides used in agriculture as sprays for crops can give rise to dangerous poisoning through careless handling or accidental contamination. Two kinds of poisoning occur, one of which closely resembles heat stroke. In the second kind asphyxia may develop rapidly. Warning symptoms are giddiness, nausea, blurred visions and tightness of the chest. Signs may include slow pulse, contracted pupils, sweating, blueness of the face and lips, unconsciousness and possible convulsions.

Treatment: Artificial respiration, which may have to be repeated or continued for a long time. As the doctor may wish to give a special antidote by injection, the first aider should give the suspected causes of the condition when sending for medical aid.

Common Poisons in India

Arsenic and opium account for the largest number of deaths from poisoning in India. Arsenical poisoning is the more common of the two, except in Bengal, which is an opium eating country. Arsenic is the chief homicidal poison, while opium is the favorite of suicides.

Arsenic Poisoning

Common white arsenic in the crude form, appears as lumps resembling white earthen ware and is easily obtainable in bazaars all over India. It is imported from the Persian Gulf and is used for preserving skins and wood work, for destroying vermin and as a medicine. It is powdered down and being practically tasteless it is easily mixed with sweets and food. Being fatal in small doses it is the most common homicidal poison.

Symptoms: Are those of a violent irritant in which there is always an interval of half to one hour after taking before symptoms appear. Burning pain in the stomach with vomiting and purging of blood stained matter come on, followed by numbness and cramps in the muscles. After large doses, collapse and shock precede death from coma.

Treatment: General rules for poisons. Give an emetic white of egg or warm ghee to drink. In severe cases, give treatment for shock, i.e. hot bottles and stimulants.

Datura Poisoning

Datura poisoning is the third most common poison in India coming, however, a long way after arsenic and opium in frequency. Datura or thorn apple, is common in India and the crushed seeds are administered in food and drink by criminals, with intent to rot rather than to kill.

Symptoms: Are those of Belladonna poisoning, coming on fairly rapidly after partaking. Dryness of the throat, flushing of the face with a hot dry skin, and widely dilated and fixed pupils are typical. Difficulty in swallowing occurs with restlessness. Purposeless movements with muttering delirium lead on to conditions of coma; with death from failure of heart and respirations. The pupils remain widely dilated throughout and for days after recovery which may take place.

Treatment

General rules for poisoning: Give an emetic; prevent hypnosis by flicking with towels or cold douching. Stimulate by hot coffee or a tablespoon-full of brandy. Apply warmth and artificial respiration if necessary.

Indian Hemp Poisoning

Indian hemp is easily procured in Indian bazaars in the form of (1) Bhang, which is the powdered leaves and small stalks (2) Ganja the dried flowering tops which are smoked in a pipe, and (3) as charas which is the resinous juice, expressed from leaves and branches. This is often mixed with alcoholic drinks or with sugar in sweets. In Egypt and Saudi Arabia it is termed Hashish. It is not a common cause of death and is used as an individual vice, and as an intoxicant preparatory to robbery. The effects are those of a brain stimulant followed by narcosis. In the stage of stimulation mental excitement is produced with hallucinations said to be pleasant. Laughing, singing and wild delirium are common results, while in some cases, there are violent homicidal tendencies, in which addicts run amok. The drug is sometimes taken by assassins to induce courage, or administered to them for the same purpose.

Symptoms: The pupils are dilated; the pulse full and slow, and there is general tingling of the skin. Giddiness gives place to stupor, coma and death.

Treatment: The same as for Datura poisoning.

Aconite Poisoning

Aconite is a most virulent poison, but fortunately not commonly employed in India. It is readily obtainable in Indian bazaars, and sold as the dried shriveled root of the plant. It is used by native Hakims (or medicine men) for certain fevers and it is sometimes added to some of the country spirits as an extra intoxicant. Primitive hill tribes use aconite as dressing for their poisoned arrows. When poisoning by aconite is met with, it is usually accidental, but homicidal poisoning is not unknown. The crushed root is mixed with tea, or cooked with food in these cases. The effect is first to stimulate sensory and motor nerves, with paralyzing effect later, in which the centers for the heart and respiration become involved. The mind remains unaffected.

Protective Measures

In children the accidental poisoning occurs generally due to the intake of attractive substances, in anxiety or ignorance and in adults it occurs due to carelessness. The toxic effects of various types of medicines and intoxicating substances if taken in excessive amount can be seen. The normal dose given to adult person can be toxic to children. Therefore, following rules should be observed:

- Medicine bottles and packets should be clearly labeled. Medicines of unlabelled bottles should not be used and should be destroyed.
- Write the word 'poison' on the toxic medicines and household insecticides. Keep them in locked almirah.
- Never take medicines from the unclearly labeled bottles. Do not take them in dark room.
- The label on the bottle should be read before taking the medicine, during measuring the dose and while keeping the bottle back to the place.
- Caustic soda or potash solution used for cleaning the floor appear like water and by mistake it is drunk as water when one feels thirsty. Therefore clear label should be put on the bottle.
- Empty bottles are filled with some acids, like acid used in the batteries, acids used in cleaning sink, wash basins, toilet, etc. and are sold in the market, in which sometimes the original label is not taken out from the bottle. Therefore the original label should be removed and the new label of the filled substance should be put and the bottles should be kept beyond the reach of the children.

- To avoid food poisoning food should be prepared with cleanliness and kept covered. Flies should be prevented to sit on the cooked food. Vegetables should be washed and boiled properly, and in suspected case boiled water must be consumed.

FIRST AID IN CONVULSIONS

Convulsions or fits are caused by irritation of the nerve cells in the brain. In the disease called epilepsy the cause of the irritation is not known. In other cases the irritation may be due to toxins or poisons in the blood.

Epileptic fit: This may occur at any time in persons who are subject to them. The person suddenly becomes unconscious and falls down. He goes stiff all over, the breath is held and the eyes turn up. His face may turn red and then blue. After about half a minute the muscles start twitching, and then there will be rhythmical movements of arms, legs, head and jaw, and deep breathing with foaming at the mouth. The tongue may be bitten and head or limbs injured.

First aid treatment: The aim is to prevent the patient from hurting himself. Quickly get ready a spatula or some hard object wrapped in a piece of cloth, to place between his teeth well back on one side, as soon as he opens his mouth after the rigid stage (to prevent biting of the tongue). Loosen any tight clothing, turn the head to one side, and wipe away any froth. Do not try to stop the convulsive movements except to prevent injury. Keep the environment quiet, and after the fit allows the patient to sleep quietly. When he recovers he should be taken to a doctor. Infantile convulsions: Infants may have fits due to teething, stomach or chest trouble, intestinal worms, or at the beginning of an infectious illness. There may be only twitching of muscles and holding of the breath, or it may' be like an epileptic fit.

Treatment: Reassure the mother and get her to wrap the child in a blanket and lay him down quietly on his side. If he has teeth and may bite his tongue, place a gag (as for epileptic fit) between the teeth. The child should be taken to a doctor. If the fits continue and a doctor is not available, the child may be put into a bath of warm water. This will usually bring about relaxation. Then wrap the child immediately in a towel and gently dry him. Keep him warm and quiet.

FAINTING

A faint is a brief loss of consciousness of no more than momentary duration caused by a temporary reduction in the flow of blood to the brain. Recovery is usually rapid and complete. It may be a nervous reaction to pain or fright; or the result of an emotional upset, exhaustion or lack of food. It is, however, more common after long periods of physical inactivity, especially in warm atmosphere, where lack of muscular activity causes a large volume of blood to collect in the lower part of the body and legs. This reduces the amount of blood available to the circulation, e.g. as in a soldier standing on Parade.

Signs and symptoms: Pulse will be slow at first (this is an important clue) and weak.
- Casualty may be very pale
- The skin is cold and clammy
- The breathing is shallow.

Aim: Position the casualty so that gravity helps to increase the flow of blood to the brain.

Prevention: If the casualty is on parade or standing in a crowd, advise him (or) her to flex the leg muscles and toes to aid circulation. If the casualty feels unsteady, make her sit down and help her to learn forward with her head between her knees and advise her to take deep breaths.

Treatment

- When a casualty faints, lay her down with her legs raised, and maintain an open airway.
- Loosen any tight clothing at her neck, chest and waist, to assist circulation and breathing.
- Make sure that the casualty has plenty of fresh air; place her in a current of fresh air and fan air on her face. If necessary, place her in the shade.
- Reassure her whilst she is regaining consciousness; gradually raise her to a sitting position.
- Check for and treat any injury that she may have sustained on falling.
- Check breathing rate, pulse and level of responsiveness until fully recovered.

If the casualty does not begin to regain consciousness rapidly, open her airway and check breathing.

Complete the ABC of resuscitation if required and place her in the recovery position. Summon medical aid and seek other causes for unconsciousness.

EPISTAXIS

- Bleeding occurs from the blood vessels inside the nostrils.
- Bleeding coming from Nose is also a sign of fractured skull.
- Make the causality to sit with the head bent forward, loosen the tight clothing around the neck.
- Allow the blood to drain from the nostrils.

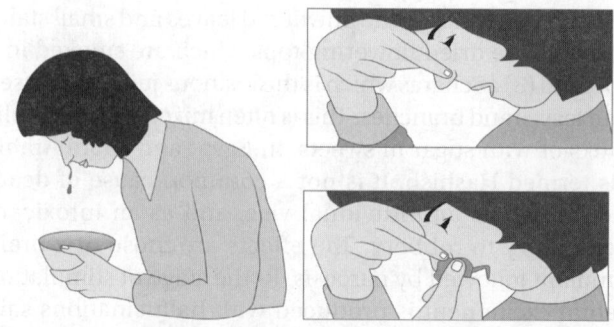

Fig. 30.44: First aid for epistaxis.

- Ask the causality to breathe through her mouth and to pinch the soft part of the nostril for 10 minutes
- If the bleeding restarts tell the casuality to reapply pressure.
- If bleeding follows a head injury, the blood may appear thin and watery. It is a serious sign because it indicates skull fracture.
- Tell the casualty to pinch her nose.
- Advise her not to speak, swallow, cough spit because she may disturb the blood clots that have formed in the nose.
- Give her clean cloth to wipe off the dribbling.
- Advise the casualty to rest quietly for few hours. Avoid exertion, blowing of nose at least four hours so as to not to disturb the clot.
- If after 30 minutes also bleeding persists or recurs, seek medical aid.

ELECTRIC SHOCK

Severe injury may be caused by the passage through the body of an electric current. This may be due to contact with a line and nacked wire, cable or rail or from a stroke of lightning. The immediate effect is shock which may be relatively mild or so severe as to cause death (electrocution) depending on the strength of the current and on the path it takes in passing to arch through the body. Another result is burning and the burns may be severe and deep, especially with higher voltages.

Electric Injuries

a. In houses and offices, firm domestic apparatus with voltages up to 450 (alternating current).
b. In factories from equipment with voltages as high as 1,100 (alternating current).
c. Contact with a live-rail voltage in the region of 1,000 (direct current).
d. From over head lines with high voltages of well over 100,000 (alternating current).
e. From lightning where the strength of the current is immeasurable and the voltage may be many millions, e.g. standing under trees (or) in contact with metal railings (or) golf clubs. Alternating currents are more dangerous than direct currents as the muscles are thrown into spasm causing the casualty to remain fixed in contact with the current.

Moisture is a powerful conductor of electricity and when present, will facilitate the passage of the current. If the skin at the point of contact of earth is wet even the lower voltages may be dangerous. More important than the actual strength of the current is the path it takes through the body in finding its way to earth. Thus a very strong current passing to earth through the lower limb might be less dangerous than a much weaker current crossing the chest as unfortunately it is likely to do if it enters through the hand and arm. In these cases there may be immediate fatal paralysis of the heart or more commonly a sudden stoppage of breathing from paralysis of the muscles of respiration. If the nerves controlling the heart and circulation escape, the heart may continue to function even though the breathing has stopped.

It is for this reason that in electrical injuries the face is blue (asphyxia) rather than white and that artificial respiration may have to be carried on for a very long time. As long as the heart beats life may be saved.

Treatment

Electric injury is an emergency calling for prompt and intelligent action: (i) Prompt action if the casualty's life is to be saved. (ii) Intelligent action if two casualties instead of one are to be avoided.

- Switch off the current if the switch cannot be found immediately and the supply is through a flexible cable the current may be cut off by removing the plug (or) even breaking the cable or wrenching it free. Do not attempt to cut the cable with a knife or scissor. It is impossible to switch off or break the current.
- Remove the casualty from contact with the current the greatest care is necessary; insulating materials must be used and they must be dry. With ordinary domestic apparatus rubber gloves are good and a dry cap, coat or other garment or a folded newspaper give fair protection. If possible the rescuer should stand on some insulating material such as rubber-soled shoes or boots or piles of new papers. With very high voltage, e.g. overhead lines, danger may exist even if the casualty is not actually in contact because the current may jump the gap (arcing). In these cases the rescue should, if possible, be left to a properly trained electrical man although there is no danger if the current is switched off. If expert help is not available, approach with great caution and keep as far away from any part of the electrical equipment as possible. Drag the casualty away with some nonconducting implement such as a dry walking stick, a dry board or dry rope.
- Unless the casualty is breathing normally give artificial respiration, for some hours if necessary.
- Treat for shock.
- Treat any burns.
- Transfer to hospital or seek medical aid.

Even after apparent recovery the casualty should be seen by a doctor to ensure that all is well as causalities suffering from electrical injuries are liable to rephase even when the effect have seemed to be mild.

HANGING, STRANGLING AND THROTTLING

Pressure on the outside of the neck by hanging, strangling or throttling squeezed the airway shut and blocks off the flow of air to the lungs. Hanging involves suspension of the body by the neck from a nose. Strangling involves cutting off the air supply by a tight constriction around the neck.

Throttling involves cutting off the air supply by intentional squeezing of the person's throat, as in an assault. The first two conditions may occur accidentally, e.g. a tie may become caught in machinery.

Symptoms and Signs

- Body may still be suspended.
- General symptoms and signs of asphyxia.
- Congestion of the face and neck with the veins becoming prominent.
- Constriction may still be visible around neck (e.g. a scarf), or it may be hidden in the folds of the skin (e.g. wire).
- There may be marks around the casualty's throat or neck where a constriction has been removed.

Aim: Restore adequate breathing and arrange removal to hospital.

Treatment

- Remove the constriction from around the casualty's neck immediately, supporting the weight of her body if she is

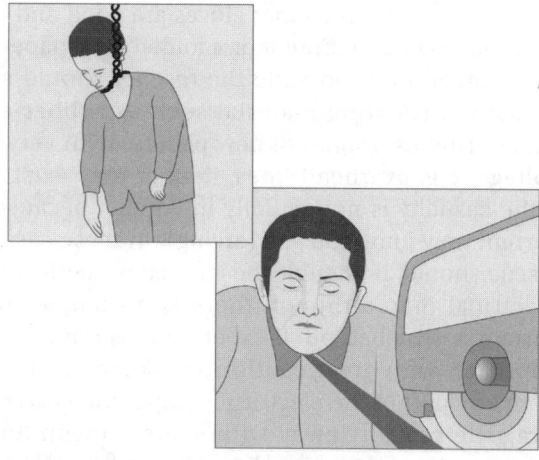

Fig. 30.45: Airway obstruction by hanging, strangling or throttling.

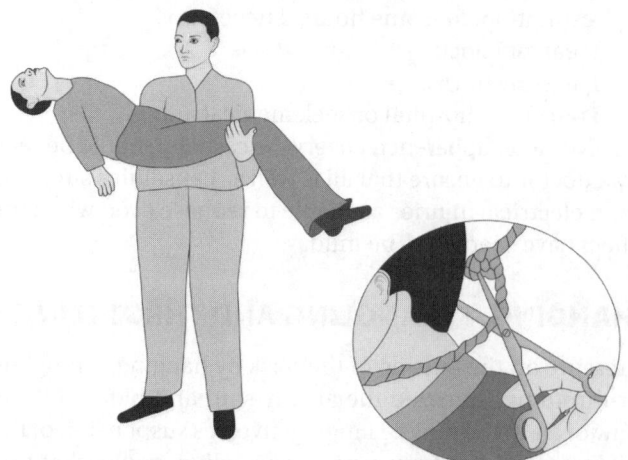

Fig. 30.46: First aid measures of hanging, strangling or throttling.

hanging. If there is a knot, cut below it (a knot is difficult to cut and it may be useful evidence).
- If the casualty is unconscious, open her airway and check breathing. Complete the ABC of resuscitation if required and place the casualty in the recovery position.
- Arrange the removal to hospital. Note: Seek medical aid even if recovery seems complete.

BANDAGING FIRST AID

A bandage is any gauze or cloth material used for any of the purpose to support to hold or to immobilize the body part.

Bandaging is a technique of application of specific roller bandages to different parts of body.

Purpose of Bandaging

- To control bleeding by pressure
- To immobilize sprained or fractured limb.
- To hold a dressing or compress in place.
- To secure splints in case of fracture of deformity
- To protect open wound from contaminants.
- To provide support and aid in case of varicose veins or impaired circulation.

General Principles

- The patient should be placed in a comfortable position and it should be convenient for the nurse.
- The position of the part to be band aged should be well supported and elevated if necessary.
- The nurse should stand directly in front of the patient or facing part to be bandaged.
- A bandage should accomplish its purpose. It may be used to hold dressing in place, to support a part or to immobilize.
- Apply and fix bandage at least two circular turns around part is its smallest diameter, so that it can stay in place.
- Skin surfaces should be separated. They may be separated by either gauze or cotton. In the application of casts, special padding is used over bony prominences.
- Always bandage to the right.
- Exert even pressure as far as possible. The bandage should be done in the direction of the venous circulation.
- Do not cover the ends of the finger or toes, unless it is necessary in order to cover the injury. It is necessary to observe circulatory changes.
- Never apply a wet bandage as when is applied, it tends to shrink and become tight as it dries.
- Do not apply a bandage too loosely because it may slip and expose the wound.
- All turns of bandage should be made clockwise unless there is some special reason for doing otherwise, the roll should be held in the palm of the hand, with the free end of the bandage coming from the part of the roll.
- Applying bandage, secure terminal extremity by pinning with safety pins or strapping adhesive.

- Remove bandages by gathering folds in a loose mass. Passing mass from one hand to the other.
- Examine the bandage part frequently for pain, swelling, etc.

TYPES OF BANDAGES (FIG. 30.47)

- **Circular bandage:** The bandage is wrapped around the part with complete overlapping of the previous bandage turn. This is used primarily for anchoring a bandage where it is begun and where it is terminated.
- **Spiral bandage:** The bandage ascends in a spiral manner so that each turn overlaps the preceding one by one half or two-thirds the width of the bandage. The spiral turn is useful for the wrist, the finger and the trunk.
- **Figure-of-eight:** The figure-of-eight turn consists of making oblique overlapping turns that ascend and descend alternatively. It is effective for use around joints, such as knee, elbow and ankle.
- **Recurrent-stumps bandage:** After a few circular turns to anchor the bandage the initial end of the bandage is placed in the center of the body part being bandaged, well back from the tip to be covered. Recurrent bandages are used for gingers for the hand and for the stump of an amputated limb.
- **T-bandage:** It is used to secure rectal or perineal dressing. The double 'T' bandage is used for males and single 'T' bandages is for the females. The strips of the 'T' bandage are brought between the patients leg and is pinned to the waist band in front.

Materials Used for Bandage

- Gauze
- Muslin

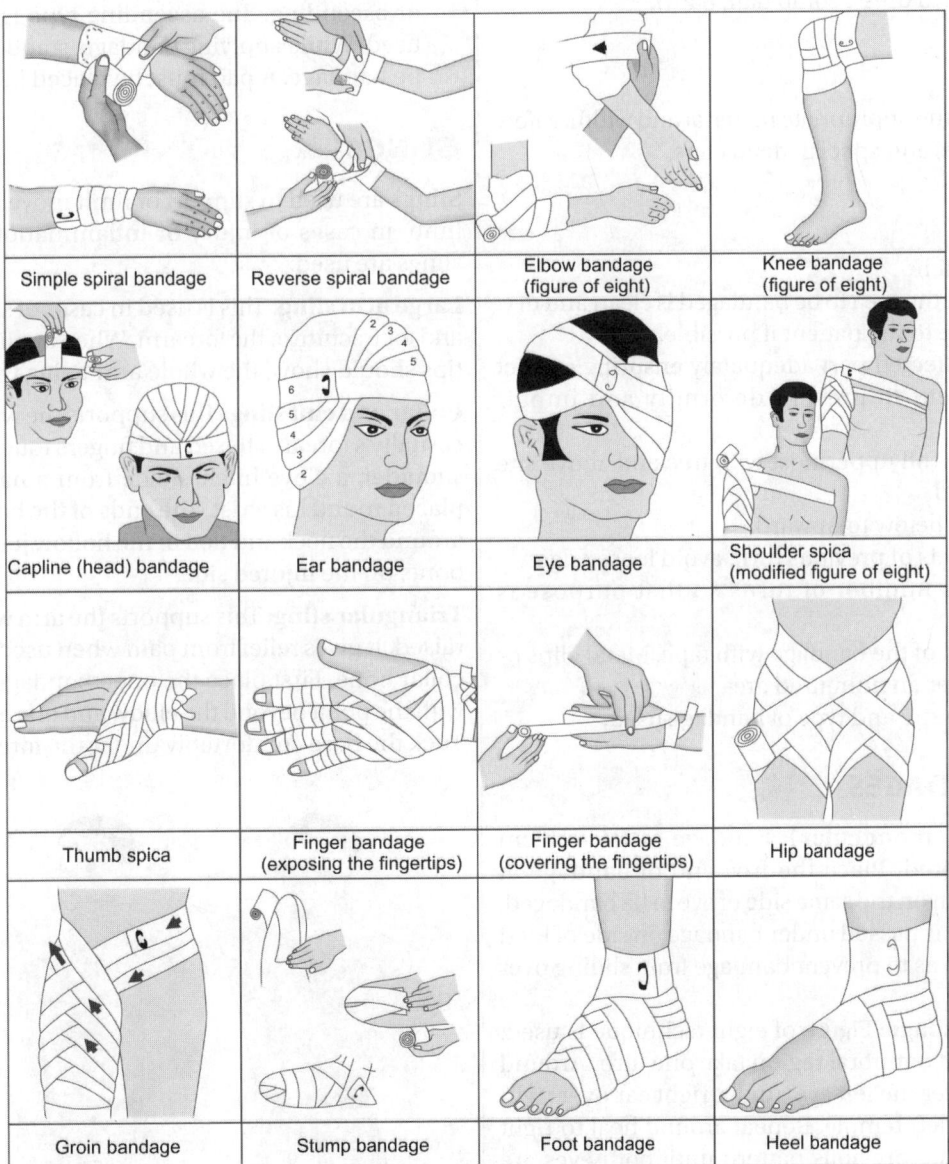

Fig. 30.47: Types of bandages.

- Rubber
- Elastic
- Flannel
- Crinoline for plaster
- Adhesive.

Assessing before Applying Bandage

- Inspect and palpate the area for swelling.
- Inspect for the presence of and status of wounds.
- Note the presence of drainage (amount, color, odor and velocity).
- Inspect and palpate for adequacy of circulation (skin temperature, color and sensation)
- Ask the patient about any pain experienced (location, intensity, onset and quality).
- Assess the ability of the patient to reapply the bandage when needed.
- Assess the capabilities of the patient regarding activities of daily living (to dress, comb hair, bath).

Equipment

Clean bandage of the appropriate material and width, safety pin, adhesive tape, and special metal clips.

Procedure

- Explain to patient.
- Make sure that the area to be bandaged is clean and dry.
- Stand opposite to the patient if possible.
- Support the affected part adequately ensuring correct body alignment to prevent deformity and impair circulation.
- Keep bandage roll uppermost with free and above site to be bandaged.
- Bandage from below to upward.
- Cover two-thirds of previous turn, avoid loose edges.
- Take requires number of turns so that purpose is achieved.
- Secure the end of the bandage with tape. Metal clips or a safety pin over an uninjured area.
- Document the site and type of bandage used.

SPECIAL BANDAGES

- **Eye bandage (monocular):** Bandage of 1½ to 2 cm width is required. Place the free end of bandage at temporal region on the same side of eye to be bandaged. A piece of tape is passed under bandage on side of food eye and tied so as to prevent bandage from sliding over good eye.
- **Bioccular bandage:** Figure of eight technique is used. Start form right temporal region take one turn. Around head, down over the left eye, under right ear over right eye to right to left temple. Repeat around heal to right temple following previous pattern until both eyes are covered.
- **Ear-mastoid bandage:** Bandage with 2 feet width and 5 yards length is required make circular turns around head above ears, beginning on affected side. Follow with circular turns. The first turn is taken beneath occiput, and carried high over to opposite side of head below ear.
- **Jaw barton bandage:** Used in fracture of lower jaw and to hold dressing on chin. Bandage of 2 inches width and 5 to 6 yards length is required. Begin at nape of neck below occiput, carry bandage obliquely up, behind and close to ear, then under chin and up in front of left ear to top of head.
- **Cape line bandage (head bandage):** A double roller bandage of 2 feet width and 8 yards length is required. Place centre of bandage in middle of forehead and carry roller in opposite direction to occipital. Cross rollers one over other. The roller in inferior position in brought over head to middle of forehead.
- **Shoulder spica:** A bandage of 2½ inches width and 8 yards is required. The spica may be either descending or ascending. The ascending type is most commonly used. While applying bandage, stand at side which is to be bandage. A pad must be placed in axilla.

SLINGS

Slings are used to support or limit movement of the upper limb, in cases of injury or inflammation. Three types of slings are used:

Large arm sling: This is used in cases of simple rib fracture and for fracture of the forearm. When applied, only the finger tips should show, the whole arm being well supported.

Collar and cuff sling: This supports the wrist only. With the casualty's forearm flexed and fingers touching the opposite shoulder, a clove hitch, made from a narrow bandage, is placed round his wrist. The ends of the bandages are taken around the neck and tied in the hollow just above the collar bone, on the injured side.

Triangular sling: This supports the arm with the hand well raised. It gives relief from pain when used in fracture of the collar bone. First place the open bandage across the chest with the point beyond the elbow and one end over the hand. Tuck the base comfortably under the forearm.

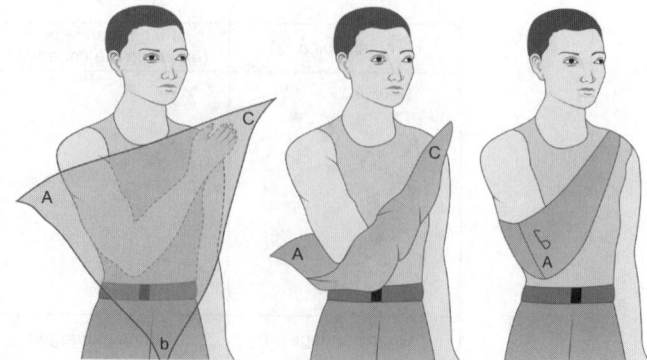

Fig. 30.48: Triangular sling application technique.

Take the end behind the elbow across the back and tie to the first end with the knot just in front of the shoulder, on the uninjured side. Fold in the point and fix the bandage with the safety pin.

Improvised slings: The lower edge of the casualty's coat or shirt may be turned up and pinned to support the arm, or the hand may be passed inside a buttoned up coat. A muffler, tie or other suitable cloth may be used to support the arm.

Bandage for the scalp: Place the open bandage on the head with the point at the back. Fold a narrow hem at the base, place it just above the eyebrows, then take the two ends backwards, cross them below the occiput with the point underneath, then back to the forehead where they are tied. Draw the point down and then upwards, and fix it with a safety pin.

BINDER

Abdominal support is made from extra-strong, single wide panel of elastic containing heat resistant rubber with high modulous of elasticity. Hook loop closures provide perfect fitting of the belt around the waist, controlled compression, its quick, easy application and removal. Flexi nylon splints ensure no wrinkles, no buckling and no rolling over of the belt. It doesn't show up from the clothes because of its sleek construction. After a number of surgical procedures, surgeons may also advocate the use of an abdominal binder. The compression of the binder is thought to help keep organs in place and promote better breathing function. Hospitals generally choose binders that allow for putting in drainage tubes to surgery sites if needed. Sometimes the surgical area is merely wrapped closely in stretchy fabrics or fabrics like gauze and this material can be cut in places to allow for tube placement if needed.

Definition

A binder bandage is designed for a specific body part for example; the triangular binder (sling) fits the arm. Binders are used to support large areas of the body such as the abdomen, arm or chest.

Binders are special wide bandages used for supporting specific parts of body and large dressings. Binder (abdominal) also called many tailed bandage. It is a rectangular piece of strong cloth with many tails attached to either sides of its. It is commonly used as abdominal binder for the support of the abdominal musculature.

Purpose of Binder

It is applied after paracentesis and child births in order to maintain the intra-abdominal pressure and to prevent shock and collapse.
a. To hold dressing in place.
b. To support abdomen and prevent would dehiscence following abdominal surgery.

Types of Binder

- **T- binders:** Are used to secure dressing on the rectum and perineum and in the groin. The single T-binder is used for female patients and the double T-binder is used for male patients.
- **Sling:** A sling is used to support and arm. Most healthcare agencies use commercial strap slings or sleeve slings.
- **Straight binders:** A straight binder is a straight piece of material, usually about 15 to 20 cm (6 to 8 inches) wide and long enough to more than circle the torso. It is used for the chest and the abdomen.
- **Breast binder:** To provide pressure on the breast (e.g. when drying up the milk flow after childbirth) or to support the breast (eg. after surgery).

Equipment

- Appropriate binder, abdominal pads as required
- For pads and safety pins/clips/velcro.

Procedure

- Collect equipment and assemble at bedside.
- Explain procedure to patient.
- Place patient in comfortable lying or sitting Position, supporting the area as appropriate.
- Clean and dry the area. Place the dressing pad adequately on would.
- Apply the binder in appropriate manner:
  Abdominal binder: Keep the patient in a supine position, so that the patient is flat in the bed. The patient should lie on the binder with tails equally extended to either side.
  T-binder: Secure waist strap in front by using pin or tie. Bring single or double T-straps between patient's legs and secure over strap in middle using a second pin.
  Breast binder: Encircle chest with binder, overlap and secure in middle of chest. Pull shoulder straps tight and secure in front just below shoulder line. Place patient in comfortable position.
- Document in nurses record date and time, type, area and reason for applying binder.

COMMUNITY EMERGENCIES

Disasters are sudden, catastrophic events that disrupt patterns of life and in which there is possible loss of life and property in addition to multiple injuries. Disasters can

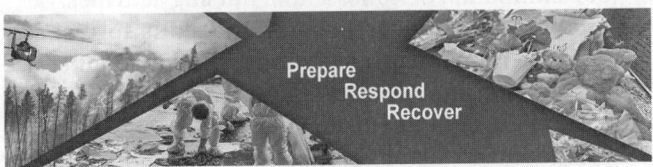

Fig. 30.49: Disaster management process.

be either natural or man-made. The extent of disruption of services and administration of emergency care during a disaster depends on the extent of the disaster and the preparedness of the community. Disasters are not confined to a particular part of he world, they can occur anywhere and at any time.

Major emergencies and disasters have occurred throughout history and as the world's population grows and resources become more limited communities are increasingly becoming vulnerable to the hazards that cause disaster. Disaster is catastrophic occurrence that invariably has profound implication of public health. It is a destructive event that results in the need for a wide range of emergency resources to assist and ensure the survival of the disease stricken. Any disaster is an emergency situation and the health sector alone cannot tackle it in isolation. Local community civil defence, army, police, fire brigade, government organization, non-governmental bodies and voluntary organizations should combine to reverse the effects of disaster management.

Goals of Disaster Nursing

The overall goal of disaster nursing is to achieve the best possible level of health for the people and the community involved in the disaster.

Other goals of disaster nursing are the following:
- To meet the immediate basic survival needs of populations affected by disasters (water, food, shelter, and security).
- To identify the potential for a secondary disaster.
- To appraise both risks and resources in the environment.
- To correct inequalities in access to health care or appropriate resources.
- To empower survivors to participate in and advocate for their own health and well-being.
- To respect cultural, lingual, and religious diversity in individuals and families and to apply this principle in all health promotion activities.
- To promote the highest achievable quality of life for survivors.

Principles of Disaster Nursing

The basic principles of nursing during special (events) circumstances and disaster conditions include:
- Rapid assessment of the situation and of nursing care needs.
- Triage and initiation of life-saving measures first.
- The selected use of essential nursing interventions and the elimination of nonessential nursing activities.
- Adaptation of necessary nursing skills to disaster and other emergency situations. The nurse must use imagination and resourcefulness in dealing with a lack of supplies, equipment, and personnel.
- Evaluation of the environment and the mitigation or removal of any health hazards.
- Prevention of further injury or illness.
- Leadership in coordinating patient triage, care, and transport during times of crisis.
- The teaching, supervision, and utilization of auxiliary medical personnel and volunteers.
- Provision of understanding, compassion, and emotional support to all victims and their families

Types of Disaster

Disasters are classified in various ways, on the basis of its origin/cause:
- Natural disasters
- Man-made disasters

And on the basis of speed of onset:
- Sudden onset disasters
- Slow onset disasters

Natural Disasters

A serious disruption triggered by a natural hazard (hydrometeorological, geological or biological in origin) causing human, material, economic or environmental losses, which exceed the ability of those affected to cope. Natural hazards can be classified according to their (1) hydrometeorological, (2) geological or (3) biological origins.

- **Hydrometeorological disaster:** Natural processes or phenomena of atmospheric hydrological or oceanographic nature. Phenomena/Examples: Cyclones, typhoons, hurricanes, tornados, storms, hailstorms, snowstorms, cold spells, heat waves and droughts.
- **Geographical disaster:** Natural earth processes or phenomena that include processes of endogenous origin or tectonic or exogenous origin such as mass movements, Permafrost, snow avalanches. Phenomena/Examples: Earthquake, tsunami, volcanic activity, mass movements landslides, surface collapse, geographical fault activities etc.
- **Biological disaster:** Processes of organic organs or those conveyed by biological vectors, including exposure to pathogenic, microorganism, toxins and bioactive substances. Phenomena/Examples: Outbreaks of epidemics diseases, plant or animal contagion and extensive infestation etc.

Human-induced Disasters

A serious disruption triggered by a human-induced hazard causing human, material, economic or environmental losses, which exceed the ability of those affected to cope. These can be classified into: (1) Technological disaster and; (2) Environmental degradation.
- **Technological disaster:** Danger associated with technological or industrial accidents, infrastructure failures or certain human activities which may cause the loss of life or injury, property damage, social or economic disruption or environmental degradation,

sometimes referred to as anthropological hazards. Examples include industrial pollution, nuclear release and radioactivity, toxic waste, dam failure, transport industrial or technological accidents (explosions fires spills).

- **Environmental degradation:** Processes induced by human behaviors and activities that damage the natural resources base on adversely alter nature processes or ecosystems. Potentials effects are varied and may contribute to the increase in vulnerability, frequency and the intensity of natural hazards. Examples include land degradation, deforestation, desertification, wild land fire, loss of biodiversity, land, water and air pollution climate change, sea level rise and ozone depletion.

Levels of Disaster

Goolsby and Kulkarni (2006) further classify disasters according to the magnitude of the disaster in relation to the ability of the agency or community to respond. Disasters are classified by the following levels:

Level I: If the organization, agency, or community is able to contain the event and respond effectively utilizing its own resources.

Level II: If the disaster requires assistance from external sources, but these can be obtained from nearby agencies.

Level III: If the disaster is of a magnitude that exceeds the capacity of the local community or region and requires assistance from state-level or even federal assets.

Disaster Management of Health Sector in India

- **National organization:** Under the Indian federal system, disaster management is a responsibility of state governments. Research survey guidelines and provisions of financial assistance to the state are the responsibilities of the central government. There is crisis managements group headed by the cabinet secretary and consisting of nodal ministers for nature disaster. In this event of a disaster a multi disciplinary central government team, at the invitation of the affected state conducts a disaster assessment and also makes recommendation for assistance.
- **State level organization:** Disaster preparedness as response in this state is usually delegated to relief and rehabilitation department or the department level is headed by the chief secretary of the government with participation of all other related agencies and departments.

  District level of organization: A district level coordination and review committee is constituted and headed by the collector as chairman with participation of all other related agencies and departments.
- **Community level helpers (CLHs):** Any community when faced with a disaster, the response to the situation by local people or group who immediately come forward to help. They are called the community level helpers (CLHs). They are a vital link between the affected population and the helping agencies (individuals, nongovernmental organization and governmental organizations)
- **Community level helpers** can provide psychological intervention through daily visits. During such visits the can talk about the survivors feeling and experiences impart health education, discuss health problems, motivate individuals to hold group meetings and organize educational activities. Community level helpers therefore have to educate the survivors about common stress reaction following a disaster and ways to cope with stress and the available resource.

Steps of Safety Measures during Disaster

The American Red Cross and the Federal Emergency Management Agency (FEMA), two well known authorities on disaster preparedness, response and recovery have devised a personal checklist to help individuals and families prepare for disaster they strike.

Step-1

- Find out what could happen to you?
- Determine what types of disaster are most likely to happen.
- Learn about your communities warning signals.
- Ask about postdiaster pre care (shelters usually will not accept pets).
- Review the disaster plans at your workplace, school and other places where your family spends time.
- Determine how to help elderly or disabled family members and neighbors.

Step-2

- Create a disaster plan
- Discuss the types of disaster that are most likely to happen and review what to do in each case.
- Pick two places to meet, including outside your home and outside your neighborhood.
- Choose an out of state friend to be your Family contact", It is easier to call long distance.
- Review evaluation plans, including care of pets. Identify ahead of time where to go if evaluation is necessary.

Step-3

- Complete this checklist
- Post-emergency phone numbers by phones
- Teach everyone how and when to call 911.
- Determine when and how to turn off water, gas and electricity at the main switches.
- Check adequacy of insurance coverage
- Local and review use of fire extinguisher
- Install and maintain smoke detectors.

- Conduct a home hazard hunt and fix potential hazards.
- Stock emergency supplies and assemble a disaster supplies.
- Become certified in first aid and cardiopulmonary resuscitation
- Locate all escape routes from your home, find two ways out of each room.
- Find the safe spots in your home for each type of disaster.
- Review plan for every 6 months.
- Conduct fire and emergency evaluation drills.
- Replace stored water every 3 months and stored food every 6 months.
- Test and recharge fire extinguisher according to manufacturer's instructions
- Test your smoke detectors monthly and change the batteries at least once a year.

CONCLUSION

First aid is the provision of initial care for an illness or injury. It is usually performed by a non-expert person to a sick or injured person until definitive medical treatment can be accessed. Certain self-limiting illnesses or minor injuries may not require further medical care past the first aid intervention. It generally consists of a series of simple and in some cases, potentially life-saving techniques that an individual can be trained to perform with minimal equipment. First aid is the initial assistance or treatment given to causality for any injury or sudden illness before the arrival of an ambulance, doctor or qualified person.

First aid is a skill based knowledge, training and experience. Practice of first aid is sometimes messy, smelly and distasteful and the first aider may be afraid that you will not be able to cope with unpleasantness. Certain skills are considered essential to the provision of first aid and are taught ubiquitously. Particularly the "ABC"s of first aid, which focus on critical life-saving intervention, must be rendered before treatment of less serious injuries. ABC stands for airway, breathing, and circulation.

BIBLIOGRAPHY

1. Alice L Price. The Art, Science and Spirit of Nursing. Philadelphia, WB Saunders Company, 3rd edition; 1968.
2. Harkness-Hood G, Dincher, JR. Total Patient Care: Foundations and Practice of Adult Health Nursing, 8th edition. St. Louis: Mosby-Year Book, Inc; 1992.
3. Kozier Barbara B, Du Gas Beverly Witter. Fundamentals of Patient Care: A Comprehensive Approach to Nursing. WB Saunders Company; 1967.
4. Kurzen CR. Contemporary Practical/Vocational Nursing, 2nd edition. Philadelphia: JB. Lippincott; 1992.
5. Potter PA, Perry AG. Fundamentals of Nursing Concepts, Process and Practice, 3rd edition. St. Louis: Mosby-Year Book, Inc;1993.
6. Shafer Kathleen, et al. Medical-Surgical Nursing, 6th edition. Saint Louis, C V Mosby Co; 1975.
7. Shakuntala Sharma 'Birpuri'. Principles and Practice of Nursing. Jaypee Brothers Medical Publishers (P) Ltd, New Delhi; 1997.
8. Sr. Nancy. Principles and Practice of Nursing, Vol. 1, 3rd edition. NR Brother's Indore; 1992.
9. Taylor C, Lillis C, LeMone P. Fundamentals of Nursing: The Art and Science of Nursing Care. Philadelphia: JB. Lippincott; 1993.
10. Thresvamma CP. Fundamentals of Nursing, Procedure Manual for General Nursing Course. PC Mathew, Kottayam, Kerala; 1992.
11. Timby BK, Lewis LW. Fundamental Skills and Concepts in Patient Care, 5th edition. Philadelphia: JB Lipcpincott, Co; 1992.
12. Virginia Henderson. Principles and Practice of Nursing. New York, MacMillan Publishing Co; 1970.

REVIEW QUESTIONS

Long Essays

1. Define first aid, explain the aims. Objectives and principles of first aid.
2. Define wounds, explain the types and first aid measures of wounds.
3. Explain different techniques and methods of transporting causalities.

Short Essays

1. Golden rules of first aid.
2. Hemorrhage: Types and first aid.
3. Shock: Types and first aid.
4. Fracture: Types and first aid.
5. First aid in injuries to joints and muscles.
6. Respiratory emergencies types and first aid.
7. Burns and scalds.
8. Basic cardiac life support.
9. First aid for foreign bodies in the eye, ear, nose, and throat.
10. General rules for the treatment of poisoning.
11. First Aaid in convulsions.
12. Epitasis.
13. Hanging, strangling and throttling.
14. Bandaging first aid.
15. Principles of disaster nursing.
16. Community emergencies.

Short Answers

1. Advanced life support (ALS).
2. Basic life support (BLS).
3. Importance of first aid.
4. First aid kit.
5. Dislocation.
6. Lifting casualties.
7. Fireman's lift.
8. Asphyxia.
9. Types of bandages.
10. Slings.
11. Types of binder.

CHAPTER 31
Meeting Needs of Perioperative Patients

LEARNING OBJECTIVES

- Definition and concepts of perioperative nursing
- Preoperative phase: Preparation of patient for surgery
- Intraoperative phase: Operation theater set-up and equipment and role of nurse
- Postoperative phase: Recovery unit, postoperative care
- Wounds: Types, classification, wound healing process, factors affecting wound healing, complications of wound, surgical asepsis, care of wound types, equipment, and procedure and special considerations
- Dressing: Suture care
- Care of drainage

TERMINOLOGY

- **Perioperative care:** Perioperative care is the care that is given before, during and after surgery. It takes places in hospitals, in surgical centers attached to hospitals, in freestanding surgical centers or health care providers' offices. This period is used to prepare the patient both physically and psychologically for the surgical procedure and after surgery.
- **Perioperative nurse:** Perioperative nurses are registered nurses (RN) who work in hospital surgical departments, day surgery unit (also called ambulatory surgery) clinics and physician's office. They work closely with the surgical patients, family members and other health care professionals to help plan, implement and evaluate treatment.
- **Perioperative nursing:** Perioperative nursing includes those activities performed by the professional registered nurse in the preoperative, intraoperative and postoperative phases of surgery.
- **Operation room nurse:** Operation room (OR) nurse are referred to as perioperative nurse to meet accurately reflect their specialized duties.
- **Scrub nurse:** Selecting and passing instruments and supplies used for the operation to maintain a safe and comfortable environment.
- **Postoperative period:** The postoperative period begins after the transfer to the PACU and terminates with the resolution of the surgical sequelae. It is quite common for this period to end outside of the care of the surgical team.
- **Preoperative phase:** This phase begins when the decision for surgical intervention is made and ends when the patient is transferred from the operating room.
- **Intraoperative phase:** This phase begins when the patient is admitted or transferred to the surgery department and ends when he or she is admitted to the recovery area.
- **Nursing process:** The nursing process is cyclical, that is the component of the nursing process follows a logical sequence, but more than one component may be involved at any given time. The nursing process provides a framework for accountability in nursing.
- **Ectomy:** A suffix denoting removal or excision of a structure e.g. hysterectomy (removal of the uterus).
- **Orrhaphy:** A plastic or repair operation, e.g. perineorrhaphy (repair of the perineum). The ending plasty is also used, to describe a plastic operation where the aim is to rebuild and restore tissue destroyed by injury or disease.
- **Oscopy:** Inspection of the interior of an organ or passage by means of special instruments, usually carrying a light, e.g. cystoscopy (examination of the bladder by means of a cystoscope).
- **Ostomy:** Constructing an artificial opening into an organ, e.g. gastrostomy (makes an opening from the stomach on to the surface of the abdomen).
- **Otomy:** Incising or dividing a structure, e.g. laparotomy (incising and opening the abdomen), tenotomy (dividing a tendon).
- **Sterile supply room:** The sterile supply room is a clean area and houses all sterilized and packaged instruments and supplies needed for surgery.
- **Scrub sink areas:** Scrub sink areas are found in various locations close to the operating suites. Caps, masks, antiseptic soap, scrub brushes and eyeglass defogging agents are located at each scrub station.

- **Equipment room:** The equipment room is used to store large apparatus, such as the operating microscope, image intensifier and laser machine.
- **Housekeeping supply room:** The housekeeping supply room is area where supplies used to decontaminate the surgical suites and those used in general operating room cleanup are stored.
- **Anesthesia supply room:** As the name suggests, the anesthesia supply room is where all equipment needed by the anesthesiologists is stored. Anesthesia machines, hoses, catheters, airway devices, and other equipment are located in this area.
- **Substerile rooms:** Substerile rooms are located between one or more operating suites. These rooms typically contain a refrigerator for small tissue grafts, medications, and solutions.
- **Post-anesthesia care unit** The post-anesthesia care unit (PACU) is located immediately adjacent to the operating room and is supervised by that department and nursing and administrative personnel. Patients are taken to the PACU immediately following surgery so that they can be continuously monitored while emerging from general or light anesthesia.
- **Ablative surgery:** Surgery performed to remove a diseased organ or other tissue.
- **Biopsy:** The removal and examination of tissue from the living body.
- **Constructive surgery:** Surgery to repair a malformed organ or tissue.
- **Elective surgery:** Surgery performed for a person's well-being, but not absolutely necessary for life.
- **Exploratory surgery:** Surgery performed to confirm the extent of the pathologic process and sometimes to confirm a diagnosis.
- **Frozen section:** A technique used in biopsy procedures where tissue specimens are removed from a patient with a microtome, are rapidly frozen, and then examined for a possible malignancy.
- **Palliative surgery:** Surgery performed to relieve the symptoms of a disease process, e.g. removal of portions of a cancerous brain tumor which will help relieve a patient of some symptoms, but will not lead to a cure because total removal is not possible.
- **Reconstructive surgery:** Surgery performed to repair tissues whose function or appearance is damaged, e.g. plastic surgery.
- **Aseptic technique:** Methods and practices that prevent cross-contamination in surgery.
- **Closed gloving:** Method of donning sterile gloves when a surgical gown is worn.
- **Fallout contamination:** Contamination of a sterile surface by particles arising from a source above it.
- **Open gloving:** Method of donning sterile surgical gloves when a gown is not worn.
- **Strikethrough contamination:** Contamination of a sterile surface by moisture that has originated from a nonsterile surface and penetrated the protective covering of the sterile item.
- **Surgical scrub:** Precise method by which all team members who will be working in sterile attire scrub their hands and arms before performing an operation.
- **Anesthesia:** Loss of feeling sensation, especially loss of the sensation of pain with loss of protective reflexes in a part or in the whole of the body, usually induced by drugs.
- **Anesthesiologist** is a specialist in the science or art of anesthesia.
- **Nurse anesthetist** is a nurse who is specially trained and obtained certificate of anesthesiology.
- **Anesthetic agent:** It is a drug or agent used to induce anesthesia.
- **Extubation:** Removal of endotracheal tube.
- **General anesthesia** is a type of anesthesia that works by putting the entire body to sleep. It is most often used during emergency or extensive surgery. Medications are used to prevent pain, relax the muscles, and regulate body functions. When the surgery is over, medications are given to reverse the process.
- **Intubation:** This is the process of inserting one end of a tube, called an endotracheal tube, into airway.
- **Patient-controlled analgesia (PCA):** Analgesia simply means relief of pain. PCA is a method by which the patient controls the amount of pain medicine (analgesia) he/she receive.

INTRODUCTION

Perioperative nursing includes activities performed by the registered nurse during preoperative, intraoperative and postoperative phases of the patient's surgical experiences. Surgery became a medical specialty, because often the treatment of a wide variety of illness and injuries include some types of surgical interventions. Surgery is an invasive method of treatment that may be planned or unplanned, major or minor, and that may involve any body part or system. Care for the client during all phases of the surgical experience needs to be continuous, and integrated surgical procedures require physical and psychosocial adaptations and are stressors for both the client and the family. The client's recovery from a surgical procedure requires skillful and knowledgeable nursing care whether the surgery is of outpatient or in the hospital setting. Nurses working in both settings must understand the principles of caring for surgical clients.

DEFINITION AND CONCEPT OF PERIOPERATIVE NURSING

- Perioperative nursing refers to the role of the nurse during the preoperative, intraoperative and postoperative phases of a client's surgical experience. The concept

of perioperative nursing stresses the importance of providing continuity of care.
- A perioperative nurse is defined as the registered nurse, who, using the nursing process, designs, coordinates and delivers care to meet the identified needs of the clients whose protective reflexes or self-care abilities are potentially compromised because they are under the influence of anesthesia during operative or other invasive procedures.
- Perioperative nurse possesses and applies knowledge of the procedure and the client's intraoperative experience throughout the client-care continuum. And also they assess, diagnose, plan, intervene and evaluate the outcome of interventions based on criteria and support of a standard care targeted towards the population.
- The perioperative nurse addresses the changing physiological, pathophysiological, sociocultural and spiritual responses of the client that have been initiated by the prospect of performance of the invasive procedure.

Objectives of Perioperative Nursing

The nurse must have a basic understanding of operating room techniques. She plays an important role to plan and manage the care during different phases in order to meet individualized needs. She must have the knowledge about the operative site and procedure, effect of the anesthesia and the operative trauma to the patient. The nurse can participate in perioperative nursing.
- To apply nursing process to nursing actions.
- To promote an understanding of the patient's total surgical experience by demonstrating the ability to assess physiologic, psychologic and sociologic patient needs.
- To reinforce basic knowledge of the total patient experience as a basis for management of preoperative patient's anxiety related to body image and postoperative pain related to intraoperative procedure.
- To assist the patient to relieve anxiety preoperatively and by assessing their needs for psychologic support.
- To recognize the effects of preoperative medications, anesthesia, positioning at procedure as the basis for planning the patient's postoperative recovery and rehabilitation.
- To become an effective communicator with patients through preoperative and postoperative teaching based on the knowledge of the intraoperative procedure.

Phases of Perioperative Nursing

- **Preoperative phase:** This is the phase of the patient's surgical experience begins when the decision is made to undergo surgical intervention. This phase ends when the patient is transferred to the operating table. During this phase, the nurse gathers data by doing assessment and plan components of nursing process. The nurse identifies the patient's physiologic, psychologic and spiritual needs and finds existing or potential problems. Nursing activities range from a baseline assessment of the client during the preoperative interview and continues with assessment in the preadmission unit, client room, holding area, or induction room on the day of surgery. Before surgery, the nurse prepares the client and family for the surgery, performs diagnostic tests, and assesses the client in preparation for the operation.
- **Intraoperative phase:** This phase begins with transfer of the patient to the operating table and extends to the time the patient is admitted to the recovery area. In this phase, nursing interventions range from communicating the clients plan of care, identifying nursing activities, necessary for expected outcome and establishing priorities for nursing actions. During surgery, the nurse assists surgeons and other operating room nurses to ensure that the client receives optimal care. The nurse also coordinates client needs with team members and personnel's from other disciplines, coordinates the use of the supplies and equipment, controls the environment, prepares for potential emergencies, and communicates and documents the client's plan of care.
- **Postoperative phase:** This phase begins with admission of the patient to the recovery area which includes post-anesthesia care unit or an intensive care unit. This phase ends when the surgeon discontinues follow-up-care. It begins with the client's transfer to an area for recovery and ends with client's recovery from surgery. Nursing activities range from communicating pertinent information about the client's surgery, to assist the client to improve physical stability and wakefulness and institute measures to help the client achieve maximum recovery.

Classifications of Surgical Procedures

Surgery can be defined as the art and science of treating diseases, injuries and deformities by operation and instrumentation. The surgical procedure involves the interaction of the patient, the surgeon, and the nurse. Surgical procedures usually are classified on the basis of urgency, degree of risk, and purposes.
- **Based on urgency:** Surgery may be classified as elective surgery, urgent surgery and emergency surgery.
    - **Elective surgery:** It is preplanned and performed on the basis of client's choice. It is not essential and may not be necessary for health and delay in surgery has no ill effects, can be scheduled in advance based on the choice of client. The purposes of elective surgery are as follows:
        - To remove or repair a body part
        - To restore function
        - To improve health
        - To improve self-concept.

For example, tonsillectomy, hernia repair, cataract extraction and lens implant, hip prosthesis, hemorrhoiditis, etc.
- **Urgent surgery** in which the surgery is the necessity for the client's health, but not an emergency. This is performed for the purposes as in elective surgery and to prevent further tissue damage. For example, removal of gallbladder, coronary artery, removal of tumor, etc.
- **Emergency surgery:** When surgery must be done immediately to preserve the client's life, remove or repair body part, restore function, improve health and self concept. For example, control of hemorrhage, repair of trauma, perforated ulcer, intestinal obstruction, tracheostomy, cesarean section.
- **Based on degree of risk or seriousness:** Surgery has been classified as major or minor on the basis of risk for the client:
  - **Major surgery:** It involves extensive reconstruction or alteration in body parts poses great risks to wellbeing. It requires hospitalization usually prolonged to well-being; has a high degree of risk; involves major body organs, life threatening situations and potential postoperative complications. Major surgery may be elective, urgent, or emergency. For example, nephrectomy, cholecystectomy, colostomy, hysterectomy.
  - **Minor surgery:** It is primarily elective; it is usually a brief, carries low-risk and results in few complications. It can be performed in clinics, outpatient clinic and minor operation theaters. For example, teeth extraction, removal of warts, skin biopsy, laparoscopy, dilatations and curettage.
- **Based on purpose:** Surgical procedures based on purpose include diagnostic, ablative, palliative, reconstructive, transplant, constructive.
  - **Diagnostic:** It is surgical exploration that allows physician to make or to confirm diagnosis, may involve removal of tissue for further diagnostic testing. For example, breast biopsy, laparoscopy, bronchoscopy, exploratory laparotomy (incision in peritoneal cavity to inspect abdominal organs).
  - **Ablative:** It is excision or removal of diseased body part. For example, appendicectomy, subtotal thyroidectomy, partial gastrectomy, colon resection, amputation, cholecystectomy, etc.
  - **Palliative surgery:** It is performed to relieve or reduce intensity of an illness or disease symptoms will not produce cure. For example, colostomy, nerve root resection (rhizotomy) debridement of necrotic tissue, balloon angioplasty, arthroscopy, etc.
  - **Reconstructive surgery:** It is performed to restore function to traumatized or malfunctioning tissues and to improve self-concept. For example, scar revision, plastic surgery, skin graft, internal fixation of fractures, breast reconstruction.
  - **Transplant:** It is performed to replace organs or structures that are diseased or malfunctioning. For example, kidney, cornea, liver, heart, joints, total hip replacement.
  - **Constructive surgery:** It is performed to restore function lost or reduced as a result of congenital anomalies. For example, repair of cleft palate, closure of atrial defect in heart.

PREOPERATIVE NURSING

Preoperative nursing is based on the nurses understanding of several important characteristics including high quality multidisciplinary team work, effective and therapeutic communication and collaboration with the client, client's family and the surgical team.

Purpose

- Preoperative nursing care is the care given to the patient before surgery.
- The preoperative period for different type surgery is different, e.g. for emergency surgery preoperative period is very short, for a planned surgery time for surgery is fixed with the mutual consent of the surgeon and the patient.
- Preoperative care of the patient begins as soon as the surgeon makes with diagnosis and decides that an operation is necessary for the patient.

Preparation of the Patient on the Evening before Operation

- Remove all jewellery and hand over them to the relatives.
- Remove the lipstick and nail polish.
- Shave the area to be operated.
- After shaving ask the patient to have a thorough bath and dress in clean clothes.
- The patient should be reassured to prevent anxiety and fear of operation.

Preparation of the Patient on the Day of Surgery

- Help the patient to go to toilet and for mouth care.
- Remove hairpins, clips, ornaments, false teeth, etc.
- Comb and tie hair with a ribbon.
- Remind the patient and his relatives about the fasting before surgery.
- Check the orders for bowel preparation.
- Clean the operation site with soap and water thoroughly, dry the area with clean towel.
- Cover the site with sterile towel and fix if by means of bandages.

- Introduce nasogastric tube, urinary catheter if ordered.
- Stop all medications unless specifically ordered by the surgeon.
- **Psychological preparation:** Discuss with the patient to give full information about the surgery, such as:
  - Type of surgery
  - Consequences of surgery (if it is done and if it is not done).
  - The problems to be faced (disabilities expected)
  - Expected duration of hospitalization
  - Expected time of resuming duty (if employed)
  - Cost of surgery
  - Treatment/investigations done before surgery and its purpose
  - Necessary arrangements to be made about the family, financial matters, work, hospitalization, etc.

  Eradicate fear of operation from the patient:
  - Allow the patient to ask questions and clear all his doubts.
  - Introduce to the patient someone who had similar surgeries and successfully recovered from the symptoms.
  - Explain what happens during anesthesia.
  - Explain how to get rid of pain after surgery.
  - Tell the patient when he can have meals.
  - Answer all questions asked by the patient in a language he can understand, so that the patient will have confidence to undergo surgery.
  - Let the patient see the persons, places and equipment involved in his operation.
  - Always start the procedures with an explanation, so that it will inspire confidence in the medical team. The patient has to feel that he will be safe in the hands of the competent people during surgery.
  - For many patients, their admission to the hospital is a first experience in their lives. In such situation, the nurses should make them feel at home by eradicating their fear.
- **Meet the spiritual needs of the Patient**
  - Let the patient meet the ministers of his religion, if requested.
  - Obtain inform consent.
  - Build up the general health.
  - Preoperative teaching.
  - Surgical preparation.
  - Preparation of the patient on the evening before operation enema and bowel wash.
  - Preparation of the patient on the day of the surgery.
  - Sending the patient to operating room

Preparation of Skin

Preliminary Assessment

- Check the doctor's orders for the diagnosis and the orders for operation.
- Check the type of the operation to be done and the area to be prepared.
- In doubt, clarify with the surgeon, or at least with the seniors.
- Check the orders for specific precautions.
- Check the operative area for any skin lesion.
- Check the cleanliness of the skin to be prepared.
- Check the abilities and the limitations of the patient.
- Check the consciousness of the patient and the ability to follow instructions.
- Check whether the patient is getting any treatment and can be discontinued till the skin preparation is complete.
- Check whether the equipment are in working order. Check the equipment in the patient's unit.

Equipment

- Clean razor with sharp blade in a container.
- A bowl with the disinfectant.
- Shaving cream or soap jelly.
- Cotton tipped applicators.
- Scissors.
- Kidney tray and paper bag.
- Mackintosh and towel.

Equipment for Cleaning the Area and Dressing the Skin Area

- Basin with warm water.
- Wash clothes.
- Soap with soap dish.
- Spirit, mercurochrome, iodine
- Binders and safety pin
- A sterile tray containing sponge, holding forceps, cotton balls, dressing towel and gloves.

Purpose

- To shave the skin without scratches.
- To disinfect the razor after shaving.
- To lather the skin area for a wet shaves. The skin is soft when it is wet.
- To smear the cream on the area.
- To cut long hair, if any, and to cut short the nails.
- To receive the wastes.
- To protect the bed and garment. Dressing the skin area.
- To clean the area after the shave.
- To use as antiseptics on the skin.
- To secure the dressing towel in place.
- To clean and to paint the area.
- To cover the area after cleaning.
- To maintain the aseptic technique when dressing the area.

Preparation of the Patient and the Environment

- Identify the patient and explain the procedure to win his confidence and cooperation.

- Explain the sequence of the procedure and tell him how he can cooperate with you.
- Provide privacy with curtains, and drapes.
- Place the patient in a comfortable and relaxed position according to the part to be prepared.
- Give proper support to the body parts, if the patient has to raise it from mattress and hold it in a position for a considerable time.
- Arrange the equipment conveniently at the bedside.
- Close the doors and windows to prevent drought.
- Adjust the height of the bed according to the comfortable working of the nurse. Bring the patient to the edge of the bed.
- Fold back the upper bedding towards the foot end of the bed leaving a sheet or bath blanket over the patient. Expose the parts as necessary.
- Protect the bed with a mackintosh and towel.
- Remove the ornaments and the cosmetics used on the area to be prepared.
- Inspect the finger and toe nails. If long, cut short.

Procedure

- Wash hands to prevent cross infection
- Lather the area for the easy removal of the hair. The skin will be soft when it is wet.
- Shave the skin by holding the skin taut and the razor held at 45° angle to the skin and moved in the direction the hair is growing. Use short, firm but gentle strokes.
- This approach decreases the skin irritation and ensure complete removal of hairs.
- Rinse the area with soap and water and then with water alone, using the wash clothes. Thorough cleaning will remove the dirt and soap residue from the skin.
- Repeat the steps 2 to 4 times until the entire area has been prepared clean and no hair is visible. Dry the area.
- Discard the razor into the bowl with antiseptic. Disinfect the razor.
- Put on gloves, if available. Clean the area with spirit starting from the center to the periphery. Paint the area with either iodine or mercurochrome spirit, iodine and mercurochrome are antiseptics. If iodine is used special care should be taken to prevent blistering.
- Cover the operative area with the sterile towel and secure with binders.

After Care of the Patient and the Equipment

- Put on fresh gown.
- Adjust the position of the patient in bed. Rearrange the bed clothes.
- Remove the mackintosh and towel.
- Take all equipment to the utility room. Remove the razor from the disinfectant solution, discard the blade, clean it thoroughly, dry it and replace it in its proper place. All the equipment are cleaned, dried and replaced in their proper places.
- Wash hands
- Record the procedure on the nurse's notes with date and time.
- Record the area prepared and the condition of the skin.
- If there is time, send the patient for a thorough bath after shaving of the skin but before he is prepared for operation.
- Always entrust the patient to someone who will take responsibility of the patient while he is in the operation theater.

Obtain Informed Consent

- The nurses should get an informed consent from patient/guardian for each operation.
- Never compel them to give their consent.
- They should understand the language used in the consent form.
- Explain the complications that may occur in the period of anesthesia.

Sending the Patient to Operating Room

- Administer the premedications to the patient one hour before surgery.
- Check the vital signs.
- Write the patients name, age, sex, ward, bed no. diagnosis, hospital no. etc. on an identification card and fasten it on the dress or on arm to prevent mistaken identity.
- Ask the patient to void just before sending to operating room.
- Transfer the patient on to a patient trolley and cover him with clean sheets to prevent draught.
- Never leave the patient alone on trolley.
- Always send the patient charts with all reports.

Nurse's role and responsibilities: The nurse is responsible for the preparation and safety of the client on the day of surgery.

- **Skin preparation:** The skin is cleaned by scrubbing the operative site one or more times with an antiseptic soap or solution to remove bacteria. This can be done by the client while taking a bath or shower. Ideally, a shower is taken in the evening before the morning of surgery. Shampooing the hair and the cleaning of the fingernails also help to reduce number of organisms present. The incision area usually is shaved before surgery because hair serves as a reservoir of bacteria. Usually the operative area is washed before surgery with an antiseptic such as povidone iodine (Betadine) to clean and disinfect the skin.
- **Elimination:** The gastrointestinal tract needs special preparation on the evening before surgery to:
  - Reduce the possibility of vomiting and aspiration during anesthesia
  - Reduce the possibility of a bowel obstruction, and
  - Prevent contamination from fecal material during intestinal tract or bowel surgery.

Emptying the bowel in no longer routine procedure before surgery, but the nurse should use preoperative assessment to determine the need for an order of bowel elimination. If the client is scheduled for surgery of the GI tract, cleansing enema usually ordered. Insertion of an indwelling urinary catheter may be ordered before surgery, especially in clients having pelvic surgery, to prevent bladder distention or accidental injury. If an indwelling catheter is not in place, the client should void immediately before receiving premedication to ensure an empty bladder during surgery.

- **Nutrition and fluids.** Preparation involves restricting food and fluid. If a client undergoing surgery is to receive a general anesthesia, foods and fluids are restricted 8 to 10 hours before the operation. This restriction significantly reduces the possibility of aspirations of gastric contents, which can cause aspiration pneumonia. Most clients have an NPO status after midnight.
- **Rest and sleep:** These are important components in reducing stress before surgery and in healing and recovery after surgery. The nurse can facilitate rest and sleep in the immediate preoperative period by meeting psychological needs, carrying out teaching, providing a quiet environment, and administering prescribed bedtime sedative medication.

The nurse's responsibility on the day of surgery will include the following:

- Note allergies according to institutional policy.
- Take and record the vital signs, assess and report the abnormalities for elevated temperature.
- Check the identification band to make sure it is legible, accurate and securely fastened to the client.
- Be sure that informed consent has been obtained and is clearly documented.
- If a skin preparation has been ordered, check that it has been completed accurately and thoroughly.
- Check for carry out any special orders, such as administering enema or starting on line, recurred previous records, inserting nasogastric tube, giving medications.
- Verify that the client has not eaten for the last 8 hours. Check that fluids have been restricted although sometimes the physician will order clients to take their usual oral medication with a small sip of water.
- Ask the client to void measure and record the amount of urine (if indicated).
- Assist the client with oral hygiene if necessary. Help the client to remove jewellery to prevent loss or injury from swelling, during or after surgery. Many facilities allow the client to keep wedding band or mangala suthra (tali) on as long as they are taped securely. If Jewellery is removed, it should be stored according to policy or given to authorized member of her family.
- Remove all hairpins or hairpieces. This prevents injury to the client during surgery as well as possible loss or hairpieces or wigs.
- Remove colored nail polish from at least one nail for the pulse oximeter to allow intraoperative and postoperative assessment of skin and nail beds for circulation and oxygenation of tissues.
- If the client is wearing hearing aid, notify the operating room nurse.
- Remove all prosthesis, such as dentures, or partial plates, eye glasses, contact lenses and artificial limbs and store them safely (dentures may cause respiratory distress).
- Give the preoperative medications that are prescribed, either at a scheduled time or "on call". The commonly ordered medications are:
  - Sedatives and tranquilizers to alleviate anxiety and facilitate anesthesia induction, e.g. diazepam.
  - Anticholinesterase to decrease pulmonary and oral secretions, to prevent laryngospasm, e.g. atropine.
  - Narcotic analgesics to facilitate client's sedation and relaxation and to decrease the amount of anesthetic agent need, e.g. morphine.
  - Neuroleptic agents to cause a general state of calmness and sleepiness.

To prevent omissions and preoperative nursing intervention, most facilities supply nurses with a preoperative checklist. As each intervention on the list is completed, the nurse initials it. Documents through checklists and narrative charting, the nursing intervention carried out.

- Assist in moving client from the operating room stretcher when it is time to transport the client to surgery, ensuring accurate identification.

INTRAOPERATIVE PHASE: THREATER-SET-UP, EQUIPMENT AND ROLE OF NURSE

Intraoperative phase begins when the client enters the surgical site and ends with admission to the recovery area. Nursing care during this phase focuses on the client's emotional wellbeing, as well as on physical factors such as safety positioning, maintaining asepsis and controlling the surgical environment **(Fig. 31.1)**. The nurses are the client's advocates upon induction of anesthesia.

In the surgical holding area, the nurse is responsible for reviewing the record for completeness, ensuring proper identification of the client, client's safety and providing emotional support. It is important to deal with the fears and concerns of a frightened or agitated client. A relaxed client undergoes anesthetic induction easier than who is anxious. If the client still seems anxious despite sedation and reassurance, notify the surgeon or anesthesia personnel. Here the anesthesiologist sees the client, IV fluids starts

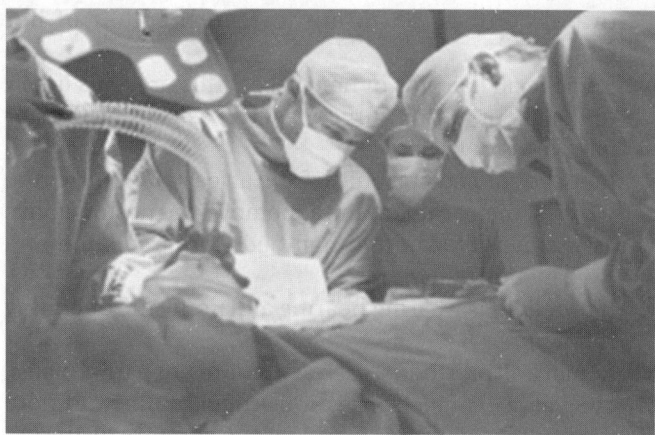

Fig. 31.1: Intraoperative care.

time him or her or nurse anesthetist. Nurse anesthetist also can administer medication needed during surgery. The procedures vary among institutions of heath care.

Definition: The term "intraoperative" refers to the time during surgery. Intraoperative care is patient care during an operation and ancillary to that operation. Activities such as monitoring the patient's vital signs, blood oxygenation levels, fluid therapy, medication transfusion, anesthesia, radiography, and retrieving samples for laboratory tests, are examples of intraopreative care. Intraopreative care is provided by nurses, anesthesiologists, nurse anesthetists, surgical technicians, surgeons, and residents, all working as a team.

Purpose of intraoperative care: The purpose of intraopreative care is to maintain patient safety and comfort during surgical procedures. Some of the goals of intraopreative care include maintaining homeostasis during the procedure, maintaining strict sterile techniques to decrease the chance of cross-infection, ensuring that the patient is secure on the operating table, and taking measures to prevent hematomas from safety strips or from positioning.

Anesthesia: Anesthesia means the absence of pain (Greek: an without + esthesis = feeling). Anesthesia is an artificially-induced state of partial or total loss of sensation, with or without loss of consciousness. Anesthesia produces muscle relaxation, blocks transmission of nerve impulses and suppresses reflexes. There are two types of anesthesia, i.e. general anesthesia and regional anesthesia.

General anesthesia: General anesthesia is a drug-induced depression of the central nervous system (CNS) that is reverted either by metabolic elimination in the body or by pharmacologic means. General anesthetic agents produce analgesia, amnesia and unconsciousness, characterized by loss of reflexes and muscle tone. There are four stages of anesthesia. Brief explanation and nursing intervention in these stages are as follows:

Onset starts from anesthetic administration to loss of consciousness. In this stage, client may be drowsy or dizzy and may experience auditory or visual hallucinations. Nursing action in this stage will include, close operating room doors, keeping room quiet, and stand by to assist client.

Excitement: Starts from loss of consciousness to loss of eyelid reflexes. Here there will be increase in automatic activity, irregular breathing. In such a case client may struggle.

Surgical anesthesia: This stage starts with loss of eyelid reflexes, to loss of motor reflexes and depression of vital functions. Here client is unconscious, muscles are relaxed and no blink or gag reflexes. In this stage, begins preparation (if indicated) only when anesthetists indicate stage III has been reached and client is under good control.

Danger (death) stage: Vital functions too depressed may lead to respiratory and circulatory failure. In this stage, client is not breathing and he may or may not have a heartbeat. If arrest occurs, nurse responses immediately to assist establishing airway, provides cardiac arrest tray, drugs, syringes, long needles, assist surgeon with closed or open cardiac massage.

General anesthesia can be administered by inhalation or intravenously. The selections of anesthetic agents are according to decision of the anesthesiologist. But continuous monitoring of side effects of the drugs and vital signs are essential.

Regional anesthesia: Regional anesthesia blocks the pain stimulus at the origin. Regional anesthesia produces a loss of painful sensation in only one region of the body and does not result in unconsciousness. The client may receive sedative that produces drowsiness.

The regional anesthetic agents block the conduction of impulses in nerve fiber without depolarizing the cell membrane are: Local agents and topical agents. An example of local agents is Bupivacaine HCL (Marcaine HCL) (Xylocaine) and examples of topical agents will include Benzocaine, Ethylchloride spray, Tetracaine HCL. All these agents have their own side effects. Contraindication for children. Test dose can be given prior to use, of these agents to know any allergies to these agents.

The types of regional anesthesia are as follows:
- Topical anesthesia
- Local infiltration anesthesia
- Field block anesthesia
- Peripheral nerve block anesthesia
- Spinal anesthesia
- Epidural anesthesia
- Caudal anesthesia.

The other types of anesthesia are used in modern drugs acupuncture, cryothermia and hypnoanesthesia. The type of anesthesia chosen depends on the surgery performed and level of unconsciousness desired.

Nursing care during surgery Nursing care during surgery will include providing emotional care, assisting the client with positioning (as require and for type of surgery). Maintaining safety, maintaining surgical asepsis, prevent client's heat loss, monitoring malignant hyperthermia, assisting with surgeon to perform surgery by providing proper equipments and supplies, assisting with wound closure, assessing drainage, and transferring client to recovery room.

Intraoperative Nursing Interventions

Nursing assessment of the intraopreative patient involves obtaining data from the patient and the patient's record to identify variables that can affect care and serve as guidelines for developing an individualized plan of patient care. The intraopreative nurse uses the focused preoperative nursing assessment documented on the patient record. This includes assessment of physiologic status (e.g. health-illness level, level of consciousness), psychological status (e.g. anxiety level, verbal communication problems, coping mechanisms), and physical status (e.g. surgical site, skin condition, and effectiveness of preparation; immobile joints), and ethical concerns.

Based on the assessment data, some major nursing diagnoses may include the following:
- Anxiety related to expressed concerns due to surgery or Operating room (OR) environment.
- Risk for perioperative positioning injury related to positioning in the OR
- Risk for injury related to anesthesia and surgery.
- Disturbed sensory perception (global) related to general anesthesia or sedation.

Based on the assessment data, potential complications may include the following:
- Nausea and vomiting
- Anaphylaxis
- Hypoxia
- Unintentional hypothermia
- Malignant hyperthermia
- DIC
- Infection.

Goals for care of the patient during surgery include reducing anxiety, preventing positioning injuries, maintaining safety, maintaining the patient's dignity and avoiding complications.

POSTOPERATIVE NURSING

The postoperative phase of surgery is final phase of the surgical experience. Nursing plays a critical role in returning the client to an optimal level of functioning. The postoperative period can be divided into two phases, i.e. immediate post-anesthesia and postoperative period, and later in postoperative phase.

Immediate Postoperative Phase

Immediate postoperative phase is the first few hours after surgery when the client is recovering from the effect of anesthesia. Here the nurse has to keep all emergency equipment and drugs, etc. for the use of patient's recovery from anesthesia and on admission to postoperative unit, the nurse performs the following (**Table 31.1**):
- Assess airway patency and support as needed, and assess for the presence of hoarseness, cramp, stridor, wheezes or decreased breath sounds
- Applies humidified oxygen via nasal cannula or facemask (unless otherwise ordered)
- Records vital signs (blood pressure, heart rate, strength and regularity, respiratory rate and depth, oxygen saturation, skin color, and temperature)
- Assess the client's level of consciousness, muscle strength and ability to follow commands
- Observe the client's IV infusions, dressings, drains and special equipment
- Remain at the client's bedside, continuing close observations of the client's conditions. After the client has been positioned safely and the baseline vital signs status has been ascertained, the nurse receives verbal report regarding surgery in detail, i.e. type of surgery, time of incision, patient's condition during surgery, type of anesthesia, sedative, all untoward incident happened and everything about surgery and documents the reliable and retainable information for further care that follow surgeon's and anesthetist's instructions for patient's recovery.

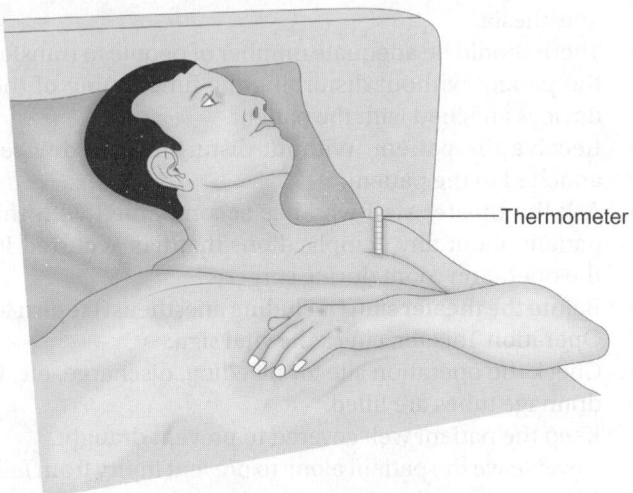

Fig. 31.2: Temperature measurement of postoperative patients.

TABLE 31.1: Postanesthetic assessment.

Sl. No.	Parameter	Assessment
1.	Airway	Patency, presence/adequacy of artificial airway
2.	Vital signs	Respiratory rate: depth, character, heart rate (pulse, pulse oximeter or cardiac monitor), blood pressure (cuff or arterial line)
3.	Pressure reading	Pulmonary artery wedge pressure, central venous pressure (CVP), intracranial pressure
4.	Level of consciousness	Ability to follow commands, sensation and ability to move extremities following regional anesthesia
5.	Patient position	Position to facilitate breathing, to prevent pressure on body parts or invasive lines and to promote comfort
6.	Tissue oxygenation	Skin: Color, temperature, moisture. Nail beds: Color, capillary refill. Lips/Oral mucosa: Color, pulse oximetry peripheral pulses: Presence strength
7.	Dressing/Suture lines	Dressing: Dry or minimal drainage, suture lines (if visible): Color approximation of wound edges
8.	Fluid lines/Tubes	Intravenous fluids: Rare, amount in bottle/bag/infusion site. Other lines (example, CVP line, arterial lines); patency, connection, character and amount of drainage. Ryle's tube drainage, urine output, quality and color. Note and record fluids coming out of dressing.

Preparation of Postanesthetics Bed and Reception of Tile Patient

- After sending the patient to operating room prepare a bed to receive the patient undergone surgery and anesthesia.
- There should be adequate number of people to transfer the patient without disturbing the functioning of the devices attached with the patient.
- Receive the patient. Without disturbing the devices attached to the patient.
- Ask the theater staff who has accompanied with the patient about any complications that has accurred in the operation room during surgery.
- Before the theater staff (including anesthetist) return to Operation Theater, check the vital sign.
- Check the operation site for bleeding, discharge, etc. if drainage tubes are filled.
- Keep the patient well covered to prevent draught.
- Never leave the patient alone to prevent injury from fall.
- Observe the patient for swallowing reflexes.
- Quickly observe the functioning of all devices and make sure they are in its functioning order.
- Check the doctor's order for other instruction and treatment.

Care of Patient Who is under the Effects of Anesthesia

- Patient needs close and diligent observation, until the patient fully recovers from anesthesia.
- A noisy breathing is indicative of airway obstruction that can occur due to the tongue falling back and obstructing the pharynx, apply suction immediately.
- Keep the patient in a suitable position that will be helpful to drain out the vomits, blood, secretions collected.
- The oropharyngeal airway left in the mouth of the patient should be removed as soon as the patient has required cough and swallowing reflexes.
- If the patient is cyanosed administer oxygen inhalation.
- In order to prevent injury from falls from bed, put a side rails on the bed.
- Keep the family informed of the successful completion of surgery, transfer of the patient from the operating room to recovery room, etc.

Observation of the Patient in the Postoperative Period

- Close and diligent observation by the nurses is important to detect complications in the early stages, and thus, save the patient.
- On the first day (postoperative) the patient need close and frequent observation.

The main points that should be observed are:
- Vital signs—BP, pulse rate, respiratory rate.
- Intake and output—IV fluids, oral fluids.
- Urinary concept—Time and amount.
- Bowel movement.
- Sign of hypo/hypervolemia.
- Any breathing difficulties.
- Pain over the calf muscles.

Management of patients in recovery room:
- The patient airway should be regularly checked.
- Monitor oxygen saturation more than 95%.
- Breathing should be normal.
- Temperature should be normal
- Pain relief is mandatory.
- Check the pressure areas.
- IV cannula should be at hand and fit well.
- Any medicine given should be recorded with time.
- If central venous line is present this should be handled in a strict aseptic way and clearly labeled.
- All tubes and catheter should be cared and should be properly fixed.
- Before sending the patient in ward, patient must be fully awake with all the verbal response.
- Pulse, BP, respiration and temperature should be normal (PTRBP Charting).
- The effect of muscle relaxants must be completely reversed. Patient should be able to cough, lift the head and protrude the tongue.

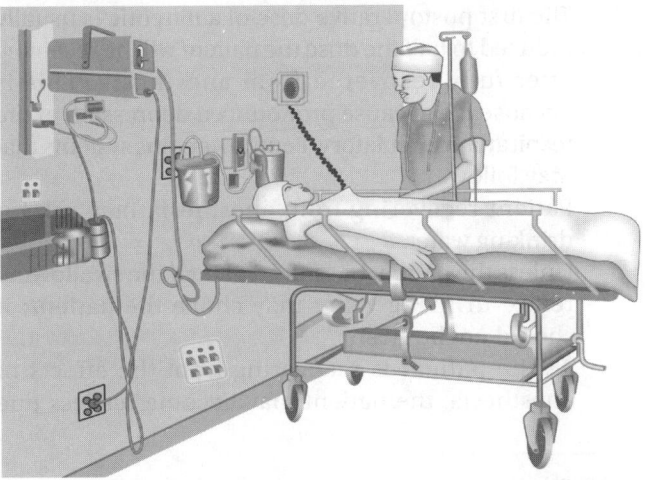

Fig. 31.3: Postanesthetics care unit observations.

- Dressing (incision site) should be rechecked and if there is bleeding, inform the doctor and redress it after achieving homeostasis.
- Antiemetic drugs should be given if needed.
- Take a green signal from anesthetist before sending to ward.
- Urine output, amount of drain, nasogastric aspiration should be recorded.

Postoperative Care (in General)

- **Preparation of postanesthetic bed and reception of the patient.**
  - After sending the patient to operating room prepare a bed to receive the patient undergone surgery and anesthesia.
  - There should be adequate number of people to transfer the patient without disturbing the functioning of the devices attached with the patient, such as: i.v. infusion set, self retaining suction set, blood transfusion sets, nasogastric tube, oxygen, urinary catheter, cardiac monitoring, water seal drainage system, plaster casts, traction sets.
  - Receive the patient without disturbing the devices attached to the patient. The recovery room nurse-in charge may give the necessary instructions to the personnel before transferring the patient.
  - Ask the theater staff who has accompanied with the patient about any complications that has occurred in the operation room during surgery.
  - Before the theater staff (including anesthetist) return to operation theater, check the vital signs: blood pressure, pulse rate, respiration, color of the skin and nails for any cyanosis, etc. Compare it with the baseline data recorded before sending to operation theater.
  - Check the operation site for bleeding, discharge etc., if drainage tubes are fitted.
  - Keep the patient well covered to prevent draught.
  - Never leave the patient alone to prevent injury from falls.
  - Observe the patient for swallowing reflexes. If not present, keep the patient in a side lying position to prevent the tongue falling back and obstructing the airway. After tonsillectomy, the patient may be kept in prone position to prevent blood aspirating in the lungs. The patient who had spinal anesthesia, the foot it may be raised on bed blocks.
  - Quickly observe the functioning of all devices and make sure that they are in its functioning order, e.g. the drainage tubes connected with the drainage bottle, the IV sets are patent.
  - Check the doctor's orders for other instructions and treatment.

- **Care of the patient who is under the effects of anesthesia**
  - Patient needs close and diligent observation until the patient fully recover from anesthesia. This will help to detect the early signs of complications after surgery and the nurse will be able to respond immediately.
  - A noisy breathing is indicative of airway obstruction that can occur, due to the tongue falling back and obstructing the pharynx, or fluid collected in the airway passages or fluids aspirated into the lungs. Apply suction immediately, send and call the surgeon and the anesthetist.
  - Keep the patient in a suitable position that will be helpful to drain out the vomitus, blood and secretions collected in the mouth and will prevent them aspirating into the lungs. This position is maintained until protective reflexes are returned.
  - The oropharyngeal airway left in the mouth of the patient should be removed as soon as the patient has regained the cough and swallowing reflexes.
  - Excessive secretions in the mouth or anywhere in the respiratory passage can lead to airway obstruction. It should be sucked out. If intratracheal auctioning is necessary, always use sterile technique.
  - If the patient is cyanosed, administer oxygen inhalation. At the same time, find out the cause and remove the cause. Prolonged oxygen therapy should be guided by arterial blood gas determinations.
  - A weak thready pulse with a significant fall in blood pressure may indicate circulatory failure. It may also indicate blood loss from the body. The surgeon and the anesthetist should be informed.
  - In order to prevent injury from falls from bed put on the side rails on the bed. Till the patient recover from the effects of anesthesia, the nurse should not leave the patient alone. Even, when the patient has recovered from the effects of anesthesia, entrust the patient to someone responsible for the care.
  - While awakening from anesthesia, patients need frequent orientation as to where they are, what has

been done to them, and reassurance that they are safe in the hands of the medical team. They also need to know that the operation is over and they are recovering from anesthesia.

– Although these patients, while they are under the effects of anesthesia, appear to be unconscious, the nurses should be careful, not to make any statement about the patient or his disease conditions that may create anxiety in the patient.

– When the patients under the effects of anesthesia complain pain in the operation site, the narcotics/sedatives may be ordered by the surgeon and it should be given with caution.

– The first postoperative dose of a narcotic is usually reduced to half the dose the patient will be receiving after fully recovered from anesthesia. This is because it can cause pronounced depression of the respiratory/circulatory/central nervous systems that may follow.

– Patient recovering from anesthesia may ask for drinking water.

– Unless the patient has fully regained the swallowing reflex, drinking water may choke the patient; it should not be given.

– As the patient is recovering from the effects of anesthesia, the patient may become restless due

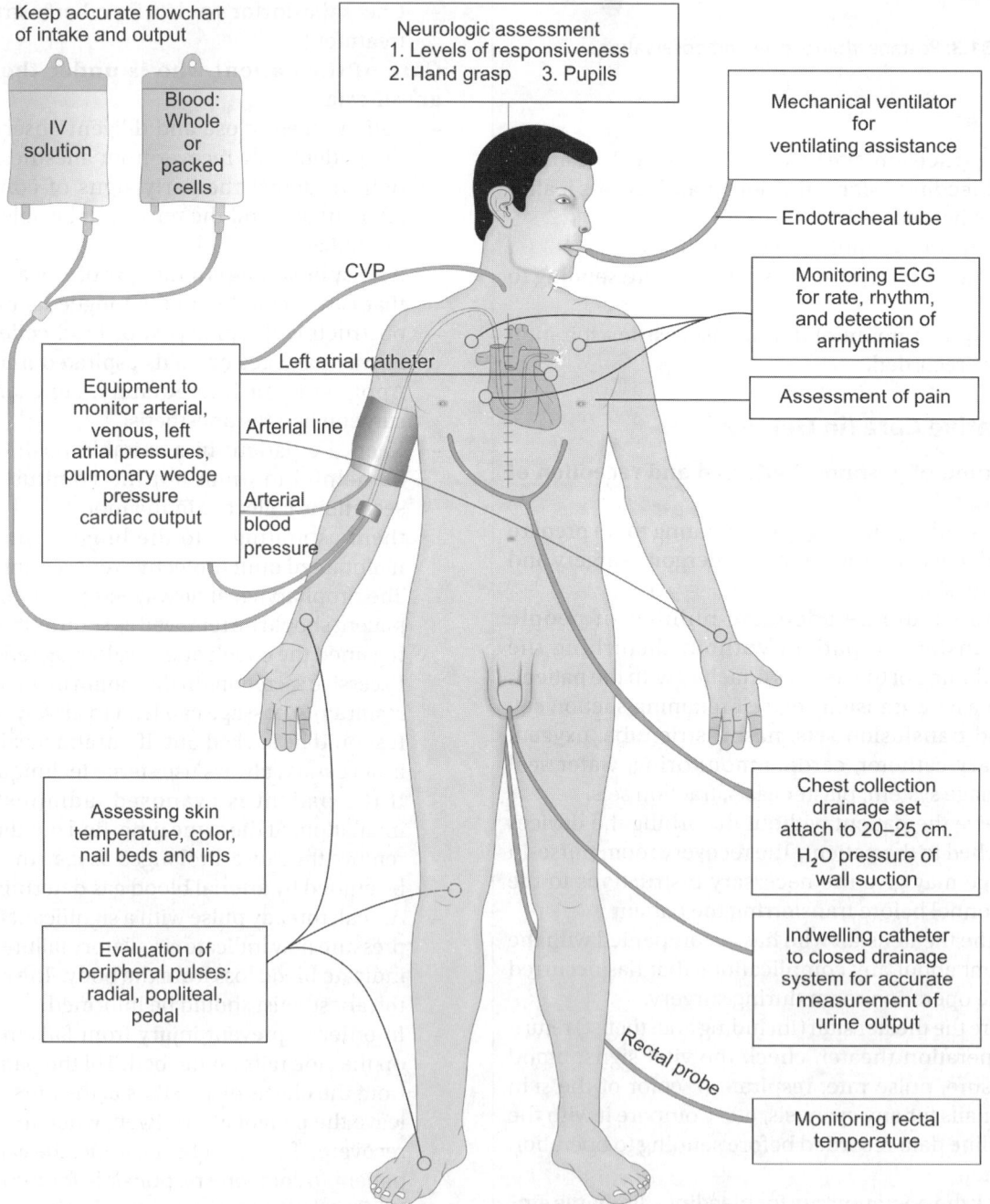

Fig. 31.4: Tubes and catheters of postoperative patient.

to the discomfort caused by the presence of those devices attached to the patient, such as IV sets, urinary catheters, drainage tubes, etc.
- The nurse should help the patient by giving adequate explanations.
- Keep the family informed of the successful completion of surgery, transfer of the patient from the operating room to recovery room, etc. These informations will reduce their anxiety.
- If possible, allow the relatives to meet surgeon to clear their doubts.

- **Observation of the patient in the postoperative period**
  - Close and diligent observation by the nurses are important to detect complications in the early stages, and thus, save the patient.
  - On the first postoperative day the patient needs close and frequent observations: e.g. the vital signs are checked every 15 minutes or more frequently (during the period when the patient is in the recovery room).
  - Once the vital signs are stabilized, the observations may be made every 2 hourly or 4 hourly according to the progress made by the patient.
  - The main points that should be observed are:
    - Vital signs—blood pressure, pulse rate, respiratory rate, skin color, skin temperature.
    - Intake and output—IV fluids, oral fluids taken by the patient, nasogastric aspiration, wound drainage, blood loss.
    - Abdominal girth in patients with abdominal distension.
    - Urinary output- time and amount.
    - Bowel movements.
    - Signs of hypo/hypervolemia.
    - Any breathing difficulties.
    - Pain over the calf muscles.
    - Operation site for bleeding, drainage.
    - Any specific observation as told by the surgeon and according to the operation done: e.g. vaginal discharge in patients who had hysterectomy, any arrhythmias in patients who had cardiac problem, motor and sensory functions in a patient with neurological problems.

- **Diet of the patient**
  - All patients, except patients who had abdominal surgery, may start the normal diet, if desired so, on the first day. Remember to exclude nausea and vomiting due to the effect of anesthesia.
  - Patient who had abdominal surgery, but did not involved the intestine or stomach, can have the clear fluids on the day after the surgery.
  - Gradually, it can change into soft diet and then normal diet.
  - Patients who are with specific diseases, for which, they were taking special diets, should continue to observe the control of their diet as ordered by the doctor (e.g. a diabetic patient).
  - Remember, the patients who had undergone any type of surgery, need a diet rich in vitamins and minerals.

Postoperative health teaching: All patients need health teaching according to the educational background of the patient. Teach the patient following points:
- Maintenance of personal hygiene.
- Diet that is allowed for the patient; any control on the diet.
- Ambulation; activities that are permitted, as well as restricted.
- Any adjustments to be made in the occupation of the patient.
- Any drugs to be taken postoperatively; the side effects and precautions.
- Date on which the patient may resume duty.
- Learning of any particular procedure to be carried out postoperatively, e.g. care of the colostomy. When the patient is unable to perform the procedure, teach the patient's relatives.

POSTOPERATIVE COMPLICATIONS

Postoperative complications can range from minor, self limiting problems to major life threatening ones depending on the nature of the surgery and the organ operated upon. Complication can be due to anesthesia or surgery or a reaction to the stress of surgery itself. Some complications are general and apply to all procedures and some are specific that apply to only that procedure. Common complications include fever, chest infection, pneumonia, wound infection, bleeding or deep vein thrombosis. Most of the complications manifests after the first few days of surgery—usually 1 to 3 days.

Types of complications: Postoperative complications generally fall in one or more of the three broad categories:
- Anesthesia related complications
- Complications common to any procedure
- Complications common to specific procedure

Depending on the severity of the complications they can again be broadly categorized as major or minor.

Minor complications: Dryness of the mouth and throat, sore throat, drowsiness, shivering, vomiting, dizziness, and giddiness are common side effects of the medicines used during anesthesia. They are self-limiting and do not persist beyond an hour or two. Fatigue, feeling weak, headache are also common and could be attributed to the fasting that is often required before and after a surgery. Under normal circumstances these symptoms vanish in a day or two. Some people also experience bloated feeling, constipation and urine retention following an operation and these resolve spontaneously. Fever can occur as a reaction to the intravenous fluid transfused during an operation.

Major complications: These complications can be serious and sometimes even life-threatening. They prolong the recovery period and stay in the hospital. The complications may happen during surgery or in the postoperative period.

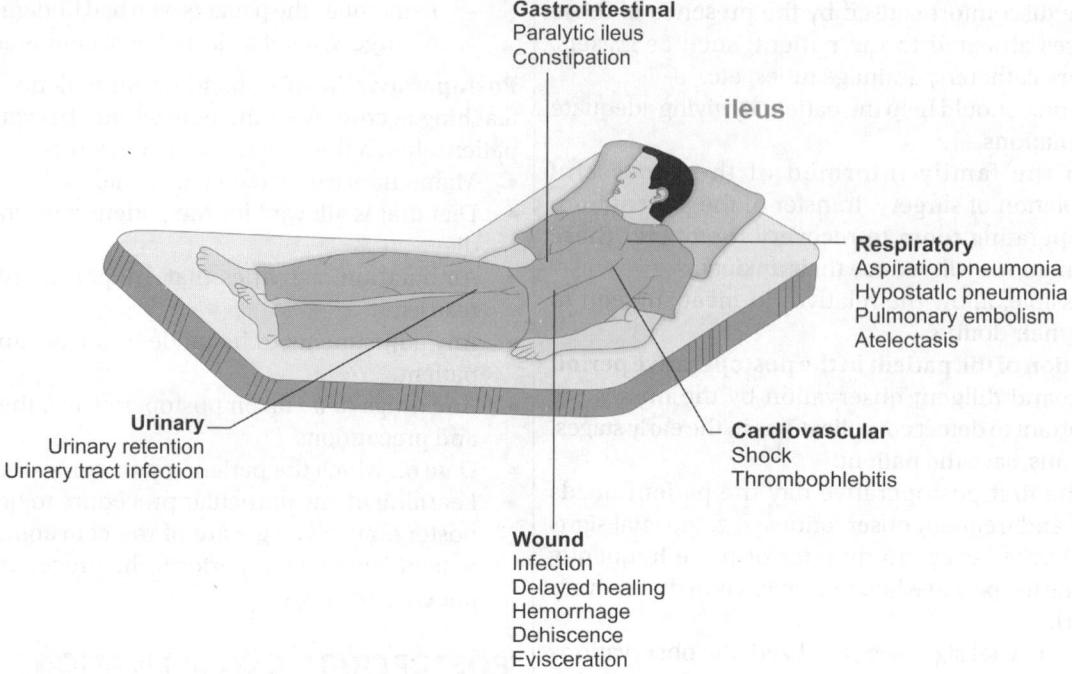

Fig. 31.5: Postoperative complications.

Prevention of Postoperative Complications

- **Wound complications:** Meticulous surgical techniques, Perioperative antibiotics for clean-contaminated wounds, delayed closure of dirty wounds.
- **Respiratory complications:** Avoid smoking in advance of elective surgery, encourage coughing and deep breathing, sufficient but not excessive analgesia, early postoperative ambulation.
- **Oliguria:** Adequate intravenous fluids, assure outflow.
- **Hypotension:** Avoid hypovolemia, monitor for arrhythmias, early recognition and treatment of infection, titrate medication doses carefully.
- **Bleeding:** Meticulous operative technique, screen for factor deficiencies, platelets and fresh frozen plasma for massive blood loss, avoid DIC by preventing infections/treating early, keep gastric pH neutral.
- **Alimentary tract dysfunction:** Use nasogastric tube, stool softeners, and cathartics when necessary.
- **Hyperglycemia:** Avoid large infusions of glucose, monitor diabetics carefully, and administer insulin.
- **Adrenal insufficiency:** Provide stress doses of corticosteroids when adrenals are chronically suppressed.
- **Thyroid storm:** Control hyperthyroidism prior to surgery.
- **Alterations in cognitive function:** Avoid hypoxia and electrolyte imbalance, titrate carefully.

PERIOPERATIVE NURSING PROCESS

Perioperative nursing is a nursing specialty that works with patients who are having operative or other invasive procedures. Perioperative nurses work closely with surgeons, nurse anesthetists, surgical technologists and nurse anesthetists and nurse practitioner. They perform preoperative, intraoperative, and postoperative care primarily in operation theaters, stress test evaluations, cardiac monitoring, vascular monitoring, and health assessments. Perioperative nurses typically have Basic Life Support and Advanced Cardiac Life Support certification.

Steps in nursing process: The nursing process consists of five steps or components. These five steps of the nursing process are assessment, nursing diagnosis, planning, implementation and evaluation. The scientific nursing activities and responsibilities are associated with each steps of the nursing process.

Sl. No.	Steps	Description
1.	Assessment	It is collecting, verifying and organizing data about the client's health status. Data about physical, emotional, developmental, social, cultural, intellectual and spiritual aspects of the client's are obtained from a variety of sources and are the basis for actions and decisions taken at a subsequent phases.
2.	Nursing diagnosis	It is a process of making a clinical judgment about a client's potential or actual health problem. Nursing diagnosis is the statement of the judgment. In this phase, the nurse sorts, clusters the data and analyzes, what are the actual and potential health problems for which the client needs nursing assistance and what may be the contributing factors to this problem?

Contd...

Contd...

Sl. No.	Steps	Description
3.	Planning	It involves a series of steps in which the nurse and client set priorities, formulate goals or expected outcomes and establish a written care plan for nursing interventions. The plan to resolve or minimize the identified problems of the client and to coordinate the care provided by all the health team members.
4.	Implementation	It is putting the nursing care plan into action. During the implementation phase, the nurse continues to collect data and carries out the prescribed nursing activities or delegates the care to an appropriate person who validates the nursing care plan.
5.	Evaluation	It is assessing the client's response to nursing interventions and then comparing the response to predetermined standards. These standards are often referred to as 'outcome criteria'. The nurse determines the extent to which the goals are predetermined and the outcomes of care that have been achieved, partially achieved or not met.

WOUNDS

Wounds (injury to tissues) vary from minor lacerations to severe crushing injuries. Life-threatening problems, such as airway obstruction, hemorrhage, and shock, must be dealt with before the wound is treated. A wound is an injury in which the skin is cut or penetrated. For instance a knife, bullet, ice pick or wood splinter may inflict a wound. If the wound is deep, severe bleeding may occur or there may be serious damage to structures within the body, such as the stomach, lungs or brain. Depending on how they are caused, e.g. by blunt force, sharp weapon or firearm.

Classification of Wounds

Wounds may be classified in two different ways, i.e. according to the mechanism of injury and the degree of wound contamination at the time of surgery.

- **Mechanism of injury**
  Wounds may be described as incised, contused, lacerated, or puncture.
  - **Incised wounds:** These are made by a clean cut with a sharp instrument, e.g., those made by the surgeon in every surgical procedure. Clean wounds (those made aseptically) are usually closed by sutures after all bleeding vessels have been ligated carefully.
  - **Contused wounds:** These are made by blunt force and are characterized by considerable injury of the soft part, hemorrhage, and swelling.
  - **Lacerated wounds:** These are with jagged, irregular edges, such as would be made by glass or barbed wire.
  - **Puncture wounds:** These result in small openings in the skin, e.g. those made by bullets or knife steps.
- **Degree of Contamination:** Wounds may be described as clean, clean-contaminated, contaminated, or dirty or infected.
  - **Clean wounds:** These are uninfected surgical wounds in which there is no inflammation and the respiratory, alimentary, genital, or uninfected urinary tracts are not entered. Clean wounds are usually sutured closed; if necessary, a closed drainage system (e.g. Jackson Pratt) is inserted. The relative probability of wound infection is 1 to 5%.
  - **Clean-contaminated wounds:** These are surgical wounds in which the respiratory, alimentary, genital and urinary tract are entered under controlled conditions; there is no unusual contamination. The relative probability of wound infection is 3 to 11%.
  - **Contaminated wounds:** These include open, fresh, accidental wounds, and surgical procedures with major breaks in aseptic technique or gross spillage from the gastrointestinal tract; included in this category are incisions in which there is acute, nonpurulent inflammation. The relative probability of wound infection is 10 to 17%.
  - **Dirty or infected wounds:** These are those in which the organisms that caused postoperative infection were present in the operative field before surgery. These include old traumatic wounds with retained devitalized tissue and those that involve existing clinical infections or perforated viscera. The relative probability of wound infection is over 27%.

Wound Healing Process

Various continuous and overlapping cellular processes contribute to the restoration of a wound; cell regeneration, cell proliferation, and collagen production. The response of tissue to injury goes through several phases, i.e. inflammatory, proliferative and maturation.

Inflammatory phase: Vascular and cellular responses occur immediately when tissue is cut or injured. Vasoconstriction of vessels occurs and a fibrinoplatelet clot forms in an attempt to control bleeding. This reaction lasts from 5 to 10 minutes and is followed by vasodilation of the Veins. Microcirculation loses its vasoconstriction ability because norepinephrine is destroyed by the intracellular enzymes. Also histamine is released, which increases capillary permeability.

When the microcirculation is damaged, blood elements such as antibodies, plasma proteins, electrolytes, complement and water permeate the vascular space for

2 to 3 days, causing edema, warmth, redness and pain. Neutrophils are the first leukocytes to move into damaged tissue. Monocytes that transform to macrophages engulf the debris and transport it from the area. Antigen-antibodies also appear. Basal cells at the wound edges undergo mitosis, and the resulting daughter cells migrate.

With this activity, proteolytic enzymes are secreted and dissolve the base of blood clots. The gap between both sides eventually meets in 24 to 48 hours. At this point, cell migration is enhanced by hyperplastic bone marrow activity.

Phases of Wound Healing

Phases	Length of time	Events
Inflammatory (also called lag or exudative phase)	1–4 days	Blood clot forms wound and it becomes edematous Dabris of damaged tissue and blood clot are phagocytized
Proliferative (also called fibroblastic or connective tissue phase)	5–20 days	Collagen produced granulation tissue forms, Wound tensile strength increases
Maturation (also called differentiation, resorptive, remodeling or plateau phase)	21 days to months or even years	Fibroblasts leave wound, tensile strength increases Collagen fibers reorganize and tighten to reduce scar size

Proliferative phase: Fibroblasts multiply and form a lattice framework for migrating cells. Epithelial cells from buds at the edges of the wound; these buds develop into capillaries, the nutritional source for the new granulation tissue.

Collagen is the primary component of replaced connective tissue. Fibroblasts initiate the synthesis of collagen and mucopolysaccharides. In a period of 2 to 4 weeks, amino acid chains form into fibers of increasing length and diameter; these fibers become a well-structured pattern of packed bundles. The synthesis of collagen causes capillaries to decrease in number. Thereafter, collagen synthesis decreases in an attempt to balance the amount of collagen that is destroyed. Such synthesis and lysis result in increased tensile strength.

After 2 weeks, the wound has only 3 to 5 percent of the original skin strength. By the end of a month, only 35 to 59 percent of wound strength has been reached. Never more than 70 to 80% of strength is regained. Many vitamins, particularly vitamin C, aid in the metabolic process involved in wound healing.

Maturation phase: About 3 weeks after injury, fibroblasts begin to leave the wound. The scar appears large, until collagen fibrils reorganize into tighter positions. This, along with dehydration, reduces the scar but increases its strength. Such tissue maturation continues and reaches maximum strength in 10 or 12 weeks, but it never reaches the original strength of the prewound tissue.

Factors Affecting Wound Healing

Factors	Rationales	Nursing assessment/Interventions
Age of patient Handling of tissues Hemorrhage	The older the patient, the lesser resilient the tissues. Rough handling causes injury and delayed healing. Accumulation of blood creates dead spaces as dead cells that must be removed. The area becomes a growth medium for infection.	Handle all tissues gently. Handle tissues carefully and evenly. Monitor vital signs, observe incision site for evidence of bleeding and infection.
Hypovolemia	Insufficient blood volume leads to vasoconstriction and reduced oxygen and nutrients available for wound healing.	Monitor for volume deficit (cirulatory impairment). Correct by fluid replacement as prescribed.
Local factors edema	Reduces blood supply by exerting increased interstitial pressure on vessels.	Elevate part; apply compresses.
Inadequate dressing technique Too small	Permits bacteria invasion and contamination.	Follow guidelines for proper dressing technique.
Too tight	Reduces blood supply carrying nutrients and oxygen	Follow guidelines for proper dressing technique.
Nutritional deficits	Insulin secretion may be inhibited, causing blood glucose to rise. Protein-calorie depletion may occur.	Monitor blood glucose levels. Administer vitamin A and C supplements as prescribed
Foreign bodies	Foreign bodies retard healing.	Keep wounds free of dressing threads and talcum powder from gloves
Oxygen deficit tissue oxygenation inssifficient	Insufficient oxygen may be due to inadequate lung and cardiovascular function as well as localized vasoconstriction.	Encourage deep breathing, turning, controlled coughing.

Contd...

Contd...

Factors	Rationales	Nursing assessment/Interventions
Drainage collection	Accumulated secretions hamper healing process. Institute measures to remove accumulated secretions.	Monitor portable and other closed drainage system for proper functioning.
Medications Steroids Anticoagulants Broad-spectrum/specific antibiotics	May mask presence of infection by impairing normal inflammatory response. May cause hemorrhage Effective if administer immediately before surgery for specific pothology or bacterial contamination If administered after wound is closed, ineffective because of intravascular coagulation.	Be aware of action/effect of medications patient is receiving.
Patient overactivity	Prevents approximation of wound edges. Resting favors healing.	Utilizes measures to keep wound edges approximated: taping, bandaging, splints Encourage rest.
Sysemic disorders Hemorrhagic shock	These are depressants of cell function that directly affect wound healing.	Be familiar with the nature of the specific disorder.
Acidosis Hypoxia Renal failure	— — —	Administer prescribed treatment. Cultures may be indicated to determine appropriate antibiotics.

Forms of Wound Healing

In the surgical management of wound healing, wounds are described as healing by first, second, or third intention.

- **Healing by first intention (primary union):** Wounds made aseptically, with a minimum of tissue destruction, and properly closed, as with sutures heal with little tissue reaction by first intention. When wounds heal by first intention, granulation tissue is not visible and scar formation is minimal.
- **Healing by second intention (granulation):** In wounds in which pus formation (suppuration) has occurred or in which the edges have not been approximated, the process of repair is less simple and takes longer.
  When an abscess is incised it collapses partly, but the dead and the dying cells forming its walls are still being released into the cavity. For this reason, drainage tubes or gauze packing is often inserted into the abscess pocket to allow drainage to escape easily. Gradually, the necrotic material disintegrates and escapes easily and the abscess cavity fills with a red, soft, sensitive tissue that bleeds very easily. This tissue is composed of minute, thin-walled capillaries and buds that later form connective tissue.
  These buds called granulations enlarge until they fill the area left by the destroyed tissue. The cells surrounding the capillaries change their round shape to become long, thin, and intertwined with each other to form a scar or cicatrix. Healing is complete when skin cells (epithelium) grow over these granulations. This method of repair is called healing by granulation, and it takes place whenever pus is formed or when loss of tissue has occurred for any reason.
- **Healing by third intention (secondary suture):** If a deep wound either has not been sutured early or breaks down and then is resutured later, two opposing granulation surfaces are brought together. This results in a deeper and wider scar.

Complications of wound: The nurse must know when to suspect complications that necessitate inspection of the wound.
- Continued presence of pain.
- Swelling and/or redness around the wound.
- Persistent rise of temperature and/or an increasing pulse rate.
- Presence of toxemia, indicated by the onset of vomiting, diarrhea, loss of appetite and increasing pallor.
- Discharge from the wound.
- Any symptoms of tetanus—very rare nowadays.
- Any symptoms of too tight a plaster or dressing, e.g. pain, tingling or cyanosis of the tips of the fingers or toes.

The following complications can occur in a wound

Hematoma (Hemorrhage): The dressings are inspected for hemorrhage at frequent intervals during the first 24 hours after surgery. Any undue amount of bleeding is reported. At times, concealed bleeding occurs in the wound, beneath the skin. This hemorrhage usually stops spontaneously but results in clot formation within the wound. If the clot is small, it will be absorbed and need not to be treated. When the clot is large, the wound usually bulges somewhat, and healing will be delayed unless it is removed. After several sutures are removed by the physician, the clot is evacuated and the wound is packed lightly with gauze. Healing occurs usually by granulation, or a secondary closure may be performed.

Infection (Wound Sepsis) or surgical wound infections: These are the second most frequent nosocomial infection in hospitals. The most important area of prevention lies in meticulous wound management and surgical technique. In addition, cleanliness and disinfection are important. Nosocomial infection accounts for many postoperative wound infections. Other infections may result from *Escherichia coli, Proteus vulgaris*, Aerobacter aerogenes, Pseudomonas aeruginosa, and other organisms.

When the inflammatory process occurs, it usually causes symptoms in 36 to 48 hours. The patient's pulse rate and temperature increase, the WBC count rises, and the wound usually becomes swollen, warm and tender with incisional pain. Local signs may be absent when the infection is deep. When a diagnosis of wound infection in a postoperative wound is made, the surgeon usually removes one or more sutures and, under aseptic precautions, separates the wound edges with a pair of blunt scissors or a hemostat. Once the incision is opened, a drain is inserted.

Cellulites: It is a bacterial infection that spreads into tissue planes. All the manifestations of inflammation are evident; Streptococcus is frequently the responsible organism. Systemic antibiotics are usually effective. If an extremity is the site of the infection, elevation reduces dependent edema and the application of heat promotes local blood circulation. Rest decreases muscular contractions that could introduce the offending organisms into the circulatory system.

Abscess: It is a localized bacterial infection characterized by a collection of pus (bacteria, necrotic tissue, and WBCs). Usually a "point" develops that is tender. Because the area is under pressure, there is a tendency for the infection to seed bacteria that may invade adjacent tissues (cellulites) or vascular spaces (bacteremia, sepsis). Treatment is surgical drainage or excision and the administration of antibiotics. Recurrence is prevented by allowing the treated wound to drain. Rest, elevation of the part and heat are helpful.

Lymphangitis: It is a spread of infection from a cellulitis or abscess to the lymphatic system. This is treated by rest and antibiotics.

Dehiscence and evisceration: The complications of dehiscence (disruption of surgical incision of wound) and evisceration (protrusion of wound contents) are especially serious when they involve abdominal incisions or wounds. These complications result from sutures giving way, from infection, and, more frequently, after marked distention or strenuous cough. They may also occur because of increasing age, poor nutritional status, and the presence of pulmonary or cardiovascular disease in patients who undergo abdominal surgery.

When the wound edges separate slowly, the intestines may protrude gradually, or not at all, and the earliest sign may be a push of bloody (serosanguineous) peritoneal fluid from the wound. When the rupture of a wound occurs suddenly coils of intestine may push out of the abdomen. Frequently, the patient may say that "something gave way". The evisceration causes pain and can be associated with vomiting.

When disruption of a wound occurs, the surgeon is notified at once. The protruding coils of intestine are covered with sterile dressings moistened with sterile saline.

An abdominal binder, properly applied, is an excellent prophylactic measure against an evisceration of this kind, and often it is used along with the primary dressing, especially for surgery on patients with weak or pendulous abdominal walls, or when rupture of a wound has occurred. Vitamin deficiency or lowered serum protein or chloride may require correction.

DRESSING: SUTURE CARE

Wound care is defined as cleaning, monitoring and promoting healing in a wound that is closed with sutures, clips or staples.

Purpose of Dressing

- Provide physical, psychological and aesthetic comfort.
- Remove necrotic tissue.
- Prevent, eliminate or control infection.
- Absorb drainage.
- Maintain a moist wound environment.
- Protect the wound from further injury.
- Protect the skin surrounding the wound.
- Promote homeostasis as in a pressure dressing.
- Prevent contamination from feces, urine, vomitus, etc.
- For splinting or immobilization of wound.

Types of Dressing

Dry dressing: Clean wounds are dressed by the application of 4 to 8 layers of gauze folded into suitable size and shape. The surrounding of the wound is cleansed by some antiseptic and dried and dry dressing is applied after the application of medicine to the wound.

Wet dressing: It is used if wounds are infected and there is pus. The wet dressing compresses the hot, it stimulated the supportive process. The dressing is made of many layers of gauze or cotton pad covered with gauze.

Pressure dressing: It is done when there is bleeding or oozing from the wound. The dressing consists of thick pad of sterite gauze applied over the wound with a firm bandage and binder.

General Instructions

- Maintain aseptic technique to prevent cross infection to the wound and to the ward.
- All the material touching the wound should be sterile.
- Wash hands before and after each dressing to avoid cross infection.
- All equipment should be disinfected thoroughly, so that they will be free from pathogens.
- Use masks, sterile gloves and gown for large dressing to minimize the wound contamination.
- Dressing is changed at least 15 minutes after the room has been cleaned and avoids meal timings.

- Clean wound should be dressed before infected or discharging wounds.
- Wounds that are draining freely should be dressed frequently, according to the doctor's order.
- Avoid coughing, sneezing and talking when the wound is opened.
- While dressing avoid contamination with patients skin. Clothing and bed linen with soiled instruments and dressings.
- Clean the wound from cleanest area to the less clean area, e.g. clean the wound from is center to the periphery.
- If the dressings are adherent to the wound due to drying of the secretions or blood, wet it with normal saline before it is removed from the wound.
- While dressing, keep the wound edges as near as possible to promote healing.
- Measure the amount of discharge from the wound. Note the color, amount and consistency of the drainage.
- Before doing the dressing, inspect the wound for any complication and if it is present, report immediately to avoid further complications.

Preliminary Assessment

- Check the doctor's order for specific instructions.
- Identify the correct patient, bed number and general condition.
- Check the nurse's record to note the condition of the wound in previous dressing.
- Check the abilities of the patient for self-help understanding and limitation.
- Check the availabilities of the equipment.

Equipment: A sterile tray containing: Artery forceps-1, Dissecting forceps-2, Scissors-1, Sinus forceps-1. Probe-1, Small bowl-1, Safety pin-1, Gloves, Masks and Gowns, cotton balls, gauze pieces, cotton pads and dressing towels.

A trolley containing: Cleaning solutions as necessary, ointments and powders as ordered, Vaseline gauze in sterile containers, Roller gauze in sterile container, Chittle forceps in a solution, sterile gauze, cotton and pad drum, bandages, adhesive plaster, pins and scissors, mackintosh and draw sheet, kidney tray and covered bucket to put soiled dressing.

Procedure

- Explain the procedure to the patient, using sensory preparation.
- Inspect the wound for redness, swelling or signs of dehiscence or evisceration.
- Observe the characteristics of any drainage.
- Clean the area around the wound with an appropriate cleansing solution.
- Swab from clean area towards the less clean area. (Clean the wound from the center to periphery).
- Apply medications if ordered.
- Apply sterile dressing-apply gauze pieces first and then the cotton pads.
- Remove the gloves and discard it in to the bowl with lotion.
- Secure the dressing with bandage or adhesive tapes.

After Care

- Assess the patient to dress up and to take a comfortable position.
- Change the garments if soiled with drainage.
- Remove the mackintosh and towel. Replace the bed linen.
- Take all equipment to the utility room. Discard the soiled dressing in to a covered container and send for incineration.
- Wash hands and record the procedure on the nurse's record with date and time.
- Teach the patient/family about wound care and signs and symptoms of infection.

SUTURING THE WOUND

Materials and equipment: If the ideal suture existed it would be biologically inert and cause no tissue reaction. It would be very strong but simply dissolve in body fluids and lose strength at the same rate that the tissue gains strength. It would be easy for the surgeon to handle and knot reliably, as well as being reasonably priced. It would neither cause nor promote complications. However, despite great improvements in suture materials, no single suture is ideal in all circumstances. Regardless of its composition, suture material is a foreign body to human tissue and will elicit a foreign body reaction to some degree.

Suture materials can conveniently be divided into two broad groups: absorbable and non-absorbable. Two major mechanisms of absorption result in the degradation of absorbable sutures. Sutures of biological origin, such as catgut, are gradually digested by tissue enzymes. Sutures manufactured from synthetic polymers are principally broken down by hydrolysis in tissue fluids and are the preferred material. Non-absorbable sutures, such as nylon, are made from a variety of non-biodegradable materials, and are ultimately encapsulated or walled off by fibroblasts.

The sizes and tensile strengths of all suture materials are standardized. Size denotes the diameter of the material—the smaller the diameter, the less tensile strength it will have. Stated numerically, the higher the first number, the smaller the diameter of the suture. Examples of suture size used are: Trunk and lower limbs 3/0, Scalp 2/0, 3/0 or 4/0, Upper limbs 4/0, Most wounds 4/0, Face 5/0, 6/0.

SURGICAL DRESSING

A dressing is a protective covering applied to a wound. The goal of a wound care is to promote tissue repair and regeneration, so that skin integrity is restored. Dressing is used as a protective cover over the wound which helps meet the goal of wound care. Most dressings especially for the surgical wounds consist of three layers. The dressings applied directly over the wound called contact layer, allows drainage to pass into the middle layer. This layer should be able to remove without causing further tissue damage. This middle layer dressing absorbs the drainage and the outer layer keeps the two inner layers in place.

Purposes of dressings: There are many different types of dressings, but all have essentially the same purposes as follows:
- Remove necrotic tissue
- Prevent, eliminate, or control infection
- Absorb drainage of discharge
- Control bleeding
- Apply medication
- Maintain a moist wound environment
- Promote quick healing
- Provide comfort
- Protect the wound from further injury
- Protect the skin surrounding the wound.

Advantages of Dressings

Dressings have advantages and disadvantages. The advantages of wound dressing are as follows:
- Dressings absorb drainage to help promote wound healing
- Dressings protect the wound from mechanical injury
- Dressings when used as a pressure dressing or with elastic bandages promote homeostasis help prevent hemorrhage, and aid in wound edge approximation
- Dressing splint or immobilize the wound, facilitating healing and preventing further trauma
- Dressings prevent contamination from the external environment
- Dressings provide physical, psychological and esthetic comfort.

The nurse prepares the client for the dressing change by explaining what will be done before starting the procedure. Proper screening is used to provide privacy. The client is assisted to a position that is comfortable and also convenient for the person changing the dressing. The area is exposed while maintaining proper draping. It is important to use appropriate aseptic techniques when changing the dressings to prevent nosocomial infections.

Purposes of an Effective Dressing

As stated earlier, a dressing is applied to a wound for one or more of the following reasons:
- To provide a proper environment for wound healing.
- To absorb drainage.
- To splint or immobilize the wound.
- To protect the wound and new epithelial tissue from mechanical injury.
- To protect the wound from bacterial contamination and from soiling by feces, vomitus, and urine.
- To promote hemostasis, as in a pressure dressing.
- To provide mental and physical comfort for the patient.

In some instances, dressings are eliminated during the immediate postoperative period. Circumstances in which dressings are not necessary, are facial lacerations, pedicle flaps, or skin grafts on a smooth surface.

When the initial dressing on a clean, dry incision is removed, often it is not replaced. Generally, initial dressings on clean, dry incisions are left in place until the wound edges are sealed and the wound is healing (usually 24 hours).

The advantages of not using any dressings include the following:
- The conditions that promote growth of organisms (warmth, moisture, and darkness) are eliminated.
- The wound can be readily observed.
- Bathing is easier.
- Reactions to tape are avoided.
- Patient's comfort and activity are increased.
- Costs for dressings are reduced
- Psychological impact of the surgical incision is reduced.

General Instructions

- The Procedure of changing dressings, examining and closing the wound, uses principles of asepsis.
- The initial dressing change in frequently done by the physician especially for craniotomy, orthopedic or thoracotomy procedures; subsequent dressing changes are the nurse's responsibility.

Equipment

Sterile
- Gloves—Disposable
- Scissors, forceps
- Appropriate dressing materials
- Sterile saline
- Cotton dipped swabs
- Culture tubes
- For draining wound add extra gauze and packing material, absorbent, pad and irrigation set.

Unsterile
- Gloves
- Plastic bag for discarded dressings
- Tape proper size and type
- Pads to protect patient bed
- Gown for nurse if wound is infected.

Procedure

Pre-Preparation
- Inform the patient of dressing change. Explain procedure and have patient lie in bed.

- Avoid changing dressing at meal time.
- Ensure privacy by drawing the curtains or closing the door. Expose dressing site.
- Respect patient modesty and prevent patient from being chilled.
- Wash hands thoroughly.
- Place dressing supplies on a clean, flat surface.
- Place clean towel or plastic bag under part of the body where wound in located.
- Cut off pieces of tape to be used in dressing change.
- Place disposable bag nearby to collect soiled dressings.
- Determine what types of dressing are necessary.

Cleaning the Surgical Wound

- Use aseptic technique.
- Open package of sterile gloves; open sterile cleaning, sterile supplies.
- Wear sterile gloves.
- Clean along wound edges using a small circular motion from one end of incision to the other, do not scrub back and forth across the incision line.
- Sterile saline in the cleansing agent of choice. Topical antiseptics (alcohol based may be used on intact skin surrounding the wound but should never be used within the wound.
- Repeat same process with drain site separately.
- Discard used cleaning supplies in disposable.
- Pad the incision site and drain site dry with a sterile dressing sponge.

Dressing the Wound

- Maintain asepsis with use of sterile gloves
- After wound in dry apply appropriate dressing.
- Tape dressing, using only the amount of tape required for secure attachment of dressing.
- When dressing the drain site.
  - Use pre made drain sponge (Can be prepared by making 5 cm slit with sterile scissors in 4x4 inch gauze sponge)
  - Gently slip sponge around drain repeat with second drain sponge, placing it at right angle to other sponge.

Dressing the drainage tube insertion site: Be sure that one sponge in place at a right angle to the second sponge. So the slits are going in different direction, if drainage is heavy, a sterile absorbent pad or extra gauze may be placed overall.
- When dressing an excessive draining wound
  - Consider need for extra dressings and packing materials.
  - Use Montgomery straps if frequent dressing is required.
  - Protect skin surrounding wound from copious or irritating drainage by applying some types of skin barriers.

After Care (Follow-up Care)

- Assess patient's tolerance to the procedure and help patient more comfortable.
- Discard disposable items according to hospital protocol and clean equipment that is to be recessed.
- Wash hands.
- Record nature of procedure and condition of wound, as well as patient reaction.

SUTURE REMOVAL

Suture removal is a process removing materials used to secure wound edges or body parts together from healed wound without damaging newly formed tissue.

The timing of suture removal depends on the shape, size and location of the sutured incision.

The sutures may be removed by the surgeon or by the nurse. In all cases the surgeon gives the written order for the removal of the sutures.

Purpose

- Sutures are foreign bodies and if they are not removed they are capable of causing local inflammation.

Principle

- Never pull the visible portion of the suture through underlying tissue.
- Suture line is cleansed before and after suture removal.
- No part of the stitch which is above the skin level enter and contaminate the tissue under the skin.

The Usual Timing

- Scalp: 2-5 days
- Abdominal wounds: 7-10 days
- Lower limbs: 10-14 days.

Factors affecting the Suture Removal

- Type of suture
- Wound bedding.

Types

- Removing staples: To remove staples, the nurse simply inserts the tips of the staple remover under each wire staples. Squeezes are center of the staple with the tips, freeing the staples from the skin.
- Intermittent suture: The surgeon tied each individual suture made in the skin.
- Continuous suture: It is the series of sutures with only two knots.
- Retentions suture: They were placed deeply than skin sutures.

General Instructions

- Confirm the doctor's order for the removal of the sutures.
- The suture removal is done in conjunction with the dressing charge.
- The suture line is cleaned before and after suture removal.
- When removing interrupted it sutures alternate ones are removed first.
- Suture material left beneath the skin acts as a foreign body and clients the inflammatory response.
- If wound dehiscence occurs during the removal of sutures, inform the surgeon immediately.
- After removing the sutures, even if the wound is dry, the small dressing is applied for the day or two to prevent infection.
- If wound discharge occurs, the patient should be instructed to contact the surgeon.
- Abdominal belts or many tailed bandages may be applied as the abdomen after removal of abdominal sutures in obese patients to prevent wound dehiscence and evisceration.

Preliminary Assessment

- Check the physician's order.
- Assess the general candidates of the patient.
- Check the specific precautions if any.
- Check the consciousness of the patient and his ability to follow instructions.

Preparation of Patient and Environment
- Explain the procedure to the patient.
- Provide privacy, if needed.
- Clean the area before and after the procedure.

Equipment

- Water proof thrash bag.
- Adjustable light.
- Clean gloves, if the wound is dressed.
- Sterile gloves.
- Sterile forceps.
- Normal saline solution.
- Sterile gauze pads.
- Antiseptic cleaning agent.
- Sterile curve tipped suture scissors.
- Povidone iodine sponges.
- Optional adhesive butterfly strips and compound benzoin tincture or other skin protectant.

Procedure

- To remove the interpreted sutures grasp the suture at the knot with a toothed forceps and pull it gently to expose the portion of the stitch under the skin.
- Cut the suture with a sharp scissors between the knot and the skin on one side either below the knot or apposite the knot. Then pull the thread out of one piece.
- The suture which is already above the skin should not be drawn under the skin. After removal of sutures every suture should be examined for completeness.
- Mattress sutures have no threads underlying the skin. The visible suture opposite the knot should be cut and the suture is removed by putting in the direction of the knot.
- If a continuous suture is applied, it is cut through, close at each skin orifice on one side and the cut sections are removed through the opposite side by gentle traction.

Post-procedure Care

- After the removal of any suture we should clear the area.
- We can give dressing also the area to prevent infection.
- Tell the patient to keep the area clean.
- Document the status of the wound, after suture removal.
- Care of drainage

CARE OF DRAINS

- To drain fluid which has collected or is expected to collect, e.g. blood, serum, pus, bile.
- As a safety valve to an anastomosis or suture line, e.g. the duodenal stump after gastrectomy or the ureter after removal of a stone.

In the first case, the drain is removed when drainage has become negligible or has ceased. This is often within 1-3 days.

In the second case, the drain is removed once the danger of leakage has passed. This is usually 4-5 days.

The drain is usually brought out through a small incision separate from the main wound, to avoid both- interference with healing and contamination of the wound. Sometimes it is brought out through the wound, while in certain circumstances the wound itself requires drainage.

Wherever a drain is inserted it should be covered with a sterile dressing or, if a tube, its exit from the skin is surrounded with such a dressing.

Types of Drain

- **Tubing:** Fenestrated or split plastic, latex or rubber.
- **Corrugated:** Plastic or rubber sheeting.
- **Penrose tubing:** Soft, thin, flat latex tubing
- **Other drains for specific** purposes, e.g. catheters for certain cavities, T-tubes for the common bile duct. The drain is stitched to the skin. A safety pin should be put into a corrugated drain to prevent it slipping deep to the skin.

Wound Drainage

After surgery, some patients require wound drains. The wound drain is inserted while the patient is in the operating room receiving general anesthesia. The purpose of the drain is to remove fluid and/or blood from the surgical site. This helps the healing process. Not all patients need wound drains following surgery. Wound drains are usually made of plastic. One end is placed within the wound to be drained and the other end is connected to a suction collection device. The fluid may be collected in a drainage bag, plastic bulb, and plastic carton or onto a dressing.

Types of Surgical Drain

Open

- Directly on to dressings.
- Into an adhesive plastic bag stuck to the skin around the drain.

Closed

- Tube or catheter into a sealed sterile disposable bag.
- Chest tube to an under fluid seal.
- Suction tube attached to a low grade suction machine or to a sealed vacuum apparatus. The practical details of the management of such drains vary with the maker of drain used.

In closed drainage, organisms from the air are excluded, the discharge can be measured and the main wound can be kept dry.

Management of Drain

The nature and quantity of drainage should be carefully noted. The quantity of fluid draining can be measured accurately if it is collected into a bag or suction apparatus. This should be recorded every 24 hours or more frequently, if there is a large quantity. Some surgeons advocate that drains should be shortened gradually by pulling them out a little and cutting off the excess, so that the drainage track can heal from the bottom, and that tube drains should be rotated so that they do not adhere to the tissues. However, many simply remove the drain when it has ceased to fulfil a useful function.

The following complications may arise if a tube is left in situ for too long a period:
- Infection
- Intestinal obstruction
- Erosion of a blood vessel causing a secondary hemorrhage
- Perforation of an organ causing a fistula
- Adhesions
- Incisional hernia.

Care of wound drainage: The nurse must connect and maintain the tubes to the ordered suction device, must avoid introduction of microorganisms into wound or drainage system, and must also avoid dislodging tubes. The procedures are as follow.
- Wash hands and assemble all equipment.
  - Suction unit (Hemovac, electric or wall vacuum continuous unit, intermittent suction).
  - Graduated container.

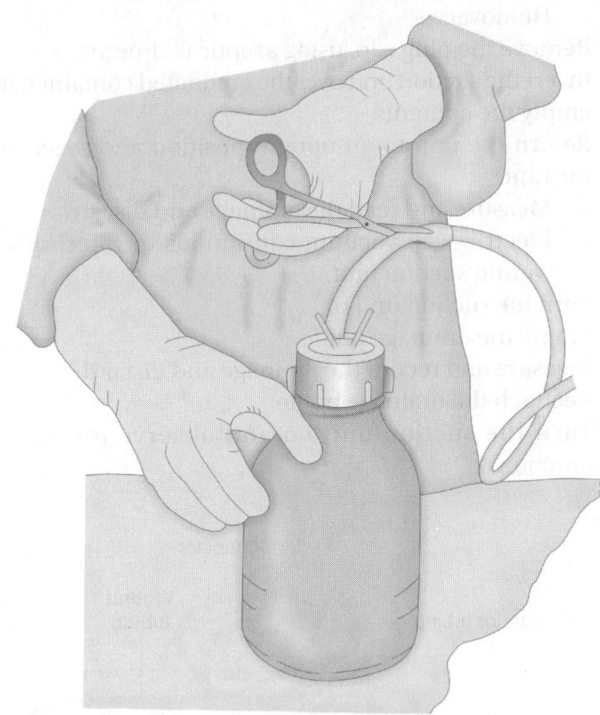

Fig. 31.6: Care of drainage tubes and bottle.

- Verify physician's order.
- Identify and approach the patient, explain what you are going to do, and gain his cooperation.
- Provide for the patient's privacy and position the patient to facilitate access to the drainage tube.
- Provide adequate lighting.
- Wash your hands.
- Activate the appropriate/ordered tube drainage/suction unit.
  - Hemovac (wound drainage tube suction).
- Remove the plug cap aseptically and place the portable suction unit upright on a firm surface.
- Compress the suction unit as flat as possible.
- Replace the plug cap immediately.
- Position the suction unit to prevent kinking of the tubes or dropping of the unit.
- Observe the suction unit for proper compression and patency.
  - Electric or wall vacuum continuous or intermittent wound/gastrointestinal suction unit.
- Plug the unit into an electrical outlet or attach to a wall system vacuum.
- Connect the suction tube to the patient's drainage tube, using aseptic technique.
- Tape the connection. Ensure that the tubing is not pulling on the drainage tube.
- Turn the suction unit on "Low" unless specifically ordered differently.
- Observe the suction system for proper functioning.

- Empty the drainage collection device, as necessary.
  - Hemovac.
- Remove the plug cap, using aseptic technique.
- Invert the suction unit over the graduated container and empty the contents
- Return the unit to an upright position and reactivate the unit.
  - Measure and read the drainage and discard
  - Electric wall vacuum continuous or intermittent wound suction unit.
- Turn the suction unit off.
- Empty the drainage bottle.
- Measure and record the drainage and discard.
- Reattach the drainage bottle.
- Turn the suction unit on and observe for proper function.

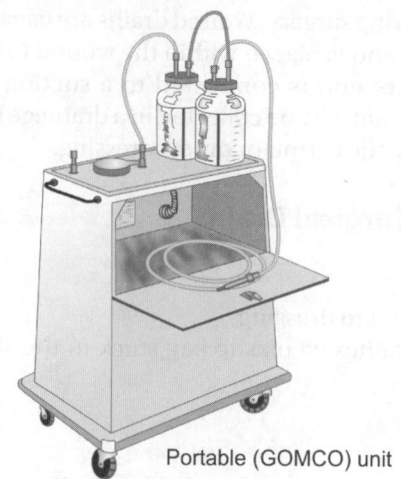

Fig. 31.10: Wound/gastrointestinal suction portable unit.

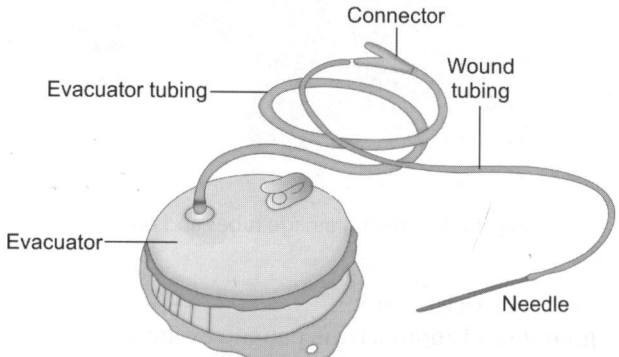

Fig. 31.7: Hemovac.

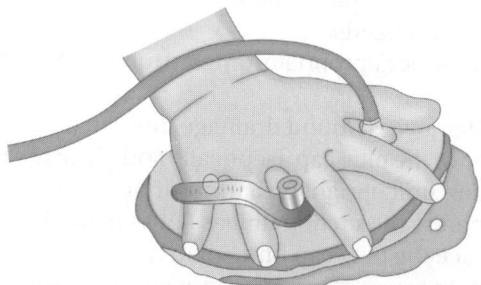

Fig. 31.8: Compressing unit to form vacuum.

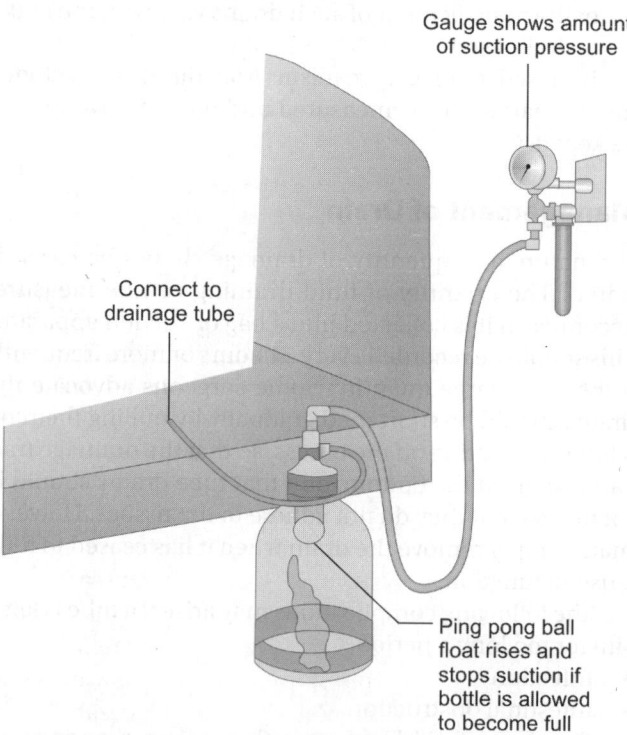

Fig. 31.11: Wound/gastrointestinal suction wall unit.

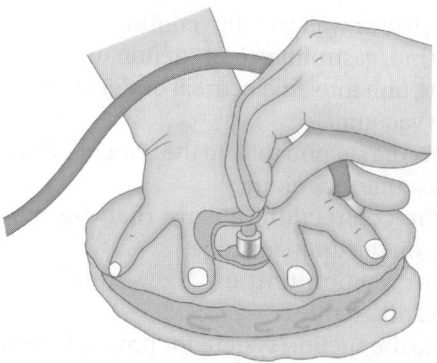

Fig. 31.9: Replace plug in outlet to retain vacuum.

- Discard equipment or return it to the appropriate location.
- Wash your hands.
- Record procedure and report significant observation to the Charge Nurse.
  - Type of wound catheter and suction.
  - Amount, color, characteristics, and odor of drainage.
  - The patient's reaction to the procedure.
  - Function of suction system.
  - Any observations of the wound area or dressing.
  - All patient teaching done and the patient's apparent level of understanding.

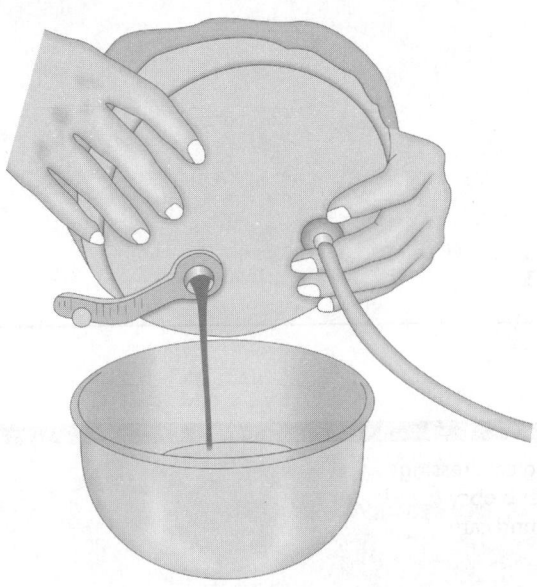

Fig. 31.12: Opening outlet to remove drainage.

CONCLUSION

Perioperative Nurses provide for the surgical patient's needs, by assessing, planning and implementing nursing care patient receives preoperatively, intraoperatively, and postoperatively. Nursing activities performed by the perioperative nurse include patient assessment, creating and maintaining a sterile and safe environment, preoperative and postoperative teaching, monitoring physiologic and psychological status, integration and coordination of care across settings and among disciplines, patient advocacy, and efficient provision of resources. Surgery is described as the treatment of diseases, injury or deformity by a manual or instrumental procedure. Different nurses care the surgical client during each phase of surgical experience. The nurse's major responsibility is to provide safe, consistent and effective nursing care during each phase of surgery. Preoperative phase begins when the client decides to have surgery and ends when the client is transferred to the operating room. Intraoperative phase begins when the client is transferred to the operating room and ends when the client is admitted to the post-anesthesia room. Operating room nurses required special abilities to take responsibilities with the emergencies of their different roles like scrubbing up nurse, circulatory nurse, etc. postoperative phase begins with the transfer of the client to the post-anesthesia room/postoperative ward and ends with the discharge of the client from the hospital or facility providing continuing care.

BIBLIOGRAPHY

1. Harkness-Hood G, Dincher JR. Total Patient Care: Foundations and Practice of Adult Health Nursing, 8th Edition. St. Louis: Mosby-Year Book, Inc., 1992.
2. Kurzen CR. Contemporary Practical/Vocational Nursing, 2nd Edition. Philadelphia: JB Lippincott, 1992.
3. Potter PA, Perry AG. Fundamentals of Nursing Concepts, Process and Practice, 3rd Edition, St. Louis: Mosby-Year Book, Inc., 1993.
4. Taylor C, Lillis C, LeMone P. Fundamentals of Nursing: The Art and Science of Nursing Care, Philadelphia: JB Lippincott, 1993.
5. Timby BK, Lewis LW. Fundamental Skills and Concepts in Patient Care, 5th Edition. Philadelphia: JB Lippincott, Co., 1992.

REVIEW QUESTIONS

Long Essays

1. Define perioperative nursing, explain the objectives and phases of perioperative nursing.
2. Define postoperative complications, explain detail about immediate and late postoperative complications.
3. Explain in detail about perioperative nursing process.

Short Essays

1. Classifications of surgical procedures.
2. Preoperative nursing: objectives, principles and procedures.
3. Preparation of the patient on the day of surgery.
4. Intraoperative phase: theater-set-up, equipment and role of nurse.
5. Immediate postoperative phase.
6. Postoperative nursing: objectives, principles and procedures.
7. Prevention of postoperative complications.
8. Wound healing process.
9. Factors affecting wound healing.
10. Suturing the wound.
11. Dressing: suture care.
12. Suture removal.
13. Care of drains.

Short Answers

1. Elective surgery.
2. Reconstructive surgery.
3. Informed consent.
4. Classification of wounds.
5. Types of dressing.
6. Types of drain.
7. Wound drainage.

CHAPTER 32
Surgical Procedures

LEARNING OBJECTIVES
- Abdominal paracentesis
- Thoracentesis
- Lumbar puncture
- Bone marrow biopsy and aspiration
- Surgical dressing
- Liver biopsy
- Wound care

ABDOMINAL PARACENTESIS

Abdominal paracentesis is defined as the removal of fluid from the peritoneal cavity. Abdominal paracentesis or peritoneal tap is defined as the insertion of needle or cannula with trocar into the peritoneal space through the abdominal wall to remove peritoneal fluid.

Purpose

- To relieve pressure on the abdominal and chest organs if a transudate collects as a result of renal, cardiac or liver diseases.
- To study chemical, bacteriological and cellular composition of the peritoneal fluid for the diagnosis of diseases.
- To drain exudates in peritonitis.
- To remove fluid and instill air to create artificial pneumoperitoneum as a treatment for pulmonary tuberculosis affecting the base of the lungs.
- To remove blood or pus.
- To use as a prelude to other procedures like X-ray, peritoneal dialysis or surgery.

Indications

- **Diagnostic:** To diagnose the nature of fluid, transudate or exudates, Koch's ascites, spontaneous bacterial peritonitis and malignancy.
- **Therapeutic:** Ascites with cardiopulmonary embarrassment, ascites refractory to medical line of treatment and ascites causing abdominal discomfort.

Contraindications

- **Primary:** Bleeding and severe jaundice with impending hepatic coma because tapping may precipitate hepatic coma.
- **Secondary:** Multiple previous abdominal operations but can be done under ultrasound guidance and presence of dilated bowel.

General Instructions

- Abdominal paracentesis should be done with strict aseptic technique to prevent introduction of infection into the peritoneal cavity.
- Ask the patient to void five minutes before the procedure to prevent injury to the bladder.

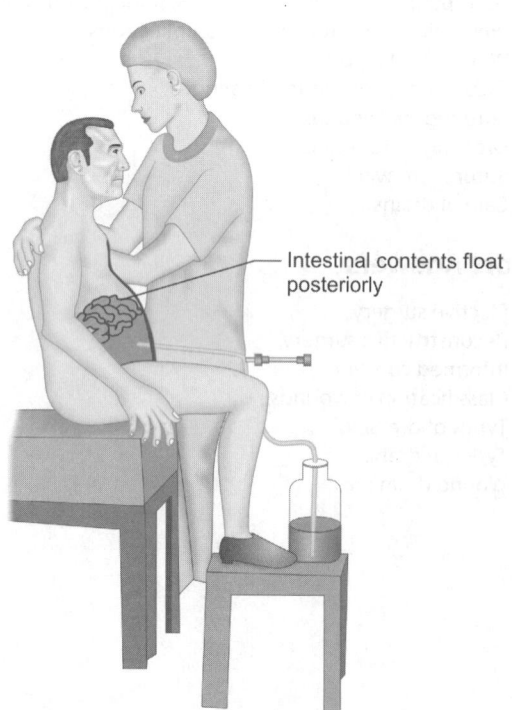

Fig. 32.1: Patient positioned for abdominal parencentesis.

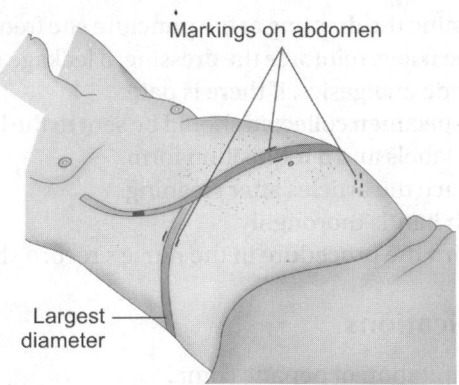

Fig. 32.2: Measuring the abdominal girth to conform the fluid collection.

- Keep the patient warm and comfortable to prevent chills.
- Withdrawing fluid should be done slowly and small quantity at a time.
- Use a tapping needle or trocar of smaller gauge possible. This will reduce the puncture wound as small as possible and thereby reduce the chance of fluid leaking from the peritoneal cavity after the procedure is over.
- The flow of fluid can be controlled by the application of clamps on the tubing.
- The nurse should remain with the patient throughout the procedure to observe the patient's general condition.
- The puncture wound should be sealed immediately after the procedure to prevent infection and leakage of peritoneal fluid.
- The specimens collected should be sent to the laboratory without delay.

Routine Investigations

- Specific gravity, cell count, bacterial count, protein concentrations, culture and acid test strain.
- In most disorders, the fluid is clear and straw colored. Turbidity suggests infection.
- Anguinous fluid usually signals neoplasm or tuberculosis.
- A protein concentration <3 g/100 mL suggests liver diseases or systemic disorders.
- Higher protein content suggests exudates cause such as tumor or an infection.

Preliminary Assessment Check

- The doctors order for any specific precautions.
- The general condition and diagnosis of the patient.
- Self-care ability of the patient.
- Condition of the abdomen.
- Articles available in the unit.

Preparation of the Patient and Environment

- Explain the procedure to the patient and his relatives.
- Obtain a written consent from the patient or relatives.

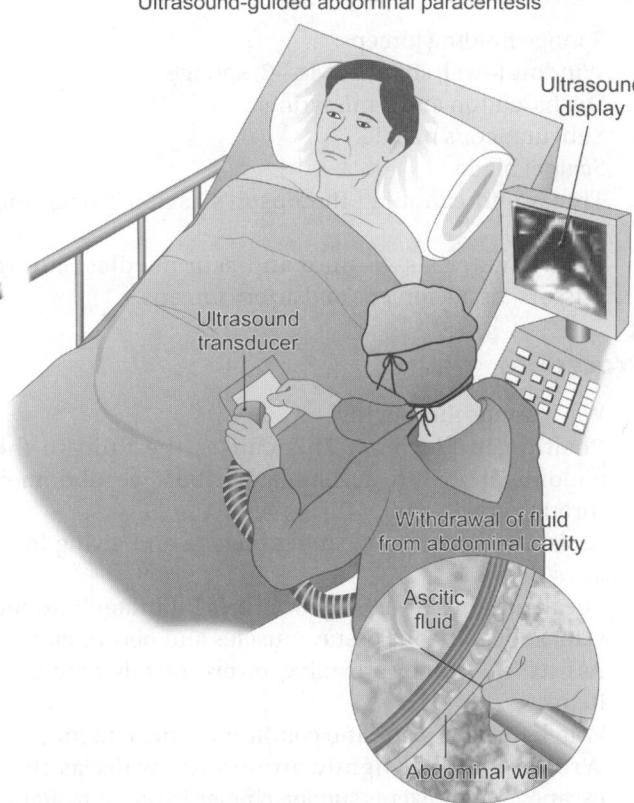

Fig. 32.3: Ultrasound guided abdominal parencentesis.

- Prepare the skin as for a surgical procedure.
- Empty the bladder just before the procedure.
- Maintain privacy with screens.
- Protect the bedding with a mackintosh and towel.
- Arrange the article at the bedside.

Site and Position

- **Premedication:** Inj. atropine sulphate 0.65 mg, intramuscularly half an hour procedure is given to the patient.
- **Selecting a site:** The primary object of selecting a site is to avoid injury to the urinary bladder and other abdominal organs. In the flank at midpoint below anterior superior iliac spine and umbilicus.

Position: The patient is positioned in Fowler's position supported by back rest and pillow near the edge of the bed.

Equipment

An unsterile tray containing:
- Mackintosh and towel.
- Sterile gloves and masks.
- Tincture iodine, spirit and tincture benzoin.
- Novocaine 1 to 2%/Xylocaine 2%.
- Adhesive tape and scissors.
- Kidney basins, pint measure, bucket.
- IV bottles, back rest and abdominal binder.

A Sterile Tray Containing

- Sponge holding forceps.
- Window towel, small bowls—2, sponge.
- Swabs, cotton and 2 mL syringe.
- Subcutaneous needle.
- Scalpel blade.
- Trocar and cannula (Thompson's ascites trocar and cannula).
- Suture materials—Suture and skin needles, suture scissors, tissue forceps and artery forceps.

Procedure

- Wash hands thoroughly.
- Position in Fowler's: This causes the fluid in the abdominal cavity to accumulate in the lower abdomen through gravity pull.
- Assist the doctor in cleaning the site and giving local anesthesia.
- Local anesthesia—2% lignocaine is infiltrated into the skin, subcutaneous tissue, muscles and peritoneum.
- Assist the doctor by providing towels and other required items.
- Watch the vital signs and condition of the patient.
- Wrap the binder tightly around the waist as fluid escapes. This prevents sudden change in pressure. Rapid change in pressure causes distention of abdominal veins, reducing blood in the heart. This may cause heart failure.
- Collect the required amount in a pint measure or bucket.
- Usually a pint to one liter of fluid is removed. Avoid rapid removal of fluid. Sudden withdrawal of a large quantity of fluid at one setting may change the intra-abdominal pressure.
- After finishing withdrawal of fluid, seal the puncture wound with tincture benzoin and cover with a pad to prevent leakage of fluid.

Post-procedure Care

- Apply abdominal binder tightly from top to bottom. It helps to maintain intra-abdominal pressure.
- Monitor the patient's general condition. Any change in the color, pulse, respiration and blood pressure should be reported immediately.
- Examine the dressing at the puncture site frequently for any leakage, reinforce the dressing, if leakage is present.
- Provide analgesics, if there is pain.
- The specimen collected should be sent to the laboratory with labels and a requisition form.
- Replace the articles after cleaning.
- Wash hands thoroughly.
- Record the procedure in the nurse's record sheet.

Complications

- Precipitation of hepatic coma.
- Fainting, if large amount of fluid is removed too rapidly. This can be prevented by applying abdominal binder.
- Peritonitis.
- Perforation of viscus.
- Depletion of proteins.

THORACENTESIS

Thoracentesis is defined as introducing a hollow needle into pleural cavity and aspirating fluid, using aseptic technique.

Thoracentesis refer to the puncture by needle through the chest wall into the pleural space for the purpose of removing pleural fluid (blood, serous fluid, pus, etc.) and or air (pneumothorax).

Thoracentesis or pleural aspiration or pleural tap is the insertion of needle into the pleural space through the chest wall to remove the pleural fluid or possibly air.

Purpose

- To remove excessive pleural fluid (serous fluid, blood or pus).
- To drain fluid/air from pleural cavity for diagnostic or therapeutic purposes.
- To introduce medications.

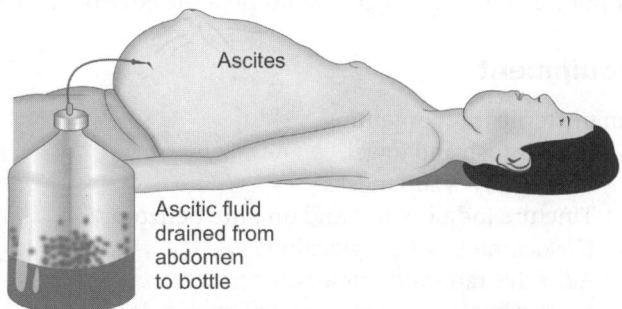

Fig. 32.4: Aspiration of fluid from the abdomen.

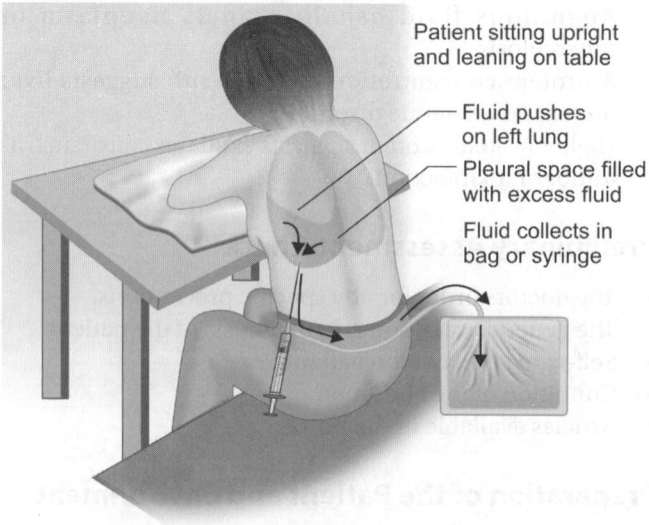

Fig. 32.5: Thoracentesis procedure.

- To aid in full expansion of lung.
- To obtain specimen for biopsy.
- To take pleural biopsy for diagnostic examination.
- To relieve pain.
- To relieve breathlessness caused by accumulation of fluid or air in the pleural space.
- To aid in diagnosis and treatment (chemical, bacteriological, cellular, composition and malignancy).

General Instructions

- The patient should be prepared physically and psychologically for the procedure.
- Thoracentesis is indicated in case of pleural effusion due to infection, traumatic injury, cancer or cardiac diseases, etc.
- Common site for thoracentesis is just below the scapula at the seventh or eighth intercostals space.
- The patient should be warned that any sudden movements during the procedure may cause injury to the lungs, blood vessels, etc.
- The level of the aspiration needle should be short to prevent pricking of the lungs.
- Usually upright position is used during the procedure as it helps to collect the pleural fluid at the base of the pleural cavity and hence facilitates to remove the fluid easily.
- Maintain strict aseptic technique to prevent introduction of infection into the pleural space.
- The 3 way adaptor should be fitted with the needle before it is introduced into the chest cavity.
  The adaptor should be in a closed position to prevent the entry of air in to the pleural cavity.
- The nurse should check the syringes and needle for airtightness. If these are not air-tight, air may be entering the pleural cavity and collapse.
- Remove the fluid slowly and not more than 1000 mL at a time, if the tap is therapeutic to prevent mediastinal shift.
- Use water seal drainage system, if pleural fluid is purulent and difficult to drain.
- The specimen should be sent to the laboratory soon after it collected.

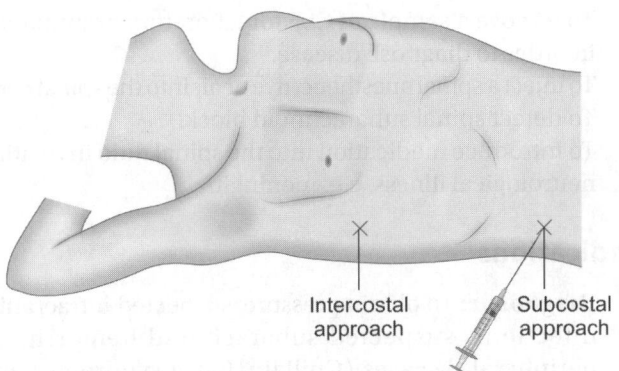

Fig. 32.6: Thoracenthesis position and site.

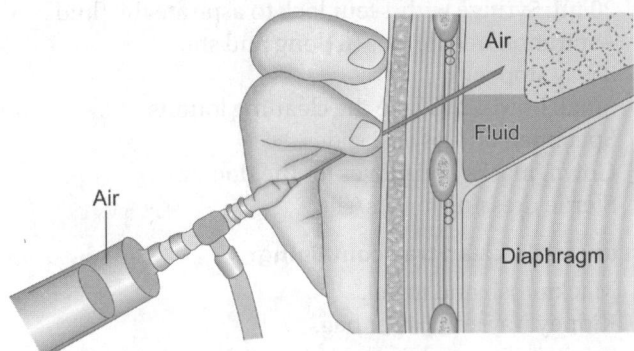

Fig. 32.7: Aspiration of air from the pleural cavity.

- The aspiration should be discontinued, if any signs of complications are noted such as sharp pain, respiratory distress, excessive coughing, crepitus, hemoptysis, circulatory collapse, etc.

Preliminary Assessment Check

- Doctors order for any specific instructions.
- Written informed consent of the patient or relatives.
- General condition and diagnosis of the patient.
- Review fresh erect chest X-ray.
- Confirm the diagnosis, location and extent of the pleural air/fluid/pus.
- Acute respiratory insufficiency (tension pneumothorax, rapidly developing effusion without dyspnea) may demand thoracocentesis without X-ray.
- Mental status of the patient to follow instructions.
- Articles available in the unit.

Preparation of the Patient and Environment

- Explain the sequence of the procedure.
- Provide privacy.
- Chest X-ray should be taken before thoracentesis is done to diagnose the location.
- Check the vital signs and record it on the nurse's record for reference.
- A mild sedation may be given to the patient before starting the procedure.
- Maintain the desired position during the procedure.
- The nurse should remain near the patient to observe him and to remind him not to move during the procedure.
- Arrange the articles at the bedside or in the treatment room.
- Premedication inj-Atropine sulphate 0.65 mg, intramuscularly or intravenously half an hour before procedure.

Equipment

A sterile tray containing:
- Sponge holding forceps-1.
- Dissecting forceps-1.
- Syringe (5 mL) and 2 needles for giving local anesthesia.

- 20 mL Syringe with 1 leur lock to aspirate the fluid.
- Aspiration needle No. 16 (long and short).
- 3 way stopcock.
- Small bowls-2 to take the cleaning lotions.
- Specimen bottles and slides.
- Gown, masks and gloves for the doctor.
- Sterile dressing towels/slit.

An unsterile/clean tray containing:
- Mackintosh and towel.
- Kidney tray and paper bag.
- Spirit, iodine and tincture benzoin.
- Lignocaine 2%.
- Suction apparatus with water seal drainage system.

Procedure

- Position the patient in Fowler's. Bring patient to one-side of bed with feet supported, arms and head leaning forward on cardiac table with pillows.
- Unite gown to expose site for aspiration.
- Instinct patient to avoid coughing and to remain immobile during procedure.
- Explain that a feeling of deep pressure will be experienced while fluid is being aspirated from pleural space.
- Provide sterile gloves to doctor.
- Open sterile set and assemble 20 mL, 50 mL syringes, 20 to 22 G needles and aspiration needle.
- Pour antiseptic solution to clean site.
- After showing label to doctor clean top of local anesthetic bottle and assist to withdraw.
- Reassure patient and instruct to hold breath during insertion of aspiration needle.
- As physician does procedure, observe for signs and symptoms of complications.
- After fluid is withdrawn from pleural space, transfer to specimen container.
- After needle is withdrawn, apply pressure over puncture site. Assist in sealing site with tincture benzoin swab.

After Care

- Instruct patient to lie on nonaffected site for 1 hour. Ensure bed rest for 6 to 8 hours.
- Monitor vital signs every half hour until stable.
- Observe patient for signs and symptoms of hemothorax, tension pneumothorax, subcutaneous emphysema and air embolism.
- Administer analgesics and antibiotics as prescribed.
- Instruct patient to carry out deep breathing exercises.
- A chest X-ray may be taken to determine the effects of the procedure.
- The puncture site should be treated aseptically to prevent contamination of the wound.
- The container with aspirated fluid should be labeled and sent to the laboratory with requisition form.
- Replace the articles after cleaning.
- Wash hands thoroughly.
- Record the procedure in the nurse's record sheet.

Complications

- **Pneumothorax and hemothorax:** Sudden rise of sharp pain in the chest, persistent cough, shortness of breath, fall in blood pressure, rapid pulse, anxiety, restlessness and faintness, profuse sweating, pallor and cyanosis.
- **Tension pneumothorax:** Marked dyspnea, cyanosis, reduced or absence of breath sounds and decreased movement of chest on respiration on the affected site. Acute chest pain, increased pulse and respiratory rates. Shifting of the trachea to the unaffected side.
- **Mediastinal shift:** Cyanosis, severe dyspnea, deviation of larynx and trachea from their normal midline position towards the unaffected side, shifting of the heart beat position of maximum impulse and distended neck veins.
- **Pulmonary edema:** Blood tinged frothy sputum:
   a. Coughs, wheezing, severe dyspnea
   b. Cyanosis, tachycardia, tachypnea, distended neck veins
   c. Signs of heart failure, peripheral edema
   d. Altered level of consciousness.

LUMBAR PUNCTURE

Lumbar puncture is the insertion of a needle into the subarachnoid space of the spinal canal to withdraw cerebrospinal fluid. Lumbar puncture or spinal tap or spinal puncture is the insertion of a needle into the lumbar region of the spine for removal of cerebrospinal fluid.

Lumbar puncture is an aspiration of cerebrospinal fluid (CSF) from the subarachnoid space (lumbar cistern) by puncturing the space between the spinous process of L3/L4 or L4/L5.

Purpose

- To test the pressure of CSF.
- To relieve pressure by removing CSF.
- To remove fluids such as CSF, blood, pus, etc. contained in the subarachonid space, thereby reduce the intracranial pressure.
- To remove a sample of CSF for laboratory examination in order to diagnose disease.
- To inject a spinal anesthetic, dye or air into the spinal cord.
- To detect spinal subarachnoid block.
- To introduce medication into the spinal fluid in treating neurological illness, e.g. meningitis.

Indications

- **Diagnostic:** To obtain pressure, suspected intracranial infections, suspected subarachnoid hemorrhage, peripheral diseases (Guillain–Barré syndrome) and peripheral vascular diseases.

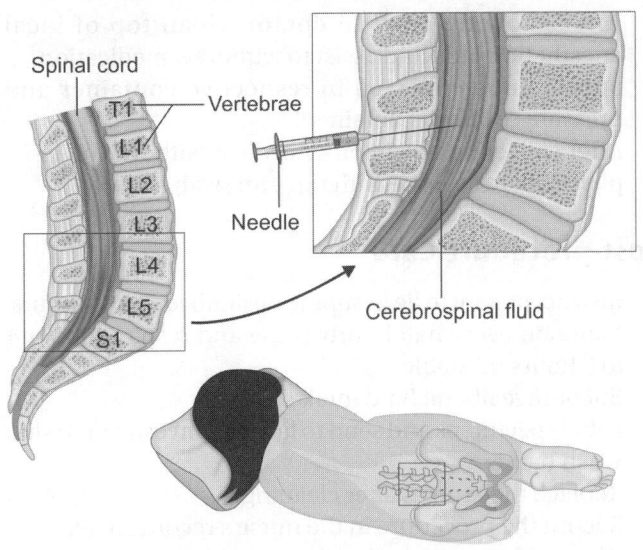

Fig. 32.8: Lumbar puncture procedure.

- **Therapeutic:** Intrathecal drug administration Inj. hydrocortisone 50 to 100 mg in spinal arachnoiditis, tuberculous meningitis to prevent late fibrotic strictures. Inj. crystalline penicillin in pyogenic meningitis. Inj. methotrexate in acute lymphatic leukemia.
- **Anesthetic:** Inj. lignocaine 50 mg and inj. bupivacaine 1% in spinal anesthesia.
- **Radiological:** To do a myelogram/myelography/ myodil dye injection.

Contraindications

- Gross spinal tension with obvious neurological damage because of danger of complete transvere lesion.
- Sepsis in skin at or near the proposed puncture site or osteomyelitis.
- Papilledema or other signs of raised intracranial pressure or focal neurological signs, until intracranial mass is ruled out.
- Bleeding diathesis or anticoagulant therapy.

General Instructions

- Site used for lumbar puncture is between third and fourth or between fourth and fifth lumbar vertebrae in adults and still lower in children.
- Strict aseptic techniques are to be followed. Since any infection introduced into the spinal cavity would be fatal for the patient.
- The position used is side lying position with the knees drawn to the chin or a sitting position with the head and neck flexed is maintained during the procedure.
- The patient should be placed near the edge of the bed or table for the convenience of the doctor.
- The lumbar puncture needles should be sharp, small in size and not curved.
- The pressure reading of the CSF is taken when the patient is relaxed and the fluid level remains fairly constant in the manometer.
- The flow of CSF varies in different conditions, when the intracranial pressure is high the fluid may spurt out in jets, when the tension is low as in case of dehydration.
- The patient's vital sign should be checked frequently during and after the procedure to detect the early signs of complications.
- Drug to be injected must be warmed to body temperature and it should be injected very slowly.
- The amount of CSF withdrawn is equal to the volume of fluid to be introduced or is sufficient for the laboratory investigations planned.
- If a 'Queckenstedt's test is to be carried out during the procedure. The nurse is asked to compress the jugular vein first on one side, then on the other side and finally on both sides at the same time.
- When the 'Queckenstedt's test is normal, there is a sharp rise in the pressure followed by a full as the compression is released. If the test is negative, one must conclude, that a block exists between the ventricles of the brain and the spinal canal which might be caused by spinal tumor, dislocation or fracture of the vertebrae, etc.
- Queckenstedt's test is control indicated in the presence of intracranial disease particularly in the presence of intracranial pressure and intracranial hemorrhage.
- At the end of the procedure, the puncture site is sealed to prevent leakage of fluid from the spinal cavity and infection, entering into the spinal cavity.
- After the lumbar puncture, the patient should lie flat on the bed.

CSF Analysis Done to Detect

- **Physical findings:** Color and appearance normally the CSF is crystal clear. Turbulence indicate infection, blood indicates hemorrhage.
- **Cell count:** Normally there is no RBC found in CSF. Presence of RBC indicates hemorrhage in the CNS. Increased number of WBC indicates infection somewhere in the CNS.
- **Sugar count:** Bacterial infections such as tuberculosis meningitis often lower the sugar content from the normal level of 40 to 60 mg per 100 mL.
- **Chloride level:** Bacterial infection also reduces the chloride level from the normal 720 to 750 mg per 100 mL.
- **Protein level:** In the presence of degenerative diseases and brain tumors, the protein content is increased from the normal level of 30 to 50 mg per 100 mL.
- **Serological test:** Serological test for syphilis may be positive in the CSF even when the blood serology is negative.

Preliminary Assessment

- The doctor's order for specific instructions.
- General condition and diagnosis of the patient.

- Self-care ability of the patient.
- Mental status to follow directions or instructions.
- Specimen bottles available to collect sample.
- Equipment available in the unit.

Preparation of the Patient and Environment

- Explain the sequences of the procedure.
- Provide privacy.
- Warn the patient that any movement.
- Monitor the vital signs before the procedure starts.
- Prepare the skin as for as a surgical procedure.
- Arrange the articles that are necessary for lumbar puncture at the bedside.
- Protect the bed with mackintosh and towel.
- The nurse should stand near the patient throughout the procedure observing the general condition and helping him to maintain the desired position.
- Provide a stool for the doctor to sit comfortably during the procedure.

Equipment

An unsterile tray containing:
- Mackintosh drapes and towel.
- Cleaning articles, tincture, iodine, spirit.
- Local anesthetic 2% Xylocaine.
- Tincture benzoin.
- Mask, apron.
- Kidney tray or plastic bag.
- Monometers, specimen container, lab requisition forms.

A sterile tray containing:
- LP needles-2 sizes with their stilette.
- Sponge holding forceps.
- Syringe (5 mL) with needles to give local anesthesia.
- Small bowl to take cleaning lotion.
- Specimen bottles.
- Cotton balls, gauze pieces and cotton pads.
- Gloves, gown and masks.
- Dressing towels or slit.
- The 3 way adapter, manometer and tubing to measure the pressure of CSF.

Procedure

- Position patient on left side with pillow under head and between legs.
- Make the patient to lie on firm surface with spine parallel to edge of bed.
- Place the patient in fetal position to that chin touches knee and assist patient to maintain this posture throughout procedure.
- Cover the patient with top sheet and expose back.
- Wash hands thoroughly.
- Provide sterile gloves to doctor.
- Open a LP set and assists in preparing site.
- Open 5 mL, 2 ml syringe, 20 or 22 G needles and place one by one into sterile tray.
- After showing label to doctor, clean top of local anesthetic bottle and assist to withdraw medication.
- Specimen is collected in respective container and pressure reading is obtained.
- After collecting specimens, needle is withdrawn. Assist physician to seal site with tincture swab.

Post-procedure Care

- Instruct patient to lie in supine position for 6 to 24 hours.
- Maintain every half hourly pulse and respiration for 4 to 5 hours till stable.
- Encourage liberal fluid intake.
- Label specimens and send to lab with investigation slip.
- Wash hands.
- Replace the articles after cleaning.
- Record the procedure in the nurse's record sheet.
- Observe for any complication.
- Check the puncture site frequently for CSF leak.

Complications

- Injury to the spinal cord and spinal nerves.
- Infection introduced into the spinal cavity which may rise to meningitis.
- Leakage of CSF through the puncture site and lowering the intracranial pressure and cause post-puncture headaches.
- Damage to intervertebral disks.
- Pain radiating to the things due to tumor of the spinal nerves.
- Herniation of the brain structures into the foramen magnum due to sudden reduction in the intracranial pressure.
- Temperature elevation.
- Local pain, edema and hematoma at the puncture site.
- Sixth cranial nerve palsy caused by removal of large volume of CSF with traction on the sixth nerve.

BONE MARROW BIOPSY AND ASPIRATION

Aspiration is defined as sucking a small amount of tissue in to the needle by applying suction with syringe.

Biopsy is defined cutting and removing a small amount of tissue from an area for examination.

Bone marrow aspiration is a diagnostic procedure performed in blood dyscrasias in which a specimen of bone marrow is taken from the sternum, iliac crest posterior superior iliac spine or tibia (children) by means of a hollow thick needle.

Purpose

- To diagnose blood dyscrasia such as aplastic anemia, leukemia, thrombocytopenia, etc.
- To diagnose metastatic neoplasm.
- To diagnose deficiency states of *vit-biz*, folic-acid, iron, pyridoxine, etc.

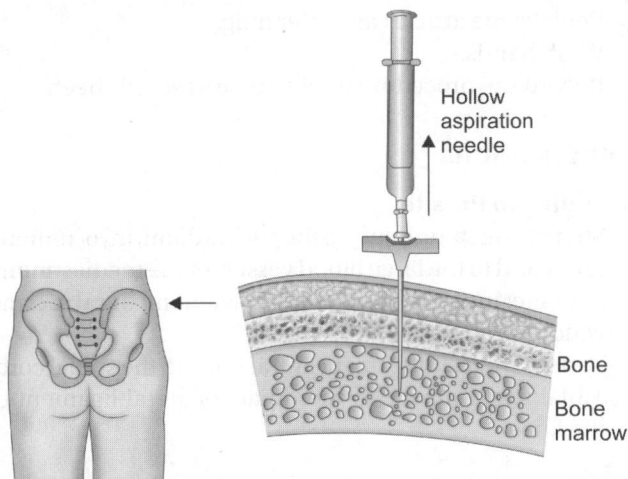

Fig. 32.9: Bone morrow aspiration procedure.

- To diagnose toxic states producing bone marrow depression or destruction.
- To determine the number, size and shape of red cells, white cells and platelets.
- To follow course of disease and patient's response to treatment.

Indications

Diagnostic: Bone marrow examination is essential for the diagnosis of a plastic, megaloblastic anemia, multiple myeloma, myelofibrosis, myelosclerosis and aleukemic leukemia. Bone marrow examination is helpful but not essential for diagnosis of anemia, leukemia, thrombocytopenic purpura, agranulocytoma, tropical diseases; malaria, kala-azar, etc.

Prognostic: Agranulocytosis, leukemia and anemia,

Therapeutic: Bone marrow transplant.

Site and Position of the Patient

Sternal puncture: The usual puncture site is either the manubrium sterni or the upper part of the body of sternum. The patient lies in the dorsal recumbent position (Supine) with a pillow under the shoulders to raise the chest.

Iliac puncture: The bone marrow biopsy is taken from the iliac crest 2 cm posterior and 2 cm interior to the anterior superior iliac spine. Alternately, the posterior iliac spine is also used. For iliac puncture, the patient lies either on his side or abdomen.

Spinous process aspiration: In the spinous process of the lumbar vertebrae, usually L3 or L4 is the puncture site. The patient is placed in the lumbar puncture position.

Tibial puncture in children: In children up to the age of two years the proximal end of tibia, just below the tibial condyles and medial to the tibial tuberosity is selected.

General Instructions

- The procedure should be done under very strict aseptic technique, since the infection can be introduced into the bone cavity through the puncture site.
- The penetration of the needle beyond the bone cavity is prevented by a guard attached to the needle.

Preliminary Assessment Check

- The doctors order for any specific instructions.
- General condition and diagnosis of the patient.
- Self-care ability of the patient.
- Mental status to follow instructions.
- Availability of articles in the unit.
- Location and type of insertion.

Preparation of the Patient and Environment

- Explain the sequence procedure to the patient.
- Provide privacy.
- A thorough preparation of skin to prevent infection introduced in to the bone cavity.
- Place the patient in a correct position according to the site used.
- Sedation may be given to the patient.
- Arrange the articles at the bedside or in the treatment room.
- Check the vital signs of the patient and record it in the nurse's record sheet.
- The nurse should remain with the patient to reassure him and to observe him during the procedure.

Equipment

A sterile tray containing:
- Sponge holding forceps—1.
- Dissecting forceps—2.
- The complications should be watched for injury to associate organs.
- The vital signs should be checked throughout the procedure and reassure the patient.

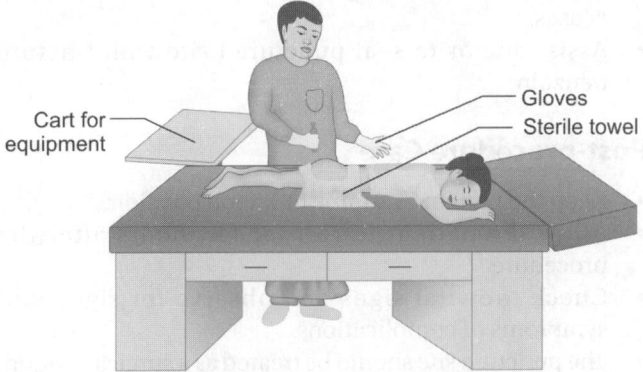

Getting ready for the bone marrow test

Fig. 32.10: Positioning the child for bone marrow aspiration.

- The nurse should remain with the patient throughout the procedure and observe for signs of complications.
- Smear is made on 3 to 4 slides. Specimens are sent to the laboratory without delay.
- Marrow puncture needle with obturator—1.
- Aspiration syringe—1.
- Syringe for local anesthesia—1, needle—2.
- Small bowls—2, to take cleaning solutions.
- Cotton swabs, gauze pieces, cotton pads, etc. in containers.
- Dressing towels or slit to create a sterile field.
- BP handle with blade—1, to make a small incision on the skin.
- Slides to make smears.

An unsterile tray containing:
- Mackintosh and towel.
- Lignocaine 2%.
- Adhesive tape and scissors.
- Kidney tray and paper bag.
- Spirit, iodine, tincture benzoin, etc.

Procedure

- Transfer the patient from bed to treatment room.
- Position the patient and assess the doctor to locate and mark the site.
- Open small dressing pack and slides, syringes, needles and scalpel blade into pack.
- Assist the doctor to clean site with antiseptic solution and drape with sterile towels.
- A small incision may be made with scalpel blade. Bone marrow needle with stylet is introduced through incision and marrow is aspirated.
- Inform patient that a brief episode of sharp pain during aspiration will be experienced.
- Syringe with aspirated marrow is handed over to technician and collect into various containers as indicated.
- Collect bone marrow tissue in small bottle containing FAA solution.
- Apply pressure over punctured site until bleeding ceases.
- Assist doctor to seal punctured site with tincture benzoin.

Post-procedure Care

- Keep the patient in supine or lateral position.
- Allow the patient to rest for few hours after the procedure.
- Check the vital signs and observe for signs and symptoms of complications.
- The puncture site should be treated as a surgical wound. The dressing should be done under strict aseptic techniques.
- Give mild analgesics, if needed.
- Label specimen and send to laboratory.
- Replace the articles after cleaning.
- Wash hands.
- Record the procedure in the nurse's record sheet.

Complications

According to the site
- Sternal puncture: Injury to the pericardium, myocardium, lungs and to the large blood vessels of the mediastinum.
- Iliac site: Injury to the sacroiliac ligament, dural sac and cauda equina.
- Vertebral site: Injury to the dural sac and the spinal cord.
- Tibial site: Damage to the tibial collateral ligament of the knee.

Other Complications

- Bleeding from puncture site. The causes are thromocytopenia and bleeding diathesis. Bleeding can be prevented by local pressure.
- Perfection of aorta, due to penetration of posterior side of sternum, if too much force is applied.
- Infection (osteomyelitis).

SURGICAL DRESSING

Surgical dressing is a sterile technique used to promote wound healing. It is a protective covering placed on the wound.

Purpose

- To protect the wound from mechanical injury.
- To splint or immobilize the wound.
- To absorb drainage.
- To prevent contamination from bodily discharges (feces, urine).
- To debride the wound by combining capillary action and the end of necrotic tissue and in its mesh.
- To inhibit or kill microorganisms by using dressings with antiseptics, antimicrobial properties.
- To provide a physiologic environment conducive to healing.
- To provide mental and physical comfort for the patient.

Types of Dressing

- **Dry-to-dry dressing**
  - Offers good wound protection, absorption of drainage.
  - Disadvantage: They adhere to wound surface when drainage dries, removal can cause pain and disruption of granulation tissue.
- **Wet-to-dry dressing**
  - They are particularly useful for untidy or infected wounds that must be debrided and closed by 2 degree.

- Gauze saturated with sterile saline or an antimicrobial solution is packed into the wound, eliminating dead space.
- The wet dressings are then covered by dry dressings.
- As drying occurs, wound debris and necrotic tissue are absorbed into the gauze dressing by capillary action.
- The dressing is changed when it become dry.
• **Wet-to-wet dressings**
  - Used on clean open wounds as on granulating surfaces, sterile saline as an antimicrobial agent may be to saturate the dressings.
  - Provide a more physiologic environment, which can enhance the local healing process as well as ensure greater patient comfort.
  - Disadvantage: Surrounding tissues can become macerated, the risk of infection may rise and bed linens become damp.

General Instructions

- The procedure of changing dressings, examining and closing the wound, uses principles of asepsis.
- The initial dressing change is frequently done by the physician especially for craniotomy, orthopedic or thoractomy procedures; subsequent dressing changes are the nurse's responsibility.

Equipment

Sterile

- Gloves—disposable
- Scissors, forceps
- Appropriate dressing materials
- Sterile saline
- Cotton dipped swabs
- Culture tubes
- For draining wound add extra gauze and packing material, absorbent pad and irrigation set.

Unsterile

- Gloves
- Plastic bag for discarded dressings
- Tape proper size and type
- Pads to protect patient bed
- Gown for nurse if wound is infected.

Procedure

Pre-preparation

- Inform the patient of dressing change. Explain procedure and have patient lie in bed.
- Avoid changing dressing at mealtime.
- Ensure privacy by drawing the curtains or closing the door. Expose dressing site.
- Respect patient modesty and prevent patient from being chilled.
- Wash hands thoroughly.
- Place dressing supplies on a clean, flat surface.
- Place clean towel or plastic bag under part of the body where wound in located.
- Cut-off pieces of tape to be used in dressing change.
- Place disposable bag nearby to collect soiled dressings.
- Determine how many and what types of dressings are necessary.

Cleaning the Surgical Wound

- Use aseptic technique.
- Open package of sterile gloves; open sterile cleaning sterile supplies.
- Wear sterile gloves.
- Clean along wound edges using a small circular motion from one end of incision to the other do not scrub back and forth across the incision line.
- Sterile saline in the cleansing agent of choice. Topical antiseptics alcohol, basically may be used on intact skin surrounding the wound but should never be used within the wound.
- Repeat same process with drain site separately.
- Discard used cleaning supplies in disposable.
- Pad the incision site and drain site dry with a sterile dressing sponge.

Dressing the Wound

- Maintain asepsis with use of sterile gloves.
- After wound in dry apply appropriate dressing.
- Tape dressing, using only the amount of tape required for secure attachment of dressing.
- When dressing the drain site.
  - Use premade drain sponge (Can be prepared by making 5 cm slit with sterile scissors in 4x4 inch gauze sponge).
  - Gently slip sponge around drain repeat with second drain sponge, placing it at right angle to other sponge.

  Dressing the drainage tube insertion site: Be sure that one sponge in place at a right angle to the second sponge. So, the slits are going in different direction, if drainages in heavy, a sterile absorbent pad or extra gauze may be placed overall.
- When dressing an excessive draining wound:
  - Consider need for extra dressings and packing materials.
  - Use Montgomery straps, if frequent dressings are required.
  - Protect skin surrounding wound from copious on irritating drainage by applying some type of skin barriers.

After Care (Follow-up Care)

- Assess patient's tolerance to the procedure and help patient more comfortable.

- Discard disposable items according to hospital protocol and clean equipment that is to be recessed.
- Wash hands.
- Record nature of procedure and condition of wound, as well as patient reaction.

LIVER BIOPSY

Definition

It is the removal of a bit of liver tissue particularly for histological examination.

Purpose

- Diagnostic purpose.
- Morphologic studies.
- Biochemical studies.
- Bacteriologic studies.
- Immunologic studies.
- To get information regarding progression of disease.
- Response to therapy.

Indication

- Cirrhosis of liver.
- Hepatic malignancies.
- Granulomas.
- Reticuloendothelial diseases, e.g. Leukemia.

Contraindication

- Bleeding disorders, e.g. thrombocytopenia.
- Infection in liver, peritoneum, biliary tract.
- Severe form of hepatocellular jaundice.
- Gross ascites.
- Suspected hemangioma of liver.

Site: Needle is inserted at eighth and ninth intercostals space.

Position

- Position the patient on the right side near to the edge of bed.
- After procedure position patient supine.

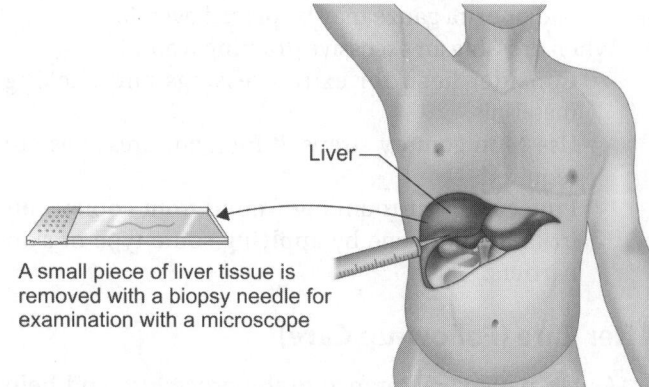

Fig. 32.11: Liver biopsy.

General Instruction

- Aseptic technique to be followed.
- Investigate clotting time, bleeding time and prothrombin time.
- Explain the need of procedure in a simple way.
- Watch for complications during and after the procedure.
- Keep 2U of blood available for emergency.
- After procedure patient should take 24 hours strict bed rest.

Preliminary Assessment

- Check the doctor's order for specific instructions.
- Check age, sex, name and diagnosis of patient.
- Check investigation report from laboratory.
- Check patient's ability to obey orders.
- Check patient's self-care ability.
- Check if all articles are available in the unit.

Preparation of Patient and Environment

- Explain the procedure to minimize fear and anxiety.
- Provide privacy.
- Position the patient.
- Teach the patient breathing exercise.
- Vitamin K is injected to prevent hemorrhage.
- Informed consent is obtained from the patient.
- Shave the area and clean it with antiseptic agent.
- Arrange articles at bedside.
- Monitor vitals before, during and after the procedure.
- Maintain nil per OS (NPO), hours before procedure.

Equipment Needed

An Unsterile Tray

- Solutions- Surgical spirit, tincture benzoin, iodine.
- Mackintosh with towel
- K-basin
- Paper bag
- Xylocaine 2%.

Sterile Tray

- Formalin 10% solution in a container.
- Sponge holding forceps.
- Dissecting forceps.
- Small 2 bowls to receive solutions.
- 5 mL syringe with needle.
- Liver biopsy needle with stylet.
- Specimen bottles with formalin and stopcock.
- Sterile dressing towels.
- Dressing materials—5 cotton balls, 2 Pads, 3 Gauges.
- Gloves, mask, gown.

Procedure

- Procedure by the physician.
- Give adequate instructions (not to move during procedure).

- Position the patient on the examination table.
- Wear gown, face mask and gloves.
- Open the sterile pack and pour the solution into small bowls.
- Surgical cleaning is done by doctor.
- Instruct the patient to take a deep breath.
- Needle is inserted to the area for taking biopsy.
- Hold the puncture site with left hand and remove needle with right hand.
- Apply mild and gentle pressure over the area.
- Sent the liver biopsy to laboratory with written instruction.

After Care

- Place patient in comfortable position.
- Instruct client to take rest for 12 to 24 hours.
- Check for complications such as bleeding, hematoma formation.
- Monitor vital signs.
- Replace articles after washing and sent to CSSD.
- Keep patient NPO for 4 hours.
- Wash hands thoroughly.
- Recording and reporting.
- Documentation.

Complications

- Pain due to irritation of liver cells.
- Hemorrhage.
- Damage to neighboring organs.
- Peritonitis.
- Infection the needle site.
- Shock.
- Pneumothorax.

WOUND CARE

Chronic wounds such as bed sores, ulcers, and abscesses are often an important part of wound care nursing. Wound care nurses can also care for ostomy sites, as well as the areas around feeding tubes, ports, and recent surgeries. Most work in a hospital setting, treating patients who require acute care; although some travel as home health consultants, or work in nursing homes and other residential facilities. Wound care nurses may need to consult with doctors to discuss the need for antibiotics, surgical drains, or surgical debridement in the case of serious wounds. They also work with other patient caregivers to educate them about wound care and handling the patient's case. For example, in an elderly person with bed sores, regular rotation of the patient and the use of specialized pillows to relieve pressure on the sores may be an important part of patient care.

Definitions: Wound care is defined as cleaning, monitoring and promoting healing in a wound that is closed with sutures, clips or staples.

Purpose of Dressing

- Provide physical, psychological and anesthetic comfort.
- Remove necrotic tissue.
- Prevent, eliminate or control infection.
- Absorb drainage.
- Maintain a moist wound environment.
- Protect the wound from further injury.
- Protect the skin surrounding the wound.
- Promote homeostasis as in a pressure dressing.
- Prevent contamination from feces, urine, vomitus, etc.
- For splinting or immobilization of wound.

Types of Dressing

Dry dressing: Clean wounds are dressed by the application of 4 to 8 layers of gauze folded into suitable size and shape. The surrounding of the wound is cleansed by some antiseptic and dried and dry dressing is applied after the application of medicine to the wound.

Wet dressing: It is used if wounds are infected and if there is pus. The wet dressing compresses, it stimulated the supportive process. The dressing is made of many layers of gauze or cotton pad covered with gauze.

Pressure dressing: It is done when there is bleeding or oozing from the wound. The dressing consist thick pad of sterile gauze applied over the wound with a firm bandage and binder.

General Instructions

- Maintain aseptic technique to prevent cross infection to the wound and to the ward.
- All the material touching the wound should be sterile.
- Wash hands before and after each dressing to avoid cross infection.
- All articles should be disinfected thoroughly, so that they will be free from pathogens.
- Use masks, sterile gloves and gown for large dressing to minimize the wound contamination.
- Dressing is changed at least 15 minute after the room has been cleaned and avoid meal timings.
- Clean wound should be dressed before infected or discharging wounds.
- Wounds that are draining freely should be dressed frequently, according to the doctor's order.
- Avoid coughing, sneezing and talking when the wound is opened.
- While dressing avoid contamination with patients skin. Clothing and bed linen with soiled instruments and dressings.
- Clean the wound from cleanest area to the less clean area, e.g. clean the wound from its center to the periphery.
- If the dressings are adherent to the wound due to drying of the secretions or blood, wet it with normal saline before it is removed from the wound.

- While dressing, keep the wound edges as near as possible to promote healing.
- Measure the amount of discharge from the wound. Note the color, amount and consistency of the drainage.
- Before doing the dressing, inspect the wound for any complication and if it is present, report immediately to avoid further complications.

Preliminary Assessment

- Check the doctor's order for specific instructions.
- Identify the correct patient, bed number and general condition.
- Check the nurse's record to note the condition of the wound in previous dressing.
- Check the abilities of the patient for self-help, understanding and limitation.
- Check the availabilities of the articles.

Equipment

A sterile tray containing: Artery forceps-1, dissecting forceps-2, scissors-1, sinus forceps-1, probe-1, small bowl-1, safety pin-1, gloves, masks and gowns, cotton balls, gauze pieces, cotton pads and site or dressing towels.

A trolley containing: Cleaning solutions as necessary, ointments and powders as ordered, Vaseline gauze in sterile containers, roller gauze in sterile container, Cheatle forceps in a solution, sterile gauze, cotton and pad drum, bandages, adhesive plaster, pins and scissors, mackintosh and draw sheet, kidney tray and covered bucket to put soiled dressing.

Procedure

- Explain the procedure to the patient, using sensory preparation.
- Inspect the wound for redness, swelling or sign of dehiscence or evisceration.
- Observe the characteristics of any drainage.
- Clean the area around the wound with an appropriate cleansing solution.
- Swab from clean area towards the less clean area (clean the wound from the center to periphery).
- Apply medications if ordered.
- Apply sterile dressing—Apply gauze pieces first and then the cotton pads.
- Remove the gloves and discard it in to the bowl with lotion.
- Secure the dressing with bandage or adhesive tapes.

After Care

- Assess the patient to dress up and to take a comfortable position.
- Change the garments if soiled with drainage.
- Remove the mackintosh and towel. Replace the bed linen.
- Take all articles to the utility room. Discard the soiled dressing in to a covered container and send for incineration.
- Wash hands and record the procedure on the nurse's record with date and time.
- Teach the patient/family about wound care and signs and symptoms of infection.

CONCLUSION

Medical surgical nurses provide basic medical care to patients of all ages suffering an extensive variety of ailments. Preoperatively: Preparation of patients for their procedure involves ensuring premedication is administered, the patient/guardian has given written consent, the required blood-tests have been done, identification labels and identification bracelets are correct, all allergies have been recorded in the patient's notes and that the patient has been fasted appropriately. Post-operatively: Postoperatively the patient must be closely observed for signs of shock, arrest. The surgical nurse also ensures the wound created by the surgery is intact, and must be knowledgeable in wound care and the care of surgical drains. Surgical nurses are responsible for the management of pain and postoperative nausea and vomiting, which are common postoperative side effects. The surgical nurse is also responsible for the discharge of the patient and giving the patient information on support systems and measures necessary to their recovery.

BIBLIOGRAPHY

1. Alice L. Price. The Art, Science and Spirit of Nursing. Philadelphia: WB Saunders Company, 3rd Edition, 1968.
2. Kozier Barbara B, Du Gas, Beverly Witter. Fundamentals of Patient Care: A Comprehensive Approach to Nursing. WB Saunders Company, 1967.
3. McClosky JC, Grace HK. Current Issues in Nursing, 4th Edition. St. Louis: Mosby Year Book, Inc., 1994.
4. Mitchell PR, Grippando GM. Nursing Perspectives and Issues, 5th Edition. Albany, New York: Delmar Publishers, Inc., 1993.
5. Potter P, Perry A. Fundamentals of Nursing-Concepts, Process and Practice, 3rd Edition. Mosby Year Book, 1993.
6. Shafer, Kathleen, et al. Medical-Surgical Nursing, 6th Edition. Saint Louis: CV Mosby Co., 1975.
7. Shakuntala Sharma 'Birpuri'. Principles and Practice of Nursing. Jaypee Brothers Medical Publishers (P) Ltd., New Delhi, 1997.
8. Sr. Nancy. Principles and Practice of Nursing; Vol. 1, 3rd Edition. NR Brothers, Indore, 1992.
9. Taylor C, Lillis C, LeMone P. Fundamentals of Nursing: The Art and Science of Nursing Care. Phila-delphia: JB Lippincott, 1993.

10. Thresvamma CP, Mathew PC. Fundamentals of Nursing. Procedure Manual for General Nursing Course, Kottayam, Kerala, 1992.
11. Virginia Henderson. Principles and Practice of Nursing. New York: MacMillan Publishing Co, 1970.

REVIEW QUESTIONS

Long Essays

1. Define liver biopsy; explain the purpose, indication and procedure.
2. Define lumbar puncture; explain the purpose, indication and procedure.

Short Essays

1. Abdominal paracentesis: Indication and procedures.
2. Thoracentesis: Indication and procedures.
3. Bone marrow biopsy and aspiration.

Short Answers

1. Sternal puncture.
2. Iliac puncture.
3. Dry-to-dry dressing.
4. Wet-to-dry dressing.

APPENDIX 1

Abbreviations and Symbols

ABG: Arterial blood gas
Ab: Antibody
ABCDE: Airway, breathing, circulation, disability, expose and examine
AC: Before meal (ante cibum)
ACTH: Adreno corticotrophic hormone
AD: As desired
ADL: Activities of daily living
AIDS: Acquired immunodeficiency syndrome
AI: Adequate intake
AM: Morning
AMALG: Amalgam filling
AMA: Against medical advice
A and P: Auscultation and percussion
APC: Aspirin, phenacetin and caffeine
AP: Apical pulse or antero-posterior
AQ: Aqueous
A-R: Apical radial pulse
AROM: Active range of motion; artificial rupture of membrane
Ax: Axillary
BID: Twice a day (bis in die)
BM: Bowel movement
BMR:. Basal metabolic rate
BP: Blood pressure
BPM: Beats per minute
BRP:. Bathroom privilege
BUN: Blood urea nitrogen
C: Centigrade
CBC: Complete blood count
CC: Cubic centimeter
CNS: Central nervous system
CO_2: Carbon dioxide
CSF: Cerebrospinal fluid

CXR: Chest X-ray
D and C: Dilatation and curettage
DNS: Dextrose in normal saline
DPT: Diphtheria, pertussis, tetanus
D/W: Dextrose in water
Dx: Diagnosis
EEG: Electroencephalogram
EENT: Eye, ear, nose, throat
ECG: Electrocardiogram
F: Fahrenheit
FBS: Fasting blood sugar
FHB: Fetal heartbeat
GI: Gastrointestinal
G or Gm: Gram
Gr: Grain
Gt: Drop (gutte)
Gtt: Drops
GU: Genitourinary
GYN:. Gynecology
HCL: Hydrochloric acid
Hb: Hemoglobin
HS: At bed-time (hours of sleep)
H_2O: Water
IV:. Intravenous
IVP: Intravenous pyelogram
KI:. Potassium iodide
LP: Lumbar puncture
NaCl: Sodium chloride
NOCTE: At night
NPO: Nothing by mouth (nothing by os)
OPD: Outpatient department
OR:. Operating room
PM: Afternoon

PRN: As needed, when necessary
Pt: Patient
Q: Every
QD: Every Day
QH:. Every Hour
QID:. Four times a day
QN: Every night
QOD: Every other day
RBC: Red blood count or red blood cell
Rh: Rhesus factor
Rx: Prescription, take
Sol: Solution

SOS: If necessary
STAT: Immediately -at once
SC: Subcutaneous
TID: Three times a day
TPR:. Temperature, pulse, respiration
Tsp: Teaspoon, tablespoon
ULQ: Upper lower quadrant
UR:. Upper right
URQ: Upper right quadrant
UTI: Urinary tract infection
WBC: White blood cells
Wt: Weight

APPENDIX 2
Temperature Conversion Table

TEMPERATURE

Degree-C: means temperature in degrees Celsius (degree C × 9/5 + 32 = degree F)

Degree-F: means temperature in degrees Fahrenheit (degree F- 32 × 5/9 = degree C)

°C	°F	°C	°F
34.0	93.2	38.6	101.5
34.2	93.6	38.8	101.8
34.4	93.9	39.0	102.2
34.6	94.3	39.2	102.6
34.8	94.8	39.4	102.9
35.0	95.0	39.6	103.3
35.2	95.4	39.8	103.6
35.4	95.7	40.0	104.0
35.6	96.1	40.2	104.4
35.8	96.4	40.4	104.7
36.0	96.8	40.6	105.2
36.2	97.2	40.8	105.4
36.4	97.5	41.0	105.9
36.6	97.9	41.2	106.1
36.8	98.2	41.4	106.5
37.0	98.6	41.6	106.8
37.2	99.0	41.8	107.2
37.4	99.3	42.0	107.6
37.6	99.7	42.2	108.0
37.8	100.0	42.4	108.3
38.0	100.4	42.6	108.7
38.2	100.8	42.8	109.0
38.4	101.1	43.0	109.4

APPENDIX 3
Laboratory Values

Normal Values

Test	Normal values	Test	Normal values
• FBS	70–100 mg%	Calcium	8.5–105 mg%
• RBS	80–120 mg%	• Phosphorus	2.5–5 mg%
• PPBS	100–140 mg%	LIPID PROFILE	
• Urine sugar	Nil	• Cholesterol	150–250 mg%*
• Glyocsylated Hb	4.5–8 mg%	• HDL cholesterol	30–70 mg%*
• Urea	10–45 mg%	• Triglyceride	10–160 mg%
• Creatinine	0.7–1.5 mg%	• VLDL	6–40 mg%
		• LDL	180 mg%
• Uric acid	3–7 mg%	• Acid phosphatase	0–3 KAU/dL
• Sodium	133–143 mEq/L	• Amylase	25–125 U/dL
• Potassium	3.9–5.3 mEq/L		
• Chloride	98–108 mEq/L		
• Blood non-protein nitrogen (NPN)	20–40 mg%	*Better to keep serum cholesterol level below 200 mg%	
LIVER FUNCTIONS TEST		IRON PROFILE	
• Total Protein	6–8 g/dL	• Iron	60–205 µg/dL
• Albumin	3.4–5 g/dL	• TIBC	230–380 µg/dL
• A/G ratio	1.2–1.7	• Transferrin	1.2–2 g/dL
• Total bilirubin	0.2–1.2 mg%		
• Conj. bilirubin	0.1–0.4 mg%	URINE	
• SGOT (AST)	5–50 IU/L	• Creatinine	1.0–1.8
• SGPT (ALT)	5–50 IU/L	• Reducing sugars	100 mg/day
• Alkaline phosphatase	100–250 IU/L	• Urea	30 g/day
• Gamma GT (GGT)	10–45 IU/L	• Uric acid	0.8 g/day
• CPK	0–192 IU/L	• Chloride	10–15 g/day
• CPK-B	0–13 IUL	• Urobilinogen	0.4 g/day
• CPK-MB	0–25 IU/L	• Ketone bodies	1 mg/day
• LDH	200–400 IU/L	• Phosphorus	10 g/day
		• Titrable acidity	200–400 mL

Glossary

- **Acidosis:** Abnormal accumulation of acid in or loss of base from the body, with pH less than 7.35.
- **Activities of daily living (ADL):** All the activities an individual carries out to maintain physical integrity.
- **Acute phase of illness:** Time when therapy and nursing care are directed toward assisting the patient to recover from disabling disease or injury with a minimum of superimposed impairment—social, psychological, or physical.
- **Adaptation:** The work expended by the body in attempting to maintain homeostasis and to ward off the effects of stressors. Adaptive behaviors are those that promote adaptation.
- **Adolescence:** Period between the onset of puberty and the cessation of physical growth, the passage from childhood to adulthood.
- **Airway management:** Corrects positioning of the airway, appropriate interventions used to ensure potency of the airway and adequate oxygenation and ventilation.
- **Airway:** Name given to the passages which connect the lungs to the atmosphere outside the body.
- **Alkalosis:** Abnormal accumulation of base in or loss of acid from the body, with pH greater than 7.45.
- **Angina:** Pain produced by the heart; a severe crushing pain in the center of the chest or strangling sensation in the throat.
- **Antitoxin:** A particular kind of antibody produced by the body in response to the presence of a toxin.
- **Anuria:** Absence of urine formation, usually indicative of kidney failure but may be secondary to severe dehydration.
- **Apoplexy:** Old fashioned name for a stroke or bleeding in the brain.
- **Artery:** Blood vessel which takes blood from the heart to the rest of the body.
- **Artificial respiration:** Method of helping the victim to breath; this is best done by the mouth to mouth method.
- **Asphyxia:** Out of date term for breathing with difficulty, which leads to shortage of oxygen, an excess of carbon dioxide in the blood and eventual suffocation.
- **Assessment:** A dynamic, ongoing process that uses observations and interactions to collect information, recognize changes, analyze needs and plan care.
- **Assessments:** The evaluation and interpretation of short and long-term measurements to provide a basis for decision making and to enhance public health officials' ability to monitor disaster situations.
- **Asthma:** Condition which makes breathing difficult, often accompanied by a wheeze.
- **Atelectasis:** A collapsed or airless state of the lung that may involve all or part of the lung.
- **Atresia:** Absence or abnormal closure of a normal body orifice or passage.
- **Auscultation:** Elicitation and evaluation of sounds produced by the body, frequently by using a stethoscope to magnify body sounds.
- **Auscultation:** Observation by listening with the stethoscope to organ sounds within the body.
- **Autonomy:** The governing of one's self according to one's own system of morals and beliefs or life plan.
- **Bacteriostasis:** The process of preventing the growth and reproduction of microorganisms by the use of chemicals or heat.
- **Bandage:** Strip of cloth or other material used to bind up a wound.
- **Baseline data:** Information gathered about pre-illness states from initial contact used to measure changes in the patient's condition.
- **Basic human needs:** Physical and psychological needs common to all people that create tension and anxiety if not met.
- **Basic life support:** It includes noninvasive measures used to treat unstable patients, such as extraction of airway obstructions, cardiopulmonary resuscitation, care of wounds and hemorrhages, and immobilization of fractures.
- **Basis four food groups:** One pattern for devising a balanced diet including milk group, meat group, vegetable-fruit group, and bread-cereal group.
- **Bladder training:** Program to assist the incontinent patient to control urination without catheter and without retention.
- **Bland diet:** Similar to a general diet but excludes highly seasoned, fried, and fatty foods and foods high in roughage. Also called light diet.
- **Blood:** Red fluid which circulates in the arteries and veins of the body transporting oxygen and food stuffs and removing waste materials.
- **Body alignment:** The position in which the various parts of the body are held while sitting, standing, walking, and lying.
- **Body mechanics:** Efficient use of the body as a machine and as a means of locomotion, balance, and stability.
- **Bowel training:** Program to assist incontinent patient in achieving bowel control, allowing controlled bowel movement every 1 to 3 days.
- **Brachial artery:** The main blood vessel of the arm.
- **Bronchial drainage:** Treatment to assist removal of retained bronchial secretions. Usually follows intermittent positive pressure or nebulizer treatment. Includes special positioning and use of percussion and vibration techniques.
- **Capillary:** Minute blood vessels between the ends of the arteries and the beginnings of the veins.
- **Carbon dioxide:** Waste gas produced by the body and exhaled through the lungs and air passages.
- **Carbon monoxide:** Poisonous gas produced by car and other internal combustion engines and in some domestic gas supplies. It is extremely dangerous and, if inhaled, can kill.
- **Cardiopulmonary resuscitation (CPR):** Protocol performed when an individual's respiratory and cardiovascular system require support to maintain vital functions, airway management, ventilation and chest compressions are provided to improve tissue perfusion until definitive care is available.

- **Carotid artery:** Main artery in the neck.
- **Case definition:** Standardized criteria for deciding whether a person has a particular disease or health related condition; often used in investigations and for comparing potential cases; case definitions help decide which disaster-specific conditions should be monitored with emergency information surveillance systems.
- **Case finding:** A set of activities used by the nurse working in community settings that identifies clients who are not currently receiving health care, but who could benefit from such care.
- **Case management:** A systematic process used by nurses to ensure that client's multiple health and service needs are met. These include assessing client needs, planning and coordination services, referring to other appropriate providers and monitoring and evaluating process.
- **Case management:** Case management is the collaborative process that assesses, plans, implements, coordinates, monitors, and evaluates the options and services required to meet an individual's health needs.
- **Casualty:** Any person suffering physical and/or psychological damage that leads to death, injury, or material loss.
- **Celsius:** Metric temperature measurement with 0°C being the freezing point of water and 100°C being the boiling point. Normal body temperature is 37°C.
- **Chronic illness:** A condition or illness that is long-term and either without cure or has a residual effort that limits activities of daily living.
- **Circulation:** System through which blood moves in the body.
- **Clean wound:** One that has not been invaded by pathogenic microorganisms; one that heals without infection.
- **Clear liquid diet:** Includes only broth, tea, clear or strained juices, and gelatin.
- **Clinical nurse specialist:** A well prepared nurse with a specific clinical expertise who assumes accountability for quality nursing care including leadership and management.
- **Closed wound:** Has no break in the continuity of the overlying skin or mucous membrane.
- **Collaborative nursing function:** Those activities carried out as a health team member, giving and receiving assistance to and from other health team members in the care of the patient.
- **Coma:** Unconscious state from which it is impossible to wake a, person.
- **Communication:** A verbal and nonverbal process for exchanging messages between individuals in person-to-person relationships.
- **Community assessment:** The process of determining the real perceived needs of defined community of people.
- **Community health problem:** The health need identified in community assessment.
- **Community profile:** The characteristics of the local environment that are prone to a chemical or nuclear accident (these characteristics include population density; age distribution; number of buildings; and local relief agencies).
- **Community resources:** A collection of health care providers or supportive care providers who share common interest or a sense of unity.
- **Community-based nursing:** Nursing care within the context of the clients family and community with a prevention focus that enhances the client's ability for self-care, a collaborative effort to maintain continuity of care.
- **Complementary therapies:** Interventions that focus on body, mind and spirit integration, may be used in addition to conventional therapies.
- **Concept:** A view or idea we hold about something, ranging from something highly concrete to something highly abstract.
- **Conduction:** Means of heat transfer in which molecular collision produces transmission; direct contact between warmer and cooler object required.
- **Constructed survey:** A time-consuming and expensive method of collecting information about a community with a valid and reliable survey, using a random sample of a targeted population where the data collected are analyzed for patterns and trends.
- **Consultation:** An interaction problem solving process between the nurse and the client.
- **Contaminated wound:** One in which the potential for infection is relatively great, such as in a wound occurring under accidental conditions without the benefit of aseptic technique.
- **Contamination:** An accidental release of hazardous chemicals or nuclear materials that pollute the environment and place humans at a risk of contamination.
- **Contingency plan:** An emergency plan developed in expectation of a disaster; often based on risk assessments, availability of human and material resources, community preparedness, and local and international response capabilities.
- **Continuity of care:** Coordination of services provided to clients before they enter a health care setting, during the time they are in the setting, and after they leave the setting.
- **Contract:** A term sometimes used to describe the fiduciary relationship in professional ethics which is grounded in promises or pledges.
- **Convulsion:** Fit or sudden loss of consciousness often associated with shaking of whole or part of the body.
- **Coordinate care:** The coordination of interdisciplinary sources of care and support to provide successful continuity of care.
- **Coordination:** A systematic exchange of information among principal participants in order to carry out a unified response in the event of an emergency.
- **Covenant:** A solemn agreement made between two or more parties that, as related to health care, emphasizes the moral and social character of the bond between professional and patient.
- **Crackles:** An abnormal discontinuous, non-musical sound heard on auscultation, primarily during inhalation, also called rales.
- **Crisis management:** Administrative measures that identify, acquire, and plan the use of resources needed to anticipate, prevent, and/or resolve a threat to public health and safety (e.g. terrorism).
- **Cultural assessment:** Considers the cultural beliefs, values and practices of an individual, group or community to determine needs and interventions within a specific cultural context.
- **Cultural care:** Health care in a cultural context, acknowledging the client's cultural beliefs about disease and treatment.
- **Cultural knowledge:** Familiarity with a culturally or ethnically diverse group's world view, beliefs, values, practices, life styles and problem solving strategies.
- **Cultural skill:** The ability to collect relevant cultural data regarding the client's health history.
- **Cyanosis:** Blueness of the lips or fingertips produced by shortage of oxygen in the blood, or poor blood circulation.
- **Decontamination:** The removal of hazardous chemicals or nuclear substances from the skin and/or mucous membranes

by showering or washing the affected area with water, or by rinsing with a sterile solution.
- **Delegation:** A management principle used to obtain desired results through the work of others, and a legal concept used to empower on person to act for another.
- **Development task:** The usual and expected psychosocial, cognitive or psychomotor skill at certain periods in life, failure to master the developmental task can lead to unhappiness and difficulty with later tasks.
- **Development:** Changes that occur over time in function and psychosocial and cognitive behavior.
- **Developmental tasks:** Identified physical, psychological and social changes occurring at various stages from the prenatal stage through the older years.
- **Diabetes:** Disease in which the body's ability to use sugar is impaired due to insufficient insulin. This results in a high concentration of sugar in the blood and urine.
- **Diagnosis:** Process of deciding on the nature and name of the condition or disease from which person is suffering.
- **Digestion:** Breaking up of food substances in the gut before absorption into the body.
- **Disaster epidemiology:** The study of disaster related deaths, illnesses, and injuries in humans; also includes the study of the factors and determinants that affect death, illness, and injury following a disaster (methodology involves identifying and comparing risk factors among disaster victims to those who were left unharmed. Epidemiologic investigations provide public health professionals with information on the probable public health consequences of disasters).
- **Disease:** Any condition that actually or potentially hinders individual function.
- **Dislocation:** Bones that are out of joint.
- **Documentation:** The process of obtaining and recording information used for communication, references and legal issues.
- **Dressing:** Sterile or very clean piece of material for application directly onto a wound.
- **Drug:** Another word for a medicine or substance intended for healing; not all drugs are addictive.
- **Dysphagia:** Inability to swallow or difficulty in swallowing.
- **Edema:** Presence of abnormally large amounts of fluid in the intercellular tissue spaces of the body.
- **Elective surgery:** Surgery needed by the patient but in which scheduling can be performed when it is convenient and beneficial to the patient, contrasting with emergency surgery.
- **Elimination:** One means by which the body, through the integumentary, respiratory, urinary, and gastrointestinal systems, maintains homeostasis related to temperature, chemical composition, and osmotic pressure.
- **Emergency:** Psychologic, medical or traumatic condition that requires immediate care or care within 1 hour to prevent further deterioration.
- **Emetic:** Substance to make a casualty vomit (such as salt and water or Ipecac syrup).
- **Employee wellness programs:** Plans that focus on keeping employees healthy and preventing illness and accidents.
- **Environment:** The sum of people, things, conditions, or influences surrounding persons.
- **Environmental assessment:** Evaluation of the client's home and neighborhood environment.
- **Epidemic:** The occurrence of any known or suspected contagion that occurs in clear 'excess of normal expectancy, (a threatened epidemic occurs when the circumstances are such that a disease may reasonably be anticipated to occur in excess of normal expectancy).
- **Epidemiology:** The study of health, illness and the factors that determine health and illness in a selected population.
- **Epidemiology:** The study of the various factors and conditions that determines the occurrence and distribution of health, disease, defect, disability, and death among group of individuals.
- **Epilepsy:** Disease in which the sufferer suddenly loses consciousness or' has a fit.
- **Esophagus:** Tube of muscular tissue connecting the mouth to the stomach.
- **Ethics:** An evaluation of actions, rules, or the character of persons, especially as it refers to the examination of a systematic theory of right or wrong at the ultimate level.
- **Evaluation research:** The application of scientific methods to assess the effectiveness of programs, services, or organizations established to improve a patient's health or prevent illness.
- **Evaluation:** A detailed review of a disaster relief program designed to determine whether program objectives were met, to assess the program's impact on the community, and to generate "lessons learned"
- for the design of future projects (evaluations are most often conducted at the completion of important milestones, or at the end of a specified period)
- **Exposure surveillance:** To look for exposure to risk (in a disaster setting, exposure may be based on the physical or environmental properties of the disaster event; also known as a risk factor variable; predictor variable, or independent variable).
- **Exposure:** Condition produced when the body's temperature regulation mechanism fails and the person becomes too hot or too cold.
- **Extracellular fluid:** Fluid found outside the cell, composing approximately one-third of the body's fluid in older children and about one-half of the body's fluid in infants.
- **Faint:** Weak, dizzy feeling followed by a short loss of consciousness due to poor blood supply to the brain.
- **Family health:** How well the family functions together as a unit, the family's ability to carry out usual and desired daily activities.
- **Family structure:** The characteristics of individuals (age, gender, number) who make up the family unit.
- **Femoral Artery:** The main blood vessel in the leg.
- **Fidelity:** The state of being faithful, which includes obligations of loyalty and the keeping of promises and commitments. Also the principles that actions are right insofar as they demonstrate such loyalty.
- **First responder:** Local police, fire, and emergency medical personnel who arrive first on the scene of an incident and take action to save lives, protect property, and meet basic human needs.
- **Fistula:** An abnormal passage or communication between two organs or tissues.
- **Fit:** Loss of consciousness due to an electrical discharge in the brain.
- **Formalism:** The view that actions are right or wrong based on their formal characteristics rather than their consequences (often a synonym for deontologist).
- **Fracture:** Break or crack in a bone.
- **Functional assessment:** Determination of level of health defined by one's ability to carry out usual and desired daily activities.

- **Functional inspired oxygen (FIO$_2$):** The measure of oxygen concentration being taken into the respiratory system (especially in supplemental oxygen therapy).
- **Gastric lavage:** Irrigation of the stomach, usually by means of a tube inserted through the nose or mouth, to remove poisons or irritating matter from stomach, to prepare for surgery, or to relieve nausea and vomiting.
- **General adaptation syndrome:** Three stages of physiologic changes in response to stress identified by Selye; the alarm reaction, stage of resistance, and state of exhaustion.
- **Gerontology nursing:** The nursing care of older adults, particularly those older than 65 years.
- **Grief:** The emotional response to loss. Definite stages of typical reactions have been identified as panic, emotional response, negotiation, commitment, and completion.
- **Growth:** Measurable physical and physiological changes that occurs over time.
- **Hematemesis:** Vomiting of bright red blood or denatured blood that looks like coffee grounds, usually represents a bleeding source proximal to the jejunum.
- **Hemoglobin:** Red pigment in the blood cells which combines readily with oxygen.
- **Hazard:** The probability that a disaster will occur (hazards can be caused by a natural phenomenon, e.g. earthquake, tropical cyclone, by an uncontrolled human activity, e.g., conflict, overgrazing).
- **Health behavior:** Activities a person engages in when feeling healthy; to take measures to prevent disease and illness or to detect them before symptoms occur.
- **Health care system:** All services that provide promotion of health, prevention of disease, detection and treatment of disease, follow-up service, and rehabilitation.
- **Health indicator:** Reflects the major public health concerns and illuminates factors that affect the health of individuals and communities.
- **Health promotion:** Activities that enhance the well being of an already healthy individual.
- **Health protection:** Environmental or regulatory measures that confer protection on large population groups.
- **Health:** A state of complete mental, physical, and social well-being, which maximizes the individual's ability to function in a normal manner.
- **Health:** State of physical, mental and social well being and not merely the absence of disease or infirmity.
- **Health-illness continuum:** A complex, dynamic process that includes physical, psychological, and social components that affects the level of wellness or illness at a given point in time.
- **Health-illness continuum:** Health described in a range of degrees from optimal health at one end to total disability or death at the other.
- **Heart attack:** Sudden crushing pain in the chest, due to inadequate blood supply to the heart muscle.
- **Holism:** A way of viewing the person as an integrated whole of mind, body and spirit, reflects the interactive process that occurs in all of us.
- **Holistic assessment:** Considers not only physical and psychosocial factors, but also cultural, functional, nutritional, environmental and spiritual aspects of the client.
- **Home health care:** Components of comprehensive health care whereby health services are provided to individuals and families in their places of residence for the purpose promoting, maintaining or restoring health.
- **Home visit:** Assessment, diagnosis, planning and evaluation of nursing care in the client's home.
- **Hospice care:** A system of comprehensive care that provides support and assistance to clients and families affected by terminal illness. Providing respectful, non-invasive care, pain and symptom control and emotional, physical, psychologic and spiritual support.
- **Hospice care:** Holistic service provided to dying persons and their loved ones to prove a more dignified and comfortable death.
- **Hygienic care:** Those nursing measures affording personal cleanliness, comfort, rest, and exercise.
- **Hypocapnia:** Decreased levels of carbon dioxide in the blood.
- **Hypothermia:** Cooling of body temperature to subnormal levels, temperature levels considered to be dangerous to infants and children are core body temperature below 35.6°C (96°F).
- **Hypothermia:** Loss of body heat producing a severe fall in body temperature.
- **Hypoxia:** Decreased oxygenation of cells and tissues.
- **Hysteria:** An uncontrolled emotion occurring in immature people.
- **Illness behavior:** Activities a person engages in when feeling ill that will lead to the defining of the state of health and gain help.
- **Immunity:** Resistance of the body to the effects of a harmful organism or its toxin.
- **Immunodeficiency:** A defect in the immune system leading to increased susceptibility to multiple and repeated infections.
- **Incontinence:** The involuntary voiding of urine or the involuntary defecation of feces or both.
- **Infected wound:** Also called septic wound, one in which the invasion of pathogens is too great for the resistance of the first line of internal body defenses, causing clinical symptoms of infection to develop.
- **Infection control:** Utilization of standards established to monitor infections, trace sources and patterns of disease spread and institute measures to control spread.
- **Infection:** Condition resulting from invasion of the body by pathogenic or non-pathogenic organism such as bacteria, viruses, protozoa, helminths or fungi.
- **Informed consent:** A requirement both legal and ethical, that the child and the parent or guardian completely understand proposed procedures or treatments including their benefits and risks.
- **Ingestion:** Swallowing of a potentially toxic substance, such as inappropriate amounts or types of medication, petroleum products, insecticides or toxic plants.
- **Inspection:** Careful observation to identify physical findings.
- **Inspection:** Observation with the eye.
- **Insulin:** Chemical substance in the body which regulates the concentration of sugar in the blood.
- **Intake:** Measure of fluid taken into the body. Includes liquids taken orally, intravenous fluids or tube feedings, and in special situations may include estimates of water from solid foods, injections, and so on.
- **Integrated communications:** A system that uses a common communications plan, standard operating procedures, clear text, common frequencies, and common terminology.
- **Interview:** A purposeful, goal-directed conversation with patient or family.
- **Intracellular fluid:** Fluid found within the cells, composing approximately two-thirds of the body's fluid in older children and about one-half of the body's fluid in infants.

- **Joint:** Structure at which bones are joined together.
- **Justice:** A moral principle that holds that actions (or rules) are morally right insofar as they reflect a specified pattern of distribution of benefits and harms. A synonym for moral rightness; right taking into account of all moral principles.
- **Kidneys:** Pair of organs in the body which filter chemicals, retaining some and passing others out in the urine.
- **Larynx:** The voice box or Adam's apple.
- **Latrines:** A pit designed to capture and contain excreta; most often trenches with multiple platforms across them, or solitary pits surrounded by a structure.
- **Legalism:** The position that ethical action consists in strict conformity to law or rules; cf. antinomianism, rules of practice, situationalism.
- **Liaison:** An agency official who works with individual agencies or agency officials to coordinate interagency communications.
- **Ligament:** Tough tissue which binds together bodily structures such as bones.
- **Listening:** Detection of the speaker's meaning by using clues about emotional state and nonverbal cues as well as speech content.
- **Local government:** Any country, city, village, town, district, political subdivision of any state, Indian tribe or authorized tribal organization, or Alaska native village or organization, including rural communities, unincorporated towns and villages, or any other public entity.
- **Long-term illness:** Chronic illness. An illness of 3 or more months' duration.
- **Loss:** A range of adverse consequences that can impact communities and individuals (e.g. damage, loss of economic value, loss of function, loss of natural resources, loss of ecological systems, environmental impact, health deterioration, mortality, morbidity).
- **Lungs:** Two air-filled, sac-like organs in the chest through which oxygen is inhaled and carbon dioxide exhaled.
- **Melena:** Renal passage of black, tarry stools, indicating denatured blood from the upper GI tract.
- **Medical asepsis:** The prevention of the transfer of pathogenic organisms to clean areas.
- **Medical coordination:** The coordination between health care providers during the transition from the pre-hospital to the hospital phase of patient care; simplification and standardization of materials and methods is a prerequisite.
- **Medic-Alert:** Disc or bracelet worn by people with certain illnesses such as epilepsy or diabetes, which gives vital information about the person.
- **Mitigation:** Measures taken to reduce the harmful effects of a disaster by attempting to limit the disaster's impact on human health and economic infrastructure.
- **Monitoring:** A process of evaluating the performance of response and recovery programs by measuring a program's outcomes against stated objectives (monitoring is used to identify bottlenecks and obstacles that cause delays or programmatic shortfalls that require assessment).
- **Mortality data:** Information about the number of deaths used to assess the magnitude of a disaster, evaluate the effectiveness of disaster preparedness, evaluate the adequacy of warning systems, and to aid contingency planning by identifying high-risk groups.
- **Muscles:** Bundles of special fibers which change length producing movement.
- **Nasal polyps:** Semitransparent herniations of respiratory epithelium.
- **Natural disasters:** Natural phenomena with acute onset and profound effects. (e.g. earthquakes, floods, cyclones, tornadoes)
- **Nebulization:** A method of administering water or liquid drugs in which a mist like spray is produced, breaking the substances into minute particles for inhalation.
- **Negligence:** Failure to act in the way a reasonable, prudent person of similar background would act in similar circumstances.
- **Neonatal mortality rate:** Number of deaths per 1000 live birts that occur at birth or within the first 28 days of life.
- **Nerves:** Collections of fibers which carry "electrical" impulses around the body.
- **Neutralism:** A characteristics of moral or ethical evaluations in which there is general application not favoring one party.
- **Nonverbal communication:** Exchanging information by using gestures, facial expressions, posture and body movements, not necessarily intentional.
- **Normative:** The branch of ethics related with which actions are right or wrong, which states are valuable, or which character traits of persons are praiseworthy e.g. metaethics.
- **Nursing assessment:** The first step of the nursing process. The sum total of data collection, observation, communication, and the physical examination.
- **Nursing audit:** A retrospective review of patient records to evaluate written documentation of nursing care action.
- **Nursing care plan:** The individualized written guide for nursing care actions.
- **Nursing diagnosis:** The process of recognizing patient's needs, and identifying and stating the nature and extent of the related nursing problems.
- **Nursing history:** Interview, gathering data, focusing on the meaning of health and illness care to the patient and family; a basis for planning care.
- **Nursing process:** A problem solving approach to providing nursing care using four essential steps; assessment, planning, implementation, and evaluation.
- **Objective symptoms or signs:** Those that the nurse can see, hear, feel, smell, or measure.
- **Ordering:** A characteristic of moral or ethical evaluations on which a set of principles, rules, or character assessments provides a basis for ranking conflicting claims.
- **Outcome variable:** A health event, usually encompassing illness, injury or death; also known as a response variable.
- **Output:** Measure of fluid lost by body. Includes urine, emesis, drainage, and in special situations, estimates of respiratory, gastrointestinal, and perspiration amounts.
- **Oxygen:** Gas, vital to the body's production of energy, making up one-fifth of the air.
- **Pain:** An unpleasant sensory and emotional experience associated with actual or potential tissue damage or described in terms of such damage.
- **Palliative care:** Medical treatments or procedures that aim to promote comfort and quality of life rather than to cure the underlying disease.
- **Palpation:** Observation by touch, to feel a part with the fingers.
- **Palpation:** The use of touch to determine factors such as texture, temperature, moisture, organ size and location.
- **Parenteral:** Literally outside the intestinal tract. Generally any of the ways by which suitable liquid preparations of drugs are injected by needle into the tissues or directly into the bloodstream.

- **Pay surgery centers:** Ambulatory services that provide preoperative, operative and postoperative care on an outpatient basis.
- **Pediatrics:** Branch of medicine concerned with growth, development and care of children and treatment of their diseases.
- **Percussion:** Observation by hearing, elicitation of sound determined by tapping surfaces with fingers.
- **Percussion:** Tapping of the body to determine the density, location and size of organs.
- **Perineal care:** Cleansing of the vulvar and anal region in the female; the penis, scrotum, and anal region in the male.
- **Peristalsis:** Progressive, wave like movements caused by contraction and relaxation of the longitudinal and circular muscles of the GI tract, propels a bolus of food or fluid forward.
- **Pharynx:** Space at the back of the nose and mouth.
- **Physical environment:** The total of nonliving things surrounding persons such as air, water, and land.
- **Poison:** Any substance which is harmful to the body.
- **Preparedness:** All measures and policies taken before an event occurs that allow for prevention, mitigation, and readiness (preparedness includes designing warning systems, planning for evacuation and relocation, storing food and water, building temporary shelter, devising management strategies, and holding disaster drills and exercises. Contingency planning is also included in preparedness as well as planning for post-impact response and recovery.)
- **Prescriptivism:** The view that ethical utterances function to prescribe conduct rather than make cognitive claims.
- **Prevention:** Primary, secondary, and tertiary efforts that help avert an emergency; these activities are commonly referred to as "mitigation" in the emergency management model (for example, prevention activities include cloud seeding to stimulate rain in a fire; in public health terms, prevention refers to actions that prevent the onset or deterioration of disease, disability and injury).
- **Preventive rehabilitative processes:** Processes that minimize the ill effects of bed rest, inactivity, and disruption of normal patterns of activities of daily living.
- **Primary nurse practitioner:** Nurses with advanced preparation in data gathering and assessment, who provide services in the patient's first contact with the health care system; generally in ambulatory care settings. Responsible for referral and/or collaborative follow-up care.
- **Primary prevention:** Preventing the occurrence of death, injury, or illness in a disaster (e.g., evacuation of a community in a flood prone area, sensitizing warning systems for tornadoes and severe storms).
- **Prognosis:** Outlook of present illness, whether patient can be expected to return to normal daily routine; whether there will be a physical handicap; whether there must be continuous medical therapy; whether death is near.
- **Protective isolation:** Sometimes called reverse isolation; seeks to protect the patient from microorganisms in the environment.
- **PSRO (Professional Standards Review Organization):** A method of patient record evaluation to determine the effectiveness of medical diagnosis and treatment in relation to federally financed health care.
- **Puberty:** Period of time during which adolescent experience a growth spurt, develop secondary sexual characteristics and achieve reproductive maturity.
- **Publicity:** A characteristic of moral or ethical evaluations in which one must be willing to state the evaluation and the basis on which it is made publicity.
- **Pulse:** Throbbing of the arteries due to the pumping of blood by the heart.
- **Radial artery:** Main artery on the thumb side of the wrist.
- **Radiation:** Energy emitted by atoms that are unstable – radiation with enough energy to create ion pairs in matter.
- **Radiation:** Transfer of heat or energy through space as with light, infrared, or ultrasound rays.
- **Range-of-motion exercises:** Exercises whose action takes a limb c-joint through all angles of movement of which it is capable.
- **Readiness:** Links preparedness to relief; an assessment of readiness reflects the current capacity and capabilities of the organization involved in relief activities.
- **Recovery:** Actions of responders, government, and the victims that help return an affected community to normal by stimulating community cohesiveness and government involvement (One type of recovery involves repairing infrastructure, damaged buildings, and critical facilities. The recovery period falls between the onset of the emergency and the reconstruction period.)
- **Referred pain:** Pain (usually from a visceral lesion) felt in a part of the body distant from the actual lesion, usually in a surface area.
- **Rehabilitation or reconstruction:** A long-term development project that follows a disaster or emergency that reconstructs a community's infrastructure to pre-existing levels; is often associated with an opportunity to improve a community rather than to simply "reconstruct" a pre-existing system.
- **Rehabilitation:** Process of assisting a disabled person who is acutely or chronically ill or convalescent to realize particular goals in living and working to the utmost potential.
- **Relief:** Action focused on saving lives (Relief activities often include search and rescue missions, first aid, and restoration of emergency communications and transportation systems. Relief also includes attention to the immediate care of survivors by providing food, clothing, medical treatment, and emotional care).
- **Reporting unit for surveillance:** The data source that provides information for the surveillance system (Reporting units often include hospitals, clinics, health posts, and mobile health units. Epidemiologists select reporting units after they define "what a case is" because the source of data is dependent on that definition).
- **Representativeness:** The accuracy of the data when measuring the occurrence of a health event over time and its distribution by person and place.
- **Resource management:** A management style that maximizes the use of and control over assets; this management style reduces the need for unnecessary communications, provides for strict accountability, and ensures the safety of personnel.
- **Respiration:** The physical and chemical process by which oxygen and carbon dioxide are exchanged in the body. Breathing is the mechanical part of respiration.
- **Respiratory isolation:** Isolation used for diseases that are commonly spread by droplet infection and those in which the organism is present in the respiratory system.
- **Response:** The phase in a disaster when relief, recovery, and rehabilitation occur; also includes the delivery of services, the management of activities and programs designed to address

- the immediate and short-term effects of an emergency or disaster.
- **Restorative phase:** Following acute stage of illness. Long-term considerations are examined so that appropriate actions geared toward realistic goals for the patient may be instituted.
- **Resuscitation:** Attempt to restart a stopped heart or restore breathing.
- **Retention:** Inability to empty the bladder voluntarily and completely.
- **Richter scale:** A scale that indicates the magnitude of an earthquake by providing a measure of the total energy released from the source of the quake; the source of an earthquake being the segment of the fault that has slipped.
- **Rigorism:** The view that moral rules should be applied relatively rigidly .
- **Roy adaptation model:** Based on the idea that human responses fall into four broad areas of adaptation; physiologic needs, self-concept, role-function, and interdependence relations.
- **Scientific principles:** Comprehensive and fundamental laws, doctrines, truths, or sets of facts that form the basis for established rules of action.
- **Secondary sexual characteristics:** Physical characteristics of males and females influenced by reproductive hormones but having no direct role in reproduction (i.e. voice, body shape, pubic hair, distribution, breasts).
- **Shock:** Inadequate tissue perfusion, usually caused by illness or injury, that results in respiratory or cardiovascular compromise.
- **Shock:** Reaction of the body in which all the tissues are starved of oxygen.
- **Sick-role behavior:** Activities a person engages in, believing himself or herself ill.
- **Sign:** Clue noticed by a doctor or first-aider which indicates the cause of illness (c.f. symptoms).
- **Situational crisis:** Unanticipated event that poses a threat to an individual's psychosocial or psychologic well-being.
- **Situationalism:** The position that ethical action must be judged in each situation guided by, but not directly determined by, rules; cf. antinomianism, rules of practice.
- **Sling:** Material used to hold an injured limb.
- **Snellen's test:** Commonly used test of gross visual acuity; used as a screening test for visual defects.
- **Social environment:** The interpersonal relationship that exist for persons.
- **Social relativism:** The view that moral judgments are grounded only in each society's collective opinion (cf. cultural relativism)
- **Soft diet:** Made of pureed foods or those with fine texture and less cellulose or fiber content than a general diet.
- **Spiritual needs:** Those needs relating to religious and ethical/moral issues.
- **Sprain:** Stretched ligament.
- **Standards of consent:** The frame of reference upon which consent may be evaluated (see reasonable person standard, professional standard, subjective standard).
- **Sterile:** Germ-free condition.
- **Sterilization:** The process of destroying all microorganisms.
- **Strain:** Stretched muscle or tendon.
- **Stress:** Any situation or condition positive, or negative requiring adjustment on the part of the individual, family or group.
- **Strict isolation:** Isolation used to prevent spread of highly communicable disease by contact and airborne routes of transmission.
- **Stridor:** A shrill, harsh sound that can be heard during inspiration, expiration or both, produced by the flow of air through a narrowed segment of the respiratory tract.
- **Stroke:** Illness produced by the loss of blood supply to an area of the brain.
- **Stupor:** A level of unconsciousness in which only pain produces a reaction.
- **Subcutaneous:** Loose areolar tissue just beneath the layers of the skin.
- **Subjective symptoms:** Those symptoms that the patient tells about (the patient's perspective).
- **Support systems:** Resources the patient has available to provide caring and concern; helpful in meeting needs for warmth and reassurance.
- **Supportive nursing measures:** Nursing measures that have as their objective the meeting of physiologic and psychological needs of the patient rising from the stresses imposed by illness or injury.
- **Surgical asepsis:** The methods employed to maintain sterility of an area.
- **Surveillance:** The ongoing and systematic collection, analysis, and interpretation of health data essential to the planning, implementation, and evaluation of public health practice; systems are designed to disseminate data in a timely manner and often include both data collection and disease monitoring.
- **Technological hazard:** A potential threat to human welfare caused by technological factors (e.g. chemical release, nuclear accident, dam failure. Earthquakes and other natural hazards can trigger technological hazards as well).
- **Terminal:** Used to designate patient for whom death is inevitable though dying may not have begun.
- **Theory:** A set of interrelated constructs (concepts), definitions, and propositions that present a systematic view of phenomena by specifying relations among variables, with the purpose of explaining and predicting the phenomena.
- **Therapeutic play:** Guided play that promotes the child's psycho physiologic well-being.
- **Total communications:** Method for teaching, hearing, handicapped people involving maximum use of residual hearing with aids, learning of special listening techniques, use of speech, reading and sign language.
- **Toxicological disaster:** A serious environmental pollutant that causes illness by a massive, accidental escape of toxic substances into the air, soil, or water; these disasters affect humans, animals, and plants.
- **Trauma:** Injury from an external cause, such as motor vehicle collision, fall, gunshot wound or stabbing may be self-inflicted, may be deliberately inflicted or accidental and may be physical or psychologic.
- **Triage:** Sorting process used to decide the urgency of an individual's illness or injury and allocate appropriate resources ill or injured. People receive the appropriate level of care, before those with less urgent or emergent conditions.
- **Universality:** A characteristic of moral or ethical evaluations in which an action or character trait should be evaluated the same by all people.
- **Victim distribution:** A victim distribution plan defines the transport distribution of victims among neighboring hospital according to their hospital treatment capacity; these plans often avoid taking victims to the nearest hospital since walking victims will overcrowd hospitals closest to the disaster site.

- **Voluntary agency (VOLAG):** A nonprofit, non-governmental, private association maintained and supported by voluntary contributions that provides assistance in emergencies and disasters.
- **Vulnerability analysis:** The assessment of an exposed population's susceptibility to the adverse health effects of a particular hazard.
- **Vulnerability:** The susceptibility of a population to a specific type of event; it is also associated with the degree of possible or potential loss from a risk that results from a hazard at a given intensity (the factors that influence vulnerability include demographics, the age and resilience of the environment, technology, social differentiation, and diversity as well as regional and global economics politics).

Index

Page numbers followed by *f* refer to figure and *t* refer to table.

A

Abdomen 103, 284
    examination of 105
Abdominal binder 693
Abdominal girth 723*f*
Abdominal thrusts 642, 672
Abdominal trauma, first aid for 653*f*
Abortion 28, 576
    pill 576
Abrasion 642, 649
Abscess 714
Absolute bone conduction test 537
Absolute stressors 596
Absorption 468, 495
Abstain 589
Abstinence 576
Accident 92, 218
    report 83
    triangle 218
Accidental falls 218
Accidental injuries 177
Accidental report 78
Accurate technique 100
Acetaminophen 642
Acetone 394
Acid-base
    balance 464, 465, 482
    imbalances 482
Acidosis 483, 741
Acinetobacter baumannii 170
Aconite poisoning 687
Acquaintance rape 576
Acquired immunodeficiency syndrome 588
Activate emergency medical services 679
Active coping 594
Active euthanasia 28, 547, 560, 561
Active listening 54
Active transport 466
Acuity records 79
Acute care physiologic monitoring system 148
Acute illness 1
Adaptation 1, 594, 599, 741
    levels of 599
Adaptive coping 594
Administer drug 511
Administering oral medications, technique for 508
Admission and discharge 239
Admission assessment 86, 93
Admission nursing history forms 79
Admission procedure 238
Admission to hospital unit 236
Admission, types of 237, 238
Adoptive theories 632
Adrenal gland 468
Adrenal insufficiency 710
Adrenal venography 415
Adrenocorticotropic hormone 469, 597
Advance care planning 546
Advanced life support 642
Adventitious breath sounds 138, 445
Adverse reaction 495
Advocacy skills 41

Affective disorders 249
Agent-host-environmental model 5, 5*f*
Age-specific spiritual interventions 623
Agnosticism 608
Agricultural poisons 686
Air
    and water mattresses 205, 205*f*
    contamination 189
    cushion 206, 206*f*
        care of 152
    embolism 521
    from pleural cavity, aspiration of 725*f*
    hunger 139
    lock method 514
    mattress 152
    movement 220
    purity of 221
    tight drainage system, maintenance of 455
Airbag 642
Airborne 171
    precautions 180
    transmission 173
Airway 94, 460, 642, 653, 741
    assessment 444
    maintain 671
Airway management 438, 741
    nursing intervention for 445
    nursing process in 444
Airway obstruction
    by hanging 690*f*
    by strangling 690*f*
    by throttling 690*f*
Alanine transaminase 382
Alarm reaction 594, 597
Albumin 382
    test 359, 394
Algor mortis 556, 557
Alimentary system 118
Alimentary tract dysfunction 710
Alkaline phosphatase 382
Alkalosis 483, 741
Allergic contact dermatitis 163
Allergic reaction 492, 496, 521
Allergies 92
Ambu bag 152, 460*f*
Ambulating clients 254
Ambulatory surgical centers 16
American Heart Association 642
American Hospital Association 240
American Nurses Association 32
American Red Cross and Federal Emergency Management Agency 695
Amikacin 512
Aminophylline 513
Ampicillin 512
Amputation bed 202
Anabolism 464
Analgesia, patient-controlled 698
Anaphylactic shock 655
Anaphylaxis 642
Anecdotal records 78
Anemia, diet in 330
Anemic hypoxia 432

Anesthesia 396, 698, 704
    general 698, 704
    supply room 698
    topical 704
Anesthetic agent 698
Anger 549-551, 605
Angina 642, 741
Angiocardiography 378
Angiography 378, 412
    types of 412
Animism 608
Ankle, fracture of 660
Ankylosis 251
Anorexia 321, 326
    nervosa 326
    signs of 326*f*
    symptoms of 326*f*
Anosmia 528
Anoxia 425
Antagonist 496
Anthropometric indices 324
Anthropometry measurement 324*t*
Antibiotics 512
Antibody 163
Anticipated life transitions, crisis of 601
Anticipatory grief 546, 549
Antidiuretic hormone 468
Antigen 163, 169
Antihelmentic enema 367
Antimicrobial soap 163
Antiseptic 163
    hand
        rub 163
        wash 163
Antitoxin 741
Anuria 343, 346, 741
Anxiety 549
Aortography 412
Aphasia 534, 534*f*
Apical pulse 108
Apnea 139, 425, 429
    monitor 148
Apneustic breathing 425
Apoplexy 741
Apothecaries fluid measure 501
Apothecaries system 500, 501
Appetite, factors affecting 324
Aqueous humor 528
Arms 284
Arsenic poisoning 687
Art of nursing 32, 41
Arterial bleeding 654
Arterial blood gases, monitor 445
Arterial embalming 562
Arterial lines 147
Artery 741
    forceps 457*f*
Artificial airway 535
    management 442
Asceticism 608
Asepsis 163, 177
    principles of 177
    types of 177

Aseptic technique 177, 178f, 698
Aspartate transaminase 382
Asphyxia 139, 140, 673, 741
　　cause of 673
　　signs of 674
　　symptoms of 674
　　treatment of 674
　　types of 674
　　vicious cycle of 673f
Aspirate 333
Aspiration 728
　　pneumonia 544
Aspirin 379
Assisted death 546
Assisted oral care 280f
Asthma 741
　　attack 431
Asthmatic breathing 425
Astringent enema 367
Atelectasis 251, 741
Atheism 608
Atmospheric pressure, changes in 137
Atmospheric temperature 220
Atresia 741
Attention 67
Attitude 55, 275, 611
Audience knowledge 53
Audition 528
Auditory deficits 532
Auscultate lungs 445
Auscultation 86, 90, 96, 97, 741
Autoclave 159
　　machine 159f
Autonomy 34, 43, 61, 546, 741
Autopsy 559, 561
　　considerations 562
Auxiliary nurse midwife 38
Avoirdupois system 501
Axillary temperature 115
　　measuring 116f

B

Back 103, 284
　　care 286
　　massage 286, 287f
　　rest 203, 204f, 224
　　rub 286, 287f
　　　techniques, steps of 287f
Bacteremia 172
Bacterial infections 363
Bacteriostasis 741
Balanced crystalloid 464
Balanitis 576
Bandage 741
　　circular 691
　　first aid 690
　　materials used for 691
　　purpose of 690
　　types of 691, 691f
Barium enema 373, 378
　　procedure 374f
Barium meal 378
Barium swallow 378
Barium X-ray 378
Barrier protection 177
Barrier techniques infection control 174
Basal gastric analysis 340
Basic attitudes 623
Basic cardiac life support 678
Basic communication skills 54
Basic food groups 323
Basic human needs 741
Basic life support 642, 643, 678, 680f, 741

steps of 678
symbol of 678f
Basic nursing principles 33
Bathroom
　　bath 282
　　care of 157
Bed bath 282
Bed blocks 206
Bed cradle 194, 205, 205f, 224
Bed making 194, 195
　　procedure steps 197f
　　purpose of 196
Bed rails
　　potential benefits of 229
　　potential risks of 230
Bed rest 231
Bed ridden patient, hair washing for 293f
Bed shampoo 293
Bed steads 224
Bed, types of 196f
Bedding and bed linens 147, 226
Bedpan
　　and urinals 146, 225
　　care of 152, 153
　　types of 365, 365f
　　use of 365
Bedside
　　commode 146, 225
　　locker 146, 225
　　table 146, 225
Bedsore, care of 289
Bee sting 685
Behavior, reinforcement of 604
Behavioral changes 13
Behavioral determinants 3, 8
Benedict's test 360f
Bereavement 546, 548
Betty Neuman systems model 638f
Bicarbonate 465, 474
Bigotry 609
Bile pigments 360, 394
Bile salts 360, 394
Bilirubin 382
Binder
　　purpose of 693
　　types of 693
Biofeedback
　　technique 215, 216
　　types of 215
Biological adaptation 599
Biological disaster 694
Biological environment 9
Biomedical waste 187, 190f
　　ill effects of 188
　　management 184, 189
　　　elements of 189
Biopsy 377, 379, 698
Biopsychosocial aspects 7
Biopsychosocial model 7f
Biot's respiration 139, 425, 429
Birth control, barrier methods of 576
Bites and stings 684
Black color stool 371
Bladder and urethra, visual examination of 404f
Bladder irrigation 351, 352f
　　nurses assisting in 353f
　　system 352f
Bladder training 348, 741
Bland diet 741
Bleeding 397, 710
　　control 655
　　external 655
　　internal 655

Blindness, prevent 536
Blisters 684
Blocked airway 397
Blood 168, 741
　　borne pathogens 163
　　brain barrier 513
　　circulation time of 511
　　culture 390
　　oxygen level, acute diseases affect 431
　　smear 390
　　transfusion 490, 491f
Blood pressure 93, 140, 586
　　alterations in 141
　　cuff application technique 140f
　　diastolic 141
　　factors influencing 141
　　measuring 90f
　　monitor device 140f
　　systolic 141
Blood sugar
　　level 93
　　measurement procedure 386f
Body after death, care of 558
Body alignment 255, 741
　　assessment of 255
Body areas 86, 100
Body building foods 323
Body cast 264
Body changes, impact on 13
Body fluid 464
　　disturbances 471
　　physiology of 466
　　regulation of 466
Body heat 111, 113
Body image 564, 569
　　factors affecting 569f
Body language 277
Body mass index, measuring 102
Body mechanics 254, 741
　　elements of 255
　　meaning of 254
　　nursing process in 256
　　principles of 256
　　techniques of 256
Body movements 56
Body position 253, 259
Body substance isolation 176
　　types of 176
Body system 252
Body temperature 110
　　assessment of 112
　　factors affecting 111f
　　measure 116f
　　regulation of 111, 119
Bolus injection 488
Bone marrow 169
　　aspiration 729f
　　　procedure 729f
　　biopsy 377, 728
Boric acid 649
Botox treatment 348
Bowel elimination 253, 361
　　factors affecting 361, 361f
　　problems in 362
　　role of nurse in 375
Bowel irrigation, methods of 370
Bowel movement 671
Bowel training 741
Bowel wash 369
　　procedure 370f
Braces 247
Brachial artery 741
Brachial pulse 108

Braden scale 287-289
  risk factors 288
Braden score 289
Bradycardia 108, 136
Bradypnea 139, 425, 429
Breast 586, 587
  binder 693
Breastfeeding 337
  contraindication for 337
Breath
  patterns, types of normal 429t
  sounds types, normal 138
Breathing 94, 460, 642, 643, 653
  mechanics of 427
  patterns, types of abnormal 429t
  problems with 557
Bronchial drainage 741
Bronchial sound 138
Bronchography 378, 411
Bronchopulmonary dysplasia 431
Bronchoscopy 377, 397
  instrument, parts of 398f
  procedure 398f, 411f
Bronchovesicular sound 138
Bruise 643, 651
Buffer systems 482
Bulk-forming agents 363
Burn 172, 643, 681, 682
  causes of 681
  classification of 683
  depth of 684
  dry 682
  intermediate 684
  superficial 684
  types of 682
Burn injury 682f
  degrees of 681f
  first aid for 682f
  management of
    first degree 683f
    second degree 683f

C

Calcium 465, 473
  loss of 473
  regulation of 473
Calendar method 576
Canadian Nurses Association 32
Cancer assessment 474
Candida albicans 588
Candidiasis 588
Cape line bandage 692
Capillary bleeding 654
Capillary blood glucose, monitoring 384
Carbolic acid 649
Carbon dioxide 741
Carbon monoxide 741
Carcinogen 218
Cardiac bed 201
Cardiac catheterization 378, 416
  procedure 417f
Cardiac massage, external 461f
Cardiac monitors 147
Cardiac output 108
Cardiac table 146, 206f, 225
Cardiopulmonary resuscitation 459, 459f, 642, 643, 741
Cardiovascular physiology 426
Cardiovascular pressure 586
Cardiovascular system 250, 586, 587
  clinical examination of 98f
Care
  continuity of 24, 308, 546, 742
  principles of 151, 153

Carminative enema 367
Carotid artery 742
Carotid pulse 108
Cast 247
  application of 265
  material 264
  purpose of 263
  types of 263
Casualty 742
Catabolism 464
Catharsis 604
Catheter
  and drainage tube 148f
  care 353
  method 368
Catheterization
  procedure 351f
  right-side 416
  types of 351
Caudal anesthesia 704
Cavity embalming 562
Ceftazidime 512
Ceftriaxone 512
Cell count 727
Cellulites 714
Census report 78
Centers for Disease Control and Prevention 192
Central nervous system 528, 556, 704
Central venous catheter 148
Cephalosporins 512
Cerebral angiography 378, 412, 413, 413f
Cerebral tissue perfusion, ineffective 541
Certified nurse-midwife 42
Cervical
  biopsy 378
  fracture management 662f
Chair method 667
Checking pulse, sites for 136f
Chemical burns 682
Chemical disinfectants 160
  mechanism of 160
Chemical sterilant 163
Chemoreceptor 528
Chest 103, 284
  circumference 324
  examination of 105
  pain 643
  X-ray 409, 409f
Chest catheter
  proper placement of 455
  removal 458
Chest drainage
  bottles in 456f
  factors affecting 455
  system 454f
    two bottle 455f, 556
    types of 455f, 456
Chest tube 148
  drainage system 454f
Chest wound 654
  first aid measures for 654
Cheyne-Stokes respiration 139, 425, 429
Child, first aid for 673
Chlamydia 588
  trachomatis 588
Chloride 465, 473
  level 727
  regulation of 474
Choking 643, 671, 672f, 674
  first aid in 672
  infants, first aid for 673
Cholecystography 378, 420
  procedure 420f

Chronic pain 211
  treatment 213f
Circulation 460, 642, 653, 742
  and breathing, assessment of 461f
Circulatory overload 492, 521
Circulatory system 118, 252, 253, 556
Cisternal puncture 378
Civil law 47
Clamping drainage tube 457f
Cleaning sharp instruments, steps of 154
Cleaning, types of 226
Cleanliness, principles of 226
Cleansing bath, types of 282
Clear fluid diet 330
Clear liquid diet 742
Clinical death, signs of 557
Clinical nurse specialist 42, 742
Clinical thermometer 114
Clitoris 586
Closed chest underwater seal drainage 457
Closed gloving 698
Clostridium
  difficile 170
  perfringens 588
Clove-Hitch restraint 228, 228f
Coarse sounds 445
Cochlea 528
Cognitive function, alterations in 710
Cold
  burns 682
  dry 130
  enema 367
  pack 134
  stage 123
  test 360, 394
Cold application 124, 130
  complications of 131
  contraindications of 131
  physiological effects of 130
  types of 131f
Cold compress 131
  application 132f
Collaborative nursing function 742
Collar and cuff sling 692
Colle's fracture 659
Collision 643
Colloid 464
Colloidal osmotic pressure 468
Colon, examination of 399f
Colonoscope, parts of 400f
Colonoscopy 377, 399
Colostomy
  irrigation 372, 373f
    solutions for 372
    technique 372f
  types of 372
Coma 546, 742
  classification of 669
Common bowel elimination problems 362
Common cold 168
Common hair scalp problems 292
Common hospital-acquired infections 172
Common legal issues 47
Common medication mistakes 504f
Common poisons and antidotes 686
Common vehicle transmission 173
Communicable disease 166
Communicated fracture 657
Communication 41, 50, 66, 76, 581, 584, 742
  barriers in 57, 58f
  forms of 53
  importance of 52
  in hospital 66

in nursing 65
kinds of 52
levels of 52
nature of 51
principles of 52
process 53
  elements of 53f
  factors affecting 54, 55f
  model 51f
purpose of 52, 66
skills 54f, 65
strategies 535
system 67
types of 51f
Communicator, ability of 54
Community 1
  approach 80
  areas, nurses working in 38
  assessment 742
  based nursing 742
  development block 2
  emergencies 693
  health 1
    nurse 1, 2, 37, 38
    problem 742
    workers 38
  legal approaches in 80
  level helpers 695
  profile 742
  resources 742
Complementary alternative medicine 214
Complementary therapy 742
  uses of 214
Complete blood count 379, 380
Complete drug history 512
Compound fracture 657
Comprehensive health care 2
Compression fracture 657
Computer-aided teaching 272
Computerized documentation 79
Computerized miniature pumps 524
Conception 576
Conceptual framework 631f
Condom 576
Conductive hearing loss, treatments of 537
Condylomata lata 588
Cone photoreceptor 528
Confidentiality and autonomy 33, 39
Confidentiality and privacy 591
Congestive heart failure 492
Connecting suction catheters, method of 446f
Connective tissue disorders 258
Consciousness, level of 481
Constant fever 118
Constipation 362, 543, 544
  management of 363
  signs of 362
  symptoms of 362
  treatment 362f
Constructed survey 742
Contact lens
  care of 298, 299f
  handling 298
Contact transmission 172
Contamination 742
  degree of 711
Contraception 582
Contractures 543, 544
  prevention of 671
Controlling bleeding, method of 655f
Contusion 643
Convection 111
Conventional angiography, uses of 412
Conventional pulmonary angiography 412

Convulsion 742
  first aid in 688
Corneal blink reflex, absence of 542
Coronary angiography 412
Corrigan's pulse 136
Corticotropin releasing hormone 597
Coughing 430
  impaired 251
  techniques 445
Cow milk 337
Cradle method 645, 666
Crash cart 149
Crib-net restraint 228
Crifla vine 649
Criminal law 47
Crisis 118, 120, 622
  and resolution, concept of 600
  counseling 602
  development, phases in 601
  intervention 601, 602
    centers 605
    modalities of 604
    techniques of 602, 604
  management 742
  phases of 600
  reflecting psychopathology 602
  resolution of 601
  response 600
  signs of 601
  symptoms of 601
  types of 600, 601
Critical thinking
  components of 302
  importance of 302
  levels of 302f, 305
  meaning of 302
  skills required for 303f
Crush injuries 660
Crystalline penicillin 512
Crystalloid 464
Cuffs 442
Cultural assessment 742
Cultural assimilation 610
Cultural awareness 608
Cultural background 11
Cultural barrier 273
Cultural beliefs 276, 562
Cultural care 742
Cultural competence 608, 610
Cultural diversity 609, 612, 613
  and spirituality 608
  impact of 613
Cultural humility 609
Cultural influences 7
Cultural knowledge 742
Cultural nursing practice, scope of 615
Cultural progressive care model 611f
Cultural sensitivity 609
Culturally congruent care 615
Culturally diverse nursing care 615
Culturally responsive care 611
Cushing's traid 541
Cyanosis 139, 425, 430, 459, 643, 742
Cystic fibrosis 431
Cystoscope 377, 404
Cystoscopy
  instrument, parts of 405f
  procedure 404f, 405f
  purpose of 404
Cytotoxic damage 434

D

Daily living, activities of 276f, 741
Daily water input 466

Data analysis and organization 318
Data assessment 318
Data collection 309, 318
  guideline for 310
  methods of 310
Data retrieval 86
Data, sources of 309
Datura poisoning 687
Dead body care 557, 558
  hygienic 558
  purpose of 558
Death 556
  and dying, responsibility for 48
  anxiety, management of 555
  documentation of 559
  pronouncement of 559
  signs of 555
  stage 704
Deep breath 598
Deep burns 684
Deep vein thrombosis 543
Defecation reflex 361
Dehydration 363
Denture
  care of 280f, 296, 297f
  cleaning procedure 297f
Depressed fracture 657
Depression 550, 551, 605
Dermatitis 218
Descriptive theories 632
Developing illness, risk factors for 10
Development crisis 602
Diabetes 743
  control and complications trial 384
Diabetic diet 330
Diagnostic testing, salient features of 379
Dialysis 467, 519
  catheters 148f
Diarrhea 362, 363, 363f, 375
  causes of 363
  signs of 363
  symptoms of 363
Diastolic pressure 140
Diet on health, effects of 328f
Diet therapy, principles in 329
Diffusion 466, 467, 519, 608
Digestion 743
Dilution formula 227
Dimensional analysis method 502
Direct contact transmission 164, 172
Direct laryngoscopy 395, 396
Direct pressure 655
Disability 94, 249, 653
  limitation 18
Disaster
  epidemiology 743
  geographical 694
  human-induced 694
  levels of 695
  management process 693f
  nursing
    goals of 694
    principles of 694
  response 604
  types of 694
Discharge
  instructions 272
  planning 243, 313
  plans 319
  prescriptions 272
  procedure 244
  reasons for 243
  teaching 458
    goals 244

Discomfort 194
  causes of 195
Disease transmission, modes of 166
Disinfectant, choice of 160
Disinfection 164
Dislocation 643, 660, 661, 743
Disposable
  equipment 146
    syringes and needles 509
    thermometer 114
Disposal drainage systems 456
Dispositional crisis 601
Distant stressors 597
Distraction 215
Distress 594
Diversity 218, 609
Dobutamine 513
Documentation 74, 74f, 258, 743
  and reporting 74
Dog bite 685
Dopamine 513
Doppler ultrasound stethoscope 108
Dorsal gluteal site 514
Dorsal recumbent position 208, 208f
Drag method 666
Drain
  care of 718
  management of 719
  types of 718
Drainage
  apparatus, proper placement of 455
  lack of 459
Drainage tubing
  accidental disconnection of 459
  and bottle, care of 719f
  length of 455
  maintaining patency of 455
Dressing 743
  advantages of 716
  drainage tube insertion site 717
  purpose of 714, 716, 733
  suture care 714
  types of 714, 730, 733
  wound 717, 731
Drinking glasses 147, 225
Droplet infection 167
Droplet precautions 180, 181
Droplet transmission 172
Drowning 674
Drug 743
  abuse 496
  allergies 512
  calculation formula 502f
  cumulative action of 499
  dependence 496
  formulary 497
  habituation 496
  information sources 497
  interaction 496
  rules regarding recording of 506
  sources of 496, 496f
  tolerance 496
Drug administration 497
  legal aspects of 507
  nurses responsibility in 506
  parenteral route of 519f
  routes of 499f
Dry dressing 714, 733
Dry heat 124
Dry inhalation 448
Dry-to-dry dressing 730
Dying person, care of 554, 557
Dying, signs of 554
Dyspepsia 321

Dysphagia 325, 743
  types 325
Dysphasia 321
Dyspnea 139, 140, 425, 429, 430
  management 430
  nursing care of 430
Dysrhythmia 108
Dysuria 343, 346

E

Ear 99, 103, 285
  care of 279, 284
  drops, instillation of 524
  examination of 105
  external 528
  foreign body in 677
  mastoid bandage 692
Eating and drinking, problems with 557
Eating disorders 564
Ectomy 697
Edema 743
Educational program, elements of 271
Elbow
  dislocation 662
    types of 662
  restraint 228, 228f
Electric injuries 689
Electrical burns 682
  and shock, first aid treatment for 684
Electrical hazards 222f
Electrocardiogram 378, 413
Electroencephalogram 378
Electrolyte 471, 472
  description 465
  imbalances 474
  importance of 472
  measurement of 381
  movement 467
Electromyelography 379
Electromyography muscle biofeedback 215
Electronic charting, advantages of 79
Electronic thermometer 114
Electronystagmogram 537
Elimination, problems with 557
Embalming 562
  chemicals 563
  concept of 562
  process, steps of 562
Emergency 643, 743
  admission 237
  code 643
  department 643
    care of 241f
  medical technique 642
  oxygen 643
Emollient enema 368
Emollient stool softeners 363
Emotional attachment 578
Emotional changes 13
Emotional channels, support with 57
Emotional intelligence 564
Emotional stress 596
Emotions 56, 137
Empathy 27, 62
Employee wellness programs 743
Empty urine collection bag 354
Enamel bed pan and urinal 153f
Enamel ware, care of 152
End stage renal disease 492
Endocrine 120
Endometrial biopsy 378
Endoscopic fiberoptic instruments 154f

Endoscopic retrograde cholangiopancreatography 377, 421
Endoscopic unit and equipment 155f
Endoscopy 377, 394
  procedure 394f
Endotoxin 164
Endotracheal tube 148, 441
  and inserting technique 442f
Enema 366, 367f, 368
  administration 368f
  classification of 367
  types of 368f
Energy yielding foods 323
Enteroscopy 379
Enuresis 343, 346
Environment 8, 32, 38, 56, 221, 345, 639, 743
  and adaptation 600
  assessment of 599
  preparation of 93, 103
Environmental assessment 743
Environmental barrier 273
Environmental degradation 695
Environmental determinants 3, 7
Environmental factors 531
Environmental hazards 188
Environmental issues 231
Environmental manipulation 604
Environmental sanitation 10
Environmental stressors 595
Enzyme 169
Epidural analgesia administration 513
Epidural anesthesia 704
Epilepsy 743
Epileptic fit 688
Epiphyseal fracture 658
Episodic acute stress 596
Epistaxis 688
  first aid for 688f
Equipment 38, 237, 238, 280
  maintenance
    cleaning of 145
    concept of 145
    disinfection of 145
  preparation of 103, 111, 113, 456
  room 698
  safe use of 146
Erikson's theory 568
Eroticism, sexual health concerns to 578
Erythromycin injection 512
Escherichia coli 714
Esophageal dysphagia 325
Esophagogastroduodenoscopy 377, 408, 408f
Esophagus 743
Esthetic factor 221
Ethic 743
  Committees 27
Ethical decision making 45
Ethical dilemmas 45
Ethical principles 43
Ethnic 609
  and religious sensitivity 33, 40
Ethnocentrism 609
Eustress 594
Euthanasia 546, 560, 561
  passive 547, 560, 561
Evacuant enema 523
Evaporation 111
Excitement 586, 704
  phase 586
Excretion 495
Exercise 137
  and activity tolerance 250
  benefits of 248
  effects of 250

Exhaustion, stage of 595, 597
Exogenous 171
Experience, lack of 312
Expiration 425
Explanatory theory 632
Exposure 653, 743
    surveillance 743
External environment, influence of 220
Extracellular fluid 743
    volume 464
Extreme cold, effects of 123
Extremities 103
Extubation 698
Eye 99, 102, 285
    arteries, angiography of 412
    care of 279, 284, 284f
    chemical burns of 676
    contact 56
    dryness of 542
    examination of 105, 408f
    foreign body in 676
    hygiene of 676
    injury hazards 189
    wounds 651

F

Face 283
    fracture of 658
    mask 152
Facial appearance 557
Facial expressions 56
Facial protection 184
Facilitate mourning 553
Facilitated diffusion 467
Facilitating attitudes 55
Factor-isolating theory 632
Fainting 643, 688, 743
Fairness 305
Faith
    healing 608
    loss of 622
    questioning of 622
Fall from bicycle 657f
Fall risk assessment 230
Fallout contamination 698
False crisis 118, 120
Family
    assessment of 599
    dynamics, impact of 14
    folder 74
    health 743
    history 92
    practices 11
    records 78
    roles, impact of 13
    structure 743
    theory 632
Fastigium 118, 120
Fasting 608
    blood glucose level 384
    plasma glucose 384
Fear 623
    and pain 249
Febrile convulsion 643
Fecal impaction 362
Fecal incontinence 362
Feces
    abnormal characteristics of 371, 388
    normal characteristics of 371, 388
Feeding infant 337
Feeding pump 334f
Feeding techniques, types of 339f
Feeding, artificial 337

Feelings 549
Feet, care of 285, 286f
Female health workers 38
Femoral artery 743
Femur, fracture of 659
Fever 118, 121, 169
    care of 119
    causes of 120
    continuous 118, 120
    control 121
    irregular 119
    measurement of 119f
    stages in course of 120
    types of 118, 120
Fiber 363
Fiberoptic
    care of 154
    laryngoscope 395, 396, 396f
FICA spiritual assessment 620t
Fidelity 45, 743
Field block anesthesia 704
Fight-or-flight response 594f
Figure-of-eight 691
Fire
    precautions 218
    prevention 218
Fireman's lift 645, 666
    and carry 665
First aid 122, 123, 218, 644, 645f, 656, 659, 660, 684
    and emergencies 642
    equipment 648f
    general rules for 644
    golden rules of 647
    importance of 645
    kit 648
    measures 658, 684, 685
    objectives of 644
    principles of 644, 645
    scope of 644
    treatment 657, 685, 688
Fistula 743
Fixing shoulder dislocation, tips for 662
Flange 442
Flatulence 362, 364
    causes of 364f
Flatus tube 365, 365f
    insertion of 364
Flexible fiberoptic bronchoscope, parts of 398
Florence Nightingale
    contributions of 31
    history of 30
Flucloxacillin 512
Fluid 511
    and electrolyte
        movement of 466
        status 470
    and food intake 345
    calculations 339
    from abdomen, aspiration of 724f
    imbalances 469
    injected, composition of 510
    intake 465
    movement, factors affecting 467, 519
    pressure 468
    rate calculation 521
    restriction 492
    volume excess 470, 471
Fluid balance
    factors affecting 466
    maintaining 540
Fluid loss
    mild 470

    moderate 470
    severe 471
Fluid volume deficit 470
    signs of 470
    symptoms of 470
Fluoroscopy 406
    procedure 406f
Flush out, care of 157
Folding sponge cloth, technique of 282f
Food
    allergy 321
    exchanges 321
    functions of 322
    guide pyramid 323f
    habits 10
    intolerances and sensitivities 363
    physiological functions of 323
    poisoning 321
    psychological functions of 323
    social functions of 323
Foot drop 194
    prevention of 671
Footboard 204f
Footrests 204
Fore-and-aft
    carry 667
    method 665
Foreign bodies in ear, first aid for 675
Foreign bodies
    in eye, first aid for 675, 676f
    in nose, first aid for 675
    in throat, first aid for 675
    removal from ear, hospital-based 677f
Fortum 512
Fowler's position 210, 210f
Fracture 643, 657, 743
    bed 202, 202f
    causes of 657
    complicated 657
    management, Rice method of 660f
    pan 365
Freud's anal stage 579
Freud's genital stage 581
Freud's oral stage 579
Freud's phallic stage 580
Friction 138, 290
Frostbite 123, 643
Frozen section 698
Functional bowel disorders 363
Functional extracellular fluid 492
Functional inspired oxygen 744
Fundoscopy 377, 407, 407f
Fundus of eye, examination of 407f
Funduscope, types of 407
Funnel and catheter method 368
Futile measures 547

G

Gait 250
    belt 537
Gallstones, choledochoscopic removal of 422f
Gamma-glutamyltransferase 382
Gas
    poisoning 685
    sterilization 160
Gastric analysis 340
Gastric gavage 334
    principles in 335
Gastric lavage 744
Gastric secretions, constituents of 340
Gastroenteritis 170
Gastrointestinal infections 172
Gastrointestinal system 251-253, 556

Gastrointestinal therapeutic system 524
Gastrointestinal tract 469
Gastrojejunostomy feeding 335, 335f, 336f
Gauntlet cast 263
Gender identity 581
Gender role 581
General adaptation syndrome 594, 597, 744
General cold application 130
General sense 528
Generic approach 604
Genetic inheritance 8
Genitourinary system 556
Gentamicin 512
Gention violet 649
Gerontology nursing 744
Gestation 528
Giger and Davidhizar's transcultural assessment model 617, 617f
Glasgow coma scale 539
Glass instruments, care of 156
Glass syringes 508
Gloves 152, 177, 184
Gloving technique 181f
Glucometer random blood sugar 384
Glycated hemoglobin 384
Glycerin
  enema 367
  syringe 368
Gonorrhea 588
Good communication 67
Good first-aider, qualities of 644
Good housekeeping, principles of 226
Good workmanship 33
Gowns 179, 184
Graduate nurse 38
Greenstick fracture 657
Grief
  and loss, theories of 551
  complicated 549
  five stages of 551
  manifestations of 549
  normal 548
  physical sensations of 549
  resolution of 605
  stages of 550, 605
  Tonkin's model of 551
  types of 548
  uncomplicated 548
Grieving, four tasks of 551
Gross motor skills 96
Growth 744
  and development 95
  hormone releasing hormone 597
Guilt 549
Gustatory receptor cells 528

H

Habits 275
Hair
  care of 278, 291
  combing 292
  factors affecting 292
  factors influence on 292
  shampoo technique 293f
  wash 293
Hair care 291f
  aspects of 291
  problems of neglected 279
  types of 278
Halitosis 543
Hand
  care of 285
  hygiene 164

seats 665
sensitive parts of 89
Hand washing
  and gloving 173
  prevents disease transmission 170f
  technique 173f
Handling casualty, pick-a-back method of 665f
Handling laparoscopic instruments, method of 403f
Hanging 674
  first aid measures of 690f
  strangling and throttling 689
Hartmann's solution 464
Hays test 360, 394
Hazard 218, 744
Hazardous event 218
HbA1c blood test 384
Head
  and face 102
  bandage 692
  circumference 93, 324
  nurse 37
  tilt-chin lift position 679f
  to toe
    care 278
    examination 102
Healing by first intention 713
Healing by second intention 713
Healing by third intention 713
Healing environment, goals of 222
Health 1, 2, 32, 634, 639, 744
  alternative therapies of 214
  and child development 3
  and disease, cultural factors in 10
  and people cooperation 3
  and sexual reproduction 581
  behavior 1, 275, 744
  concept of 2, 11, 17
  determinants of 7, 11f
  deviation self-care requisites 636
  dimensions of 3, 3f
  education 605
  educator, competencies of 268
  factors affecting 87, 10f
  factors influencing 8
  food tips 330f
  for all 2, 17
  for peace and security 3
  fundamental right 3
  gain for all 3
  hazards 188, 189
  history 90
  indicator 744
  personnel 310
  programmes 20
  promoting behavior 1
  protection 744
  sector, disaster management of 695
  services 9, 16
  wellness model 5, 5f
Health and health
  allied resources 9
  care 3
  information 3
Health and illness 7
  continuum 1, 4, 5f, 744
  models of 5
Health assessment 86, 106, 237f
  principles of 87
  recording of 105
  responsibilities of nurse in 87
  role of nurse in 105

Health belief
  and motivation 276, 277
  model 1, 5, 6f
Health care 308
  agency 21
    types of 21
  attorney for 27
  delivery system 3, 8, 16, 19, 19f, 34f
  environment 218
    safety in 219
  infections 233
  levels of 18
  organizations 22
  secondary 19
  services 19, 20
  system 19, 744
  team 2, 20
    members 21f
  workers, body mechanics for 256
Health problems 19
  chronic 249
Health promotion 1, 18, 20, 744
  diagnosis 311
  model 6, 6f
Health related
  factors 567
  services 9
Health teaching
  importance of 71
  postoperative 709
Healthy bladder 346f
Hearing
  assessment of 537
  impaired 538
  impairment 537
Hearing aid
  and earmolds, cleaning 298
  care and maintenance of 298
  care of 298, 298f
Hearing loss
  bilateral progressive 538
  conductive 537, 538
  fluctuating sensorineural 538
  mixed 537
  treatments for mixed 538
  types of 537
Heart
  and blood vessels 469
  and respiratory diseases 258
  attack 643, 744
  blood circulation in 426f
  failure, late-stage 431
  monitors 147
  rate 93, 586, 587
Heat and fire hazards 189
Heat cramps 120, 122
Heat exhaustion 120, 122
Heat loss, factors influences 111, 111f, 113
Heat production 110
  factors influences 111, 111f, 113
Heat stroke 109, 120, 122
Heat, application of 510
Hectic fever 119
Height and weight 102
Heimlich maneuver 672f
Hematemesis 744
Hematocrit 380
Hematoma 713
  formation 521
Hematuria 343
Hemoglobin 380, 744
Hemoptysis 425
Hemorrhage 459, 643, 654, 713
  control 655f

effects of 654
types of 654, 655f
Hemorrhoids 362
Hemothorax 726
Henderson's theory 634
　application of 635f
　components of 635f
Heparin lock 487
Hepatitis
　B 588
　　infection 588
Heritancy 346
Hernia, abdominal 678
Herpes viruses 588
Heterosexual 584
Hiccough 429
High protein diet 330
Hiking 606
Histotoxic hypoxia 432
Holism 621, 744
Holistic assessment 744
Holistic health 1
Home health care 744
Home oxygen therapy 438
Home visit 744
Homeostasis 425, 594
Homophobia 609
Homosexual 584
　behavior 580
Hornet sting 685
Hospice 547
　care 16, 21, 744
Hospital
　bed 194
　classification of 24, 25f
　cleaning 222
　equipment 175
　functions of 24
　furnitures 157
　objectives of 23
　scope of 23
Hospital admission 236
　and discharge 236
Hospital diet 329
　types of 331f
Hospital patient safety 220
　culture 234
Hospital waste
　classification of 186
　segregation of 185f
Hospital-associated infections, types of 172
Hot air oven 159, 159f
　mechanism of 159
Hot application 124,
　complications of 125
　contraindications of 125
　physiological effects of 124
　principles of 125
　types of 124f
Hot fomentation procedure 127, 127f
Hot stage 123
Hot test 359, 394
Hot water
　bag 125, 125f
　bottle 152
House fly 167f
Household waste 187
Housekeeping supply room 698
Huff coughing 445
Human biology 8
Human crutch 645, 665, 666
Human functioning, aspects of 556
Human growth hormone 597

Human immunodeficiency virus 588
Human milk 337
Human relation skills 54
Human response 312
Humerus, fracture of 659
Humility 305
Hydration 94
Hydrogen peroxide 649
Hydrometeorological disaster 694
Hydrostatic pressure 466-468, 519
Hygiene 275
　practices, factors influencing 276
　types of 275
Hygienic care 744
Hypemic hypoxia 432
Hypercalcemia 479
Hypercapnia 425
Hyperextension 247
Hyperglycemia 643, 710
Hyperkalemia causes 474, 477
Hypermagnesemia 480
Hypernatremia 474, 475
Hyperphosphatemia 481
Hyperpnea 425, 429
Hyperpyrexia 119
Hypertension 141
　causes of 141, 142
Hyperthermia 109, 118, 120, 121
Hyperventilation 139, 425, 430
Hypervolemia 470, 471
Hypnosis 216
Hypocalcemia 474, 478, 478
Hypocapnia 744
Hypodermic embalming 563
Hypoglycaemia 643
Hypokalemia 477
Hypomagnesemia 479
Hyponatremia 475
Hypophosphatemia 481
Hypostatic pneumonia 250, 543, 544
Hypotension 142, 710
　signs of 142
　symptoms of 142
Hypothalamic center 542
Hypothalamus 468
Hypothermia 109, 118, 120, 744
Hypoventilation 139, 425, 430
Hypovolemia 470, 471
Hypovolemic shock 655
Hypoxemia 425
Hypoxia 425, 430, 432, 744
　histologic 432
　stages of 432
Hypoxic hypoxia 432
Hysteria 744
Hysteron-salphingography 378

I

Iatrogenic disease 496
Ice 661
　cap 132, 132f
　　application procedure 133f
　collar 132
Idiosyncratic reaction 496
Iliac and femoral angiography 412
Iliac puncture 729
Illness
　acute phase of 741
　behavior 12f, 744
　　stages of 12, 12f
　causes of 11f
　chronic 742
　concepts of 12

　prevention 20
　levels of 17
　stage 168
Illness-illness behavior 12
Imbalanced nutrition 543
Immobility 247
　complications of 254
　degrees of 247, 249
　high risk of 250
　problems with 557
Immune
　response 169
　system 248
Immunity 164, 169, 744
Immunization 164
Immunodeficiency 744
Immunological diseases 120
Impaired tissue integrity cornea, risk for 542
Inadequate care 623
Inappropriate care 623
Incident report 74, 80, 83
　purpose of 83
Incision 643
　pain 459
Incontinence, types of 347
Indoor games 606
Indoor recreational options 606
Induce stress 595
Industrial hygiene 276
Industrial nurse 37
Infection 120, 397, 713, 744
　agent 166
　and infection process 165
　at needle site 521
　chain of 166f, 167
　control 163, 164, 181, 744
　　policy 174
　　role of nurse in 181
　course of 168
　defenses against 168
　healthcare associated 164
　hospital-acquired 170, 174
　nature of 164
　process 165
　sources of 171
　transmission of 167f
　types of 165
Infectious agent 165f, 167
Infectious diseases, transmission of 492
Infertility 576
Infibulation 576
Infiltration 521
Inflammation 169
Inflammatory phase 711
Informed consent 27, 74, 80, 744
Infrared therapy 126, 126f
Infusion pump 149
Ingestion 744
Inhalations, types of 448
Injection 509
　complications of 511
　selection of site for 511
　types of 509
Injured person, transport of 645, 663
Injury 643
　mechanism of 711
　risk for 541
Inner cannula 442
Instilling nasal drops 525
Instrument care, general principles of 145
Insulin 744
Intact penis 576
Integrated communications 744

Integumentary system 86, 100, 118, 251-252, 253
Intense concern 550
Intense feelings 603
Intensive care 602
Intercourse 576
Intermittent feeding 336
Intermittent fever 120
Intermittent gravity drip 336
Intermittent infusion 488
International Federation of Clinical Chemistry 384
International Red Cross Society 22
Interneuron 528
Interpersonal relationship
    principles of 60
    role of nurse in 61
    skills 59, 60, 60*f*
Interpersonal theory and nursing process 633
Interstitial fluid volume 464
Intestinal diseases 363
Intimacy 62, 581
Intimate relationship 63
Intra-aortic balloon pump 149
Intra-articular injections 513
Intracardiac injections 513
Intracellular fluid 492, 744
    volume 464
Intracranial pressure monitor 148
Intradermal injection 516, 517
Intramuscular injection 513
    administration 514*f*
    sites of 514, 514*f*
Intraoperative care 704*f*
    purpose of 704
Intraoperative nursing interventions 705
Intrapleural brain falls out 459
Intrapleural drain 459
Intrathecal injections 513
Intravenous bolus dose administration 488*f*
Intravenous cannulation, care of 487*f*
Intravenous catheter 520*f*
    insertion 483, 485*f*
    sites 484*f*
Intravenous cutdown 488
Intravenous fluid administration system 522*f*
Intravenous infusion 518
    therapy 520*f*
Intravenous injection 517
Intravenous pyelography 423
Intubation 698
Inverse fever 118, 120
Involuntary euthanasia 547, 561
Iodine 649
Iontophoresis 523
Isolation 173
    hospitals 25
    nursing 174
    room 175*f*
    technique 182
    unit 175
    ward 175
    waste 187

J

Jacket restraint 228
Jaw Barton bandage 692
Jellyfish sting 685
Jet injection 523
Job satisfaction 308
Joint 745
    and muscles
        first aid in injuries to 663
        injuries to 663

    deformity 544
    dislocations of 660
    mobility 247, 248, 249
Jugular catheter insertion, external 484*f*

K

Kegel's exercises 348
Kidney 469, 745
    role of 482
    tray 146, 225
Kitchen, care of 156
Knee-chest position 210*f*
Knowledge, lack of 312
Kubler-Ross five stages 551
Kussmaul's respirations 139, 425, 429

L

Labia 586
Laparoscope, types of 403
Laparoscopic instrument, types of 403*f*
Laparoscopic procedure, method of 404*f*
Laparoscopy 377, 402, 403
    tubes 402*f*
Large arm sling 692
Laryngoscope
    application technique 395*f*
    care of 155
    purpose of 395
    types of 395
Laryngoscopy 377, 395
    indirect 395
Larynx 745
    anatomical structure of 395*f*
    examination of 395*f*
Latrines 745
Laugh 598
Law and nurse 47
Law, types of 47
Leadership role 634
Leaning environment components 220*f*
Learning process 623
Legal records 80
Legalism 745
Legs 284
Leininger's sunrise model 616, 617*f*
Lethal effects 496
Leukocyte 379
Liaison 745
Life after death 608
Life saving equipment 149*f*
Life, loss of 548
Life-sustaining treatment 547
Lift with leg muscles 259
Lifters and moving, general principles of 259
Lifting and transferring 258
Lifting casualty 666
    in wheelchair 667
Lifting criteria 259
Lifting technique 666
Ligament 745
Linen
    and bandages 156
    care of 150
    types of 150
Lipid profile 383
Lipoprotein profile 383
Liposomes 524
Liquid diets 329
Liquid medical waste 187
Listening 745
    check 298
    improve 59
    skills 54, 60

Lithotomy position 208, 208*f*
Liver
    aspiration 378
    biopsy 378, 732, 732*f*
    function test 382
Living will 547, 560
Livor mortis 557
L-lactate dehydrogenase 382
Loading stretcher 664
Local adaptation
    syndrome 597
    system 598
Local bath 128, 128*f*
Local cold application 130
Local heat applications 124
Local infiltration anesthesia 704
Local inspection 88
Log rolling 261
    technique 262*f*
Long arm cast 263
Long leg cast 264
Lordotic position 411
Loss, categories of 547
Love and belongingness 4
Low calorie diet 329
Low fat diet 329
Low protein diet 329
Low pyrexia 119
Low self-esteem 571
Low temperature 109
Lower extremity venography 414
    ascending 415
    descending 415
    procedure 414*f*
Lower extremity, care of 282*f*
Lower lobes 451
Low-oxalate diet 321
Lumbar puncture 377, 726
    procedure 727*f*
Lung 397*f*, 469, 745
    affected lobes of 449*f*
    diseases 410*f*
    gas exchange process in 440*f*
    role of 482
    segments, examination of 397*f*
Lymphangitis 714
Lymphatic system 169

M

Mackintoshes 152
Magnesium 465, 473
    losses of 473
    regulation of 473
Maintain urinary 671
Makirational loss 548
Maladaptive coping 594
Maladaptive grief responses 605
Manipulation 90, 604
Mask 179
Maslow's hierarchy 4, 4*f*, 314*f*
Massage 216, 510
Material media 496
Maturation phase 712
Maturational crisis 600, 602
Mechanical soft diet 331
Mechanical suction on water seal drainage system, application of 456
Mechanical ventilation 445
Mechanisms controlling fluid 467
Mechanoreceptor 528
Mediastinal shift 726
Medical advice, discharge against 243
Medical and nursing research 24

Medical asepsis 179f, 745
  guidelines for maintaining 177
Medical care contact 12
Medical coordination 745
Medical device 144
Medical education and training 24
Medical equipment 144
Medical hand washing 178, 182
Medical records 310
Medical waste, categories of 187f
Medication action
  factors influencing 498
  types of 498
Medication administration 496
  errors in 503
  rights of 502, 503f
Medication dosage, factors influence 499
Medication dose calculation 501
Medication errors 233, 499
  causes of 503
  types of 503
Medication into ear, administration of 524f
Medication into nose, administration of 525f
Medication management 430
Medication stock checking 506f
Medication, administration of 495
Medication, forms of 497
Medicine
  and medicine cupboard, care of 505
  indigenous systems of 19
  purpose of 497
  rules for administration of 506
Medicolegal cases, role of nurse in 240
Medicolegal issues 239, 559
  nurses responsibility in 560
Meditation 216
Melena 745
Membranes, selective permeability of 467, 520
Menstrual hygiene 275
Mental health 275
  assessment 92
Mental illnesses 92
Mental preparation 93, 104
Mental status 102, 534
  assess changes in 445
Message, completeness of 59
Metabolic acidosis 483
Metabolic alkalosis 483
Metabolic system 248, 250, 252, 253
Metabolism 251, 495
Metaparadigm 627
Methicillin-resistant Staphylococcus aureus 170
Metric system 500
Mid upper arm circumference 325
Military hospitals 21
Military nurse 37
Milk formula, preparation of 337
Minimize auditory clutter 224
Minimize hospital room clutter 224
Mitigation 173, 219, 745
Mobile crisis programs 604
Mobility
  and immobility 247
  effects of 250
  factors affecting 249
Moist cold 130
Moist heat 124, 158, 682
Monoclonal antibodies 524
Mortality data 745
Mosquitoes 167f
Motion exercise, range of 258
Motor neuron 528
Mouth
  and pharynx 103

breathing 543
care, complication of neglected 281, 281f
examination of 105
wash 279
Movement, regulation of 255
Mummification procedure 228f
Mummy device 227
Mumps 168
Muscle 745
  atrophy 251
  injuries 657
  mass 253
  tone and activity 345
  wasting 544
Muscular system 586, 587
Musculoskeletal injury 657
  acute 661
Musculoskeletal system 118, 248, 250-253
Myelography 378, 422
  procedure 423f
Myotonia 585

N

Nails, care of 285
Narayanasamy's access model 616
Narcotic 219
Nasal cannula 434, 434f
Nasal catheter 435, 435f
Nasal polyps 745
Nasal suctioning 446
Nasogastric tube
  feeding 334f
  insertion 332, 334f
  measurement technique 333f
Nasopharyngeal airway 440
  insertion technique 441f
Nasopharyngeal suctioning procedures 446f
Nasotracheal tubes
  advantages of 441
  problems with 441
National Sexuality Education Standards 592
Natural disasters 694, 745
Nausea 321, 326
Nebulization 745
Neck 103
  examination of 105
  plate 442
Needle
  care of 154
  parts of 509f
Neisseria gonorrhoeae 588
Neonatal intensive care equipment 149
Neonatal mortality rate 745
Neoplasms 120
Nervous system 118, 251
Neuman's theory 637
Neural mechanism 469
Neural pathway 530f
Neurogenic shock 655
Neurological assessment 95f
Neurological observations 95
Neurological system 94
Neurological tests 103
Neuromuscular defects 249
Neuromuscular irritability 480
Neutralism 745
Nightingale's pledge 30
Nitrofurazone 649
Nocturia 343, 346
Noise 189, 221
  respiration 429
Nonmaleficence 27, 44
Non-pharmacological therapies 215

Nonrebreather mask 436
Nonverbal communication 54, 56, 60, 745
  types of 56f
Nonverbal skills 591
Non-voluntary euthanasia 547, 561
Normal hospital diet 328f
Normal movement, basic elements of 248
Normal respiratory, types of 137
Normal sensation 530
Normothermia 109
Norton scale 287, 288
Nose 99, 103, 285
  care of 279, 284
  examination of 105
  foreign body in 677
Nosocomial infection 170, 174f
  causes of 170
  transmission of 172
  types of 171
Numbness 549
Nurses
  administrators 42
  and co-worker 43
  and practice 42
  and profession 43
  and society 43
  anesthetics 27
  client helping relationship 67
  community relationship 67
  competences 617
  educator 42
  extended role of 42
  family relationship 68
  feeding helpless patient 332f
  functions of 35
  health team relationship 68
  patient relationship 50, 61f, 68, 633
  practitioner 27, 42
  professional etiquettes for 46
  researcher 42
  responsibilities of 36f, 77, 78, 241, 245, 250, 259, 507, 524, 587, 588, 702, 703
  role of 35, 36f, 61f, 62, 71, 192, 214, 216, 241, 245, 273, 278, 326, 589, 602, 614, 702
  sheet 78
  theorists 628
  vital role of 75f
Nursing 1, 27, 31, 32, 634, 639
  agency 636
  and medical diagnosis 311f
  approach 80
  audit 745
  care 265, 558
  concept of 32
  director 37
  education, nursing personnel in 38
  ethics 42
  evaluation 315, 316f
  history of 27, 28, 745
  homes 16, 24
  implementation 314, 314f
  intervention 121, 541, 550, 574, 606
  legal issues in 47
  management 121, 253, 347, 670
  objectives of 32
  philosophy of 32
  planning 313, 313f
  postoperative 705
  procedures 38
  profession 34
  professional standards of 40f
  roles 315, 634
  science 33
  scope of 36

spiritual dimensions of 623
superintendent 36
supervisor 36
Nursing assessment 68, 309, 309f, 572, 745
    purpose of 309
Nursing care plan 317, 317t, 536, 540, 745
    purpose of 318
    types of 317
Nursing diagnosis 68, 212, 253, 301, 307, 310, 312, 312f, 710, 745
    classifications 311
    problem-focused 301
    purpose of 311
Nursing metaparadigm 628, 630
    components of 629f
Nursing personnel
    categories of 37
    responsibilities of 227
Nursing practice 66
    theoretical models of 631
Nursing process 301, 307f, 570, 697, 745
    advantages of 307
    assessment 69f
    benefits of 308
    characteristics of 307
    critical thinking to 304t
    evaluation in 315, 315f
    meaning of 306
    purpose of 307
    steps in 87f, 306f, 307, 710
Nursing service 37
    administrative positions 37
    nursing personnel in 37
Nursing system 636
    theories of 636
    types of 636
Nursing theories 627, 631
    components of 630, 630f
    development of 633
    history of 628
    levels of 632f
    values and goals of 627f
Nutrient 321
    enema 368
Nutrition 94, 671
    and fluids 703
    and health 322
    status 322
Nutritional assessment 324
Nutritional needs 540
Nycturia 346

O

Obesity 321
Observation and reporting, responsibility for 47
Obstructive pulmonary disease, chronic 431
Obturator 442
Occupational safety and health administration 163, 192
Odor 371, 388, 393
Oil enema 367
Olfaction 528
Olfactory bulb 528
Olfactory sensory neuron 528
Oliguria 343, 346, 710
Oliguric phase 321
Oncotic pressure 468
Open airway 461, 679f
Open bed 199
Open fracture 657
Open gloving 698
Open victim's airway 679
Opening stretcher 668

Operation bed 201
Operation
    eradicate fear of 701
    room nurse 697
    theater 178f, 201f
Optic disc 528
Optic nerve 528
Optimum environment 220, 226
Oral care, partially assisted 280f
Oral cholecystography 420
Oral dysphagia 325
Oral glucose tolerance test 384
Oral hygiene 279
    complication of neglected 278
Oral medication 507
    administration of 507
Oral mucous membrane 543
Oral report 78
Oral route 172
Oral suctioning 446
Oral temperature 114
    measurement techniques 115f
Orem's concept, relationship of 636
Orem's theory 636, 637f
Organ donation 560-562
    counseling for 560
Organ systems 86, 100
Organization function 23f
Orgasm phase 586
Oropharyngeal airway 438
    application procedure 439f
    parts of 438f
    types of 439f
Orotracheal tubes, problems with 439
Orrhaphy 697
Orthopnea 139, 140, 425, 429
Orthostatic albuminuria 343
Oscopy 697
Osmolality 467
Osmolarity 467
Osmoreceptor 529
Osmosis 464, 466, 467, 519
Osmotic pumps 524
Osteoporosis 251
Ostomy 697
Otomy 697
Over bed table 146, 224, 225
Overflow incontinence 347
Own spiritual quest, awareness of 623
Oxygen 745
    administration 434, 434f, 436f
    cylinder
        and connections 434f
        care of 433
    delivery system 433f
    levels, monitoring 433
    mask 435
    saturation 93
    status, factors affecting 428f
    tent 436
    therapy 430, 431, 433
        dangers of 434
    transducers, types of 453
Oxygenation
    alterations in 432
    factors affecting 431
    needs 425

P

Packed cell volume 380
Pain 93, 94, 211, 745
    acute 211
    assess for 445

    causes of chronic 213f
    clinical manifestation of 211
    components of 211
    experiences 212
    perception, factors influencing 211, 211f
    types of 211, 211f
Palpation 88, 96, 97, 99, 745
Panoptic ophthalmoscope 408
Papilledema 541
Paplau's theory 633
Paracentesis, abdominal 377, 722, 722f
Paradigm 627
Parasites 363
Parathyroid gland 469
Parathyroid hormone 469
Parenteral administration 499
Parenteral nutrition 321
Parenteral route 172
Passive transport 466
Past sexual activity 588
Patella, fracture of 659
Patency, assess airway for 444
Patent airway, maintaining 540
Pathogenic organisms, pressure of 290
Patient and environment, preparation of 125, 257, 260, 283, 295, 515, 701
Patient care
    equipment 146, 147f, 150
    standards 74
    unit, terminal cleaning of 245
Patient centered care 38, 39f, 270, 270F
Patient centered collaborative team 40f
Patient education 267, 269
    importance of 269
    methods 272
    record 79
Patient lifting technique 260f
Patient monitoring devices 147f
Patient teaching
    purpose of 71
    role of nurse in 72
Patient vomiting, nursing care of 327f
Patient's bill of rights 240
Patient's health status 11
Pediatric blade 396f
Pediculi, types of 294
Pediculosis
    dangers of 294
    prevention of 294
Pediculosis treatment 294, 294f
    medications for 294
Pelvic floor exercises 348
Pelvis, fracture of 659
Penetrating chest wounds 652, 652f
    management of 653f
Penicillin
    drug interaction of 512
    test 517
Perceived loss 548
Percussion technique 451, 451f
Percutaneous tibial nerve stimulation 348
Perform rescue breathing 681
Perfusion 425
Pericardial aspiration 377
Perineal care 296f, 746
Perineum care 295
Periodic breathing 140
Perioperative care 697
Perioperative nursing
    phases of 699
    process 710
Peristalsis 746
Personal cleaning tip 223

Personal commitment 32, 41
Personal hygiene 10, 275, 276, 278
    factors influences on 277
    importance of 277
    maintain 671
    principles of 277
    purpose of 277
Personal protecting equipment 184, 191
    types of 184f
Personal protective clothing 191
Peumoecephalography 378
Pharmacokinetics 495
Pharmacological management 602
Pharmacopeias 496, 497
Pharmacotherapeutics 495
Pharyngeal dysphagia 325
Pharyngeal reflex, absence of 543
Pharynx 746
Philosophy 1, 627
Phlebotomy procedure 379f
Phosphate 465, 474
Photoisomerization 529
Photoreceptor 529
Physical adaptation 599
Physical assessment 93, 534
Physical barriers 168
Physical comfort 270
Physical condition 276, 277
Physical environment 8, 221, 746
    factors 221f
Physical examination 88f, 89f, 91f, 310
    instruments 104f
    methods of 88
    procedure 100
    techniques 101f
Physical hazards
    reduction of 223
    types of 222f
Physical preparation 104
Physical stress 596
Physical techniques 430
Physiologic homeostasis 598
Physiological and sexual response 586
Physiological changes after death 556
Physiological stressors 595, 596
Pilot balloon 442
Pituitary gland 468
Planned hospital discharge 243
Plasmalyte 464
Plaster cast 263, 265
    application 264f
Plaster of Paris 264
Plastic syringes 509
Plateau phase 586
Platelet
    count 380
    volume, mean 380
Pleuralism 623
Pneumaturia 343
Pneumonia 431
    hospital-acquired 170
Pneumothorax 726
Poison 644, 685, 746
Poisoning, treatment of 686
Political system 3, 8, 9
Pollution
    control 219
    prevention 219
Polydipsia 321
Polyphagia 321
Polyuria 321, 343, 346
Poor sexual health, consequences of 584
Portable suction apparatus 155f

Portal venography 415, 416
Position unresponsive victim 679
Positive health concept 565
Positive self-concept, characteristics of 565
Positive stress 594
Postanesthesia care unit 698
Postanesthetic assessment 706t
Postanesthetic care unit observations 707f
Postmortem care 561
Postoperative complications, prevention of 710
Postprandial plasma glucose 384
Postrenal condition 345, 346
Postural drainage 430, 449, 450f
    techniques 451
Posture 248
    and gait 56
Potassium 465, 472
    functions of 472
    losses of 473
    permanganate 648
    regulation of 473
Practice specific relaxation techniques 598
Practice-level nursing theories 632
Prerenal conditions 344, 346
Prescriptivism 746
Present health status 91
Pressure areas, care of 671
Pressure dressing 714, 733
Pressure points 655
    care of 289
Pressure sore 290f, 543
    cause of 290
    clinical manifestation of 290
    degrees of 291
Pressure ulcers, assessment of 287
Preventive medicine 276
Preventive rehabilitative processes 746
Primary health care 2, 18
Primary Health Center 2
Primary nurse practitioner 746
Primary nursing 2
Privacy, maintenance of 103
Problem-solving therapy 602
Prodromal stage 168
Professional communication, elements of 60, 67
Professional development 33, 40
Professional growth 308
Professional nurse
    characteristics of 34
    quality of 34
    values of 33, 39
Professionalism in nursing, concept of 41
Progestasert 524
Prokinetics 363
Prostate-specific antigen 346
Protective and regulatory foods 323
Protective isolation 746
Protective measures 687
Protective mechanism, normal 168f
Protein
    level 727
    total 382
Proteinuria 343
Proteus vulgaris 714
Protoscopy 377
Proxy consent 28
Pseudomonas aeruginosa 170, 172
Pseudo-resolution 601
Psychiatric emergencies 602
Psychiatric illnesses 92
Psychodynamic nursing 633
Psychogenic pain 211
Psychological alterations 252, 253

Psychological barrier 272
Psychological factors 250, 345
Psychological preparation 701
Psychological stressors 596
Psychomotor skill 314
Psychosocial assessment 612
Psychosocial care and assessment 612
Psychosocial functioning 251
Psychosocial technique 430
Psyllium 363
Puberty 746
    and pre-puberty 580
Pubic region 284
Public facilities 181
Public hospitals 21, 24
Public sector 19
Pulmonary angiography 378, 412, 413, 413f
Pulmonary edema 726
Pulmonary system 250
Pulse 108, 135, 746
    abnormal 136
    absence of 557
    characteristics of 136
    checking 135f
    common sites for checking 135
    deficit 108
    factors affect 136
    oximeter 108, 147, 453
    oximetry probe, placement of 453f
    oxymetry and settings 453f
    pressure 108
    rhythm 108
    volume 108
Puncture 644
    wounds 650, 711
Pupil 529
Pyrexia 109, 118
    high 119
    moderate 119
Pyrogenic reactions 492, 521

Q

Quality assurance 144
Quality care 2
Quality clients care 308
Quality control, responsibility in 47
Queckenstedt's test 727
Quotidian fever 118

R

Racism 609
Radial artery 746
Radiation 111, 746
    burns 682
    errors 233
Radiological studies 409
Rales sound 138
Random blood glucose level 384
Range of motion 247, 249, 250
    exercise 257, 257f, 746
    types of 257
Rapid shallow breathing, signs of 459
Rapidly acting lubricants 363
Rapport 62
Reasoning
    deductive 312
    inductive 312
Rebreather mask, partial 436
Receptor cell 529
Record keeping and reporting, responsibility for 48
Record maintenance, legal implication in 80
Record writing, principles of 77

Records and report
 legal implications of 80
 meaning of 75
 principles of 76
Recovery room, management of 706
Recreation and diversional therapies 606
Rectal drip method 368
Rectal rectum 523
Rectal temperature 117
 measurement of 117f
Rectum 586, 587
Recurrent-stumps bandage 691
Red blood cell
 count 380
 indices 380
Re-engineer hospital discharges 234
Referred pain 211, 746
Reflexes, testing of 90
Regional anesthesia 704
 types of 704
Regular bedpan 365
Rehabilitation 18, 20, 321, 746
 care 21
Reinvest emotional energy 552
Relapsing fever 119, 120
Relative stressors 596
Relaxation techniques 216
Religious beliefs 562
Religious problems 622
Relinquish old attachments 552
Remittent fever 118, 120
Removing causality 674f
Removing obstruction 680f
Renal biopsy 378
Renal condition 345, 346
Renal venography 415
Replacing chest drainage bottles 458
Report and records, importance of 75
Reporting incidents, tips for 83
Reproduction, sexual health concerns to 578
Reproductive system, infection of 588
Research consumer 36
Resistance reaction 597
Resorption 468
Resource management 746
Respiration 137, 427, 746
 abnormal 139
 abnormalities in 429
 alterations in 139
 artificial 741
 characteristics of 137, 429
 external 137, 429
 factors influences 137, 427
 internal 137, 429
 regulation of 137, 429
 times of 137
 types of 429
Respiratory acidosis 483
Respiratory alkalosis 483
Respiratory arrest 139
Respiratory complications 710
Respiratory depression 474
Respiratory distress syndrome 431
Respiratory emergencies 671
Respiratory functioning
 alterations in 430
 factors affecting 427
Respiratory infection 172
Respiratory isolation 746
Respiratory mechanism 674
Respiratory physiology 427
Respiratory rate 93
 classification 137t

Respiratory rhythm, abnormal 138f
Respiratory status 254
Respiratory system 96, 118, 248, 250, 252, 253, 556
 clinical examination of 97f
 functions of 427
 physiology of 427
Respiratory tract 673
Responsibility, sense of 35
Rest and sleep 137, 703
Restraints
 hazards of 229
 principles of 227
 types of 227
Resuscitation 464, 747
Retention enema 523
Retina 408, 529
Retrograde pyelograpgy 378
Reusable equipment 146
Rhonchi 86
 sound 138
Rhythms, abnormal 136
Rice treatment 661
Richter scale 747
Rigor
 care in 119
 mortis 556, 557
 pathophysiology of 123
 stages of 123
Rigorism 747
Ringer's lactate 464
Rinne's test 537
Robotic systems 403
Rochin 512
Rocking movements 259
Rod photoreceptor 529
Roentgenogram 419
Rogers theory 638
Rothera's test 360, 394
Routine admission 237
Roy's adaptation model 639f, 747
Roy's theory 639
Rubber articles, care of 151
Rubber bed 152
Rubber gloves, care of 151
Rubber tube and catheters 152
Rule of nines 682
 in burn's assessment 681f
Rules regarding
 administration 506
 labels 506
 measuring medicine 506
Rupture, abdominal 678

S

Sadness 549
Safe and clean environment, role of nurse in 234
Safety and health issues 191
Safety belts 229
Safety devices 227
Safety inspections 144
Safety measures during disaster, steps of 695
Safety needs 4
Salt free diet 330
Sand bags 205, 205f
Sanitary annexes, care of 156
Savlon 648
Scalds 681, 682
Scalp, bandage for 693
School health records 81
School hygiene 275, 276
Scientific principles 158, 747
Scoop stretcher 668

Scorpion
 bite 684
 sting 685
Scrotum 586, 587
Scrub nurse 697
Scrub sink areas 697
Scuba diving 606
Sea urchin sting 685
Sedative enema 367
Seeing and hearing 271
Seizures 96
Selecting nursing interventions 319
Self and image, concept of 566f
Self-actualization needs 4
Self-administered bath 282
Self-awareness 564, 566
Self-care deficit 543
 theory of 636
Self-colostomy irrigation 372f
Self-concept 564, 566
 components of 568, 569f
 concept of 564
 development of 566
 disorders of 571
 disturbance 571
 domains of 565
 impact of 14
 influences to 567f
 theory 567
Self-efficacy 566
Self-esteem 56, 564, 566, 570, 582
 domains of 565f
 increasing 604
Self-injury 564
Self-monitoring 321
Selye's theory 597
Semiquantitative interpretation 360f
Senior staff nurse 38
Senna 363
Sense organs, problems with 557
Sensorineural defects 538
Sensorineural hearing loss 537, 538
 irreversible 538
 sudden 538
 treatment of 538
Sensorium 529
Sensory
 alterations 532
 history 534
 assessment 531, 531f
 importance of 532
 deficits 532
 deprivation 533
 signs of 533
 symptoms of 533
 experience
 components of 530
 perception 530
 function 96
 factors influencing 530
 integration, concept of 529
 needs 528
 neuron 528
 organs, functioning of 529
 overload 533
 signs of 533
 symptoms of 533
 reaction 530
 receptors 530
 stimulation 540
Sepsis 233
Septic shock 655
Septicemia 172

Serological test 727
Serum
　electrolytes 381, 465
　glucose 384
　glutamic
　　oxaloacetic transaminase 382
　　pyruvic transaminase 382
　hepatitis 521
　sickness, hook for 474
Service orientation 34
Severe fever, management of 120
Sewage disposal 221
Sex 576
　acute 596f
　addiction 577
　and marriage 10
　assignment 577
　cell 577
　change operation 577
　chromosomes 577
　chronic 596f
　drive 577
　flush 577
　negative 577
　positive 577
　selection 577
　therapy 577
　worker 577
Sexism 577, 609
Sexology 577
Sexophobia 577
Sexual abuse 577, 590
Sexual arousal 577
Sexual assault 577
Sexual characteristics, secondary 747
Sexual development
　milestones in 579f
　throughout life 579f
Sexual dysfunction 577
Sexual harassment 577
　prevention of 590
Sexual health 275, 577, 583f
　characteristics of 581, 582
　concerns 578
　education 591
　importance of 583
　improve 585
　nurses responsibility in 592
　problems 585
　services, advantages of nurses in 592
Sexual history
　collecting 587
　components 587
Sexual identity 577, 581
Sexual intercourse 577
Sexual minority 577
Sexual norms 577
Sexual orientation 577, 584
　sexual health concerns to 578
Sexual preference 577
Sexual response cycle 577, 585
Sexual safety 578, 583
Sexuality 576, 577, 579, 580
　components of 581
　model, circles of 581
Sexualization 581
Sexually healthy person, characteristics of 583f
Sexually transmitted disease 577, 589
　prevention of 589
Sexually transmitted infection 577, 589
Sharp instruments, care of 154
Shock 549, 644, 655, 747
　and denial 550

and disbelief 550
causes of 656
clinical features of 656f
electric 689
first aid in 657
types of 655
Shoulder
　dislocation 661
　spica 692
　　cast 264
Shunt tubes 148f
Sick person, transport of 645
Sick role, assumption of 12
Sickness, diet in 328
Sick-role behavior 747
Sighing hunger 139
Sight, speech and hearing 557
Sigmoidoscopy 377, 379, 401
　procedure 401f
　types of 401
Simple face mask 436, 436f
Simple fracture 657
Sims' position 209, 209f
Situational crisis 600, 747
Situational loss 548
Situational low self-esteem 571
　nursing intervention for 573
Sitz bath 129
　indications of 129f
　procedures 129f
　solutions for 129
Skateboarding 606
Skeleton-muscular defects 249
Skene's glands 577
Skiing 606
Skills 611
Skin 94, 99, 586, 587
　and hygienic care 265
　care 336
　conditions 102
　factors affecting 282
　integrity, maintaining 540
　musculoskeletal system 557
　preparation 701, 702
　warm and dry 542
Skull
　circumference 105
　fracture of 658
Skydiving 606
Sleep 254
　apnea 431
Sling 692, 693, 747
Smegma 577
Smell 531
Smiths test 360, 394
Snake bite 684
Snellen's test 747
Soak bath 128, 128f
Soap water enema 367
Social adaptation 599
Social communication 52
Social crisis 600
Social environment 9, 747
Social hygiene 275
Social interaction 531
Social practices 276, 277
Social relationship 63
Social relativism 747
Social stressors 595
Socio cultural background 56
Socioeconomic determinants 3, 8
Socioeconomic factors 11
Socioeconomic status 276, 277

Sodium 465, 472
　losses of 472
　regulation of 472
Sodomy 577
Soft diet 321, 331, 747
Soft tissue management, method of 663f
Solid medical waste 187
Solid wastes 186
Solution, temperature of 370
Sonogram 577
Sonorous percussion 90
Sore 644
Sound, characteristics of 89, 90
Space occupying lesions 669
Special drug delivery systems 523
Special foot care 286
Special sense 529
Specimen collection 385
Speculum 578
Speech therapy 538
Sperm 578
Spinal anesthesia 704
Spinal fracture 658
Spinous process aspiration 729
Spiral bandage 691
Spiral fracture 657
Spiritual distress 624
　dealing with 624f
　indicators 624f, 625
　manifestations of 625
　meaning of 624
　signs of 624
　symptoms of 624
Spiritual health
　factors affecting 621, 622f
　lifespan consideration in 619
Spiritual need 621, 747
Spiritual quest 621
Spiritual well-being 621, 623
Spirituality 582, 608
　and nursing 618
　and religion 619
　characteristics of 621
Splinters 675
Splints 247
Sprain 644, 660, 747
Sputum
　characteristics of 389
　culture 389
　cup 146, 225
　　care of 153
Staff nurse 36, 38
Stagnant hypoxia 432
Stainless steel instruments 153f
　care of 153
　list of 153
Standard radiographical positions 411
Standard stretcher 667
Standard universal precautions 177
Standardized care plans 79
Staphylococcus aureus 170
Steam inhalation 448
Stenotrophomonas maltophilia 170
Sterile 747
　supply room 697
　tray 405, 732
Sterilization 747
　chemical method of 158
　methods of 157f, 158
　natural method of 158
　physical methods of 158, 158f
　radiation method of 160
　techniques 157

Index

Sternal puncture 729
Sterofundin 464
Stertorous breathing 140
Stick method 666
Stimulant enema 367
Stimulant laxatives 363
Stimulation gastric analysis 340
Stimulation test 341
Stimuli, amount of 531
Stomach
   and duodenal problems, diagnosis of 408*f*
   foreign body in 678
Stool, white colored 371
Strain 747
Stress 594, 595, 747
   acute 596
   and adaptation 594
   chronic 596, 597
   incontinence 347
   management
      nursing intervention for 599
      role of nurse in 599
      strategies of 598
   meaning of 595
   negative 594
   sources of 595
   symptoms of 595
   theories 631
   types of 596
Stressful events sequences 597
Stressor 594
   types of 596
Stretcher 666, 667
   exercise 664
Strict isolation 747
Stridor 140, 425, 747
   respiration 139
Strikethrough contamination 698
Stroke 644, 747
Structure and functions 249
Structured communication 52
Stupor 747
Subcutaneous emphysema 459
Subcutaneous injection site 515, 516, 516*f*
Subnormal temperature 118
Substances, addition of 511
Substerile rooms 698
Suction catheters 149*f*
Suction machine, care of 155
Suctioning procedure 445
Suffocation 674
   first aid for 675
Sugar
   count 727
   test 359, 393
Sun stroke 122
Support systems 747
Supportive educative nursing system 636
Supportive nursing measures 747
Suprapubic catheterization 347*f*
Surgery
   ablative 698
   constructive 698, 700
   elective 698, 743
   emergency 700
   exploratory 698
   minor 700
   nursing care during 705
   palliative 698, 700
   reconstructive 698, 700
Surgical and diagnostic procedure 345
Surgical anesthesia 704
Surgical asepsis 178, 179*f*, 747
   principles of 178, 179

Surgical aseptic
   procedures 179
   technique 178*f*
Surgical drain, types of 719
Surgical dressing 715, 730
Surgical fomentation 127
Surgical hand washing 178, 179*f*
Surgical procedures 722
   classification of 699
Surgical scrub 698
Surgical sharp instruments, care of 154
Surrogate decision making 547
Surrogate role 634
Suture removal, factors affecting 717
Swan-Ganz catheter 147
Sweating stage 123
Swimming 607
Sx's minor bleeding 474
Synthesis 306
Syphilis 588
Syphon method 335
Syringe
   and needle, selection of 483, 516, 518
   method 335
   parts of 509*f*
System wise complications 251*f*
Systemic circulation pathway 427
Systems thinking 33, 40
Systolic pressure 140

T

T- binders 693
Tachycardia 109, 136
Tachypnea 139, 425, 429
Taking pulse, sites of 135
Taking vital signs, timings of 110
Tarry black stools 371
T-bandage 691
T-binder 693
Technical skill 315, 511
Technological disaster 694
Technological hazard 747
Tegaserod 363
Tele-health 16
Telephone contacts 604
Temperature 93, 739
   alterations 120
   biofeedback 215
   conversion table 739
   regulation 121
Tension pneumothorax 726
Terminal cleaning, guidelines for 245
Terminal sedation 547
Tertiary health care 19
Testes 586, 587
Testing stretcher 667
Theater dress 179
Theater headwear 179
Theoretical nursing models, goals of 631
Theory, types of 632
Therapeutic bath 282
Therapeutic communication 52, 62
   phases 64
   techniques 63
Therapeutic diet 321, 329
   functions 329*f*
   modifications of nutrients in 328
Therapeutic effectiveness 33, 221
Therapeutic modalities 249
Therapeutic nurse-patient relationship 61
Therapeutic patient education 267
Therapeutic play 747
Therapeutic procedures 148*f*

Therapeutic relationship 62, 63
Therapeutic touch 216
Thermal process 191
Thermometer 114, 114*f*
   care of 114, 156
   parts of 114
   scales of 114
   types of 114
Thoracentesis 377, 724
   position and site 725*f*
   procedure 724*f*
Three bottle system 456
Throat 99
   examination of 105
   foreign body in 678
   swab 391
Thrombocyte count 380
Thrombophlebities 521
Throttling, first aid measures of 690*f*
Thyroid
   stimulating hormone 597
   storm 710
Thyrotropin releasing hormone 597
Tibia and fibula, fracture of 659
Tibial puncture 729
Time-limited stressors, acute 596
Tissues within throat, swelling of 674
Toe
   and nails, care of 278*f*
   pleat 194
   types of 200
Toilet articles 147, 225
Total body water 464
Total communications 747
Total incontinence 347
Total parenteral nutrition
   method 338, 339*f*
   role of professionals in 339
   side effects of 339
Toxic 219
   effects 495
Toxicological disaster 747
Toxin 219
Tr. benzoin inhalation, indication of 448
Tracheal suctioning 446
Tracheostomy 425
   suctioning procedure 447, 447*f*
   tube 149, 441, 442*f*, 535*f*
Transcultural healthcare 615
Transcultural nursing 614, 615, 616*t*
   care, factors influencing 615
   concept of 614
   models of 616
   roles and duties of 615
Transdermal adhesive units 524
Transdermal route 522
Transesophageal echocardiography 418
Transverse fracture 657
Trauma 120, 249, 644, 747
Traumatic injuries 92
Traumatic stress 596
   crisis resulting from 602
Trendelenburg's position 210, 210*f*
Treponema pallidum 588
Triangular sling 692
Trichomonas vaginalis 588
Trimming cast 264
True crisis 118, 120
Tub bath 282
Tube feeding
   advantages of 334
   indication for 333*f*, 334
Tube method 368
Tubeless gastric analysis 340, 341

Tuberculin test 517
Tuberculosis 170
Two handed seat 665, 667
Two rescuer handling techniques 664f
Two-way communication 67
Tympanic membrane thermometer 114

U

Ultrasound guided abdominal parencentesis 723f
Ultraviolet light sterilization 158, 160
Unconscious 644
   casualty 673
   infant, first aid in 673
   patient 668f
      first aid for 669f
      oral care for 281f
Unconsciousness 668
   causes of 668
Unit care, purpose of 226
United Nations Development Programme 22
Universal self-care requisites 636, 637
Unsafe injections practices 233
Unsafe surgical care procedures 233
Unsafe transfusion practices 233
Unwanted pregnancy, prevention of 590
Urge incontinence 347
Urinals
   care of 153
   types of 349f
Urinary bladder, catheterization of 349
Urinary catheter 148, 355f
   care of 353f
   insertion technique 351f
   types of 350f
Urinary elimination 343, 346
   factors affecting 345
   role of nurse in 361
Urinary incontinence 346, 347
   risk of 348
   types of 347f
Urinary output, monitoring 348, 348f
Urinary retention 346, 540
Urinary sample collection 355f
Urinary system 118, 251-253
   diagnostic examination of 344
Urinary tract infection 170, 172
Urine
   characteristics of 344, 344t
      abnormal 358, 393
      normal 358, 393
   collection 356, 386, 387
   culture 357, 387
   elimination
      alteration in 346
      physiology of 344, 344f
   normal 345t
      characteristics of 356, 387
   pH 360, 394
   sample collection, mid-stream 356f
   specific gravity 360, 394
   specimen, collecting 354
   test 358, 392
      methods of 358f, 359f
   types of examination of 359, 393
Uterus 586

V

Vaccine 164
Vagina 586
Vaginal smear 392
Vaginal swab 392
Vancomycin 512
Vasocongestion 585
Vastus lateralis site 514
Vector borne transmission 173
Vectorcardiogram 419
Venipuncture site 520
Venography 378, 414, 415
   complications of 416
   purpose of 414
   results of 416
   risks of 416
Venous bleeding 654
Venous thromboembolism 233, 234
Ventilation 164, 425
Ventrogluteal site 514
Venturi mask 436
Verbal communication 53, 60
Vermin and insects 225
Vertical pleat 200
Vertigo 644
Vesicular sound 138
Victim distribution 747
Victim outreach programs 604
Video education 272
Viral infections 363
Vision 529
   impairment and nursing diagnoses 536
Visual acuity 529
Visual analog 212f
Visual examination 88f
Visual impairment 535, 536
   causes of 536
   nursing care for 536
   signs of 536
Visual inspection 298
Vital signs 86, 93, 108, 110
   guidelines
      for assessing 109
      for taking 110
   measurement technique 109, 109f
   monitoring 121
   observation of 671
   principles of 110
Voice, tone of 57
Voluntary agency 748
Voluntary agreement 44
Voluntary euthanasia 547, 561
Voluntary health agencies 20
Voluntary hospitals 24
Vomiting 321, 327, 644, 541
   nursing care plan for 327

W

Waist restraint 229f
Wait and test 589
Walking cast 264
Ward in-charge 37
Wards patient unit, type of 226
Wash basins 225
Wash hair 558
Wash hands 177
Wash person's face 558
Wasp sting 685
Waste
   basket 147, 225
   concept of 185
   types of 186
Water
   daily output of 466
   flask 147, 225
   hammer pulse 136
   intake
      and output 466f
      sources of 465
   moist inhalation 448
   regulatory mechanism 469f
   requirements 465
   seal chest drainage 454
   supply 221
Wear face protection 177
Wear protective body clothing 177
Weber's test 537
Weight control 254
Wellness 301
Wet dressing 714, 733
Wet floor 223f
Wet-to-dry dressing 730
Wet-to-wet dressings 731
Wheeze 86, 139, 445
   sound 138
White blood cell 379
   types of 379
Withdrawing treatment 547
Withholding treatment 547
Wound 644, 649, 711, 720f
   abdominal 653, 654
   and skin sepsis 172
   care 733
   classification of 711
   clean 711, 742
      surgical 717, 731
   closed 742
   complications of 710, 713
   contaminated 711, 742
   contused 650, 711
   dirty 711
   drainage 718
      care of 719
   first aid measures
      in major 654
      in minor 653
   first aid techniques for 650f
   gunshot 651
   healing
      factors affecting 712
      forms of 713
      phases of 712
      process 711
   incised 649, 711
   infected 652, 711, 744
   infections, surgical 713
   lacerated 650, 711
   sepsis 713
   suturing 715
   types of 649, 649f
Writing and reading skills 54
Writing nursing care plan 317
Writing nursing diagnosis 312
   rules for 312

X

X-ray examination 378

Z

Z-tract method 514